Library Service
VA Medical Center
830 Chalkstone Avenue
Providence, RI 02908

Surgical Critical Care

Surgical Critical Care

Second Edition

edited by

Jerome H. Abrams
University of Minnesota
VA Medical Center
Minneapolis, Minnesota, U.S.A.

Paul Druck
University of Minnesota
VA Medical Center
Minneapolis, Minnesota, U.S.A.

Frank B. Cerra
University of Minnesota
Minneapolis, Minnesota, U.S.A.

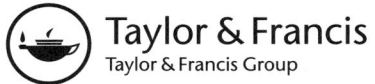

Boca Raton   London   New York   Singapore

Published in 2005 by
Taylor & Francis Group
6000 Broken Sound Parkway NW, Suite 300
Boca Raton, FL 33487-2742

© 2005 by Taylor & Francis Group, LLC

No claim to original U.S. Government works
Printed in the United States of America on acid-free paper
10 9 8 7 6 5 4 3 2 1

International Standard Book Number-10: 0-8247-5911-7 (Hardcover)
International Standard Book Number-13: 978-0-8247-5911-7 (Hardcover)

This book contains information obtained from authentic and highly regarded sources. Reprinted material is quoted with permission, and sources are indicated. A wide variety of references are listed. Reasonable efforts have been made to publish reliable data and information, but the author and the publisher cannot assume responsibility for the validity of all materials or for the consequences of their use.

No part of this book may be reprinted, reproduced, transmitted, or utilized in any form by any electronic, mechanical, or other means, now known or hereafter invented, including photocopying, microfilming, and recording, or in any information storage or retrieval system, without written permission from the publishers.

For permission to photocopy or use material electronically from this work, please access www.copyright.com (http://www.copyright.com/) or contact the Copyright Clearance Center, Inc. (CCC) 222 Rosewood Drive, Danvers, MA 01923, 978-750-8400. CCC is a not-for-profit organization that provides licenses and registration for a variety of users. For organizations that have been granted a photocopy license by the CCC, a separate system of payment has been arranged.

Trademark Notice: Product or corporate names may be trademarks or registered trademarks, and are used only for identification and explanation without intent to infringe.

Library of Congress Cataloging-in-Publication Data

Catalog record is available from the Library of Congress

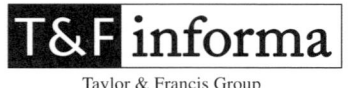

Taylor & Francis Group
is the Academic Division of T&F Informa plc.

Visit the Taylor & Francis Web site at
http://www.taylorandfrancis.com

Preface

Despite the advances in critical care in the years that have passed since the first edition of this book, achieving unambiguous diagnosis, clearly appropriate interventions, and improved patient outcomes remains elusive. The ability to acquire only static, low-dimensional, sparse data about dynamic, high-dimensional information-dense problems present constant challenges. We long for accuracy; instead we receive information with significant error. We recognize our limited understanding of critical illness, yet we cannot avoid intervening on our patients' behalf. In response to these conflicts, our goals in this second edition are the same as those of the first edition: to provide a foundation for understanding current ideas about the presentation and mechanism of the altered physiology and metabolism seen in the critically ill patient, to offer approaches to problems that are frequently encountered, and to suggest an approach when consensus about a clinical problem does not exist. The organization of this edition is similar to that of the first edition. Part I emphasizes the altered metabolism seen in the critically ill patient. Part II considers preoperative, intraoperative, and postoperative care of the critically ill patient. Part III discusses pathophysiologic conditions by organ system. Systemic pathophysiology receives emphasis in Part IV. Common procedures in the SICU are presented in Part V. Finally, measurement and interpretation of quantified data are discussed in Part VI. An introduction to the recognition, understanding and reduction of uncertainty in critical care data is provided in Part VII.

Again we are indebted to all of the contributors. We deeply appreciate their hard work, in a more difficult environment, in providing expert discussions of the problems we face daily.

Jerome H. Abrams
Paul Druck
Frank B. Cerra

Contents

Preface . . . . *iii*
Contributors . . . . *xxxi*

Part I: Altered Metabolism of Critical Illness and Shock

1. Stress Response and Multiple Organ Failure 3
Victor Lazaron and Jerome H. Abrams
Introduction *3*
Multiple Organ Failure Syndrome *5*
    Clinical Features *5*
    Pathophysiology *8*
Conceptual Hypotheses *13*
Clinical Progress *15*
Future Considerations *16*
Summary *16*
References *17*

2. Oxygen Transport 21
Jerome H. Abrams and Frank B. Cerra
Oxygen Supply and Demand *21*
Blood Flow *22*
Adequacy of Oxygen Transport *24*
    Delivery-Dependent Oxygen Consumption *24*
    Delivery-Dependent Lactate Production *26*
Treatment *27*
Summary *29*
Appendix *29*
Recommended Reading *32*

3. Lactic Acidosis 33
Paul Druck
Pathogenesis *33*
    Hyperlactatemia *33*
    Associated Acidemia *35*

Etiology *35*
Clinical Correlates *37*
Treatment *37*
Summary *40*
References *40*

4. Nutritional Support in Critical Illness *43*
Paul Druck
Introduction *43*
Physiologic Effects of Malnutrition *43*
Nutritional Assessment *44*
Providing Nutritional Support *46*
    Meeting Caloric Requirements *46*
    Meeting Protein Requirements *47*
    Meeting Micronutrient Requirements *47*
    Special Formulations, Immune-Enhancing Formulas *48*
    Choice of Delivery Route: Enteral vs. Parenteral *48*
    Timing of Initiation of Nutritional Support *51*
    Conditions Requiring Modification of
      Nutrition Regimen *52*
    Monitoring Adequacy of Nutritional Support *54*
Preoperative Nutritional Support *55*
Summary *55*
References *56*

Part II: Care of the Critically Ill Patient

A. Trauma and Injuries

5. Initial Approach to the Injured Patient *63*
Richard G. Barton
Initial Management and Stabilization *63*
    Airway *63*
    Breathing–Ventilation *64*
    Circulation *65*
    Disability *67*
Evaluation and Initial Treatment *68*
Physical Examination *69*
    Head and Neck *69*
    Chest *69*
    Abdomen *69*
    Extremities *70*
Evaluation and Treatment of Specific Injuries *70*
    Head Injury *71*
    Neck Injury *72*
    Chest Injuries *72*
    Emergency Department Thoracotomy *74*
    Abdominal Injuries *74*
    Genito-Urinary Injuries *76*
    Musculoskeletal Injuries *76*

Summary 78
References 78

6. Fractures in Blunt Multiple Trauma 81
William J. Flynn, Jr. and Larry Bone
Treatment 84
    Fracture Management 84
Summary 85
References 85

7. Burns, Electrical Injury, and Hypothermia and Frostbite 87
David H. Ahrenholz and William Mohr
Burns 87
    Fluid Resuscitation 89
    Treatment 90
    Metabolic Support 92
    Early Excision and Grafting 92
    Late Management 93
Electrical Injury 93
Hypothermia and Frostbite 94
Summary 95
References 96

B. Preoperative, Intraoperative, and Postoperative Evaluation

8. Cardiovascular Risk: Assessment and Reduction 97
Jon F. Berlauk and Jerome H. Abrams
Risk Factors 97
Guidelines for Assessing and Managing Risk 100
    PCWP > 15 mm Hg 108
    PCWP < 15 mm Hg 108
Summary 109
References 109

9. Life Support and Management of Cardiac Arrest 113
Michael D. Pasquale
Overview 113
Airway Management 113
Ventilation 114
Circulation 114
The Arrested Heart 115
Pharmacologic Approach 117
    Epinephrine 117
    Vasopressin 119
    Norepinephrine 119
    Dopamine 120
    Atropine 120

        Isoproterenol *120*
        Sodium Bicarbonate *120*
        Calcium *121*
        Amiodarone *121*
        Lidocaine *121*
        Procainamide *122*
Expectations for Resuscitation *122*
        Prearrest Factors *123*
        Arrest Factors *123*
        Other Factors *124*
        Patient Outcome *124*
Do-Not-Resuscitate Orders *124*
Summary *125*
        Pharmacologic Guidelines *126*
References *126*

10. Evaluation of Hepatic Function *129*
George M. Logan and Joseph R. Bloomer
Effects of Anesthesia and Surgery *129*
Risk Factors for Surgery *130*
        Acute Hepatitis *130*
        Chronic Hepatitis *130*
        Cirrhosis *130*
Indications for Preoperative Metabolic Support *133*
Assessment of the Preoperative Patient *134*
Summary *135*
References *136*

11. The Surgical Patient and Renal Failure *139*
Mark E. Rosenberg and Ricardo Correa-Rotter
Introduction *139*
Risk Factors and Precipitating Conditions *139*
Preoperative Evaluation of Kidney Function *140*
        Estimating GFR *141*
        Assessment of Volume Status *143*
        Assessment of Electrolytes *144*
Specific Problems *144*
        Radiocontrast-Induced ARF *144*
        Drug-Induced ARF *145*
        Cardiovascular Surgery and ARF *146*
Chronic Renal Failure *147*
        Dialysis *147*
        Anesthesia *147*
        Bleeding Disorders *148*
        Anemia *148*
        Calcium, Phosphorus, and Magnesium *148*
Summary *149*
        Preoperative Assessment *149*
        Management of the Surgical Patient with CRF *149*
Bibliography *150*

Contents

**12. Perioperative Pulmonary Complications and
Pulmonary Risk Assessment** 151
Paul Druck
Introduction *151*
Nature and Incidence of Postoperative
  Pulmonary Complications *151*
Postoperative Pulmonary Pathophysiology *152*
Estimating the Risk: Preoperative Assessment *153*
Risk Factors for PPCs *154*
  Patient-Specific Factors *154*
  Procedure-Specific Factors *154*
Modifying Pulmonary Risk *155*
  Preoperative *155*
  Intraoperative *156*
  Postoperative *156*
Summary *157*
References *157*

13. Ethical Considerations in Surgical Intensive Care 161
Melissa West
Informed Consent and Decision-Making Capacity *161*
  Informed Consent *161*
  Decision-Making Capacity *161*
  Patients Without Decision-Making Capacity *163*
Advance Directives and DNR Orders *164*
  DNR Orders *164*
  DNI Orders *165*
  The Presence of a DNR/DNI Order Does Not Imply
    Limits to Other Types of Care *166*
  If in Doubt, Err on the Side of Preserving Life *166*
Inappropriate Requests from Patients: The Futility Debate *166*
  Case Studies *167*
Professional Integrity *168*
End of Life Issues *169*
  Relief of Suffering at the End of Life *169*
  Withdrawal of Life-Sustaining Treatment *170*
Physician-Assisted Suicide *171*
Summary *172*
References *173*

14. Nursing Considerations 175
Valerie Nebel
Collaboration *175*
The Role of the Nurse *176*
Airway and Ventilator Management *176*
  Routine SICU Care *176*
  Suctioning of Patients on Mechanical Ventilation *177*
  Care of Patients with Acute Respiratory
    Distress Syndrome *178*
Wound Management and Pressure Ulcer Prevention *178*

Management of Diarrhea *180*
Management of Delirium *180*
Summary *181*
References *182*

Part III: Pathophysiologic Conditions

C. Central Nervous System Function

15. Coma 187
Frederick Langendorf
Introduction *187*
Anatomy and Physiology *187*
Differential Diagnosis *188*
    Approach to Diagnosis *188*
    Vascular Disease *188*
    Trauma *190*
    Other Structural Pathologies *191*
    Nonstructural Pathologies *191*
Approach to the Patient with Coma *191*
    History *191*
    Examination *192*
    Laboratory Examination and Other Tests *195*
    Emergency Management of Coma *198*
Prognosis *199*
    General Principles *199*
    Anoxic Encephalopathy *199*
    Traumatic Coma *200*
    Subarachnoid Hemorrhage and Other Vascular Disease *200*
    Infection *201*
Relatives of Coma *201*
    Locked-In State *201*
    Brain Death *201*
    Persistent Vegetative State *202*
Summary *203*
References *205*

16. Seizures 207
Frederick Langendorf
Introduction *207*
A Framework for Considering Seizures by Cause *207*
    Definitions *207*
    Acute Symptomatic Seizures *208*
    Remote Symptomatic Seizures *208*
    Idiopathic Seizures and Epilepsy Syndromes *209*
Seizure Types *209*
    Convulsive Seizures (Generalized Tonic–Clonic Seizures,
       Grand Mal Seizures) *209*
    Absence Seizures *210*

Contents   xi

    Myoclonic Seizures *210*
    Complex Partial Seizures *211*
    Simple Partial Seizures *211*
  Differential Diagnosis *211*
    Syncope *211*
    Transient Ischemic Attacks *212*
    Migraine *213*
    Psychiatric Disorders *214*
  Treatment *215*
    Acute Symptomatic Seizures *215*
    Remote Symptomatic Seizures *215*
    Idiopathic Seizures *215*
  Antiepileptic Drugs *216*
    AEDs in the Acute Setting *216*
    Pharmacologic Considerations *216*
    Long-Term Management *217*
  Evaluation of a First Seizure *218*
    History *218*
    Laboratory Evaluation *218*
    Imaging *218*
    Electroencephalogram (EEG) *219*
  Posttraumatic Seizures *219*
    Epidemiology and Definitions *219*
    Risk *220*
    Diagnosis *220*
    Treatment *221*
  Status Epilepticus *221*
    Definition and Epidemiology *221*
    Clinical Features of Generalized Convulsive
      Status Epilepticus *222*
    Evaluation and Management of GCSE *222*
    Nonconvulsive Status Epilepticus *223*
  Summary *224*
  References *226*

17. Head Injury **229**
 Anthony Bottini
  Basic Concepts *229*
  Skull Fractures *231*
    Linear Nondisplaced Skull Fractures *231*
    Depressed Skull Fractures *233*
    Basilar Skull Fractures *233*
  Hematomas *234*
    Epidural Hematoma *234*
    Acute Subdural Hematoma *235*
    Traumatic Intracerebral Hematoma *236*
    Delayed Traumatic Intracerebral Hematoma *237*
  Pathophysiology *237*
  Management of ICP *238*
  Posttraumatic Seizures *241*

Summary 242
References 242

18. Spinal Cord Injury 245
Anthony Bottini

Clinical Assessment 245
    Motor Examination 246
    Sensory Examination 246
Radiographic Assessment 249
Neurological Syndromes Following Spinal Cord Injury 251
    Brown–Sequard Syndrome 251
    Central Cord Syndrome 254
    Anterior Cord Syndrome 254
Stabilization and Protection of the Injured Spine 254
Medical Management 256
    Monitoring 256
    Steroids 256
    Hemodynamics 257
    Respiratory System 258
    Deep Venous Thrombosis and
      Pulmonary Emboli 260
    Autonomic Dysreflexia 261
Gastrointestinal Management 261
    Nutritional Support Following Acute
      Spinal Cord Injury 261
    Poikilothermia 262
    Skin Breakdown 262
Urinary Tract Management 262
Preparation for Rehabilitation 263
    Psychological Factors 263
Summary 264
References 266

19. Stroke: Diagnosis and Management 269
Sabrina Walski-Easton and Edward Rustamzadeh

Introduction 269
Epidemiology 269
    Unmodifiable Risk Factors 270
    Modifiable Risk Factors 270
Pathophysiology 271
    Physiology of Ischemia 272
    Cerebral Blood Flow 273
    Cerebral Autoregulation 273
Diagnosis 274
    Clinical Diagnosis 274
    Radiological/Laboratory Diagnosis 277
Medical Therapy 278
    Intensive Care Therapy 278
    Blood Pressure 279

Contents   xiii

                    Neuroprotection 281
                    Systemic Thrombolytic Therapy 281
                    Neurointerventional Therapy 282
                    Anticoagulation 282
                    Hemorrhagic Complications 283
                    Management of Cerebral Edema 284
                    Seizure Prophylaxis 285
              Surgical Management 287
                    Supratentorial Infarcts 287
                    Infratentorial Infarcts 287
              Summary 287
              References 289
              Appendix 293
                    NIH Stroke Scale 293

20. **Encephalopathy** 297
    Jodie Herk Taylor
    Emergency Causes of Mental Status Change 298
          Reassess the ABCs 298
    Summary 307
    References 307

D. Cardiovascular Function

21. **Altered Cardiac Physiology** 309
    Vivian L. Clark, James A. Kruse, and Richard W. Carlson
    Normal Physiology 309
          Heart Rate 309
          Preload 310
          Afterload 313
          Contractility 314
    Pathophysiology of Heart Failure 314
    Pericardial Tamponade 318
    Cardiac Function in Sepsis and Septic Shock 320
    Summary 320
    References 321

22. **Cardiac Arrhythmias and the Perioperative Period** 323
    Charles C. Gornick and Arthur H. L. From
    Introduction 323
    Bradyarrhythmias 324
          Sinus Node Dysfunction 324
          Etiology 324
          Treatment 324
          Abnormalities of AV Conduction 326
          Etiology 327
          Pacemaker Code 329
    Tachyarrhythmias—Primary Atrial Arrhythmias 330
          Atrial Fibrillation 330

>   Atrial Flutter *340*
>   Multifocal Atrial Tachycardia *344*
>   Other Primary Atrial Tachycardias *345*
>   Nonparoxysmal Junctional Tachycardia *346*
>   AV Nodal and AV Reentrant Arrhythmias *347*
>   AV Nodal Reentry *347*
>   AV Reentry Tachycardia and the WPW Syndrome *349*
>   Ventricular Arrhythmias *352*
>   Premature Ventricular Contractions and Nonsustained
>   Ventricular Tachycardia (NSVT) *352*
>   Sustained Ventricular Tachycardia and
>   Ventricular Fibrillation *353*
>   Antitachycardia and Defibrillator Devices *358*
>   Acknowledgments *358*
>   Summary *359*
>   References *361*

23. Myocardial Infarction 367
Steven M. Hollenberg and Sandeep Nathan
> Anatomy of Acute Infarction *367*
>   Definitions *367*
>   Pathogenesis *367*
>   Distributions of the Major
>   Coronary Arteries *368*
> Diagnosis of Acute Infarction *368*
> Thrombolytic Therapy for Acute
>   Myocardial Infarction *369*
>   Thrombolytic Agents *370*
>   Combination Fibrinolytic and Anti-Platelet
>   Therapy in Acute STEMI *371*
>   Glycoprotein IIb/IIIa Receptor Antagonists *372*
> Primary PCI in Acute Myocardial Infarction *372*
>   Coronary Stenting and Glycoprotein IIb/IIIa
>   Antagonists *373*
>   Other Indications for Angioplasty in Acute
>   Myocardial Infarction *374*
> Medical Therapy for Myocardial Infarction *375*
>   Aspirin *375*
>   Thienopyridines *375*
>   Heparin *376*
>   Nitrates *376*
>   β-Blockers *377*
>   Angiotensin-Converting Enzyme Inhibitors *377*
>   Calcium Antagonists *378*
>   Antiarrhythmics *378*
> Complications of Acute Myocardial Infarction *379*
>   Postinfarction Angina and Infarct Extension *379*
>   Ventricular Free Wall Rupture *379*
>   Ventricular Septal Rupture *379*

Contents

   Acute Mitral Regurgitation *379*
   Right Ventricular Infarction *379*
   Cardiogenic Shock *380*
 Summary *380*
 Suggested Reading *382*

24. Hypertensive Emergencies 385
 Rakesh Gupta and John W. Hoyt
 Types of Hypertensive Crises *385*
 Initial Evaluation *386*
 Management of Hypertensive Crisis *388*
 Antihypertensive Agents *388*
 Cardiac/Vascular Complications and
  Their Management *392*
 CNS Complications and Their Management *393*
 Summary *393*
 Bibliography *394*

25. Cardiopulmonary Interactions 395
 Michael R. Pinsky
 Cardiopulmonary Interactions *395*
   Intrapulmonary Gas Exchange and Work of Breathing *395*
   Changes in Lung Volume *395*
   Changes in Intrathoracic Pressure *397*
   Ventricular Interdependence *399*
 Clinical Applications of Cardiopulmonary
  Interactions *399*
 Using Cardiopulmonary Interactions to Diagnose
  Cardiovascular Insufficiency *402*
 Summary *403*
 Appendix—Case Examples *404*
   Case 1 .... *404*
   Case 2 .... *405*
 References *406*

26. Vascular Emergencies in the Surgical Intensive
 Care Unit 411
 Alexandre d'Audiffret, Steven Santilli, and Connie Lindberg
 Introduction *411*
 Acute Arterial Insufficiency *411*
   Lower Extremity Ischemia *411*
   Upper Extremity Ischemia *413*
 Acute Mesenteric Ischemia *414*
   Clinical Presentation and Differential Diagnosis *414*
   Medical and Surgical Management *414*
 Phlegmasia Cerulea Dolens and Venous Gangrene *414*
 Complications Associated with Invasive Monitoring *415*

Radial Artery Catheterization *415*
Brachial Artery Complications *415*
Axillary Artery Catheterization *415*
Access Complications *416*
Vascular Complications Associated with
Vascular Procedures *416*
Aortic Procedures *416*
Carotid Endarterectomy *416*
Hypotension/Hypertension *417*
Cervical Hematoma *417*
Hyperperfusion Syndrome *417*
Summary *417*
References *418*

E. Pulmonary Function

27. Acute Lung Injury ... 421
Larry A. Woods, Alan J. Cropp, and Bhagwan Dass
Introduction *421*
Incidence *422*
Risk Factors *422*
Mediators of ALI *422*
Pathophysiology *424*
Clinical Course *425*
Management *426*
Hypoxia *427*
Mechanical Ventilation *427*
Alternative Ventilator Strategies *428*
Pharmacologic Therapies *429*
Summary *430*
References *430*

28. Bronchospasm ... 433
Stephen Trzeciak and R. Phillip Dellinger
Pathophysiology *433*
Clinical Findings and Physical Examination *434*
Laboratory Data *435*
Traditional Medical Therapy *435*
Bronchodilator Therapy *435*
Anti-inflammatory Therapy *437*
Other Medical Therapies *437*
Considerations in the Intubated and Mechanically
Ventilated Patient *438*
Summary *440*
References *441*

29. Venous Thromboembolism ... 443
Mark D. Cipolle
Incidence *443*
Risk Factors *443*

Contents   xvii

        Diagnosis *445*
                Pulmonary Angiography *447*
                V/Q Scanning *447*
                Helical Computed Tomography *448*
                Ultrasonographic Examination of the Lower
                    Extremities for DVT *448*
                D-Dimer Assay *449*
                Combinations of Diagnostic Tests *449*
        Prophylaxis *450*
                Low-Dose Heparin *452*
                Low-Molecular-Weight Heparin (LMWH) *453*
                Oral Anticoagulants *453*
                Sequential Compression Devices *454*
                Graduated Compression Stockings (GCSs) *454*
                Vena Cava Interruption *454*
                Recommendations *454*
        Treatment *457*
                Anticoagulation *457*
                Thrombolytic Therapy *460*
                Pulmonary Embolectomy *461*
        Summary *461*
        References *462*

30. Airway Management 469
        Ian J. Gilmour
        Indications for Endotracheal Intubation *469*
        Route of Intubation and Selection of Tube *469*
        Standard Approaches to Intubation *471*
        Difficult Airway *473*
        Confirmation of Successful Intubation *474*
        Changing of Orotracheal Tube *477*
        Extubation *477*
        Tracheostomy *479*
                Tube Selection *480*
                Shape and Construction of Tube *481*
                Special Considerations with Recent Tracheostomy *481*
                Changing of TT *482*
        Pulmonary Hemorrhage/Massive Hemoptysis *484*
                All Cases *484*
                Bronchoscopy *485*
                Balloon Tamponade *485*
                Angiography/Embolization *485*
                Radionuclear Scanning *485*
                Surgery *485*
        Summary *486*
        References *487*
        Suggested Reading *488*
                Airway Management *488*
                Difficult Intubation *488*

Tracheostomy *488*
Hemoptysis *488*

31. Mechanical Ventilator Support *489*
Karl L. Yang and Guillermo Guiterrez
Gas Exchange *489*
Respiratory Mechanics *490*
Modes of Ventilation *491*
    Control Mode Ventilation (CMV) *493*
    Assist-Control Ventilation (ACV) *493*
    Intermittent Mandatory Ventilation (IMV) *494*
    Other Ventilator Variables *494*
    Other Modes of Mechanical Ventilation *497*
Summary *498*
References *498*

32. Discontinuation of Mechanical Ventilation *501*
Paul Druck
Introduction *501*
Approaches to Discontinuation of
  Ventilatory Support *502*
    The Earliest Approach: Weaning Criteria and
      T-Piece Trials *502*
    "Weaning Modes" of Ventilation: The Tapered
      Support Method *502*
    Protocol Weaning *503*
    What Constitutes an Adequate Trial of Spontaneous
      Breathing *504*
    Current Recommendations *505*
Failure to Wean *505*
    Failure to Oxygenate *506*
    Failure to Ventilate (CO_2 Retention) *506*
Summary *508*
References *508*

F. Renal Function

33. Disturbances of Acid–Base Homeostasis *511*
Jon F. Berlauk and Jerome H. Abrams
ABG Interpretation *511*
Metabolic Acid–Base Disorders *516*
    Metabolic Acidosis *516*
    Metabolic Alkalosis *518*
Respiratory Acid–Base Disorders *519*
    Respiratory Acidosis *521*
    Respiratory Alkalosis *522*
Summary *524*
References *525*

34. Acute Renal Failure 527
Mark E. Rosenberg
Introduction 527
Differential Diagnosis 527
    Prerenal ARF 527
    Intrinsic ARF 531
    Postrenal ARF 532
Prevention 533
    Mannitol and Loop Diuretics 533
    Dopamine 534
Management 534
    Fluid Balance 534
    Hyperkalemia 535
    Hyponatremia 535
    Hypocalcemia and Hyperphosphatemia 535
    Acidosis 535
    Nutrition 536
    Dialysis 536
    Bleeding 536
    Drug Dosing 536
Course and Prognosis of ARF 536
Summary 537
Suggested Reading 538

35. Support of Renal Function 539
Connie L. Manske
Hemodialysis 539
Continuous Venovenous Hemofiltration 543
Continuous Venovenous Hemofiltration with Dialysis 543
Choosing a Method of Renal Replacement Therapy 543
Summary 544
References 544

G. Gastrointestinal and Hepatic Function

36. Gut Function: Practical Considerations for the Intensivist 547
David C. Evans
The Gut Mucosal Barrier 547
    Physical Barrier Function 547
    Immunologic Barrier 548
    Bacteriologic Barrier 549
The Gut and MSOF 550
Supporting Gut Barrier Function 551
    Oxygen Transport 551
    Enhancing Gut Motility 552

Nutritional Support 552
Stress Ulcer Prophylaxis 552
Antibiotic Prophylaxis 553
Gut Failure: What Do We Mean? 554
Summary 554
References 555

37. Acute Gastrointestinal Hemorrhage 557
Jerome H. Abrams
UGI Hemorrhage 557
Common Causes 559
Mallory-Weiss Lesion 559
Esophageal Varices 559
Gastritis 561
Peptic Ulcer Disease 562
LGI Hemorrhage 563
Patient Evaluation 563
Summary 565
References 566

38. Acute Pancreatitis in the Surgical Intensive Care Unit 569
Jeffrey G. Chipman
Introduction 569
Pathophysiology 569
Etiology 569
Pathology 570
Diagnosis 571
History and Physical Information 571
Laboratory Data 573
Radiologic Data 574
Fine Needle Aspiration 574
Treatment 575
Source Control 575
Debridement and Drainage 575
Antibiotics 576
Restoration of Oxygen Transport 577
Metabolic Support 578
Outcomes 579
Future Considerations 579
Summary 579
References 580

39. Biliary Complications During Critical Illness 583
Paul Druck
Acute Cholecystitis 583
Epidemiology of Acute Cholecystitis in the Critically Ill 583

Pathogenesis of Acute Cholecystitis in
the Critically Ill 583
Diagnosis of Acute Cholecystitis in
the Critically Ill 584
Treatment of Acute Cholecystitis in
the Critically Ill 586
Obstructive and Nonobstructive Jaundice and Cholangitis 586
Initial Evaluation of the Jaundiced Patient 586
Obstructive Jaundice and Cholangitis 587
Nonobstructive Jaundice 587
Summary 589
References 589

40. Acute Abdomen 591
Michael D. Pasquale and Roderick A. Barke
History and Physical Examination 591
Resuscitation and Monitoring 594
Diagnostic Evaluation 595
Laboratory Tests 595
Radiologic Tests 596
Miscellaneous Tests 597
Diagnosis and Treatment 597
Diagnostic Difficulties in the Critically Ill Patient 599
Acalculous Cholecystitis 599
Acute Mesenteric Ischemia 599
Pancreatitis 601
Immunosuppression 601
Summary 601
Reference 602
Suggested Reading 602

**41. A Pathophysiologic Approach to Fulminant Hepatic
Failure in the Intensive Care Unit** 605
Kambiz Kosari and Timothy D. Sielaff
Introduction 605
Definitions 605
Acute-on-Chronic Liver Failure (ACLF) 605
Fulminant Hepatic Failure (FHF) 606
Hepatic Encephalopathy 606
Causes 607
Acute-on-Chronic Liver Failure 607
Fulminant Hepatic Failure 607
Pathophysiologic Features 609
Tissue Hypoxia 609
Hepatic Encephalopathy 611
Management 613
Before Transfer to a Liver Center 613
Treatment of ACLF Patients 614
Issues Regarding Patient Transfer 614
Liver Center Care 615

                Liver Transplantation 620
                Liver Assist Devices 621
                Hybrid Bioartificial Livers 622
        Conclusions 624
        Summary 624
        References 625

H. Endocrine System

42. Endocrine Emergencies 629
Paul Druck
        Adrenal Insufficiency 629
                Etiology of AI 629
                Clinical Features and Diagnosis of AI 630
                Treatment of Adrenal Crisis 631
                Prevention of Perioperative AI 632
        Thyroid Dysfunction 634
                Thyroid Storm 634
                Myxedema Coma 637
                Sick-Euthyroid Syndrome 638
        Disorders of Glucose Homeostasis 639
                Maintenance of Normoglycemia in
                    Critically Ill Patients 639
                Diabetic Ketoacidosis and Hyperglycemic
                    Hyperosmolar Nonketotic Syndrome
                    (Hyperosmolar Coma) 639
        Summary 641
                Adrenal Insufficiency 641
                Thyroid Disorders 642
                Disorders of Glucose Homeostasis 642
        References 642

43. Divalent Ions 647
Jeffrey A. Bailey and John E. Mazuski
        Calcium 647
                Hypocalcemia 648
                Hypercalcemia 650
        Magnesium 651
                Hypomagnesemia 652
                Hypermagnesemia 653
        Phosphorus 654
                Hypophosphatemia 654
                Hyperphosphatemia 655
        Summary 657
        References 658

44. Chemical Homeostasis 661
Roderick A. Barke
        Body Compartments and Distribution of Water
            and Electrolytes 661

Contents xxiii

    Effect of Stress of Surgery or Trauma on Fluid Homeostasis 662
        Evolution of Understanding of Hormonal Response 663
    Goal of Fluid and Electrolyte Therapy 664
    Hyperosmolality, Hypertonicity, and Hypernatremia 664
        Hypo-Osmolality and Hyponatremia 668
        Potassium 670
    Summary 672
    References 672
    Suggested Reading 673

I. Infectious Diseases

45. Antibiotic Resistance in the Intensive Care Unit 675
    Jan E. Patterson and Daniel L. Dent
    Introduction 675
    Epidemiology of Antimicrobial Resistance in the ICU 675
        Antibiotic Utilization in the ICU 676
        The Role of Infection Control 680
    Specific Pathogens 681
        Methicillin-Resistant *S. aureus* (MRSA) 681
        Vancomycin-Resistant Enterococci (VRE) 682
        Pseudomonas aeruginosa 683
        Enterobacter spp. 684
        Extended-Spectrum Beta-Lactamase (ESBL)-Producing
          Klebsiella pneumoniae 685
        Acinetobacter baumannii 686
    Summary 686
    References 687

46. Intra-abdominal Infection 693
    Ori D. Rotstein and Jerome H. Abrams
    Anatomy and Physiology of Abdominal Cavity 693
    Defense Against Peritoneal Infection 694
        Local Response 694
        Systemic Response 695
    Diagnosis and Management of Intra-abdominal Infection 695
        Secondary Peritonitis 695
        Intra-abdominal Abscess 698
        Tertiary Peritonitis 699
    Summary 701
    References 701
    Suggested Reading 702

47. HIV/AIDS and the Surgeon 703
    Omobosola Akinsete and Edward N. Janoff
    Introduction 703
    Epidemiology 704
    Transmission of HIV 705
    Transmission of HIV from Surgeon to Patient 707

Prevention of Occupational HIV Infection *708*
Recognizing HIV Infection *710*
Antiretroviral Therapy *712*
Complications and Outcome of Surgery Among HIV-Infected Patients *717*
HIV/AIDS: Ethical and Legal Issues *718*
Summary *719*
References *720*

48. Infection in the Immunocompromised Patient 725
Gregory A. Filice
Basic Concepts *725*
Innate Defects *728*
    Neutropenia *728*
    Complement Deficiency *730*
    Asplenia or Splenic Dysfunction *730*
    Malnutrition *731*
    Malignancy *731*
    Diabetes Mellitus *731*
    Neurological Dysfunction *731*
    Tobacco Use *732*
    Stress *732*
    Hypochlorhydria *732*
    Altered Microbial Flora *732*
Defects in Immunity *733*
    Antibody Deficiency *733*
    CMI Defects *733*
    Infection-Induced Immune Dysfunction *733*
    Transplantation *734*
Fever and Infectious Diseases in Critical Care *735*
Management *737*
Prevention *738*
Summary *739*
References *741*

Part IV: Systemic Dysfunction

J. Critical Care Pharmacology

49. Optimization of Drug Doses 745
Pamela K. Phelps and Bruce C. Lohr
Absorption *745*
Distribution *746*
Metabolism *746*
Excretion *747*
Use of Serum Concentrations *748*
    Inotropic/Vasoactive Agents *754*
    Antihypertensive Agents *767*
    Sedative Agents *776*

Contents   xxv

      Summary 779
      References 780

50. Adverse Drug Reactions and Drug Interactions in the Intensive Care Unit 783
      Douglas DeCarolis
      Cardiovascular Agents 783
          Antiarrhythmic Drugs 783
          Other Antiarrhythmic Agents 786
          Vasoactive Drugs 787
          Inotropic Agents 788
          Vasopressor Agents 788
          Sedative Agents 788
          Analgesic Agents 790
          Non-opioid Agents 791
      References 795

51. Anaphylaxis 799
      Paul Druck
      Definitions 799
      Epidemiology 799
      Inciting Agents 800
      Pathophysiology 801
          Mediators of Anaphylaxis 801
          Effects of the Principal Mediators 802
      Clinical Manifestations 802
          Respiratory Effects 802
          Cardiovascular Effects 803
          Mucocutaneous Manifestations 803
          Miscellaneous Manifestations 804
      Treatment 804
          Initial Steps and Basic Support 804
          Treatment of Respiratory Compromise 805
          Hemodynamic Compromise 806
          Adjunctive Measures and the Recovery Phase 806
      Prevention 807
          Iodine-Containing RCM 807
          Beta-Lactam Antibiotics 807
      Summary 808
      References 809

K. Coagulation and Transfusion

52. Disorders of Coagulation 811
      Aneel A. Ashrani and Nigel S. Key
      Introduction 811
      Physiology of Hemostasis 811
          Role of Platelets 811
          Role of the Coagulation Proteins:
              Secondary Hemostasis 812
          Role of Vascular Endothelium 813

Pathophysiology of Hemorrhagic and
  Thrombotic Diatheses *814*
Bleeding Disorders *814*
  Preoperative and Postoperative Management of a Patient
    with a Hemostatic Defect *817*
Special Hemostatic Challenges *820*
  Cardiopulmonary Bypass Surgery *820*
  Liver Disease *820*
  Renal Disease *822*
Thrombotic Disorders *822*
Disseminated Intravascular Coagulation *826*
Heparin-Associated Thrombocytopenia *828*
Summary *829*
References *831*

53. Transfusion Therapy 833
James R. Stubbs
Red Blood Cell Transfusion *833*
  Principles of Oxygen Delivery and
    Oxygen Consumption *834*
Plasma Transfusion *846*
  Indications *847*
  Contraindications *848*
Platelets *848*
  Platelet Selection *848*
  Prophylactic Platelet Transfusion *849*
  Therapeutic Platelet Transfusion *851*
  Platelet Refractoriness *851*
  Platelet Alloimmunization—Prevention *855*
  Contraindications *856*
Cryoprecipitate Transfusion *856*
  Indications *856*
Leukoreduced Blood Components *857*
  Febrile Nonhemolytic Transfusion Reactions *857*
  Cytomegalovirus *859*
  Immunomodulation *861*
Recombinant Factor VIIa *863*
  Massive Transfusion *867*
Transfusion-Associated Graft-vs.-Host Disease *869*
  Implicated Blood Components *871*
  Prevention *871*
  Gamma Irradiation Guidelines *871*
Noninfectious Risks of Transfusion *872*
  Acute *872*
  Delayed *874*
Infectious Risks of Blood Transfusion *874*
  West Nile Virus *875*
  Bacteria *876*
Summary *877*
References *879*

54. Agents Used for Anticoagulation *895*
   James R. Stubbs
   Warfarin *895*
   Unfractionated Heparin and LMWH *897*
   Summary *900*
   References *900*

Part V: Common SICU Procedures

55. Bronchoscopy *905*
   Marshall I. Hertz and Paul Gustafson
   Overview *905*
   Indications *906*
      Suspected Pneumonia *906*
      Atelectasis *907*
      Hemoptysis *907*
      Foreign Body *908*
      Suspected Tracheobronchial Disruption *908*
      Smoke Inhalation *908*
      Difficult Intubation *908*
   Contraindications *908*
   Bronchoscopy and Bronchoalveolar Lavage
      with Intubation *909*
      Supplemental Oxygen *909*
      Bronchoscope *909*
      Ventilator Management *910*
      Monitors *910*
      Medications *910*
      Bronchoalveolar Lavage Technique *910*
   Complications *912*
   Summary *914*
   References *914*

56. Vascular Access *915*
   Thomas Wozniak and Larry Micon
   Central Venous Access *915*
      Indications for Catheterization *915*
      Subclavian Vein Catheterization *916*
      Internal Jugular Approach *918*
      Femoral Vein Cannulation *919*
   Pulmonary Arterial Access *920*
   Systemic Arterial Catheterization *923*
      Technique *924*
      Complications *924*
      Doppler-Guided Catheterization *925*
   Summary *925*
   References *925*

57. Care of Central Lines *929*
   Steven D. Eyer
   Catheter-Related Sepsis *929*
      Incidence *929*
      Causes *929*
   Aseptic Technique *930*
   Catheter Removal or Exchange *931*
      Central Venous Catheters *931*
      Pulmonary Artery Catheters *932*
      Samples for Culture *932*
      Replacement of Lines *932*
      Clinical Reasons for Replacement *933*
      Guidewire Exchange *934*
   Catheter-Related Thrombosis *934*
   Summary *934*
   Suggested Reading *935*

58. Percutaneous Tracheostomy *937*
   Jeffrey G. Chipman
   Introduction *937*
   Background *937*
   Indications and Contraindications *938*
   Technique *938*
      Location *938*
      Personnel *939*
      Equipment *939*
      Method *939*
   Pitfalls *943*
   Conclusions *943*
   Summary *943*
   References *944*

59. Lumbar Puncture, Thoracentesis, Thoracostomy, and Paracentesis ... *947*
   Sharon Henry
   Lumbar Puncture *947*
      Anatomy *947*
      Positioning *947*
      Procedure *947*
      CSF Analysis *948*
      Complications *949*
   Thoracentesis *950*
      Procedure *950*
      Complications *951*
      Fluid Analysis *951*
   Thoracostomy *951*
      Procedure *951*
      Complications *953*
      Drainage Systems *954*
      Chest Tube Removal *955*

Contents   xxix

           Sclerosis 955
           Maintaining Chest Tube Patency 955
    Paracentesis 955
        Procedure 955
        Diagnostic Tests 956
        Complications 956
    Open and Closed Peritoneal Tap and Lavage 957
        Closed Procedure 957
        Open Procedure 958
        Semi-open Procedure 958
        Results 958
    Summary 958
    References 959

Part VI: Measurement and Interpretation of Data

60. Blood Pressure Monitoring 963
    Jerome H. Abrams
    Damped Oscillating Systems: Resonance 963
    Measuring Damping Coefficient 965
        Theory 965
        Clinical Application 966
    Summary 970
    References 970

61. Cardiac Output 973
    Jerome H. Abrams
    The Fick Principle 974
    Other Methods of Measurement 977
    Summary 978
    References 978

62. Respiratory Monitoring 981
    Ian J. Gilmour
    Monitoring Lung Volumes 984
    Monitoring Gas Exchange 987
    Pulse Oximetry 989
    Monitoring Carbon Dioxide Removal 990
    Summary 993
    References 994
    Suggested Reading 994

Part VII: Approaches to Complex Problems

63. Responding to Uncertainty in the Intensive Care Unit: Some Unanswered Questions in Critical Care and How They Got That Way 997
    Jerome H. Abrams
    Resolving Degeneracy-Distinguishing Response Variables
       from Control Variables 998

Use of Dynamical Systems *1005*
Joint Probabilities *1008*
Use of Statistical Ensembles *1011*
Summary *1017*
References *1017*

Index *1019*

Contributors

Jerome H. Abrams *Department of Surgery (112), VA Medical Center, Minneapolis, Minnesota, USA*

David H. Ahrenholz *Department of Surgery, The Burn Center Regions Medical Center, St. Paul, Minnesota, USA*

Omobosola Akinsete *Department of Medicine, VA Medical Center, Minneapolis, Minnesota, USA*

Aneel A. Ashrani *Division of Hematology, Oncology and Transplantation, University of Minnesota, Minneapolis, Minnesota, USA*

Jeffrey A. Bailey *Department of Surgery, St. Louis University School of Medicine, St. Louis, Missouri, USA*

Roderick A. Barke *Department of Surgery (112), VA Medical Center, Minneapolis, Minnesota, USA*

Richard G. Barton *Department of Surgery, University of Utah School of Medicine, Salt Lake City, Utah, USA*

Jon F. Berlauk[†]

Joseph R. Bloomer *Department of Internal Medicine, University of Alabama, Birmingham, Alabama, USA*

Larry Bone *Department of Orthopedics, Erie County Medical Center, Buffalo, New York, USA*

Anthony Bottini *Centracare Clinic—Neurosurgery, St. Cloud, Minnesota, USA*

Richard W. Carlson *Department of Medicine, Maricopa Medical Center, Phoenix, Arizona, USA*

Frank B. Cerra *Childrens Rehab Center, University of Minnesota, Minneapolis, Minnesota, USA*

[†]Deceased

Jeffrey G. Chipman Surgical Critical Care, VA Medical Center, Minneapolis, Minnesota, USA

Mark D. Cipolle Lehigh Valley Hospital, Allentown, Pennsylvania, USA

Vivian L. Clark Cardiac Catheterization Lab, Henry Ford Hospital, Detroit, Michigan, USA

Ricardo Correa-Rotter Department of Nephrology, Instituto Nacional de la Nutricion, Salvador Zubbiran, Mexico City, Mexico

Alan J. Cropp Critical Care Medicine, St. Elizabeth Hospital Medical Center, Youngstown, Ohio, USA

Alexandre d'Audiffret Vascular Surgery Service (112K), VA Medical Center, Minneapolis, Minnesota, USA

Bhagwan Dass Critical Care Medicine, St. Elizabeth Hospital Medical Center, Youngstown, Ohio, USA

Douglas DeCarolis Pharmacy Service (119), VA Medical Center, Minneapolis, Minnesota, USA

R. Phillip Dellinger Section of Critical Care Medicine, Cooper University Hospital, Camden, New Jersey, USA

Daniel L. Dent Department of Surgery, University of Texas Health Science Center at San Antonio, San Antonio, Texas, USA

Paul Druck Surgical Service (112), VA Medical Center, Minneapolis, Minnesota, USA

David C. Evans Critical Care, McGill University Health Care, Montreal, Quebec, Canada

Steven D. Eyer Trauma, St. Mary's Medical Center, Duluth, Minnesota, USA

Gregory A. Filice Infectious Disease Section (111F), VA Medical Center, Minneapolis, Minnesota, USA

William J. Flynn, Jr. Department of Surgery, Erie County Medical Center, Buffalo, New York, USA

Arthur H. L. From Department of Medicine, VA Medical Center, Minneapolis, Minnesota, USA

Ian J. Gilmour Anesthesia Associates of Martinsville, Inc., Martinsville, Virginia, USA

Charles C. Gornick Cardiac Electrophysiology, Minneapolis Heart Institute, Minneapolis, Minnesota, USA

Guillermo Guiterrez Pulmonary Medicine Department, University of Texas Medical School, Houston, Texas, USA

Rakesh Gupta Department of Critical Care, St. Francis Medical Center, Pittsburgh, Pennsylvania, USA

Paul Gustafson Cardiopulmonary Services, University of Minnesota, Minneapolis, Minnesota, USA

Contributors

Sharon Henry Shock Trauma Center, University of Maryland, College Park, Maryland, USA

Marshall I. Hertz University of Minnesota, Minneapolis, Minnesota, USA

Steven M. Hollenberg Cooper University Hospital, Camden, New Jersey, USA

John W. Hoyt Department of Critical Care, St. Francis Medical Center, Pittsburgh, Pennsylvania, USA

Edward N. Janoff Infectious Disease Section (111F), VA Medical Center, Minneapolis, Minnesota, USA

Nigel S. Key Department of Medicine, University of Minnesota, Minneapolis, Minnesota, USA

Kambiz Kosari Department of Surgery, University of Minnesota, Minneapolis, Minnesota, USA

James A. Kruse Pulmonary and Critical Care Medicine, Detroit Receiving Hospital, Detroit, Michigan, USA

Frederick Langendorf Department of Neurology, Hennepin County Medical Center, Minneapolis, Minnesota, USA

Victor Lazaron Department of Surgery, University of Minnesota, Minneapolis, Minnesota, USA

Connie Lindberg Vascular Surgery Service (112K), VA Medical Center, Minneapolis, Minnesota, USA

George M. Logan Park Nicollet Clinical Gastroenterology, Minneapolis, Minnesota, USA

Bruce C. Lohr College of Pharmacy, University of Minnesota, Minneapolis, Minnesota, USA

Connie L. Manske Adult Dialysis, University of Minnesota, Minneapolis, Minnesota, USA

John E. Mazuski Department of Surgery, Washington University School of Medicine, St. Louis, Missouri, USA

Larry Micon Tower Surgical, Indianapolis, Indiana, USA

William Mohr The Burn Center Regions Medical Center, St. Paul, Minnesota, USA

Sandeep Nathan Department of Medicine and Department of Cardiology, Rush–Presbyterian–St. Luke's Medical Center, Chicago, Illinois, USA

Valerie Nebel Surgical Service (112), VA Medical Center, Minneapolis, Minnesota, USA

Michael D. Pasquale Department of Surgery, Lehigh Valley Hospital, Allentown, Pennsylvania, USA

Jan E. Patterson University of Texas at San Antonio, San Antonio, Texas, USA

Pamela K. Phelps College of Pharmacy, University of Minnesota, Minneapolis, Minnesota, USA

Michael R. Pinsky Department of Critical Care Medicine, University of Pittsburgh Medical Center, Pittsburgh, Pennsylvania, USA

Mark E. Rosenberg Department of Medicine, University of Minnesota, Minneapolis, Minnesota, USA

Ori D. Rotstein Department of Surgery, University of Toronto, Toronto, Ontario, Canada

Edward Rustamzadeh Neurosurgery Department, University of Minnesota, Minneapolis, Minnesota, USA

Steven Santilli Vascular Surgery Service (112K), VA Medical Center, Minneapolis, Minnesota, USA

Timothy D. Sielaff Department of Surgery, University of Minnesota, Minneapolis, Minnesota, USA

James R. Stubbs Department of Pathology, University of South Alabama Medical Center, Mobile, Alabama, USA

Jodie Herk Taylor University of Minnesota and Hennepin County Medical Center, Minneapolis, Minnesota, USA

Stephen Trzeciak Department of Emergency Medicine, Cooper University Hospital, Camden, New Jersey, USA

Sabrina Walski-Easton Neurosurgery Department, University of Minnesota, Minneapolis, Minnesota, USA

Melissa West ECC (11L), VA Medical Center, Minneapolis, Minnesota, USA

Larry A. Woods Critical Care Medicine, St. Elizabeth Hospital Medical Center, Youngstown, Ohio, USA

Thomas Wozniak Cardiothoracic and Vascular Surgery, Indianapolis, Indiana, USA

Karl L. Yang Herman Hospital, Louisville, Kentucky, USA

Part I
Altered Metabolism of Critical Illness and Shock

1
Stress Response and Multiple Organ Failure

Victor Lazaron
University of Minnesota, Minneapolis, Minnesota, USA

Jerome H. Abrams
VA Medical Center, Minneapolis, Minnesota, USA

INTRODUCTION

When adaptive, the intricate interplay of metabolism, physiology, and immunity can surmount devastating injuries or illnesses and allow individuals to return to a life of quality. When maladaptive, this response produces sequential failure of all major organ systems. The jaundiced, comatose patient requiring the assistance of a ventilator and the support of dialysis may remain suspended between recovery and further deterioration. Recovery becomes more remote as each day passes, and no progress is seen. With the advances of modern intensive care medicine patients, who in past years would have died of their illnesses, are routinely resuscitated and supported. This triumph has produced many new problems in clinical care and has exposed a "natural history" of critical illness in which each stress to normal physiology and the corresponding host response to that stress combine to produce a new homeostatic set point for each organ system and for the patient as a whole. The level of exogenous support required to sustain the patient without further deterioration determines whether each successive set point is closer or farther from a state of health.

Many terms are used to describe this phenomenon. An early descriptor, hypermetabolism, refers to the elevation of cardiac output, oxygen consumption, increased energy demands, and catabolic metabolism of these patients (1). Table 1 lists definitions developed by the American College of Chest Physicians and the Society of Critical Care Medicine in 1992 to describe various components of this complicated clinical state. Although an expert panel reviewed these definitions in 2003, the 2003 consensus conference did not provide any new definitions. Rather, an expanded list of signs and symptoms was developed to overcome the "overly sensitive and nonspecific" criteria in the 1992 conference (2) and to better "reflect clinical bedside experience" (Table 2). Specific definitions of organ system failure (OSF) that have been used to establish prognosis were elaborated by Knaus and Wagner (3) and are listed in Table 3. Presently, the accepted definition of multiple organ failure (MOF) is "the presence of altered organ function in an acutely ill patient such that homeostasis cannot be maintained without intervention" (4,5). A recent review of ICU

Table 1 Definitions

Infection: microbial phenomenon characterized by an inflammatory response to the presence of microorganisms or the invasion of normally sterile host tissue by those organisms.

Bacteremia: the presence of viable bacteria in the blood.

Systemic inflammatory response syndrome (SIRS): the systemic inflammatory response to a variety of severe clinical insults. The response is manifested by two or more of the following conditions: (1) temperature $>38°C$ or $<36°C$; (2) heart rate >90 beats/min; (3) respiratory rate >20 breaths/minute or $PaCO_2$ <32 mm Hg; and (4) white blood cell count $>12,000$ per mm^3, <4000 per mm^3, or $>10\%$ immature (band) forms.

Sepsis: the systemic response to infection, manifested by two or more of the following conditions as a result of infection: (1) temperature $>38°C$ or $<36°C$; (2) heart rate >90 beats/min; (3) respiratory rate >20 breaths/minute or $PaCO_2$ <32 mm Hg; and (4) white blood cell count $>12,000$ per mm^3, <4000 per mm^3, or $>10\%$ immature (band) forms.

Severe sepsis: sepsis associated organ dysfunction, hypoperfusion, or hypotension. Hypoperfusion and perfusion abnormalities may include, but are not limited to, lactic acidosis, oliguria, or an acute alteration in mental status.

Septic shock: sepsis induced hypotension despite adequate fluid resuscitation along with the presence of perfusion abnormalities that may include, but are not limited to, lactic acidosis, oliguria, or an acute alteration in mental status. Patients who are receiving inotropic or vasopressor agents may not be hypotensive at the time the perfusion abnormalities are measured.

Sepsis induced hypotension: a systolic blood pressure <90 mm Hg or a reduction of ≥ 40 mm Hg from baseline in the absence of other causes for hypotension.

Multiple organ dysfunction syndrome (MODS): presence of altered organ function in an acutely ill patient such that homeostasis cannot be maintained without intervention.

Source: From Bone RC, Balk RA, Cerra FB, Dellinger RP, Fein AM, Knaus WA, Schein RMH, Sibbald WJ. Definitions for sepsis and organ failure and guidelines for the use of innovative therapies in sepsis. Chest 1992; 101:1644–1655.

patient outcomes by Marshall et al. (6) showed a marked increase in mortality with each additional OSF (Table 4). Several scoring systems used in critical care medicine reflect this reality in their weighting of OSF by the level of clinical support required (7,8).

MOF is seen more commonly in the elderly, in patients with a comorbid medical diagnosis, and in patients with the largest initial physiologic derangement (3,9). MOF is more common in medical than in surgical patients. The most frequent precipitating diagnoses are sepsis, pneumonia, congestive heart failure, cardiac arrest, and gastrointestinal bleeding (10). In surgical patients, MOF is associated with operation for both ruptured and elective aortic aneurysm, for gastrointestinal perforation, and for gastrointestinal malignancy. Multiple trauma, especially head trauma, is associated with increased frequency of MOF. Current data support a gender and genetic heterogeneity that determines the likelihood of developing organ failure in response to a specific insult (11).

In a retrospective review of patients, the number of Gram-negative infections per patient was not significantly different in patients who survived, compared to patients who died (12). Discriminators of survival were arterial partial pressure of oxygen (PaO_2)/fraction of inspired oxygen (FIO_2) on day 1, serum lactate concentration on day 2, serum bilirubin on day 6, and serum creatinine on day 12 (Table 5). Plasma transferrin concentration, AST, and alkaline phosphatase were not discriminators. Patients who survived were younger, spent less time undergoing mechanical ventilation, and had shorter stays in the SICU. Total hospital days were not significantly different in both the groups.

Table 2 Revised Diagnostic Criteria for Sepsis (Infection, Documented or Suspected, and Some of the Following)

General variables
   Fever (core temperature >38.3°C)
   Hypothermia (core temperature <36°C)
   Heart rate >90 beats/min or >2 SD above the normal value for age
   Tachypnea
   Altered mental status
   Significant edema or positive fluid balance (>20 mL/kg over 24 h)
   Hyperglycemia (plasma glucose >120 mg/dL or 7.7 mmol/L) in the absence of diabetes
Inflammatory variables
   Leukocytosis (WBC count >12,000 cells/μL)
   Leukopenia (WBC count <4,000 cells/μL)
   Normal WBC with >10% immature forms
   Plasma C-reactive protein >2 SD above the normal value
   Plasma procalcitonin >2 SD above the normal value
Hemodynamic variables
   Arterial hypotension (SBP <90 mm Hg, MAP <70 mm Hg, or an SBP decrease
     >40 mm Hg in adults or <2 SD below normal for age)
   Mixed venous oxygen saturation >70% in adults
   Cardiac index >3.5 L/min per m^2
Organ dysfunction variables
   Arterial hypoxemia (PaO_2/FIO_2 <300)
   Acute oliguria (urine output <0.5 mL/kg per hour or 45 mmol/L for at least 2 h)
   Creatinine increase >0.5 mg/dL
   Coagulation abnormalities (INR >1.5 or a PTT >60 s)
   Ileus (absent bowel sounds)
   Thrombocytopenia (platetet count <100,000 cells/μL)
   Hyperbilirubinemia (plasma total bilirubin >4 mg/dL or 70 mmol/L)
Tissue perfusion variables
   Hyperlactatemia (>1 mmol/L)
   Decreased capillary refill or mottling

MULTIPLE ORGAN FAILURE SYNDROME

Clinical Features

MOF syndrome does not involve isolated organ failure. Rather, it is the sequential and accumulated failure of all the major organ systems of the body, which occurs until significant and concomitant dysfunction is seen in the lung, liver, kidneys, and nervous system. A stereotypical pathway leading to the development of MOF or multi-organ dysfunction syndrome (MODS) was originally described by Skillman et al. (13). In their series of patients with stress ulceration of the stomach, they described a clinical syndrome of respiratory failure, hypotension, sepsis, and jaundice. Later, Tilney et al. (14) presciently termed the phenomenon, "an unsolved problem in postoperative care," an apt description to this day.

    The typical progression is an inciting event, acute lung injury, hypermetabolism, and finally MOF syndrome. The hypermetabolism is manifested in elevated cardiac output, increased oxygen consumption, and pronounced nitrogen losses. In some individuals, the inciting injury is massive. In others, especially those who may be recovering from

Table 3 Definitions of Organ System Failure (Presence of One or More of the Following Values During a 24 h Period Defines OSF)

  I. Cardiovascular system
   a. Heart rate ≤54
   b. Mean arterial blood pressure ≤49 mm Hg
   c. Ventricular tachycardia or fibrillation
   d. pH ≤7.24 with $PaCO_2$ ≤49 mm Hg
 II. Respiratory system
   a. Respiratory rate ≤5 or ≥49
   b. $PaCO_2$ ≥50 mm Hg
   c. $AaDO_2$ ≥350 mm Hg
   d. Ventilator dependence beyond initial 72 h of OSF
III. Renal system
   a. Urine output ≤479 mL/24 h or ≤159 mL/8 h
   b. BUN ≥100 mg/dL
   c. Creatinine ≥3.5 mg/dL
 IV. Hematologic system
   a. WBC ≤1000 per mm^3
   b. Platelets ≤20,000 per mm^3
   c. Hematocrit <20%
  V. Neurologic system
   a. Glasgow coma scale ≤6 (in absence of sedation)
 VI. Hepatic system
   a. Prothrombin time >4 s above control (without anti-coagulation)
   b. Bilirubin >6 mg%

Source: Adapted from Ref. (3).

another insult, the inciting injury may be one that is generally well tolerated. Shock, ischemia/reperfusion, significant soft tissue injury, necrotic tissue, and pancreatitis have been associated with MOF (15).

Once the source of injury has been controlled, the patient initially responds to supportive measures, such as intravenous fluids and ventilator therapy. After several

Table 4 30-Day Survival Rates in ICU Patients as a Function of Number of Organ Systems in Failure

Number	Mortality (%)
0	0.8
1	6.8
2	26.2
3	48.5
4	68.8
5	83.3

Source: Adapted from Ref. (6).

Table 5 Discriminators of Survival

	SICU day	Mean value in survivors	Mean value in nonsurvivors
PaO_2/FIO_2	1	311 ± 25	233 ± 14
Lactate (mmol)	2	1.1 ± 0.2	3.4 ± 0.7
Bilirubin (mg/dL)	6	2.2 ± 0.6	8.5 ± 2.2
Creatinine (mg/dL)	12	1.9 ± 0.6	3.9 ± 0.3

days, low-grade fever, tachycardia, and dyspnea appear. The chest X-ray reveals bilateral, diffuse, patchy infiltrates. The patient's mental status may be altered. Respiratory distress progresses, and intubation and mechanical ventilation may prove necessary. At this point, although the patient demonstrates hemodynamic stability, as measured by heart rate and by urine output, the characteristic features of the systemic inflammatory response syndrome (SIRS) are already present (Tables 1 and 2). The cardiac index is typically elevated, the oxygen consumption is increased, and the systemic vascular resistance is low. Progression of SIRS leads to the MOF syndrome.

The primary overall response to MOF is an increase in oxygen consumption. The patient must maintain adequate arterial oxygen saturation and increased cardiac output to provide the increased oxygen delivery necessary for survival. A pathologic condition of the lungs may interfere with arterial oxygen saturation. The lung may demonstrate a primary pathologic state in the form of pneumonia. Secondary lung involvement, acute lung injury, can occur not only from a primary lung infection but also from hemorrhagic shock, systemic shock, pancreatitis, multiple trauma, and ischemia/reperfusion injury. One characteristic of acute lung injury is the increase in dead-space ventilation. The tissue injury and, perhaps, pulmonary therapy with increased airway pressures, cause progressive mismatch between ventilation and blood flow, with increased numbers of nonperfused but ventilated alveoli. Patients with this condition develop an increased minute ventilation to excrete carbon dioxide. In these patients, the work of breathing demand, a result of the need for high minute ventilation, may exceed the patient's work of breathing reserve (1).

Cardiac response may be limited by inadequate preload, previous cardiac disease, or acquired cardiac dysfunction. Inadequate resuscitation and redistribution of the body fluid compartments can lead to a decrease in preload. Preexisting cardiac valvular or coronary vascular disease may limit the patient's ability to respond to increased cardiac output. Acquired cardiac malfunction can arise from malnutrition or the presence of soluble myocardial depressant factors (see Chapter 3). Experimental and clinical evidence demonstrate decreased ejection fraction in sepsis (16,17).

The clinical herald of MOF is jaundice. After 7–10 days, the bilirubin concentration exceeds 3 mg/dL. At the time jaundice appears, the biliary tree is dilated, cholestasis is present, and sludge is usually evident on ultrasound examination. These changes are mirrored by deterioration in other hepatic functions: hepatic protein synthesis of albumin, transferrin, prealbumin, and retinol-binding protein falls. Development of jaundice is temporally associated with measurable changes in other metabolic variables. Oxygen consumption rises, and cardiac output increases. Evidence for hepatic failure includes progressive jaundice, decreasing amino acid clearance, reduction in hepatic protein synthesis, unrestricted ureagenesis in the absence of protein administration, and decreased triglyceride clearance. In late MOF, mitochondrial dysfunction in the liver is reflected by an increased ratio of the concentrations of beta hydroxybutyric acid to acetoacetate (BOHB/AcAc). Terminally, hypoglycemia occurs.

In the transition to late organ failure, a concomitant decrease in SVR is typically observed. Wound healing deteriorates, and pressure lesions of the skin are common. The patient becomes thrombocytopenic. As organ failure progresses, increased intravascular volume is needed to maintain preload, and inotropes are frequently required to maintain adequate cardiac output and oxygen delivery. In late organ failure, blood, urine, or sputum cultures often demonstrate the presence of *Candida* organisms and viruses. Between hospital days 14 and 21, renal failure worsens, and dialysis may be necessary.

Energy expenditure is increased during the hypermetabolic and the MOF phases. Although both oxygen consumption and carbon dioxide production are elevated, the respiratory quotient (R/Q) usually is 0.8–0.9, a value consistent with a mixed fuel source. Carbohydrate, fat, and amino acids are used for high-energy phosphate production. Adequate metabolic support should include a mixture of carbohydrate, fat, and amino acids. Total body protein catabolism is increased and exceeds the protein synthetic rate. The catabolism of the lean body mass has been termed autocannabalism, and urinary nitrogen excretion can exceed 20 g/day (18). The amino acids derived from catabolism of the lean body mass are used in sites of active protein synthesis, in wounds for oxidation, and for conversion to other substrates. With protein loading, the uptake of amino acids by skeletal muscle is suppressed, but hepatic amino acid uptake is increased. The liver can synthesize increased amounts of acute phase reactants, while albumin and transferrin synthesis is down-regulated. The increased urea production and associated azotemia reflect the increased amino acid turnover.

Although the metabolic signals that cause catabolism are not suppressed by exogenous amino acid administration, the protein synthetic rate is increased with amino acid loading. When the synthetic rate equals the catabolic rate, nitrogen equilibrium is achieved. If metabolic support is absent or inadequate, hepatic protein synthesis fails, and the patient has a higher mortality risk.

In late organ failure, protein synthesis fails, and catabolism is unabated. Clearance of all amino acids, including branched-chain amino acids, is reduced. In addition, in late MOF, the endogenous R/Q exceeds one, a value that indicates net lipogenesis. Further details of metabolic support are discussed in Chapter 3.

Although the stereotypic failure of each major organ system suggests that a "final common pathway" exists in response to physiologic and inflammatory insults of various types, many questions remain (19,20). Are molecular and cellular injuries amplified to cause systemic illness and organ failure? Is injury to tissue, an organ, or the human as a whole converted to cellular injury? Are pathways from the molecular to the macroscopic and from the macroscopic to the molecular at work simultaneously? The remainder of this chapter will review some of the recent progress that has been made at the cellular and molecular levels in understanding the initiation of inflammation, and discuss hypotheses that may eventually lead to an understanding of why organ systems fail and why they recover. Data from recent clinical trials conducted on populations of patients with severe sepsis and organ failure provide new insights.

Pathophysiology

Survival requires the host, first, to detect either tissue invasion or tissue damage and, second, to repel the invaders or to repair the damage. The autonomic nervous system functions as a "sixth sense" to detect invasion of microbes or evidence of trauma, and serves as the surveillance system that sets the stress response in motion (21). The autonomic nervous system treats trauma and infection as the same emergency (22) and can be activated by a variety of stimuli. Hypotension, a consequence of reduced cardiac output in shock, has long been known to activate secretion of the classical stress hormones. When activated, the autonomic nervous system produces arteriolar constriction, venous capacitance vessel constriction, increased heart rate, and augmented contractility. It stimulates both the renin angiotensin system and the secretion of epinephrine and other medullary adrenal hormones. Renin enzymatically produces angiotensin I. Angiotensin I is converted to angiotensin II by angiotensin converting enzyme. Although angiotensin II increases release of aldosterone from the adrenal cortex, its role in early shock is the increase of arteriolar tone in the mesentery. In addition, arginine vasopressin is released by the posterior pituitary. Arginine vasopressin also increases tone in splanchnic beds (23).

Peripheral tissue inflammation can directly stimulate the hypothalamus (24). Stimulation of the hypothalamus releases catecholamines, glucagon, and glucocorticoids. Catecholamines, epinephrine, and norepinephrine are important in increasing inotropy, chronotropy, and vasoconstriction. In addition, epinephrine potentiates glycogenolysis.

Glucagon raises serum concentrations of glucose by stimulating glycogenolysis. Secretion of glucagon increases with secretion of epinephrine and cortisol. Glucocorticoids also stimulate gluconeogenesis and glycogen deposition. The glucocorticoids are implicated in protein catabolism, in which amino acids become substrates for hepatic gluconeogenesis. These stress hormones are implicated in the relative hyperglycemia observed in physiologic stress states (25,26).

Other important stimuli that activate the inflammatory response include pain, damage to tissues, and microbial invasion. Pain causes neurons to release active peptides. Injury to cells releases formed proteins that stimulate release of cytokines. Included in this group are high mobility group B1 (HMGB1) proteins and heat shock proteins. Microbial products are detected by binding to both soluble and cell surface receptors. The response is rapid. As Nathan observes, "A rapid response requires sentinel cells pre-stationed in the tissues. Mast cells and macrophages fulfill this function" (22).

Trauma or infection can release neuropeptides that stimulate local mast cells, which, in turn, stimulate other mast cells, nerve endings, endothelium, and neutrophils through G protein receptors. One consequence of this mechanism is the release of platelet activating factor (PAF) by neutrophils. Elaboration of PAF is associated with invasion of extravascular tissues by neutrophils. Neutrophils also are activated by tumor necrosis factor (TNF) and leukotrienes produced by the mast cells. Products of neutrophil activation, including elastase, expose integrins and allow binding of neutrophils to extracellular matrix proteins. Of importance, the combined signals of integrin binding plus binding of TNF, C5a, or other cytokines are required for release of enzymes that cause tissue destruction.

If allowed to proceed without regulation, the inflammatory response can produce tissue destruction that is detrimental to the host. This unchecked destruction of tissue is typically prevented by the regulatory steps that are present even in the early stages of inflammation. At a cellular level, pro-inflammatory agents may change function as the inflammatory response persists. For example, pro-inflammatory products are transformed to anti-inflammatory lipoxins. COX2 converts arachidonate to PGE2, a substance associated with increased capillary permeability. An increase in PGE2 concentrations then provides negative feedback and inhibits COX2. The requirement that combined signals are necessary for release of neutrophil products provides an important level of control. As

Nathan (22) observes, "Ongoing infection [is required] to avoid defaulting to the resting state. Each newly recruited cell generally commits to release pro-inflammatory signals only after integrating aspects of both host and microbial origin." This observation has a counterpart in immunology. B cells need antigen receptor binding plus T cell signals to function. T cells need antigen receptor binding plus antigen presenting cell (APC) signals, and APCs require cytokines plus microbial products, or microbial products plus necrotic host cell products, for the initial inflammatory response to develop into the immune response.

Controls on the inflammatory process are exerted through the central nervous system. The cholinergic anti-inflammatory pathway inhibits macrophage activation. Experimentally, direct stimulation of the vagus nerve inhibits TNF production in organs innervated by the vagus, including liver, lung, spleen, kidney, and gut. Release of acetylcholine has been demonstrated to inhibit activation of the macrophages (27).

When ordered, the inflammatory response can limit the spread of infection, limit tissue damage, and repair tissues. The forces that convert the ordered and regulated inflammatory process into one that produces ongoing tissue damage are not well understood. A model for the understanding of organ failure is sepsis. Current understanding of the pathogenesis of organ failure in sepsis involves several steps: host recognition of microbes or foreign tissue, signal amplification, the counter-inflammatory response, and the coagulation cascade (28).

Recognition of Microbes or Foreign Tissue

Many endogenous and exogenous mediators of inflammatory states have been studied in human, experimental animal, and *in vitro* systems. The generalized Shwartzman reaction provides an important clue. In the generalized Shwartzman reaction, two doses of endotoxin are administered to the same animal, usually a rabbit, 24 h apart. If both doses are given intravenously, a shock state may be produced that is often accompanied by disseminated intravascular coagulation. If the first dose is given intradermally, and the second dose given intravenously, a hemorrhagic reaction occurs at the site of the dermal injection, the local Shwartzman reaction. The observation that enterobacteriaceal endotoxin [lipopolysaccharide (LPS)] was the mediator of the shock state seen in the generalized Shwartzman reaction led to the identification of the signaling receptor complex for endotoxin, which consists of toll-like receptor 4 (TLR4), LPS-binding protein, and the opsonic receptor CD14 (29,30). Remarkably, members of the toll-like receptor family bind a wide range of ligands and have proved to be the primary signaling molecules for most inflammatory stimuli, including Gram-negative and Gram-positive bacterial toxins, bacterial DNA, fungal elements, and even endogenous products of cellular injury and death (Table 6). These acts of immune recognition of toxic nonself products are fundamental to the innate immune system and act prior to the organization of cellular or humoral immunity.

Indeed, the recognition of nonself by the macrophage (mediated ultimately through the toll-like receptor system) acts to stimulate and coordinate the development of cellular and humoral responses to a significant infectious challenge. Thus, the physiologic pathway that mediates inflammatory signaling in response to and clearance of LPS may serve as a model for understanding the response to an inflammatory challenge. Figure 1 illustrates the known components of cell surface recognition of LPS.

Experimental models, both *in vitro* and *in vivo*, have demonstrated that alteration of function of any of a number of proteins in the extracellular serum or at the cell surface will perturb physiologic inflammatory signaling by TLR4 in response to LPS. In animal

Table 6 Toll-like Receptors and Their Ligands

TLR1	Lipoteichoic acid, lipopeptide, and certain species of LPS
TLR2	Lipoarabinomannan, lipopeptide, peptidoglycan, fungal cell wall, and heat shock proteins
TLR3	Double stranded DNA (viral)
TLR4	LPS and viral proteins
TLR5	Bacterial flagellin
TLR6	Zymosan
TLR 7, 8	Unknown
TLR9	Bacterial DNA (nonmethylated CpG)
TLR10	Unknown

survival studies, significant inflammatory blockade achieved by directed immune modulation resulted in increased survival in response to *toxic* challenge with LPS, but decreased survival in response to an *infectious* challenge, such as experimental peritonitis. These studies indicate that intact innate immune signaling is required for a vigorous host response to infection but may become deleterious with prolonged exposure to a toxic stimulus. Genetic polymorphisms of TLR4 and the associated protein, CD14, have both been associated with altered susceptibility to Gram-negative infection and septic shock, a finding that supports the importance of this pathway in clinically significant disease.

Signal Amplification

From the activation of TLR4 at the macrophage cell surface, the inflammatory signal is transduced to the nucleus via a series of protein–protein interactions that alter gene transcription and production of inflammatory mediators (31,32). Mononuclear cells produce interleukin-1 (IL-1), IL-6, and TNFα in addition to other cytokines. These pro-inflammatory cytokines are released early, mimic many features of LPS administration, and stimulate inflammatory cell migration into tissues. Several of these mediators, such as (TNFα) and IL-1, have been extensively studied, but immune modulatory strategies aimed at blocking these mediators in patients with severe sepsis or septic shock have been unsuccessful.

Two other macrophage derived products may prove to be useful clinical targets for therapy. HMGB1 is a nonhistone chromosomal protein that is implicated in stabilizing nucleosomes, gene transcription, and modulating steroid receptors. Antibody to HMGB1 was protective in LPS-induced shock in animals. Migration inhibitory factor (MIF) is a pro-inflammatory cytokine. Antibody to MIF was beneficial in cecal ligation and puncture (28).

Counter-Inflammatory Response

After initial inflammatory activation, the release of mediators produces activated neutrophils that can swarm to the site of infection to eradicate the invaders. These cells produce toxic proteins, peptides, and reactive oxygen species that not only kill pathogenic organisms but also can cause collateral damage to host cells. Activated neutrophils also are trapped in pulmonary capillary beds, as well as in post-capillary venules of other tissues. Damage to these tissues attracts additional immune cells, and the unregulated amplification of this process may lead to organ failure distant from the site of the original infection. The down-regulation of these activated neutrophils is believed to be related to neutrophil apoptosis (33). Pro- and counter-inflammatory signals within the activated neutrophil are targets of study (34).

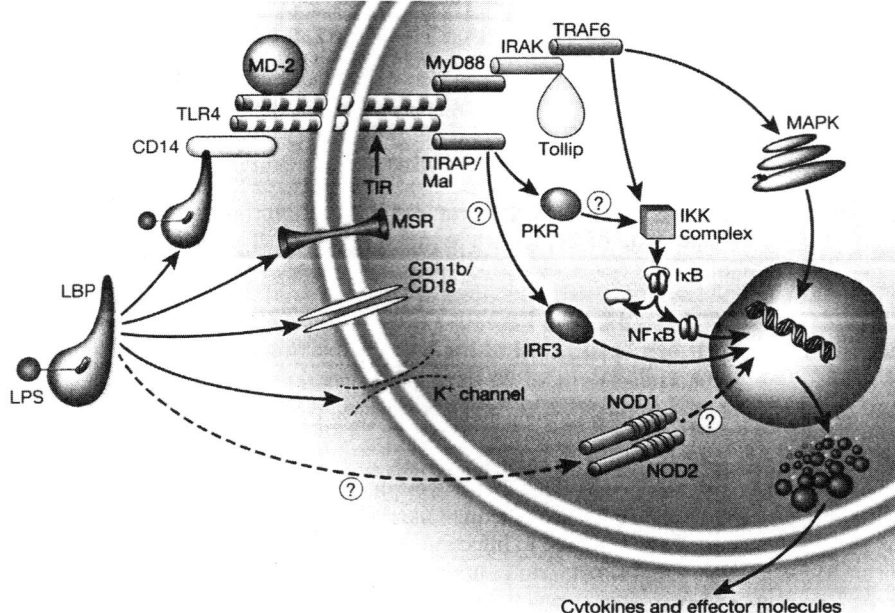

Figure 1 Cell-surface recognition of LPS. The principal mechanism by which LPS is sensed is via an LPS-binding protein (LBP)–LPS complex and then signalling through the TLR4–MD-2 complex. However, other cell surface molecules also sense LPS; these include the macrophage scavenger receptor (MSR), CD11b/CD18 and ion channels. Intracellular signalling depends on binding of the intracellular TLR domain, TIR (Toll/IL-1 receptor homology domain) to IL-1 receptor-associated kinase (IRAK), a process that is facilitated by two adapter proteins, MyD88 (myeloid differentiation protein 88) and TIRAP [TIR domain-containing adapter protein; also called MyD88-adapter-like protein (Mal)], and inhibited by a third protein Tollip (Toll-interacting protein). Note that there is also an MyD88-independent pathway by which TIRAP/Mal signals through an RNA-dependent protein kinase (PKR) and interferon regulatory factor (IRF)-3. Recently, it has been proposed that cells may also be able to respond to LPS by intracellular receptors called NOD proteins (for nucleotide-binding oligomerization domain). NOD1 (also called caspase-recruitment domain 4) was identified originally on the basis of structural homology to the apoptosis regulator, Apaf-1. The NOD proteins have some similarities to the resistance (R) genes in plants that are involved in pathogen recognition; in common with TLRs and R genes, NODs have leucine-rich repeats. Expression of NOD1 and NOD2 confer responsiveness to Gram-negative LPS but not to lipoteichoic acid, which is found in Gram-positive bacteria. The mechanism by which NOD may recognize LPS in the cytosol is unknown. [Reproduced by permission from Ref. (28).]

IL-10, an anti-inflammatory mediator, has been studied in animal models and in clinical trials with mixed results. These investigations indicate that the timing of IL-10 production (or administration) is crucial to its effectiveness—too early or too late in relation to an infectious challenge and the effect is counter-productive (35,36).

The Coagulation Cascade

With local and systemic inflammation comes microvascular coagulation. Endothelial damage exposes tissue factor (TF) to intravascular factor VII with resultant activation of the extrinsic pathway of coagulation (Fig. 2). Sepsis drives expression of TF on

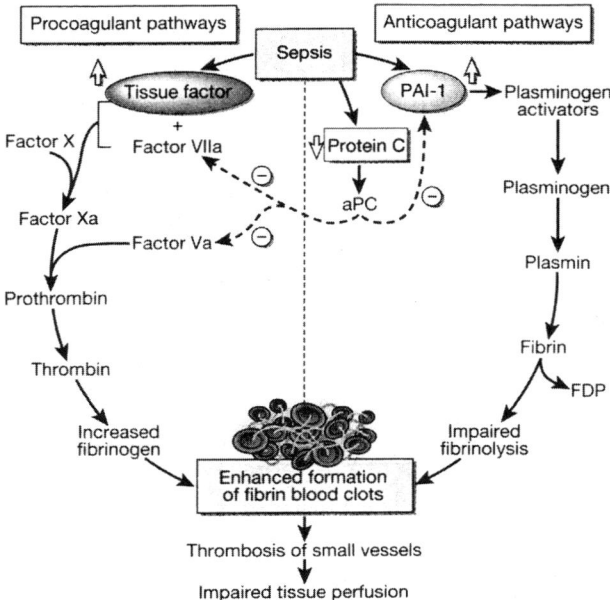

Figure 2 Sepsis disturbs the normal homeostatic balance between procoagulant and anticoagulant mechanisms. Tissue factor expression is enhanced leading to increased production of prothrombin that is converted to thrombin, and that in turn generates fibrin from fibrinogen. Simultaneously, levels of the plasminogen-activator inhibitor-1 (PAI-1) are increased, resulting in impaired production of plasmin and thus failure of normal fibrinolytic mechanisms by which fibrin is converted to degradation products (FDP). Sepsis also causes a fall in the levels of the natural anticoagulant protein C (and also antithrombin and the tissue factor pathway inhibitor, TFPI, not shown). The activated form of protein C, aPC, dissociates from the endothelial protein C receptor to inactive factor Va and VIIa and inhibit PAI-1 activity; hence reduced levels of protein C result in further procoagulant effect. The net result is enhanced formation of fibrin clots in the microvasculature, leading to impaired tissue oxgenation and cell damage. [Reproduced by permission from Ref. (28).]

endothelial and monocyte cell surfaces, a process that amplifies microvascular procoagulant signaling. Down-regulation of this system is largely mediated by anti-thrombin and by activated protein C (aPC). Failure of the down-regulatory mechanisms can lead to the spectacular morbidity seen in Meningococcal *purpura fulminans* and, presumably, to much of the organ dysfunction seen in patients with adult respiratory distress syndrome and acute renal failure. The recent clinical trial of aPC in patients with severe sepsis and organ dysfunction produced a measurable improvement in mortality (37,38).

CONCEPTUAL HYPOTHESES

As briefly outlined earlier, our understanding of the molecular and cellular events leading from an infectious or inflammatory stimulus to local and systemic host injury have been vastly expanded over the last decade (28). Yet the progression from a single illness or injury to MOF often occurs without clear cause. Figure 3 shows some of the parallel

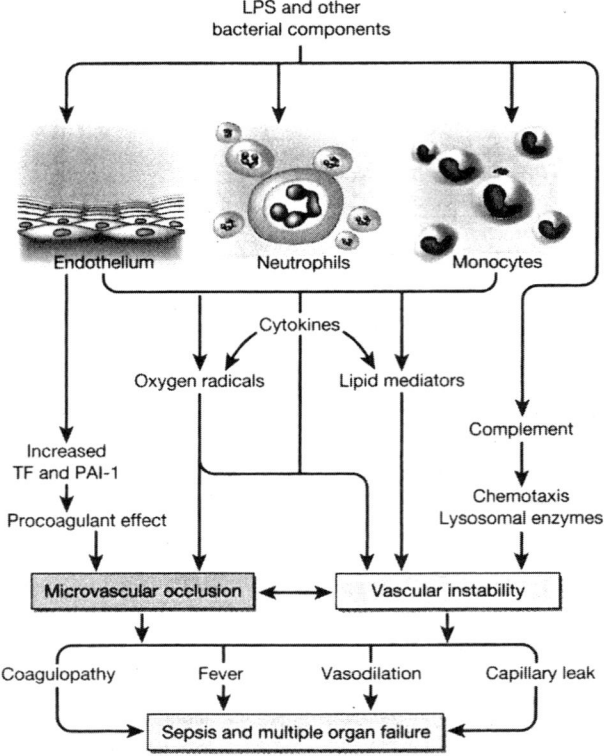

Figure 3 Pathogenetic networks in shock. LPS and other microbial components simultaneously activate multiple parallel cascades that contribute to the pathophysiology of adult respiratory distress syndrome (ARDS) and shock. The combination of poor myocardial contractility, impaired peripheral vascular tone and microvascular occlusion leads to tissue hypoperfusion and inadequate oxygenation, and thus to organ failure. [Reproduced by permission from Ref. (28).]

pathways that function simultaneously to produce shock. Several hypotheses have been proposed to account for the development of the syndrome of MOF in such patients.

The two-hit hypothesis reflects the clinical and experimental observations that a single inflammatory insult may prime the host response and make the host response to the next challenge exaggerated and potentially counter-productive (39). For example, pneumonia or an episode of catheter sepsis that might ordinarily be well tolerated produces a profound inflammatory response with progressive organ failure. This hypothesis grew from observations in trauma patients with early and late MOF. Early MOF resulted from a massive injury; whereas, late MOF appeared to develop after a significantly lesser perturbation in a patient who had already suffered a primary injury (40). Specific modifications of current therapy may influence the amount of "priming" that takes place and leave patients less vulnerable to subsequent nosocomial infection. For example, the use of hypertonic saline for resuscitation may be beneficial (41). Improved understanding of the molecular mechanisms of priming may allow prophylactic immunomodulation in patients who have already suffered a first "hit."

The gut translocation hypothesis states that the alimentary tract serves as a repository for vast quantities of bacteria, fungi, and microbial toxins that access the systemic circulation under conditions of increased intestinal permeability during critical illness (42,43). This phenomenon results in ongoing systemic infection and inflammation via toxins that produce MOF. This hypothesis is quite controversial. Selective decontamination of the GI tract with oral antibiotics in hopes of decreasing the nosocomial infections that were thought to emanate from the gut have not consistently improved mortality. Meta-analyses suggest a mortality benefit of ~10%, despite a decrease in hospital acquired infection, in combined medical and surgical intensive care populations (44). Another recent meta-analysis suggests that gut decontamination may be beneficial in surgical patients (45). In a series of studies, Deitch (46) has shown that mesenteric lymph collected after hemorrhagic shock is an inflammatory stimulus and can cause neutrophil activation and endothelial injury. Furthermore, division of the thoracic duct attenuates observed lung injury in experimental hemorrhagic shock and thermal injury. These data support a potential role for the gut as a "motor of sepsis" that does not depend on ongoing translocation of pathogenic microorganisms to the systemic circulation.

The immune paralysis hypothesis states that an inflammatory insult produces both a systemic inflammatory response and a compensatory anti-inflammatory response. Under certain conditions, the anti-inflammatory response is excessive and leads to immune failure and heightened susceptibility to nosocomial infection (47). This hypothesis is supported by many clinical data, including the observation that anergy to delayed hypersensitivity skin testing strongly correlates with susceptibility to sepsis and mortality from septic complications in surgical patients (48). Other potential markers of immune failure in trauma patients include decreased immunoglobulin levels, decreased opsonization activity of plasma, and suppressed MHC class 2 antigen expression on circulating monocytes (49). These findings correlate with a shift in T cells toward the Th2 phenotype, which is predominantly anti-inflammatory (50). The degree to which this phenotypic shift in T lymphocyte activity is adaptive, and how much may represent overcompensation and immune failure, is not presently known. Studies are ongoing to examine and potentially modulate the molecular mechanisms responsible for this shift.

CLINICAL PROGRESS

The roles of tissue hypoxia, blood sugar control, corticosteroid administration, and the use of aPC in clinical outcomes have been recently subjected to clinical trials. A recent study by Rivers et al. (51) demonstrated improved survival with early restoration of oxygen transport in septic patients. Strategies for increasing oxygen delivery are discussed in Chapters 2 and 63. Van den Berghe et al. (52) studied the benefit of intensive control of blood sugar in critically ill patients. With intensive control of blood sugar in a group of primarily post-operative cardiac surgery patients, mortality was improved. The mechanism producing benefit is not clear. Low-dose corticosteroids were shown to reduce mortality in highly selected patients. These findings suggest that adrenal insufficiency may be a part of the organ failure syndrome. Perhaps, corticosteroids are vital for the counter-inflammatory response (53). The importance of the coagulation cascade in producing MSOF is suggested by the aPC trial. In a randomized controlled trial, a survival benefit was observed in patients with sepsis who received aPC (37).

FUTURE CONSIDERATIONS

Basic science research has made remarkable strides in determining the pathways at the cellular, protein, and gene levels, which regulate both the initial and the secondary inflammatory responses to infection, toxin, or ischemia. Several lines of investigation are working their way toward clinical trials. However, none of the organizing hypotheses alone adequately explains the clinical phenomena observed in critically ill patients. Rather, they are conceptual frameworks that serve well to organize research data at a reductionist level, but, when applied to complex clinical situations, the shortcomings of a single unifying hypothesis are strikingly apparent. One difficulty is the concept of sepsis and MOF as a single disease entity. By the 1991–1992 Consensus Conference criteria, both an 80-year-old with fecal peritonitis and an 8-month-old with otitis media can be said to have "sepsis" (4). Should both be entered in the same clinical trial? Yet clinical trials in "sepsis" patients are by nature beset with extreme selection bias problems. Identification of a statistically identifiable benefit hidden in a sea of patients who will get well without the intervention, and patients who will sicken and die with or without the intervention, poses formidable difficulties. Clearly, identifying the appropriate patient population for trials, as well as for each of the therapies we already possess, will be essential to improving care. A 2001 conference re-examined the definitions of sepsis, and proposed a model of categorizing response to infectious challenge modeled on the TNM staging system used by oncologists (54) and designated as the PIRO model. In this formulation, P is patient disposition and reflects genetic susceptibility to infection and inflammation; I is infection and includes site, extent, and organism(s) responsible; R is response and quantifies the characteristics of the patient response to infection (by measurement of mediators and markers of inflammation) both with regard to an expected time course and extent based on population studies; and O represents organ dysfunction. The hope is to produce a hypothesis-generating schema by staging each patient with sepsis/MOF in a way that reflects the clinical picture seen daily in ICUs, leads to more focused use of current therapies, and produces better designed clinical trials. The difficulties with restaging patients as they progress clinically and keeping the model from becoming too cumbersome for useful application will be challenging, but as a first step in clearly defining patient populations for clinical trials, the model is worthy of a strong effort.

SUMMARY

- MOF is defined as the presence of altered organ function in an acutely ill patient such that homeostasis cannot be maintained without intervention.
- MOF is the sequential and accumulated failure of all the major organ systems.
- Characteristics of MOF include an increase in oxygen consumption, acute lung injury, and an increase in dead-space ventilation.
- Energy expenditure is increased during the hypermetabolic and MOF phase. The respiratory quotient is usually 0.8–0.9 and reflects a mixed fuel source.
- Total body catabolism is increased and exceeds protein synthetic rate. The liver synthesizes increased amounts of acute phase reactants.
- Pathogenesis of organ failure involves host recognition of microbes or foreign tissue, signal amplification, the counter-inflammatory response, and the coagulation cascade.

- Members of the toll-like receptor family are the primary signaling molecules for most inflammatory stimuli.
- The signal resulting from activation of the toll-like receptor is transduced to the nucleus, and gene transcription is altered. Pro-inflammatory mediators are released early and include TNF, IL-1, and IL-6.
- The counter-inflammatory response may down-regulate migration of activated neutrophils to organs, and limit the effects of toxic proteins, peptides, and reactive oxygen species that are produced to kill pathogens, but may damage host tissue.
- Local and systemic inflammation stimulate microvascular coagulation. Down-regulation of procoagulant signaling is mediated by anti-thrombin and aPC.
- Current mechanisms of organ failure are hypothesized to include: the two-hit hypothesis, gut translocation, and immune paralysis.
- Current strategies to prevent MOF include: source control, increased oxygen delivery, intensive control of serum blood sugar concentration, low-dose corticosteroid therapy, and prevention of microvascular coagulation.

REFERENCES

1. Cerra FB. Multiple organ failure syndrome. In: Bihari DS, Cerra FB eds. New Horizons. Multiple Organ Failure. Fullerton, CA: Society of Critical Care Medicine, 1989; 1–24.
2. Levy MM, Fink MP, Marshall JC, Abraham E, Angus D, Cook D, Cohen J, Opal S, Vincent J-L, Ramsay G. 2001 SCCM/EISCM/ACCP/ATS/SIS International Sepsis Definitions Conference, Crit Care Med 2003; 31:1250–1256.
3. Knaus WA and Wagner DP. Multiple systems organ failure: epidemiology and prognosis. Crit Care Clin 1989; 5:221–232.
4. Society of Critical Care Medicine Consensus Conference Committee. American College of Chest Physicians/Society of Critical Care Medicine Consensus Conference: definitions for sepsis and organ failure and guidelines for the use of innovative therapies in sepsis. Crit Care Med 1992; 20:864–874.
5. Bone RC, Sibbald WJ, Sprung CL. The ACCP-SCCM Consensus Conference on sepsis and organ failure. Chest 1992; 101:1481–1483.
6. Marshall JC, Cook DJ, Christou NV, Bernard GR, Sprung CL, Sibbald WJ. Multiple organ dysfunction score: a reliable descriptor of a complex clinical outcome. Crit Care Med 1995; 23:1638–1652.
7. Rosenberg AL. Recent innovations in intensive care unit risk-prediction models. Curr Opin Crit Care 2002; 8(4):321–330.
8. Vincent JL, Ferreira F, Moreno R. Scoring systems for assessing organ dysfunction and survival. Crit Care Clin 2000; 16(2):353–366.
9. Knaus WA et al. Prognosis in acute organ system failure. Ann Surg 1985; 202:685–693.
10. Zimmerman JE, Knaus WA, Sun X, Wagner DP. Severity stratification and outcome prediction for multisystem organ failure and dysfunction. World J Surg 1996; 20:401–405.
11. Wichmann MW, Inthom D, Andress HJ, Schildberg FW. Incidence and mortality of severe sepsis in surgical intensive care patients: the influence of patient gender on disease process and outcome. Intensive Care Med 2000; 26(2):167–172.
12. Cerra FB, Negro F, Eyer S. Multiple organ failure syndrome: patterns and effect of current therapy. Update Intensive Care Emerg Med 1990; 10:22–31
13. Skillman JJ, Bushnell LS, Goldman H, Silen W. Respiratory failure, hypotension, sepsis, and jaundice. Am J Surg 1969; 117:523–530.

14. Tilney NL, Bailey GL, Morgan AP. Sequential system failure after rupture of abdominal aortic aneurysms: an unsolved problem in postoperative care. Ann Surg 1973; 178:117–122.
15. Barton R and Cerra FB. The hypermetabolism multiple organ failure syndrome. Chest 1989; 96:1153–1160.
16. Parrillo JE, Burch C, Shelhamer JH, Parker MM, Natanson C, Schuette W. A circulating myocardial depressant substance in humans with septic shock. Septic shock patients with a reduced ejection fraction have a circulating factor that depresses in vitro myocardial cell performance. J Clin Invest 1985; 76:1539–1553
17. Cunnion RE, Parrillo JE. Myocardial dysfunction in sepsis. Crit Care Clin 1989; 5:99–118.
18. Cerra FB, Siegel JH, Coleman B, Border JR, McMenamy RR. Septic autocannibalism: a failure of exogenous nutritional support. Ann Surg 1980; 192:570–580.
19. Fry DE. Multiple organ system failure. Surg Clin North Am 1988; 68:107–122.
20. Cerra FB. Multiple organ failure syndrome. Dis Mon 1992; 38:843–947.
21. Blalock JE. The immune system as a sensory organ. J Immunol 1984; 132:1067–1070.
22. Nathan C. Points of control in inflammation. Nature 2002; 420:846–852.
23. Fink MP. Shock: An overview. In: Rippe JM, Irwin RS, Fink MP, Cerra FB, eds. Intensive Care Medicine 3rd ed. NY: Little Brown and Company, 1996:1861.
24. Besedovsky H, Sorkin E, Felix D, Haas H. Hypothalamic changes during the immune response. Eur J Immunol 1977; 7:323–325.
25. Zaloga GP. Hormones: vasopressin, growth hormone, glucagon, somatostatin, prolactin, G-CSF, GM-CSF. In: Chernow B. The Pharmacologic Approach to the Critically Ill Patient. Philadelphia: Williams and Wilkins, 1994:705.
26. Chin R, Eagerton DC, Salem M. In Chernow B. The Pharmacologic Approach to the Critically Ill Patient. Philadelphia: Williams and Wilkins, 1994:718.
27. Tracey KJ. The inflammatory reflex. Nature 2002; 420:853–859.
28. Cohen J. The immunopathogenesis of sepsis. Nature 2002; 420:885–891.
29. Lazaron V and Dunn DL. Molecular biology of endotoxin antagonism. World J Surg 2002; 26(7):790–798.
30. Beutler B. TLR4 as the mammalian endotoxin sensor. Curr Top Microbiol Immunol. 2002; 270:109–120.
31. Takeda K and Akira S. Toll receptors and pathogen resistance. Cell Microbiol. 2003; 5(3):143–153.
32. Means TK, Golenbock DT, Fenton MJ. The biology of Toll-like receptors. Cytokine Growth Factor Rev 2000; 11(3):219–232.
33. Akgul C, Moulding DA, Edwards SW. Molecular control of neutrophil apoptosis. FEBS Lett 2001; 487(3):318–322.
34. Abraham E. Neutrophils and acute lung injury. Crit Care Med. 2003; 31(4 Suppl): S195–S199.
35. Remick DG, Garg SJ, Newcomb DE, Wollenberg G, Huie TK, Bolgos G. Exogenous interleukin-10 fails to decrease the mortality or morbidity of sepsis. Crit Care Med 1998; 26(5):895–904.
36. Song GY, Chung CS, Chaudry IH, Ayala A. What is the role of interleukin 10 in polymicrobial sepsis: anti-inflammatory agent or immunosuppressant? Surgery 1999; 126(2):378–383.
37. Bernard GR, Vincent JL, Laterre PF, LaRosa SP, Dhainaut JF, Lopez-Rodriguez A, Steingrub JS, Garber GE, Helterbrand JD, Ely EW, Fisher CJ Jr. Recombinant human protein C Worldwide Evaluation in Severe Sepsis (PROWESS) Study Group. Efficacy and safety of recombinant human activated protein C for severe sepsis. N Engl J Med 2001; 344(10):699–709.
38. Dhainaut JF, Laterre PF, Janes JM, Bernard GR, Artigas A, Bakker J, Riess H, Basson BR, Charpentier J, Utterback BG, Vincent JL, Recombinant human protein C Worldwide Evaluation in Severe Sepsis (PROWESS) Study Group. Drotrecogin alfa (activated) in the treatment of severe sepsis patients with multiple-organ dysfunction: data from the PROWESS trial. Intensive Care Med 2003; 29(6):894–903.

39. Rotstein OD. Modeling the two-hit hypothesis for evaluating strategies to prevent organ injury after shock/resuscitation. J Trauma 2003; 54(5 Suppl):S203–S206.
40. Faist E, Baue AE, Dittmer H, Heberer G. Multiple organ failure in polytrauma patients. J Trauma 1983; 23(9):775–787.
41. Ciesla DJ, Moore EE, Zallen G, Biffl WL, Silliman CC. Hypertonic saline attenuation of polymorphonuclear neutrophil cytotoxicity: timing is everything. J Trauma 2000; 48(3):388–395.
42. Moore FA. The role of the gastrointestinal tract in postinjury multiple organ failure. Am J Surg 1999 Dec; 178(6):449–453.
43. Marshall JC, Christou NV, Meakins JL. The gastrointestinal tract. The "undrained abscess" of multiple organ failure. Ann Surg 1993; 218(2):111–119.
44. Ramsey G and van Saene RH. Selective gut decontamination in intensive care and surgical practice: where are we? World J Surg 1998; 22:164–170.
45. Nathens AB, Marshall JC. Selective decontamination of the digestive tract in surgical patients: a systematic review of the evidence. Arch Surg 1999 Feb; 134(2):170–176.
46. Deitch EA. Role of the gut lymphatic system in multiple organ failure. Curr Opin Crit Care 2001; 7(2):92–998.
47. Bone RC. Sir Isaac Newton, sepsis, SIRS, and CARS. Crit Care Med. 1996; 24(7):1125–1128.
48. Pietsch JB, Meakins JL, MacLean LD. The delayed hypersensitivity response: application in clinical surgery. Surgery 1977; 82(3):349–355.
49. Cheadle WG, Mercer-Jones M, Heinzelmann M, Polk HC Jr. Sepsis and septic complications in the surgical patient: who is at risk? Shock 1996; 6(Suppl 1):S6–S9.
50. Faist E, Schinkel C, Zimmer S. Update on the mechanisms of immune suppression of injury and immune modulation. World J Surg 1996; 20(4):454–459.
51. Rivers E, Nguyen B, Havstad S, Ressler J, Muzzin A, Knoblich B, Peterson E, Tomlanovich M, Early Goal Directed Therapy Collaborative Group. Early goal directed therapy in the treatment of severe sepsis and septic shock. N Engl J Med 2001; 345:1368–1377.
52. Van den Berghe G, Wouters P, Weekers F, Verwaest C, Bruyninckx F, Schetz M, Vlasselaers D, Ferdinande P, Lauwers P, Bouillon R. Intensive insulin therapy in critically ill patients. N Engl J Med 2001; 345:1359–1367.
53. Annane D, Sebille V, Charpentier C, Bollaert PE, Francois B, Korach JM, Capellier G, Cohen Y, Azoulay E, Troche G, Chaumet-Riffaut P, Bellisant E. Effects of treatment with low doses of hydrocortisone and fluodrocortisone on mortality in patients with septic shock. J Am Med Assoc 2002; 288: 862–871.
54. Levy MM, Fink MP, Marshall JC, Abraham E, Angus D, Cook D, Cohen J, Opal SM, Vincent JL, Ramsay G. 2001 SSSM/ESICM/ACCP/ATS/SIS International Sepsis Definitions Conference. Crit Care Med 2003; 31(4):1250–1256.

2
Oxygen Transport

Jerome H. Abrams
VA Medical Center, Minneapolis, Minnesota, USA

Frank B. Cerra
University of Minnesota, Minneapolis, Minnesota, USA

Restoration of oxygen transport as an endpoint of resuscitation remains controversial. The available literature investigating this idea supports widely disparate conclusions. The following discussion views restoration of oxygen transport as one of the foundations of modern critical care. When successfully achieved, along with source control and metabolic support, improved mortality can be demonstrated. An analysis of this controversy and critical review of the literature leads to a model that supports our perspective. The interested reader can refer to Chapter 63 for a detailed discussion. Despite the controversy surrounding oxygen transport, the initial priorities of managing a patient admitted to the surgical intensive care unit are well defined. Once the airway has been safely secured, source control becomes the next priority. Hemorrhage must be stopped. Abscesses must be drained, since even small amounts of undrained pus can produce grave systemic consequences. Other infections must be treated as specifically as possible. When adequate source control has been established, the next mandate, although controversial, is restoration of oxygen transport. After oxygen transport has been restored, appropriate metabolic support becomes the next goal (see Chapter 3 for a discussion of metabolic support).

OXYGEN SUPPLY AND DEMAND

Restoration of oxygen transport requires supplying adequate oxygen to tissues to satisfy demand. Consequently, the critical care physician must be able to identify both the supply of oxygen to tissues and the demand for oxygen by tissues (Table 1).

The clinical determinants of oxygen supply are well defined and may be measured routinely. The components of oxygen demand are less direct and reflect changes in oxygen use as a consequence of alterations in oxygen supply. Intuitively, increased use of oxygen with increased supply means that tissues are consuming oxygen to meet increased metabolic demands. The situation may be more complicated, as discussed in Chapter 63.

Table 1 Components of Tissue Oxygen Supply and Demand

Component	Clinical variable
Oxygen supply	
Oxygen carrier	Hb concentration
Oxygen carrier saturation	Hb saturation
Oxygen carrier delivery	$DO_2 = CO \times$ arterial oxygen content
	$= (1.36 \times Hb \times \% \, Sat + 0.034 \, PaO_2) \times CO \times 10$
Oxygen demand	
Tissue oxygen demand	Flow-dependent oxygen consumption, delivery-dependent lactate production or lactate/pyruvate > 16.5
Oxygen consumption	$\dot{V}O_2 = CO \times DVO_2 \times 10$
	$= [CO \times (1.36 \times Hb(\%\,\text{arterial sat} - \%\,\text{venous sat})] \times 10$
	$+ 0.034\,(PaO_2 - PVO_2)$

Note: DO_2, oxygen delivery; PaO_2, partial pressure of arterial oxygen; $\dot{V}O_2$, oxygen consumption; PVO_2, partial pressure of mixed venous oxygen; DVO_2, arteriovenous oxygen content difference.
From Abrams JH. Indications for hemodynamic monitoring. In: Najarian JS, Delaney JP, eds. Progress in Trauma and Critical Care Surgery. St. Louis: Mosby–Year Book, 1992:278.

Providing sufficient hemoglobin, the physiologic carrier of oxygen, is an efficient way of improving oxygen transport. Oxygen delivery (DO_2) is approximated by the relationship:

$$DO_2 = [1.36 \times Hb(g/dL) \times \%\text{arterial saturation} + 0.034\,PaO_2] \times \text{cardiac output (L/min)} \times 10$$

As this relationship indicates, providing an appropriate concentration of oxygen carriers is one of the most important ways of augmenting oxygen delivery. For a constant cardiac output, increasing hemoglobin concentration from 7 to 10 g/dL would increase DO_2 by approximately 40%. Changing the arterial oxygen partial pressure from 60 to 90 mm Hg would increase the arterial oxygen saturation from 88% to 95%, with a resultant increase in DO_2 of only 7%. This example emphasizes that increasing the hemoglobin concentration is a very effective means of increasing DO_2. The appropriate hemoglobin concentration depends on the clinical context. In practice, the risks and benefits of transfusion must be carefully balanced. An elderly patient with coronary artery disease, tachycardia, ST–T changes on the electrocardiogram, and abdominal sepsis may require hemoglobin concentrations in excess of 8 g/dL. In contrast, a well-trained athlete with excellent cardiovascular conditioning may tolerate a lower hemoglobin concentration. Chapter 53 provides a comprehensive review of transfusion therapy.

The target for saturation of hemoglobin is 90%. In an SICU, supplementary oxygen generally is required. For some patients, oxygen administered by face mask may be sufficient. For other patients, positive pressure ventilatory support may be necessary. Strategies for ensuring adequate oxygenation can be challenging and are discussed in Chapters 30 and 31.

BLOOD FLOW

Once sufficient hemoglobin is available and saturated, it must flow throughout the tissues. Providing an adequate cardiac output considers preload, afterload, and contractility. Table 2 lists the determinants of cardiac output.

Table 2 Determinants of Cardiac Output

Component	Clinical variable	Clinical target
Preload	PCWP	12–15 mm Hg
Afterload	SVR = (MAP − CVP/CO) × 80	<1000 dynes/s per cm^5
Contractility	Undefined	Undefined

Note: PCWP, pulmonary capillary wedge pressure; SVR, systemic vascular resistance; MAP, mean arterial pressure; CVP, central venous pressure.

Preload, afterload, and inotropic support are each evaluated in turn to minimize increases in myocardial oxygen consumption. A useful clinical target for preload is the pulmonary capillary wedge pressure (PCWP). In SIRS states, oxygen needs are increased. To meet these needs, a CO greater than normal is generally necessary. Normal filling pressures may not be sufficient to produce increased cardiac flow. Rather, as noted by Cunnion and Parillo, a PCWP of 12–15 mm Hg may be necessary. Note that pressure measurements are not volume measurements. Figure 1 shows the hysteresis involved in volume loading and unloading in the vascular system. As the figure suggests, a given pressure may correspond to two different left ventricular end-diastolic volumes. Similarly, a given volume may correspond to two different ventricular pressures. At the extremes of pressure and volume, a single pressure may map to a single volume. Most patients' cardiac performance curves are not at the extremes. Nonetheless, PCWP is a useful clinical guide, because a large amount of clinical experience is attached to this measurement.

Once preload is sufficient, afterload is addressed. A clinical target of systemic vascular resistance (SVR) of approximately 1000 dynes/s per cm^5 is typical. SVR is a proportionality constant that relates flow and pressure and has the same role as resistance in Ohm's law ($V = IR$). When preload is adequate, a vasodilator may be added, if the SVR is elevated and a need for increased CO exists. Sodium nitroprusside, used with nitroglycerin, has been useful. Sodium nitroprusside has a short half-life and, consequently, may be rapidly adjusted. If used, the critical care physician must be alert to its potential for toxicity. Frequently, afterload reduction may cause a measurable decrease in preload and a need for additional preload replacement.

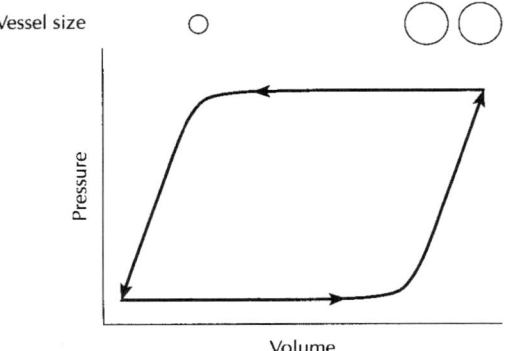

Figure 1 Relationship between volume loading and volume unloading in vascular system. (From Cerra FB. Manual of Critical Care. St. Louis: CV Mosby, 1987:80.)

If criteria addressed in the remaining discussion suggest that greater CO is necessary, and if preload and afterload are in the target range, inotropic support is considered. Cunnion and Parillo have shown decreased ejection fraction in a model of synchronously beating cultured myocardial cells. When perfused with serum from patients with SIRS, the cells demonstrated reduced amplitude of contraction. Contraction returned to normal values when cells were perfused with normal serum. The authors concluded that a soluble myocardial depressant factor was present in the serum of individuals with SIRS. Patients may have a need for augmented contractility in such states. Dobutamine or dopamine both may be useful inotropes.

ADEQUACY OF OXYGEN TRANSPORT

How does the critical care physician decide when oxygen transport is sufficient? How can the critical care physician decide if a patient requires increased cardiac output? Variables that traditionally have been used to assess resuscitation (i.e., blood pressure, pulse, urine output, capillary refill, and mental status) do not comprehensively describe oxygen transport. If inadequate oxygen transport is defined as shock, most historical definitions of shock do not allow the critical care physician to easily develop an approach to restoring oxygen transport. Nearly all definitions emphasize a mismatch between existing blood volume and the volume of the vascular tree. As early as 1917, Archibald and McLean observed: "While low blood pressure is one of the most consistent signs of shock, it is not the essential thing, let alone the cause of it."

What other information would help the physician to decide when oxygen transport is restored? Since this discussion relates to the general idea of shock, the following definition of shock is offered: Shock is a distribution of states in which tissue oxygen demand exceeds tissue oxygen supply for a single mechanism or for a combination of mechanisms. This definition has three components. One indicates that a patient may be in a greater or lesser degree of shock. Shock is not a binary phenomenon: one is not in shock or out of shock. Patients may be partially resuscitated and, consequently, partly in shock. Understanding the distribution enables the physician to identify the need for additional resuscitation. Chapter 63 provides a detailed derivation of this distribution, a three-dimensional response surface. The response surface may be derived from variables that reflect aerobic and anaerobic energy production. Another component of the definition identifies the mechanisms of shock as single or multiple. For example, a patient with usually well-compensated congestive heart failure might be involved in a motor vehicle crash. The result might be combined hemorrhagic shock and cardiogenic shock. In a similar manner, a hypovolemic patient may acquire sepsis and demonstrate a combination of septic shock and hypovolemic shock.

The last component of the definition requires further discussion. How does one decide if tissue oxygen demand exceeds tissue oxygen supply? Clearly, a "tissue oxygen demandometer" would be invaluable. Since no such device exists, clinical variables must be found to identify this potential mismatch. Two clinical criteria have been used in practice: (1) delivery-dependent oxygen consumption and (2) delivery-dependent lactate production (or its equivalent condition, an abnormal lactate/pyruvate ratio).

Delivery-Dependent Oxygen Consumption

Delivery-dependent oxygen consumption has generated controversy for many years. Figure 2 is a graphical representation commonly invoked to describe the relation of

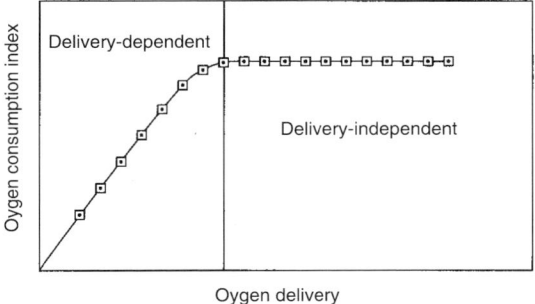

Figure 2 Idealization of flow-dependent oxygen consumption. (From Abrams JH. Indications for hemodynamic monitoring. In: Najarian JS, Delaney JP, eds. Progress in Trauma and Critical Care Surgery. St. Louis: Mosby–Year Book, 1992:275.)

oxygen delivery to oxygen consumption. In this formulation, the steeply varying part of the curve is the delivery-dependent portion. The flat part of the curve is the delivery-independent component. A patient who falls on the delivery-independent portion of the curve is protected against sudden catastrophic decreases in oxygen consumption when oxygen delivery may be diminished. For example, if the patient, assumed to be on the flat part of the curve, were to develop hypovolemia and cardiac output decreased, no significant changes in oxygen consumption would occur. Several studies support this concept of delivery-dependent oxygen consumption; nonetheless, controversy exists about whether delivery-dependent oxygen consumption can be demonstrated in humans. Part of the controversy results from the way in which oxygen consumption and oxygen delivery are measured. In clinical practice, the Fick principle is used:

$$\dot{V}O_2 = CI \times DVO_2$$

where $\dot{V}O_2$ is the oxygen consumption; CI, the cardiac index; and DVO_2 is the arterio-venous oxygen content difference.

Oxygen delivery is the cardiac index multiplied by the arterial oxygen content (CaO_2):

$$DO_2 = CI \times CaO_2$$

Since the hemoglobin concentration, the arterial saturation of the hemoglobin, and the cardiac index are factors in both the dependent and the independent variables, the possibility of spurious correlation has been raised by Archie. Stratton and colleagues concluded that the amount of correlation observed is not explained by coupling of variables. Another part of the controversy arises from the graphical representation of Fig. 2. In our view, use of oxygen delivery and oxygen consumption as the coordinates raises several concerns, which are discussed in detail in Chapter 63. In that chapter we argue that a three-dimensional analysis is necessary for adequate description of the structure of this problem and that state variables, variables that are path independent, are necessary for logical analysis. The graphical relation in Fig. 2 remains a reasonable heuristic device, if not a logically sound one. Its value is in providing a geometric interpretation of the controversial questions at issue.

Delivery-Dependent Lactate Production

The idea of delivery-dependent oxygen consumption addresses the first criterion of adequate oxygen transport. Why is the second criterion necessary? The need for determining delivery-dependent lactate production, or the ratio of lactate to pyruvate, is equivalent to asking if one can imagine a situation in which delivery-dependent oxygen consumption appears to be absent, but the aerobic metabolism of the cell remains abnormal. Such a situation could occur if global extraction, as measured by the arteriovenous oxygen content difference (DVO_2), is limited in certain pathologic states. The critical care physician then would see a fixed, narrowed DVO_2, and the oxygen consumption would vary only with the change in CO. A common finding in SIRS, adult respiratory distress syndrome, or liver failure is a decreased DVO_2. In Fig. 3, using the heuristic of Fig. 2, a graphic equivalent of this question is demonstrated. Is it possible that the patient needs to be on curve A but has been able to achieve only the oxygen consumption of curve B? The use of the serum lactate concentration (or the lactate/pyruvate) is helpful in deciding whether a gap exists between the patient's oxygen delivery and tissue oxygen demand. In the formulation of Chapter 63, the use of the lactate/pyruvate results in a three-dimensional response surface, rather than a family of curves. If extraction of oxygen, as measured by DVO_2, is limited, the anaerobic metabolic pathways may be important. The use of serum lactate concentration guides the decision to supply additional delivery of oxygen.

The use of the lactate–pyruvate ratio provides additional information. A normal lactate–pyruvate ratio helps to identify the situation in which the concentration of lactate may be abnormally high, in the range of 2.5–3.5 mmol, but the aerobic metabolism of the cell is adequate. This finding suggests the phenomenon of aerobic glycolysis, represented in Fig. 4. In inflammatory-mediated states, pyruvate dehydrogenase is down regulated. Entry of pyruvate into the tricarboxylic acid cycle is decreased, and increased lactate production occurs. Nonetheless, the lactate/pyruvate remains normal. The aerobic capabilities of cells are functioning, because other carbon sources, including fats and amino acids, especially the branched-chain amino acids, find increased use as sources of oxidative fuel. The lactate/pyruvate is useful in identifying those patients

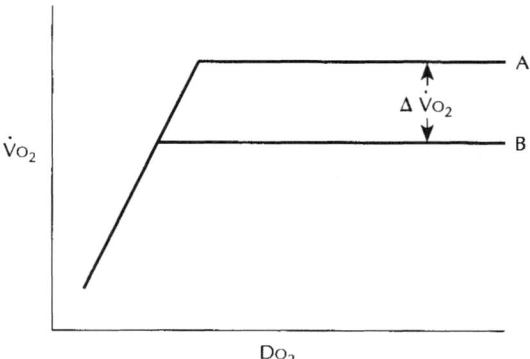

Figure 3 Flow-dependent lactate production. (Modified from Abrams JH. Indications for hemodynamic monitoring. In: Najarian JS, Delaney JP, eds. Progress in Trauma and Critical Care Surgery. St. Louis: Mosby–Year Book, 1992:276.)

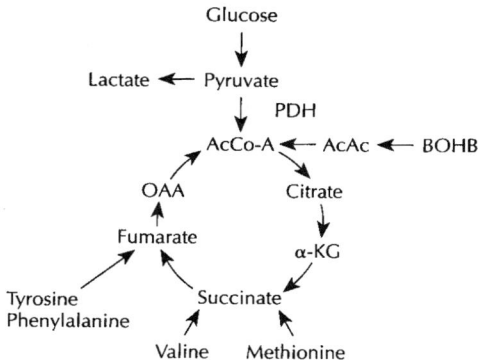

Figure 4 Aerobic glycolysis. (From Abrams JH. Indications for hemodynamic monitoring. In: Najarian JS, Delaney JP, eds. Progress in Trauma and Critical Care Surgery. St. Louis: Mosby–Year Book, 1992:277.)

with moderately elevated lactate concentrations, which persist despite increased oxygen delivery, in whom aerobic metabolism is still an adequate source of energy production.

TREATMENT

Invasive hemodynamic monitoring is necessary to accomplish restoration of oxygen transport with currently available technology. A controversial body of evidence indicates that survival is increased, if patients are resuscitated by oxygen transport standards early in their clinical course. The major indication for invasive hemodynamic monitoring, then, becomes restoration of oxygen transport. From the pulmonary artery catheter, PCWP, cardiac index, and mixed venous blood samples are obtained. Arterial blood is sampled to determine arterial oxygen content. With arterial oxygen content, DO_2 may be calculated, and with the addition of mixed venous oxygen content, DVO_2 and the oxygen consumption index may be derived. Note that mixed venous blood is sampled from the pulmonary artery. A serum lactate concentration should be considered a mandatory part of the data obtained. Other calculated quantities, such as SVR, can be derived.

With the combined approach of source control, restoration of oxygen transport, and metabolic support, a decrease in mortality can be demonstrated. Review of the literature investigating outcomes produced by increasing oxygen delivery yields conflicting conclusions. We reserve a review of the literature and an analysis of the controversy for Chapter 63.

Figure 5 presents an algorithm for restoration of oxygen transport. The initial decision point addresses the presence or absence of a known cause of shock. For example, a patient experiencing massive hemorrhage requires transfusion of packed red blood cells as the highest priority. Another important decision node is the presence or absence of SIRS. Does the patient have an inciting pathology that can produce SIRS? Does the patient have sepsis, pancreatitis, adult respiratory distress syndrome, or multiple trauma? If the answer is yes, monitoring with a pulmonary artery catheter receives serious consideration. If the clinical setting does not suggest SIRS, but suspicion is high for

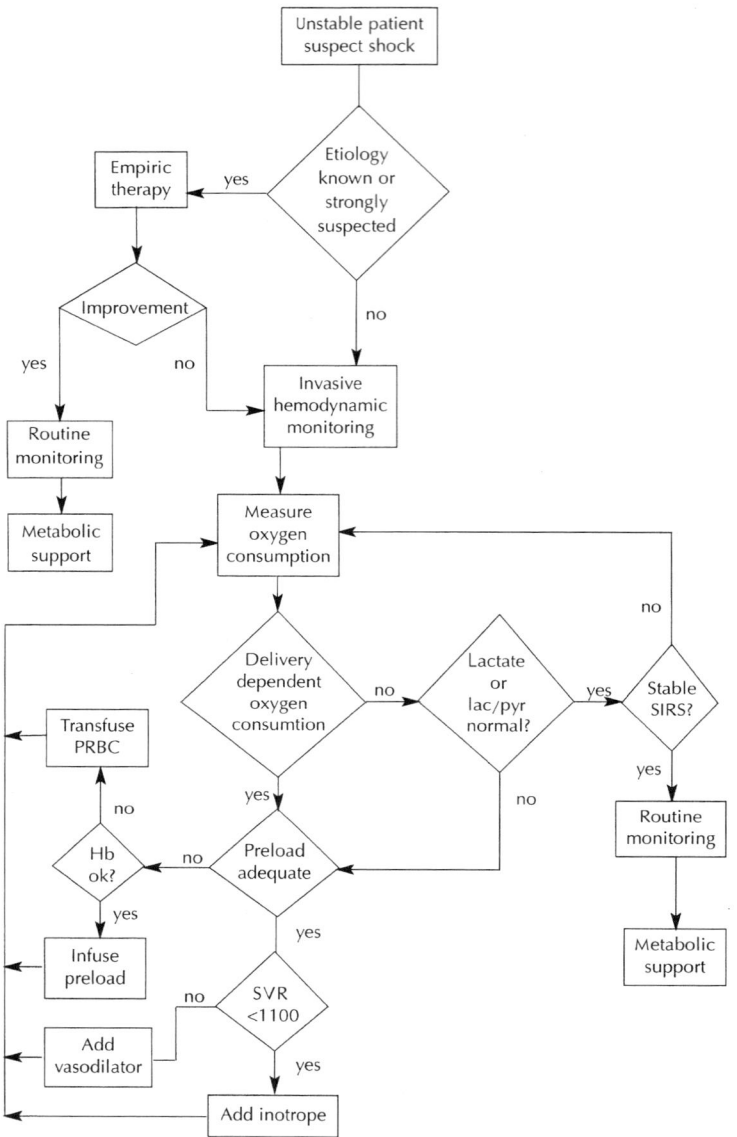

Figure 5 Approach to restoration of oxygen transport.

inadequate oxygen delivery by another mechanism, the physician can then determine the serum lactate concentration. If elevated, oxygen delivery should be increased with the use of invasive hemodynamic monitoring, as needed. The physician should then measure CO, arterial and mixed venous blood gases, and serum lactate. In the case of persistent but moderate hyperlacticacidemia, lactate/pyruvate, if available, is of use. Oxygen consumption is then calculated. If the oxygen consumption is below expected values, the serum lactate concentration (or lactate/pyruvate) is elevated, or the arteriovenous oxygen content difference is significantly widened, oxygen delivery is increased. The oxygen consumption and lactate are again determined, and the arteriovenous oxygen content difference is again noted. Oxygen delivery is increased until clinical targets of normal serum lactate concentration and an arteriovenous oxygen content difference of approximately 4.0–4.5 vol% are met. For most patients, the CI is elevated, the PCWP is in the range of 10–15 mm Hg, the oxygen consumption is 20–100% increased over that of the resting human, the DVO_2 is less than 4.5 vol%, and the serum lactate concentration is normal. A general approach has been outlined earlier. The risks and benefits of each intervention at each decision point must be analyzed for each patient. As an example, the appendix applies the algorithm suggested in Fig. 5 to a specific clinical situation.

SUMMARY

- Source control, restoration of oxygen transport, and metabolic support, when successfully addressed, have been shown to reduce mortality in the critically ill.
- Clinical indicators of inadequate oxygen transport are delivery-dependent oxygen consumption and delivery-dependent lactate production. The lactate/pyruvate, if available, is useful in identifying patients who demonstrate aerobic glycolysis.
- Components of oxygen delivery include hemoglobin concentration, hemoglobin oxygen saturation, and cardiac output.
- Cardiac output is augmented by addressing preload, afterload, and contractility.

APPENDIX

A 39-year-old woman was admitted for elective cholecystectomy for symptomatic cholelithiasis. Laparoscopic cholecystectomy was performed without complication. The patient's estimated blood loss was negligible, and the bile obtained from the gall bladder was sent for Gram's stain and culture. The patient had no significant medical history and was taking no medications preoperatively. She was extubated in the post-anesthesia recovery unit. During the first postoperative night, she received family visitors, who noted that she was progressing well.

You are telephoned at 0300 h of the first post-operative night, because the patient was disoriented for time and place. You immediately see the patient and confirm that she is oriented for person, but disoriented for time and place. At this time, her temperature is 101.2 °F, the blood pressure is 120/80, the heart rate is 110 beats per min, and the respiratory rate is 28 breaths/min. The lungs are clear to percussion and auscultation, the cardiac examination is normal, and the abdominal examination is remarkable only for the presence of the laparoscopic port sites. The sites are examined carefully, and no erythema, undue tenderness, or crepitus is noted. A detailed neurologic examination reveals no additional focal neurologic deficit.

The appearance of disorientation and tachypnea in this patient is worrisome. Disorientation with tachypnea and acute respiratory alkalosis are the earliest signs of Gram-negative sepsis. Although a Gram's stain and culture of the bile were obtained at the time of the surgical procedure, no information is available at this time. With a diagnosis of Gram-negative sepsis, you should administer intravenous fluid replacement and institute antibiotic therapy with agents effective against the pathogens of the biliary tree.

Lactated Ringer's solution infusion is begun, and ticarcillin/clavulonic acid is administered. Results of the Gram's stain are available and demonstrate many Gram-negative rods in the bile. Despite the administration of 2L of lactated Ringer's solution over 45 min, the patient's blood pressure decreases from 120/80 to 90/60. In addition, the heart rate increases to 140. The temperature rises to 102.7 °F. An arterial blood gas study confirms the suspicion that a respiratory alkalosis is present. The pH is 7.52, the $PaCO_2$ is 28 mm Hg, the PaO_2 is 110 mm Hg, and the serum bicarbonate concentration is 22.5 mg/dL, while the patient is breathing 2L/min oxygen via a nasal cannula. Blood samples are sent for CBC, electrolytes, and coagulation studies. Cultures of the blood and urine are obtained.

These findings are all consistent with Gram-negative septic shock. Fluid replacement should begin immediately. Although controversy exists about the relative advantages of crystalloid compared with those of colloid, all agree that physiologic endpoints should guide volume replacement therapy. You decide to transfer this patient to the SICU for the further management of septic shock, especially resuscitation by oxygen transport standards. In this case resuscitation means not simply maintenance of blood pressure and reduction of the pulse, but an oxygen consumption appropriate for an individual with septic shock and absence of delivery-dependent lactate production, or normalization of the lactate/pyruvate. With currently available monitoring, invasive hemodynamic monitoring with a pulmonary artery catheter is necessary for assessing oxygen transport.

With crystalloid infusion ongoing, the patient is transferred to the SICU. A pulmonary artery catheter and an arterial line were placed. By this time, several laboratory test results are available. The hemoglobin is 11.5 gm/dL, electrolytes are normal, and coagulation studies are normal. The following variables were measured:

P	110 beats/min
BP	82/52
UO	40 mL/h
CI	3.2 L/min per m^2
PCWP	4 mm Hg
DO_2	826 mL/min
DVO_2	2.9 vol%
$\dot{V}O_2$	93 mL/min per m^2
SVR	766 dyne/s per cm^5
Hb	11.5 g/dL
Lac	6.2 mmol

These data suggest that this patient requires additional preload. Although the patient's PCWP is in the range of low normal, she demonstrates inadequate oxygen transport. The calculated $\dot{V}O_2$ is less than that expected for the clinical diagnosis, and the lactate concentration is elevated at 6.2 mmol. The arteriovenous oxygen content difference is below normal. This finding is consistent with sepsis and is characteristic of a global oxygen extraction deficit. The SVR also is consistent with septic shock.

With an elevated serum lactate concentration and the question of whether delivery-dependent oxygen consumption is present, you should increase oxygen delivery and evaluate the changes. The most efficient intervention in augmenting oxygen delivery is

Oxygen Transport

providing sufficient hemoglobin concentration. In this patient, the hemoglobin concentration is adequate. Increasing cardiac output is the next step appropriate for increasing oxygen delivery. Cardiac output manipulation should address preload, afterload, and contractility. The patient's PCWP is currently 4 mm Hg. With sepsis, myocardial dysfunction may be present. Increasing preload may augment cardiac output.

Additional crystalloid was infused until the PCWP reached 14 mm Hg. At this point, another hemodynamic profile was obtained:

P	92 beats/min
BP	90/55
UO	45 mL/h
CI	4.2 L/min per m^2
PCWP	12 mm Hg
DO$_2$	1071 mL/min
DVO$_2$	2.8 vol%
$\dot{V}O_2$	119 mL/min per m^2
SVR	655 dyne/s per cm^5
Hb	11.4 g/dL
Lac	4.1 mmol

The increase in preload produces an increase in oxygen delivery. With the increased oxygen delivery, the patient's oxygen consumption also increases. The lactate concentration remains high. This patient does not yet meet the criteria for resuscitation by oxygen transport standards. She has an elevated serum lactate concentration and an oxygen consumption less than that expected for an individual with septic shock. Could this represent the presence of delivery-dependent oxygen consumption? Once again, you should increase the oxygen delivery and evaluate the changes in oxygen consumption. Preload now meets the target value. Afterload is the next decision point. Afterload, as measured by the SVR, is below the usual clinical target, a finding consistent with Gram-negative sepsis. Additional afterload reduction is not likely to be tolerated by the patient. The use of an α-agonist to increase the SVR should be considered in the setting of end organ dysfunction that arises from an inadequate perfusion pressure. Routine use of an α-agonist may produce reduced splanchnic blood flow. With adequate cardiac and renal function, an α-agonist is not selected at this time. Rather, an inotropic agent is considered.

Dobutamine infusion is begun. A new hemodynamic profile is obtained at an infusion rate of 10 μg/kg per min.

P	84 beats/min
BP	98/58
UO	45 mL/h
CI	6.7 L/min per m^2
PCWP	14 mm Hg
DO$_2$	1747 mL/min
DVO$_2$	2.8 vol%
$\dot{V}O_2$	188 mL/min per m^2
SVR	550 dyne/s per cm^5
Hb	11.4 g/dL
Lac	1.8 mmol

With increased contractility, both oxygen delivery and oxygen consumption increase. A concomitant decrease in the serum lactate concentration is observed. The patient's global oxygen extraction deficit had been present during this period of resuscitation, as demonstrated by the arteriovenous oxygen content difference, which did not vary significantly.

RECOMMENDED READING

Abrams JH, Barke RA, Cerra FB. Quantitative evaluation of clinical course in surgical ICU patients: The data conform to catastrophe theory. J Trauma 1984; 24:1028–1037.

Archibald EW, McLean WS. Observations upon shock, with particular reference to the condition as seen in war surgery. Ann Surg 1917; 66:280–286.

Archie JP. Mathematic coupling of data. Ann Surg 1981; 193:296–303.

Cerra FB. Hypermetabolism, organ failure, and metabolic support. Surgery 1987; 101:1–14.

Cerra FB. The multiple organ failure syndrome. Crit care state of the art 1988; 9:107–128.

Clowes GHA, Vucinic M, Weidner MG. Circulatory and metabolic alterations associated with survival and death in peritonitis: clinical analysis of 25 cases. Ann Surg 1966; 163:869–885.

Cunnion RE, Parillo JE. Myocardial dysfunction in sepsis. Crit Care Clin 1989; 5:99–118.

Danek SJ, Lynch JP, Weg JL, Dantzker DR. The dependence of oxygen uptake on oxygen delivery in the adult respiratory distress syndrome. Am Rev Respir Dis 1980; 122:387–395.

Edwards JD, Brown GCS, Nightingale P, Slater RM, Faragher EP. Use of survivors' cardiorespiratory values in therapeutic goals in septic shock. Crit Care Med 1989; 17:1089–1103.

Kaufman BS, Rackow EC, Falk JL. The relationship between oxygen delivery and consumption during fluid resuscitation of hypovolemic and septic shock. Chest 1984; 85:336–340.

Patel TB, Olson MS. Regulation of pyruvate dehydrogenase complex in ischemic rat heart. Am J Physiol 1984; 246:H858–H864.

Schofield PS, McLees DJ, Kerbey AL, Sugden MC. Activities of cardiac and hepatic pyruvate dehydrogenase complex are decreased after surgical stress. Biochem Int 1986; 12:189–197.

Shoemaker WC. Hemodynamic and oxygen transport patterns in septic shock. In: Sibbald WJ, Sprung CL, eds. Perspectives in Sepsis and Septic Shock. Fullerton, CA: New Horizons, 1986:203–234.

Shoemaker WC, Appel PL, Bland R. Use of physiologic monitoring to predict outcome and to assist in clinical decisions in critically ill postoperative patients. Am J Surg 1983; 43:146–150.

Shoemaker WC, Appel PL, Bland R, Hopkins JA, Chang P. Clinical trial of an algorithm for outcome prediction in acute circulatory failure. Crit Care Med 1982; 10:390–397.

Shoemaker WC, Montgomery ES, Kaplan E, Elwyn DH. Use of sequential cardiorespiratory variables in defining criteria for therapeutic goals and early warning of death. Arch Surg 1973; 106:630–636.

Stratton HH, Feustel PJ, Newell JC. Regression of calculated variables in the presence of shared measurement error. J Appl Physiol 1987; 62:2083–2093.

Waxman K, Nolan LS, Shoemaker WC. Sequential perioperative lactate determination. Physiological and clinical applications. Crit Care Med 1982; 10:96–99.

Weil MH, Afifi AA. Experimental and clinical studies in lactate and pyruvate as indicators of the severity of acute circulatory failure (shock). Circulation 1970; 41:989–1001.

3
Lactic Acidosis

Paul Druck
VA Medical Center, Minneapolis, Minnesota, USA

Lactic acidosis indicates a severe metabolic derangement, with significant associated mortality. The term "lactic acidosis" actually embodies two separate pathologic processes: *hyperlactatemia* and *metabolic acidemia*. Because the most common cause of hyperlactatemia, cellular hypoxia, may simultaneously cause acidemia, the combined term lactic acidosis is commonly used to describe any condition of increased lactate levels. Despite this usage, many causes of hyperlactatemia are *not* associated with acidemia.

PATHOGENESIS
Hyperlactatemia

Lactate is a metabolic "dead end," as it is derived exclusively from pyruvate (a rare exception will be noted later) and must be converted back to pyruvate to be utilized. Lactate and pyruvate exist in a cytosolic equilibrium catalyzed by lactate dehydrogenase (LDH) and regulated by the concentrations of reactants and products:

$$\text{Pyruvate} + \text{NADH} + \text{H}^+ \longleftrightarrow \text{Lactate} + \text{NAD}^+$$

Lactate concentration thus depends on (1) NADH/NAD^+ ratio and (2) pyruvate concentrations. Basal lactate production averages 20 mmol/kg per day (1400 mmol/day at 70 kg) (1). Normal plasma lactate concentrations are 1–2 mmol/L, and the normal lactate/pyruvate ratio is approximately 10–20 : 1.

Effect of the NADH/NAD⁺ Ratio

Normally, NAD^+ is regenerated from NADH indirectly via mitochondrial oxidative phosphorylation. Impairment of oxidative phosphorylation, by cellular hypoxia or other causes of mitochondrial dysfunction, causes the NADH/NAD^+ ratio to rise. The lactate/pyruvate equilibrium is shifted toward lactate, and the lactate concentration rises. Reduction of pyruvate to lactate during cellular hypoxia actually may be useful, because it produces NAD^+, which is necessary for ongoing glycolysis. The NADH/NAD^+ ratio also may be increased by the reduction of NAD^+ to NADH during the metabolism of large amounts of other substrates such as ethanol. Mechanisms such as these cause hyperlactatemia with an elevated lactate/pyruvate ratio (normal = 10–20 : 1).

Effect of Pyruvate

Increased pyruvate concentrations may result in increased lactate production. Pyruvate concentrations, in turn, reflect relative rates of utilization and production (see Fig. 1). Pyruvate may be used for gluconeogenesis or may be oxidized to acetyl CoA by the pyruvate dehydrogenase complex (PDH). Acetyl CoA may undergo further oxidation in the tricarboxylic acid (TCA) cycle or be used for the biosynthesis of fatty acids, cholesterol, and other substances. Sepsis specifically inhibits PDH, thereby interfering with cellular energy production and pyruvate utilization (2). The principal disposal route for pyruvate under this circumstance of down-regulation of PDH is gluconeogenesis via the Cori cycle, which occurs in the liver and kidney only. When inhibition of PDH directs accumulating pyruvate to gluconeogenesis, glycolysis returns the three carbon moities back to the expanding pyruvate pool for eventual repeated gluconeogenesis (futile cycling) and further lactate buildup.

Pyruvate overproduction is a minor contributor to hyperlactatemia. The principal sources of pyruvate are glycolysis and deamination of gluconeogenic amino acids (especially alanine). Glycolysis may be accelerated by hypoxia, because a falling ATP/ADP, AMP ratio stimulates phosphofructokinase. Hypoxia also stimulates glycogenolysis by rapidly activating glycogen phosphorylase, the activity of which provides increased substrate for glycolysis. Alkalosis stimulates glycolysis at the phosphofructokinase level, but its effect on lactate production may be partially offset by a shift in the lactate/pyruvate equilibrium toward pyruvate. Sepsis and hypermetabolism drive protein catabolism with mobilization of large quantities of gluconeogenic amino acids, which ultimately contribute to the pyruvate pool. Mechanisms such as these cause hyperlactatemia with a normal lactate/pyruvate ratio (normal = 10–20 : 1).

Clearance of Lactate

Normally, the liver clears up to 70% of a lactate load (largely through gluconeogenesis), and the kidneys clear 20–30% (via gluconeogenesis and oxidation). Hepatic extraction follows saturable, second order kinetics, with a V_{max} equal to 5.72 mmol/kg$^{0.75}$ per h (~3300 mol/day at 70 kg), as determined in lactate loading studies in animals (3). Hepatic dysfunction from acidosis, ischemia, hypoxia, or underlying parenchymal disease can markedly impair extraction. Renal excretion is minimal with a tubular

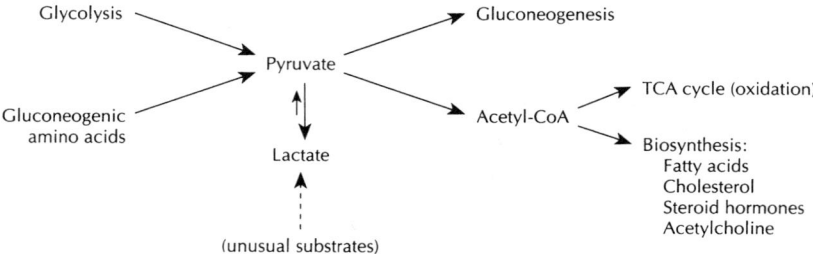

Figure 1 Overview of lactate and pyruvate metabolism.

transport maximum of 6–10 mmol/L. Other tissues, such as skeletal and cardiac muscle can also utilize lactate (1).

Associated Acidemia

The principal endogenous source of H^+ is ATP hydrolysis:

$$ATP + H_2O \rightarrow ADP + P_i + H^+$$

This H^+ is not consumed during the reverse reaction, ADP phosphorylation to ATP. Instead, this H^+ is eliminated in the final step of mitochondrial electron transport:

$$2H^+ + 2e^- + \frac{1}{2}O_2 \rightarrow H_2O$$

Impaired electron transport function, as a result of cellular hypoxia or cytochrome antagonists such as cyanide, interferes with this clearance of H^+, and acidemia results. When excess lactate is produced from cellular hypoxia or other causes of mitochondrial dysfunction (increased $NADH/NAD^+$ ratio: see the earlier section on Effect of the $NADH/NAD^+$ Ratio), acidemia occurs as well—true lactic acidosis. Note that endogenously produced lactate is the weak conjugate *base* of lactic acid; lactic *acid* is not produced, and is not the source of the acidemia in so-called lactic acidosis. Thus, hyperlactatemia may be accompanied by acidemia when the underlying etiology is mitchondrial dysfunction and will not be accompanied by acidemia (unless another acid/base disturbance is present) when the etiology is pyruvate overproduction or impaired pyruvate utilization.

ETIOLOGY

The traditional classification scheme of Cohen and Woods, which categorizes lactic acidoses as Type A (evidence of tissue hypoxia) and Type B (no evidence of tissue hypoxia) is still useful (see Table 1) (4). The most common cause is inadequate tissue oxygen delivery, either global (shock) or compartmental (e.g., extremity or mesenteric ischemia). Anemia itself rarely causes lactic acidosis, unless the anemia is unusually severe. More commonly, anemia exacerbates cellular hypoxia caused by perfusion deficits by further impairing oxygen delivery.

Sepsis is associated with down-regulation of PDH activity and can cause parallel increases in pyruvate and lactate levels. If sepsis is complicated by regional or global hypoperfusion, acidosis with further increases in lactate and an increased lactate/pyruvate ratio may occur (2). A large number of drugs and toxins can cause elevated serum lactate concentrations as a consequence of their metabolism, their effects on glucose metabolism, or liver injury. The metabolism of large quantities of short-chain alcohols may consume intermediates (NAD^+) necessary for pyruvate utilization and produce an expansion of the pyruvate pool. Ethylene glycol and propylene glycol may be converted directly to lactate without pyruvate intermediates; ethylene glycol also causes acidemia through the production of glyoxylic and oxalic acids. Propylene glycol is a vehicle for certain water-insoluble drugs such as lorazepam. If administered in sufficiently high doses, particularly in a patient with preexisting liver disease, it can cause hyperlactatemia (5,6).

Table 1 Etiologies of Lactic Acidosis

Type A (tissue hypoxia present)
   Shock (cardiogenic, hypovolemic, septic)
   Regional ischemia (extremity, mesenteric)
   Severe hypoxemia
   Severe anemia
   Asthma exacerbation
   Carbon monoxide poisoning
   Cyanide poisoning (including cyanide toxicity in nitroprusside therapy)
   Generalized seizures
   Congenital disorders of oxidative phosphorylation
Type B (no evidence of tissue hypoxia)
   Sepsis with no evidence of inadequate tissue oxygen delivery
   Drugs and toxins
      Acetaminophen overdose
      Antiretroviral therapy of HIV
      Biguanides (metformin, phenformin)
      Ethanol or methanol intoxication
      Ethylene glycol poisoning
      Propylene glycol (drug vehicle) in large quantities
      Fructose (in large quantities)
      Isoniazid
      Salicylate overdose
      Various sugar alcohols, e.g., sorbitol, xylitol
   Severe deficiencies of thiamine or biotin
   Fulminant liver failure
   Diabetic ketoacidosis
   Hematologic malignancies and metastatic small cell carcinoma
   Short bowel or blind intestinal loop syndrome (D-lactic acidemia)
   Inborn errors of metabolism
      Glucose-6-phosphatase deficiency
      Fructose-1,6-diphosphatase deficiency
      Pyruvate carboxylase deficiency
      Pyruvate dehydrogenase deficiency

An emerging etiology is antiretroviral therapy (ART) for HIV with nucleoside analog reverse transcriptase inhibitors, such as zidovudine. These agents have been shown to cause mitochondrial dysfunction along with clinical manifestation of myopathy, neuropathy, myelotoxicity, and possibly liver injury, associated with lactic acidosis and an elevated lactate/pyruvate ratio (7). Measurement of the lactate/pyruvate ratio has been advocated to monitor patients for ART-related toxicity (8). Lactic acidosis also has been reported in HIV patients not receiving ART. Carnitine has been proposed as a possible treatment, because it acts as an acceptor for acyl groups from acyl CoA, thus increasing the concentration of free CoA, which in turn stimulates the PDH complex (9). Case reports have described decreases in serum lactate concentrations with carnitine administration, but no prospective trials have evaluated the impact on survival (10).

Vitamin deficiencies are usually exacerbating factors in stressed patients with other causes of hyperlactatemia. Thiamine is a necessary cofactor for PDH; biotin is neccesary for pyruvate carboxylase, which catalyzes the first step in gluconeogenesis from pyruvate

Lactic Acidosis

(see section on Effect of Pyruvate). Hyperlactatemia also is associated with certain hematologic and solid tissue malignancies, especially small cell carcinoma with extensive hepatic metastases. The large burden of tumor cells producing lactate is responsible (11). Hepatic insufficiency rarely causes hyperlactatemia in unstressed patients unless very profound hepatic failure is present. However, it will prolong the half-life of a lactate load produced during a metabolic insult, particularly if accompanied by hypoxia, acidosis, or splanchnic hypoperfusion, which can further impair hepatic clearance. In general, lactic acidosis in a patient with liver disease has the same clinical significance as in a patient with normal liver function (12) (see Table 1, Fig. 2).

CLINICAL CORRELATES

Lactic acidosis has been associated with weakness, malaise, anorexia, vomiting, changes in mental status, hyperventilation, tachycardia, hemodynamic instability, mild hypochloremia, hyperphosphatemia, and hyperuricemia. Some data also support an independent deleterious effect of lactate as a negative inotrope (13–15). In general, the manifestations of lactic acidosis are those of the underlying disorder (1).

A correlation exists between the magnitude of lactic acidosis and the prognosis (16–18). The rate and magnitude of response to therapy and the etiology of the lactic acidosis are probably better indicators of prognosis and adequacy of treatment.

If pyruvate determinations are available, the lactate/pyruvate ratio may be indicative of the predominant class of derangement. A normal ratio (<20) is associated with sepsis and certain metabolic disorders. An elevated ratio (>20) is consistent with hypoperfusion, hypoxemia, compartmental ischemia, or interference with mitochondrial oxidation (19) (Fig. 2). Mixed disorders may occur.

TREATMENT

As hyperlactatemia, with or without metabolic acidemia, is a consequence of a severe underlying metabolic disorder, and not an independent disease state, treatment should be directed at identifying and correcting the underlying disorder. As this disorder improves, the lactic acidosis will resolve. Specific therapy and general supportive care will be dictated by the patient's diagnosis and general condition.

Inadequate tissue oxygen delivery should be corrected by improving cardiac performance, blood oxygen content, and regional perfusion (see Chapter 2). Compartmental ischemia (extremity or splanchnic) may require restoration of arterial or venous patency or resection. If sepsis is suspected, it should be treated by elimination of the infectious source, administration of antibiotics, and restoration of adequate tissue oxygen delivery. The presence of toxins should be considered and excluded. Preexisting metabolic disorders, such as diabetes mellitus or thiamine deficiency, should be addressed.

Signs of resolving hyperlactatemia and acidemia indicate metabolic improvement, but occult hypoperfusion can still exist in the face of a normal or near-normal lactate concentration. Acidemia in particular is a *late* consequence of tissue hypoxia. The principles of establishment of flow-independent oxygen consumption should be considered (see Chapter 2).

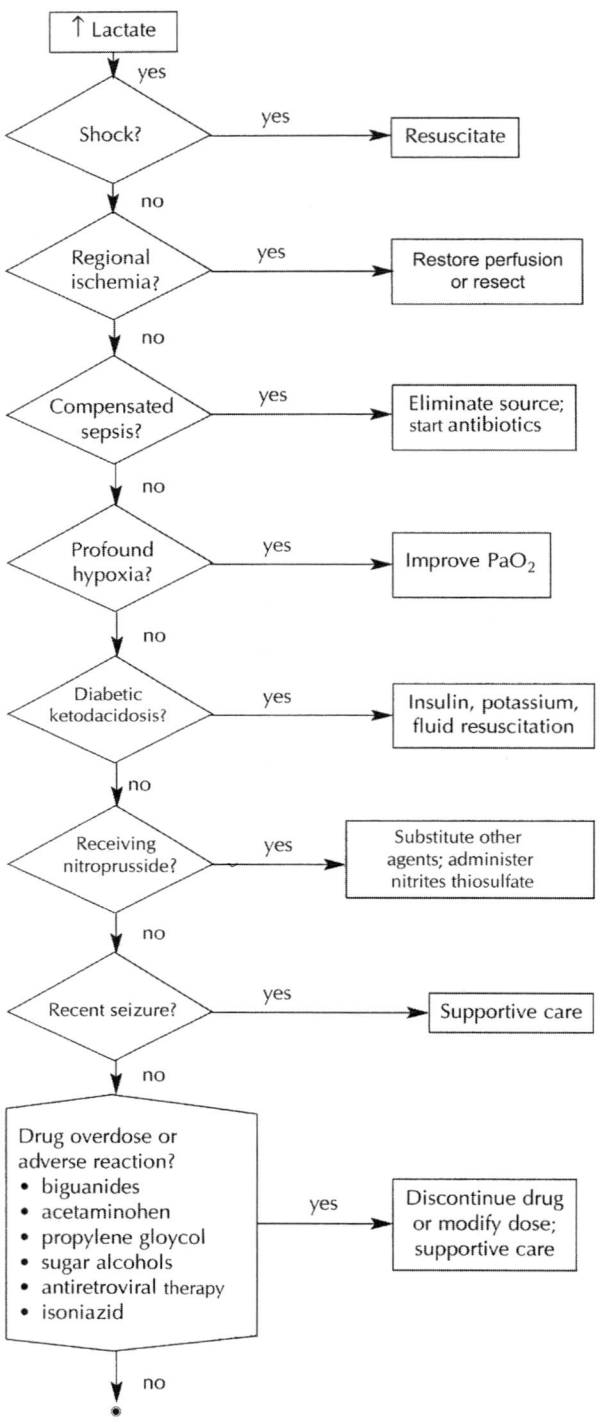

Figure 2 Algorithm for determination of etiology of elevated serum lactate. (*Continued*)

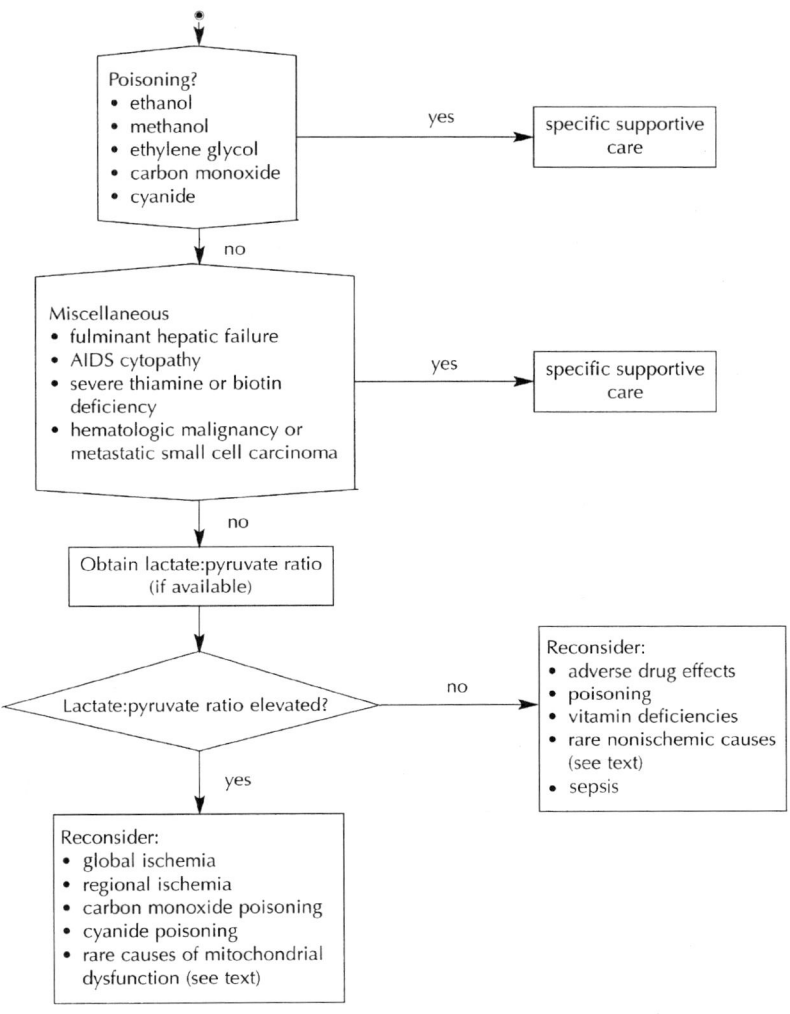

Figure 2 *Continued.*

The management of severe metabolic acidemia is controversial. The basic strategy always should be correction of the underlying derangement and restoration of adequate perfusion. A growing body of evidence suggests that alkali therapy (bicarbonate) is deleterious, as it causes intracellular acidosis with paradoxical worsening of hyperlactatemia, a shift in the oxyhemoglobin dissociation curve to the left with impairment of tissue oxygenation, increased susceptibility to cardiac dysrhythmias, and in patients with congestive heart failure, sodium and fluid overload. Clinical evidence indicates that even severe acidemia (pH < 7.2) does not significantly affect hemodynamics, nor does bicarbonate administration result in improvement (20). Hemodialysis or peritoneal dialysis may be useful in severe lactic acidosis associated with renal insufficiency or congestive heart failure (1). Dichloroacetic acid (DCA) stimulates PDH activity and can lower blood lactate concentration, but in a randomized trial failed to improve survival (21).

SUMMARY

- Lactic acidosis usually represents a severe metabolic derangement and is associated with significant mortality.
- True lactic acidosis (hyperlactatemia accompanied by metabolic acidemia) is a result of mitochondrial dysfunction secondary to tissue hypoxia or specific mitochondrial toxins.
- Hyperlactatemia without acidemia may be caused by a wide variety of metabolic conditions, drugs, or toxins.
- Lactate is primarily cleared by the liver and kidneys; therefore, renal and especially hepatic dysfunction may magnify the effects of a lactate-producing insult.
- The treatment of lactic acidosis is the treatment of the underlying disorder that led to the lactic acidosis. Specific attempts to correct the acidemia or reduce the lactate levels alone have not been shown to be clinically useful.

REFERENCES

1. Madias NE. Lactic acidosis. Kidney Int 1986; 29:752–774.
2. Vary TC, Seigel JH, Nakatani T, et al. Effect of sepsis on activity of pyruvate dehydrogenase complex in skeletal muscle and liver. Am J Physiol 1986; 250:E634–640.
3. Naylor JM, Kronfeld DS, et al. Hepatic and extrahepatic lactate metabolism in sheep: effects of lactate loading and pH. Am J Physiol 1984; 247:E727–E755.
4. Cohen RD, Woods HF. Clinical and Biochemical Aspects of Lactic Acidosis. Boston: Blackwell Scientific, 1976.
5. Cate JC, Hedrick R. Propylene glycol intoxication and lactic acidosis. N Engl J Med 1980; 303:1237.
6. Christopher MM, Eckfeldt JH, et al. Propylene glycol ingestion causes D-lactic acidosis. Lab Invest 1990; 62(1):114–118.
7. Shaer AJ, Rastegar A. Lactic acidosis in the setting of antiretroviral therapy for the acquired immunodeficiency syndrome. Am J Nephrol 2000; 20:332–338.
8. Chariot P, Monet I, et al. Determination of the blood lactate : pyruvate ratio as a noninvasive test for the diagnosis of zidovudine myopathy. Arthritis Rheum 1994; 37(4):583–586.
9. Stacpoole PW. Lactic acidosis and other mitochondrial disorders. Metabolism 1997; 46(3):306–321.
10. Claessens Y, Cariou A, et al. Detecting life-threatening lactic acidosis related to nucleoside-analog treatment of human immunodeficiency virus-infected patients, and treatment with L-carnitine. Crit Care Med 2003; 31(4):1042–1047.
11. Spechler SJ, Esposito AL, Raymond S, et al. Lactic acidosis in oat cell carcinoma with extensive hepatic metastases. Arch Int Med 1978; 138:166–1664.
12. Kruse JA, Zaidi SAJ, Carlson R, et al. Significance of blood lactate levels in critically ill patients with liver disease. Am J Med 1987; 83:77–82.
13. Yatani A, Funini T, Kinoshita K, et al. Excess lactate modulates ionic currents and tension components in frog atrial muscle. J Mol Cell Cardiol 1981; 13:147–161.
14. Jurkowitz M, Scott KM, Altschuld RA, et al. Ion transport by heart mitochondria: retention and loss of energy coupling in aged heart mitochondria. Arch Biochem Biophys 1974; 165:98–113.
15. Mochizuki S, Kobayashi K, Neely JR, et al. Effect of L-lactate on glyceraldehyde-3-phosphate dehydrogenase in heart muscle. Recent Adv Stud Cardiol Struct Metab 1976; 12:175–182.

16. Weil MH, Afifi AA. Experimental and clinical studies on lactate and pyruvate as indicators of the severity of acute circulatory failure (shock). Circulation 1970; 41:989–1001.
17. Vitek V, Cowley RA. Blood lactate in the prognosis of various forms of shock. Ann Surg 1971; 173:308–313.
18. Peretz DI, Scott HM, Duff J, et al. Significance of lactic acidemia in the shock syndrome. Ann NY Acad Sci 1965; 119:1133–1141.
19. Seigel JH, Cerra FB, Coleman B, et al. Physiological and metabolic correlations in human sepsis. Surgery 1979; 86:163–193.
20. Forsythe SM, Schmidt GA. Sodium bicarbonate for the treatment of lactic acidosis. Chest 2000; 117(1):260–267.
21. Stacpoole PW, et al. A controled clinical trial of dichloroacetate for treatment of lactic acidosis in adults. N Engl J Med 1992; 327(22):1564–1569.

4
Nutritional Support in Critical Illness

Paul Druck
VA Medical Center, Minneapolis, Minnesota, USA

INTRODUCTION

Malnutrition is prevalent among hospitalized patients, and contributes significantly to morbidity and mortality. Retrospective reviews implicate malnutrition as the cause of a two- to four-fold increase in morbidity and a three- to six-fold increase in mortality (1–4). Malnutrition is an independent risk factor for gastrointestinal (GI) anastomotic leakage (5). Critically ill patients have accelerated and pathologic metabolism ("hypermetabolism") that aggravates this problem. Prompt recognition of malnutrition and institution of metabolic support is a cornerstone of critical care.

PHYSIOLOGIC EFFECTS OF MALNUTRITION

The different forms of malnutrition include protein calorie deficiency (marasmus), predominantly protein deficiency (kwashiorkor), and specific micronutrient deficiency syndromes, which usually accompany global malnutrition. Malnutrition is associated with a wide variety of physiologic derangements (Table 1). Some, such as immune system depression and delayed wound healing, are observed after only moderate degrees of depletion and are the abnormalities best appreciated by, and of greatest concern to, most physicians. Changes that reflect extensive loss of functional protein, such as skeletal muscle wasting, loss of GI mucosa, reduction of cardiac mass, and respiratory insufficiency, are usually the result of more severe malnutrition. The derangements and findings of specific micronutrient deficiency syndromes (vitamins, minerals, trace elements) are too numerous to describe here (Table 2). A comprehensive textbook of nutrition that describes these syndromes is an invaluable resource for any physician, particularly the intensivist.

Malnutrition adversely affects virtually all aspects of the immune system. Total lymphocyte counts and lymphocyte proliferation are decreased, and atrophy of the spleen, thymus, and lymph nodes can occur. Leukocyte chemotaxis, phagocytosis, intracellular killing, and antibody response by B-lymphocytes are impaired. The GI mucosal barrier

Table 1 Physiologic Consequences of Malnutrition

Impaired immune competence
Impaired wound healing
Respiratory insufficiency
Anemia
GI mucosal atrophy (loss of barrier function, immune function, and absorptive function)
Skeletal muscle wasting
Hepatic dysfunction
Anasarca
Loss of cardiac muscle mass
Renal cortical atrophy
Specific micronutrient deficiency syndromes (Table 2)

is compromised, and the gut-associated lymphoid tissue (GALT), which accounts for ~80% of the body's lymphoid tissue, is reduced (see later).

NUTRITIONAL ASSESSMENT

Malnutrition, except in its most advanced forms, may not always be immediately apparent. Any patient with risk factors for malnutrition (Table 3) should undergo nutritional assessment. Historical indicators of malnutrition include unplanned loss of 10% or more of body weight in the past 6 months (6,7) or symptoms of micronutrient deficiencies (Table 2). Physical findings of malnutrition include evidence of significant weight loss (redundant skin, wasted appearance, ill-fitting clothes), which can be unreliable in obese patients; signs of micronutrient deficiencies; or wasting of muscles such as the temporalis muscle or intrinsic muscles of the hand, which are normally preserved even in inactive patients (in the absence of stroke or neuromuscular disease). Unexplained congestive heart failure, edema, neuropathy, anemia, coagulopathy, osteoporosis, or other signs of micronutrient deficiency syndromes should also raise suspicion. Focused clinical evaluation has been shown to correlate well with a variety of objective measurements (8).

The measurement of visceral protein serum concentrations (e.g., albumin, prealbumin, transferrin; see later) has assumed a prominent role in nutritional assessment, but interpretational difficulties can arise. Anthropometry, including weight vs. height tables, skin fold thickness, and the creatinine-height index, may be confounded by inherent variability, differences in baseline status (with respect to body fat or muscle mass), and renal function (9). Lean body habitus, which is detected anthropometrically, does not increase risk as does functional impairment secondary to inadequate nutrient intake (10). A number of indices incorporating historical, clinical, and laboratory measurements are in common use and are the bases of patient stratification in many modern studies of the effect of nutritional status on outcome (Table 4) (11,12).

Visceral proteins (including albumin, transferrin, prealbumin, and retinol-binding protein) are serum proteins synthesized by the liver. Reduced serum concentrations are frequently a consequence of malnutrition, but other mechanisms may be the cause. For example, reduced hepatic synthetic capacity and sepsis or inflammation, which "reprioritizes" hepatic synthesis away from visceral proteins in favor of acute phase reactants, will

Table 2 Micronutrient Daily Requirements and Deficiency Syndromes in Adults

Vitamin A (retinol) (5000 IU)	Nyctalopia (night blindness), xerosis, keratomalacia
Vitamin B₁ (thiamine) (22 mg)	Beriberi—high-output cardiac failure, Wernicke's encephalopathy, Korsakoff syndrome, peripheral neuropathies
Vitamin B₂ (riboflavin) (1.2–1.7 mg)	Dermatitis, glossitis, keratitis, stomatitis, altered metabolism of certain drugs
Vitamin B₁₂ (cyanocobalamin) (3.0 μg)	Enteritis, macrocytic anemia
Vitamin B₆ (pyridoxine) (2.2 mg)	Dermatitis, glossitis, cheilosis, peripheral neuritis, seizures
Vitamin C (ascorbic acid) (60 mg)	Scurvy—anemia, coagulopathy with purpura and hemarthroses, dermatitis, poor wound healing, loosening of teeth
Vitamin D (500 IU)	Osteomalacia (if long term)
Vitamin E (5–10 mg)	Peripheral neuropathy, increased platelet aggregation, hemolysis, hemolytic anemia
Vitamin K (70–140 μg)	Coagulopathy
Folate (400 μg)	Pancytopenia, dermatitis, stomatitis, diarrhea, fetal neural tube defects
Niacin (13–18 mg)	Pellagra—dermatitis, diarrhea, encephalopathy, or dementia
Essential fatty acids (4% of calories as linoleic acid; 1% as linolenic acid)	Dermatitis, thrombocytopenia, anemia, possibly impaired wound healing and increased susceptibility to infection
Calcium (800 mg)	Paresthesias, tetany
Chromium (5–200 μg)	Impaired glucose tolerance, peripheral neuropathy, encephalopathy
Copper (2–6 mg)	Microcytic anemia
Iron (10–20 mg)	Microcytic anemia
Selenium (50–200 μg)	Cardiomyopathy, skeletal muscle abnormalities, and myalgias
Zinc (15–20 mg)	Dermatitis, diarrhea

decrease visceral protein serum concentrations and cause an overestimation of malnutrition (13,14). On the other hand, albumin, which has a long half-life (20 days), may not decrease rapidly enough to reflect early malnutrition. Albumin serum concentrations also are sensitive to changes in intravascular volume and capillary permeability (15,16). The half-life of transferrin (8–9 days), although shorter than that of albumin, likewise makes transferrin an insensitive indicator of early malnutrition. Serum concentrations of transferrin also are affected by changes in iron stores (17). Thyroid-binding prealbumin has a half-life of only 2–3 days, a property that makes it more sensitive to early changes in nutritional

Table 3 Risk Factors for Malnutrition

Decreased intake: Anorexia, debility, inability to chew, dysphagia, chronic postprandial pain, nausea, vomiting or diarrhea, s/p obesity surgery or gastrectomy, fad diets
Maldigestion/malabsorption: Bowel obstruction, chronic vomiting or diarrhea, intestinal fistula, infectious enteritis, sprue, inflammatory bowel disease
Miscellaneous: Malignancy, cirrhosis, nephrosis, large body surface area burns, chronic hemodialysis

Table 4 Assessment of Nutritional Status

History: risk factors or indicators (Table 3), recent onset of unexplained congestive heart failure, or neuropathy; new onset coagulopathy, anemia, osteoporosis, or other micronutrient deficiency syndrome

Physical examination: redundant skin, unexplained loss of muscle mass, unexplained edema

Measurement of visceral proteins: albumin, transferrin, prealbumin, retinol-binding protein (see text for caveats)

Nutritional indices (see Nutritional Assessment, p. 44)
1. Subjective global assessment (12) (estimates degree of malnutrition):
   Weight loss in past 6 months
   Changes in dietary intake
   GI symptoms persisting for more than 2 weeks
   Functional capacity
   Disease and its relation to nutritional requirements
   Physical findings: loss of subcutaneous fat, muscle wasting, ankle edema, sacral edema, ascites
   Rating: subjective ranking based on individual rating of above factors as: well nourished, moderately malnourished, or severely malnourished
2. Prognostic nutritional index (PNI) (estimates surgical risk ascribable to malnutrition):

   PNI = 158 − 16.6 (albumin g/dL) − 0.78 (triceps skin fold mm)
      − 0.20 (transferrin g/dL) − 5.8 (cutaneous hypersensitivity score: nonreactive = 0, <5 mm induration = 1, ≥5 mm = 2)

   Predicted risk of complications after upper GI surgery:
      PNI < 40 predicts low risk; 40–49: intermediate; >49: high

---

status. Serum concentrations may be affected by intravascular volume and distribution. In addition, clearance is decreased by renal failure (18,19). Finally, retinol-binding protein has an extremely short half-life (12 h) but is affected by vitamin A levels. Like prealbumin, retinol-binding protein undergoes renal clearance. While normal serum concentrations of visceral proteins generally indicate adequate nutrition, and depressed serum concentrations generally indicate malnutrition, considerable room for misinterpretation exists. Visceral protein determinations should be interpreted within the clinical context and not viewed as diagnostic "gold standards."

Assessing nutritional status in critically ill patients is more difficult and complex for several reasons. Key historical data may be unobtainable, edema may obscure certain physical findings, visceral protein analysis may reflect altered intravascular volume, capillary integrity, hepatic function (see earlier), and multisystem dysfunction. Loss of lean body mass, often seen during critical illness, may mimic malnutrition. Nutritional support should be instituted for any hemodynamically stable, critically ill patient who appears to be malnourished at presentation, who has not received adequate nutrient intake in the last 5–7 days, or who is unlikely to resume adequate nutritional intake in 5–7 days.

PROVIDING NUTRITIONAL SUPPORT

Meeting Caloric Requirements

Ideally, energy requirements are determined by measuring actual energy expenditure with indirect calorimetry. If this measurement is unavailable, energy expenditure may be

Nutritional Support in Critical Illness

estimated by the Harris–Benedict equations (derived from calorimetric measurements in healthy volunteers). Calculation by this method tends to overestimate requirements, particularly when "correction factors" are applied (20). The Harris–Benedict equations for basal energy expenditure (BEE) and "correction factors" are (21–24):

Males:
  Kcal = 66 + [13.7 × Wt (kg)] + [5 × Ht (cm)] − [6.8 × age]
Females:
  Kcal = 655 + [9.6 × Wt (Kg)] + [1.7 × Ht (cm)] − [4.7 × age]
Corrections:
  1. Add 20% for minimally stressed, sedentary patient.
  2. Add 50% for severely stressed patient (sepsis, injury).
  3. Add up to 100% for large body surface area burns (>40% BSA).
  4. Add up to 100% for unstressed, malnourished patient in whom repletion and weight gain are desired.
  5. Consider 120 kg to be "current weight" for morbidly obese patients.

The daily energy requirement is approximately 20–25 kcal/kg current body weight per day but may be increased to 30 kcal/kg per day or more by sepsis, injury, burns, or respiratory distress. This caloric requirement should be provided by a combination of carbohydrates (glucose in the case of TPN) and lipids. The relative proportions may be adjusted to minimize substrate intolerance, such as hyperglycemia or hypertriglyceridemia. At least 7% of total calories must be provided as omega-6 polyunsaturated fatty acids (PUFAs) to prevent essential fatty acid deficiency, although administration of 15–30% of total calories as lipid is considered ideal (25).

Meeting Protein Requirements

In healthy individuals, protein normally is required at a rate of 0.9–1.0 g/kg current body weight per day. Lean body mass lost from pre-existing malnutrition should be repleted by increasing the daily protein delivery to 1.2–1.5 g/kg per day. Severe sepsis or injury may require 1.5 g/kg per day or more. The adequacy of protein administration may be assessed by nitrogen balance studies and by response of visceral protein levels (see Monitoring Adequacy of Nutritional Support, p. 54). Note that in sepsis, cytokine-driven proteolysis results in markedly negative nitrogen balance that is not reversed by nutrient intake (26–28). The goal of protein administration during sepsis is not necessarily to achieve positive nitrogen balance, but rather to support ongoing protein synthesis to achieve the least negative nitrogen balance.

Meeting Micronutrient Requirements

Micronutrients (vitamins, minerals, and trace elements) should be provided at the normally required daily rate to prevent deficiency from inadequate administration or toxicity from excessive administration. Vitamin K must be provided as well; hepatic stores will be depleted in 30 days or fewer, and coagulopathy may result in the absence of oral intake and, especially, with antibiotic alteration of colonic flora. Zinc and magnesium can be lost in large amounts in lower GI output and should be further supplemented in patients with diarrhea or large volume fistula output (25). Water-soluble vitamins are not stored in appreciable quantities, and malnourished patients may have severe pre-existing deficiencies. Thiamine is required for carbohydrate metabolism, and 100–200 mg should be given at the start of refeeding, and for several days thereafter.

Special Formulations, Immune-Enhancing Formulas

A number of micronutrients perform specialized functions in support of the immune system or metabolism; only some have been studied individually. Most clinical data come from studies of two commercially available enteral feeding formulas that utilize combinations of these nutrients. *Impact* is supplemented with omega-3 PUFAs, arginine, and RNA; *Immun-aid* is supplemented with omega-3 PUFAs, arginine, RNA, glutamine, and branched-chain amino acids (BCAAs). Seventeen randomized, controlled trials of these or similar formulas compared with standard enteral formulas have been conducted and show trends toward reduction in infectious complications and length of stay. Only one study (29) demonstrated a significant reduction in mortality. Two meta-analyses have demonstrated significant reductions in infectious complications, duration of mechanical ventilation, and hospital length of stay. No differences in ICU length of stay or mortality were demonstrated (30,31). Recently, omega-3 PUFAs (32), and glutamine (as a stable dipeptide) (33) have become available in parenteral form, where they appear to exert beneficial effects similar to those seen with enteral forms.

PUFAs are incorporated into cell membranes where they act as precursors of leukotrienes and prostglandins. Omega-6 PUFAs (corn oil, soybean oil) are metabolized to the immunosuppressive, thrombotic, and proinflammatory 4-series leukotrienes and 2-series prostaglandins, which include the potent immunosuppressive PG_{E2}, thromboxane A_2, and platelet-activating factor. Omega-3 PUFAs (fish oil, some minor vegetable sources), on the other hand, produce the 5-series leukotrienes and 1- and 3-series prostaglandins, which support lymphocyte function but are less proinflammatory and thrombotic (34).

Arginine supports lymphocyte function via increased expression of IL-2 protein and receptor, is a precursor for synthesis of polyamines that help to regulate DNA replication and cell cycle, and, as a nitric oxide precursor, supports natural killer cell activity (35).

Glutamine is a key energy substrate for enterocytes, hepatocytes, lymphocytes, and macrophages. It helps to maintain integrity of the GI mucosal barrier and GALT, enhances leukocyte phagocytosis and intracellular killing, and enhances proliferation of immune cells via support of nucleotide synthesis (36).

Exogenous nucleic acids can be used in the synthesis of new nucleotide-containing molecules such as DNA and RNA, and thus support rapidly proliferating tissues, such as immune cell clones (37).

BCAAs are mobilized from skeletal muscle in large quantities during sepsis, but supplementation has been found to produce only modest improvements in nitrogen balance without improvement in overall outcome (38). They have, however, been found to produce a more rapid return to baseline of neurological function after critical illness-induced worsening of hepatic encephalopathy (39).

Choice of Delivery Route: Enteral vs. Parenteral

Patients unable to receive oral nutrition may receive support enterally or parenterally. Each route has its own specific advantages, complications, indications, and contraindications. When compared with parenteral nutrition, enteral nutrition is generally associated with fewer complications, decreased expense, and a lower incidence of septic complications. It is, therefore, the preferred route. Parenteral nutrition is generally reserved for patients unable to tolerate enteral feeding. Patients unable to tolerate full support by the enteral route may still benefit from some advantages of enteral nutrition by administration of low volumes of enteral nutrients during predominantly parenteral nutrition (40).

Enteral Nutrition

Theoretical advantages of the enteral route include preservation of the structural integrity and function of GI mucosa, which are adversely affected by fasting, with or without parenteral nutrition. TPN (lack of enteral nutrients) has been shown to lead to increased intestinal permeability to large molecules, possibly including endotoxin, and to bacterial translocation in animals. These observations fuel unproven speculation that increased intestinal permeability and translocation are mechanisms of continued sepsis, hypermetabolism, and multiple system organ failure in humans (41). While increased intestinal permeability and bacterial translocation have been documented in humans after trauma or critical illness and brief fasting (42–44), such a causal relationship has not been proven (45). Lack of enteral nutrition also has been shown to lead to decreased intestinal mucosal thickness and villus height (46), to reduce the mass of gut-associated lymphoid tissue, and to decrease GI and respiratory IgA levels (47). Gut-associated lymphocytes sensitized to micro-organisms in the GI tract disseminate and are associated with resistance to pneumonia caused by the same organisms (48). This phenomenon may explain the increased rates of pneumonia seen with TPN as opposed to enteral nutrition (49).

The principal complications of enteral feedings are vomiting, aspiration, abdominal distention, intractable diarrhea, possible misplacement of nasal or transcutaneous feeding tubes with intrabronchial or intraperitoneal delivery of feeding formula (both are uncommon), possible precipitation of bowel ischemia, and failure to deliver intended volumes (see later). Specific contraindications to enteral feeding are bowel obstruction, marked abdominal distention, repeated regurgitation or vomiting, intractable diarrhea, presence of a GI fistula whose output increases unacceptably during enteral feeding or which is causing failure to absorb adequate nutrients, short bowel syndrome (although continued infusion of small amounts of trophic nutrients may enhance hypertrophy), and ileus (relative contraindication—enteral feeding may still be tolerated). Another important contraindication is bowel ischemia, whether secondary to vascular obstruction or to splanchnic hypoperfusion (low-flow state, hypotension, use of vasoconstrictive agents). Some conditions such as severe inflammatory bowel disease or radiation-induced enteritis may cause a combination of these problems and require parenteral nutrition.

Aspiration, often subclinical, occurs in at least 40% of patients receiving enteral nutrition who do not have endotracheal tubes and in up to 75% of endotracheally intubated patients. A number of factors are associated with increased risk of aspiration (Box 1). The likelihood of an aspiration event causing pneumonia is related to the volume and character of the aspirate; larger volumes, more particulate nature, and less physiologic pH are all associated with a higher risk of pneumonia.

Placing the feeding tube in the post-pyloric position decreases the risk of ventilator-associated pneumonia from 36% to 27% and reduces the interval for reaching the goal rate of delivery (50). That the rate of regurgitation, aspiration, or pneumonia is lower for nasojejunal (beyond ligament of Treitz) than for nasoduodenal delivery has not been conclusively proven. The risk of aspiration also may be reduced by keeping the head of

Box 1 Risk Factors for Aspiration During Enteral Feeding

Increased tendency for gastroesophageal reflux
   (pre-existing reflux disease)
   Presence of nasogastric tube
   Supine or Trendelenberg's position
   Opiates or anticholinergic drugs
Delayed gastric emptying
   Generalized ileus or diabetic gastroparesis
   Hyperglycemia
   Sepsis
   Drugs such as dopamine, propofol, and opiates
   Electrolyte abnormalities
Diminished airway protection mechanisms
   Altered mental status
   Recent or current tracheal airway device

---

the bed elevated at least 30° and by correcting hyperglycemia and electrolyte abnormalities. Concern about the risk of aspiration has prompted the practice of measuring gastric residual volumes and discontinuing infusion, if a threshold is exceeded. This practice is largely responsible for the frequent failure to achieve nutritional goals in enterally fed patients. While those patients who do not tolerate enteral, and especially gastric, feeding are likely to have high residual volumes, a recent review of studies of the measurement and use of gastric residual volumes failed to detect a correlation between residual volume and actual gastric volume, gastric emptying, regurgitation, or aspiration (51). A recent consensus statement recommends: (1) stop infusion for overt regurgitation or vomiting; (2) if the residual volume is >500 mL, withold feedings and reassess tolerance; (3) gastric residual volumes <500 mL do not necessarily contraindicate continued feeding, but should be interpreted in conjunction with clinical evaluation; (4) residual volumes <500 mL should be reinfused if no clinical evidence of regurgitation, distention, or intolerance is present (52).

If regurgitation occurs: (1) a prokinetic agent such as metoclopramide or erythromycin may be added; (2) the need for dopamine, narcotics, and sedatives should be reassessed, if they are being administered; (3) a search for occult sepsis should be undertaken; and (4) the feeding tube should be positioned more distally (if possible) with simultaneous tube decompression of the stomach. If regurgitation cannot be prevented by these maneuvers, the rate of infusion will need to be decreased or even terminated. Parenteral nutrition may then be added or substituted.

Parenteral Nutrition

Parenteral nutrition is reserved for those patients who cannot receive or tolerate enteral nutrition. This group includes patients in whom a feeding tube cannot be positioned properly (rare), who continually remove such tubes, or have one or more of the contraindications to enteral feedings described earlier (see Enteral Nutrition). The complications of parenteral nutrition involve insertion and maintenance of the central venous catheter and physiologic and metabolic complications related to the composition and route of delivery of the nutrients.

Catheter-related complications include pneumothorax, hemothorax, arterial injury, brachial plexus injury, hydrothorax, air embolism, catheter sepsis, central vein thrombosis, perforation of the superior vena cava or right atrium, and cardiac arrhythmia (53). Metabolic complications, many of which may be avoided by careful attention to composition and rate of delivery, include hyperglycemia, hypertriglyceridemia, electrolyte abnormalities, deficiency syndromes from failure to provide micronutrient supplementation (Tables 2 and 5), hepatobiliary complications such as steatosis and cholestasis (54–56), and pathologic changes in the GI mucosa (see earlier). Transient two- to three-fold elevations in transaminases generally resolve spontaneously. Persistent elevations associated with hepatic dysfunction require reducing total calories delivered, reducing glucose to less than 5 g/kg per day, using lipids for a mixed calorie source, and progressing to enteral feeding as soon as feasible (53,57). Accelerated gallstone formation with risk of cholecystitis is often referred to as "TPN-associated cholecystitis," although it is the NPO state, not the delivery of intravenous nutrients, that predisposes to gallstone formation (58,59). Administration of small amounts of enteral nutrition, enteral lipids, or cholecystokinin will prevent this complication (60). Intrahepatic cholestasis is occasionally seen and is possibly due to the toxic effects of lithocholic acid (produced by intestinal bacteria from chenodeoxycholic acid). Treatment with metronidazole or ursodeoxycholic acid has been suggested (61).

Timing of Initiation of Nutritional Support

Traditionally, nutritional support is begun within 7 days of fasting to prevent immunosuppression and loss of lean body mass. Interpretation of the results of studies of very early initiation of support is confounded by variables involving route (enteral vs. parenteral), composition (standard vs. immune-enhancing), and definitions of "early" (8 h to 3 days).

Table 5 Providing Nutritional Support—The Basics

Nonprotein calories:
  20–25 kcal/kg usual weight per day
  Ratio of carbohydrate-to-lipid depends on substrate tolerance
  Hypermetabolic critical illness may necessitate ≥ 30 kcal/kg per day
  Number of nonprotein calories delivered should be based on measured or
    estimated energy expenditure and readjusted regularly. Avoid overfeeding
Protein:
  0.9–1 g/kg usual weight per day is basal requirement in nondepleted patient
  Pre-existing malnutrition may necessitate ≥ 1.2 g/kg per day
  Sepsis, multiple system organ failure, profound protein malnutrition may
    necessitate ≥ 1.5 g/kg per day
  Follow nutritional variables and response to therapy; adjust as needed
Micronutrients:
  Monitor electrolytes and adjust as needed
  Provide vitamins (including vitamin K), minerals, trace elements at
    normally recommended doses to avoid toxicity. Correct thiamine deficiency
    with 100–200 mg/day for several days, then continue at maintenance doses
Essential fatty acids: at least 7% total calories as omega-6 PUFAs
Consider supplemental Zn, Mg for above average GI output

Despite evidence of very rapid development of GI mucosal dysfunction in critically ill patients (42,62), data regarding the clinical benefit of early initiation of nutritional support (enteral *or* parenteral, as opposed to enteral *vs.* parenteral) in critically ill patients are sparse. Early postoperative enteral nutrition, compared with crystalloid fluids, reduced infectious complications, but not mortality, in patients with peritonitis in one study (63) but was associated with *increased* infectious morbidity and ICU and hospital lengths of stay in mechanically ventilated, medical ICU patients in another study (64). Patients who could be classified as critically ill on the basis of extensive upper GI resections for maligancy (esophagectomy, gastrectomy, pancreatectomy) did not benefit from early postoperative enteral nutrition (65).

Conditions Requiring Modification of Nutrition Regimen

A number of medical conditions require modification of standard nutritional support regimens. A brief description of some of the most common follows.

Glucose intolerance may be worsened by rapid infusion of simple sugars (glucose), parenteral delivery, and the presence of an underlying critical illness. Reducing the rate of delivery and concentration of glucose, and compensating for lost calories by adding additional lipid calories are helpful. Insulin may be required, and if so, continuous infusion is best suited for the demands of continuous glucose infusion. Regular insulin may be added directly to the TPN solution. Enteral feedings cause less severe hyperglycemia and are preferred. If patients are receiving continuous rather than bolus enteral feedings, they may require some form of continuously available insulin—either intravenous infusion or long acting preparations with intermittent short-acting insulin coverage as needed.

Hypertriglyceridemia ($>$400 mg/dL) should be addressed by reducing lipids to not more than 7% of caloric requirements and by substituting carbohydrate calories.

Respiratory insufficiency with CO_2 retention requires care to avoid administering carbohydrate and/or protein calories in excess of the caloric requirement, which will cause lipogenesis with increased CO_2 production and minute ventilation requirement. Alteration of the carbohydrate-to-lipid ratio of appropriately fed patients does not make a large difference in RQ or CO_2 production.

Congestive heart failure may require fluid and sodium restriction, both of which are difficult with TPN. Minimizing other fluids, carefully assessing the minimal amount of TPN necessary, reducing the sodium concentration, and using diuretics as needed are important. Again, enteral feedings, especially with calorically dense formulations, are better tolerated. The same caveats exist for renal failure, with the additional need to limit azotemia. Protein should be limited to the amount that is absolutely essential, but adequate calories still must be provided or protein will be deaminated and utilized for gluconeogenesis. If allowed to occur, this response will increase the urea load and worsen azotemia, and protein will be unavailable for synthetic purposes. Potassium and magnesium should be limited, especially in anuric or oliguric patients, and calcium and phosphorus serum concentrations need close monitoring.

Liver failure is often associated with malnutrition, and improvement of nutritional status is associated with improvement in liver function. Unfortunately, nutritional support can also exacerbate features of liver failure. Encephalopathy may be precipitated or worsened by a protein load. If encephalopathy is observed, protein should be restricted to basal amounts (1.0 g/kg per day), if possible. New encephalopathy or encephalopathy that has worsened from baseline during a critical illness may resolve faster if protein is provided with a BCAA supplemented formula (available enterally or parenterally) (39). Ascites will be worsened by sodium and fluid overload and may be reduced by using the enteral route if possible, reducing the sodium content of the feedings, limiting the total volume of feeding to the minimum necessary, and using spironolactone and loop diuretics as tolerated.

Acute pancreatitis: Controversy exists regarding the role of nutritional support in the management of acute pancreatitis. Specific issues are: (1) when should the patient be fed; does early nutritional support improve outcome? (2) should the patient receive parenteral or enteral nutrition? (3) does enteral or parenteral nutrition exacerbate pancreatitis? (4) if pancreatitis is worsened by nutrition, can this be ameliorated? (5) are the newer immune-enhancing nutrients beneficial in pancreatitis? (6) should the severity of pancreatitis influence these decisions?

Patients with pancreatitis who are unable to tolerate oral feedings should receive nutritional support after $\sim$7 days to prevent malnutrition. In severe pancreatitis, or pancreatitis complicated by sepsis or other stressful conditions, catabolism and increased resting energy expenditure accelerate the development of malnutrition. The only randomized trials of early nutrition vs. no nutritional support [one of enteral nutrition in severe acute pancreatitis (66) and one of parenteral nutrition in predominantly mild to moderately severe pancreatitis (67)] failed to demonstrate improved outcome with early initiation of nutritional support.

Two of three randomized trials of enteral vs. parenteral nutrition demonstrated reduction in septic complications (68) or organ failure (69) with enteral feeding. The third study in patients with mild pancreatitis demonstrated no difference in outcome but greater expense with parenteral nutrition (70). The hypothesis that pancreatic necrosis becomes infected as a result of translocation of intestinal bacteria makes enteral nutrition, with its potential to preserve the gut mucosal barrier (see Enteral Nutrition) attractive, but this benefit has not been proven.

Concerns that intravenous lipids exacerbate pancreatitis appear to be based on cases of pancreatitis associated with extreme hypertriglyceridemia. For patients whose triglyceride serum concentrations are kept below 400 mg/dL, no evidence of harm has been demonstrated (71). Enteral nutrition delivered distal to the ligament of Treitz (jejunum) does not appear to exacerbate or complicate the course of pancreatitis (68,72,73). Consensus exists that gastric or duodenal feeding can exacerbate pancreatitis, although there are inconsistencies in the data (74).

No evidence supports a specific benefit of the immune-enhancing nutrients on the course of pancreatitis, other than the general observation of reduced nosocomial infections in critically ill patients, and the theoretical consideration that by reducing the number of nosocomial infections, contamination of sterile pancreatic necrosis may be prevented.

In summary, patients with pancreatitis should receive nutritional support if they appear malnourished at presentation or are unable to resume oral intake after 7 days. Preliminary data suggest that enteral nutrition distal to the ligament of Treitz may be superior to parenteral nutrition in *severe* pancreatitis. Parenteral nutrition, including intravenous lipids, is well tolerated if jejunal feedings are not feasible or not tolerated, and if hypertriglyceridemia is avoided. Immune-enhancing nutrients may reduce nosocomial infections and length of stay in that group of patients who are critically ill as a consequence of pancreatitis.

Short bowel syndrome, the result of massive resection of small intestine after infarction or inflammatory bowel disease, results in intolerance of enteral nutrients with diarrhea, massive fluid and electrolyte loss, and malnutrition. The minimum length of small intestine required to be able to survive on enteral nutrition alone depends on age, region of small intestine remaining, presence or absence of ileocecal valve and colon, and functional integrity of remaining intestine. In general, adults with less than 50 cm of small intestine but intact colon, or with less than 100 cm of small intestine, but with a jejunostomy, require either full or partial parenteral support (75).

In the postoperative period, the patient will require parenteral nutrition, but small amounts of enteral formula should be provided, because enteral nutrients are an important trophic stimulus for postresection hypertrophy. Diarrhea, even in the absence of enteral input, can result in severe fluid and electrolyte losses, including hypocalcemia. Eventually, trials of oral or enteral feeding must begin, with inevitable malabsorption and worsening of diarrhea and fluid and electrolyte losses. Tolerance of oral/enteral nutrition can be improved with antiperistaltic, antidiarrheal agents, but avoid doses sufficiently large to cause ileus. Elemental diets are often not well tolerated, because their high osmolality leads to massive osmotic diarrhea. Complex diets, if tolerated, may need to be supplemented with medium chain triglycerides, which are more easily digested than long chain fats. Increased dietary fiber also may be helpful. Gastric hypersecretion may occur and should be managed with H_2-receptor antagonists or proton pump inhibitors. Sufficient parenteral nutrition must be provided throughout this period to prevent malnutrition. Recent studies with growth hormone, glutamine, and a high fiber diet have demonstrated enhanced nutrient absorption, even if begun well after the acute postresection phase (76,77). Even if the patient is unable to become completely independent of parenteral nutrition, continued modified oral/enteral feeding, as tolerated, will minimize the amount of parenteral nutrition required, and thus improve life style.

Refeeding syndrome may occur with abruptly refeeding severely malnourished patients and may precipitate life-threatening metabolic complications. Severe malnutrition causes profound depletion of potassium, phosphorus, and magnesium stores, although serum concentrations may be in the normal range. Refeeding-induced anabolic metabolism causes rapid utilization of these electrolytes and leads to dangerous reductions in serum concentrations. Serious symptoms of hypophosphatemia, which usually occur only at phosphorus serum concentrations <1 mg/dL, include cardiac and respiratory failure; neuromuscular dysfunction including mental status depression, weakness, and rhabdomyolysis; and erythrocyte, leukocyte, and platelet dysfunction. The cardiac dysfunction may be exacerbated by thiamine and selenium deficiency, pre-existing cardiomyopathy of severe malnutrition, and sudden expansion of the extracellular fluid compartment. Initially, nonprotein calories should be administered at no more than estimated BEE. Glucose-induced hyperinsulinemia accounts for many of the symptoms of refeeding; glucose administration should be limited to not more than 200 g per day for the first few days. Protein is well tolerated and may be administered at repletion doses (1.5 g/kg per day). Careful attention must be paid to repleting phosphorus, magnesium, potassium, and trace elements. Additional thiamine, 100–200 mg/day, should be added immediately and continued for several days (78,79).

Monitoring Adequacy of Nutritional Support

In addition to monitoring serum concentrations of electrolytes and observing for substrate intolerance (see Conditions Requiring Modification of Nutrition Regimen), one should monitor the metabolic response to nutritional support and make appropriate adjustments.

As discussed in the section Nutritional Assessment, visceral protein analysis is subject to many non-nutritional effects, particularly during critical illness. Prealbumin appears to be most sensitive to adequacy of nutritional support (80,81). Nitrogen balance studies accurately reflect net protein gain or loss for the collection period and are excellent monitoring tools. Zero nitrogen balance during maintenance or positive balance during repletion are desirable. During sepsis or severe inflammation, cytokine-driven proteolysis will result in negative nitrogen balance despite provision of protein (26–28). Excessive amounts of protein should not be administered in an attempt to achieve positive nitrogen balance under these circumstances. Rather, the least negative nitrogen balance possible should be sought. With resolution of the acute phase of illness, visceral proteins should be expected to normalize, if adequate nutritional support is provided.

PREOPERATIVE NUTRITIONAL SUPPORT

Immune compromise and impaired wound healing associated with malnutrition are of particular concern for the surgical patient. The rate of GI anastomotic leaks is significantly increased in malnourished patients (5). While early studies of preoperative nutritional support failed to demonstrate benefit, largely because of failure to stratify patients according to nutritional status, evidence that certain subsets of patients might benefit was observed (3). A large, multicenter, randomized trial of 1 week of preoperative TPN in malnourished patients demonstrated a reduction in the rate of complications in severely malnourished patients. Patients with lesser degrees of malnutrition had a decrease in wound and anastomotic complications, but this beneficial effect was counterbalanced by an increase in rates of IV catheter sepsis and pneumonia (82). From these findings, providing preoperative nutritional support (parenteral, or enteral if possible) to *severely* malnourished patients about to undergo major surgical procedures is prudent, if the brief delay is acceptable.

SUMMARY

- Malnutrition is associated with three- to four-fold increases in morbidity and mortality among hospitalized patients.
- The diagnosis of malnutrition is based on history and physical examination and may be corroborated by visceral protein measurements. Several multimodality nutritional indices are in common use.
- Nutritional support should be provided for any patient who has not received adequate nutrient intake for 5–7 days and is unlikely to do so imminently. Nutrition should be provided via the enteral route, if possible, if the patient is hemodynamically stable and if the patient tolerates the feedings. If enteral feedings are not feasible, parenteral nutrition should be instituted.
- Basic nutritional requirements are (1) non-protein calories as determined by indirect calorimetry, Harris–Benedict estimation, or 20–25 kcal/kg per day, with a combination of carbohydrates and lipids; (2) protein at 0.9–1.2 g/kg per day; and (3) micronutrients (vitamins, minerals, trace elements, and essential fatty acids). Stressful conditions such as sepsis, trauma, burns, and severe inflammation may increase requirements.

- Enteral nutrition is associated with fewer complications than parenteral nutrition. It has theoretical advantages of better preservation of the gut mucosal barrier and GALT, which should decrease rates of nosocomial infections. Contraindications include bowel obstruction, vomiting and aspiration, abdominal distention, high-output intestinal fistula, intractable diarrhea, and suspicion of inadequate bowel perfusion.
- The immune-enhancing enteral formulas are supplemented with combinations of glutamine, arginine, BCAAs, omega-3 PUFAs, and nucleotides, and are associated with preservation of immune function, reduced rates of nosocomial infection, and shorter hospital stays.
- Parenteral nutrition is associated with complications of catheter insertion and maintenance, such as pneumothorax, catheter sepsis, and central vein thrombosis, and with pathological changes in GI mucosal structure and function if no simultaneous enteral nutrition is provided.
- Patients receiving nutritional support should be monitored for metabolic response and nutritional status. Substrate intolerance and complications such as hyperglycemia, hypertriglyceridemia, and electrolyte imbalances should be monitored and addressed. In addition, for enteral feeding, regurgitation/aspiration, abdominal distention, and diarrhea must be monitored. For parenteral nutrition, fluid overload, hepatic dysfunction, and catheter complications, such as sepsis, must be monitored.
- Preoperative nutritional support may reduce the risk of complications in the subset of patients with *severe* malnutrition.

REFERENCES

1. Seltzer MH, Bastidas JA, et al. Instant nutritional assessment. J Parenter Enteral Nutr 1979; 3:157–159.
2. Reinhardt GF, Myscofski JW, et al. Incidence and mortality of hypoalbuminemic patients in hospitalized veterans. J Parenter Enteral Nutr 1980; 4:357–359.
3. Detsky AS, Baker JP, et al. Perioperative parenteral nutrition: a meta-analysis. Ann Intern Med 1987; 107:195–203.
4. Reilly JJ, Hull SF, et al. Economic impact of malnutrition: a model system for hospitalized patients. J Parenter Enteral Nutr 1988; 12:371–376.
5. Golub R, Golub RW, et al. A multivariate analysis of factors contributing to leakage of intestinal anastomoses. J Am Coll Surg 1997; 184:364–372.
6. Blackburn GL, Bistrian BR, et al. Nutritional and metabolic assessment of the hospitalized patient. J Parenteral Enteral Nutr 1977; 1:11–22.
7. Mughal MM, Meguid MM. The effect of nutritional status on morbidity after elective surgery for benign gastrointestinal disease. J Parenter Enteral Nutr 1987; 11:140–143.
8. Baker JP, Detsky AS, et al. Nutritional assessment. A comparison of clinical judgement and objective measurements. N Engl J Med 1982; 306:969–972.
9. Jeejeebhoy K. Nutritional assessment. Nutrition 2000; 16:585–590.
10. Hill GL. Body composition research: implications for the practice of clinical nutrition. J Parenter Enteral Nutr 1992; 16:197–218.
11. Buzby GP, Mullen JL, et al. Prognostic nutritional index in gastrointestinal surgery. Am J Surg 1980; 139:160–167.
12. Detsky AS, McLaughlin JR, et al. What is subjective assessment of nutritional assessment? J Parenter Enteral Nutr 1987; 11:8–13.

13. Manelli JC, Bdetti C, et al. A reference standard for plasma proteins is required for nutritional assessment of adult burn patients. Burns 1998; 24:337–345.
14. Spanga G, Seigel JH, et al. Reprioritization of hepatic plasma protein release in trauma and sepsis. Arch Surg 1985; 120:187–189.
15. Klein, S. The myth of serum albumin as a measure of nutritional status. Gastroenterol 1990; 99:1845–1846.
16. Franch-Arcas, G. The meaning of hypoalbuminaemia in clinical practice. Clin Nutr 2001; 20:265–269.
17. Roza AM, Tuitt D, et al. Transferrin: a poor measure of nutritional status. J Parenter Enteral Nutr 1984; 8:523–528.
18. Tuten MB, Wogt S, et al. Utilization of prealbumin as a nutritional parameter. J Parenter Enteral Nutr 1985; 9:709–711.
19. Mears E. Outcomes of continuous process improvement of a nutritional care program incorporating serum prealbumin measurements. Nutrition 1996; 12:479–484.
20. Foster GD, Knox LS, et al. Caloric requirements in total parenteral nutrition. J Am Coll Nutr 1987; 6:231–253.
21. Harris JA, Benedict FG. A Biometric Study of Basal Metabolism in Man. Publication No. 279. Washington, DC: Carnegie Institute, 1919.
22. Rutten T, Blackburn GL, et al. Determination of optimal hyperalimentation infusion rate. J Surg Res 1975; 18:477–483.
23. Long CL, Schaffel N, et al. Metabolic response to illness and injury: estimation of energy and protein needs from indirect calorimetry. J Parenter Enteral Nutr 1979; 3:452–456.
24. Heimburger DC, Weinsier RL. Handbook of Clinical Nutrition. 3rd ed. St. Louis: Mosby, 1997:211–214.
25. Cerra FB, Benitez MR, et al. Applied nutrition in ICU patients. A consensus statement of the American College of Chest Physicians. Chest 1997; 11:769–778.
26. Clowes GHA, Heideman M, et al. Effects of parenteral alimentation on amino acid metabolism in septic patients. Surgery 1980; 88:531–543.
27. Shaw JHF, Wildbore M, et al. Whole body protein kinetics in severely septic patients. Ann Surg 1987; 205:288–294.
28. Hasselgren P, Pedersen P, et al. Current concepts of protein turnover and amino acid transport in liver and skeletal muscle during sepsis. Arch Surg 1988; 123:992–999.
29. Galban C, Montejo JC, et al. An immune-enhancing enteral diet reduces mortality rate and episodes of bacteremia in septic intensive care unit patients. Crit Care Med 2000; 28:643–648.
30. Heys SD, Walker LG, et al. Enteral nutritional supplementation with key nutrients in patients with critical illness and cancer: a meta-analysis of randomized controlled clinical trials. Ann Surg 1999; 229:467–477.
31. Beale RJ, Bryg DJ, et al. Immunonutrition in the critically ill: a systematic review of clinical outcome. Crit Care Med 1999; 27:2799–2805.
32. Chen W-J, Yeh S-L. Effects of fish oil in parenteral nutrition. Nutrition 2003; 19:275–279.
33. Tremel H, Kienle B, et al. Glutamine dipeptide-supplemented parenteral nutrition maintains intestinal function in the critically ill. Gastroenterology 1994; 107:1595–1601.
34. Kinsella JE, Lokesh B, et al. Dietary polyunsaturated fatty acids and eicosanoids: potential effect on the modulation of inflammation and immune cells: an overview. Nutrition 1990; 6:24–44.
35. Daly JM, Reynolds J, et al. Immune and metabolic effects of arginine in surgical patients. Ann Surg 1988; 208:515–523.
36. Hall JC, Heel K, et al. Glutamine. Br J Surg 1996; 83:305–312.
37. Daly JM. Specific nutrients and the immune response: from research to clinical practices. J Crit Care Nutr 1995; 2:24–29.
38. Bower RH, Muggia-Sullam M, et al. Branched chain amino acid-enriched solutions in the septic patient. A randomized prospective trial. Ann Surg 1986; 203:13–20.

39. Naylor CD, O'Rourke K, et al. Parenteral nutrition with branched-chain amino acids in hepatic encephalopthy. A meta-analysis. Gastroenterology 1989; 97:1033–1042.
40. Omura K, Katsuyasu H, et al. Small amount of low residue diet with parenteral nutrition can prevent decreases in intestinal mucosal integrity. Ann Surg 2000; 231:112–118.
41. Carrico J, Meakins JL. Multiple organ failure syndrome. Arch Surg 1986; 121:196–208.
42. Kompan L, Krezmar B, et al. Effects of early enteral nutrition on intestinal permeability and the development of multiple organ failure after multiple injury. Int Care Med 1999; 25:157–161.
43. Hadfield RJ, Sinclair DG, et al. Effects of enteral and parenteral nutrition on gut mucosal permeability in the critically ill. Am J Resp Crit Care Med 1995; 152:1545–1548.
44. Alverdy JC, Aoys E, et al. Total parenteral nutrition promotes bacterial translocation from the gut. Surgery 1988; 194:185–190.
45. Lemaire LC, van Lanschott JJ, et al. Bacterial translocation in multiple organ failure: cause or epiphenomenon still unproven. Br J Surg 1997; 84:1340–1350.
46. Buchman AL, Moukarzel AA, et al. Parenteral nutrition is associated with intestinal morphologic and functional changes in humans. J Parenter Enteral Nutr 1995; 19:453–460.
47. King BK, Li J, et al. A temporal study of TPN-induced changes in gut-associated lymphoid tissue and mucosal immunity. Arch Surg 1997; 132:1303–1309.
48. King BK, Kudsk KA, et al. Route and type of nutrition influence mucosal immunity to bacterial pneumonia. Ann Surg 1999; 229:272–278.
49. Moore FA, Feliciano DV, et al. Early enteral feeding, compared with parenteral, reduces postoperative septic complications. The results of a meta-analysis. Ann Surg 1992; 216:172–183.
50. Heyland DK, Drover JW, et al. Optimizing the benefits and minimizing the risks of enteral nutrition in the critically ill: role of small bowel feeding. J Parenter Enteral Nutr 2002; 26:S51–S57.
51. McClave SA, Snider HL. Clinical use of gastric residual volumes as a monitor for patients on enteral tube feeding. J Parenter Enteral Nutr 2002; 26:S43–S50.
52. McClave SA, DeMeo MT, et al. North American summit on aspiration in the critically ill patient: consensus statement. J Parenter Enteral Nutr 2002; 26:S80–S85.
53. Maroulis J, Kalfarentzos F. Complications of parenteral nutrition at the end of the century. Clin Nutr 2000; 19:295–304.
54. Spiliotis J, Kalfarentzos F. Total parenteral nutrition-associated liver dysfunction. Nutrition 1994; 10:255–260.
55. Freund H. Abnormalities of liver function and hepatic damage associated with total parenteral nutrition. Nutrition 1991; 7:1–6.
56. Gaddipati K, Yang P. Hepatobiliary complications of parenteral nutrition. Gastroenterologist 1996; 4:98–106.
57. Buchmiller CE, Kleiman-Wexler RL, et al. Liver dysfunction and energy source: results of a randomized clinical trial. J Parenter Enteral Nutr 1993; 17:301–306.
58. Messing B, Bories C, et al. Does total parenteral nutrition induce gallbladder sludge formation and lithiasis? Gastroenterology 1983; 84:1012–1019.
59. Roslyn JJ, Pitt HA, et al. Gallbladder disease in patients on long term parenteral nutrition. Gastroenterology 1983; 84:148–154.
60. Sitzmann JV, Pitt HA, et al. Cholecystokinin pevents parenteral nutrition induced biliary sludge in humans. Surg Gynecol Obstet 1990; 170:25–29.
61. Lindor KD, Burnes J. Ursodeoxycholic acid for treatment of home parenteral nutrition associated cholestasis: a case report. Gastroenterology 1991; 101:250–253.
62. Hernandez G, Velasco N, et al. Gut mucosal atrophy after a short enteral fasting period in critically ill patients. J Crit Care 1999; 14:73–77.
63. Singh G, Ram RP, et al. Early postoperative enteral feeding in patients with nontraumatic intestinal perforation. J Am Coll Surg 1998; 187:142–146.

64. Ibrahim EH, Mehringer L, et al. Early versus late enteral feeding of mechanically ventilated patients: results of a clinical trial. J Parenter Enteral Nutr 2002; 26:174–181.
65. Heslin MJ, Latkany L, et al. A prospective randomized trial of early enteral feeding after resection of upper gastrointestinal malignancy. Ann Surg 1997; 226:567–580.
66. Powell JJ, Murchison JT, et al. Randomized controlled trial of the effect of enteral nutrition on markers of the inflammatory response in predicted severe acute pancreatitis. Brit J Surg 2000; 87:1375–1381.
67. Sax HC, Warner BW, et al. Early total parenteral nutrition in acute pancreatitis: lack of beneficial effects. Am J Surg 1987; 153:117–124.
68. Kalfarentzos F, Kehagias J, et al. Enteral nutrition is superior to parenteral nutrition in severe acute pancreatitis: results of a randomized prospective trial. Brit J Surg 1997; 84:1665–1669.
69. Windsor ACJ, Kanwar S, et al. Compared with parenteral feeding, enteral feeding attenuates the acute phase response and improves disease severity in acute pancreatitis. Gut 1998; 42:431–435.
70. McClave SA, Greene LM, et al. Comparison of the safety of early enteral vs. parenteral nutrition in mild acute pancreatitis. J Parenter Enteral Nutr 1997; 21:14–20.
71. Silberman H, Dixon NP, et al. The safety and efficacy of a lipid-based system of parenteral nutrition in acute pancreratitis. Am J Gastroenterol 1982; 77:494–497.
72. Vu MK, van de Meek PPJ, et al. Does jejunal feeding activate exocrine pancreatic secretion? Eur J Clin Invest 1999; 29:1053–1059.
73. Nakad A, Piessevaux H, et al. Is early nutrition in acute pancreatitis dangerous? About 20 patients fed by an endoscopically placed nasogastrojejunal tube. Pancreas 1998; 17:187–193.
74. Eatock FC, Brombacher GD, et al. Nasogastric feeding in severe acute pancreatitis may be practical and safe. Int J Pancreatol 2000; 28:23–29.
75. Wilmore DW, Lacey JM, et al. Factors predicting a successful outcome after pharmacologic bowel compensation. Ann Surg 1997; 226:288–293.
76. Byrne TA, Morriset TP, et al. Growth hormone, glutamine, and a modified diet enhance nutrient absorption in patients with severe short bowel syndrome. J Parenter Enteral Nutr 1995; 19:296–302.
77. Scolapio JS, Camilleri M, et al. Effect of growth hormone, glutamine, and diet on adaptation in short-bowel syndrome: a randomized, controlled study. Gastroenterology 1997; 113:1074–1081.
78. Apovian CM, McMahon MM, et al. Guidelines for refeeding the marasmic patient. Crit Care Med 1990; 18:1030–1033.
79. Brooks MJ, Melnik G. The refeeding syndrome: an approach to understanding its complications and preventing its occurrence. Pharmacotherapy 1995; 15:713–726.
80. Nataloni S, Gentili P, et al. Nutritional assessment in head injured patients through the study of rapid turnover visceral proteins. Clin Nutr 1999; 18:247–251.
81. Bauer P, Charpentier C, et al. Parenteral with enteral nutrition in the critically ill. Intens Care Med 2000; 26:893–900.
82. The Veterans Affairs Total Parenteral Nutrition Cooperative Study Group. Perioperative total parenteral nutrition in surgical patients. N Engl J Med 1991; 325:525–532.

Part II
Care of the Critically Ill Patient

A. Trauma and Injuries

5
Initial Approach to the Injured Patient

Richard G. Barton
*University of Utah School of Medicine,
Salt Lake City, Utah, USA*

INITIAL MANAGEMENT AND STABILIZATION

As in any immediately life-threatening situation, the management of a trauma patient begins with the establishment or maintenance of the *airway*, the assurance of adequate *breathing* or ventilation, and restoration of the *circulation*. As part of this initial resuscitation effort, a brief survey of the patient should be performed to identify and treat immediately life-threatening injuries such as tension pneumothorax, hemothorax, or brisk external hemorrhage. Additionally, the patient must be managed in such a way as to prevent permanent *disability*, which initially involves protection and immobilization of the cervical, thoracic, and lumbar spines. Finally, a comprehensive *evaluation* of the patient's injuries should be accomplished with a detailed physical examination, laboratory tests, and appropriate X-ray and diagnostic procedures.

Although the basic algorithm for the initial management of trauma is a simple one, the key to successful trauma management is continuous reassessment and reorganization of priorities as the clinical condition of the patient changes

Airway

Initial airway management will vary, depending on the presence or absence of shock, respiratory compromise, maxillofacial injuries, the mental status of the patient, and the potential for neurologic or cervical spine injury. A patient who is alert, talking, breathing comfortably, and hemodynamically stable may require only mask or nasal cannula oxygen. Frequently, in the multiple trauma patient, a need exists to establish an airway, protect an existing airway (depressed mental status, oropharyngeal blood or vomitus, extensive facial fractures, expanding neck hematoma, and facial or other large burns), or provide ventilatory support in the setting of existing or impending respiratory failure. Tracheal intubation is frequently required. Clinical signs of respiratory failure include tachypnea, shallow labored breathing, use of accessory muscles, stridor, paradoxical chest wall movement as in the setting of flail chest, cyanosis, confusion, or abnormal arterial blood gases ($PO_2 < 60$ mm Hg or $PCO_2 > 50$ mm Hg, particularly with pH < 7.30). Apnea or cardiopulmonary arrest mandate immediate intubation, and intubation should be considered in the setting of ongoing hemorrhage and hemodynamic instability, particularly when surgery is anticipated. If tracheal intubation can be performed semi-electively, a cross-table lateral cervical spine X-ray should be taken first to identify obvious cervical spine fractures; however, an adequate airway must take precedence over all other potential problems, and intubation should be performed immediately, if necessary.

Orotracheal intubation with axial stabilization is the most reliable method of intubation and is the method of choice. Standard orotracheal intubation usually requires manipulation of the head and neck and should be avoided in the setting of known or suspected cervical spine injury.

Blind nasotracheal intubation requires minimal head and neck manipulation and is perhaps the tracheal intubation method of choice in the spontaneously breathing patient with known or suspected cervical spine injury. In experienced hands, it can be performed successfully in 90% of cases (1). Nasotracheal intubation should be avoided when midfacial fractures or basilar skull fractures are suspected, and is not possible in the apneic patient.

The laryngeal mask airway (LMA) and particularly, the intubating laryngeal mask airway (ILMA), are used by anesthesiologists and paramedical transport personnel for the "difficult airway" (2). Unfortunately, placement of a nasogastric tube when the LMA is in place may be difficult, and the LMA alone may not provide adequate protection against aspiration of blood or gastric contents. The surgeon or intensivist needs to recognize the wire-reinforced endotracheal tube used with the LMA and communicate effectively with transport personnel, such that the LMA is not removed haphazardly from a patient with a difficult airway.

The esophageal–tracheal Combitube® is a redesigned version of the esophageal obturator airway. It is introduced blindly; if it is introduced into the esophagus (most common), then a distal balloon is used to occlude the esophagus, a proximal balloon is used to occlude the pharynx, and the patient is ventilated via side ports above the vocal cords and between the two balloons. If the device is inserted into the trachea (uncommon), then the trachea can be ventilated directly. The Combitube is recommended by the American Society of Anesthesiologists as an alternative airway rescue device (2).

Cricothyroidotomy has replaced tracheostomy as the surgical procedure of choice for emergency airway access in all but a few cases, such as laryngeal fracture or complete tracheal disruption. Cricothyroidotomy is particularly appropriate in patients with obvious maxillofacial injuries and suspected cervical spine injury. In an adult patient, a size 6 tracheostomy tube, a size 6 endotracheal tube, or even a 12 gage angiocath can usually be placed through the cricothyroid membrane. If appropriate connectors are not available, a 5 mL plastic syringe barrel can be cut in half and the luer tip inserted into the angiocath hub. The ventilator tubing is then connected to the cut end of the syringe barrel.

Airway management is summarized in Table 1 and discussed in more detail in Chapter 30.

Breathing–Ventilation

Bag and mask ventilation should be continued until airway access has been obtained. Even after intubation, bagged ventilation by hand may be appropriate until the cardiopulmonary status of the patient has been stabilized. Ventilatory support to obtain PCO_2 and pH in the normal range and oxygen saturation >90% are the goals of mechanical ventilation. In the past, patients with closed head injury were hyperventilated to reduce intracranial pressure (ICP). It is now recognized that hyperventilation and hypocarbia reduce

Table 1 Airway Management in the Trauma Patient

	Advantages	Disadvantages
Orotracheal intubation	Reliable Usually easy Method of choice in cardiopulmonary arrest	Requires manipulation of head and neck Relatively contraindicated with known or suspected cervical spine fracture
Blind nasotracheal intubation	Does not require neck manipulation Can be done in the awake patient	Requires considerable experience Requires that patient is breathing (air flow or vapor in tube) Contraindicated in setting of midfacial or basilar skull fracture Sinusitis with long-term use
Laryngeal mask airway	Minimal neck manipulation Appropriate choice if other methods unsuccessful	Difficult to place NG tube May not prevent aspiration
Cricothyrotomy	Method of choice when cervical spine and facial fractures present Technically easier than tracheostomy	Requires surgical procedure
Tracheostomy	Good long term airway access (ventilator weaning, secretion control) More comfortable than cricothyrotomy Appropriate in laryngeal fracture, laceration	Technically demanding, particularly in emergency situation (bleeding, poor lighting, etc.)

ICP by causing vasoconstriction, which in turn may reduce cerebral perfusion pressure (CPP) (3). Hyperventilation to reduce ICP should be avoided in the majority of head injured patients.

Circulation

Having secured the airway and ensured ventilation, the next priority is restoration or support of the circulation. In the seriously injured patient, at least two large bore (14 gage) peripheral IV cannulae should be placed, preferably in the antecubital veins in an uninjured upper extremity. When IV access cannot be established percutaneously, cut-down catheterization is appropriate and is usually performed in the saphenous vein at the ankle or the cephalic vein in the antecubital fossa. Many physicians are now more comfortable with the placement of central venous catheters than with cut-down IV access, and central lines are used with increasing frequency in the initial management of trauma. Subclavian lines are easier to dress and care for and may be more comfortable for the patient, but they carry the risk of pneumothorax, which may further complicate the resuscitation of the critically ill trauma patient. The internal jugular catheter may be difficult to place when a cervical collar is in place. Femoral lines are often the most practical, if for no other reason than the area around the groin is usually less crowded than the area near the head and chest of the seriously injured patient. When the femoral vein is used for access, it should be punctured below the inguinal ligament to avoid the complication of retroperitoneal hemorrhage. If central lines are placed for rapid fluid administration, the relatively short, large-bore introducers such as Cordis® or Arrow® should be placed using a dilator via the Seldinger technique. These large-bore introducers also can be placed into large peripheral veins by "rewiring" previously placed IV catheters. Procedures for central venous access are discussed in Chapter 56. External hemorrhage should be controlled with direct manual pressure, and tourniquets generally should be avoided.

Fluid resuscitation usually is initiated with crystalloid (lactated Ringer's) at a rate that is commensurate with the degree of shock but may exceed several liters per hour. Normal saline usually is used for resuscitation of the head injured patient. Colloid solutions can be used as an adjunct to crystalloid and are more efficient for the expansion of intravascular volume. The disadvantages of colloid solutions in general include expense, viscosity (flow slowly through IV tubing), and the fact that most are packaged in glass bottles, preventing the use of pressure bags or powered infusion systems for rapid infusion. Five percent albumin, particularly when used early in the course of shock resuscitation, may be associated with worse outcomes than crystalloid alone (4).

Traditionally, indications for blood transfusion have included massive or ongoing hemorrhage and persistent hypotension or shock after crystalloid infusion exceeding 2–4 L (50 mL/kg of body weight). With the recognition of the problems associated with hemodilution and dilutional coagulopathy, the American College of Surgeons, in its Advanced Trauma Life Support (ATLS) course recommends that blood be considered after 2 L of crystalloid infusion in the patient who remains unstable (5). If cross-matched blood is not yet available, type-specific or O-negative blood may be appropriate, particularly in the setting of ongoing hemorrhage or hemodynamic instability. In the more stable patient, the benefits of blood transfusion should be weighed carefully against the expense, availability, and risk of transfusion-associated viral infections. A young healthy patient, in whom hemorrhage has been arrested, will generally tolerate a hematocrit of 20–25%; whereas, the older patient with underlying cardiopulmonary disease should generally be transfused to maintain a hematocrit of 27–30% (6). Transfusions are discussed in more detail in Chapter 53.

In the setting of ongoing hemorrhage, decisions to transfuse platelets or clotting factors (fresh frozen plasma and cryoprecipitate) should generally be based upon the results of standard clotting tests and platelet counts. "Automatic" replacement of clotting factors and platelets is probably not indicated, except perhaps in the setting of "massive" transfusions, exceeding 8–10 units of packed red blood cells. Disorders of coagulation are discussed in more detail in Chapter 52.

Vasopressors have little, if any place, in the management of shock in the trauma patient. Use of vasopressors may produce adverse effects on peripheral tissue perfusion. CPR is appropriate for the trauma patient in cardiopulmonary arrest, although the prognosis in the trauma patient requiring chest compressions is usually grim. Persistent hypotension or cardiac arrest in the trauma patient is usually a consequence of exsanguinating hemorrhage, but it may result from one of several treatable causes.

The most common cause of intractable shock in the trauma patient is ongoing hemorrhage. Patients with massive hemorrhage (brisk external bleeding and expanding abdomen) should be triaged to the operating room within minutes of arrival in the emergency room. Less obvious but equally lethal sources of ongoing hemorrhage include extremity and pelvic fractures. Depending on the severity of the injury, the hematoma from a femur fracture may contain 2–4 units of blood, and pelvic fractures may be responsible for 6–20 units of blood.

Other treatable causes of intractable shock include flail chest, tension pneumothorax, hemothorax, or pericardial tamponade. Flail chest, caused by four or more ribs fractured in two places in a single hemithorax or by a similar number of ribs fractured anterolaterally in both hemithoraces, presents as discordant chest wall movement in the spontaneously breathing patient. Classically treated with intubation and positive pressure ventilation, current management allows for selective intubation, as intubation appears to be associated with a higher incidence of pneumonia (7).

Tension pneumothorax presents as diminished breath sounds and hyperresonance to percussion in the affected hemithorax with deviation of the trachea to the opposite side. The neck veins may be distended. Chest X-ray, which should be taken early in the management course of the trauma patient, will confirm the diagnosis, but treatment should not be delayed in the deteriorating patient if the diagnosis is suspected. If tension pneumothorax is suspected, a 16–18 gage angiocatheter or needle can be inserted into the pleural space anteriorly through the second intercostal space at the midclavicular line as a temporary life-saving measure. The definitive treatment is the placement of a chest tube.

Tension hemothorax presents with diminished breath sounds and dullness to percussion in the affected hemithorax. Treatment includes placement of a large (36–40 french) chest tube directed from the mid-axillary line into the posterior or dependent portions of the pleural space. Continued bleeding from a tube thoracostomy may warrant surgical exploration and repair of the injured lung or blood vessels.

Pericardial tamponade is suspected in the presence of persistent hypotension and dilated neck veins, particularly in the presence of a penetrating injury to the chest. Muffled heart sounds and pulsus paradoxus are classic signs of pericardial tamponade, but they may be difficult to appreciate in a noisy emergency department. Ultrasonography, done as part of the Focused Assessment for the Sonographic examination of the Trauma patient (FAST), is an excellent screening tool (8–10) and is highly sensitive and specific for the diagnosis of pericardial tamponade in the patient with precordial or transthoracic wounds (8). Definitive treatment of pericardial tamponade involves throracotomy or median sternotomy to drain the blood-filled pericardium and to repair the source of pericardial blood. Needle pericardiocentesis via a subxyphoid approach can be life saving, but it must be considered a temporizing measure in the trauma patient. A significant hemodynamic improvement should be noted after 50–75 mL of blood (usually nonclotting) are withdrawn from the pericardium, if pericardial tamponade is the cause of unexplained hypotension. In the patient undergoing laparotomy, a pericardial window through the membranous portion of the diaphragm can be used to establish the diagnosis and provide initial relief of the tamponade, but may not allow definitive treatment of the source of bleeding.

Disability

Simultaneously addressed with the initial management of airway, breathing, and circulation is the prevention of long-term or permanent neurologic disability. The spine, in particular the cervical spine, must be carefully protected and stabilized until adequate diagnostic maneuvers have been completed. In the awake, cooperative, neurologically intact patient, the lack of neck pain, tenderness, or neurologic deficit may be sufficient evidence to forego X-ray evaluation. However, cervical spine X-rays are mandatory in the patient who complains of neck, shoulder, or back pain; in the patient with cervical spine tenderness or neurologic deficit; in any patient with penetrating neck trauma; and in any blunt trauma patient unable to cooperate with the examination, such as the head injured or intoxicated patient. A mechanism of injury associated with an increased risk of cervical spine injury, such as a high speed motor vehicle crash, also must be considered an indication for cervical spine X-ray examination. A cross-table lateral cervical spine X-ray film, demonstrating all seven cervical vertebrae adequately, will allow identification of the majority of unstable cervical spine fractures, but the cervical spine should not be considered to be uninjured until adequate anteroposterior, odontoid, and oblique views have been obtained. Although the cross-table lateral film does provide some assurance of cervical spine stability, particularly when airway management and diagnostic or surgical procedures are top priorities, the neck should be maintained in a hard cervical collar until the full cervical spine X-ray series has been completed and interpreted as normal. Once the neck has been radiographically "cleared," it should be cleared "clinically" before the cervical collar is completely removed. If the posterior cervical midline is nontender to palpation, the patient should be asked to move his/her neck, carefully at first, and ultimately through flexion, extension, and axial rotation, to evaluate the possibility of ligamentous injury. The collar can be removed when the patient's neck is nontender and range of motion is full and without pain.

Criteria for X-ray evaluation of the thoracic and lumbar spines are similar to the criteria for cervical spine X-ray but are of secondary priority. Taking the time to obtain all the X-rays in the radiology department during this acute phase is frequently associated with complications. The patient at risk should be placed supine on a firm surface and log-rolled as needed until appropriate anteroposterior and lateral X-ray views or CT scan with sagittal and coronal reconstructions have been obtained.

EVALUATION AND INITIAL TREATMENT

Once the airway has been secured, breathing or ventilation established, and resuscitation of the circulation underway, a thorough and comprehensive evaluation of the patient's injuries is initiated. Such an evaluation is precluded only when the patient requires immediate triage to the operating room for hemodynamic instability or for emergency neurosurgical intervention.

Early in the emergency department phase of a patient's care, blood samples should be sent for appropriate laboratory tests, including type and cross-match, CBC, electrolytes, BUN, creatinine, amylase, coagulation studies, and arterial blood gas analysis. A urinalysis should be obtained for any penetrating wound to the trunk and for all cases of significant blunt trauma.

A nasogastric tube should be placed in the patient with chest or abdominal trauma, in the intubated patient, or in the patient with a depressed mental status. If extensive mid-face or basilar skull fracture is suspected, then an orogastric tube is appropriate.

In the seriously injured patient, a Foley catheter should be placed, both to obtain urine for diagnostic purposes and to assess the adequacy of resuscitation. Blood at the urethral meatus or a "high riding prostate" noted on digital rectal examination suggests urethral injury. In this situation, a retrograde urethrogram should be obtained before attempting Foley catheter placement.

In the multiply injured patient, anterior–posterior chest, anterior–posterior pelvis, and lateral cervical spine radiographs should be obtained early in the course of the evaluation, as processing of these films will take several minutes. Radiographs of the pelvis may be deferred in the patient in whom a CT scan of the abdomen and pelvis is anticipated (11). Other radiographs and diagnostic procedures are obtained on the basis of the history and physical examination.

PHYSICAL EXAMINATION

If hemodynamic stability permits, the patient should be disrobed to undergo a thorough physical examination. As much as possible, a complete medical history should be obtained simultaneously with the examination of the patient, with particular attention given to the mechanism of injury and to medications, allergies, and the possibilities of alcohol or drug abuse.

Head and Neck

In addition to the usual eye, ear, nose, and throat examination, the head and neck examination should include careful palpation of the cranium and facial bones for tenderness or deformity suggestive of fractures. Dental occlusion should be assessed. Hemotympanum, otorrhea, rhinorrhea, or "racoon's eyes" are suggestive of basilar skull fracture. A thorough cranial nerve examination, including pupillary light responses and fundoscopic examinations, should be performed. In the alert, cooperative patient, the posterior cervical spine should be palpated carefully to assess tenderness or bony deformity. In penetrating neck trauma, a pulse deficit or expanding hematoma should be sought as evidence of a major vascular injury. Crepitus in the neck suggests esophageal or laryngeal injury. Hoarseness, unilateral hypoventilation, or upper extremity neurologic deficit are all suggestive of significant skeletal or nerve injury.

Early in the course of the evaluation, the Glasgow Coma Score and its three individual subscores (see Chapter 17) should be obtained and recorded (Table 2), both for communication with other health care professionals and as a baseline for comparison in patients with a changing neurologic status.

Chest

Examination of the chest should include inspection of the chest wall for penetrating injuries or contusions and palpation of bony prominences for evidence of fracture. Tenderness to anterior–posterior or lateral compression suggests sternal or rib fractures. Any abnormalities in the heart and lung examination (e.g., murmurs, rubs, gallops, and dysrhythmias) or signs of congestive heart failure should be noted. Pneumothorax, hemothorax, and flail chest should be identified and treated as previously described. An upper extremity or carotid artery bruit or pulse deficit may suggest an unsuspected great vessel injury.

Abdomen

Inspection may reveal abdominal wall hematoma or contusion, which can suggest possible injury to underlying solid organs. Tenderness, particularly in the upper abdomen, may

Table 2 Glasgow Coma Scale

Test	Response	Score
Eye opening	Spontaneous	4
	To verbal command	3
	To pain	2
	None	1
Best motor response (arm)	Obedience to verbal command	6
	Localization of painful stimulus	5
	Flexion withdrawal response to pain	4
	Abnormal flexion response to pain (decorticate rigidity)	3
	Extension response to pain (decerebrate rigidity)	2
	None	1
Best verbal response	Oriented conversation	5
	Disoriented conversation	4
	Inappropriate words	3
	Incomprehensible sounds	2
	None	1
Total		3–15

suggest liver or spleen injury; whereas signs of peritoneal irritation suggest hemoperitoneum or hollow viscus injury. The back and flanks should be inspected. "Log-rolling" of the patient, as previously described, may be required. An expanding abdomen may be a sign of exsanguinating intra-abdominal hemorrhage.

In a patient in cardiopulmonary arrest, an expanding, tympanitic abdomen suggests esophageal placement of the endotracheal tube. The pelvis should be examined for stability and tenderness to anteroposterior and lateral compression. Rectal and vaginal examinations are performed in any patient with injuries to the abdomen, pelvis, or perineum and in any patient with significant blunt trauma. Pelvic fractures often are associated with vaginal and rectal tears, and injuries to the male urethra are suggested by a "high riding" or hematoma-surrounded prostate.

Extremities

The extremities should be inspected for obvious deformities, contusions, and hematomas and palpated for bony tenderness or deformity. A detailed neurovascular examination should be performed in all cases, particularly with extremity injuries or suspected spinal cord injury. If major skeletal injuries are not suspected, passive and active range of motion should be tested and joint ligamentous integrity assessed. Joint dislocation, particularly with a distal pulse deficit, requires emergency relocation and vascular evaluation to minimize further compromise of perfusion distal to the joint.

EVALUATION AND TREATMENT OF SPECIFIC INJURIES

A detailed discussion of all potential injuries, diagnostic procedures, and therapeutic interventions is beyond the scope of this chapter. Although the initial steps in the management of trauma, as described here, are relatively standard, the treatment of specific problems is much more controversial. As a result, even the diagnostic approach for the evaluation of specific injuries may be controversial. Some commonly encountered problems are discussed subsequently.

Head Injury

Patients requiring immediate neurosurgical evaluation and treatment are those with evidence of brain stem dysfunction from transtentorial (uncal) herniation. Usually an expanding intracranial mass lesion causes the herniation. Transtentorial herniation is suggested by the triad of abnormal pupillary light reflex, depression of consciousness, and asymmetric motor signs. Pupillary dilation, the most reliable localizing sign, is ipsilateral to the lesion in 95% of patients. CT scan is the diagnostic procedure of choice in the head-injured patient and should be performed urgently to localize surgically correctable lesions. Emergency burhole exploration is still performed by some neurosurgeons, particularly when CT scan is unavailable (3). In the absence of signs of brain stem compression, head CT scan can usually be delayed until chest and abdominal injuries have been evaluated. General indications for head CT scan in the trauma patient are included in Table 3.

Although plain skull radiographs may be appropriate for trauma patients in the pediatric population (up to ∼2 years of age), they are of little value in the adult trauma population, especially if head CT is available. The identification of a skull fracture, even though such a fracture is associated with an increased risk of intracerebral injury, does not establish the diagnosis of intracerebral injury; nor does the lack of a skull fracture rule out the presence of an intracerebral injury. Even when a depressed skull fracture is noted (a diagnosis that usually requires surgical intervention and can be made with skull radiographs), the patient should still undergo a CT scan to evaluate the brain for associated injuries.

Initial therapy in the head injured patient is directed at control or prevention of secondary injury due to compression of, or swelling within, the normal brain tissue. Urgent neurosurgical intervention may be required to control bleeding, drain mass lesions, establish ICP monitoring, or perform ventriculostomy for monitoring and treating cerebral edema. If increasing ICP is suspected on the basis of clinical or CT scan criteria (compressed ventricles, midline shift, and loss of sulci and gyri), initial management should include elevation of the head of the bed, isotonic fluid administration, and intravenous mannitol with an initial dose of 0.5–1.0 gm/kg. Intravascular volume and blood pressure should be maintained to support CPP. In selected patients, neurosurgeons may

Table 3 Indications for Head CT Scan in the Trauma Patient

Decreased or decreasing level of arousal
Change in mental status
Unilateral dilation of a pupil
Cranial nerve VI nerve palsy
Hemiparesis
Seizures
Suspected depressed or open skull fracture
Penetrating head injury
Glasgow coma score ≤ 10
History of prolonged loss of consciousness

use vasopressors to support CPP, but vasopressors should not be considered part of the initial management of the head-injured patient. Hyperventilation, once the mainstay of the acute management of elevated ICP, should be avoided because it reduces cerebral perfusion (3). Phenytoin and benzodiazapines are appropriate for control of seizures. Phenytoin, given prophylactically to patients with intracerebral blood observed on head CT scan, may reduce the incidence of seizures in the immediate post-traumatic period (12). A more detailed discussion of the management of head injuries is included in Chapter 17.

Neck Injury

Suspected cervical spine injury is managed with a hard cervical collar and immobilization of the head and torso. Evaluation requires a full set of cervical spine X-rays, including lateral, odontoid, anteroposterior, and, in some cases, oblique views. All seven cervical vertebrae, as well as the cephalad extent of the first thoracic vertebral body, need to be visualized. If necessary, a swimmer's view is obtained. After neurosurgical consultation, CT scan with coronal or sagittal reconstructions may further delineate the extent of fractures. CT angiography can be used to evaluate the vertebral arteries when cervical spine fractures involve the inter-vertebral foramina. In the absence of identifiable fracture, neck pain or tenderness warrant further evaluation with flexion–extension radiographs or magnetic resonance imaging (MRI) to evaluate soft tissue injury. The hard cervical collar must be left in place until fractures or ligamentous injury have been excluded or until other therapy (e.g., traction or operative stabilization) is undertaken. Spinal cord injury is discussed further in Chapter 18.

The evaluation and management of penetrating neck injuries is controversial (13). Mandatory vs. elective exploration of penetrating (through the platysma) neck injuries continues to be debated. If a policy of mandatory exploration is followed, all patients with penetrating injuries are explored in the operating room immediately. The only diagnostic study obtained preoperatively is a cervical spine X-ray.

If a policy of selective exploration is observed, the patient undergoes early exploration for signs of significant injury (e.g., airway compromise, expanding hematoma, pulse deficit suggesting a major vascular injury, or air in the soft tissues suggesting an esophageal, laryngeal, or tracheal injury) or for evidence of nerve injury. Patients who do not meet the criteria for immediate exploration are admitted to the hospital and observed. Further controversy exists regarding the need for further diagnostic evaluation in patients selected for observation. Suspected esophageal injury is best evaluated with a water soluble contrast esophagram, as esophagoscopy may not detect small perforations. Angiography can be used to exclude major vascular injury and is particularly helpful in penetrating injuries above the angle of the mandible and at the thoracic inlet. Fiberoptic laryngoscopy or bronchoscopy are appropriate for identification of tracheal and laryngeal injuries.

Chest Injuries

High velocity, penetrating wounds to the heart or great vessels are usually lethal and consequently rarely require evaluation. On the other hand, patients sustaining stab wounds or other low velocity penetrating injuries often survive to be evaluated in the emergency department. Chest X-ray is the primary diagnostic study required. Pneumothorax or hemothorax from suspected injury to the lung or intercostal vessels can often be managed by tube thoracostomy as the only mode of treatment. The "sucking chest wound" is managed by covering the wound with a sterile, occlusive dressing and placing a chest tube through a separate incision. Surgical intervention is generally indicated for an initial chest tube output exceeding 1000 mL, continued bleeding exceeding 200–300 mL/h, or for a total chest tube output exceeding 1500–2000 mL of blood in the adult patient. Suspected penetrating injury to the heart or great vessels requires surgical intervention.

Serious chest injuries after blunt trauma include pulmonary contusion, myocardial contusion, septal injury, cardiac tamponade, valvular injuries, and injuries to the aorta and great vessels. Laceration or free rupture of the great vessels usually is associated with death at the scene of the accident. Contained ruptures or leaks of the aorta and great vessels should be suspected on the basis of characteristic chest radiograph findings, some of which are listed in Table 4. Similar X-ray findings, a carotid or upper extremity pulse deficit, or bruit often are present with great vessel injury. Although CT angiography is becoming widely accepted for the evaluation of injuries to the aorta, arch aortogram with great vessel run-off remains the standard (14–16). Transesophageal echocardiography, performed in the emergency department or in the operating room, is both sensitive and specific for the diagnosis of aortic injury and more rapidly done than angiography (17). In the stable patient, CT angiography or standard angiography should be performed before the patient is transferred to the operating room for evaluation and treatment of other injuries. In the unstable patient, the immediately life-threatening injuries should be addressed first. An aortic arch injury with free rupture is rapidly, almost instantaneously lethal. Gradually decreasing blood pressure usually is the result of other injuries, such as intra-abdominal hemorrhage.

Pulmonary contusion is diagnosed with chest X-ray. Typical findings are a new infiltrate associated rib fractures or overlying soft tissue injury. Cardiac contusion can be diagnosed with ECG (any new abnormalities) and serial cardiac enzymes (Troponin I) (18,19). In most cases, treatment involves 24 h of observation with cardiac monitoring and management of dysrhythmias. Cardiogenic shock, if it occurs, requires rapid identification and resuscitation. Echocardiography usually can be reserved for evaluation of cardiac dysfunction or new murmurs. Cardiac contusion does not appear to have the same adverse effect on perioperative mortality as recent myocardial infarction. The presence of cardiac contusion should not preclude necessary surgical intervention for other injuries (20).

Table 4 Chest Radiograph Findings Consistent with Injury of the Aorta and Great Vessels

Mediastinal widening (>8 cm)
Deviation of the trachea or NG tube to the right
Left pleural cap
Left pleural effusion
Depression of the left main stem bronchus
Indistinct aortic knob
Obscuration of the aortopulmonary window
First and second rib fractures[a]
Fractured scapula[a]

[a]Suggest deceleration injury of sufficient magnitude to result in aortic injury.

Emergency Department Thoracotomy

Penetrating injury to the chest in a rapidly deteriorating or moribund patient is the primary indication for emergency department thoracotomy. When the left chest has been opened via an anterolateral thoracotomy, pericardial tamponade can be relieved by opening the pericardium, and cardiac bleeding controlled by direct digital pressure until suture repair can be performed. The phrenic nerve should be avoided as the pericardium is incised. Massive bleeding from the lung can be controlled by cross-clamping the pulmonary hilum after division of the inferior pulmonary ligament. Injuries of the great vessels are controlled with finger pressure until suture repair can be accomplished. In collected reviews, meaningful survival after emergency department thoracotomy is reported to be ~8% (21). In one large series, survival after emergency department thoracotomy was 19.8% for stab wounds isolated to the chest, 3.4% for gunshot wounds, and 3.8% for blunt trauma (21). As few as 1% of patients undergoing emergency department thoracotomy for blunt trauma will have "meaningful" survival. Emergency thoracotomy should not be performed if ECG activity or pupillary light reflexes are absent. Emergency department thoracotomy generally is not recommended for blunt chest or abdominal trauma, and should be performed only if vital signs are present in the emergency department (21).

Abdominal Injuries

The management of penetrating abdominal injuries, like that of penetrating neck injuries, is somewhat controversial. General agreement exists that gunshot wounds require surgical exploration. Stab wounds have been managed with local exploration, laparotomy, or by observation, with or without peritoneal lavage. In general, the author favors surgical exploration for any stab wounds suspected of penetrating the peritoneal cavity. Laparoscopy can be used to confirm penetration of the peritoneal cavity, although the author favors open exploration if violation of the peritoneum is confirmed.

Diagnostic procedures for the evaluation of blunt abdominal trauma include ultrasonography, abdominal CT scan, or peritoneal lavage, either by percutaneous or open techniques. Plain abdominal radiographs have little value in blunt abdominal trauma. Ultrasonography can be used for the evaluation of hemoperitoneum in addition to hemopericardium, hemothorax, and sternal fracture. FAST is a surgeon-performed, rapid diagnostic procedure for evaluation of injuries to the trunk. It involves the sequential examination of the pericardium and dependent areas of the abdomen, including the right upper quadrant, left upper quadrant, and pelvis. Several authors have verified the accuracy of FAST in hypotensive trauma patients (8,22,23). In a study of 1540 patients FAST was 100% sensitive and 100% specific in hypotensive blunt trauma patients (8). Surgeon-performed ultrasonography also has been used successfully to diagnose traumatic pleural effusions, nontraumatic pleural effusions (24), and sternal fractures (25). It is a good screening tool for hemopericardium (9). Because FAST is both sensitive and specific for blood in the abdomen, the hypotensive blunt trauma patient with a positive FAST should be taken directly to the operating room. Because FAST will often miss the specific injuries responsible for the blood and because many patients with solid organ injuries are managed non-operatively, the stable patient with a positive FAST should probably undergo CT scan of the abdomen.

The use of CT scanning for the evaluation of abdominal trauma was popularized in the mid-1980s (26,27). Prior to the development of sonographic evaluation of the abdomen, CT scan became the most widely used diagnostic procedure for the evaluation of abdominal trauma. Although FAST has become the principle screening tool for the evaluation of abdominal trauma in major trauma centers, CT scan remains the "gold standard" noninvasive procedure for the evaluation of abdominal trauma. Advantages to CT scan include the ability to assess the presence and severity of solid organ injuries and the ability to evaluate retroperitoneal structures including duodenum, pancreas, and kidneys. Expense, time required to perform a study, and the need for interpretation by surgeons or radiologists with extensive experience reading CT scans in trauma patients are some disadvantages. Ideally, scans should be performed with intravenous contrast and delayed images to assess ureters and bladder. Although many radiologists would favor the use of oral contrast to improve study quality, it is rarely needed to evaluate traumatic injury of the abdomen. Because of the risk of aspiration in the trauma patient, oral contrast generally should be avoided. CT scan is appropriate in any patient in whom physical examination is unreliable, including the patient with head injury, intoxication, or spinal cord injury. It is recommended for any patient in whom the diagnosis of abdominal trauma is equivocal and in patients with unexplained hemodynamic instability or a falling hematocrit. As mentioned previously, CT scan can be used to evaluate the stable patient with a positive FAST.

Peritoneal lavage has largely been replaced by ultrasonography for the rapid evaluation of the unstable blunt trauma patient. Like FAST, peritoneal lavage is most useful for the identification of blood in the peritoneal cavity, but it does not provide information about the etiology or significance of the blood. It can be used as a screening tool when FAST is not available. We have used peritoneal lavage to evaluate the neurosurgical or orthopedic trauma patients that become unstable in the operating room. The percutaneous peritoneal lavage technique is reported to have a complication rate in the range of 0–5%; whereas, the complication rate of the open technique is approximately half that of the percutaneous technique (28–30). Peritoneal lavage by either technique should identify 95–98% of intra-abdominal surgical pathology. The incidence of false positive lavages (leading to negative laparotomies) is <6% (28–30). Generally accepted criteria for a positive peritoneal lavage in blunt trauma are included in Table 5. Prior to peritoneal lavage, a nasogastric tube and Foley catheter should be placed to decompress stomach and bladder, respectively, and to minimize the risk of puncturing these organs. Whereas peritoneal lavage is usually

Table 5 Criteria for "Positive" Peritoneal Lavage (PPL)

Immediate aspiration of gross intraperitoneal blood
Lavage fluid containing:
  RBC $\geq 100,000/mm^3$
  WBC $\geq 500/mm^3$
  Any bile
  Any bacteria
  Meat fibers or food particles
Special considerations:
  Retroperitoneal hematoma from pelvic fractures may confound results; consider supraumbilical lavage
  Place nasogastric tube and Foley catheter prior to lavage
  Abdominal surgical scars are relative contraindication to PPL
  Must retrieve 600–700 mL of 1000 mL lavage fluid

done in an infra-umbilical location, the supra-umbilical position should be considered in the patient with pelvic fracture. Extreme care should be used when considering peritoneal lavage in the pregnant patient or in the patient with previous abdominal surgery. Contraindications to FAST, CT scan, or peritoneal lavage are peritonitis and a rapidly expanding abdomen.

Genito-Urinary Injuries

CT scan with IV contrast provides excellent visualization of the kidneys and collecting system and has largely replaced the intravenous pyelogram (IVP) for the evaluation of the upper urinary tract in both blunt and penetrating trauma (31,32). CT cystography or standard cystography is appropriate for evaluation of the urinary bladder. Although rarely used, a "one shot" IVP, performed in the emergency department or on the operating table, provides limited but very important information in the patient with gross hematuria who must be explored urgently to control intra-abdominal hemorrhage. Specifically, the single shot IVP provides information about the number of functioning kidneys within the abdomen, findings which may be important in intraoperative decisions regarding renal exploration, renal repair, or nephrectomy.

Angiography, historically done when a kidney failed to visualize on IVP, has been largely replaced by CT angiography for the evaluation of the devascularized kidney. Because of prolonged warm ischemia time to the injured kidney and the association of other serious injuries, devascularized kidneys are rarely salvaged.

Suspected urethral trauma requires a retrograde urethrogram and a voiding cystourethrogram for evaluation. When a urethral injury is suspected, a retrograde urethrogram should be obtained before Foley catheterization is done. Signs of urethral injury include blood at the urethral meatus or a high riding prostate noted on a digital rectal examination.

Musculoskeletal Injuries

Pelvic fractures, which are common in blunt trauma, can be extremely variable, in terms of severity, morbidity, and even mortality. Whereas anterior fractures (pubic symphysis and rami) can often be managed non-operatively, acetabular fractures and sacro-ileac joint disruption generally require operative stabilization. Posterior fractures can result in exsanguinating hemorrhage. Initial management of these life-threatening pelvic fractures is aimed at reducing pelvic volume. In our institution, a bedsheet is tied tightly about the hips to provide compression and early orthopedic consultation is obtained. The pneumatic anti-shock garment (MAST) (33,34) has been used effectively to provide pelvic compression, and externally applied pelvic clamps have been designed for the same purpose (35). The next step in the control of exsanguinating hemorrhage from pelvic fractures is external fixation (36–38). Angiography may be particularly useful in extensive pelvic fractures with major hemorrhage, both as a diagnostic and as a therapeutic procedure. Angiographic embolization of bleeding sites within the pelvis usually is favored over surgical repair of such injuries and should be done early (39–43). Embolization of identified arterial bleeding sites is often quite successful; whereas, blind embolization of hypogastric arteries to control venous bleeding is less successful.

Suspected extremity fractures require appropriate plain X-rays when time and the patient's condition permit. Suspected fractures are immobilized with appropriate splints until definitive therapy can be undertaken. Open fractures require operative

Initial Approach to Injured Patient

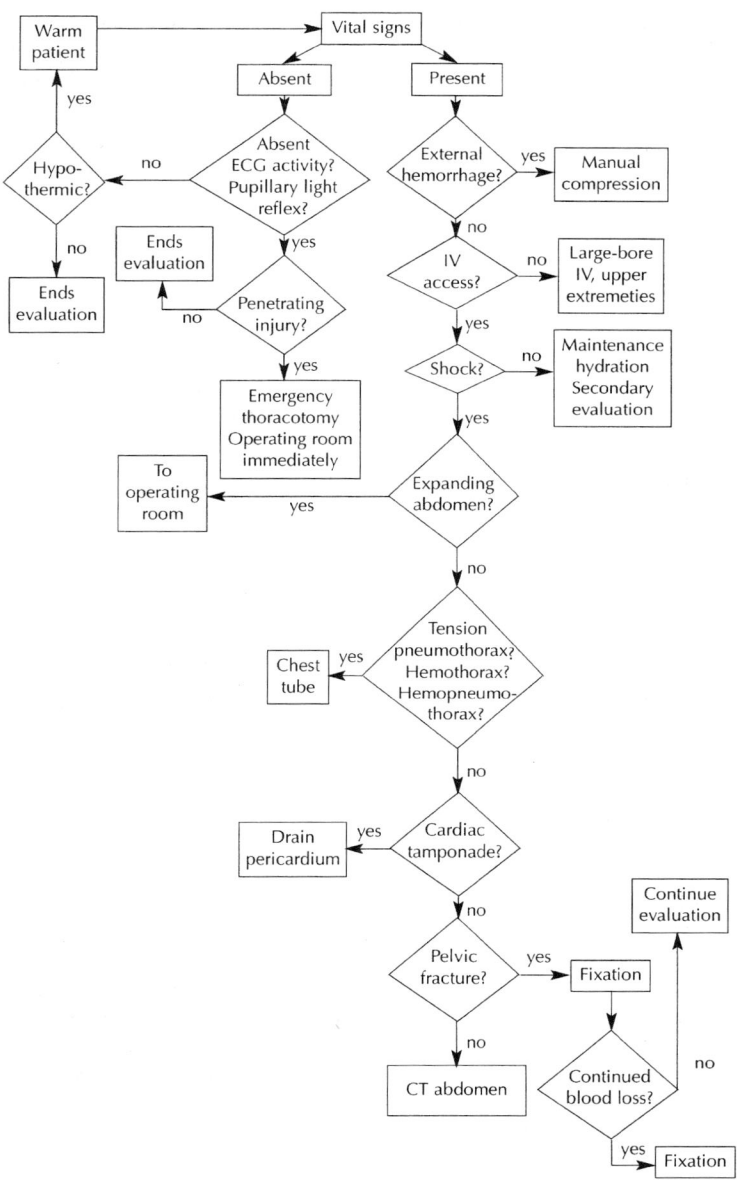

Figure 1 Initial decision-making about trauma after an airway has been established in the injured patient.

irrigation and debridement, and plain films of open fractures or joint injuries should be obtained to identify foreign body or unsuspected fractures. Bones proximal and distal to a joint injury should be evaluated radiographically.

Duplex ultrasonography or angiography is appropriate when a pulse deficit or neurovascular compromise is associated with blunt extremity trauma. The place of angiography in the management of penetrating extremity trauma with suspected vascular injury is less clear. When the diagnosis and location of vascular injury is obvious, many surgeons explore the wound and associated vessels immediately. Intra-operative angiography may be performed. Others favor angiography in the stable patient. The diagnosis must be made early, and treatment initiated rapidly, as a devascularized extremity will tolerate only 4–6 h of ischemia before irreversible injury occurs. Angiography is generally favored when extensive or multiple extremity wounds are present, such as a shotgun wound. The management of extremity injuries is covered in more detail in Chapter 6.

SUMMARY

- The initial management of trauma begins with the ensurance of an adequate airway, establishment of adequate ventilation, and resuscitation of the circulation, all of which are accomplished simultaneously with a cursory initial survey to identify and allow treatment of immediately life-threatening injuries, such as tension pneumothorax or hemothorax, flail chest, pericardial tamponade, or brisk external bleeding.
- When or if hemodynamic stability is achieved, a thorough physical examination is performed and appropriate diagnostic studies obtained.
- Care must be taken to protect the patient from permanent neurological disability during the entire process.
- The successful management of trauma demands that immediately life- and limb-threatening problems receive top priority and that the patient is continuously re-evaluated and problems re-prioritized as conditions change.
- Finally, it is imperative that trauma victims receive appropriate surgical evaluation and treatment as soon as possible.

REFERENCES

1. Moore FA, Moore EE. Trauma Resuscitation. In: Wilmore DW, Brennan MF, Harken AH, Holcroft JW, Meakins JL, eds. Care of the Surgical Patient. New York, NY: Scientific American, Inc., 1989; Vol. 1, Section I, Chapter 2, 1–15.
2. Practice guidelines for management of the difficult airway—A report by the American Society of Anesthesiologists Task Force of Management of the Difficult Airway. Anesthesiology 1993; 78:597–602.
3. Miller JD, Dearden NM, Piper IR, et al. Control of intracranial pressure in patients with severe head injury. J Neurotrauma 1992; 9:S317–326.
4. Cochrane Injuries Group Albumin Reviewers: Human albumin administration in critically ill patients: systematic review of randomized controlled trials. Br Med J 1998; 317:235–240.
5. American College of Surgeons Committee on Trauma: Shock in Advanced Trauma Life Support for Doctors® Instructor Manual. Chicago, IL: American College of Surgeons, 1997; Chapter 3, 99–115.
6. Hebert PC, Wells G, Blajchman MA, Marshall J, Martin C, Pagliarello G, Tweeddale M, Schweitzer I, Yetisir E. A multicenter, randomized, controlled clinical trial of transfusion

requirements in critical care. Transfusion Requirements in Critical Care Investigators. Canadian Critical Care Trials Group. N Engl J Med 1999; 340:409–417.
7. Richardson JD, Adams L, Flint LM. Selective management of flail chest and pulmonary contusion. Ann Surg 1982; 196:481–487.
8. Rozycki GS, Gallard RB, Feliciano DV, Schmidt JA, Pennington SD. Surgeon performed ultrasound for the assessment of truncal injuries: Lessons learned from 1,540 patients. Ann Surg 1998; 228:557–567.
9. Rozycki GS, Feliciano DV, Schmidt JA, Cushman JG, Sisley AC, Ingram W, Ansley JD. The role of surgeon performed ultrasound in patients with possible cardiac wounds. Ann Surg 1996; 223:737–746.
10. Rozycki GS, Feliciano DV, Ochsner MG, Knudson MM, Hoyt DB, Davis F, Hammerman D, Figueredo V, Harviel JD, Han DC, Schmidt JA. The role of ultrasound in patients with possible penetrating cardiac wounds: a prospective multicenter study. J Trauma 1999; 46(4):543–552.
11. Guillamondegui OD, Pryor JP, Gracias VH, Gupta R, Reilly PM, Schwab CW. Pelvic radiography in blunt trauma resuscitation: a diminishing role. J Trauma 2002; 53:1043–1047.
12. Haltiner AM, Newell DW, Temkin NR, Dikmen SS, Winn HR. Side effects and mortality associated with use of phenytoin for early posttraumatic seizure prophylaxis. J Neurosurg 1999; 91:588–592.
13. Carducci B, Lowe RA, Dalsey W. Penetrating neck trauma: Consensus and controversies. Ann Emerg Med 1986; 15:208–215.
14. Gavant ML, Menke PG, Fabian T, Flick PA, Graney MJ, Gold RE. Blunt traumatic aortic rupture: detection with helical CT of the chest. Radiology 1995; 197:125–133.
15. Dyer DS, Moore EE, Mestek MF, Bernstein SM, Ikle DN, Durham JD, Heinig MJ, Russ PD, Symonds DL, Kumpe DA, Roe EJ, Honigman B, McIntyre RC Jr, Eule J Jr. Can chest CT be used to exclude aortic injury? Radiology 1999; 213:195–202.
16. Downing SW, Sperling JS, Mirvis SE, Cardarelli MG, Gilbert TB, Scalea TM, McLaughlin JS. Experience with spiral computed tomography as the sole diagnostic method for traumatic aortic rupture. Ann Thorac Surg 2001; 72:495–501.
17. Kearney PA, Smith DW, Johnson SB, Barker DE, Smith MD, Sapin PM. Use of transesophageal echocardiography in the evaluation of traumatic aortic injury. J Trauma 1993; 34:696–701.
18. Collins JN, Cole FJ, Weireter LJ, Rible JL, Britt LD. The usefulness of serum troponin levels in evaluating cardiac injury. Am Surg 2001; 67:821–825.
19. Velmahos GC, Karaiskakis M, Salim A, Toutouzas KG, Murray J, Asensio J, Demetriades D. Normal electrocardiography and serum troponin I levels preclude the presence of clinically significant blunt cardiac injury. J Trauma 2003; 54:45–50.
20. Flancbaum L, Wright J, Siegel JH. Emergency surgery in patients with posttraumatic myocardial contusion. J Trauma 1986; 26:795–803.
21. Feliciano DV, Bitondo CG, Cruse PA, Mattox KL, Burch JM, Beall AC, Jordan GL. Liberal use of emergency center thoracotomy. Am J Surg 1986; 152:654–660.
22. Boulanger BR, McLellan BA, Brenneman FD, Wherrett LJ, Rizoli SB, Culhane J. Emergent abdominal sonography as a screening test in a new diagnostic algorithm for blunt trauma. J Trauma 1996; 40:867–874.
23. Wherrett LJ, Boulanger BR, McLellan BA, Brenneman FD, Rizoli SB, Culhane J, Hamilton P. Hypotension after blunt abdominal trauma: the role of emergent abdominal sonography in surgical triage. J Trauma 1996; 41:815–820.
24. Sisley AC, Rozycki GS, Ballard RB, Namias N, Salomone JP, Feliciano DV. Rapid detection of traumatic effusion using surgeon-performed ultrasound. J Trauma 1998; 44:291–297.
25. Fenkl R, von Garrel T, Knaepler H. Emergency diagnosis of sternum fracture with ultrasound. Unfallchirurg 1992; 95:375–379.

26. Peitzman AB, Makaroun MS, Slasky S, Ritter P. Prospective study of computed tomography in initial management of blunt abdominal trauma. J Trauma 1986; 26:585–592.
27. Fabian TC, Mangiante EC, White TJ, Patterson CR, Boldreghini S, Britt LG. A prospective study of 91 patients undergoing both computed tomography and peritoneal lavage following blunt abdominal trauma. J Trauma 1986; 26:602–608.
28. Pachter HL, Hofstetter SR. Open and percutaneous paracentesis and lavage for abdominal trauma. Arch Surg 1981; 116(3):318–319.
29. Lazarus HM, Nelson JA. Technique for peritoneal lavage without risk or complication. Surg Gynecol Obstet 1979; 149:889–892.
30. Fischer RP, Bryce CB, Engrav LH, Benjamin CI, Perry JF Jr. Diagnostic peritoneal lavage: fourteen years and 2,586 patients later. Am J Surg 1978; 136:701–704.
31. Bretan PN, McAninch JW, Federle MP, Jeffrey RBJ. Computerized tomographic staging of renal trauma. J Urol 1986; 136:561–565.
32. McAndrew JD, Corriere JN. Radiographic evaluation of renal trauma: Evaluation of 1103 consecutive patients. Br J Urol 1994; 73:352–354.
33. Batalden DJ, Wickstrom PH, Ruiz E, Gustilo MD. Value of the G suit in patients with severe pelvic fracture. Arch Surg 1974; 109:326–328.
34. Flint Lm, Brown A, Richardson JD. Definitive control of bleeding from severe pelvic fractures. Ann Surg 1979; 189:709–716.
35. Ganz R, Kroshell RJ, Jakob RP, Kuffer J. The anti-shock pelvic clamp. Clin Ortho 1991; 126:71–78.
36. Gylling SF, Ward RE, Holcroft JW. Immediate external fixation of unstable pelvic fractures. Am J Surg 1985; 150:721–724.
37. Mears DC, Fu FH. Modern concept of external fixation of the pelvis. Clin Orthop 1980; 151:65–72.
38. Peltier LF. Complications associated with fractures of the pelvis. J Bone Joint Surg 1965; 47-A:1060–1069.
39. Gilliland MG, Ward RE, Flynn TC. Peritoneal lavage and angiography in the management of patients with pelvic fractures. Am J Surg 1985; 144:744–747.
40. Moreno C, Moore EE, Rosenberg A, Cleveland HC. Hemorrhage with major pelvic fracture: a multispecialty challenge. J Trauma 1986; 26:987–994.
41. Agolini SF, Kamalesh S, Jaffe J, Newcomb J, Rhodes M, Reed JF III. Arterial embolization is a rapid and effective technique for controlling pelvic fracture hemorrhage. J Trauma 1997; 43:395–399.
42. Wong YC, Wang LJ, NG CJ, Tseng IC, See LC. Mortality after successful transcatheter embolization in patients with unstable pelvic fractures: rate of blood transfusion as a predictive factor. J Trauma 2000; 49:71–75.
43. Velmahos GC, Toutousas KG, Vasiliu P, Sarkisyan G, Chan LS, Hanks SH, Berne TV, Demetriadeset D. A prospective study on the safety and efficacy of angiographic embolization for pelvic and visceral injuries. J Trauma 2002; 53:303–308.

6
Fractures in Blunt Multiple Trauma

William J. Flynn, Jr. and Larry Bone
Erie County Medical Center, Buffalo, New York, USA

Management of fractures in patients with multiple traumatic injuries occurs within the context of the American College of Surgeon's Advanced Trauma Life Support (ATLS) algorithm (1). The physician who initially evaluates the patient seeks to identify life-threatening conditions and begins prompt resuscitation. Research has demonstrated a hierarchy of potentially lethal conditions beginning with airway problems and extending to life-threatening thoracic conditions, hypovolemia, and intracranial injuries. Definitive fracture management is considered after addressing these life-threatening conditions.

Cerebral anoxia may be fatal within 3–5 min (2). Establishing a secure airway is the first priority in resuscitation. Oral intubation with stabilization of the cervical spine is performed as indicated by mental status and evidence of airway obstruction. Emergent cricothyroidotomy may be necessary if intubation is not successful or possible. Persistent hypotension, distended neck veins, and unilateral absence of breath sounds suggest tension pneumothorax. Decompression via needle thoracentesis is followed by tube thoracostomy. Pericardial tamponade, although rare in blunt trauma patients, should be considered in a patient with persistent hypotension, distended neck veins, equal breath sounds, and distant heart sounds. Subxyphoid or transthoracic ultrasound is helpful in establishing the diagnosis (3). Percutaneous subxyphoid needle decompression may be life saving prior to open decompression and definitive management in the operating room. Hemorrhage control and restoration of intravascular volume is addressed next. Chest X-ray, abdominal ultrasound, or CT scan directs intervention as indicated. The orthopedic surgeon becomes involved in resuscitation if hemodynamic instability is attributed to pelvic or femur fracture. External stabilization, traction, or arteriographic embolization is employed to control bleeding (4,5). After hemostasis and restoration of intravascular volume, life-threatening intracranial lesions are addressed. Craniotomy, evacuation of hematomas, and ventriculostomy for monitoring trends in intracranial pressure are performed.

After the initial survey and resuscitation, diagnostic tests, directed by the physical examination and the mechanism of injury, are performed. After the patient has been resuscitated and associated injuries identified, fracture management is addressed. Management of fractures in the multiply injured patient has evolved over the past two decades. Fractures have a significant effect on the metabolic and physiologic outcome of the multiply injured patient. As early as the late 1970s, reports indicated that patients with long bone fractures, especially femur fractures, who had early fracture stabilization had a significant reduction in fat emboli syndrome (6–8). These retrospective studies were important, but a prospective randomized study by Bone et al. (9) clearly showed a significant advantage to fracture stabilization within 24 h. The patients with early fracture fixation, generally an intramedullary (IM) rod, had a significant reduction in ventilator days, length of ICU stay, and hospital stay. More significant was the reduction in the rate of adult respiratory distress syndrome, pulmonary dysfunction, pneumonia, and fat emboli syndrome (Table 1). Numerous subsequent studies have agreed with this study (10–12).

Early fracture stabilization, especially with reamed IM nailing, in the multiply injured patient with severe chest or head injury raises an important concern. In the chest-injured patient, clinicians speculated that the reaming of the femoral canal and the fat embolization that occurs during this procedure would worsen the chest condition (13,14). Studies demonstrated that the incidence of adult respiratory distress syndrome is no greater in these patients who have the fracture nailed when compared to those in whom it is plated. Bosse et al. (15) have shown an incidence of ARDS of 2.6% in 235 femur fractures associated with chest injuries treated with IM nailing. This rate is comparable to an ARDS rate of 2% in 219 patients with femur fractures associated with chest injuries that were treated with plating. Additional studies have confirmed a comparable ARDS rate in patients treated with IM nailing when compared with plating (Table 2). These findings suggest that the chest injury is the etiology of the ARDS. Incidence of ARDS is independent of the femur fracture treatment, as long as the femur fracture is stabilized early (16–20).

Early fracture fixation allows the patient to be mobilized out of bed and helps prevent pulmonary complications of lying supine for prolonged periods. Early mobilization is especially relevant in patients who have an associated blunt thoracic injury and pulmonary contusion. Pulmonary contusion is frequently complicated by hypoxia as a result of ventilation/perfusion (V/Q) mismatching. V/Q mismatching is exacerbated by prolonged periods of supine positioning that result from decisions to delay fracture fixation.

Treatment of pulmonary contusion is initially directed at increasing the concentration of oxygen in ventilated alveolar units and re-expanding alveoli that have become atelectatic as a result of bleeding and mucus plugging. Associated rib fractures produce pain on inspiration, splinting, poor cough, retained secretions, absorptive atelectasis, and possibly pneumonia. Treatment is directed at pain control through a combination of

Table 1 Comparison of Early and Late Fracture Fixation

	Early ISS (>18)	Late ISS (>18)
Number	45	37
Age	27.9	29.4
ISS	31.0	31.3
Ventilatory days	2.4	6.9
ICU days	2.7	7.6
Hospital days	17.5	26.6
Pulmonary complications	1/45 (2.2%)	14/37 (37.8%)
ARDS, pulmonary dysfunction	1/45	8/37

Table 2 Comparison of ARDS in Patients with Femur Fractures and Chest Injuries Treated with IM Nails or Plates (15)

	Number	ARDS (%)
Nails	235	2.6
Plates	219	2.0

Source: From Ref. (15).

oral and IV narcotics, nonsteroidal anti-inflammatory agents, and intercostal and thoracic epidural blockade (21).

Hemothorax is treated initially by tube thoracostomy to evacuate blood and expand the compressed lung. Pulmonary parencyhmal bleeding from low-pressure vessels usually stops with re-expansion of the lung following chest tube placement. Bleeding from lacerated intercostal arteries, perfused with systemic arterial pressure, may require thoracotomy for control. Evacuation of blood from the thorax before it clots not only re-expands the lung and improves oxygenation, but also removes a potential source of infection. Mechanical ventilation with positive end expiratory pressure (PEEP), postural drainage, and bronchoscopy is used to improve oxygenation. Recent advances in ventilator management, including permissive hypercapnea, tracheal oxygen insufflation, and the open lung technique (22,23), have been used to treat ARDS in these severely injured patients.

For patients with femur fractures and head injuries, studies indicate a trend toward a better outcome of the head injury when femur fractures are fixed early (24–26). Fracture management in patients with traumatic brain injury is complicated by the potential effect of surgery on intracranial pressure (ICP) and potential changes in cerebral perfusion pressure (CPP). The injured brain swells, and subsequent brain injury is related to the effects of edema that produce cerebral ischemia. Intraoperative hypotension may worsen cerebral ischemia and exacerbate cerebral edema. The relationship between mean arterial pressure (MAP) and ICP pressure is expressed as CPP, defined as the difference between MAP and ICP (27).

$$CPP = MAP - ICP$$

Increased CPP is achieved by maintaining MAP and minimizing ICP. Adequate intravascular volume is necessary to maintain MAP. Draining CSF through the ventriculostomy can decrease ICP. Refractory elevations in ICP require mannitol to induce an osmotic diuresis to decrease cerebral edema. Chapter 17 describes management details in head-injured patients. Decisions regarding fixation of fractures in head-injured patients are predicated on the ability to control ICP and maintain CPP. These patients with significant head injury should have ICP monitored, with careful control of ventilation and meticulous fluid balance. Surgery should be performed with the least amount of blood loss to avoid increasing the possibility of cerebral anoxia with hypotension. The presence of traumatic coma is not a contraindication to fracture fixation, if CPP can be maintained.

A successful outcome in these critically ill patients depends on restoring hemodynamic stability and adequate oxygen delivery preoperatively. These goals can be achieved by admission to the surgical ICU preoperatively for resuscitation prior to fracture fixation. Resuscitation consists of restoring circulating blood volume, rewarming, and administering packed red blood cells (PRBCs) as needed to increase the oxygen content of blood.

Fresh frozen plasma (FFP) and platelet concentrates are given to correct coagulopathy and ensure adequate hemostasis. Patients who are under-resuscitated need to be properly resuscitated prior to their fracture fixation. Hypothermia or coagulopathy require correction prior to fracture stabilization. Both hypothermia and coagulopathy are not uncommon in the blunt, multiply injured patient who requires thoracic or abdominal cavity surgery for life-threatening injuries prior to fracture management. Open coelomic cavities and blood loss cause these patients to be cold and coagulopathic. Core temperature should be restored and coagulopathy should be corrected. These patients then should have their fractures stabilized within 48 h. Studies (28) have shown that secondary surgery after 72 h from the time of injury can cause a significant increase in pulmonary, hepatic, and renal failure in these patients. Patients with decreased platelets (<180,000), neutrophil elastase >85 ng/dL, and C reactive proteins >11 ng/dL are at risk for secondary organ failure.

TREATMENT

Fracture Management

The management of fractures in the blunt trauma patient needs to be coordinated with the services of neurosurgeons, thoracic surgeons, general surgeons, and anesthesiologists. Life-threatening injuries are addressed first. Multiple teams performing simultaneous surgery may be necessary and feasible in special circumstances. An open tibia fracture that requires urgent debridement can be treated at the same time neurosurgeons are performing craniotomies. Below the knee orthopedic procedures can often be performed at the same time as abdominal surgery. Generally, most fractures are treated after procedures in coelomic cavities are finished. Again, adequate oxygenation, adequate resuscitation, and correction of coagulopathy and hypothermia are necessary to increase the probability of a successful outcome.

The only emergency orthopedic procedure (28) is the stabilization of pelvic injuries, fractures, and/or dislocations that are complicated by significant hemorrhage into the pelvic cavity. The placement of a pelvic external fixator to close the open book pelvis, to reduce the volume of the pelvic cavity, and to stabilize the pelvic ring can be life saving. In the patient with severe pelvic injury, the fixator should be placed prior to exploration of the abdominal cavity. Although preferably done in the operating room, the fixator can be placed in the emergency department.

After pelvic injuries, urgent orthopedic injuries with high priority are open fracture debridement and stabilization; reduction of joint dislocations, especially dislocated hips and knees; stabilization of long bone fractures, especially those of the femur and tibia; and decompression and stabilization of spine fracture dislocations when an increased neurologic deficit is present. When possible, two orthopedic teams can stabilize upper and lower extremity injuries simultaneously.

Stable pelvic, acetabulum, and spine fractures are generally treated between 24 and 48 h after injuries. This interval allows time for specialized studies such as CT scans and for soft tissue injury and bleeding to stabilize prior to orthopedic surgery. The complexities of these bone injuries are usually best managed when the operating team is rested and hospital resources are most available.

Fractures in the multiply injured patient must be managed in a coordinated, systematic fashion. With stabilization of the skeleton, the patient may sit up in bed or, with appropriate support, be moved out of bed, even while the patient requires a ventilator.

Fracture stabilization reduces pain, continued soft tissue trauma at the fracture site, and the metabolic and physiologic consequences of these injuries.

SUMMARY

- Fracture management is addressed after resuscitation, identification of associated injuries, and treatment of life-threatening injuries.
- Fractures affect the metabolism and physiology of the multiply injured patient. Early fracture stabilization reduces the rate of pulmonary complications, fat emboli syndrome, ventilator days, and ICU length of stay.
- Early fracture fixation allows early mobilization of the patient and avoids the complications of the supine position.
- For rib fractures, pain control with oral and IV narcotics, NSAIDS, intercostal blocks, and thoracic epidural blockade is the main treatment goal. Inadequate pain control leads to pain on inspiration, splinting, poor cough, retained secretions, and atelectasis.
- Patients with head injuries have a better outcome with early fixation of femur fractures.
- Successful outcomes in multiply injured patients with fractures require adequate resuscitation. Prior to fixation of fractures, resuscitation should be accomplished, core temperature restored, and coagulopathy corrected. Fracture fixation within 48 h of injury produces optimal outcomes.
- Pelvic injuries complicated by hemorrhage are emergencies. Placement of an external fixator can be life saving.
- Other high priority orthopedic treatments are open fracture debridement and stabilization, reduction of joint dislocations, stabilization of long bone fractures, and decompression and stabilization of spine fracture dislocations.
- Fracture stabilization reduces pain, continued soft tissue trauma from the fracture site, and metabolic and physiologic stress.

REFERENCES

1. American College of Surgeons. Advanced Trauma Life Support. American College of Surgeons, 6th ed. 1997:21–46.
2. Chen R, Bolton CF, Young B. Prediction of outcome in patients with anoxia coma: a clinical and electrophysiologic study. Crit Care Med 1996; 24(4):672–678.
3. Carrillo EH, Guinn BJ, Ali AT, Boaz PW. Transthoracic ultrasound as an alternative to subxyphoid ultrasound for the diagnosis of hemopericardium in penetrating precordial trauma. Am J Surg 2000; 179(1):34–36.
4. Starr AJ. Use of C-clamps and pelvic packing to control hemorrhage after pelvic fracture. J Orthop Trauma 2002; 16(5):362–363.
5. Nicholson BL, Borsa J. Successful resuscitation with sacral embolization after traumatic unstable pelvic fracture. Am J Roentgenol 2001; 176(3):796.
6. Riska E, Bonsdorff H, Hakkinen S. Primary operative fixation of long bone fractures in patients with multiple injuries. Injury 1976; 6:110–116.

7. Risk E, Myllynen P. Fat embolism in patients with multiple injuries. J Trauma 1982; 22:894–895.
8. Grois R, Gimbrere J, Van Niekerk J. Early osteosynthesis and prophylactic mechanical ventilation in the multiple trauma patient. J Trauma 1982; 22:895–903.
9. Bone L, Johnson K, Weigelt J, Scheinberg R. Early versus delayed stabilization of femoral fractures. J Bone Joint Surg 1989; 71A:336–340.
10. Johnson K, Cadambi A, Seibert G. Incidence of adult respiratory distress syndrome in patients with multiple musculoskeletal injuries: effect of early operative stabilization of fractures. J Trauma 1985; 25:375–384f.
11. Seibel R, LaDuca J, Hassett J, Babikian G, Mills B, Border J. Blunt multiply Trauma (ISS-36), femur traction, and the pulmonary failure septic state. Ann Surg 1985; 202:283–295.
12. Behrman S, Fabian T, Kulsk K, Taylor J. Improved outcome with femur fractures: early vs. delayed fixation. J Trauma 1990; 30:792–798.
13. Pape HC, Auf'm'Kolk M, Paffrath T, et al. Primary intramedullary femur fixation in multiple trauma patients with associated lung contusion: a cause of post-traumatic ARDS? J Trauma 1993; 34:540–548.
14. Pape HC, Regel G, Strum JA, Tscheim H. Influence of thoracic trauma and primary femoral intramedullary nailing on the incidence of ARDS in multiple trauma patients. Injury 1993; 24(suppl 3):S82–S103.
15. Bosse MJ, MacKenzie EJ, Riemer BL, et al. Adult respiratory distress syndrome, pneumonia and mortality following thoracic injury and a femoral fracture treated either with intramedullary nailing with reaming or with a plate. J Bone Joint Surg 1997; 79-A:799.
16. Charash WE, Fabian TC, Croce MA. Delayed surgical fixation of femur fractures in a risk factor for pulmonary failure independent of thoracic trauma. J Trauma 1994; 37:667–672.
17. Bone LB, Babikian G, Stegemann PM. Femoral canal reaming in the polytrauma patient with chest injury: A clinical prospective. Clin Orthop 1995; 318:91–94.
18. Bone LB, Anders MJ, Rohrbacher BJ. Treatment of femoral fractures in multiple injured patients with thoracic injury. Clin Orthop 1998; 347:57.
19. Van Os J, Roumea R, Schott F, Heystraten F, Goris R. Is early osteosynthesis safe in multiple trauma patients with severe thoracic trauma and pulmonary contusion? J Trauma 1994; 36:495–497.
20. Brundage S, McGhan R, Jurkovich G, Mach C, Maier R. Timing of femur fracture fixation: effect on outcome in patients with thoracic and head injuries. J Trauma 2002; 52:200–307.
21. Ullman DA, Fortune JB, et al. Treatment of patients with multiple rib fractures using continuous thoracic epidural narcotic infusion. Regional Anesthesia 1989; 14(1):43–47.
22. Hirvela ER. Advances in the management of acute respiratory distress syndrome: protective ventilation. Arch Surg 2000; 135(2):126–135.
23. Shapiro MB, Anderson HL 3rd, Bartlett RH. Respiratory failure: conventional and high-tech support. Surg Clin N Am 2000; 80(3):571–583.
24. Giannoudic P, Veysi V, Pape HC, Krittek and Smith M. When should we operate on major fractures in patients with severe head injuries? Am J Surg 2002; 183:261–267.
25. McKee MD, Schemitsch EH, Vincent LO, et al. The effect of a femoral fracture on concomitant closed head injury in patients with multiple injuries. J Trauma 1997; 42:1041–1045.
26. Wozasek GE, Simon P, Redl H, et al. Intramedullary pressure changes and fat extravization during intramedullary nailing: an experimental study in sheep. J Trauma 1994; 36:202.
27. Guidelines for the Management of Severe Head Injury, Brain Trauma Foundation, 1995.
28. Bone L. Management of polytrauma trauma. In: Chapman M. ed. Operative Orthopaedics. Philadelphia: Lippincott, 2002:417–430.

7
Burns, Electrical Injury, and Hypothermia and Frostbite

David H. Ahrenholz and William Mohr
The Burn Center Regions Medical Center, St. Paul, Minnesota, USA

BURNS

Burns are a major cause of morbidity and mortality in the USA. In 2001 fires caused injuries to 1 million persons; more than 21,000 patients required hospitalization for treatment of burns, and 6200 burn-related deaths occurred (1). Among burn patients, death is most commonly caused by carbon monoxide poisoning during a house fire.

Four types of energy cause burn wounds: thermal, electrical, chemical, and radiation. Thermal injury accounts for 85–90% of burns in the USA. Chemical and electrical injuries comprise the vast majority of the remainder.

The severity of any burn is determined by the age of the patient, the depth of the burn, and the size of the wound measured as a percentage of total body surface area (TBSA). Burns are described as first-, second-, or third-degree (Fig. 1). A first-degree burn involves only the epidermis. This type of burn is erythematous but does not blister, and it heals in 3–6 days without sequelae. Sunburn is a typical first-degree burn. A superficial second-degree burn involves the entire epidermis and superficial portions of the dermis. The skin is blistered with a moist and weeping base. In children under 10 years, a superficial second-degree burn will heal in <2 weeks; in adults, healing takes <3 weeks. Superficial second-degree burns produce minor color changes but not hypertrophic scarring. Patients with first-degree and superficial second-degree burns <10% TBSA are usually treated as outpatients.

A deep second-degree burn extends through the epidermis and into deeper dermis. After blister removal, it is usually dry and demonstrates an ivory or mottled red base. This type of burn requires >3 weeks to heal spontaneously and results in very significant scar formation. A third-degree burn destroys the entire thickness of the epidermis and dermis. A third-degree burn >3 cm in diameter will not heal spontaneously over its entire surface. Because both deep second-degree and third-degree burns produce marked scars, early excision and grafting is indicated after initial fluid resuscitation (2). Burns <10% TBSA may not require formal fluid resuscitation.

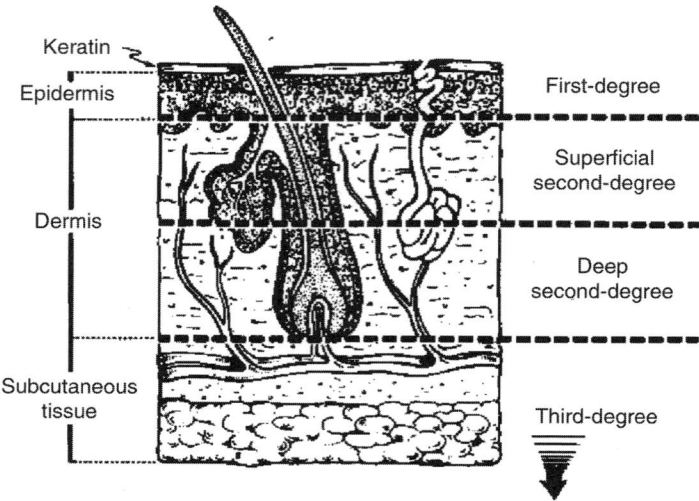

Figure 1 Simplified diagram of skin burn depth.

Initially, the burn patient's ABCs (airway, breathing, and circulation) are evaluated in the same manner as any trauma patient (4). After the evaluation of ABCs and the primary survey, a history is obtained. The medical history should include current medications, allergies, past and present medical illnesses, smoking history, use of drugs and/or alcohol, and the status of tetanus prophylaxis.

Next, a secondary head-to-toe examination is performed. Accidents can produce associated injuries that range from minor abrasions and lacerations, tympanic membrane rupture, or corneal abrasions to severe intra-abdominal, thoracic, and skeletal injuries. A burn injury alone does not acutely alter the patient's level of consciousness. Patients in a state of confusion or coma immediately after injury must be evaluated for significant smoke inhalation, closed head injury, or intoxication with alcohol or other drugs.

The initial description of the burn includes an estimation of the percent of TBSA for second- and third-degree burns (first-degree burns are always excluded). Three methods can be used to calculate burn size: the "rule of the palm," the "rule of nines," and the Lund and Browder chart. For evaluation of small or scattered burns, the rule of the palm states that the patient's palm, including the fingers and the thumb, equals ~1% of the patient's TBSA. According to the rule of nines, the major body surfaces can be expressed as multiples of 9% of TBSA in adults (Fig. 2). The head and the neck comprise ~9%, each arm and hand together represent 9%, the anterior and the posterior trunk are 18% each (two nines), each leg is 18% (two nines), and the perineum comprises 1%. Since the rule of nines is very inaccurate for children under the age of 10, the Lund and Browder chart is a better tool for estimating burn size in that age group (Fig. 3) (3).

Initial laboratory evaluation for a major burn includes complete blood count (with platelet count), electrolytes, BUN, creatinine, liver function tests, and urinalysis. Measurements of arterial blood gases (ABGs) and carbon monoxide concentration are obtained for patients with suspected inhalation injury or a history of pulmonary dysfunction. Patients with a major burn injury (>40% TBSA in patients <60 years old and all patients >60 years old) require continuous cardiac monitoring.

Burns, Electrical Injury, Hypothermia, Frostbite

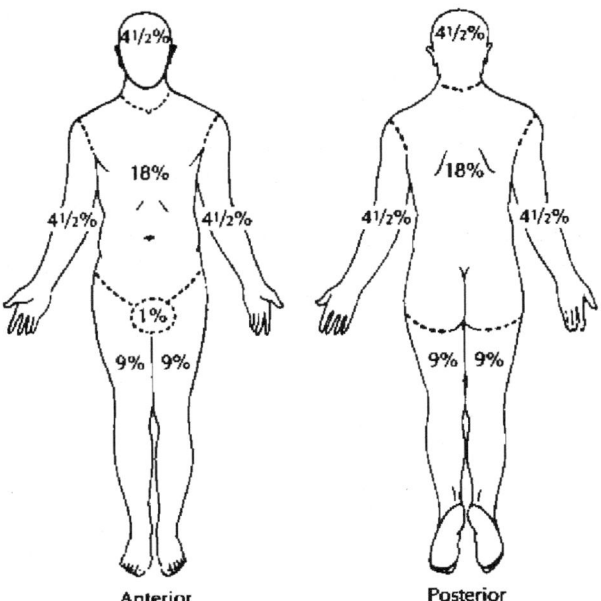

Figure 2 The "rule of nines" is easy to remember but inaccurate for use in children.

Fluid Resuscitation

During the initial assessment of the patient, two large-bore intravenous catheters are inserted, preferably in an unburned upper extremity (Fig. 4). Lower extremity intravenous catheters or cutdowns should be avoided, because they are associated with a high incidence of septic phlebitis (5). We prefer that central venous catheter sites be reserved for later use.

Patients with a significant burn (>20% TBSA) require placement of a Foley catheter for monitoring of fluid resuscitation and urinary output. A nasogastric tube should be

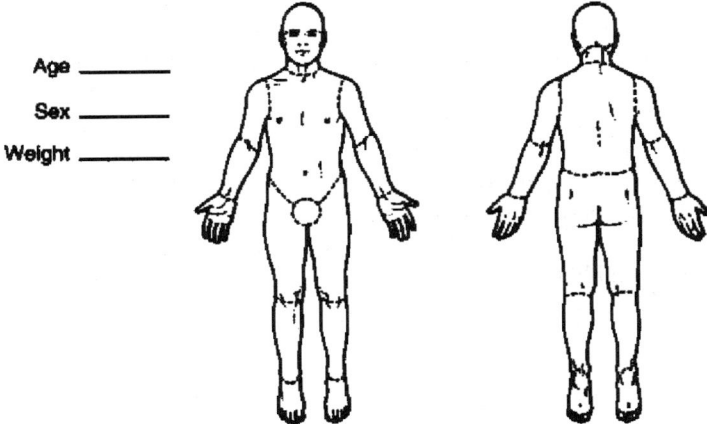

Figure 3 The Lund and Browder diagram estimates burn size, especially in children <10 years old. [From Ref. (3).]

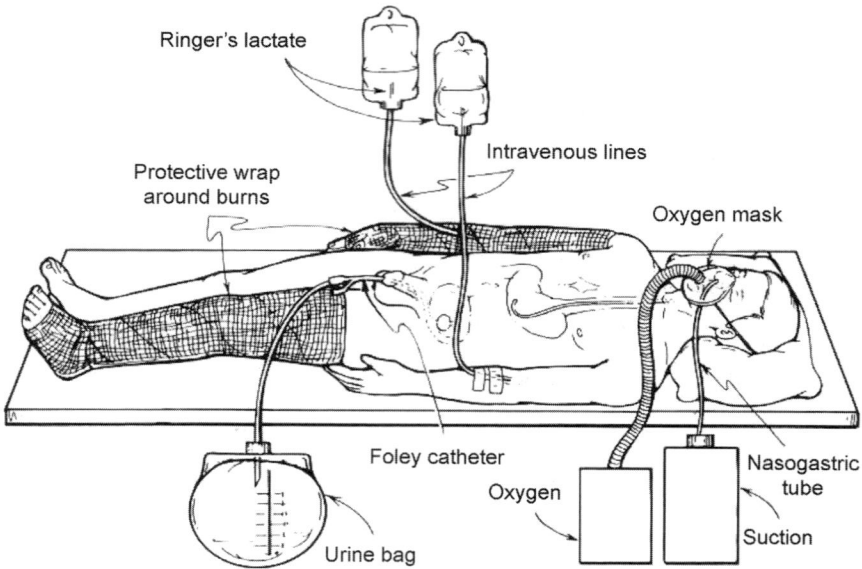

Figure 4 Patient prepared for burn treatment and/or transfer.

placed in patients with burns >25–30% of TBSA, because such patients frequently develop an ileus and are at risk for vomiting and aspiration.

Patients with second- and third-degree burns that are >10% of TBSA usually require fluid resuscitation. The Parkland formula is the most widely used, although several others are also very satisfactory. With the Parkland formula, 2–4 mL Ringer's lactate/kg/% TBSA burn is infused during the first 24 h, with half given in the first 8 h. The fluid infusion is titrated to maintain a urine flow of 0.5–1 mL/kg/h.

Patients with >40% TBSA burns, significant inhalation injury (carboxyhemoglobin >10%), facial burns, or circumferential neck burns are at risk for developing airway compromise. Early endotracheal intubation will protect the patient's airway and reduce the risk of sudden airway occlusion by edema (Fig. 5).

The initial fluid resuscitation with Ringer's lactate solution is complete at 24 h. The IV fluids are then changed to D_5W at a maintenance rate. Plasma replacement has been advocated in the first 8 h of the second 24-h period, with 0.3–0.5 mL colloid/kg/% burn to replace the plasma losses of the first 24 h. Because of the costs and the risk of infection associated with blood products, colloid replacement is not widely used.

Urine output, blood pressure, and pulse are monitored hourly during fluid resuscitation. Because all invasive monitoring is associated with infectious complications, it should be used sparingly (6). During the first 2 days of therapy, the white blood cell count should be repeated every 6 h, as leukopenia often occurs in the first 48 h in patients treated with topical silver sulfadiazene (7).

Treatment

The wound should be washed gently, and all blisters should be debrided. Silver sulfadiazine is the most commonly used topical antibiotic. However, for burns of the face and

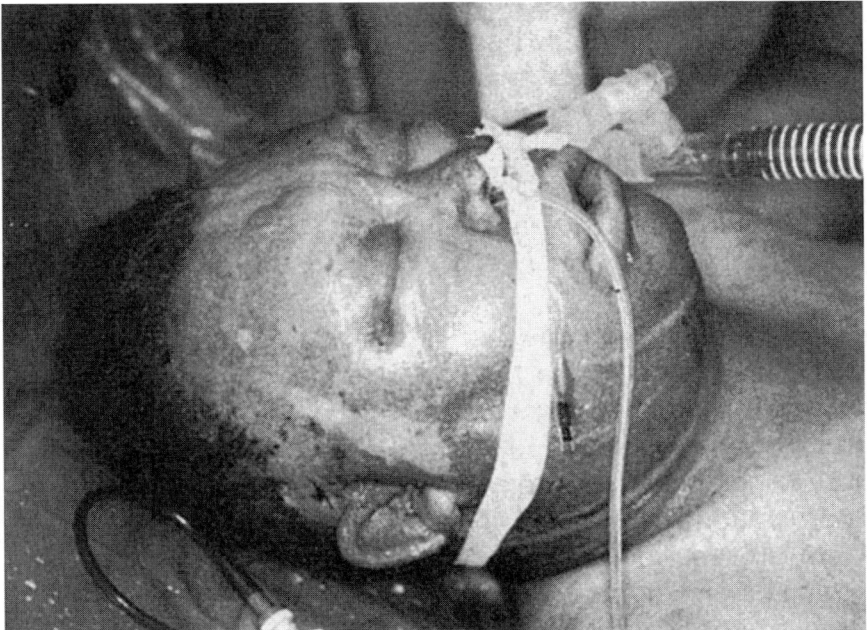

Figure 5 Facial edema 24 h after burn injury.

neck, or for small burns elsewhere, bacitracin is equally effective and less expensive. Selected superficial burns may be treated with pigskin or synthetic product (Biobrane®).

In patients with large burns, silver sulfadiazine may induce transient neutropenia. Mafenide (Sulfamylon®) is an excellent agent, but it causes metabolic acidosis and severe wound pain. Therefore, Sulfamylon is used less commonly than silver sulfadiazine. Silver impregnated fabric dressings (Acticoat®, Silverlon®) are becoming more popular as well.

Debridement and dressing of the burn wound cause severe pain, especially if the burn injury is superficial. Intravenous narcotics are used initially, because absorption of subcutaneous and intramuscular injections is unpredictable. In selected patients, oral narcotics and anxiolytic agents can be used later. Nonnarcotic analgesics are ineffective when used alone in the treatment of burn pain.

Deeply burned skin is inelastic and does not accommodate the swelling from edema fluid during resuscitation. Circumferential burns of the extremities, trunk, or neck require early escharotomy with a scalpel or electrocautery to prevent impaired ventilation or blood flow. The patient is placed in the anatomic position (palms forward). When a medial or lateral escharotomy is performed on the extremities, the escharotomy must not cross the flexor or extensor surface of the joints (Fig. 6). On the dorsum of the hand, an escharotomy paralleling the extensor tendons should overlap a forearm escharotomy at the wrist to avoid constriction. Escharotomies of the index, long, and ring fingers are placed on the ulnar side of the fingers and the radial side of the small finger. An escharotomy on the thumb may be placed on either the radial or the ulnar side. Incisions must divide all deep dermal bands to allow the involved part to swell freely.

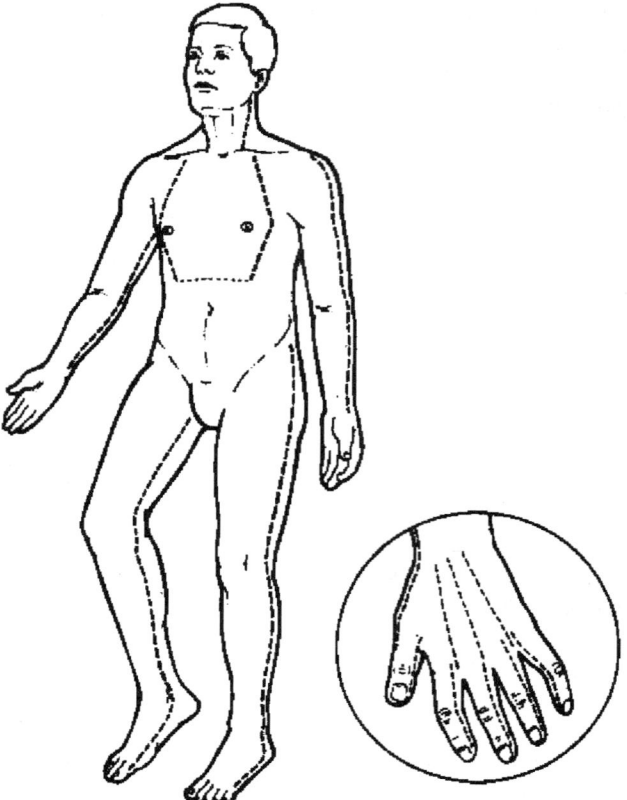

Figure 6 Recommended placement of escharotomies.

Metabolic Support

Nutritional support is critical to the survival of the patient with major burns (8). Radiographic placement of a nasojejunal tube allows early enteral feeding without the complications of parenteral alimentation. Aggressive nutritional support improves survival, reduces infection, and prevents Curling's ulcer (9). We estimate energy needs with the Harris–Benedict and Curreri formulas, measure serum albumin and prealbumin concentrations, measure nitrogen losses, add estimated wound losses, administer a calorie/nitrogen ratio feeding of 120 to 150:1, and chart nitrogen balance and body weight (10,11). Enteral feedings are preferred, but parenteral supplementation is used for patients with marked ileus or diarrhea.

Early Excision and Grafting

Wounds that are so deep that they will not heal within 3 weeks in the adult or 2 weeks in the child are best treated by early excision and grafting (2). Excision (with a tourniquet placed) and immediate autografting or homografting have significantly reduced blood losses in grafting burns of the extremities. The deepest burns require excision to fascia, but the cosmetic results are poor.

The largest burns are treated with a dermal regeneration template (Integra®, often called "artificial skin") (12). This material permits regeneration of a dermis substitute before autografting with widely meshed thin skin grafts. Cultured epidermal autografts have been used, but are extremely costly and lack long-term durability.

Late Management

Once the wound has fully epithelialized, lengthy follow-up by the burn team is required to control hypertrophic burn scars. The use of continuous pressure garments and orthoses combined with an aggressive therapy program provide optimal functional and cosmetic outcome (12). Grafting should not be performed by a team unable to provide such long-term care.

Itching and skin dryness are major problems associated with burns, since burned skin or donor sites do not produce adequate natural oils and moisturizers. Commercially available lotions significantly reduce pruritus. Antihistamines (e.g., diphenhydramine hydrochloride) also reduce itching. Low-dose doxepin hydrochloride also can be helpful. More severe itching may respond to the use of a mechanical vibrator.

Skin hyperpigmentation is commonly associated with repeated injury (sunburn, windburn, or frostbite) in the first year after burn injury. Patients are advised to avoid any sun exposure while the burn areas remain erythematous, as sunscreen agents do not completely prevent skin hyperpigmentation.

Burns often cause severe psychologic effects, and early intervention is always indicated. Prompt return of the patient to their normal activities, including self-care, school, vocational activities, and avocational interests, is crucial.

Aggressive treatment of hypertrophic burn scars minimizes the need for further surgical treatment. Reconstruction of the burn, when indicated, is best undertaken after the hypertrophic scar has matured, usually at 18–24 months after healing. If of an appropriate age, the patient should direct the timing and scope of these interventions (13).

ELECTRICAL INJURY

Electrical burns can result from conduction of electrical energy through tissue or from heat released as the current arcs through the air. Current arcs generate temperatures as high as 3000°C, secondarily ignite clothing, and add surface thermal injury to the conduction injury.

Low-voltage current can cause fatal cardiac dysrhythmias. Characteristically, survivors of injury caused by low-voltage current have minimal internal injuries. The current is concentrated at the entrance and exit sites; at these points, tissue may be charred. High-voltage current may damage tissue anywhere along its route, but the most severe damage typically occurs in the digits and distal extremities.

Serum creatinine kinase (CK) is a sensitive indicator of total muscle damage after electrical burns (14). In our series of 116 patients, patients with a total CK >2500 IU were at risk for major amputation. The intermediate risk group of 400–2500 IU of CK had a less predictable course. Of the 32 patients with a total CK >10,000 IU, 84% suffered major amputation or permanent neurologic deficits. Myocardial injury is uncommon and must be diagnosed with serum troponin levels, ECG, and clinical criteria (15).

The patient with an electrical injury requires the usual evaluation of ABCs (3), insertion of large-bore intravenous lines, and placement of a Foley catheter. Adequate fluid resuscitation is begun immediately to maintain urine output at 75–100 cc/h. Myoglobinuria, detectable as brown or blackish urine, is treated with adequate fluid resuscitation, alkalinization of the urine, and, if necessary, intravenous administration of mannitol. Fasciotomy and operative wound debridement are performed immediately, and devitalized muscle is operatively debrided. Carpal tunnel releases are performed on involved forearms. Early guillotine amputation, with care taken to salvage as much skin and subcutaneous tissue as possible, is required for extremities that remain nonperfused after fasciotomy. Wounds are packed open and debrided every 48–72 h until only viable tissue remains. Skin grafts can be used to achieve closure of most wounds, but free tissue flaps may be necessary to cover exposed bone, tendons, joints, or neurovascular structures. This protocol minimizes tissue loss, avoids renal failure, results in early wound closure, and speeds rehabilitation. Despite these measures, many patients have prolonged psychologic and neurologic complications.

HYPOTHERMIA AND FROSTBITE

Hypothermia is a clinical condition in which body temperature falls below 95°F (35°C). Moderate (<90°F or 32°C) to severe hypothermia (<82°F or <28°C) causes severe physiologic changes, including depression of mental function, cold diuresis, decreased circulating blood volume, and increased blood viscosity. Hypothermia causes no long-term morbidity; whereas frostbite, in which tissue has been frozen, results in significant morbidity (15).

Treatment of hypothermia is outlined in Box 1. Mild hypothermia responds to external rewarming, but moderate and severe hypothermia respond best to immersion in a warm whirlpool or to internal warming measures, including peritoneal or thoracic lavage. Unstable patients have been salvaged with cardiopulmonary bypass rewarming. Electrolytes, glucose, and blood gases (corrected for temperature) should be monitored during rewarming.

Frostbite occurs commonly in winter months, especially among homeless persons. The risk is increased with substance abuse or psychiatric illness. Acute frostbite injuries are treated with rapid local rewarming after correction of systemic hypothermia. Gentle local wound care and the use of antiprostaglandin agents (e.g., oral ibuprofen) are indicated (Box 2). Bone scans will aid in identification of poorly perfused digits at

Box 1 Emergency Treatment of Hypothermia

Mild hypothermia: >90°F (32°C)
   Remove wet clothing
   Cover trunk with warm blankets
   Administer warm liquids by mouth
Moderate or severe hypothermia: ≤90°F (32°C)
   Infuse warmed IV fluids
   Begin peritoneal lavage with warm fluid (104–108°F) (40–42°C)
   Consider extracorporeal bypass warming

Source: Modified from Ahrenholz DH. Frostbite. In: Copeland EM III, Howard RJ, Warshaw AL, Levine BS, Sugarman H, eds. Current Practice of Surgery. New York: Churchill Livingstone, Vol II (15); 1993: 1–11.

Box 2 Frostbite Treatment Protocol

1. Admit to hospital
2. Rewarm affected areas by immersing in 104–108°F water (40–42°C)
3. Deflate ruptured blisters. For exposed dermis, apply aloe vera q6h. (Many physicians substitute daily bacitracin or silver sulfadiazine dressing changes.)
4. Elevate and splint affected parts; place lamb's wool between digits
5. Tetanus prophylaxis
6. Narcotic analgesics
7. Ibuprofen 12 mg/kg PO every day for 1 week
8. Penicillin for evidence of infection
9. Daily wound cleansing
10. No smoking
11. Physical therapy once edema has resolved
12. Treatment of alcohol and drug addiction if present

Source: Modified from McCauley RL, Hing DN, Robson MC, et al. Frostbite injuries: a rational approach based on the pathophysiology. J Trauma 1983; 23:143.

risk for amputation, although tissue mummification usually takes several weeks (15). We have used an experimental protocol of catheter directed thrombolytic agents to restore blood flow in selected frostbite injuries (unpublished data). Amputation is always delayed until the tissue demarcates, unless infection supervenes. Following recovery, most patients have recurrent vasomotor symptoms in cold weather.

SUMMARY

- Four categories of energy cause burn injuries: thermal, electrical, chemical, and radiation.
- Burns are first-degree, superficial second-degree, deep second-degree, or third-degree (see Fig. 1).
- The rule of the palm, the rule of nines, or the Lund and Browder chart may be used to estimate the percent of total body surface area occupied by second- or third-degree burns.
- Patients with confusion or coma must be evaluated for significant smoke inhalation, closed head injury, intoxication, or poisoning.
- Patients with >10% TBSA burns require fluid resuscitation. A urinary bladder catheter should be placed in patients with >20% TBSA burn. A nasogastric tube should be used in patients with >25% TBSA burns.
- The Parkland formula provides adequate fluid replacement. Infuse 2–4 mL Ringer's lactate/kg/% TBSA burn during the first 24 h. Half of the estimated volume is infused in the first 8 h. Titrate fluid to maintain urine output of 0.5–1 mL/kg/h.
- Silver sulfadiazine is the most commonly used topical antibiotic for burns.
- Circumferential burns of the extremities, trunk, or neck require early escharotomy.

- Nutritional support is critical to patient survival, and enteral feedings are effective in providing such support.
- In electrical injuries, serum CK concentrations are sensitive indicators of total muscle damage.
- Hypothermia causes no long-term morbidity. Frostbite causes significant morbidity. Boxes 1 and 2 describe treatment of hypothermia and frostbite.

REFERENCES

1. Karter MJ. Fire Loss in the United States. National Fire Protection Association. Quincy: MA, September 2002.
2. Herndon D, Barrow R, Rutan R, et al. A comparison of conservative versus early excision. Ann Surg 1989; 209:547.
3. Lund CC, Browder NC. The estimation of areas of burns. Surg Gynecol Obstetr 1944; 79:352.
4. Advanced Burn Life Support Course. American Burn Association: Chicago, IL, 1999.
5. Pruitt BA, Stein JM, Foley FD, et al. Intravenous therapy in burn patients: Suppurative thrombophlebitis and other life-threatening complications. Arch Surg 1970; 100:399.
6. Ehrie M, Morgan A, Moore F, et al. Endocarditis with the indwelling balloon-tipped pulmonary artery catheter in burn patients. J Trauma 1978; 18:664.
7. Jarrett F, Ellerbe S, Demling RH. Acute leukopenia during topical burn therapy with silver sulfadiazine. Am J Surg 1978; 135:818.
8. Mochizuki H, Trocki O, Dominioni L, et al. Mechanism of prevention of postburn hypermetabolism and catabolism by early feeding. Ann Surg 1984; 200:297.
9. Watson L, Abston S. Prevention of upper gastrointestinal hemorrhage in burn patients. Burns 1987; 13:194.
10. Curreri PW. Assessing nutritional needs for the burned patient. J Trauma 1990; 30(suppl 12):S20.
11. Herndon DN (ed.). Total Burn Care, 2d ed., London: WB Saunders, 2002.
12. Heimbach D, Luterman A, Burke JF, et al. Artificial dermis for major burns: a multi-center randomized clinical trial. Ann Surg 1988; S208:313.
13. Rivers E, Fischer SV. Rehabilitation for burn patients. In: Kottke FJ, Lehmann JF, eds. Krusen's Hand Book of Physical Medicine and Rehabilitation. Philadelphia: WB Saunders, 1990: 1070.
14. Ahrenholz DH, Schubert W, Solem LD. Creatinine kinase as a prognostic indicator in electrical injury. Surgery 1988; 104:741.
15. Ahrenholz DH. Frostbite. Probl Gen Surg 2003; 20:129.

B. Preoperative, Intraoperative, and Postoperative Evaluation

8
Cardiovascular Risk: Assessment and Reduction

Jon F. Berlauk[*]

Jerome H. Abrams
VA Medical Center, Minneapolis, Minnesota, USA

Heart disease, especially coronary artery disease (CAD) is the primary health care problem in the USA. Nearly one out of every two deaths in this country can be attributed to cardiovascular disease. Therefore, it is not surprising that CAD is also the major cause of morbidity [myocardial infarction (MI), unstable angina, congestive heart failure (CHF), or serious dysrhythmia] and mortality after surgery. In 1988, noncardiac surgical procedures were performed in 25 million patients in all age groups. One million of these patients had diagnosed CAD, and another 2–3 million were estimated to be at risk for the disease. Many of these patients were elderly, who now constitute the fastest growing segment of our population. In 1988, 25 million (10%) were over 65 years old. The figure is projected to grow to 66 million by the year 2055. In 1988, elderly patients comprised 25% (6 million) of the noncardiac surgery group, and this figure is expected to grow to 35% (12 million) within 30 years (1). The implied magnitude of the problem of CAD is enormous. In the aging surgical population, how can the preoperative patient who is at high risk for perioperative cardiac morbidity (PCM) be identified? Can the patient's risk be reduced? For the past 35 years, clinical studies have focused primarily on the factors involved in cardiac risk assessment, but in recent years more emphasis has been devoted to risk reduction. This chapter provides a framework for assessing and reducing the risk of PCM in the surgical patient. It will emphasize that directed history and physical examination are vital for evaluating risk. As will be seen in the following discussion, the patient's functional capacity has the same weight in estimating risk as a history of MI.

RISK FACTORS

Over several decades, investigators have studied thousands of surgical patients in order to determine which preoperative risk factors can be used to predict perioperative morbidity and mortality (1). Several historical risk factors have been identified and are supported by

---
[*]Deceased. Dr. Berlauk's contribution to the first edition was updated by Dr. Abrams.

Box 1 Historical Predictors of Surgical Risk

> Age
> Recent MI (<6 months)
> Old MI (>6 months)
> Angina
> CHF
> Hypertension
> Diabetes mellitus
> Dysrhythmia
> Peripheral vascular disease
> Valvular heart disease
> Previous coronary artery bypass graft surgery

Source: From Ref. (1).

the majority of studies (Box 1). As might be expected, because of the number of studies involved, few of these risk factors are undisputed. Nevertheless, two factors consistently have been found to predict poor outcome following surgery: recent MI and current CHF.

In 1964, Topkins and Artusio (2) reported the first comprehensive, large-scale study describing the risk of previous MI in relation to subsequent noncardiac surgery. They found that the incidence of postoperative MI in patients without a previous MI was 0.66%, when compared with 6.5% in patients who had a known preoperative MI. The mortality rate following this postoperative MI was high (26.5%) in patients without a previous MI but was worse (72%) in patients who had a prior MI. In addition, these authors found that the rate of reinfarction was 54.5% in patients who had an MI <6 months before surgery, compared with only 4.5%, in patients in whom MI occurred >6 months before surgery (Table 1). This landmark study alerted physicians and surgeons that, depending on the timing, a prior MI placed a surgical patient at extraordinary risk for reinfarction and death. Such findings did not change appreciably over the next 20 years despite dramatic advances in surgery and anesthesia. Even today the reinfarction rate within the first 3 months of a prior MI is generally estimated to be 30%; between 3 and 6 months, it is ~15%; and after 6 months, it is about 5%. Overall risk of postoperative reinfarction is 6–8%, with associated mortality in several series exceeding 50% (Table 1).

In 1983, Rao et al. (12) confirmed these reinfarction rates in a retrospective study of 364 patients. Subsequently, in a second group of 733 prospectively studied patients, a significant decrease in reinfarction rate was demonstrated for each period of time following prior MI. This decrease was achieved by implementing invasive hemodynamic monitoring and by aggressively treating cardiovascular variables that deviated from normal. These authors found that reinfarction occurred in only 1.9% of all patients with a previous MI (Table 1) if two conditions were met: these patients had arterial and pulmonary artery (PA) catheters placed intraoperatively, and the postoperative period included extended postoperative SICU care. On the basis of these findings, some have inferred that preoperative optimization of the patient's status, aggressive monitoring and therapy, and an extended SICU stay may reduce the risk of reinfarction. However, further confirmation of the findings of Rao et al. (12) is necessary in order to substantiate the clinical and financial implications of this approach for all patients with a previous MI.

CHF is also a reliable predictor of perioperative risk. In 1988, 2.3 million people in the USA were found to have CHF. Its incidence doubles in each decade of life after 45 years of age, and CHF is now the leading diagnosis-related group in hospitalized patients older than

Table 1 Studies of Perioperative MI

	Year	No. of patients	Previous MI	Reinfarction (%) 0–3 months	Reinfarction (%) 3–6 months	Reinfarction (%) >6 months	Patients with reinfarction (%)	Reinfarction mortality (%)
Knopp et al. (3)	1962	8,984	427	100	100	4.5	6.1	58
Thompson et al. (4)	1962	*	192	*	*	*	5.7	63
Topkins and Artusio (2)	1964	12,712	658	54.5	54.5	4.5	6.5	72
Arkins et al. (5)	1964	1,005	267	11	7.5	7.5	7.9	81
Tarhan et al. (6)	1972	32,877	422	37	16	3	6.6	54
Steen et al. (7)	1978	73,321	587	27	11	5.4	6.1	69
Goldman et al. (8)	1978	1,001	101	4.5	4.5	2.5	3	33
Eerola et al. (9)	1980	2,063	89	*	*	*	6.7	50
von Knorring (10)	1981	12,654	157	25	25	12	15.9	28
Schoeppel et al. (11)	1983	981	53	0	0	4.5	3.8	50
Rao et al. (12) historical control group	1983	*	364	36	26	5	7.7	57
Rao et al. (12) prospective monitoring group	1983	*	733	5.8	2.3	0.8	1.9	36

Note: *Indicates data not provided.

65 years (1). After 40 years of clinical studies, only one study (13) has not found CHF to be a major risk factor for PCM. This discrepancy arises from efforts to objectively define CHF. Greater controversy exists about the predictive value of specific markers of heart failure than about the condition itself. As CHF is a constellation of clinical symptoms rather than a specific disease, such controversy is understandable. Goldman et al. (14) assigned an S_3 gallop or jugular venous distention the highest point weight in their cardiac risk index (CRI). Cardiomegaly was not a significant variable in their study, but Charlson et al. (15) disagree. Detsky et al. (16) used "alveolar pulmonary edema" in their modification of the CRI. Using multivariate analysis, Foster et al. (17) found that only dyspnea on exertion and left ventricular wall motion abnormality (during angiography) were predictors of PCM. Less qualitative measures of left ventricular performance have fared no better. In some studies, left ventricular ejection fraction (LVEF) by angiography has been shown to be the best prognostic indicator of survival in nonsurgical patients with CAD (18). Several studies have validated LVEF that is <50% of normal to be a predictor of poor outcome in patients undergoing noncardiac surgery (19,20); however, Kopecky et al. (21) and Franco et al. (22) have not confirmed the predictive value of resting or exercise LVEF. In summary, although controversy exists about how to best identify the condition, CHF is a reliable predictor of PCM.

Although MI and CHF are good predictors of PCM, they are by no means the only variables that determine outcome. In 1977, Goldman et al. (14) used multivariate analysis of 39 clinical variables in 1001 surgical patients to select nine variables that were predictors of PCM. A point score was given to each variable to reflect its statistical weight in the analysis, and the CRI was formulated (Table 2). Detsky et al. (16) later modified this index to include severe and unstable angina. More recently, Shah et al. (13) used stepwise logistic regression to analyze 24 preoperative variables in 688 patients with cardiac disease. They found that eight risk factors could be used to predict outcome. Only two of these factors, chronic stable angina and ischemia on ECG, do not have a counterpart in the CRI, a finding that underscores the validity of this index. Currently the CRI is the most widely used and best validated risk assessment index. It was derived from an unselected patient group undergoing noncardiac surgery. Therefore, if the CRI is not used to predict risk in a highly selected patient group with either unusual medical conditions or high baseline risk, it appears to be useful to stratify, if not accurately predict, risk (23).

GUIDELINES FOR ASSESSING AND MANAGING RISK

Clearly, surgical patients who have either clinically overt or occult ischemic heart disease with or without left ventricular dysfunction are at greatest risk for perioperative complications. Who should be screened for these conditions? Which tests should be used? Is the expense justified? Guidelines for perioperative cardiac evaluation have been in evolution. A comprehensive review of the evidence regarding the clinical evaluation and noninvasive testing of patients and guidelines derived from this review were published by the American College of Physicians (ACP) in 1997 (24,25). The ACP emphasized that the evaluation should begin with collecting those variables that discriminate low risk, intermediate risk, and high risk. To accomplish this initial risk stratification, the modified CRI was used (Table 2) (16). This assessment assigns statistical weight to variables obtained from history and physical examination along with baseline blood chemistries and ECG. Although such a traditional approach to risk assessment may seem antiquated as dependence on high technology increases, a thorough clinical history may be the best indicator

Table 2 Modified Multifactorial Index (16)

Variables	Points
Coronary artery disease	
MI within 6 months	10
MI >6 months	5
Canadian Cardiovascular Society angina	
Class III	10
Class IV	20
Unstable angina within 6 months	10
Alveolar pulmonary edema	
Within 1 week	10
Ever	5
Suspected critical aortic stenosis	20
Arrhythmias	
Rhythm other than sinus or sinus and atrial premature beats on last preoperative ECG	5
More than five premature ventricular contractions at any time prior to surgery	5
Poor general medical status	
$PO_2 < 60$ mm Hg	
$PCO_2 > 50$ mm Hg	
K < 3.0 meq/L	
$HCO_3 < 20$ meq/L	
BUN > 50 mg/dL	
Creatinine > 3.0 mg/dL	
Abnormal SGOT	
Signs of chronic liver disease	
Bedridden from noncardiac causes	5
Age over 70	5
Emergency operation	10

of CAD. The sensitivity and specificity of history alone to detect the presence of CAD ranges from 80% to 91% in several studies (26). The physical examination will reveal signs of CHF, cardiac dysrhythmia, valvular heart disease, and general medical status, all important variables in currently used cardiac risk indices. In fact, history and physical examination account for 20 of 53 points in Goldman's multivariate risk index (14). Poor functional status receives half the weight of an MI within 6 months of the planned procedure. Several investigators have shown that patients who cannot exercise to low cardiac workloads or those who develop a positive ischemic response to exercise are at high risk for postoperative adverse cardiac events (1). Gerson et al. (27) found that the inability to exercise was 80% sensitive and 53% specific for PCM. Hypokalemia appears to be an independent risk predictor (13,14). Cardiomegaly that may be found with another routine preoperative test, the chest X-ray, predicts PCM. Finally, 40–70% of patients with CAD who are undergoing noncardiac surgery have an abnormal ECG (1).

A low risk classification received further attention. Although a low risk classification has been validated to identify a low probability of PCM in a population of patients, 44% of patients who sustained PCM were of low risk class in the modified CRI (16). For example, an abnormal ECG receives half the weight of a recent MI on the modified CRI. An abnormal ECG may be diagnostic of underlying CAD, but a normal resting ECG is not necessarily reassuring. Only 25–50% of old MIs can be detected by ECG.

Tomatis et al. (28) found that 38% of patients with a normal ECG and a negative history of CAD still had 50% stenosis of one or more coronary vessels. Hertzer et al. (29) found that 37% of similar patients had 70% stenosis of one or more coronary arteries. Benchimol et al. (30) found three-vessel CAD in 15% of patients with a normal ECG. A normal ECG does not preclude significant disease.

To further refine risk in the Class I (10–15 points) patients, evaluation of a group of observables collectively identified as low risk variables was recommended (Table 3) (25). Patients with zero or one of these risk features have a <3% probability of PCM and likely need no further testing before a surgical procedure. If two or more of these risk features are present, the patient is considered to be of intermediate risk, with a probability of 3–15% of PCM. Of interest, ejection fraction, either by radionuclide angiography or by transthoracic echo, and exercise stress testing have not been shown to improve risk discrimination. In the case of exercise stress testing, many patients who are candidates for major surgical procedures, especially vascular procedures, are unable to complete the exercise protocol. In those patients who are able to exercise sufficiently, an exercise stress test has not been a reliable discriminator (25).

For those patients who are candidates for vascular surgery, the ACP recommended further evaluation with a dipyridamole thallium scan or with a dobutamine stress echo (DSE). Thallium-201 is taken up by myocardial cells in proportion to their blood flow. Intravenous dipyridamole dilates coronary vessels, which increases the blood flow to myocardium supplied by nonoccluded vessels. However, myocardium supplied by significantly stenotic vessels shows poor uptake (defect) on early scintigraphic scan. Later, this defect will "fill in" (redistribution), if viable myocardium is present. An old MI will appear as a persistent defect on thallium scan. Redistribution of thallium was correlated with PCM and provided additional risk stratification in patients with clinical risk predictors including CHF, angina, previous MI, and diabetes mellitus. Later

Table 3 Low Risk Index: One or None of the Following Features

After Eagle et al.
  Age > 70 years
  Q-wave on ECG
  Any angina
  History of ventricular ectopy
  History of diabetes
After Vanzetto et al.
  Age > 70 years
  Q-wave on ECG
  Any previous MI
  Any angina
  S–T segment abnormalities on resting ECG
  Hypertension with severe left ventricular hypertrophy
  History of diabetes

Note: For both indices, risk prediction was determined for vascular surgery patients.
Source: Palda VA, Detsky AS. Clinical guideline part II: perioperative assessment and management of risk from coronary artery disease. Ann Intern Med 1997; 127:313–328.

studies identified five clinical predictors and two DPT predictors. The clinical predictors were Q-waves, ventricular ectopy, diabetes mellitus, advanced age, and angina. DPT predictors were ischemic changes on ECG during the dipyridamole infusion and redistribution of thallium (31).

Mangano et al. (32) evaluated the use of DPT prospectively in consecutive patients. Their results demonstrated limited sensitivity of DPT for the detection of perioperative ischemia and adverse cardiac outcomes. Patients with redistribution defects and patients with persistent or no defects had comparable PCM. Lette et al. (33) studied 360 consecutive patients scheduled for noncardiac surgery. They found that DPT could stratify patients into subsets with predictive value for postoperative and 1 year coronary morbidity and mortality. Vanzetto et al. (34) identified additional risk discrimination with the use of DPT scanning in a group of patients scheduled for vascular surgery. Of 457 patients who had vascular procedures, 134 had at least two of the following clinical findings: age greater than 70 years, history of MI, angina, history of CHF, diabetes mellitus, hypertension with left ventricular hypertrophy, presence of Q-waves on ECG, or S–T segment abnormalities on a resting ECG. Only these 134 patients were evaluated with DPT. A negative DPT was associated with low risk (1%), and a positive scan was associated with a higher risk (23%). The diversity of findings suggests that DPT may not be universally applicable as predictor of PCM. Available evidence suggests that DPT provides improved stratification in the population of patients who are candidates for vascular surgery. Combining 24-h Holter monitoring with DPT may improve discrimination (35).

The DSE has been studied in vascular surgery patients (36,37). If a patient had one or two of the clinical risk features identified by Eagle et al. (31) (Table 4), the DSE refined risk assessment. The subset of patients with a negative DSE, even with the presence of the risk features in Table 2, had no adverse events, a finding that suggests that the DSE is an excellent negative predictor.

If either the DPT or the DSE is positive, or if the patient is in Class II (20–30 points) or Class III (>30 points), the focus on determining the nature of the cardiac risk and its potential for reversal was recommended. The nature of the cardiac risk is divided into three categories: ischemic heart disease; modifiable causes such as valvular disease, dysrhythmia, or CHF; and nonmodifiable causes, such as age. For those patients with ischemic heart disease, revascularization is the next decision point. For those patients with nonmodifiable

Table 4 Multivariate Predictors of Postoperative Ischemic Events

Redistribution on thallium imaging
Q-wave on ECG
Ischemic ECG changes after dipyridamole infusion
Age > 70 years
History of angina
History of ventricular ectopy
Diabetes

Source: Eagle KA, Coley CM, Newell JB, Brewster DC, Darling RC, Strauss HW, Guiney TE, Boucher CA. Combining clinical and thallium data optimizes preoperative assessment of cardiac risk before major vascular surgery. Ann Int Med 1989; 110:859–866.

risk features, careful evaluation of risks and benefits may indicate that modification of the intended procedure or cancellation of the procedure is the best course. For those patients with modifiable comorbidities, optimization of cardiac function may be of value.

For those patients, with intermediate risk, who are candidates for nonvascular surgery, the ACP guidelines of 1997 made no recommendation for or against clinical assessment of functional status. Many patients who are candidates for noncardiac and nonvascular surgery fall into this category. Because screening tests, except perhaps exercise ECG stress testing, focus exclusively on the detection of ischemic heart disease, a significant population of surgical patients with left ventricular dysfunction will not be identified as "at risk." A surgical patient with suspected or proven CAD will experience increased respiratory, metabolic, and cardiovascular work demand in the postoperative period—a significant and uncontrolled stress. A patient's ability to sustain a hyperdynamic stress postoperatively has been clearly linked to survival (38,39). Further, Gerson has shown that the ability to sustain a certain level of exercise is associated with improved postsurgical outcomes (27,40). In contrast, updated guidelines jointly published by the American College of Cardiology and the American Heart Association place significant emphasis on functional capacity and further generalize noninvasive testing (41). Their recommended approach to the patient who is a candidate for noncardiac surgery employs a stepwise algorithm. In the first step, the urgency of surgery is determined. If the planned surgical procedure is not an emergency, the next step is ascertaining whether the patient sustained coronary revascularization within the last five years. If coronary revascularization were performed, and if the patient remains stable without recurrence of ischemia in the interval, no further testing is recommended. The third step recommends that, if the patient were evaluated for coronary disease with favorable findings within the last two years, and if the patient remains stable and without ischemia, no further testing is recommended. In the fourth step, the presence of major risk features is assessed. These features include unstable coronary disease, decompensated heart failure, important arrhythmias, and severe valvular disease. If these features are present, surgery may be delayed and the patient referred for cardiac catheterization. The next step, step five, assesses intermediate risk features and the risk of surgery. Intermediate clinical risk features include stable angina, previous MI, compensated heart failure, diabetes mellitus, or renal insufficiency. For these patients, functional status receives significant emphasis and, in combination with the risk of surgery, determines the need for additional testing. High risk procedures include aortic surgery, peripheral vascular surgery, and major procedures in the chest and abdomen. Low risk procedures include cataract surgery, dermatologic procedures, and breast surgery. In the intermediate category are uncomplicated chest, abdominal, urologic, and orthopedic procedures. In the sixth step, patients with moderate to excellent functional capacity who are planned to undergo intermediate risk surgery usually do not require further testing. Patients with poor functional capacity or those patients with moderate functional capacity who will undergo high risk procedures are recommended to have noninvasive testing. In the seventh step, patients with no clinical risk features and moderate to excellent functional capacity can proceed with noncardiac surgery. Patients with poor functional capacity and planned high risk surgery may require noninvasive testing. In the eighth step, the results of noninvasive testing determine the need for risk modification or for further evaluation. Figures 1(a–c) summarize this algorithmic approach.

In our experience, a select group will benefit from preoperative placement of a pulmonary artery catheter to assess cardiac function. Typically, these patients have two or more of the variables listed in the table of low risk variables and poor or indeterminate

Cardiovascular Risk

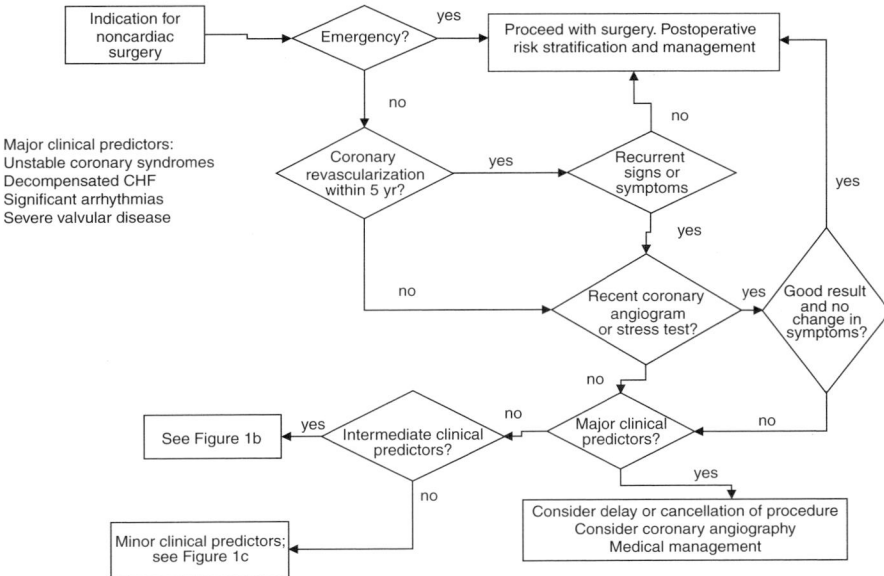

Figure 1a Approach to perioperative cardiovascular evaluation for patient requiring noncardiac surgery. Modified from Ref. (41).

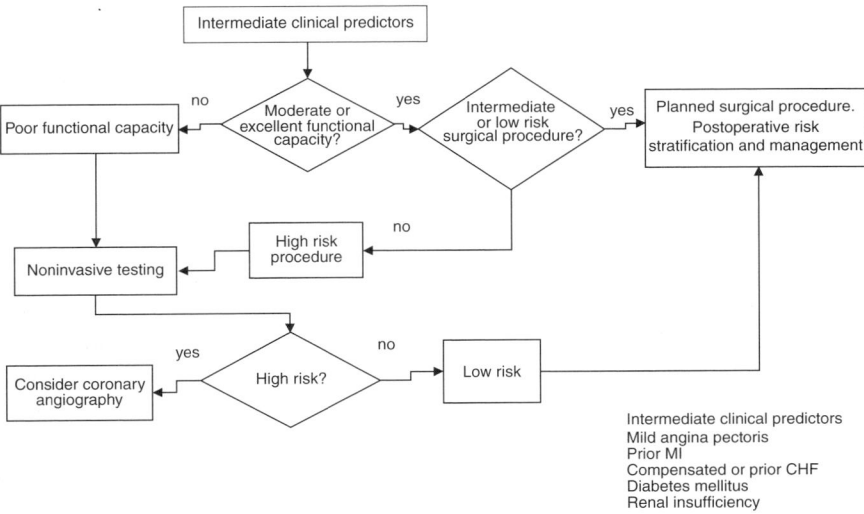

Figure 1b Approach to patient with intermediate clinical predictors. If two of the three listed intermediate factors are present, noninvasive testing is recommended. ECG exercise stress testing is recommended for the patient who can exercise. For those patients unable to exercise, a nonexercise stress test, such as a dipyridamole myocardial perfusion study or dobutamine stress echocardiography, is recommended. Modified from Ref. (41).

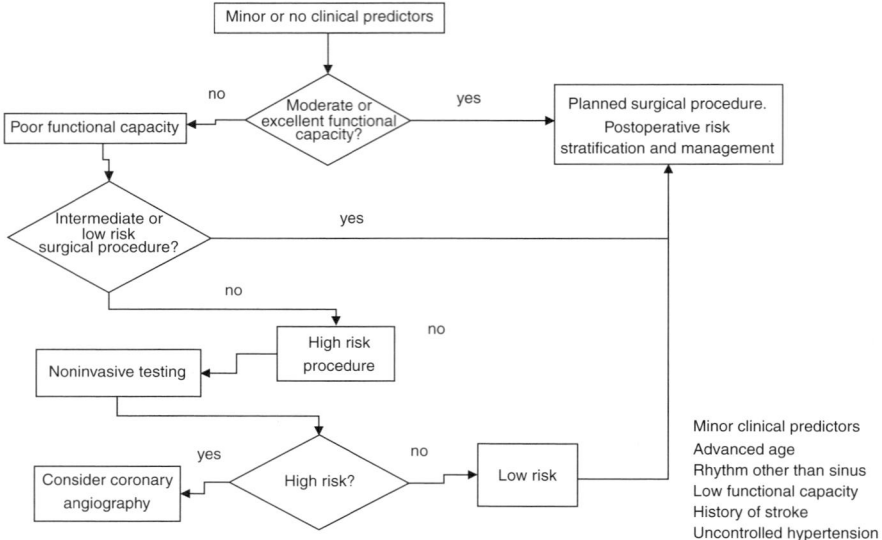

Figure 1c Approach to patient with minor or no clinical predictors. Modified from Ref. (41).

exercise tolerance. Right heart catheterization allows the ICU physician to test the patient's ability to tolerate myocardial stress under controlled conditions. We studied a group of patients with severe peripheral vascular disease who were undergoing limb salvage procedures. Such patients are recognized to be at high risk for PCM. A PA catheter was inserted preoperatively, and a preoperative cardiac physiology assessment and optimization (PCPAO) was performed. In a randomized prospective study (42), we found that optimizing left ventricular function (LVF) and oxygen transport before operation significantly reduced postoperative cardiac complications.

The patient's evaluation begins with a complete history and physical examination. Recent ECG and CXR are obtained. Antihypertensive medications, except for beta-blockers and clonidine, are discontinued. Serum electrolyte abnormalities are discontinued. Both arterial and PA catheters are generally required. Insertion of these monitoring catheters should be done with appropriate supervision. Arterial catheter sites in order of preferences are: (1) radial, (2) dorsalis pedis, (3) femoral, and (4) axillary. Brachial artery catheters should not be used routinely. Patients with arthritis, diabetes mellitus, arteriovenous shunts, peripheral vascular disease, or solid organ transplant are at high risk for complications from injudiciously placed arterial catheters. An automated sphygomanometer may be preferable in these patients. The PA catheter is usually placed via the internal jugular or subclavian veins.

The PA catheter is used to assess the patient's baseline cardiovascular status and response to intravenous fluid challenge. If cardiovascular derangements are detected, the aim of the PCPAO is to improve myocardial performance without significantly increasing the myocardial workload in order to assess a patient's ability to meet the increased tissue oxygen demands of the postoperative period. This goal is accomplished by infusing appropriate fluids, vasodilators, and inotropes to obtain a target cardiac output (Fig. 2). Target cardiac output does *not* mean maximal cardiac output. Although

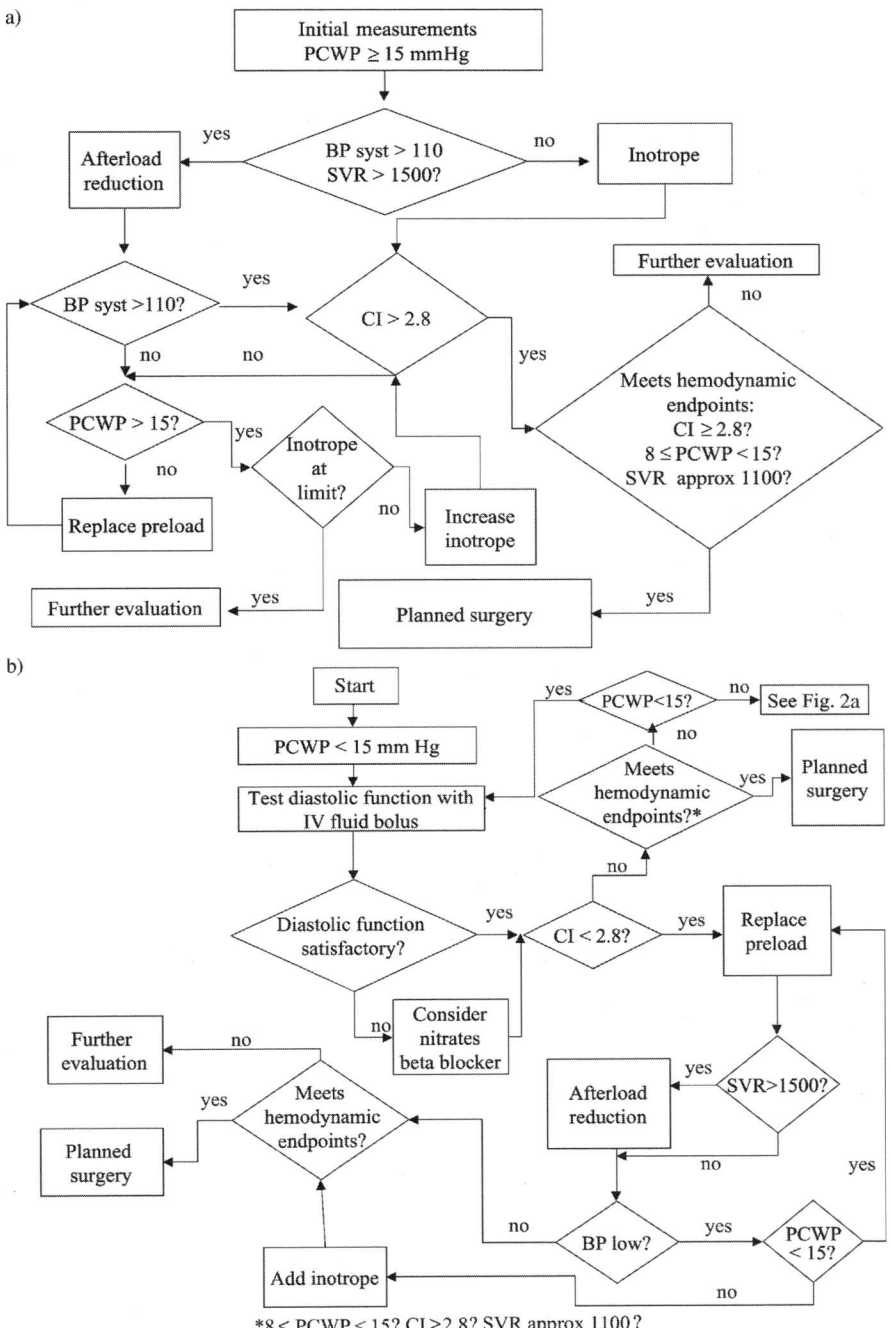

Figure 2 Preoperative cardiovascular "tune-up." Cardiovascular measurments were repeated after each intervention. Inotropes: dobutamine or dopamine; vasodilators: nitroglycerin or nitroprusside; PCWP: pulmonary capillary wedge pressure; SVR: systemic vascular resistance; CI: cardiac index. Measurement units are mmHg for pressure, dynes/sec/cm^5 for resistance, and L/min/m^2 for cardiac index. [From Ref. (42)].

certain surgical procedures do impose different levels of stress and hence create risk, the tune-up should not push the patient's limits of myocardial performance.

After baseline measurements of cardiac function, including RAP, pulmonary capillary wedge pressure (PCWP), cardiac output, and the values that may be derived from these independently measured variables, low dose nitroglycerin is administered. Nitroglycerin is used for its salutary effects on coronary arteries rather than the mild systemic venous and arterial vasodilation it produces.

Patients are classified according to their initial PCWP measurement. In preoperative patients, a few available studies suggest a clinical target of PCWP in the range of 12–15 mm Hg.

PCWP > 15 mm Hg

In general, these patients have left ventricular dysfunction. Many will require the intravenous administration of either a vasodilator agent (nitroglycerin or sodium nitroprusside) or an inotropic agent (dopamine or dobutamine) to optimize LVF (see Chapter 49 for a discussion of these agents). In patients with serious myocardial dysfunction, both vasodilator and inotropic agents may be necessary to achieve the desired hemodynamic end points. Such patients have been found to be at highest risk for postoperative complications by some investigators. Modification or postponement of the anticipated surgical procedure may be judicious in these patients. Diuretic therapy is conspicuously absent from this treatment approach. Because relative hypovolemia is a common problem in preoperative patients, improvement of myocardial function is attempted while optimal intravascular volume is maintained. Diuretics should be given only to patients in overt CHF.

PCWP < 15 mm Hg

These patients generally have inadequate intravascular volume as a consequence of chronic hypertension or dehydration. Generally they have good LVF and respond well to minimal pharmacologic intervention. Fortunately, the majority of unselected, high-risk surgical patients fall into this category. Those patients with poor LVF but a "normal" baseline PCWP (i.e., chronic compensated CHF) are identified after a fluid challenge. They demonstrate an inability to distribute an acute volume load to the left ventricle.

Appropriate colloids (albumin, hetastarch, or RBCs) rather than crystalloid are used for the fluid challenge in order to increase circulating blood volume efficiently. The majority of patients meet hemodynamic endpoint criteria with the use of fluids alone.

The following example demonstrates the type of patient who might benefit from a preoperative right heart catheterization. The patient was a 64-year-old male with cervical stenosis, and had progressive loss of strength and sensation in all extremities. The neurosurgeon's estimate was that the patient's cervical stenosis would progress and the patient would become quadriplegic. The medical history was remarkable for diabetes mellitus and two MIs at ages 53 and 59, respectively. Prior to the onset of weakness, the patient noted progressive dyspnea on exertion following the second MI. At presentation the patient's exercise was limited by extremity weakness. A chest X-ray demonstrated a mildly enlarged heart and pulmonary congestion. The ECG was consistent with an inferior MI. A cardiac echogram demonstrated an ejection fraction of 22%. The opinion of the cardiology service was ischemic cardiomyopathy with a high risk for surgical intervention. With the prospect of nearly certain quadriplegia if correction of the spinal abnormality were withheld, the patient was admitted to the ICU. A PA catheter was placed. The initial PCWP was 26 mm Hg. The cardiac index was 2.1 L/min per m^2. The patient's SVR was 2450 dynes/s per cm^5. Over the next 48 h, the patient received nitroglycerin, diuretics, and afterload reduction. The PCWP was 16 mm Hg, and the CI increased to 3.1 L/min per m^2. At that time the SVR was 1200 dynes/s per cm^5. The patient had no intraoperative and postoperative cardiac complications. At the last clinic visit, the patient reported improved sensation and strength in all extremities.

SUMMARY

- The complications of PCM are substantial and the number of patients at risk will increase in the next decades.
- A focused evaluation stratifies patients into low-, intermediate-, and high-risk categories. A CRI is useful. Heavily weighted variables include functional capacity, CHF, recent MI, and aortic stenosis.
- Low-risk patients require additional stratification. For the intermediate-risk vascular surgery patient, perform DPT or DSE.
- High-risk patients require categorization into ischemic risk, modifiable-risk, or nonmodifiable risk.
- Some patients will benefit from preoperative pulmonary catheter placement. These patients have modifiable risk features that can be identified and managed with the use of invasive hemodynamic information.

REFERENCES

1. Mangano DT. Perioperative cardiac morbidity. Anesthesiology 1990; 72:153–184.
2. Topkins MJ, Artusio JF. Myocardial infarction and surgery. Anesth Analg 1964; 43:716–720.
3. Knapp RB, Topkins MJ, Artusio JF Jr. The cerebrovascular accident and coronary occlusion in anesthesia. JAMA 1962; 182:332–334.d
4. Thompson GJ, Kelalis PP, Connolly DC. Transurethral prostatic resection after myocardial infarction. JAMA 1962; 182:908–911.
5. Arkins R, Smessaert AA, Hicks RG. Mortality and morbidity in surgical patients with coronary artery disease. JAMA 1964; 190:485–489.
6. Tarhan S, Moffitt E, Taylor WF. Myocardial infarction after general anesthesia. JAMA 1972; 220:1451–1454.
7. Steen PA, Tinker JH, Tarhan S. Myocardial reinfarction after anesthesia and surgery. JAMA 1978; 239:2566–2570.
8. Goldman L, Cladera DL, Southwick FS, Nussbaum SR, Murray B, O'Malley TA, Goroll AH, Caplan CH, Nolan J, Burke DS, Krogstad D, Carabello B, Slater EE. Cardiac risk factors and complications in noncardiac surgery. Medicine 1978; 57:357–370.
9. Eerola M, Eerola R, Kaukinen S, Kaukinen L. Risk factors in surgical patients with verified preoperative myocardial infarction. Acta Anaesthesiol Scand 1980; 24:219–223.
10. von Knorring J. Postoperative myocardial infarction: a prospective study in a risk group of surgical patients. Surgery 1981; 90:55–60.
11. Schoeppel LS, Wilkinson C, Waters J, Meyers SN. Effects of myocardial infarction on perioperative cardiac complications. Anesth Analg 1983; 62:493–498.

12. Rao TLK, Jacobs KH, El - Etr AA. Reinfarction following anesthesia in patients with myocardial infarction. Anesthesiology 1983; 59:499–505.
13. Shah KB, Kleinman BS, Rao TLK, Jacobs HK, Mestan K, Schaafsma M. Angina and other risk factors in patients with cardiac diseases undergoing noncardiac operations. Anesth Analg 1990; 70:240–247.
14. Goldman L, Caldera DL, Nussbaum SR, Southwick FS, Krogstad D, Murray B, Burke DS, O'Malley TA, Goroll AH, Caplan CH, Nolan J, Carabello B, Slater EE. Multifactorial index of cardiac risk in noncardiac surgical procedures. N Engl J Med 1977; 297:845–850.
15. Charlson ME, MacKenzie CR, Gold JP, Ales KL, Topkins M, Fairclough GP Jr., Shires GT. The preoperative and intraoperative hemodynamic predictors of postoperative myocardial infarction or ischemia in patients undergoing noncardiac surgery. Ann Surg 1989; 210:637–648.
16. Detsky AS, Abrams HB, McLaughlin JR, Drucker DJ, Sasson Z, Johnston N, Scott JG, Forbath N, Hilliard JR. Predicting cardiac complications in patients undergoing non-cardiac surgery. J Gen Intern Med 1986; 1:211–219.
17. Foster ED, Davis KB, Carpenter JA, Abele S, Fray D. Risk of noncardiac operation in patients with defined coronary disease: The Coronary Artery Surgery Study (CASS) Registry experience. Ann Thorac Surg 1986; 41:42–50.
18. Mock MB, Ringquist I, Fisher LD, Davis KB, Chaitman BR, Kouchoukos NT, Kaiser GC, Alderman E, Ryan TJ, Russell RO Jr., Mullin S, Fray D, Killip T III. Survival of medically treated patients in the coronary artery surgery study (CASS) registry. Circulation 1982; 66:562–568.
19. Pasternack PF, Imparato AM, Bear G, Riles TS, Baumann FG, Benjamin D, Sanger J, Kramer E, Wood RP. The value of radionuclide angiography as a predictor of perioperative myocardial infraction in patients undergoing abdominal aortic aneurysm resection. J Vasc Surg 1984; 1:320–325.
20. Pasternack PF, Imparato AM, Riles TS, Baumann FG, Bear G, Lamparello PJ, Benjamin D, Sanger J, Kramer E. The value of the radionuclide angiogram in the prediction of perioperative myocardial infarction in patients undergoing lower extremity revascularization procedures. Circulation 1985; 72(3 Pt 2):II–13–17.
21. Kopecky SL, Gibbons RJ, Hollier LH. Preoperative supine exercise radionuclide angiogram predicts perioperative cardiovascular events in vascular surgery [abstract]. J Am Coll Cardiol 1986; 7(suppl A):226A.
22. Franco CE, Goldsmith J, Veith FJ, Ascer E, Wengerter KR, Calligaro KD, Gupta SK. Resting gated pool ejection fraction: a poor predictor of perioperative myocardial infarction in patients undergoing vascular surgery for infrainguinal bypass grafting. J Vasc Surg 1989; 10:656–661.
23. Goldman L. Multifactorial index of cardiac risk in noncardiac surgery: status report. Cardiothorac Vasc Anesth Update 1990; 1:1.
24. Palda VA, Detsky AS. Clinical guideline part I: guidelines for assessing and managing the perioperative risk from coronary artery disease associated with major noncardiac surgery. Ann Intern Med 1997; 127:303–312.
25. Palda VA, Detsky AS. Clinical guideline part II: perioperative assessment and management of risk from coronary artery disease. Ann Intern Med 1997; 127:313–328.
26. Roizen MF. Anesthetic implications of concurrent diseases. In: Miller RD, ed. Anesthesia, 3d ed. New York: Churchill Livingstone, 1990; 825.
27. Gerson MC, Hurst JM, Hertzberg VS, Doogan PA, Cochran MB, Lim SP, McCall N, Adolph RJ. Cardiac prognosis in noncardiac geriatric surgery. Ann Intern Med 1985; 103:832–837.
28. Tomatis LA, Fierens EE, Verbrugge GP. Evaluation of surgical risk in peripheral vascular disease by coronary angiography: a series of 100 cases. Surgery 1972; 71:429–435.

29. Hertzer NR, Beven EG, Young JR, O'Hara PJ, Ruschhaupt WF III, Graor RA, Dewolfe VG, Maljovec LC. Coronary artery disease in peripheral vascular patients. A classification of 1000 angiograms and results of surgical management. Ann Surg 1984; 199:223–233.
30. Benchimol A, Harris CL, Dresser KB, Kwee BT, Promisloff SD. Resting electrocardiogram in major coronary artery disease. JAMA 1973; 224:1489–1492.
31. Eagle KA, Coley CM, Newell JB, Brewster DC, Darling RC, Strauss HW, Guiney TE, Boucher CA. Combining clinical and thallium data optimizes preoperative assessment of cardiac risk before major vascular surgery. Ann Int Med 1989; 110:859–866.
32. Mangano DT, London MJ, Tubau JF, Browner WS, Hollenberg M, Krupski W, Layug EL, Massie B. Dipyridamole thallium-201 scintigraphy as preoperative screening test: a reexamination of its predictive potential. Circulation 1991; 84:493–502.
33. Lette J, Waters D, Bernier H, Champagne P, Lassonde J, Picard M, Cerino M, Nattel S, Boucher Y, Heyen F, Dube S. Preoperative and long-term cardiac risk assessment: predictive value of 23 clinical descriptors, 7 multivariate scoring systems, and quantitative dipyridamole imaging in 360 patients. Ann Surg 1992; 216:192–204.
34. Vanzetto G, Machecourt J, Blendea D, Fagret D, Borrel E, Magne JL, Gattaz F, Guidicelli H. Additive value of thallium single-photon emission computed tomography myocardial imaging for prediction of perioperative events in clinically selected high risk patients having abdominal aortic surgery. Am J Cardiol 1996; 77:143–148.
35. Raby KE, Goldman L, Creager MA, Cook EF, Weisberg MC, Whittemore AD, Selwyn AP. Correlation between preoperative ischemia and major cardiac events after peripheral vascular surgery. N Engl J Med 1989; 321:1296–1300.
36. Poldermans D, Arnese M, Fioretti PM, Salustri A, Boersma E, Thomson IR, Roelandt JRTC, van Urk H. Improved cardiac risk stratification in major vascular surgery with dobutamine–atropine stress echocardiography. J Am Coll Cardiol 1995; 26:648–653.
37. Lalka SG, Sawada SG, Dalsing MC, Cikrit DF, Sawchuk AP, Kovacs RL, Segar DS, Ryan T, Feigenbaum H. Dobutamine stress echocardiography as a predictor of cardiac events associated with aortic surgery. J Vasc Surg 1992; 15:831–840.
38. Clowes GHA Jr., Del Guercio LR, Barwinsky J. The cardiac output in reponse to surgical trauma. A comparison between patients who survived and those who died. Arch Surg 1960; 81:212–222.
39. Bland RD, Shoemaker WC, Abraham E, Cobo JC. Hemodynamic and oxygen transport patterns in surviving and non-surviving postoperative patients. Crit Care Med 1985; 13:85–90.
40. Gerson MC, Hurst JM, Hertzberg VS, Baughman R, Rouan GW, Ellis K. Prediction of cardiac and pulmonary complications related to elective abdominal and noncardiac thoracic surgery in geriatric patients. Am J Med 1990; 88:101–107.
41. Eagle KA, Berger PB, Calkins H, Chaitman BR, Ewy GA, Fleischmann KE, Fleisher LA, Froehlich JB, Gusberg RJ, Leppo JA, Ryan T, Schlant RC, Winters WL. ACC/AHA guideline update for perioperative cardiovascular evaluation for noncardiac surgery: a report of the American College of Cardiology/American Heart Association Task Force on Practice Guidelines (Committee to update the 1996 guidelines on perioperative cardiovascular evaluation for noncardiac surgery). 2002. American College of Cardiology Web site. Available at http://www.acc.org/clinical/guidelines/perio/dirIndex.htm.
42. Berlauk JF, Abrams JH, Gilmour IJ, O'Connor SR, Knighton DR, Cerra FB. Preoperative optimization of cardiovascular hemodynamics improves outcome in peripheral vascular surgery. Ann Surg 1991; 214:289–299.

9
Life Support and Management of Cardiac Arrest

Michael D. Pasquale
Lehigh Valley Hospital, Allentown, Pennsylvania, USA

OVERVIEW

Cardiorespiratory arrest is defined as loss of pulse, blood pressure, and spontaneous respiration. This state results in cardiac output that is inadequate to sustain life. The brain and the kidneys are the organs most susceptible to irreversible ischemic damage after successful but prolonged resuscitation. With dialysis and careful medical management, the kidney often may be salvaged. However, no such protocol exists for salvage of brain function; therefore, the brain is usually regarded as the barometer of success or failure of resuscitation.

Although the means of reversing death has occupied the thoughts and efforts of man since antiquity, the technique of modern cardiopulmonary resuscitation (CPR) (i.e., effective ventilation, closed-chest cardiac massage, and external defibrillation) has evolved over only the past 40 years. The four basic principles of modern CPR are to (1) ensure airway patency, (2) ensure ventilation, (3) provide artificial circulation, and (4) restart the arrested heart (1).

AIRWAY MANAGEMENT

Management of the patient's airway is the first priority of resuscitation. It begins with ensuring airway patency and relief of airway obstruction. The most common cause of airway obstruction in the unconscious human is the tongue, which falls backward against the posterior pharynx.

Jaw-thrust or chin-lift maneuvers should be attempted before any airway adjuncts are used. In the patient with blunt trauma, the chin-lift is preferred, as it is less likely to produce injury to the spinal cord in a patient with cervical spine fracture (2). Obstructing foreign bodies always should be suspected, and blood, teeth, vomitus, secretions, or other debris, if present, should be evacuated from the airway. Abdominal thrusts may be useful in a patient with an airway that is totally obstructed by a foreign body. Once optimal positioning and removal of any foreign body have been achieved, the patient should be checked for return of spontaneous ventilation.

The presence of inspiratory stridor, gurgling, choking, hoarseness, increased respiratory effort, or difficulty with speech may be associated with partial airway obstruction, and optimization of airway patency should be pursued. A variety of airway adjuncts may be used. The oropharyngeal airway is a means of improving airway patency in unconscious patients, because it prevents the tongue from falling back onto the posterior pharynx (2). This type of airway should not be used in the conscious patient, because it may stimulate the gag reflex and induce vomiting with subsequent possible aspiration (2,3). The patient with an intact gag reflex will better tolerate a rubber nasopharyngeal airway, even though it provides a less effective route than the oropharyngeal device (2).

Endotracheal intubation (ETI) is the definitive procedure for establishing an airway and optimizing ventilation in the patient with cardiac arrest. It also provides a conduit to evacuate secretions and administer drugs for resuscitation. The trachea can be intubated by oral, nasal, or transcricoid routes. In noninjured patients without airway obstruction, the oral route is preferred. Nasotracheal intubation (NTI) can be used if the patient is breathing spontaneously (4). In the patient with trauma, if there is no need for an immediate airway, a cervical spine X-ray film can be obtained first. If this film reveals no evidence of fracture, orotracheal intubation (OTI) may be done safely (5). If there is evidence of fracture, or if an immediate airway is needed, NTI is preferred in the spontaneously breathing patient. If the patient is apneic, OTI with in-line manual cervical immobilization should be used (4,5). In a patient with severe maxillofacial injury, or one in whom orotracheal and nasotracheal techniques have been unsuccessful, a surgical airway must be established (6–8). In adults, surgical cricothyroidotomy is preferred. In children under the age of 12 years, needle cricothyroidotomy and subsequent tracheostomy should be done. Formal cricothyroidotomy should be avoided in children, because the cricoid cartilage of children provides the only circumferential support to the upper trachea and should not be damaged (6,8). A very useful procedure in ETI is the application of firm pressure over the cricoid cartilage to occlude the upper end of the esophagus (Sellick's maneuver) (9). This maneuver reduces the incidence of aspiration of gastric contents during intubation.

VENTILATION

Once airway control has been established, adequate oxygenation and ventilation should be ensured. Mouth-to-mouth or mouth-to-mask ventilation should be initiated immediately. The fractional concentration of oxygen (FIO_2) in a rescuer's exhaled air is approximately 0.16, which is sufficient to meet a victim's needs. Conversion to bag/valve/mask ventilation, when available, is done with FIO_2 of 1.0, and flow rates of 10–15 L/min. In this way an inspired oxygen concentration of ~75% can be delivered (3,7). Potential problems with this techniue include air leak, inadequate lung inflation, atelectasis, arteriovenous shunting, and hypoxemia. Also, gastric inflation secondary to high-peak inspiratory pressures and decreased lung compliance during CPR increase the risk of pulmonary aspiration. Optimal oxygenation and ventilation is achieved with ETI and subsequent bag/valve/tube respiration with 100% oxygen (3,7).

CIRCULATION

In the absence of a pulse, chest compressions are necessary. In adults, standard two person CPR involves 100 compressions per minute with a breath delivered every fifth compression (3,10,11). The generation of a forward cardiac output as a result of chest compression is a subject of controversy. Kouwenhoven (12) popularized the cardiac pump theory, which suggests that, during CPR, the heart is squeezed like a pump between the sternum and the spine. Antegrade flow is ensured by the cardiac valves (13). The relaxation phase also mimics the natural circulation with a fall in intracardiac pressures and flow of blood into the heart as the sternum returns to its normal position. Ventilation and compression are alternated so that inflation does not impede flow during compression (13,14). Interestingly, no data confirmed this assumption; however, an associated rise in venous pressure was noted during compression (15). This finding led to the speculation that the thorax was acting as the pump (thoracic pump) (15,16). This theory suggests that with sternal compression there is an abrupt increase in intrathoracic pressure that propels blood into the arterial tree (17,18). If this theory is true, then maneuvers to increase intrathoracic pressure may prove useful in resuscitation (16). Unidirectional flow is ensured via one-way valves in the superior vena cava and venous collapse, while arteries remain open (17,18). The heart is considered simply a passive conduit, and flow depends on an arteriovenous pressure gradient outside the chest.

The relative contributions of the cardiac and thoracic pumps are still unsettled. Each mechanism probably contributes to perfusion and depends on the configuration and stiffness of the chest wall, the presence of cardiac enlargement, and the method of CPR (19,20).

The blood flow established during CPR is barely life-sustaining, because cardiac output is only about 25% of normal. Although systolic pressures of 90 mm Hg are attainable, diastolic pressures are usually low (<20 mm Hg) (7). The cerebral cortex and the myocardium are inadequately perfused. The use of epinephrine, in conjunction with CPR improves pressure, but perfusion remains suboptimal. New techniques and adjuncts to external compression [i.e., simultaneous ventilation and compression CPR (SVC–CPR), abdominal binders, volume loading during CPR, interposed abdominal counterpressure during CPR] intended to harness the thoracic pump have been tried, but no conclusive evidence to suggest that they enhanced vital organ perfusion or resuscitability has been obtained (16). Efforts to recruit the cardiac pump (i.e., high-frequency, high-impulse CPR) have demonstrated increases in cardiac output, aortic diastolic blood pressure, and coronary perfusion pressure (21). Squeezing the cardiac pump appears essential for generating a coronary perfusion gradient, neurologic recovery, and increasing survival. Currently, the American Heart Association recommends compressions of moderate force and short duration to be delivered at a rate of $100-120$ min^{-1} (21).

Open cardiac massage has been show to provide a two- to threefold increase in cardiac output along with the generation of higher arterial pressures and lower venous pressures (22). These changes suggest enhanced neurologic recovery and survival, but prospective randomized clinical trials are lacking. Possible indications for open cardiac massage are failure of conventional CPR, refractory ventricular fibrillation, hypothermia-associated arrest, cardiac tamponade, massive pulmonary embolism, abdominal aortic aneurysm, hemothorax, hemoperitoneum, air embolism, flail chest, third trimester of pregnancy, postoperative state, arrest in young patients, and thoracic deformities (22).

THE ARRESTED HEART

See Figs. 1–4.

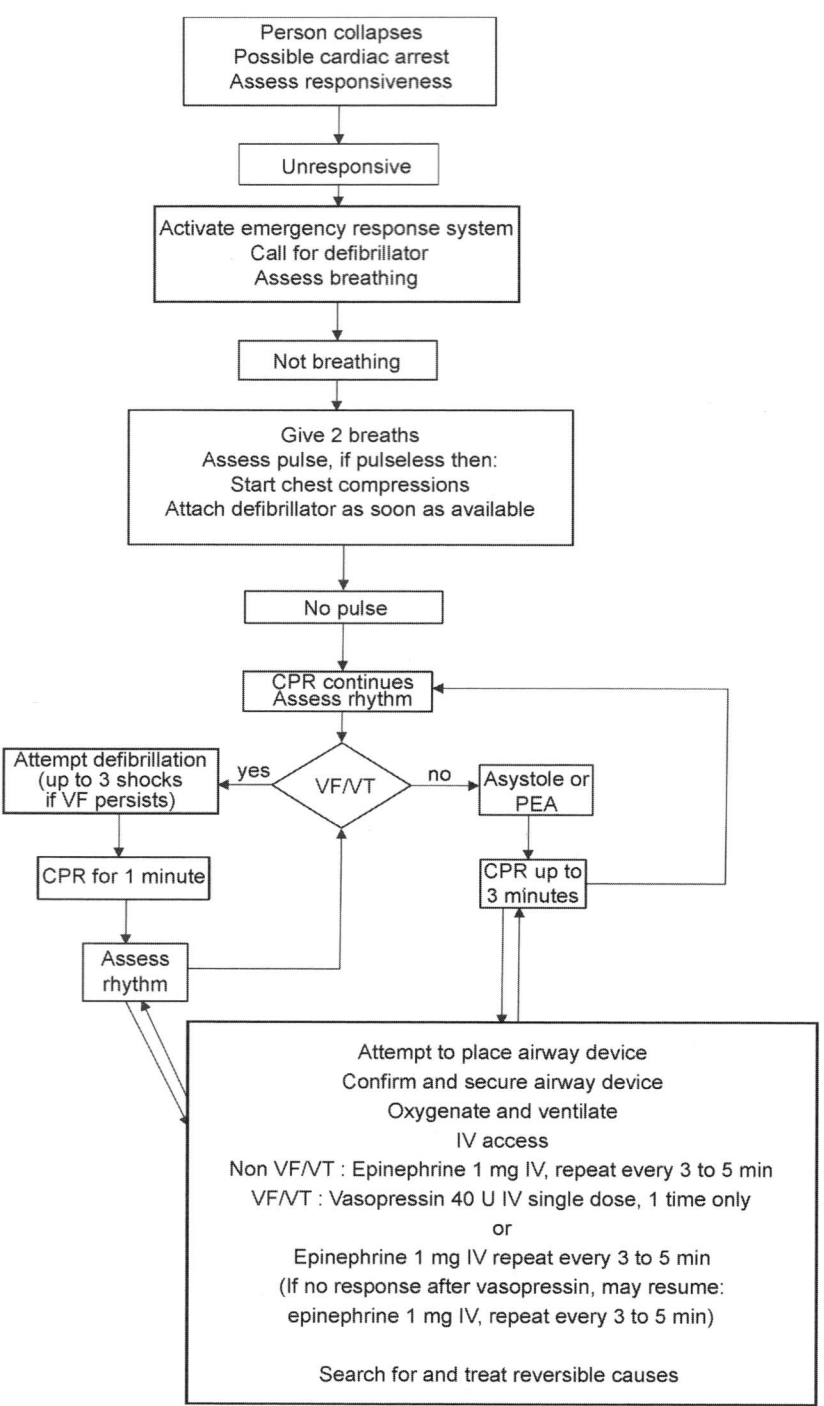

Figure 1 Approaches to possible cardiac arrest. [Adapted from Guidelines 2000 for cardiopulmonary resuscitation and emergency cardiovascular care. Circulation 2000; 102(suppl):I-144.]

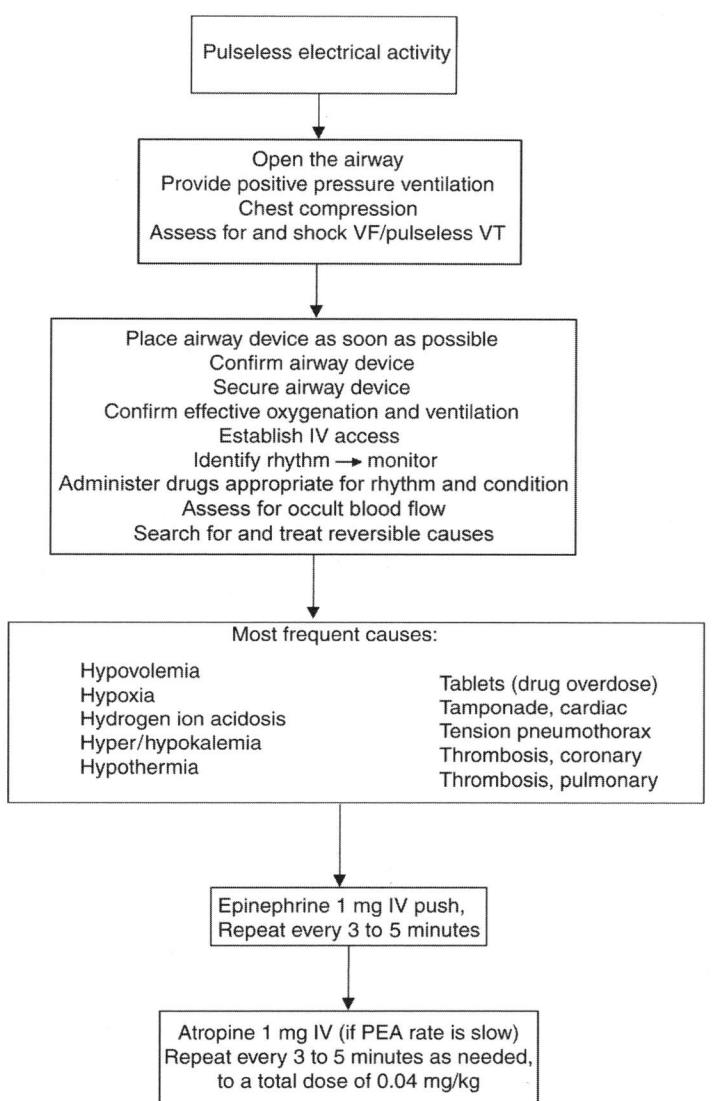

Figure 2 Guidelines for pulseless electrical activity. [Adapted from Guidelines 2000 for cardiopulmonary resuscitation and emergency cardiovascular care. Circulation 2000; 102(suppl):I-151.]

PHARMACOLOGIC APPROACH

Epinephrine

Epinephrine is an endogenous catecholamine with both alpha- and beta-receptor-stimulating actions. Despite the observation that a large body of data in animal subjects and in humans consistently show a positive benefit to the use of epinephrine in cardiac arrest, the absence of a placebo controlled trial in humans now relegates epinephrine to Class Indeterminate category (3). Epinephrine continues to be recommended for patients

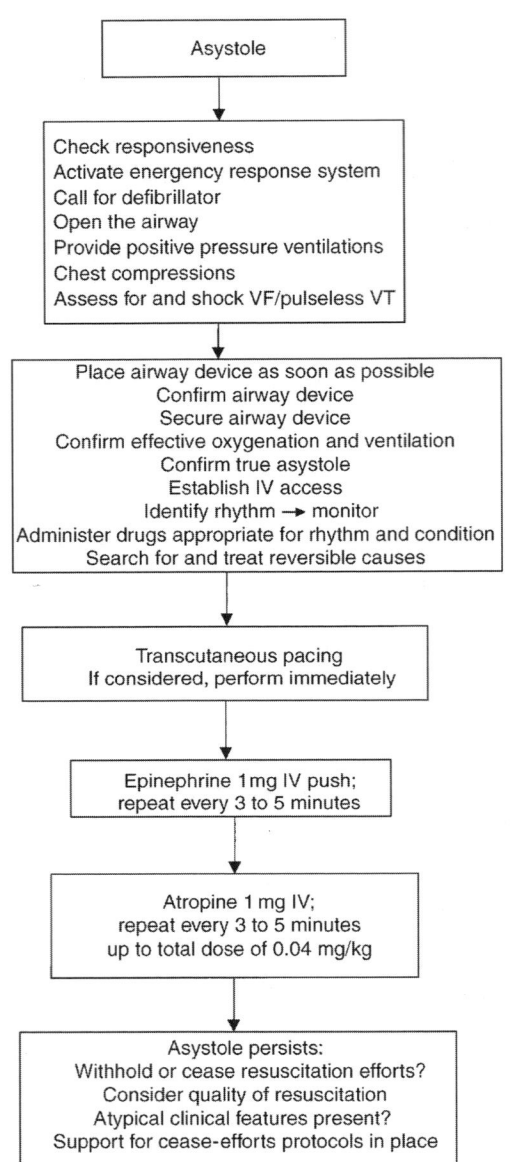

Figure 3 Guidelines for asystole. [Adapted from Guidelines 2000 for cardiopulmonary resuscitation and emergency cardiovascular care. Circulation 2000; 102(suppl):I-153.]

with cardiac arrest, ventricular fibrillation, ventricular tachycardia without a detectable pulse, pulseless electrical activity, and patients who are unresponsive to initial defibrillation attempts. The mechanism of action of epinephrine is related to its alpha vasopressor effects. Cardiovascular responses include increases in heart rate, myocardial contractile force, systemic vascular resistance, arterial blood pressure, myocardial oxygen consumption, and automaticity. Clinically, epinephrine increases perfusion pressure, improves the

Life Support and Management of Cardiac Arrest

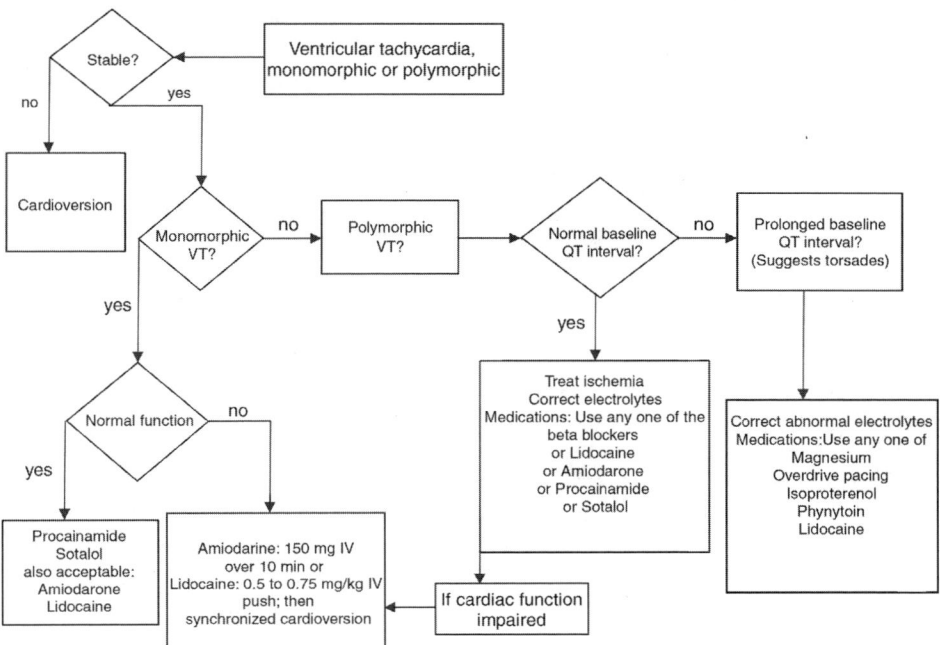

Figure 4 Guidelines for ventricular tachycardia. [Adapted from Guidelines 2000 for cardiopulmonary resuscitation and emergency cardiovascular care. Circulation 2000; 102(suppl):I-163.]

contractile state, stimulates spontaneous contraction, and increases the vigor of ventricular fibrillation. Current evidence suggests epinephrine provides higher cardiac blood flow, higher cerebral blood flow, and more favorable oxygen delivery/consumption balance than other alpha agonists (e.g., phenylephrine and methoxamine). The recommended dose of epinephrine is 1 mg intravenously (3). Because of the drug's short duration of action, this dose may be repeated at 3–5 min intervals. Epinephrine also may be given transbronchially or by direct injection into the heart.

Vasopressin

Vasopressin is currently recommended as an alternative to epinephrine for adult patients with ventricular fibrillation that is refractory to shock (3). Unlike epinephrine, vasopressin has no alpha- or beta-adrenergic activity. It exerts its effects through stimulation of smooth muscle V1 receptors. Because it has no beta-adrenergic activity, vasopressin does not cause increased myocardial oxygen consumption or skeletal muscle vasodilation during CPR. Vasopressin requires ~10 min to achieve its peak effects. When used, it should be administered immediately. In addition to shock refractory ventricular fibrillation, vasopressin may be useful in the support of patients with septic shock.

Norepinephrine

Norepinephrine is a naturally occurring catecholamine that acts as a potent alpha- and beta-receptor stimulus to increase vasoconstriction and inotropy. Significant hypotension (systolic blood pressure <70 mmHg) or cardiogenic shock is the principal indication for its use; however, substantial increases in myocardial oxygen consumption as a result of increased left ventricular wall tension may occur. Norepinephrine also has the disadvantage of causing renal and mesenteric vasoconstriction. The initial response of the coronary circulation to norepinephrine is vasoconstriction. This reponse is transient, and vasodilation usually ensues as a consequence of increased myocardial metabolic activity and increased perfusion pressures. Norepinephrine is given by continuous intravenous infusion starting at 2–4 μg/min with titration done for desired blood pressure.

Dopamine

Dopamine has strong beta-1-inotropic and alpha-adrenergic vasoconstrictor effects. In addition, specific dopaminergic receptors (DA1 and DA2) exist. Dopamine is currently recommended for patients who remain hypotensive after return of spontaneous circulation, especially if bradycardia is present (3). Dopamine is usually given as a continuous intravenous infusion of 5–20 μg/kg/min. At doses below 5 μg/kg/min, dopamine increases renal and splanchnic perfusion. In the range of 5–10 μg/kg/min, inotropy is the dominant effect. Above 10 μg/kg/min, alpha-adrenergic effects are noted, including systemic and splanchnic vasoconstriction. At doses >25 μg/kg/min, the actions of dopamine are similar to those of epinephrine.

Atropine

Atropine sulfate is a parasympatholytic drug that accelerates the rate of discharge of the sinus node and may improve atrioventricular conduction. It is currently recommended for bradycardic dysrhythmias with hypotension, high-degree atrioventricular block at the nodal level, and ventricular asystole. The recommended dosage is 0.5 mg intravenously, repeated at 5 min intervals until the desired rate is achieved (not to exceed 2 mg) (3). Atropine should not be given for atrioventricular block related to overdosage of beta blockers or calcium channel blockers. These conditions are treated with glucagon and calcium, respectively.

Isoproterenol

Isoproterenol hydrochloride is a sympathomimetic amine that is structurally related to epinephrine but acts almost exclusively on beta receptors. Because it increases myocardial oxygen consumption, decreases coronary perfusion, and predisposes to ventricular dysrhythmia, isoproterenol is not recommended as a first-line agent for cardiac arrest. It may be used with caution in patients with symptomatic bradycardia, if external pacing is not available. It also is recommended for heart transplant patients with symptomatic bradycardia. The denervated heart does not respond to atropine (3). Isoproterenol is generally given as a continuous intravenous infusion of 2–20 μg/min.

Sodium Bicarbonate

Acidemia during prolonged CPR is caused by alveolar hypoventilation and anaerobic metabolism (23). The acidosis produced exerts detrimental effects on circulation, including increased pulmonary vasoconstriction, decreased systemic vascular resistance, arteriolar dilation, venous constriction, and capillary stasis. The acidosis also decreases the vascular and cardiac responses to adrenergic amines, while enhancing the effects of vagal stimulation. Overall, decreased chronotropy, inotropy, and vascular tone occur. With a decrease in pH, the patient also is predisposed to ventricular dysrhythmias. Primary treatment of acidemia is adequate ventilation, which removes carbon dioxide. Correction of respiratory acidosis is critical, because partial pressure of carbon dioxide ($PaCO_2$) more closely reflects intracellular pH as a result of the rapid diffusibility of carbon dioxide (24,25). Recently, considerable controversy has been generated regarding the routine use of intravenous sodium bicarbonate during arrest (26). This controversy arises from the observation that, above a pH of 7.2, no direct correlation between pH and success of defibrillation or resuscitation has been demonstrated. Also, when given intravenously, sodium bicarbonate will produce carbon dioxide as it dissociates. This additional carbon dioxide passes into cells more quickly than does sodium bicarbonate and thus decreases intracellular pH (25,27,28). Current recommendations regarding administration of sodium bicarbonate are pre-existing hyperkalemia, diabetic ketoacidosis, overdose with tricyclic antidepressants, cocaine overdose, and diphenhydramine overdose. Sodium bicarbonate administration may be useful in prolonged resuscitation, if adequate ventilation is provided (3). Iatrogenic alkalosis may lead to dysrhythmias, lactate production, and cerebral and peripheral vasoconstriction. Sodium bicarbonate should be given as an intravenous bolus of 1 mEq/kg.

Calcium

Calcium is no longer recommended as first-line therapy in cardiac arrest (with the exception of cardiac arrest from hyperkalemia), as it has not been shown to be effective (3,26,29). Injection of calcium also is associated with detrimental effects, such as sinus node arrest, ventricular ectopy, and increased calcium concentrations in cytosol, which can produce mitochondrial damage (particularly in the brain and heart) (26,29,30).

Amiodarone

Amiodarone has many actions. It affects sodium, potassium, and calcium channels in addition to its effects as an alpha- and beta-adrenergic blocker. Amiodarone is currently recommended for control of rapid ventricular rate in patients with atrial arrhythmias, especially in those individuals with impaired left ventricular function or those in whom digoxin is ineffective; after defibrillation and epinephrine in individuals with pulseless ventricular tachycardia or shock refractory ventricular fibrillation; for treatment of hemodynamically stable ventricular tachycardia when cardioversion is unsuccessful; as an adjunct to electrical cardioversion of refractory paroxysmal supraventricular tachycardia; for the treatment of multifocal atrial tachycardia in patients with preserved left ventricular function; and for the treatment of atrial fibrillation, when other treatments are ineffective. Amiodarone is administered as a dose of 300 mg intravenous push in cardiac arrest. In wide complex tachycardias, 150 mg over 10 min is administered, and continuous infusion of 1 mg/min over the next 6 h is used. The maintenance infusion is then 0.5 mg/min (3).

Lidocaine

Lidocaine decreases automaticity by slowing phase 4 depolarization. In infarcted tissue, lidocaine has been shown to reduce conduction velocity and prolong the effective refractory period. Lidocaine also has been demonstrated to further depress cells that form part of a reentrant pathway in ischemic zones, while it produces little or no effect on normal or moderately depressed cells. This effect prevents emergence of a wavefront from ischemic zones and thus terminates reentrant ventricular dysrhythmias. Lidocaine also reduces the disparity in action potential duration between ischemic and normal zones and prolongs conduction and refractoriness in ischemic zones. Last, lidocaine has been shown to increase fibrillation threshold. Lidocaine has recently been given a Class Indeterminate categorization, as no study of the efficacy of lidocaine compared with that of placebo has been performed in humans. Although it remains in the algorithms for monomorphic ventricular tachycardia with normal cardiac function, monomorphic ventricular tachycardia with impaired cardiac function, polymorphic ventricular tachycardia with normal baseline QT interval, and polymorphic ventricular tachycardia with prolonged QT interval, it is now a second tier choice (3). Dosage should be a 1 mg/kg intravenous bolus followed by an infusion of 2–4 mg/min. An additional 0.5 mg/kg may be given 10 min after the initial bolus is administered, if ventricular ectopy is still present. Excessive doses of lidocaine are capable of producing myocardial and circulatory depression, and clinical indications of lidocaine toxicity primarily include CNS effects. As lidocaine is metabolized in the liver, dosages should be reduced in patients with hepatic impairment.

Procainamide

Procainamide suppresses phase 4 diastolic depolarization and, consequently, slows the rate of ectopic pacemaker discharge. It also decreases the rate of rise of phase 0 of the action potential and terminates reentrant pathways by slowing conduction in already depressed areas. Procainamide is useful in suppressing premature ventricular complexes and recurrent ventricular tachycardia, which cannot be controlled with lidocaine. It also can be used in persistent ventricular fibrillation. The dose for recurrent ventricular tachycardia or recurrent ventricular fibrillation is 20 mg/min to a maximum total dose of 17 mg/kg. Alternatively, in urgent situations, 50 mg/min may be administered up to a total dose of 17 mg/kg. For stable wide complex tachycardia, uncontrolled paroxysmal supraventricular tachycardia, or atrial fibrillation with rapid ventricular rate in Wolff–Parkinson–White syndrome, 20 mg/min is administered until dysrhythmia is suppressed, hypotension ensues, the QRS complex is widened by 50%, or a total dose of 17 mg/kg has been infused. The maintenance infusion rate is 1–4 mg/min. As procainamide is cleared by the kidney, for patients with renal impairment the maintenance dose is reduced to 1–2 mg/min. Maximum total dose also is reduced to 12 mg/kg (3). Side effects of procainamide administration include hypotension, widening of the QRS complex, lengthening of the PR and QT intervals, and atrioventricular conduction disturbances.

EXPECTATIONS FOR RESUSCITATION

Although an organized team to treat cardiac arrest produces better outcomes, only 10–20% of those patients who sustain cardiac arrest survive to be discharged to home (7). Considering the time, money, and effort allocated to resuscitation efforts, prearrest and arrest factors must be recognized for their prognostic implications in predicting outcome of cardiac arrest in the hospital.

Prearrest Factors

Age
Although Stephenson (31) noted that resuscitation was less successful in both the extremely old and the very young, most authors have not found age to significantly affect outcome (32–36). Rozenbaum and Shenkman (35) noted that patients over 65 years old had a 20% survival when compared with a 16% survival in those under 65.

Sex
No significant differences in survival have been noted based solely on the sex of the patient sustaining arrest (32,33,36).

Associated Disease
In patients with significant associated illness, most notably cancer, sepsis, pneumonia, renal failure, left ventricular dysfunction, and cerebrovascular accident with residual defect, the outcome is generally poor (32,33,36,37). In patients with one or more of these associated illnesses, Bedell et al. (33) noted a 95–100% mortality after cardiac arrest. Also, a homebound life-style was associated with a 95% mortality.

Arrest Factors

Duration of Resuscitation
Most authors concur that there is an inverse correlation between the duration of resuscitation and survival. In general, if resuscitation is accomplished in <15 min, survival is more likely (32,33,35,38). In contrast, efforts lasting longer than 30 min are almost always associated with death.

Initial Cardiac Rhythm
Patients found to be asystolic or having pulseless electrical activity are less likely to survive than those having ventricular fibrillation or ventricular tachycardia. Castagna et al. (32) noted that there were no survivors in patients whose initial rhythm was asystolic. Stiles et al. (39) noted a 6% survival for patients in asystole, compared with a 30% survival for those in ventricular fibrillation.

Recurrent Arrest
The likelihood of survival after a second or third cardiac arrest is remote, particularly in those patients with progressive metabolic or multisystem organ failure (37). DeBard (36) has noted no survival in patients having more than three cardiac arrests.

Care Setting
Rozenbaum and Shenkman, (35), Bedell et al. (33), Castagna et al. (32) DeBard (36), and Sanders (19) have shown no significant differences in survival in relation to location of care administered for cardiac arrest. Peatfield et al. (40) and Hershey and Fisher (41) have shown that survival after cardiac arrest on the ward ranges from 2% to 3%. One explanation may be that more resuscitative attempts are performed in this setting despite the presence of multiple associated diseases in these patients.

Arterial Blood Gases (ABGs)
Most studies are not conclusive regarding the use of ABGs or oxygen saturations as determinants of survival. This uncertainty results from the observation that ABGs are not

always obtained during the arrest phase. When ABGs are obtained, they are taken at different times during the resuscitation effort. Results are not correlated with whether the patient has been intubated (33,42). Sanders et al. (43) noted no significant differences in pH or $PaCO_2$ in survivors compared with nonsurvivors, but they did find that survivors tended to have a higher initial PaO_2.

Other Factors

No differences in outcome have been noted regarding time of cardiac arrest, presence of senior vs. junior members of the staff, and presence or absence of an anesthesiologist.

Patient Outcome

Of patients surviving cardiac arrest and subsequently being discharged, an annual death rate of ~10% for the first 5 years has been observed. Thereafter the death rate approaches that of the general population (7,33,44). The brain is especially vulnerable to the ischemic and anoxic insults associated with cardiac arrest. Indeed, many patients who die after cardiac arrest have ischemic brain damage as a secondary cause (45). Also, neurologic dysfunction has been noted in 2% of the long-term survivors (45).

Ischemic brain injury probably results from anoxia, which leads to a shift from aerobic to anaerobic metabolism. The ensuing lactic acidosis, besides being directly cytotoxic, leads to failure of critical membrane-bound ion pumps, notably calcium pumps. Calcium rapidly enters the neurons and leads to mitochondrial dysfunction and uncoupling of oxidative phosphorylation. Calcium also activates phospholipase and leads to generation of free fatty acids, particularly arachidonic acid. Metabolism of arachidonic acid then leads to production of oxygen free radicals, which cause further necrosis (46). Of note, ~90% of patients who are comatose after resuscitation will either regain consciousness or die within 36 h. The remaining 10% will remain in a vegetative state (45–47). Although a beneficial effect of calcium channel blockers in preventing neurologic dysfunction has been demonstrated experimentally (48,49), no beneficial effects have been confirmed clinically (50).

DO-NOT-RESUSCITATE ORDERS

In addition to moral and ethical consideration, the decision to perform CPR should be based on medical considerations, including an assessment of the expected outcome.

Recently, the Council of Ethical and Judicial Affairs (51) updated its resuscitation guidelines as follows:

1. Efforts should be made to resuscitate patients who suffer cardiac or respiratory arrest except when circumstances indicate that administration of CPR would be futile or not in accord with the desires or best interests of the patient.
2. Physicians should discuss with appropriate patients the possibility of cardiopulmonary arrest. Patients who are at risk of cardiac or respiratory failure should be encouraged to express, in advance, their preferences regarding the use of CPR. These discussion should include a description of the procedures encompassed by CPR and, when possible, should occur in an outpatient setting

Life Support and Management of Cardiac Arrest

when general treatment preferences are discussed, or as early as possible during hospitalization, when the patient is likely to be mentally alert. Early discussions that occur on a nonemergency basis help to ensure the patient's active participation in the decision-making process. In addition, subsequent discussions are desirable, on a periodic basis, to allow for changes in the patient's circumstances or in available treatment alternatives that may alter the patient's preferences.

3. If a patient is incapable of rendering a decision regarding the use of CPR, a decision may be made by a surrogate decision maker, on the basis of the previously expressed preferences of the patient or, if such preferences are unknown, in accordance with the patient's best interests.
4. The physician has an ethical obligation to honor the resuscitation preferences expressed by the patient or the patient's surrogate. Physicians should not permit their personal value judgments about quality of life to obstruct the implementation of a patient's or surrogate's preferences regarding the use of CPR. However, if, in the judgment of the treating physician, CPR would be futile, the treating physician may enter a do-not-resuscitate (DNR) order into the patient's record. When there is adequate time to do so, the physician must first inform the patient, or the incompetent patient's surrogate, of the content of the DNR order, as well as the basis for its implementation. The physician also should be prepared to discuss appropriate alternatives, such as obtaining a second opinion or arranging for transfer of care to another physician.
5. Resuscitative efforts should be considered futile if they cannot be expected either to restore cardiac or respiratory function to the patient or to achieve the expressed goals of the informed patient.
6. DNR orders, as well as the basis for their implementation, should be entered by the attending physician in the patient's medical record.
7. DNR orders only preclude resuscitative efforts in the event of cardiac arrest and should not influence other therapeutic interventions that may be appropriate for the patient.
8. Hospital medical staffs should periodically review their experience with DNR orders, revise their DNR policies as appropriate, and educate physicians regarding their proper role in the decision-making process for DNR orders.

SUMMARY

- Basic principles of management of the patient with cardiac arrest are to: (1) establish a secure, patent airway; (2) ventilate the patient; (3) provide artificial circulation; (4) restart the arrested heart
- Use jaw-thrust or chin-lift maneuvers to establish a patent airway. Endotracheal intubation is definitive. In emergencies, use oral, nasal, or transcricoid approaches. Avoid surgical cricothyoidotomy in children.
- After the airway has been established, use mouth-to-mouth resuscitation immediately, when necessary. Convert to bag/valve/mask as soon as possible.

- Begin chest compression in the absence of a pulse. Use compression of moderate force and short duration at a rate of 100–120 per min.

Pharmacologic Guidelines

Use:

- Epinephrine for cardiac arrest, ventricular fibrillation, ventricular tachycardia without a pulse, pulseless electrical activity, and patients who are unresponsive to initial defibrillatory attempts.
- Vasopressin for ventricular fibrillation that is refractory to shock. If used, administer immediately.
- Norepinephrine for significant hypotension or cardiogenic shock.
- Dopamine for patients who remain hypotensive after return of spontaneous circulation.
- Atropine for bradycardic dysrhythmias with hypotension, nodal atrioventricular block, and ventricular asystole.
- Sodium bicarbonate for patients with hyperkalemia, diabetic ketoacidosis, overdose with tricyclic antidepressants, cocaine overdose, and diphenhydramine overdose.
- Amiodarone for rapid ventricular response in patients with atrial dysrhythmias, after defibrillation and epinephrine in patients with pulseless ventricular tachycardia or shock refractory ventricular fibrillation, for hemodynamically stable ventricular tachycardia when cardioversion is unsuccessful, for atrial fibrillation when other treatments are ineffective.
- Lidocaine is now a second tier choice for suppression of ventricular dysrhythmias.
- Procainamide for suppression of PVCs and ventricular tachycardia not controlled with lidocaine.

Do not use:

- Calcium as first line therapy in cardiac arrest.

REFERENCES

1. Hermreck AS. The history of cardiopulmonary resuscitation. Am J Surg 1988; 156:430.
2. Guildner CW. Resuscitation—opening the airway. A comparative study of techniques for opening an airway obstructed by the tongue. J Am Coll Emerg Physicians 1976; 5:588.
3. Guildelines 2000 for cardiopulmonary resuscitation and emergency cardiovascular care. Circulation 2000; 102(suppl): I112–I158.
4. Iserson KV. Blind nasotracheal intubation. Ann Emerg Med 1981; 10:468.
5. Majernick TG, Bierrick R, Houston JB. Cervical spine movement during orotracheal intubation. Ann Emerg Med 1986; 15:417.
6. Attia RR, Battit GE, Murphy JD. Transtracheal ventilation. J Am Med Assoc 1975; 234:1152.
7. Dellinger RP, Mattox KL. Emergency resuscitation: what the books do not tell you. In: Civetta JM, Taylor RW, Kirby RR, eds. Critical Care. Philadelphia: JB Lippincott, 1988.
8. Kress TD. Cricothyroidotomy. Ann Emerg Med 1982; 11:197.
9. Sellick BA. Cricoid pressure to control regurgitation of stomach contents during induction of anesthesia. Lancet 1961; 2:404.
10. Shipman KH, McCrady W, Bradford HA. Closed chest cardiac resuscitation. Am J Cardiol 1962; 10:551.

11. Sykes MK, Orr DS. Cardiopulmonary resuscitation. Anaesthesia 1966; 21:363.
12. Kouwenhoven WB, Jude JR, Knickerbocker GG. Closed chest massage. J Am Med Assoc 1960; 173:1064.
13. Deshmukh NG, Weil MH, Gudpati CV, Trevino RP, Bisera J, Rackow EC. Mechanisms of blood flow generated by precordial compression during CPR. I. Studies of closed chest precordial compression. Chest 1989; 95:1092.
14. Halperin HR, Tsitlik JE, Guerci AD, Melllits ED, Levin HR, Shi AY, Chandra N, Weisfeldt ML. Determinants of blood flow to vital organs during cardiopulmonary resuscitation in dogs. Circulation 1986; 73:539.
15. Kaplin BM, Knott AP. Closed-chest cardiac massage for circulatory arrest. Arch Intern Med 1964; 114:5.
16. Ewy GA. Alternative approaches to external chest compression. Circulation 1986; 74(suppl IV):98.
17. Luce JM, Ross BK, O'Quinn, Culver BH, Sivarajan M, Amory DW, Niskanen RA, Alferness CA, Kirk WL, Pierson LB, Butler J. Regional blood flow during cardiopulmonary resuscitation in dogs using simultaneous and nonsimultaneous compression and ventilation. Circulation 1983; 67:258.
18. Martin GB, Carden DL, Nowak RM, Lewinter JR, Johnston W, Tomlanovich MC. Aortic and right atrial pressures during standard and simultaneous compression and ventilation CPR in human beings. Ann Emerg Med 1986; 15:125.
19. Sanders AB, Meislin NW, Ewy GA. The physiology of cardiopulmonary resuscitation: an update. J Am Med Assoc 1984; 252:3283.
20. Swenson RD, Weaver WD, Niskanen RA, Martin J, Dahlberg S. Hemodynamics in humans during conventional and experimental methods of cardiopulmonary resuscitaion. Circulation 1988; 19:1220.
21. Maier GW, Newton JR Jr, Wolfe JA, Tyson GS, Olsen CO, Glower DP, Spratt JA, Davis JW, Feneley MP, Rankin JS. The influence of manual compression rate on hemodynamic support during cardiopulmonary resuscitation. Circulation 1986; (suppl IV): 51.
22. Rosenthal RE, Turbiak TW. Open-chest cardiopulmonary resuscitation. Am J Emerg Med 1986; 4:248.
23. Stacpoole PW. Lactic acidosis. The case against bicarbonate therapy. Ann Intern Med 1986; 105:376.
24. Grundler W, Weil MH, Rackow EC, Falk JL, Bisera J, Miller JM, Michaels S. Selective acidosis in venous blood during human cardiopulmonary resuscitation: a preliminary report. Crit Care Med 1986; 13:153.
25. Weil MH, Rackow EC, Trevino R, Grundler W, Falk JL, Griffel MI. Difference in acid–base state between venous and arterial blood during cardiopulmonary resuscitation. N Engl J Med 1986; 315:153.
26. Schleien CL, Berkowitz ID, Traystman R, Rogers MC. Controversial issues in cardiopulmonary resuscitation. Anesthesiology 1989; 71:133.
27. Weil MH, Ruiz CE, Michaels S, Rackow EC. Acid–base determinants of survival after cardiopulmonary resuscitation. Crit Care Med 1985; 13:888.
28. Weil MH, Trevino RP, Rackow EC. Sodium bicarbonate during CPR: does it help or hinder? Chest 1985; 88:487.
29. Hughes WG, Ruedy JR. Should calcium be used in cardiac arrest? Am J Med 1986; 81:285.
30. Fiskum G. Mitochondrial damage during cerebral ischemia. Ann Emerg Med 1985; 14:810.
31. Stephenson NE. Cardiac Arrest and Resuscitation. St. Louis: CV Mosby, 1958.
32. Castagna J, Weil MH, Shubin H. Factors determining survival in patients with cardiac arrest. Chest 1974; 65:527.
33. Bedell SE, Delbanco TL, Cook EF, Epstein FH. Survival after cardiopulmonary resuscitation in the hospital. N Engl J Med 1983; 309:569.

34. Gulati RS, Bhan GL, Horan MA. Cardiopulmonary resuscitation of old people. Lancet 1983; 2:267.
35. Rozenbaum EA, Shenkman L. Predicting outcome of in-hospital cardiopulmonary resuscitation. Crit Care Med 1988; 16:583.
36. DeBard ML. Cardiopulmonary resuscitation: analysis of six years' experience and review of lieterature. Ann Emerg Med 1981; 10:408.
37. Pterson MW, Geist LJ, Schwartz DA, Konicek S, Moseley PL. Outcome after cardiopulmonary resuscitation in a medical intensive care unit. Chest 1991; 100:168.
38. Scott RPF. Cardiopulmonary resuscitation in a teaching hospital: a survey of cardiac arrests outside intensive care units and emergency rooms. Anaesthesia 1981; 36:526.
39. Stiles QR, Tucker BL, Meyer BW, Lindesmith GG, Jones JC. Cardiopulmonary arrest—Evaluation of an active resuscitation program. Am J Surg 1971; 122:282.
40. Peatfield RC, Sillett RW, Taylor D, MacNicol MW. Survival after cardiac arrest in hospital. Lancet 1977; 2:1223.
41. Hershey CO, Fisher L. Why outcome of cardiopulmonary resuscitation in general wards is poor. Lancet 1982; 1:31.
42. Snyder AB, Salloum LJ, Barone JE, Conley M, Todd M, DiGiacomo JC. Predicting short-term outcome of cardiopulmonary resuscitation using central venous oxygen tension measurements. Crit Care Med 1991; 19:111.
43. Sanders AB, Kern KB, Otto CW, Milander MM, Ewy GA. End-tidal carbon dioxide monitoring during cardiopulmonary resuscitation: a prognostic indication for survival. J Am Med Assoc 1989; 262:1347.
44. Messert B, Quaglieri CE. Cardiopulmonary resuscitation: perspectives and problems. Lancet 1976; 2:410.
45. Safar P. Cerebral resuscitation after cardiac arrest: a review. Circulation 1986; 74(suppl IV): 138, 153.
46. Seisjo BK. Mechanisms of ischemic brain damage. Crit Care Med 1988; 16:954.
47. Henneman EA. Brain resuscitation. Heart Lung 1986; 15:3.
48. Vaagenes P. Cantadore R, Safar P, Moossy J, Rao G, Diven W, Alexander H, Stezoski W. Amelioration of brain damage by lidoflazine after prolonged ventricular fibrillation cardiac arrest in dogs. Crit Care Med 1984; 12:846.
49. Winegar CP, Henderson O, White BC, Jackson RE, O'Hara T, Krause GS, Vigor DN, Kontry R, Wilson W, Shelby-Lane C. Early amelioration of neurologic deficit by lidoflazine after fifteen minutes of cardiopulmonary arrest in dogs. Ann Emerg Med 1983; 12:471.
50. Brain Resuscitation Clinical Trial 2 Study Group: a randomized clinical study of a calcium-entry blocker (lidoflazine) in the treatment of comatose survivors of cardiac arrest. N Engl J Med 1991; 324:1225.
51. Council on Ethical and Judicial Affairs. American Medical Association. Guidelines for the appropriate use of do-not-resuscitate orders. J Am Med Assoc 1991; 265:1868.

10
Evaluation of Hepatic Function

George M. Logan
Park Nicollet Clinical Gastroenterology, Minneapolis, Minnesota, USA

Joseph R. Bloomer
University of Alabama, Birmingham, Alabama, USA

The liver is involved in a wide variety of metabolic processes. Its roles include synthesis, biotransformation, and detoxification. Derangements in any of these functions can occur in the postoperative period as a result of the stress of surgery, the effects of anesthesia, or the unmasking of underlying liver disease. Patients with pre-existing liver disease are at increased risk for hepatic decompensation after surgery. The lack of controlled studies makes the precise prediction of the risk of surgery difficult in patients with liver disease. This chapter considers the evaluation of hepatic function to aid in the understanding and prediction of surgical risk.

EFFECTS OF ANESTHESIA AND SURGERY

Surgery, independent of the type of anesthesia administered, may produce transient increased concentrations in tests used to evaluate liver status. Transaminase concentrations show modest increases, usually in the range of doubling to tripling (1). These increases occur in 20% of surgical procedures. Rates as high as 61% are found in patients undergoing biliary tract surgery. Increased concentrations of alkaline phosphatase and bilirubin have been documented in 25–75% of patients after administration of most types of anesthetics (2). These findings are rarely of clinical significance.

The anesthetic agents used today for biliary tract surgery are not direct hepatotoxins, but they do reduce hepatic blood flow. Despite hepatic blood flow reduction, liver hypoxia has not been demonstrated in studies of normal volunteers undergoing general anesthesia (3). Additional intraoperative factors leading to liver dysfunction may be positive pressure ventilation, hypovolemia, and the use of vasoactive drugs. Patients with liver disease, especially those with portal hypertension, are more likely to have a decrease in hepatic blood flow during surgery. They may also have impaired metabolism of anesthetic agents and other drugs. Doses of sedatives, especially benzodiazepines and narcotics, should be reduced. In patients with decompensated liver disease, if the disease is severe, the use of sedatives should be eliminated. The metabolism of other agents also is affected. For example, the half-life of lidocaine is increased by 300% in liver disease.

RISK FACTORS FOR SURGERY

Liver dysfunction can be broadly divided into acute and chronic liver diseases. Cirrhosis is the advanced and irreversible stage of liver disease. Any of these three conditions are risk factors for hepatic surgery.

Acute Hepatitis

Acute hepatitis is associated with increases in the transaminase concentrations of aspartate aminotransferase (AST) and alanine aminotransferase (ALT), which rise to more than three times normal. Frequently, acute hepatitis is associated with increases of 10–20 times normal. Often the cause is viral. Hepatitis types A, B, or C have known viral etiologies. Currently, viral hepatitis can be diagnosed serologically. A 12-year series of more than 18,000 operations for hepatobiliary disorders at the Mayo Clinic from 1950 to 1961, a time before serologic tests were available, included 42 patients with presumed viral hepatitis (4). Of these 42 patients, 10% died postoperatively and an additional 12% had major morbidity.

In 1967, a retrospective study from the Massachusetts General Hospital reported 46,923 patients undergoing surgery and identified 73 patients with postoperative hepatic dysfunction. Of these 73 patients, 12 had unsuspected preoperative hepatic dysfunction, and 11 of the 12 patients died. In this study no distinction was made between acute and chronic liver diseases (5). Finally, Turner and Sherlock (6) reported 42% mortality and 33% hepatic decompensation in patients with acute hepatitis. In contrast, Hardy and Hughes (7) reported a series of 14 patients with acute viral hepatitis who underwent laparotomy and suffered no morbidity or mortality. These observations support the delay of elective surgery in acute viral hepatitis until the patient recovers clinically and biochemically.

Chronic Hepatitis

Chronic hepatitis is defined by an increase in serum transaminase concentrations that persists for 6 months or more. A wide variety of hepatic disorders, including alcoholic liver disease, chronic viral hepatitis, drug-induced hepatitis, autoimmune hepatitis, and primary biliary cirrhosis, are causes of chronic hepatitis.

A series of 20 patients with chronic hepatitis collected at a single institution from 1970 to 1982 is reported by Runyon (8). Runyon noted that all the patients in the series were thought to have chronic viral hepatitis, although a viral etiology was not certain in 15 of the 20 with non-A non-B hepatitis. The group was characterized by normal values or mild abnormalities in bilirubin, albumin, and prothrombin time (PT). No mortality occurred in the group after a total of 34 operations. Although some patients had transient elevations in bilirubin, the increase did not reach statistical significance.

Although this population has not been extensively studied for surgical risk, the risk of surgery, in general, would be expected to correlate with the level of impairment in hepatic synthetic function.

Cirrhosis

Cirrhosis is the irreversible stage of chronic liver disease characterized by fibrosis that disrupts the normal hepatic lobular architecture. The most common cause of cirrhosis in the USA is chronic alcoholism, but chronic hepatitis B infection is the most common cause worldwide. Less common causes include viral hepatitis C, viral hepatitis D, chronic active hepatitis of autoimmune origin, primary biliary cirrhosis, and secondary biliary cirrhosis. Secondary biliary cirrhosis is usually a result of chronic extrahepatic biliary obstructions. The inherited disorders, hemochromatosis, alpha-1-antitrypsin deficiency, and Wilson's disease, also may cause cirrhosis. In addition, cirrhosis may arise from chronic right heart failure. Those cases in which no cause is determined are called cryptogenic cirrhosis.

Patients with chronic liver disease and cirrhosis who are undergoing surgery have been the focus of several studies. A review of 429 patients undergoing cholecystectomy during a period of 8 years at the Hines VA hospital in Illinois revealed that 12.8% of patients had cirrhosis (9). The operative mortality among those patients free of liver disease was 1.1%. Among those with cirrhosis, PTs within 2.5 s of control were found in 78%. In this group operative mortality was elevated (9.3%). Operative mortality rose to 83% among those patients in whom PTs were prolonged >2.5 s above control.

Child's classification for cirrhosis and Pugh's (10) modification of this classification provide a method of predicting surgical risk in patients with cirrhosis (Table 1). Using the related Child–Turcotte–Pugh system, Poggio studied laparoscopic and open cholecystectomy in class A and class B patients (11). Of the 26 patients in the laparoscopic cholecystectomy group, only 3 required conversion to open cholecystectomy. Shorter

Table 1 Methods of Predicting Surgical Risk in Patients with Cirrhosis

Factor	A (minimal)	B (moderate)	C (advanced)
Child's classification:[a]			
Serum bilirubin (mg/dL)	<2	2–3	>3
Serum albumin (mg/dL)	>3.5	3–3.5	<3
Ascites	None	Controlled	Refractory
Encephalopathy	None	Minimal	Advanced, "coma"
Nutrition	Excellent	Good	Poor, "wasting"

Clinical/biochemical measurements	Points for increasing abnormality		
	1	2	3

Pugh's modification:[b]			
Encephalopathy	None	Minimal	Advanced
Ascites	Absent	Slight	Moderate
Bilirubin (mg/dL)	1–2	2–3	>3
Albumin (g/dL)	>3.5	2.8–3.5	<2.8
Prothrombin time (seconds prolonged)	1–4	4–6	>6
For primary biliary cirrhosis, bilirubin (mg/dL)	1–4	4–10	>10
Child–Pugh class	A	B	C
Scoring (points)	5–6	7–9	10–15

[a]Modified from Child CG III, Turcotte J. In: Child CG III, ed. The Liver and Portal Hypertension. Philadelphia: WB Saunders, 1965.
[b]Modified from Pugh RNH, Murray-Lyon IM, Dawson JL, et al. Transection of the esophagus for bleeding esophageal varices. Br J Surg 1973; 60:646–649.

surgical times and decreased transfusion requirement were observed in the laparoscopic group. The open cholecystectomy group comprised 24 patients. Both groups were similar in Child–Turcotte–Pugh class distribution; 71% of the patients were class A in the open cholecystectomy group and 85% of the patients were class A in the laparoscopic cholecystectomy group. Neither group included any class C patients. No mortality occurred in either group.

Endoscopic biliary drainage is an alternative approach to treatment of severe acute cholangitis. Lai et al. (12) reported a significantly lower mortality rate of 10% for endoscopic therapy vs. 32% for surgical drainage in patients with cholangitis and choledocholithiasis. For this procedure too, Child's classification is a prognostic factor. In a series of 52 patients with cirrhosis undergoing endoscopic therapy for obstructive biliary disease with choledocholithiasis (13), overall 5-day (early) mortality was 7.7%, and all deaths occurred in the Child's C class where the mortality rate was 22%. In contrast, a series of 69 patients with cirrhosis undergoing peptic ulcer emergency surgery for bleeding or perforation had an overall mortality rate of 54% (14). The patients were not categorized by Child–Pugh class. The risk of colectomy in patients with cirrhosis was documented by Metcalf et al. (15). Significant predictors of increased mortality were encephalopathy, ascites, low hemoglobin, and low albumin. Low risk patients had an operative mortality of 12.8%. A mortality rate of 53.3% was observed in the high-risk group. In cardiac surgery, the role of Child's class as a predictor of mortality was demonstrated by Klemperer et al. (16). In this retrospective series of 13 patients with cirrhosis, all 8 with class A liver disease survived to hospital discharge, but only 1 of 5 class B patients survived to discharge.

Garrison et al. (17) have retrospectively studied various predictors of surgical risk in a series of 100 cirrhotic patients undergoing abdominal operations other than portasystemic shunts. Predictors of surgical mortality were prolonged PT, prolonged partial thromboplastin time (PTT), pre-existing infection, depressed serum albumin, and Child's classification (Table 2). Similar findings were reported by Doberneck et al. (18) In their series of 102 patients, an increased mortality was demonstrated for a wide variety of operative procedures. The operative mortality for intraperitoneal procedures was 35%, and the overall mortality was 20%. The major risk factors identified in this study were jaundice and prolonged PT. A series of 51 patients with alcoholic cirrhosis undergoing abdominal surgery reported by Aranha and Greenlee (19) in 1986 had an overall mortality

Table 2 Predictors of Surgical Mortality in Patients with Cirrhosis[a]

Variable	Mortality (%)
Child's class	
A	10
B	31
C	76
Ascites	58
Infection	64
Prothrombin time > 1.5 s > control	63
Albumin < 3 mg/dL	58

[a]Modified from Ref. (17).

of 67%. The risk factors associated with increased mortality were PT > 2.5 s above control, emergency surgery, and ascites.

Ziser et al. (20) retrospectively reviewed 10 years of surgery on patients with cirrhosis at the Mayo Clinic. In this group of 733 patients, a mortality rate of 11.6% was observed. A multivariate analysis was performed and factors associated with mortality included: male gender, Child–Pugh score, ascites, diagnosis of cryptogenic cirrhosis, creatinine concentration, and preoperative infection.

Bariatric surgery is associated with the discovery of unanticipated cirrhosis in 1.4% of patients in the series reported by Brolin et al. (21). In this group, they found an operative mortality risk of 4% in the perioperative period and 5.6% in the late period. These rates are five times higher than those seen in patients without cirrhosis. The role of steatohepatitis progressing to cirrhosis in these patients can be estimated from the reported rates of progression to cirrhosis in nonalcoholic steatosis of 4–15% (21–24). The use of clinical and laboratory variables in the obese to predict the presence of fibrosis has shown significant predictors of age >49, a body mass index of >27.9 kg/m^2, triglycerides >1.69 mmol/L, and an ALT > 2× the upper limit of normal (25). Patients meeting one or more of these criteria are candidates for preoperative liver biopsy to identify cirrhosis.

The importance of hepatic reserve is shown in a series that assessed hepatic function via the aminopyrine breath test (26). In this study, 30 of 31 patients with a normal preoperative test survived abdominal surgery; whereas, 6 of 7 patients with depressed values died. Despite its small size, this study showed statistically significant differences in survival. The aminopyrine breath test also has been used in medical patients to predict survival. Merkel et al. (27) demonstrated a decline in aminopyrine breath test results in patients with cirrhosis in the last year of life.

The role of hepatic reserve in predicting survival also is seen in the patient undergoing hepatic resection for malignancy. Redaelli et al. (28) demonstrated improved survival in patients with higher galactose elimination capacity, another measure of hepatic capacity for metabolism. Additional reports suggest that dynamic functional testing with agents such as lidocaine and indocyanine green predicts hepatic reserve. However, none of these agents has been demonstrated in large studies to significantly improve prognosis beyond that provided by the Child–Pugh classification. Currently, their use is limited.

INDICATIONS FOR PREOPERATIVE METABOLIC SUPPORT

Patients with liver disease are at risk for nutritional deficits. In a group of 284 patients with liver disease, Mendenhall et al. (29) showed that all of the patients showed some evidence of malnutrition. Although malnutrition increases surgical risk, patients with liver disease often cannot tolerate oral repletion. Their associated malabsorption and anorexia limit oral intake. Parenteral nutrition may cause an increase in ascites and also may promote hepatic encephalopathy. However, modification of total parenteral nutrition formulas to provide branched-chain amino acids has been shown to improve hepatic encephalopathy. Fischer et al. (30,31) used an amino acid mixture, enriched in branched-chain amino acids and deficient in aromatic amino acids and methionine, along with hypertonic glucose. This approach was based on the knowledge that increased serum concentrations of aromatic amino acids occur in patients with cirrhosis. The aromatic amino acids are usually catabolized in the liver. This function is diminished in liver disease as a result of decreased functional capacity and, in patients with cirrhosis, shunting of portal blood around the liver. The branched-chain enriched amino acids stimulate protein synthesis, which results in a decrease in the circulating concentration of the aromatic amino acids. Further, the branched-chain amino acids compete with aromatic amino acids for transfer across the blood–brain barrier. This competition reduces the level of aromatic amino acids in the brain and cerebral spinal fluid and improves the aminergic neurotransmitter profile.

Prospective randomized controlled trials on protein-intolerant patients with liver disease who were resistant to standard treatments for hepatic encephalopathy have shown that infusions of branched-chain enriched amino acids produce faster and more complete recovery of patients and greater improvement in encephalopathy (32). These solutions permitted nutritional support in this group of patients, who would be otherwise intolerant of such supplementation. Two studies using enteral solutions with branched-chain amino acid enrichment showed a definite improvement in positive nitrogen balance and definite improvement in hepatic encephalopthy (33,34). Although these studies show benefit to patients by these measures, no survival benefit has been demonstrated (35). A year-long trial of daily postoperative branched-chain amino acid oral supplementation given to patients after curative resection for hepatocellular carcinoma showed significant improvement in the supplement group for asterixis, ascites, edema, and performance status (36). In this study too, there was no survival benefit of the supplementation.

Patients with encephalopathy that cannot be controlled by the usual measures of lactulose and/or neomycin administration should have metabolic support to clear the encephalopathy in the preoperative period.

ASSESSMENT OF THE PREOPERATIVE PATIENT

The history and physical examination of the preoperative patient are the most important parts of the evaluation. When the history is taken, attention should be given to inclusion of hepatitis, icteric episodes, exposure to hepatotoxins, and transfusion of blood products. Because many drugs produce deleterious hepatic effects, the use of current and recent medications (including over-the-counter agents) should be documented. Any family history of liver disease should be noted. Past and present alcohol use should be documented. Direct inquiries about arrests for driving while intoxicated and prior chemical dependency treatment should be made. Systemic symptoms of chronic liver disease, such as easy fatigue and lassitude, should be documented.

On physical examination, signs of liver disease should be sought. These signs include spider nevi, palmar erythema, gynecomastia, hepatosplenomegaly, and caput medusae. When signs of portal hypertension are present, Child's classification should be determined. This classification includes an examination for ascites, hepatic encephalopathy, and nutritional status.

Laboratory evaluation should be undertaken for patients with a history of hepatitis. Testing of these individuals should include screening for hepatitis C antibody, hepatitis A antibody IgM fraction, hepatitis A antibody IgG fraction, hepatitis B surface antigen, AST, ALT, total and direct bilirubin, alkaline phosphatase, gammaglutamyl transpeptidase (GGT), albumin, PT, and complete blood count. If these values are normal, the patient is probably not at increased risk for surgery. If the findings suggest acute hepatitis, elective surgery should be deferred until resolution of the condition is complete. In the case of significant laboratory abnormalities, a thorough evaluation for the cause should be undertaken before all but urgent surgery is done.

Patients with evidence of chronic hepatitis may require liver biopsy to determine the cause and extent of liver damage. Those with cholestasis, evidenced by increased alkaline phosphatase and confirmed by increased GGT or 5'-nucleotidase, require imaging of the biliary tree. Usually the use of ultrasonography is satisfactory, but sometimes endoscopic retrograde cholangiopancreatography is necessary to evaluate the possibility of extrahepatic ductal disease. Patients with evidence of cirrhosis should have careful evaluation of coagulation function. Many of these patients have poor nutrition and are deficient in vitamin K. If the PT is elevated, testing should be repeated 12–24 h after administration of a subcutaneous dose of vitamin K, which may be repeated if no improvement in the PT is observed. PTs that remain elevated >3 s beyond the control values after administration of vitamin K_1 may respond to infusion of fresh frozen plasma. Unfortunately, large volumes of plasma are often required and the response is transient. The splenomegaly of portal hypertension may cause thrombocytopenia. In cirrhotic patients with chronic alcohol use, direct toxic effects on the bone marrow also may reduce the platelet count.

Patients with cirrhosis should be evaluated for ascites. If present, the ascitic fluid should be tested for evidence of infection. A total white blood cell count of >500 cells/mm^3 or a polymorphonuclear cell count of >250 cells/mm^3 provide the best evidence of presumptive bacterial infection. Ascitic fluid and blood cultures should be obtained. Ascitic fluid should be sterile and controlled with diuretics to whatever extent is possible before abdominal surgery. Treatment should include salt restriction to 1 g of sodium chloride per day and a potassium sparing diuretic. Careful monitoring of serum electrolytes, weight, girth, urine sodium, and renal function all are important in the preoperative management of these patients. If the patient's volume status is uncertain, central venous pressure monitoring is helpful.

Patients with decompensated hepatic function are at risk for renal impairment. Care should be taken to avoid the use of potentially nephrotoxic drugs. Patients who are in this group appear to be at particular risk for renal toxicity from NSAIDs and aminoglycoside antibiotics. Hypovolemia should be avoided.

The patient should also be evaluated for the presence of hepatic encephalopathy. When extreme, the diagnosis is apparent. Clinical findings include confusion, asterixis, and increased serum ammonia concentration. However, mild encephalopathy can be detected by the more subtle findings of day–night reversal and psychometric testing. Hepatic encephalopathy should be treated medically prior to surgery, if possible. Therapy includes the use of oral lactulose, neomycin, or both. Lactulose acts as a laxative and creates an acidic colonic lumen in which the conversion of absorbable ammonia (NH_3) to nonabsorbable ammonium (NH_4^+) is favored. If these measures do not control the hepatic encephalopathy, or if the patient is malnourished and requires protein supplementation (which worsens the hepatic encephalopathy), nutritional support with solutions enriched in branched-chain amino acids should be administered.

SUMMARY

- Patients with liver disease have increased surgical risk.
- Surgical risk is proportional to severity of liver disease. Risk correlates with Child–Pugh classification.
- Delay all surgery, except emergency surgery, in Child–Pugh classification C cirrhosis, acute viral hepatitis, or acute alcoholic hepatitis.

- Correct reversible features of liver disease, including malnutrition, hepatic encephalopathy, coagulopathy, renal insufficiency, and ascites, before surgery.
- Evaluate ascitic fluid preoperatively for possibility of bacterial infection.
- Carefully evaluate and treat malnutrition, hepatic encephalopathy, coagulopathy, renal insufficiency, and ascites in the postoperative period for improved patient outcome.

REFERENCES

1. Ayres PR, Williard TB. Serum glutamic oxalacetic transaminase levels in 266 surgical patients. Ann Intern Med 1960; 52:1279–1288.
2. LaMont JT. Postoperative jaundice. Surg Clin North Am 1974; 54:637–645.
3. Price HL, Deutsch S, Davidson IA, et al. Can general anesthetics produce splanchnic visceral hypoxia by reducing regional blood flow? Anesthesiology 1966; 27:24–32.
4. Harville DD, Summerskill WHJ. Surgery in acute hepatitis: causes and effects. JAMA 1963; 184:257–261.
5. Dykes MHM, Walzer SG. Preoperative and postoperative hepatic dysfunction. Surg Gynecol Obstet 1967; 124:747–751.
6. Turner MD, Sherlock S. In: Smith R, Sherlock S, eds. Surgery of the Gallbladder and Bile Ducts. London: Butterworth, 1964.
7. Hardy KJ, Hughes ESR. Laparotomy in viral hepatitis. Med J Aust 1968; 1:710.
8. Runyon BA. Surgical procedures are well tolerated by patients with asymptomatic chronic hepatititis. J Clin Gastroenterol 1986; 8:542–544.
9. Aranha GV, Sontag SJ, Greenlee HB. Cholecystectomy in cirrhotic patients: a formidable operation. Am J Surg 1982; 143:55–59.
10. Pugh RNH, Murray-Lyon IM, Dawson JL, Pietroni MC, Williams R. Transection of the oesphagus for bleeding oesophageal varices. Br J Surg 1973; 60:646–649.
11. Poggio JL, Rowland CM, Gores GJ, Nagorney DM, Donohue JH. A comparison of laparascopic and open cholecystectomy in patients with compensated cirrhosis and symptomatic gallstone disease. Surgery 2000; 127:405–411.
12. Lai ECS, Mok FPT, Tan ESY, Lo C, Fan S, You K, Wong J. Endoscopic biliary drainage for severe acute cholangitis, N Engl J Med 1992; 326:1582–1586.
13. Prat F, Tennenbaum R, Ponsot P, Altman C, Pelletier G, Fritsch J, Choury A, Bernades P, Etienne J. Endoscopic sphincterotomy in patients with liver cirrhosis. Gastrointest Endosc 1996; 43:127–131.
14. Lehner T, Herfarth C. Peptic ulcer surgery in patients with cirrhosis. Ann Surg 1993; 217:338–346.
15. Metcalf AMT, Dezois RR, Wolff BG, Beahrt RW. The surgical risk of colectomy in patients with cirrhosis. Dis Col Rect 1987; 30:529–531.
16. Klemperer JD, Ko W, Krieger KH, Connolly M, Rosengart TK, Altorki NK, Lang S, Isom OW. Cardiac operations in patients with cirrhosis. Ann Thorac Surg 1998; 65:85–87.
17. Garrison RN, Cryer HM, Howard DA, Polk HC. Clarification of risk factors for abdominal operations in patients with hepatic cirrhosis. Ann Surg 1984; 199:648–655.
18. Doberneck RC, Sterling WA Jr, Allison DC. Morbidity and mortality after operation in nonbleeding cirrhotic patients. Am J Surg 1983; 146:306–309.
19. Aranha GV, Greenlee HB. Intra-abdominal surgery in patients with advanced cirrhosis. Arch Surg 1986; 121:275–277.
20. Ziser A, Plevak DJ, Wiesner RH, Rakela J, Offord KP, Brown DL. Morbidity and mortality in cirrhotic patients undergoing anesthesia and surgery. Anesthesiology 1999; 90:42–53.

21. Brolin RE, Bradley LJ, Taliwal RV. Unsuspected cirrhosis discovered during elective obesity operations. Arch Surg 1998; 133:84–88.
22. Matteoni CA, Younossi ZM, Gramlich T, Boparai N, Liu YC, McCullough AJ. Nonalcoholic fatty liver disease: spectrum of clinical and pathological severity. Gastroenterology 1999; 116:1413–1419.
23. Pinto HC, Baptista A, Camilo ME, Valente A, Saragoca A, de Moura MC. Nonalcoholic steatohepatitis. Clinicopathological comparison with alcoholic hepatitis in ambulatory and hospitalized patients. Dig Dis Sci 1996; 41:172–179.
24. Lee RG. Nonalcohlic steatohepatitis: a study of 49 patients. Hum Pathol 1989; 20:594–598.
25. Dixon JB, Bhathal PS, O'Brien PE. Nonalcohlic fatty liver disease: predictors of nonalcohlic steatohepatitis and liver fibrosis in the severely obese. Gastroenterology 2001; 121:91–100.
26. Gill RA, Goodman MW, Golfus GR, Onstad GR, Bubrick MP. Aminopyrine breath test predicts surgical risk or patients with liver disease. Ann Surg 1983; 198:701–704.
27. Merkel C, Morabito A, Sacerdoti D, Bolognesi M, Angeli P, Gatta A. Updating prognosis of cirrhosis by Cox's regression model using Child–Pugh score and aminopyrine breath test as time-dependent covariates. Ital J Gastroenterol Hepatol 1998; 30:276–282.
28. Redaelli CA, Dufour JF, Wagner M, Schilling M, Husler J, Krahenbuhl L, Buchler MW, Reichen J. Preoperative galactose elimination capacity predicts complications and survival after hepatic resection. Ann Surg 2002; 235:77–85.
29. Mendenhall CL, Anderson S, Weesner RE, Goldberg SJ, Crolic KA. Protein–calorie malnutrition associated with alcoholic hepatitis. Am J Med 1984; 6:211–222.
30. Fischer JE, Funovics JM, Aguirre A, James JH, Keane JM, Wesdorp RI, Yoshimura N, Westman T. The role of plasma amino acids in hepatic encephalopathy. Surgery 1975; 78:276–290.
31. Fischer JE, Rosen HM, Ebeid AM, James JH, Keane JM, Soeters PB. The effect of normalization of plasma amino acids on hepatic encephalopathy in man. Surgery 1976; 80:77–91.
32. Cerra FB, Cheung NK, Fischer JE, Kaplowitz N, Schiff ER, Dienstag JL, Bower RH, Mabry CD, Leevy CM, Kiernan T. Disease specific amino acid infusion (F080) in hepatic encephalopathy: a prospective, randomized, double-blind, controlled trial. J Parenter Enter Nutr 1985; 9:288–295.
33. Keohane PP, Attrill H, Grimble G, Spiller R, Frost P, Silk DB. Enteral nutrition in malnourished patients with hepatic cirrhosis and acute encephalopathy. J Parenter Enter Nutr 1983; 7:345–350.
34. Marchesini G, Dioguardi FS, Bianchi GP, Zoli M, Bellati G, Roffi L, Martines D, Abbiati R. Long-term branched-chain amino acid treatment in chronic hepatic encephalopathy. A randomized double-blind casein-controlled trial. The Italian Multicenter Study Group. J Hepatol 1991; 11:92–101.
35. Nompleggi DJ, Bonkovsky HL. Nutritional supplementation in chronic liver disease: an analytical review. Hepatology 1994; 19:518–533.
36. The San-in group of Liver Surgery. Long term oral administration of branched chain amino acids after curative resection of hepatocellular carcinoma: a prospective randomized trial. Br J Surg 1997; 84:1525–1531.

11
The Surgical Patient and Renal Failure

Mark E. Rosenberg
University of Minnesota, Minneapolis, Minnesota, USA

Ricardo Correa-Rotter
Instituto Nacional de la Nutricion,
Salvador Zubbiran, Mexico City, Mexico

INTRODUCTION

Acute renal failure (ARF) constitutes a highly lethal condition when associated with surgery or trauma (45–70% mortality) despite significant improvement in dialytic treatment in the last decades. Prevention of this complication relies on early identification of predisposing risk factors and careful preoperative evaluation of the patient's renal function. As a variety of conditions may be responsible for the development of ARF in the surgical patient, determining the etiology of ARF is imperative to provide adequate therapy. The classification of ARF into prerenal, renal, or postrenal causes is presented in Chapter 34. Acute tubular necrosis (ATN), a term often used interchangeably with ARF, is the most common form of ARF observed after trauma or surgery.

This chapter first focuses on predisposing risk factors and measures to prevent the development of ARF, with particular emphasis on the basic principles for preoperative assessment of renal function. Next, special problems often encountered in association with the development of ARF will be discussed. Finally, guidelines for the preoperative evaluation and management of the patient with known chronic renal failure (CRF) will be presented.

RISK FACTORS AND PRECIPITATING CONDITIONS

Common risk factors and precipitating conditions that favor the development of ARF are listed in Table 1. When two or more of these conditions are present in a given patient, the effect is additive, and the risk for the development of ARF is increased. In addition to the factors shown in Table 1, conditions that may favor the development of ARF are the severity of the disease leading the patient to the surgical intervention, the nature of the surgery (emergency or elective), and the presence and severity of underlying medical conditions, particularly heart failure, diabetes mellitus, and liver disease. The presence of severe Gram-negative sepsis accompanied by diminished effective circulating volume (septic shock) constitutes a common cause of ARF in the surgical patient and often may be

Table 1 Factors Associated with the Development of Acute Renal Failure in the Surgical Patient

Age over 50 years
Diabetes mellitus
Volume depletion
Nephrotoxic agents
Underlying intrinsic renal disease
Underlying vascular disease
Hypertension
Sepsis
Major cardiovascular intervention
Intravascular hemolysis
Abdominal aortic aneurysm surgery
Cardiopulmonary bypass
Long-standing obstructive uropathy

part of a syndrome of sequential multiple organ system failure. In this condition, prompt diagnosis and early aggressive treatment should be undertaken, because Gram-negative sepsis is associated with extremely high mortality.

PREOPERATIVE EVALUATION OF KIDNEY FUNCTION

An adequate assessment of the patient's renal function and fluid and electrolyte balance provides vital information for recognizing those who are prone to develop ARF in the postoperative period. A complete history and thorough physical examination provide valuable data regarding previous and current pathologic conditions, drug intake history, and estimation of extracellular volume status. Laboratory determination of glomerular filtration rate (GFR) (discussed subsequently), plasma creatinine (PCr), serum electrolytes, and urinalysis complement the preoperative evaluation.

A major initiative of the National Kidney Foundation was the publication in February, 2002 of clinical practice guidelines for chronic kidney disease (CKD). These guidelines include standardized terminology for the classification and stratification of CKD. In these guidelines "kidney" replaces "renal" in an attempt to improve the understanding by patients, families, health care providers, and the lay public. The definition of CKD as quoted directly from these guidelines is:

1. Kidney damage for ≥3 months, as defined by structural or functional abnormalities of the kidney, with or without decreased GFR, manifest by either:
   a. Pathological abnormalities or
   b. Markers of kidney damage, including abnormalities in the composition of the blood or urine, or abnormalities in imaging tests
2. GFR <60 mL/min per 1.73 m^2 for ≥3 months, with or without kidney damage

In this report, CKD was divided into stages of severity on the basis of GFR (Table 2). In Stage 1, kidney damage is present, but GFR is preserved and includes such patients as those with albuminuria or abnormal imaging studies. For example, a patient with polycystic kidney disease with cysts detected by ultrasound but with a normal GFR would be classified as Stage 1. Similarly, a patient with type 1 diabetes, normal GFR,

Surgical Patient and Renal Failure

Table 2 Stages of Chronic Kidney Disease

Stage	Description	GFR (mL/min per 1.73 m^2)
1	Kidney damage with normal or increased GFR	>90
2	Kidney damage with mild decrease in GFR	60–89
3	Moderate decrease in GFR	30–59
4	Severe decrease in GFR	15–29
5	Kidney failure	<15 or dialysis

and microalbuminuria would also be Stage 1. The definition of proteinuria and albuminuria for different collection methods is provided in Table 3. Stage 2 includes patients with evidence of kidney damage with decreased GFR (60–89 mL/min per 1.73 m^2). The gudielines recognize the fact that decreased GFR can occur in the absence of kidney damage, a condition seen in infants and older adults, individuals on vegetarian diets, patients after unilateral nephrectomy, or individuals with prerenal causes such as CHF and cirrhosis. Finally, all patients with GFR <60 mL/min per 1.73 m^2 are classified as having CKD whether or not kidney damage is present.

The staging of CKD has many advantages. Having a common classification scheme will facilitate defining the epidemiology of CKD and its complications. This classification will provide a common language for practitioners and their patients involved in the clinical care and research of CKD. The system also provides a framework for the evaluation, including the preoperative assessment, and management of patients with CKD.

Estimating GFR

A critical requirement for the accurate classification of CKD is the measurement or estimation of GFR. Serum creatinine measurement is not an accurate marker of GFR. Creatinine is not an ideal filtration marker. Because it is both filtered at the glomerulus and secreted by the proximal tubule, creatinine clearance can overestimate GFR by as much as 40% in normal individuals and even more in patients with CKD. In CKD patients, the degree of overestimation is often unpredictable. Many other factors, including protein

Table 3 Definition of Proteinuria and Albuminuria

Total protein	Value
Proteinuria	
24 h excretion	>300 mg/day
Protein/creatinine ratio	>200 mg/g
Spot urine	>30 mg/dL
Microalbuminuria	
24 h excretion	30–300 mg/day
Albumin/creatinine ratio	17–250 mg/g (men)
	25–355 mg/g (women)
Spot urine	>3 mg/dL
Albuminuria	
24 h excretion	>300 mg/day
Albumin/creatinine ratio	>250 mg/g (men)
Spot urine	>355 mg/g (women)

Table 4 Causes of Increased Serum Creatinine without a Change in GFR

Substances measured as noncreatinine chromagens with
  alkaline picrate method
    Acetoacetate and acetone
    Ascorbic acid
    Cephalosporins
Massive increase in creatinine production
  Rhabdomyolysis
Decrease in creatinine excretion (PCr increase of <0.5 mg/dL)
  Trimethoprim
  Cimetidine

intake, age, sex, ethnicity, body weight, muscle mass, diet, and drugs such as cimetidine (Table 4) influence plasma creatinine concentrations and creatinine excretion. Variation in the instrument calibration for measuring creatinine is another potential source of error. On a practical level, estimates of GFR based on serum creatinine require timed urine collections, which often can be inaccurate. Classic methods for measurement of GFR, such as inulin clearance, are cumbersome, require an intravenous infusion and timed urine collections, and are not clinically feasible for serial measurements in the clinic setting. Normal GFR based on inulin clearance and adjusted to a standard body surface area of 1.73 m^2 is 127 mL/min/1.73 m^2 for men and 118 mL/min/1.73 m^2 for women. After age 30 the average decrease in GFR is 1 mL/min/1.73 m^2/year.

Excellent alternatives to inulin clearance include the urinary clearance of radioactive filtration markers such as ^{125}I-iothalamate and ^{99m}Tc-DTPA. The plasma clearances of other markers such as iohexol or ^{51}Cr-EDTA have also been used to measure GFR but are not widely available. Other methods include creatinine clearance after cimetidine administration to block tubular secretion and the use of cystatin C.

Equations based on serum creatinine with factors for sex, age, and ethnicity are the best alternative for estimation of GFR. The most commonly used formula is the Cockcroft–Gault equation. This equation was developed to predict creatinine clearance but has been used for estimating GFR. The formula is:

$$\text{CrCl (mL/min)} = \frac{140 - \text{Age}}{\text{Serum creatinine} \times 72 \times (0.85 \text{ if female})} \quad (1)$$

The MDRD Study equation used the urinary clearance of ^{125}I-iothalamate as the standard. The formula was derived from data obtained in over 500 patients with a wide variety of kidney diseases with a GFR up to 90 mL/min/1.73 m^2. A separate group of patients was used to validate the equation. Four different versions of this formula exist and have similar accuracy. The abbreviated equation is recommended for routine use and requires only serum creatinine, age, sex, and race information. This formula is:

$$\text{GFR (mL/min/1.73 m}^2\text{)} = 186 \times (\text{SCr})^{-1.154} \times (\text{Age})^{-0.203} \times (0.742 \text{ if female}) \\ \times (1.210 \text{ if African American}) \quad (2)$$

The use of this formula clearly illustrates the inaccuracies of using serum creatinine

Surgical Patient and Renal Failure 143

to estimate GFR. As CKD is defined as a GFR <60 mL/min/1.73 m^2, then for a 50-year-old man, CKD would be defined as a serum creatinine of 1.3 mg/dL, and for a 50-year-old woman, a serum creatinine of 1.03 mg/dL. In children, GFR should be estimated using the Schwartz or Counahan–Barratt equation.

It is important to note that serum or plasma creatinine varies inversely with the GFR. This nonlinear reciprocal relation between creatinine and GFR is demonstrated in Fig. 1. As is evident from the figure, an apparently small increase in creatinine (from 1 to 2 mg/dL) can represent a loss of almost 50% of the GFR (Fig. 1). The use of serum creatinine and the GFR estimation formulas apply only to patients in steady state. For instance, a rapid fall in GFR will be followed by a delayed creatinine increase, because some time is necessary for creatinine to accumulate in plasma.

Assessment of Volume Status

Maintenance of adequate extracellular volume is mandatory, as volume depletion is a major risk factor for the development of ARF. Some of the clinical and laboratory variables useful in estimating the volume status of the patient are listed in Table 5. The history of intake/output and weight can prove to be of great value in conjunction with the physical examination. If apparent volume depletion is noted (with or without overt oliguria), urinary sodium determination, urinalysis, and urinary indices, in conjunction with GFR estimation, can aid in distinguishing prerenal azotemia from established ATN (see Chapter 34). In some patients, particularly those with sepsis and hepatic or cardiac failure, estimation of volume status may be difficult. If the volume status is in doubt, central venous pressure or pulmonary capillary wedge pressure measurements are warranted.

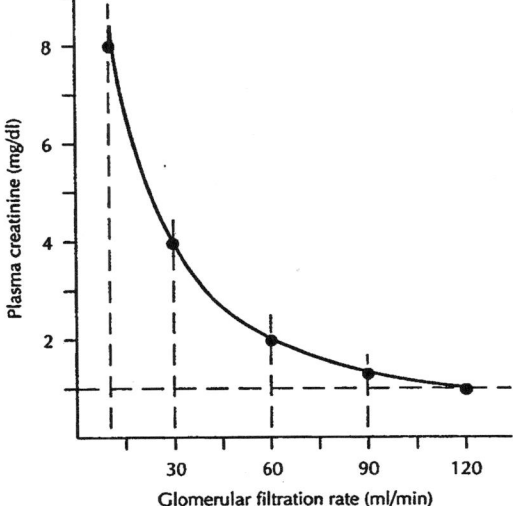

Figure 1 The reciprocal relation between GFR and PCr concentration is graphed. The hyperbolic nature of this relationship is illustrated. For example, in a patient with normal renal function, an apparently small increase in PCr from 1 to 2 mg/dL reflects a major fall in GFR (from 120 to 60 mL/min); whereas, in a patient with established renal failure, an increase in PCr from 4 to 8 mg/dL represents a relatively small reduction in GFR (from 28 to 14 mL/min).

Table 5 Estimation of Extracellular Volume Status

History
    Fluid input and output history
        decreased intake
        gastrointestinal loss (vomiting, diarrhea, hemorrhage, bowel obstruction)
        renal loss (diuretics, glycosuria, adrenal insufficiency)
        internal loss or redistribution of extracellular fluid (pancreatitis, peritonitis, severe hypoalbuminuria)
Physical examination
    Skin turgor
    Moisture of mucous membranes
    Postural blood pressure and pulse changes
    Jugular venous distension
    Chest examination (pulmonary edema, S_3 gallop, arrhythmia, pericardial rub)
    Abdominal examination (ascites, hepatomegaly)
    Peripheral edema or anasarca
    CVP or PCWP
Laboratory values
    Urinary sodium
    Urinary indices (see Chapter 34)
    BUN/Cr ratio
    Serum electrolytes

Assessment of Electrolytes

Determination of plasma electrolyte concentrations, including sodium, potassium, chloride, bicarbonate, calcium, phosphorus, and magnesium, should be part of the preoperative assessment of renal function. Identification of potentially hazardous electrolyte abnormalities, such as hyperkalemia in the patient with volume depletion or established renal insufficiency, is critical. Additionally, serum electrolyte analysis provides important information in patients suspected of having acid–base disorders, a common complication of emergency surgery. If an acid–base disorder is suspected, arterial blood gases should be obtained: an acid–base disorder cannot be accurately diagnosed on the basis of serum bicarbonate alone. The total serum calcium concentration is influenced by the serum concentration of albumin. For every 1 gm/dL decrease in serum albumin, the serum calcium is lower by 0.8 mg/dL. This correction, or measurement of ionized calcium, should be applied when interpreting plasma calcium concentrations.

SPECIFIC PROBLEMS

Radiocontrast-Induced ARF

Although noninvasive body imaging procedures such as ultrasonography, computerized tomography, and magnetic resonance imaging are in widespread use, radiographic procedures requiring infusion of a contrast medium often are required for diagnostic purposes in the surgical patient. Acute renal failure develops in a significant number of patients who receive radiocontrast material. Although ARF has been reported after exposure to a contrast medium given by various routes (oral, intravenous, or intra-arterial), its incidence following intra-arterial administration seems to be greater.

In the general population, the incidence of radiocontrast medium-induced ARF is very low (0–5%), but it is significantly higher (10–50%) in some high risk subpopulations. Identification of risk factors associated with radiocontrast medium-induced ARF plays a key role in preventing the development of this complication. Table 6 summarizes these risk factors. The principal predisposing factor for contrast nephropathy is the presence and severity of underlying renal insufficiency. Diabetic patients with normal renal function do not have an increased risk for the development of contrast nephropathy; yet, those with moderate or severe renal impairment appear to be at significantly greater risk than those with similar degrees of renal dysfunction from other causes. Exposure to large amounts or repeated doses of radiocontrast also may increase the risk and severity of contrast nephropathy. Three generations of radiocontrast agents are available for use. The first generation agents were ionic and of high osmolality (1500–1800 mOsmol/kg). The second generation agents such as iohexol, are nonionic and of lower osmolality (600–850 mOsmol/kg). The third generation agents, of which iodixanol is an example, are both nonionic and iso-osmolar to plasma (290 mOsmol/kg). The nonionic agents are associated with less nephrotoxicity in high risk patients when compared with the ionic high osmolality agents. Available data suggest that the nonionic iso-osmolal agents have the least nephrotoxicity.

Once the risk factors have been identified, the strategies in Table 7, which are aimed at preventing the development of contrast nephropathy, should be followed. Other agents such as mannitol, low dose dopamine, and furosemide have not been associated with a reduced incidence of nephrotoxicity and, in some cases, have been associated with more toxicity. Newer agents, such as fenoldopam, are being evaluated for their ability to reduce radiocontrast-induced ARF.

Drug-Induced ARF

Treatment of intercurrent medical problems (e.g., infection and analgesia) requires the use of drugs, most of which undergo renal excretion. In the patient with established renal failure, accumulation of these drugs and their metabolites will reach toxic levels unless adequate dosage adjustments are made. On the other hand, the administration of a nephrotoxic drug to a surgical patient constitutes a risk factor for the development of ARF. The addition of a nephrotoxic agent in the presence of other concomitant risk factors may have

Table 6 Risk Factors for Radiocontrast Medium-Induced ARF

Pre-existing renal failure
Diabetes mellitus
Congestive heart failure
Large dose of contrast material
Hyperosmolal ionic contrast agents
Two doses within 48 h
Volume depletion
NSAIDs
Multiple myeloma
Peripheral vascular disease

Table 7 Prevention of Radiocontrast Medium-Induced ARF

Identification of risk factors
Use of noninvasive imaging studies whenever possible
Administration of smallest possible radiocontrast dose
Use of nonionic low osmolality agents
Avoid volume depletion and NSAIDs
Saline hydration to maintain urine output 150–200 mL/h, D5W 1/2 NS at 1 mL/kg per h for 12 h prior to and 12 h after procedure
Acetylcysteine 600 mg PO bid the day prior to and the day of the procedure

an additive effect on the induction of renal dysfunction. The best way to prevent drug nephrotoxicity is to avoid using nephrotoxic drugs in the surgical patient, particularly if other risk factors are also present. Yet, this approach often is not possible. If nephrotoxic agents must be administered, keep in mind the possibility of inducing renal dysfunction in order to detect it early and adjust drug dosages. Newer, less nephrotoxic drugs such as the third generation cephalosporins and fluoroquinolones should be used when appropriate, instead of other more nephrotoxic drugs such as the aminoglycosides.

The degree of renal dysfunction directly influences the extent of drug accumulation. For proper adjustment of drug doses, the level of renal function must be determined. Endogenous CrCl or its estimation from serum creatinine [see Eq. (1)] can be used to establish the patient's renal function and provide guidelines for adjusting drug doses. If renal function is already decreasing rapidly (e.g., in ARF), PCr will overestimate renal function; therefore, drug dosages should be administered as for a patient with severe renal failure (CrCl < 10 mL/min). Dosage adjustment in these patients can be performed according to clinical course, continued monitoring of renal function, and serum drug concentrations, if available. Information regarding dosage reduction and degree of removal by dialysis for most drugs is readily available.

Cardiovascular Surgery and ARF

ARF occurs in a high percentage of patients who undergo open heart surgery (5–25%). During cardiopulmonary bypass, the kidneys are underperfused. The duration of bypass usually correlates with the severity of renal failure. Although renal circulatory compromise is the major determinant of renal dysfunction after open heart surgery, other factors participate in its pathogenesis. For example, trauma to the blood during extracorporeal circulation induces hemolysis and can activate the complement system. Other contributing factors for the development of ARF are the common occurrence of postoperative cardiac dysfunction, which leads to continued renal circulatory compromise, and the use of postoperative artificial ventilation, which may alter inferior vena cava hemodynamics by impairing venous return to the thorax. The increased intrathoracic pressure generated by positive pressure ventilation may lead to pooling of blood in the inferior vena cava and to an increase in renal venous pressure.

Adequate blood flow and perfusion pressure should be ensured during the period of extracorporeal circulation to reduce the incidence of ARF. Careful monitoring of blood pressure, maintenance of a cardiac index exceeding 2.5 L/min/m^2, and cautious use of vasodilators are recommended in the postoperative period in order to avoid significant reductions in renal flow below the kidney's autoregulatory range. Also, the period of mechanical artificial ventilation should be as short as possible to avoid hemodynamically mediated impairment of renal function.

Aortic surgery (e.g., grafting of an aortic aneurysm) poses a very high risk for the development of ARF. Suprarenal aortic clamping, a procedure sometimes necessary to perform the grafting, is responsible for temporary interruption of blood flow to the kidneys. The incidence of ARF and the degree of renal dysfunction seem to be closely related to the length of the surgical procedure. If a lengthy interruption of renal artery blood flow is expected, consideration should be given to a shunt to the distal renal artery in order to maintain kidney perfusion.

CHRONIC RENAL FAILURE

During the past two decades a significant improvement has occurred in the prognosis of patients with renal disease who subjected to elective or emergency surgery. Better dialytic procedures are probably the major element in this improved outcome, as more intensive dialysis ensures better fluid and electrolyte balance and may improve impaired clotting mechanisms, immune function, and wound healing. In addition to the routine preoperative evaluation, the renal patient will require special assessment of factors that may favor the development of perioperative complications.

Dialysis

The patient already under dialytic treatment must undergo preoperative dialysis to correct hyperkalemia and acidosis, improve volume status, and reduce the amount of uremic toxins that may be involved in the platelet dysfunction of CRF. As heparin is usually required for hemodialysis, having the patient undergo dialysis the day prior to surgery will allow sufficient time for the metabolism of the remaining heparin. If the patient is using peritoneal dialysis and is not undergoing abdominal surgery, then dialysis can be performed according to the patient's usual schedule in the preoperative period and as needed in the postoperative period. Often switching to an automated peritoneal dialysis cycler will be necessary postoperatively. Abdominal surgery in the peritoneal dialysis patient will necessitate a temporary switch to hemodialysis.

Patients with moderate kidney failure who are not yet having chronic dialysis and require surgery may undergo the surgical procedure safely with adequate conservative management of their fluid, electrolyte, and metabolic abnormalities. This subset of patients must be monitored very closely, because dialysis may need to be initiated in the event of renal function deterioration in order to prevent the appearance of uremic complications that would further complicate the patient's course. The presence of uremic manifestations as well as volume and electrolyte abnormalities unresponsive to conservative treatment are indications for immediate dialytic therapy (see Chapter 35).

Anesthesia

When the choice of a general anesthetic agent in a patient with chronic renal failure is being made, the drug's metabolism and elimination route must be taken into consideration. Metabolic acidosis may potentiate the effect of some neuromuscular blocking agents. In addition, some of these drugs (neuromuscular blockers) can favor the development of acute hyperkalemia. In general, common inhalational anesthetics such as halothane and methoxyflurorane are well tolerated by the patient with CRF, although the latter should be avoided in patients with residual renal function as it is potentially nephrotoxic.

Bleeding Disorders

Bleeding disorders are common in CRF. Platelet dysfunction and abnormal platelet–vessel interactions are the most significant clotting defects seen in uremia. These functions are adversely influenced by anemia. In most instances, platelet dysfunction will not cause excessive operative bleeding, if the patient has undergone proper dialysis and is not under the influence of chronic antiplatelet treatment sometimes prescribed to maintain patency of arteriovenous fistulas. All dialysis patients and CKD patients with GFR <50 mL/min per 1.73 m^2 are candidates for the preoperative administration of 1-deamino-8-D-arginine vasopressin (DDAVP or desmopressin) (0.3 μg/kg IV). This agent will restore hemostasis within 1 h of administration and its effect will last up to 8 h. The effects of DDAVP are attenuated with repeated dosing. Conjugated estrogens have also been shown to reduce bleeding when given at a dose of 0.6 mg/kg per day, starting 6–12 h before surgery and continued for a period of up to 5 days. Other measures include treatment with cryoprecipitate and normalization of the hemoglobin. It is critical to discontinue those drugs that interfere with platelet function, such as nonsteroidal anti-inflammatory agents or aspirin.

Anemia

Anemia is an almost universal complication of CRF. The hematocrit starts to decrease when the GFR falls below 50 mL/min. The primary mechanism of anemia is erythropoietin deficiency but other factors, such as decreased red blood cell lifespan, iron deficiency, and blood loss, may contribute to the anemia. Recombinant erythropoietin (r-HuEPO) or longer acting analogs are available to treat the anemia of renal failure in both predialysis and dialysis patients. Therapy with r-HuEPO results in a dose-dependent increase in hematocrit and obviates the need for transfusion therapy. The starting dose for r-HuEPO is usually between 50 and 150 U/kg, administered subcutaneously once per week with adjustment of dose or frequency based on patient response. Hemoglobin concentration should be monitored every 1–2 weeks at the beginning of r-HuEPO therapy or after a change in dose, and then every 4–12 weeks thereafter. BP should be monitored closely as r-HuEPO therapy has been associated with an increase in BP. To avoid true or functional iron deficiency, oral or, in some cases, parenteral iron should be administered. Transferrin saturations should be kept >20% and ferritin concentrations >100 ng/mL. In dialysis patients, r-HuEPO is administered intravenously three times per week with each dialysis session. An alternative form of erythropoietin, darbopoietin (ARANESP^{TM}), has a longer half-life when compared with r-HuEPO and allows a decreased dosing frequency.

Calcium, Phosphorus, and Magnesium

As renal function deteriorates, abnormalities in calcium, phosphorus, and magnesium homeostasis occur. (For a review of the pathophysiology the reader is referred to the

Surgical Patient and Renal Failure

references.) Lowering serum phosphorus concentration to between 3.0 and 4.6 mg/dL is a major goal of therapy in patients with CKD, both to prevent the development of secondary hyperparathyroidism and to keep the calcium–phosphorus product below 55 mg^2/dL^2 to avoid metastatic calcification. Aluminum containing antacids have been used as phosphate binders and are still the agents of choice when the calcium–phosphorus product is >70. Problems with aluminum accumulation with consequent osteodystrophy have led to a search for alternative long-term phosphate binders. At present, calcium carbonate, calcium acetate, and the non-calcium phosphate binder sevelamer are alternatives. If time permits, serum calcium and phosphorus concentrations should be normalized prior to surgery and monitored closely during the postoperative period. As magnesium balance is normally maintained by the kidney, hypermagnesemia can occur as a complication of renal failure. Magnesium concentrations should be followed closely as a general rule, and excessive magnesium intake should be avoided in the patient with end-stage renal disease. This restriction includes avoiding magnesium-containing antacids and enemas, which are rich sources of magnesium.

In the postoperative period, in addition to the usual care measures, the renal patient needs to be monitored very closely for abnormalities in intravascular volume, electrolytes, and acid–base balance, as the normal homeostatic mechanisms provided by the kidney are lacking (see Chapter 34). Increased catabolism or the systemic inflammatory response syndrome may favor a faster accumulation of nitrogenous compounds. Dialysis requirements need to be evaluated on a continuing basis as the patient recovers from the surgical procedure.

SUMMARY

Preoperative Assessment

- Identify risk factors for the development of acute renal failure to prevent complications and allow for earlier interventions.
- Assess for the presence and stage of CKD, including the calculation of estimated GFR.
- Assess volume status and the presence of fluid and electrolyte disorders by history, physical examination, and laboratory measurements.
- Recognize and minimize nephrotoxic exposures.
- Identify risk factors for radiocontrast-induced acute renal failure and institute prophylactic therapy, including minimizing the dose of contrast media, saline hydration, and acetylcysteine.
- Recognize that the nature of the surgical procedure also may increase the risk for the development of ARF (e.g., open heart surgery involving cardiopulmonary bypass and aortic surgery).

Management of the Surgical Patient with CRF

- Include in the preoperative assessment a careful assessment of extracellular volume, serum electrolytes, and acid–base status.
- Provide preoperative dialysis if indicated.

- Optimize the hemoglobin prior to the surgical procedure using recombinant erythropoietin and iron therapy as indicated.
- Optimize calcium, phosphorus, and magnesium levels prior to surgery.
- Assess bleeding risk and treat with DDAVP or other agents to minimize intraoperative bleeding.
- Adjust drug dosages to the level of kidney function.

BIBLIOGRAPHY

1. Bellomo R, Chapman M, Finfer S, et al. Low-dose dopamine in patients with early renal dysfunction: a placebo-controlled randomised trial. Lancet 2000; 356:2139–2143.
2. Conger, JD. Interventions in clinical acute renal failure: what are the data? Am J Kidney Dis 1995; 26:565–576.
3. Levey AS, Bosch J, Lewis JB, et al. A more accurate method to estimate glomerular filtration rate from serum creatinine: a new prediction equation. Ann Int Med 1999; 130:461–470.
4. Murphy SW, Barrett BJ, Parfrey PS. Contrast nephropathy. J Am Soc Nephrol 2000; 11:177–182.
5. National Kidney Foundation: K/DOQI clinical practice guidelines for chronic kidney disease: evaluation, classification, and stratification. Am J Kidney Dis 39 2002; (Suppl 1):S1–S266.
6. Schwab SJ, Hlatky MA, Pieper KS, et al. Contrast nephrotoxicity: a randomized controlled trial of a nonionic and an ionic radiographic contrast agent [see comments]. N Engl J Med 1989; 320:149–153.
7. Solomon, R, Werner, C, Mann, D, et al. Effects of saline, mannitol, and furosemide on acute decreases in renal function induced by radiocontrast agents. N Engl J Med 1994; 331:1416–1420.
8. Solomon, R. Contrast-medium-induced acute renal failure. Kidney Int 1998; 53:230–242.
9. Star RA. Treatment of acute renal failure. Kidney Int 1998; 54:1817–1831.
10. Thompson BT, Cockrill BA. Renal-dose dopamine: a siren song? Lancet 1994; 344:7–8.
11. Tepel M, Van Der Giet M, Schwarzfeld C, et al. Prevention of radiographic-contrast-agent-induced reduction in renal function by acetylcysteine. N Engl J Med 2000; 343:180.

12
Perioperative Pulmonary Complications and Pulmonary Risk Assessment

Paul Druck
VA Medical Center, Minneapolis, Minnesota, USA

INTRODUCTION

Preoperative pulmonary assessment has two goals: to help decide whether the proposed procedure is justified on the basis of its risk:benefit ratio, and to help identify features that may be improved to reduce risk. Benefit is based on an understanding of the natural history of the underlying disease to be treated and the likelihood that the proposed intervention will improve that course. The accuracy of this estimate varies considerably for different conditions and interventions. Risk is the observed incidence of complications resulting from the proposed intervention. When derived from the review of large numbers of such interventions, this risk can be predicted with great accuracy for *average populations*. However, the considerable variability among *risk subgroups* limits the usefulness of such unstratified data for the individual. Unfortunately, the enormous number of possible combinations of circumstances and comorbidities makes compilation of risk tables impractical for every possible patient. Therefore, risk assessment is always a population-derived *estimate* to be informed and guided by knowledge of individual patient variables and by sound judgment.

In the following sections, we will briefly discuss the nature of postoperative pulmonary complications (PPCs) and their underlying pathophysiology, methods available to estimate risk, variables that can affect risk estimates for the *individual*, and strategies to minimize risk.

NATURE AND INCIDENCE OF POSTOPERATIVE PULMONARY COMPLICATIONS

PPCs have been described as occurring after fewer than 5% to as many as 70% of surgical procedures. This enormous range is explained by real differences in incidence, a consequence of patient and procedure variables, as well as by variability in the definitions of complications used in the past reviews (1,2). Most current analyses restrict the term "pulmonary complication" to mean pneumonia, macroatelectasis, clinically significant gas-exchange abnormalities, pneumothorax, persistent bronchopleural fistula, and respiratory insufficiency necessitating prolonged postoperative mechanical ventilation. These complications necessitate additional treatments such as antibiotics or mechanical ventilation, affect outcome variables such as hospital or ICU length of stay and costs, and have significant impact on the patient. Past reviews predict pulmonary complications after ~10–50% of lung resection procedures (less frequently after nonresectional thoracic procedures) (3–5), 10–20% of major abdominal procedures, and <10% of extremity procedures (1,2).

POSTOPERATIVE PULMONARY PATHOPHYSIOLOGY

A number of pathologic changes in pulmonary mechanics and function occur during and after general anesthesia and surgery, which predispose the patient to PPCs. These changes are most pronounced after abdominal and thoracic surgery and are minimal in extra coelomic procedures. They include decreased static and dynamic lung volumes, decreased flow rates, altered ventilatory patterns, and impairment of intrinsic pulmonary defense mechanisms.

During general anesthesia, functional residual capacity (FRC, the sum of the residual and expiratory reserve volumes) is decreased by ~20%. If this decrease is sufficient to cause end-expiratory volume to fall below the *closing volume* (the lung volume below which airway closure occurs), atelectasis may occur (6,7). Even when such atelectasis is subsegmental and not easily appreciated on chest roentgenogram (*microatelectasis*), it can be documented and quantified on CT and accounts for at least a part of the increased intrapulmonary shunt and hypoxemia observed during and after general anesthesia (8). Increased physiologic dead space is also observed during anesthesia and may persist into the postanesthetic period (6). Despite resumption of spontaneous breathing postoperatively, the reduction of FRC, along with resultant atelectasis and hypoxemia, persists for ≥1 week (2). Deep breathing, sighing, and coughing (whose main benefit may be the deep breath preceding the cough) may be suppressed by pain as well as opioid analgesics, thus impairing the normal corrective response to atelectasis.

After abdominal surgery in particular, diaphragmatic dysfunction results in a shift in ventilatory mechanics from abdominal (diaphragmatic) breathing to ribcage (intercostal muscle) breathing (7,9,10). Resting tidal volume may decrease by as much as 20%, and forced vital capacity (FVC) and forced expiratory volume in one second (FEV$_1$) may decrease by as much as 65% after thoracic or upper abdominal surgery (2). These impairments are somewhat less for lower abdominal surgery or laparoscopic procedures. Laparoscopic cholecystectomy, for example, is associated with approximately half the postoperative loss of FVC and FEV$_1$ as that seen with open cholecystectomy (11,12). Atelectasis (mentioned earlier) decreases pulmonary compliance and further predisposes the lungs to loss of static and tidal volumes in the first days following surgery (6). Finally, mucociliary clearance may be impaired during and shortly after anesthesia, an alteration that increases the likelihood of infection (13,14). It is important to remember that these effects are temporary; pulmonary function generally returns to preoperative baseline in a week or less if pulmonary complications such as pneumonia are not superimposed.

Thoracotomy without lung resection produces changes comparable with those seen after upper abdominal surgery. The resection of lung tissue causes further impairment whose magnitude is related to the amount and functional status of lung tissue being resected. Furthermore, unlike the transient postoperative abnormalities described earlier, the loss of function secondary to lung resection is persistent. Excessive loss of ventilatory capacity may result in permanent dependence on mechanical ventilation. Approximately 90% of patients with lung cancer (the most common indication for lung resection) have some evidence of chronic obstructive pulmonary disease (COPD), and 20% have severe disease (15). Lung resection also entails a loss of pulmonary capillary bed, which increases pulmonary vascular resistance. Patients with normal cardiopulmonary function generally tolerate this increase in pulmonary vascular resistance well, but compromised patients may develop significant pulmonary hypertension.

ESTIMATING THE RISK: PREOPERATIVE ASSESSMENT

Numerous studies over several decades have noted an association among chronic pulmonary disease, abnormal spirometry [pulmonary function tests (PFTs)], and PPCs, and have, therefore, suggested using spirometry to predict the risk of complications. Extensive review demonstrates serious methodological flaws in many studies and suggests, on the basis of the remaining valid studies, that spirometry's ability to predict pulmonary complications after abdominal surgery is not superior to clinical assessment (16,17). Examples of observations that correlate significantly with pulmonary risk are: an abnormal chest roentgenogram or the need for perioperative bronchodilators (18), American Society of Anesthesiologists (ASA) Class >2, upper abdominal surgery, residual intraperitoneal sepsis, age >59, BMI >25, preoperative hospital stay >4 days, colorectal or gastroduodenal surgery (19), and mucus hypersecretion and lung hyperinflation (20). Fuso et al. (21), however, did observe predictive value of decreased FEV_1 (<61% of predicted) and of hypoxemia. FEV_1, maximum voluntary ventilation (MVV), and diffusing capacity of the lung for carbon monoxide (DLCO) have more accurately predicted complications after lung resection surgery than after abdominal surgery (22). The available data do not support an important contribution of spirometry to prediction of postoperative complications after abdominal surgery. In a 1990 consensus statement, the American College of Physicians acknowledged the lack of objective data in support of preoperative spirometry in non-lung resection surgery, but still recommended preoperative spirometry for patients with a history of smoking or dyspnea prior to thoracic or abdominal surgery (23). Some patients will already have had PFTs prior to their referral for surgery. Values that have been associated with a high risk of complications are: FEV_1 <2 L or <50% of predicted, MVV <50% of predicted, and vital capacity (VC) <70% of predicted (7,21,24,25).

Assessing the risk of lung resection surgery is more complicated, because estimating the additional functional impairment caused by loss of resected lung tissue of uncertain functional status is difficult. Preresection evaluation has evolved from simple spirometry through "split lung function studies," to "radiospirometry," which utilizes radioisotopic ventilation and perfusion scanning to estimate the functional contribution of the lung tissue to be resected. Cardiopulmonary exercise testing with measurement of VO_2 max (maximal oxygen uptake during exercise) and DLCO have also been predictive of outcome in some studies. For a more detailed discussion of controversies and current recommendations in this area, which is beyond the scope of this chapter, see a textbook of thoracic surgery or related references (3,15,26,27).

Finally, Kroenke et al. (18) and Gerson et al. (28) have noted the strong association between cardiac and pulmonary complications and suggested that preoperative *cardiopulmonary* risk assessment should be integrated. When evaluating patients preoperatively, the clinician should remember that even severe pulmonary impairment does not guarantee postoperative complications; conversely, good preoperative function does not ensure freedom from pulmonary risk.

RISK FACTORS FOR PPCs

Patient-Specific Factors

Pre-existing pulmonary disease, especially chronic obstructive disease, is the most commonly recognized factor predisposing to pulmonary complications (1,2,18,21,29–31). An important subgroup consists of those patients with active respiratory infections at the time of surgery. Respiratory infections may be exacerbated after surgery, possibly as a consequence of additional, superimposed pulmonary impairment, or the immune dysfunction that often accompanies trauma, infection, or surgery. An increased risk of wound infection in patients with pneumonia at the time of surgery has also been noted. From the standpoint of outcome analysis, a patient with a preoperative respiratory infection will emerge from surgery with the same, or an exacerbated, infection, and thus experience what amounts to a 100% pulmonary complication rate. Surgery should be deferred in such patients, if possible, until the acute infection is resolved (see the section on Treating Active Respiratory Infections).

A strong and consistent relationship between smoking and PPCs has been observed (1,2,32,33). Smoking produces a variety of pathologic changes in pulmonary function including hypersecretion of mucus and decreased mucociliary clearance (34), increased closing volume (35), decreased surfactant production and increased bronchial reactivity (36), and obstruction in small peripheral airways (37). Chronic smokers eventually develop features of COPD, the severity of which correlate with the risk of PPCs. *Asymptomatic* smokers, on the other hand, usually have no spirometric evidence of COPD but still manifest many of the effects of smoking, such as increased sputum production, decreased mucociliary clearance, and increased closing volume. Although asymptomatic smokers are generally considered to be at increased risk, little objective evidence is available (38,39).

Other factors such as poor general physical condition (19,40) and very limited exercise tolerance (29,41) are strongly associated with pulmonary complications. Although some studies find advanced age to be a significant risk factor (19,20,42,43), studies that control for actual comorbid conditions find little effect of age *per se* (18,40,44). Similarly, obesity is generally believed to increase pulmonary risk (2,19,20,45), but most studies do not confirm increased risk when they control for other factors such as the presence and magnitude of preoperative pulmonary impairment (46,47). Male gender is inconsistently associated with a higher risk of pulmonary complications (1,20,33). Although malnutrition is a known risk factor for infection and poor wound healing in general, data analyzing the influence of malnutrition on pulmonary function after surgery are inadequate.

Procedure-Specific Factors

Type and Duration of Anesthesia

The choice of anesthetic technique (general vs. regional) may be dictated by the operative procedure, thus confounding analysis of the influence of anesthesia on complication rates.

Studies that either compare site-matched procedures or randomize patients to one or the other anesthetic technique, generally fail to show differences in overall or pulmonary outcomes (48–50). A recent, large, meta-analysis (141 studies, 9559 patients) did identify an advantage of regional anesthesia with respect to mortality, overall morbidity, and pulmonary morbidity, but noted that the differences were extremely small and required the statistical power of such a large study (51).

Similarly, the duration of a surgical procedure is usually a consequence of the nature of the procedure. Although some reviews have identified increased anesthesia duration as a risk factor for pulmonary complications, especially pneumonia [>3 h (2), >4 h (33,41), or >6.5 h (40)], others have not (1,52), particularly when duration was controlled for the nature of the operation.

Site and Orientation of Incision

That the likelihood of pulmonary complications is greatest for upper abdominal surgery or thoracotomy, intermediate for lower abdominal surgery, and least for extremity procedures is a consistent observation that suggests that the distance of the incision from the diaphragm is an important factor. This observation has not been rigorously studied (1,7,22,30,31,33).

The belief that transverse abdominal incisions produce less pulmonary impairment and, therefore, fewer complications than vertical incisions is commonly held (7,53,54). However, a study of 24 patients undergoing upper abdominal surgery via upper midline vs. subcostal incisions failed to demonstrate a difference in pre- vs. postoperative spirometry or in the rate of complications for the two approaches (55). This finding may be explained by the fact that the cephalad extent (and thus proximity to the diaphragm) of upper midline and subcostal incisions is similar. On the other hand, for procedures that can be performed through a transverse incision whose distance from the diaphragm is greater than that of the upper extent of the alternative vertical incision, an advantage may be realized, not because of orientation *per se*, but because of absolute proximity to the diaphragm. This hypothesis has not been rigorously studied in a controlled, prospective manner.

MODIFYING PULMONARY RISK

Preoperative

Treating Active Respiratory Infections

Respiratory infections should be treated to resolution prior to elective surgery (see the section on Patient-Specific Factors). However, a procedure may be so urgently required that it should not be delayed, even in the face of a serious pulmonary infection. In patients with chronic bronchitis, the distinction between baseline bronchitis (which may resemble an acute infection but will not respond to antibiotic treatment) and exacerbation (which should be treated) may be difficult to make. The assistance of the patient's primary care physician or a pulmonologist may be valuable. Patients with an exacerbation of chronic bronchitis benefit from a 10-day course of antibiotics (33).

Optimizing Pulmonary Function in Patients with Chronic Pulmonary Disease

Several studies (29,49,56) have demonstrated a significant reduction in PPC in patients who began a program of deep breathing, coughing, and postural drainage, preoperatively.

Preoperative abstinence from smoking is also important (see the section on Cessation of Smoking). Decreased pulmonary complications have been observed in patients with COPD who received bronchodilators (30) or bronchodilators plus steroids preoperatively (33,49). Optimization of bronchodilator therapy is particularly important in patients with asthma (57). The advice and assistance of a pulmonologist or the patient's regular primary care provider should be sought when beginning or optimizing a bronchodilator regimen, or beginning a tapering dose of steroids prior to surgery. Airflow studies are usually needed to guide changes in regimen.

Cessation of Smoking

Many effects of smoking, such as mucus hypersecretion, decreased mucociliary clearance, and increased small airway resistance, are improved by abstinence. Whereas little change in symptoms is seen after abstinence of 1–2 weeks, progressive improvement does occur over 4–6 weeks (37,38,58). A large prospective study of patients undergoing elective coronary artery bypass demonstrated a significant decrease in pulmonary complications in patients who had abstained from smoking for 8 weeks prior to surgery as compared with those who had not (59). Whether lesser periods of preoperative abstinence, such as 4 or 6 weeks, would be useful remains unproven. Certainly, brief periods such as ≤1 week do not reduce pulmonary complications, and may needlessly delay surgical treatment. Abstaining from smoking for 24–48 h preoperatively may confer *cardiovascular* benefits, however, as a consequence of lowered carbon monoxide and nicotine levels.

Intraoperative

Once in the operating suite, final decisions regarding choice of anesthetic technique and incision may be made with the intent to minimize postoperative pulmonary impairment. The physician or surgeon should recognize that, with the exception of avoiding an upper abdominal or thoracic incision when that option exists, the impact of these choices will be slight.

Postoperative

Postoperative Analgesia

Adequate pain control is essential for maneuvers that are associated with normalization of pulmonary function postoperatively, such as deep breathing, coughing, and early ambulation. Numerous methods are available to achieve such pain relief, including intermittent parenteral opioid analgesics, patient-controlled analgesia (PCA), and epidural local anesthetics or opioids. PCA generally achieves comparable or better analgesia than intermittent bolus opioids, often with less total drug usage, but no data demonstrate fewer PPCs (60,61). Studies of epidural vs. parenteral postoperative analgesia are complicated by variable use of intraoperative epidural analgesia with light general anesthesia. Although most studies have demonstrated that epidural analgesia is associated with better postoperative spirometric parameters of lung function than parenteral analgesia, most have failed to demonstrate a corresponding reduction in pulmonary complications (62–65).

Postoperative Respiratory Therapy

The interpretation of studies comparing different postoperative respiratory care regimens is complicated by the use of different combinations of multiple modalities, and variable inclusion of a preoperative period of preparation. The following conclusions emerge. Postoperative atelectasis, with attendant hypoxia and decreased pulmonary compliance, is decreased by deep breathing maneuvers. No difference has been observed between incentive spirometry and simple, scheduled, deep breathing (66,67). Cough may be beneficial in patients with large volumes of secretions to clear, but, for other patients, coughing may offer no benefit beyond that of the preceding deep breath. The use of intermittent positive pressure breathing and continuous positive airway pressure, postoperatively, have also been studied, and, although some studies have demonstrated improved spirometry with these treatments, no decrease in the rate of PPCs has been realized (68–70).

SUMMARY

- Pulmonary complications are the most common postoperative complications, but their incidence varies widely and depends on the underlying pulmonary condition of the patient and the nature of the operative procedure.
- The most important preoperative risk factor is pre-existing pulmonary disease. Important procedural variables include proximity of the incision to the diaphragm and resection of lung tissue. Of lesser importance is type of anesthesia and duration of procedure.
- Preoperative estimation of the risk of pulmonary complications may be accomplished by a focused history and physical examination. With the exception of planned lung resections, spirometry (PFTs) adds little to this assessment, but may help in optimizing bronchodilator therapy, preoperatively.
- The likelihood of PPCs in patients with respiratory disease may be reduced by preoperative optimization. Preoperative considerations should include deep breathing exercises, optimizing or in some cases beginning bronchodilator or steroid regimens, and stopping smoking for 8 weeks preoperatively. In addition, surgery should be deferred until active infections are treated, if possible.
- Postoperative therapies associated with reduction of pulmonary complications include deep breathing exercises and adequate analgesia.

REFERENCES

1. Wightman JAK. A prospective survey of the incidence of postoperative pulmonary complications. Br J Surg 1968; 55:85–91.
2. Latimer RG, Dickman M. Ventilatory patterns and pulmonary complications after upper abdominal surgery determined by preoperative and postoperative computerized spirometry and blood gas analysis. Am J Surg 1971; 122:622–632.
3. Ferguson MK, Little L, Rizzo L, Popovich KJ, Glonek GF, Leff A, Manjoney D, Little AG. Diffusing capacity predicts morbidity and mortality after pulmonary resection. J Thorac Cardiovasc Surg 1988; 96:894–900.
4. Nagasaki F, Flehinger BJ, Martini N. Complications of surgery in the treatment of carcinoma of the lung. Chest 1982; 82:25–29.
5. Smith TP, Kinasewitz GT, Tucker WY, Spillers WP, George RB. Exercise capacity as a predictor of post-thoracotomy morbidity. Am Rev Resp Dis 1984; 129:730–734.
6. Nunn JF. Effects of anesthesia on respiration. Br J Anesth 1990; 65:54–62.

7. Tisi GM. Preoperative evaluation of pulmonary function. Am Rev Resp Dis 1979; 119:293–310.
8. Lindberg P, Gunnarsson L, Tokics L, Secher E, Lundquist H, Brismar B, Hedenstiema G. Atelectasis and lung function in the postoperative period. Acta Anesthesiol Scand 1992; 36:546–533.
9. Ford GT, Whitelaw WA, Rosenal TW, Cruse PJ, Guenter CA. Diaphragm function after upper abdominal surgery in humans. Am Rev Resp Dis 1983; 127:431–436.
10. Simonneau G, Vivien A, Sartene R, Kunstlinger F, Samic K, Noviant Y, Duroux P. Diaphragm dysfunction induced by upper abdominal surgery. Am Rev Resp Dis 1983; 128:899–903.
11. Frazee RC, Roberts JW, Okeson GC, Symmonds RE, Snyder SK, Hendricks JC, Smith RW. Open *versus* laparoscopic cholecystectomy. Ann Surg 1991; 213:651–654.
12. Rademaker BM, Ringers J, Odoom JA, de Wit LT, Kalkman CJ, Oosting J. Pulmonary function and stress response after laparoscopic cholecystectomy: comparison with subcostal incision and influence of thoracic epidural analgesia. Anesth Analg 1992; 75:381–385.
13. Sackner MA, Hirsch J, Epstein S. Effect of cuffed endotracheal tubes on tracheal mucous velocity. Chest 1975; 68:774–777.
14. Gamsu G, Singer MM, Vincent HH, Berry S, Nade JA. Postoperative impairment of mucous transport in the lung. Am Rev Resp Dis 1976; 114:673–679.
15. Olsen GN. Pulmonary physiologic assessment of operative risk. In: Shields TW, LoCicero J, et al., eds. General Thoracic Surgery, 5th ed. Philadelphia: Lippincott, Williams and Wilkins 2000:297–304.
16. Lawrence VA, Page CP, Harris GD. Preoperative spirometry before abdominal operations. A critical appraisal of its predictive value. Arch Int Med 1989; 149:280–285.
17. Zibrak JD, O'Donnell CR, Marton K. Indications for pulmonary function testing. Ann Int Med 1990; 112:763–771.
18. Kroenke K, Lawrence VA, Theroux JF, Tuley MR, Hilsenbeck S. Postoperative complications after thoracic and major abdominal surgery in patients with and without obstructive lung disease. Chest 1993; 104:1445–1451.
19. Hall JC, Tarala RA, Hall JL, Mander J. A multivariate analysis of the risk of pulmonary complications after laparotomy. Chest 1991; 99:923–927.
20. Barisione G, Rovida S, Gazziniga GM, Fontana L. Upper abdominal surgery: does a lung function test exist to predict early severe postoperative respiratory complications? Eur Respir J 1997; 10:1301–1308.
21. Fuso L, Cisternino L, Di Napoli A, DoCosmo V, Tramaglino LM, Basso S, Spadaro S, Pistelli R. Role of spirometric and arterial gas data in predicting pulmonary complications after abdominal surgery. Respir Med 2000; 94:1171–1176.
22. Markos J, Mullan BP, Hillman DR, Musk AW, Antico VF, Lovegrove FT, Carter MJ, Finncane KE. Preoperative assessment as a predictor of mortality and morbidity after lung resection. Am Rev Resp Dis 1989; 139:902–910.
23. American College of Physicians. Preoperative pulmonary function testing. Ann Int Med 1990; 112:793–794.
24. Mohr D, Lavender RC. Preoperative pulmonary evaluation. Postgrad Med 1995; 100:241–256.
25. Gass GD, Olsen GN. Preoperative pulmonary function testing to predict postoperative morbidity and mortality. Chest 1986; 89:127–135.
26. Wernly JA, DeMeester TR, Kirchner PT, Myerowitz PD, Oxford DE, Golomb HM. Clinical value of quantitative ventilation-perfusion lung scans in the surgical management of bronchogenic carcinoma. J Thorac Cardiovasc Surgery 1980; 80:535–543.
27. Olsen GN, Weiman DS, Bolton JW, Gass GD, McLain WC, Schoonover GA, Hornung CA. Submaximal invasive exercise testing and quantitative lung scanning in the evaluation for tolerance of lung resection. Chest 1989; 95:267–273.
28. Gerson MC, Hurst JM, Hertzberg VS, Baughman R, Rouan GW, Ellis K. Prediction of cardiac and pulmonary complications related to elective abdominal and noncardiac thoracic surgery in geriatric patients. Am J Med 1990; 88:101–107.

29. Lawrence VA, Dhanda R, Hilsenbeck SG, Page CP. Risk of pulmonary complications after elective abdominal surgery. Chest 1996; 110:744–750.
30. Stein M, Cassara EL. Preoperative pulmonary evaluation and therapy for surgery patients. JAMA 1970; 211:787–790.
31. Gracey DR, Divertie MB, Didier EP. Preoperative pulmonary preparation of patients with chronic obstructive pulmonary disease. Chest 1979; 76:123–129.
32. Warner MA, Divertie MB, Tinker JH. Preoperative cessation of smoking and pulmonary complications in coronary artery bypass patients. Anesthesiol 1984; 60:380–383.
33. Garibaldi RA, Britt MR, Coleman ML, Reading JL, Pace NL. Risk factors for postoperative pneumonia. Am J Med 1981; 70:677–680.
34. Lourenco RV, Klimek MF, Borowski CJ. Deposition and clearance of two-micron particles in the tracheobronchial tree of normal subjects—smokers and nonsmokers. J Clin Invest 1971; 50:1411–1419.
35. McCarthy DS, Spencer R. Measurement of closing volume as a simple and sensitive test for early detection of small airway disease. Am J Med 1972; 52:747–753.
36. Pearce AC, Jones RM. Smoking and anesthesia: preoperative abstinence and perioperative morbidity. Anesthesiol 1984; 61:576–584.
37. Martin RR, Lindsay DL, Despas P, Macklem PT, Anthonisen NR. Reversible small airway obstruction associated with cigarette smoking. Chest 1973; 63:31S.
38. Buist AS, Sexton GJ, Nagy JM, Ross BB. The effect of smoking cessation and modification on lung function. Am Rev Resp Dis 1976; 114:115–122.
39. Egan TD, Wong KC. Perioperative smoking cessation and anesthesia: a review. J Clin Anesth 1992; 4:63–72.
40. Wong DH, Weber EC, Schell MJ, Wong AB, Andersen CT, Barker SJ. Factors associated with postoperative pulmonary complications in patients with severe chronic obstructive pulmonary disease. Anesth Analg 1995; 80:276–284.
41. Williams-Russo P, Charlson ME, MacKenzie CR, Gold JP, Shires GT. Predicting postoperative pulmonary complications. Arch Int Med 1992; 152:1209–1213.
42. Klug TJ, McPherson RC. Postoperative complications in elderly surgical patients. Am J Surg 1959; 97:713–717.
43. Brooks-Brunn, JA. Predictors of postoperative pulmonary complications following abdominal surgery. Chest 1997; 111:564–571.
44. Marx GF, Mateo CV, Orkin LR. Computer analysis of postanesthetic deaths. Anesthesiol 1973; 39:54–58.
45. Putnam H, Jenicek JA, Allen CR, Wilson RD. Anesthesia in the morbidly obese. South Med J 1974; 67:1411–1417.
46. Pasulka PS, Bistrian BR, Benotti PN, Blackburn GL. The risks of surgery in obese patients. Ann Int Med 1986; 104:540–546.
47. Phillips EH, Carroll BJ, Fallas MJ, Pearlstein AR. Comparison of laparoscopic cholecystectomy in obese and nonobese patients. Am Surg 1994; 60:316–321.
48. Ravin MB. Comparison of spinal and general anesthesia for lower abdominal surgery in patients with chronic obstructive pulmonary disease. Anesthesiology 1971; 35:319–322.
49. Tarhan S, Moffitt EA, Sessler AD, Douglas WW, Taylor WF. Risk of anesthesia and surgery in patients with chronic bronchitis and chronic obstructive pulmonary disease. Surgery 1973; 74:720–726.
50. McKenzie PJ, Wishart HY, Dewar KM, Gray I, Smith G. Comparison of the effects of spinal anesthesia and general anesthesia on postoperative oxygenation and perioperative mortality. Br J Anesth 1980; 52:49–54.
51. Rodgers A, Walker N, Schug S, McKee A, Kehlet H, van Zundert A, Sage D, Futter M, Saville G, Clark T, MacMahon S. Reduction of postoperative morbidity and mortality with epidural or spinal anesthesia: results from overview of randomized trials. Brit Med J 2000; 321:1–12.

52. Forthman HJ, Shephard A. Postoperative pulmonary complications. South Med J 1969; 62:1198–1200.
53. Vaughan RW, Wise L. Choice of abdominal operative incision in patient. Ann Surg 1975; 181:829–835.
54. Halasz NA. Vertical vs. horizontal laparotomies. Arch Surg 1984; 88:911–914.
55. Williams CD, Brenowitz JB. Ventilatory patterns after vertical and transverse upper abdominal incisions. Am J Surg 1975; 130:725–728.
56. Thorens L. Postoperative pulmonary complications: observations on their prevention by means of physiotherapy. Acta Chir Scand 1954; 107:194–205.
57. Oh SH, Patterson R. Surgery in corticosteroid-dependent asthmatics. J Allergy Clin Immunol 1974; 53:345–351.
58. Camner P, Philipson K, Arvidsson T. Withdrawal of cigarette smoking. A study on tracheobronchial clearance. Arch Environ Health 1973; 26:90–92.
59. Warner MA, Offord KP, Warner ME, Lennon RL, Conover MA, Jansson-Schumacher U. Role of preoperative cessation of smoking and other factors in postoperative pulmonary complications: a blinded prospective study of coronary artery bypass patients. Mayo Clin Proc 1989; 64:609–614.
60. Welchew EA. On-demand analgesia. A double blind comparison of on-demand intravenous fentanyl with regular intramuscular morphine. Anaesth 1983; 38:19–25.
61. White PF. Use of patient-controlled analgesia for management of acute pain. JAMA 1988; 259:243–247.
62. Rawal N, Sjöstrand U, Christoffersson E, Dahlstrom B, Arvil A, Rydman H. Comparison of intramuscular and epidural morphine for postoperative analgesia in the grossly obese: influence on postoperative ambulation and pulmonary function. Anesth Analg 1984; 63:583–592.
63. Cuschieri RJ, Morran CG, Howie JC, McArdle CS. Postoperative pain and pulmonary complications: comparison of three analgesic regimens. Br J Surg 1985; 72:495–498.
64. Jayr C, Thomas H, Rey A, Farhat F, Lasser P, Bourgain JL. Postoperative pulmonary complications. Epidural analgesia using bupivacaine and opioids *versus* parenteral opioids. Anesthesiol 1993; 78:666–676.
65. Major CP, Greer MS, Russell WL, Roe SM. Postoperative pulmonary complications and morbidity after abdominal aneurysmectomy: a comparison of postoperative epidural versus parenteral opioid analgesia. Am Surg 1996; 62:45–51.
66. Celli BR, Rodriguez KS, Snider GL. A controlled trial of intermittent positive pressure breathing, incentive spirometry, and deep breathing exercises in preventing postoperative pulmonary complications after abdominal surgery. Am Rev Resp Dis 1984; 130:12–15.
67. Hall JC, Tarala R, Harris J, Tapper J, Christiansen K. Incentive spirometry versus routine chest physiotherapy for prevention of pulmonary complications after abdominal surgery. Lancet 1991; 337:953–956.
68. Sands JH, Cypert C, Armstrong R, Ching S, Trainer D, Quinn W, Stewart D. A controlled study using routine intermittent positive pressure breathing in postsurgical patients. Diseases of the Chest 1961; 40:120–123.
69. Stock MC, Downs JB, Gauer PK, Alster JM, Imrey PB. Prevention of postoperative pulmonary complications with CPAP, incentive spirometry, and conservative therapy. Chest 1985; 87:151–157.
70. Ricksten S, Bengtsson A, Soderberg C, Thorden M, Kvist H. Effects of periodic positive airway pressure by mask on postoperative pulmonary function. Chest 1986; 89:774–781.

13
Ethical Considerations in Surgical Intensive Care

Melissa West
VA Medical Center, Minneapolis, Minnesota, USA

INFORMED CONSENT AND DECISION-MAKING CAPACITY

Informed Consent

Legally and ethically a competent adult has the right to decline any medical procedure, even if this decision leads directly to death. This right to refuse life-sustaining treatment also extends to patients without decision-making capacity when the patient's prior directives explicitly decline certain treatments or when surrogate decision makers believe that the patient would refuse a certain treatment if the patient were able to communicate.

Inclusion of the following points in an informed consent discussion ensures a truly informed patient consent:

- Nature of the decision; that is, name of proposed treatment and indication for the treatment
- Alternatives available including no treatment
- Risks and benefits of each treatment option
- Assessment of the patient's understanding (generally by asking the patient to repeat the aforementioned information)
- Patient's questions
- Patient's consent or refusal

Decision-Making Capacity

Decision-making capacity is a clinical judgment usually made by a physician. Competency is a legal term that refers to an individual's ability to make rational informed decisions (1). Only a judge can declare a person incompetent and assign a guardian or conservator to make decisions for that person. Note that legally competent patients may not have decisional capacity at a given time.

No objective test to determine whether a patient has decision-making capacity exists. A certain score on a test such as the mini-mental status exam does not, by itself, indicate lack of decisional capacity.

Decision-making capacity is not an all-or-nothing phenomenon; it may change from day to day and is specific to the situation at hand. Patients who lacked decision-making capacity in the recent past may regain it. Decision-making capacity is not specific to a diagnosis. Patients with the following diagnoses may be at risk for inability to participate in decision making, but none of these diagnoses automatically excludes decisional capacity, and certainly there are patients with these diagnoses who do retain capacity:

- Cognitive impairment
- Severe depression or mania
- Psychosis
- Delirium
- Decreased level of consciousness

Definition of Decision-Making Capacity

Decision-making capacity is the patient's ability to understand and reflect on the medical issue at hand, including the consequences of agreeing to, or foregoing, a treatment, together with the ability to choose one alternative and to communicate that choice.

The following questions are helpful in assessing a patient's capacity (2):

- What is your main medical problem right now?
- What treatment was recommended for this problem?
- If you receive this treatment, what will happen?
- If you do not receive this treatment, what will happen?
- Why have you decided to (not to) receive this treatment?

When doubt about a patient's decisional capacity exists, consultation with a psychiatrist, geriatrician, or neurologist is recommended.

Case Study

An 88-year-old male was referred for evaluation of a 12 cm pelvic mass. Past medical history is significant for prostate cancer diagnosed 1 year ago (patient is currently on hormonal treatment). He is status post colectomy 4 months ago to remove an adenomatous polyp. Oncology has recommended a CT guided needle biopsy of the pelvic mass. The results might change treatment recommendations (i.e., radiation therapy to the mass if malignant). When the patient arrived in radiology, a radiologist explained the procedure and the patient signed the consent form. However, the nurse who was asked to witness the patient's signature refused, citing concerns about this patient's competency. The nurse noted the patient was oriented to himself, but not to place or date. The biopsy was canceled and an ethics consult was obtained. On exam the patient was alert, cooperative, and oriented to self. He thought he was in a nursing home (NH), was 39 years old, and lived with his mother (who was actually deceased). The patient was evaluated on two separate occasions by ethics committee members and gave similar answers in both interviews. He knew he had "something growing" inside him, that he had prostate cancer, and that "they did something to me a while back." In regard to the proposed biopsy and subsequent treatment if the mass were malignant, he stated, "I am not afraid of death because I have a strong faith; on the other hand while I'm alive I want to make the best of it. I would like the biopsy if that is what the doctor recommends." The patient is a bachelor with no children. His next of kin is his sister. When asked if the doctors could contact his sister to discuss the situation the patient said, "My sister is nosy. I don't like to tell her my business. Besides, she owes me a lot of money."

The Ethics Committee recommended proceeding with the biopsy for the following reasons: The patient showed consistency in his statements. Although confused about many aspects of his life, he clearly wished to have the biopsy. Despite his confusion about dates and locations, he was able to verbalize and to reflect on the risks and benefits of a biopsy and to arrive at a decision. He was felt competent to make this treatment decision, though not necessarily competent in all spheres.

Patients Without Decision-Making Capacity

When patients are unable to give informed consent, the appropriate decision maker is generally the proxy decision maker named by the patient in an advance directive, a court appointed conservator, or the next of kin. Some states have legislated a hierarchy of decision makers; a typical order follows (check with your institution for policies specific to hospital and state).

- Advance directive (the patients may have specified in writing whether or not they would accept a certain procedure)
- Proxy named in a durable power of attorney for health care
- Court appointed guardian or conservator
- Spouse
- Adult child
- Parent
- Adult sibling
- Grandparent
- Adult grandchild

Many institutions would add to this list a close friend who is familiar with the patient's beliefs and philosophies.

The surrogate decision maker must be given the same information about risks and benefits as would be given to the decisional patient. The role of the surrogate is then to consent to or refuse the proposed treatment using the *principle of substituted judgment.* This principle states that a surrogate attempts to decide what a patient would decide if that patient were able to do so, given that patient's attitudes and values. Exercising the principle of substituted judgment does not mean simply substituting the surrogate's judgment for that of the patient. It means using what the surrogate knows about the patient to determine what the patient would decide if the patient could speak. It is helpful to explain to surrogate families that they are not being asked to decide what they themselves want, but instead are asked to give their opinion about what the patient would say, if the patient were able to speak for him- or herself at that moment. This explanation often relieves some of the burden family members experience when they believe they are being asked to decide whether their loved one should live or die.

In the absence of an individual who knows the patient well enough to use substituted judgment, one then utilizes the *best interest standard.* Application of the best interest standard means weighing the potential benefits and burdens of the treatment options, and determining what most people would choose in the same situation.

In emergency situations the *doctrine of implied consent* states that emergency treatment should be rendered to a patient who is unable to give consent and who has no immediately available surrogate decision maker.

ADVANCE DIRECTIVES AND DNR ORDERS

An advance directive is a general term that refers to a patient's statement, oral or preferably written, about what sort of medical care the patient would want in the future. Advance directives may specify treatment preferences, appoint a proxy to speak on the patient's behalf, or both. A durable power of attorney for health care is a document that appoints a specific individual to make health care decisions for the patient, if the patient becomes unable to make those decisions him- or herself. Generally the signing of these documents is either witnessed or notarized, but preparation does not require the services of an attorney or a court. Advance directives are used when a patient is no longer able to communicate. A competent patient's current wishes override anything contained in an advance directive.

Advance directives are usually prepared by a patient with the help of a social worker and family members. By necessity, advance directives use vague, nonspecific terms, because no one is able to predict the exact medical conditions that will exist in the future. Terms such as "no reasonable expectation of recovery," "terminal condition," and "artificial means and heroic measures" can be helpful in understanding a patient's general outlook but can be difficult to interpret in a specific medical situation. For this reason, advance directives are no substitute for physician and patient discussion of end of life matters.

DNR (do not resuscitate) orders, on the other hand, are quite specific, and usually represent a decision made by patient and physician together.

DNR Orders

Physicians are often unaware of their patients' preferences regarding code status. In one study, 47% of patients' physicians did not know their patients' wishes about CPR (3). Furthermore, physicians are no better at identifying patients who would survive resuscitation than would be expected by chance alone (4). Patients often have unrealistically optimistic expectations about the success of resuscitation efforts. CPR outcomes have been documented in over 100 studies. In both the USA and Europe, average survival to discharge after in-hospital CPR is about 15% (5). Factors associated with poor survival after CPR are multiple comorbidities, organ failure, asystole (as opposed to ventricular tachycardia or fibrillation), PEA, unwitnessed arrest, and prolonged CPR (5). Discussing CPR as part of the overall treatment plan for a patient is both natural and less intimidating. A useful approach is helping the patient to identify realistic goals of treatment and, at that point, considering whether CPR is likely to further those goals. A discussion focusing on goals and expectations, rather than on one specific intervention, allows physicians to gauge better what patients would want in unforeseen circumstances.

Case Study

E.W., a 70-year-old woman, underwent a hemicolectomy for localized colon cancer. She had no immediate postoperative complications but was not able to be weaned from the ventilator as quickly as had been anticipated. On the second postoperative day, she remained on the ventilator. Her DNR/I code status had been rescinded for surgery with the order, "Suspend DNR/I while in the OR and for 48 h post-op." DNR/I status resumed automatically at 48 h. The following day, during routine suctioning, her

Surgical Intensive Care

endotracheal tube was accidentally dislodged and removed. She became tachypnic and hypotensive, and a code was called. The first responder, a third year surgical resident, noted that DNR/I was written on her identification bracelet. He was unsure about whether to proceed with intubation.

Inadvertent extubations occur occasionally in the ICU and are an example of unforeseen circumstances. The ethical principle most germane to such a situation would be "when in doubt about a patient's wishes or code status, err on the side of preserving life." Ideally, however, the patient's physician and ICU nurses would know the patient's goals of treatment and, hence, would be able to make a reasonable judgment about whether the patient would choose reintubation.

Definition of DNR

Definitions of code status or DNR orders vary from institution to institution. In general, DNR means that no chest compressions, no defibrillation, and no intubation will be performed on a patient who is found without pulse and respirations. Unless otherwise specified, the DNR designation does not preclude any other interventions (i.e., pacemakers, pharmacological therapy, and mechanical ventilation) for a patient prior to cardiac arrest. Other specific limitations of care should be designated separately.

Case Study

H.W., a 65-year-old man with increasing exertional angina while jogging, is found on catheterization to have a single 95% lesion of his LAD. He is admitted for PTCA, which is performed without immediate complication. Thirty minutes after being returned to his room, he develops bradycardia to 30 BPM and becomes unresponsive. Initial BP is 80/40. The patient has a longstanding DNR order that was not rescinded for the PTCA. Nursing calls a code. What action should the first physician on the scene take?

Using the narrow definition of DNR described earlier, the patient in this case should be treated pharmacologically and, if needed, with emergency pacing, because he is not exhibiting cardiac arrest.

DNI Orders

In some institutions, DNR orders are routinely written as DNR/DNI (do not intubate). In general, a DNI order means that, if a patient is in respiratory distress or is without respirations, endotracheal intubation will not be performed. The DNI designation does not preclude any other form of airway management, such as BIPAP or Heimlich maneuver.

Initiation of Treatment Does Not Imply Indefinite Continuation of Treatment

Difficulties arise when doctors and nurses hesitate to begin necessary treatment out of fear that the patient will not improve and will be treated indefinitely, despite futility of therapy. A useful example is endotracheal intubation. Patients with severe underlying lung disease with superimposed acute respiratory distress have sometimes not been intubated out of concern that the patient "could never come off the vent." An important principle to remember is that *stopping treatment is equivalent, morally and ethically, to never starting the treatment*. This statement does not imply they are psychologically equivalent. Withdrawing support from a ventilator-dependent patient is very different from foregoing the initial intubation. The withdrawal of ventilation should be done with the assistance of an experienced physician to ensure that patient comfort is maintained.

The Presence of a DNR/DNI Order Does Not Imply Limits to Other Types of Care

Some patients with these orders will be receiving maximal therapy; whereas, others will not. These orders *are* consistent with providing care in an intensive care unit.

Case Study

A 75-year-old retired history professor was treated with radiation therapy for prostate cancer diagnosed 8 years ago. Hormonal treatment was instituted after he developed bony metastases 3 years ago. He began chemotherapy 1 year ago for control of widespread, painful metastases. He has experienced worsening bone pain for the past few months and was admitted for pain control. While hospitalized, he developed low grade DIC. Two days later he became lethargic and hypotensive. Head CT revealed a large left frontal subdural hematoma (SDH). Evaluation by Neurosurgery indicated the patient's symptoms could be relieved by evacuation of the SDH. The patient was transferred to the ICU for monitoring and treatment of his BP until the evacuation could be performed the following day. The patient had a longstanding DNR order but no living will. Should this patient have been moved to an ICU?

Initially, several medical and nursing ICU staff were reluctant to transfer this patient with terminal disease to an intensive care bed. The attending insisted on transfer and appropriate treatment to stabilize blood pressure. The following morning the subdural was successfully evacuated, and the patient regained his usual mental status. After the evacuation, the family reported that the patient's only daughter was due to return home in several days after an extended stay abroad. The patient's last goal in life was to spend a few days with his daughter prior to his death. The patient and family expressed their gratitude for the intensive medical care that had given the patient extra days of life. Of note, after the patient's daughter arrived, the patient and physician changed his status to "comfort care, no ICU transfers."

If in Doubt, Err on the Side of Preserving Life

In an emergency situation, when confusion exists regarding an unresponsive patient's wishes, the guiding principle is always to err on the side of preserving life. As discussed earlier, treatment can be discontinued if the patient and the physician later decide that treatment is no longer wanted or appropriate.

In general, a DNR decision should be reached by the patient or surrogate decision maker in consultation with the physician. If disagreement between patient and physician occurs, the wishes of the patient generally should prevail until agreement is reached. If a consensual decision cannot be reached, one should consult the hospital ethics committee or hospital administration.

INAPPROPRIATE REQUESTS FROM PATIENTS: THE FUTILITY DEBATE

> Denial of treatment should be justified by reliance on openly stated ethical principles and acceptable standards of care ... not on the concept of futility which cannot be meaningfully defined.
>
> AMA Code of Ethics 2000–2001 (2.035)

What constitutes a futile intervention remains controversial after a decade of trying to define medical futility. Initial attempts focused on either a quantitative or a qualitative definition. The most well-known definition of quantitative medical futility stated that if an intervention had been unsuccessful in the last 100 times it was tried, then the intervention was futile and need not be offered to a patient (6). The problem with this definition was finding a series of patients whose condition matched a particular patient's medical circumstances. The qualitative approach to futility involved deciding whether the resulting quality of life after an intervention would be tolerable. The problem with this approach is that one person's assessment of tolerable quality of life may not be the same as another person's. The following points about futility are currently widely accepted:

- The patient alone should make the judgment about whether the quality of his or her life is acceptable.
- Even a remote chance of successful resuscitation may be of value to a patient.
- No consensus yet exists among physicians on what probability of survival constitutes futility.
- The lay public cannot reach consensus on this question.
- Unilateral decisions are open to bias against persons of another race, lifestyle, age, or against those who hold unfamiliar beliefs.

Is it ever acceptable for a physician to make a decision not to resuscitate:

- Without consulting the patient?
  No!
- In the face of objections from the patient or surrogate?
  No clear legal or ethical guidelines exist yet.

In a few futility cases that have come before them, the courts have ruled on narrow legal aspects; consequently, no clear legal precedent for futility decisions exists.

Case Studies

In the Baby K case, a ventilator-dependent newborn with anencephaly was discharged eventually from the NICU to a NH. Her mother insisted on all medical treatment to keep the baby alive. The hospital tried to obtain a ruling that it should not be required to provide artificial ventilation and other treatment when the baby was sent back to the hospital numerous times from the NH. The court used a narrow reading of the Emergency Medical Treatment and Active Labor Act (the so-called "anti-dumping statute") to determine that the hospital was obligated to provide necessary care (7).

In Gilgunn vs. Massachusetts General Hospital, a jury found the hospital and physicians not liable for stopping ventilator support and writing a DNR order on the basis of futility, against the wishes of Mrs. Gilgunn's daughter. Because this decision was a jury verdict, not judicial opinion, it does not set clear legal precedent (8).

Helga Wanglie, an 87-year-old woman, was hospitalized after breaking her hip. She developed pneumonia and experienced cardiopulmonary arrest. She was resuscitated and intubated but sustained severe anoxic encephalopathy. After 6 months, she remained ventilator dependent and was considered by neurology to be in a persistent vegetative state (PVS). Her husband was her surrogate decision maker. He insisted on continued support. The hospital saw the respirator as nonbeneficial because it would not restore her to consciousness. However, in the family's view, maintaining life of any kind was a worthy goal. The court did not rule directly on the benefit or futility of the ventilator. Instead, the court affirmed the right of the patient's husband to make the decision about life-sustaining treatment (9).

PROFESSIONAL INTEGRITY

> Physicians ought to "refuse to treat those who are overmastered by their disease."
>
> Hippocratic Oath

> Physicians are not ethically obligated to deliver care that, in their best professional judgment, will not have a reasonable chance of benefiting their patients. Patients should not be given treatments simply because they demand them.
>
> AMA Code of Ethics 2000–2001 (2.035)

On occasion, patient's demands may seem to compromise professional integrity. Physicians and nurses are bound to high standards of scientific and professional competence. To offer ineffective treatment or treatment that might cause harm deviates from professional standards. Physicians are justified in risking harm to patients only when a reasonable chance of benefit is also present. Health care providers have no obligation to provide treatment that is clearly ineffective or that causes harm; for example, CPR on a patient with rigor mortis or surgical treatment of a patient who could not survive anesthesia.

Most ICU conflicts involve requests for treatment that is physiologically likely to be effective, at least for the short term, but which supports a controversial end, such as continued ventilation for a patient in a PVS, where the ventilator will continue to oxygenate the lungs but will not serve to restore conscious existence.

Some medical procedures may be immoral according to the religious or personal moral tradition of some health care providers. Examples may be terminating life support or participating in the care of a patient who has stopped food and fluids. While health care workers should not be asked to violate their own moral codes, physicians ethically cannot abandon patients whose care they have assumed. Physicians are obligated to continue caring for patients until another physician willing to take over care is found.

The best strategy is preventive. Do not allow the physician–family relationship to become adversarial. Rather than starting with a discussion about the futility of resuscitation, it is helpful to define patient and family goals. Once the family or patient is able to list treatment goals, the physician can discuss the options available to help attain them. As noted earlier, for some, the goal may be organic life, even without the presence of consciousness.

The controversy surrounding medical futility needs to be addressed by society as a whole, and this process has begun. An approach that has been adopted by at least one state and several institutions is to define a process for resolving such conflicts, rather than trying to define the exact circumstances when resuscitation efforts, or other invasive treatments, might be futile (10). The process considers the following:

- The physician ascertains the patient's wishes and focuses on goals of care from the patient's perspective (such as staying alive until the arrival of an out of town relative). The determination that CPR is futile must be based on medical judgment that it cannot be expected to achieve the patient's goals.

- The physician must explain the intention to forego resuscitation to the patient or surrogate and document this discussion in the patient's record.
- If the patient disagrees, the care team meets with the family and the patient; if no agreement is reached, a formal review (as outlined in the following) is initiated.
- In the meantime, if the patient arrests before the process is complete, CPR is performed.
- A second physician must concur with the first about foregoing treatment.
- An ethics committee or equivalent group meets with the patient and care team to try to reach resolution; the committee makes a formal recommendation.
- If the patient disagrees with the recommendation, an attempt is made to transfer the patient to another physician or hospital, if such can be found.
- If there is no resolution and no transfer after 10 days, a DNR order is written over objection of patient. (The family can ask a judge to intervene during this 10-day period.)

END OF LIFE ISSUES

Frank discussion with patients and families is paramount when a patient is terminally ill. Expect the need to repeat information on several occasions, because families experiencing stress cannot always absorb large amounts of medical detail.

Relief of Suffering at the End of Life

The SUPPORT study followed 4124 terminally ill patients who died in one of the five major teaching hospitals. During the last 3 days of life, 45% of patients were unconscious. Of the 55% who were conscious:

- 40% had severe pain
- 50% had severe dyspnea
- 25% felt depressed or anxious (11)

In a study at the Durham VA Medical Center, terminally ill patients were asked their main concerns at the end of life. Freedom from noxious symptoms (pain, dyspnea), spiritual issues, and psychosocial issues were the leading concerns. Patients feared bad dying more than death itself (12).

Pain Control

In recent years, much has been written about physicians' obligation to treat pain aggressively, and nowhere is this idea more important than at the end of life. In almost all cases, physical symptoms can be treated effectively, although successful treatment may come at the expense of mental clarity. (One of the advantages of IV morphine is the capability of decreasing the dose transiently when patients want to be lucid, such as when family visits, and quickly increasing the dose when pain becomes severe.) The World Health Organization Analgesic Ladder, one of the most widely used guidelines for pain control, recommends starting with acetaminophen or other nonopioids for mild pain, adding nonsteroidals (in patients with normal renal function and without active ulcer disease) or mild opioids for moderate pain, and using narcotics for more severe pain (13). Morphine, the mainstay (as it is well tolerated and has been well studied), is available in sustained release and immediate release forms, the latter including IV, IM, subcutaneous, and concentrate for buccal surfaces. Other useful narcotics are hydromorphone, oxycodone, and fentanyl. The physician should prescribe a daily laxative whenever starting narcotics.

The Rule of Double Effect

Dosages of medications used to relieve pain, shortness of breath (SOB), or other suffering at the end of life are often high enough to depress respiration and potentially hasten death. Presuming the patient concurs, the administration of high doses of medication to relieve suffering, even to the point of respiratory depression, is considered ethical. In such cases, respiratory depression and even death may be foreseen sequelae of medication use, but the intended consequence is pain relief (or relief of other suffering such as dyspnea). This combination of benefits and risks is known as the rule of double effect. It is the distinction between intended consequence (the physician aims to relieve a particular symptom) and foreseen side effect that makes it ethical and proper to use medication doses adequate to afford relief of suffering.

Relief of Other Symptoms

Dyspnea is common at the end of life. Diuretics are useful, if volume overload is present. Opioids are as effective at relieving dyspnea as they are at relieving pain. Nausea and vomiting are common and often multifactorial in etiology. If standard antiemetics are ineffective, the combination of IV metoclopramide and dexamethasone can be helpful. Even with good control of pain and dyspnea, agitation and restlessness can occur. Remember to evaluate the patient before prescribing medication to rule out overlooked causes of agitation, such as urinary retention, constipation, or unsuspected pain. Benzodiazepines are the most commonly used drugs for agitation and can be used either intermittently or as continuous infusions (most often midazolam) for prolonged agitation.

Withdrawal of Life-Sustaining Treatment

When medical interventions are serving to only prolong the dying process, withdrawal of life-sustaining treatment should be considered.

Ventilator Withdrawal

Withdrawal from a ventilator can be technically difficult and always should be done with the help of an experienced physician to ensure patient comfort. Neuromuscular blocking agents must be stopped well ahead of extubation. Their presence would make evaluation of patient distress impossible. Generally, IV morphine or another narcotic should be infused and adjusted to relieve dyspnea while not depressing respirations more than necessary. IV benzodiazepines should be immediately available for treatment of agitation or anxiety. Two methods of ventilator withdrawal are common. The first is straightforward removal of the endotracheal tube (ET) after aggressive suctioning of the airway. An alternate approach, called terminal weaning, is more gradual. It consists of decreasing the ventilator rate, PEEP, and tidal volume in steps, while leaving the ET in place, until the physician feels patient comfort has been ensured. The ET is then removed. With either method, oxygen is provided by facemask after extubation (14).

Note that 10% of patients survive more than a few hours after ventilator withdrawal, despite physician predictions that they would die moments after extubation (15). Families must be prepared for this occurrence.

Withdrawal of Dialysis

Discontinuing dialysis usually results in death in days to a few weeks. Generally death is peaceful with patients gradually becoming lethargic as electrolyte abnormalities increase. These patients occasionally need morphine for relief of dyspnea.

Withdrawal of Other Treatments

Stopping vasoactive drugs, antibiotics, and IV fluids is less problematic for most medical personnel and families. Medication use should be considered in light of identified treatment goals. Antiepileptics are often considered comfort medications and continued until death. An example of a treatment that may or may not be used as a comfort medication is dexamethasone in a patient with brain metastases. It may be appropriate to stop the steroid for a patient who is ready for death or who is comatose. Herniation or adrenal crisis may occur, though neither condition is a certainty. Other patients for whom day-to-day existence remains meaningful, or who wish neither to hasten nor forestall death, may want to continue the medication.

If treatment is focused entirely on patient comfort, blood draws, X-rays, and frequent checking of vital signs can be discontinued.

Foregoing Food and Fluids

Anorexia occurs frequently at the end of life. Dehydration and foregoing nutrition do not appear to cause patient discomfort or distress at the end of life. For some families, and some physicians, stopping nutrition and hydration is difficult because of the symbolic value of food. Providing nutrition and hydration (whether by feeding tubes or intravenously) can present a significant burden to patients, is considered a medical treatment, and, like any other medical treatment, can be declined by patients or their surrogates.

PHYSICIAN-ASSISTED SUICIDE

Competent patients have a moral and legal right to refuse any life-sustaining treatment. Currently, in one state (Oregon), they also have the right to physician-assisted suicide (PAS). This right is limited to competent patients with an imminently terminal illness, whose decision is not driven by depression or by symptoms that could be relieved with good medical management. Physicians who believe PAS is unethical are not obliged to participate. Those who do participate write a prescription for a lethal dose of medication (typically barbiturates), but the patient is the one who decides whether or when to take the medication. (In euthanasia, which is illegal everywhere, the physician would administer the lethal medication.) Public opinion polls show a majority of US adults favor having PAS available to competent patients. Supporters cite the values of patient self-determination and well being (i.e., a patient who determines that life with a terminal illness has become so burdensome that death is preferred). Opponents contend that taking a human life, except possibly in self defense, is always wrong, that the role of physicians as healers precludes destroying life, and that legalization of PAS would lead to excesses and abuse (16).

SUMMARY

- Informed consent ideally should include:
  Nature of proposed treatment and indications
  Alternatives including no treatment
  Risks and benefits of treatment options
  Assessment of patient understanding
  Patient questions
  Patient consent or refusal
- A patient's decision-making capacity may change from day to day.
- Helpful questions in assessing a patient's decision-making capacity include:
  What is your main medical problem?
  What treatment was recommended?
  What are the consequences of treatment?
  What are the consequences of no treatment?
  Why do you wish (or refuse) treatment?
- A judge is the only individual who can declare a patient incompetent and assign a guardian or conservator to make decisions for that patient.
- Hierarchies of decision makers may be institution- or state-specific.
- The principle of substituted judgment states that a surrogate attempts to decide what a patient would decide given the patient's attitudes and values, if that patient were capable of making a decision.
- Best interest standard means weighing potential benefits and burdens of treatment options and determining what most people would choose in a given situation.
- Doctrine of implied consent states that emergency treatment should be provided to a patient who cannot give consent and for whom a surrogate decision maker is not available.
- Advanced directives often use vague, non-specific terms and are not substitutes for physician and patient discussion of end-of-life matters.
- DNR orders mean no chest compressions, no defibrillation, and no intubation will be performed on a patient with no pulse and no respiration. Other treatments may be provided unless specifically refused.
- DNI orders mean no endotracheal intubation will be performed on a patient in respiratory distress or without respirations.
- Initiation of treatment does not imply indefinite continuation of treatment.
- The presence of a DNR/DNI order does not imply limits to other types of care.
- When doubt exists, preserve life.
- When conflict about the possible futility of treatment arises or when patient demands may compromise professional integrity, the ethics committee is an important resource.
- Pain relief at the end of life is vital. The intention of relief of pain and suffering despite potential foreseen side effects, such as respiratory depression, is known as the rule of double effect and is the ethical support for pain relief.

REFERENCES

1. Farnsworth M. Evaluation of mental competency. Am Fam Physician 1989; 39:182–190.
2. Siegler M. Uncertain decision-making capacity. Intensive Ethics Education Course, Mayo Clinic, Rochester, MN, Feb 20–22, 2002.
3. The support principal investigators. A controlled trial to improve care for seriously ill hospitalized patients: the study to understand prognoses and preferences for outcomes and risks of treatments. JAMA 1995; 274:1591–1598.
4. Ebell M, Bergus G, Warbasse L, Bloomer R. The inability of physicians to predict the outcome of in-hospital resuscitation. J Gen Intern Med 1996; 11:16–22.
5. Saklayen M, Liss H, Markert R. In-hospital cardiopulmonary resuscitation. Medicine 1995; 74:163–175.
6. Schneiderman L, Jecker N, Jonsen A. Medical futility: its meaning and ethical implications. Ann Intern Med 1990; 112:949–954.
7. Annas G. Asking the courts to set the standard of emergency care—the case of Baby K. N Engl J Med 1994; 330:1542–1545.
8. Orr R. The Gilgunn case: courage and questions. J Intens Care Med 1999; 14:54–56.
9. Miles S. Informed demand for "non-beneficial" medical treatment. N Engl J Med 1991; 325:512–515.
10. Halevy A, Brody B. A multi-institution collaborative policy on medical futility. JAMA 1996; 276:571–574.
11. Lynn J. Perceptions by family members of the dying experience of older and seriously ill patients. Ann Intern Med 1997; 126:97–106.
12. Steinhauser KE, Clipp EC, McNeilly M, Christakis NA, McIntyre LM, Tulsky JA. In search of a good death: observations of patients, families and providers. Ann Intern Med 2000; 132:825–832.
13. Cancer Pain Relief: With a Guide to Opioid Availability. 2d ed. Geneva: World Health Organization; 1996.
14. Brody H, Campbell M, Faber-Langendoen K. Withdrawing intensive life-sustaining treatment—recommendations for compassionate clinical management. N Engl J Med 1997; 336:652–657.
15. Carlson RW, Campbell ML, Frank RR. Life support: the debate continues. Chest 1996; 109:852–853.
16. Brock D. Death and Dying. In: Veatch Robert, ed. Medical ethics. Sudbury, Massachusetts: Jones and Bartlett, 1997:363–394.

14
Nursing Considerations

Valerie Nebel
VA Medical Center, Minneapolis, Minnesota, USA

COLLABORATION

The care of critically ill patients requires the collaboration and contributions of a team of health care professionals. This team always includes physicians and nurses, and often also includes respiratory therapists, social workers, physical therapists, dieticians, pharmacists, and chaplains.

Studies indicate that risk-adjusted patient outcomes may be improved and length of ICU stay decreased when physicians and nurses collaborate closely in planning and carrying out the care of complex critically ill patients. In a prospective study published in 1999, Baggs et al. (1) found that units with a higher unit-level score for collaboration had better patient outcomes. They also found a positive association between nurse's reports of good nurse–physician collaboration and a lower risk of negative outcomes for patients. An earlier study by Baggs et al. (2) also demonstrated improved risk-adjusted patient outcomes when nurses reported a greater degree of physician–nurse collaboration. Knaus et al. (3) developed the acute physiology and chronic health evaluation (APACHE) tool to stratify severity of illness in 13 ICUs that were studied. They concluded that staff interaction and coordination were the critical factors in accounting for differences in predicted to actual mortality in those ICUs. Nurses and physicians have unique and different perspectives on patients' clinical courses. Patients benefit when both perspectives are included in making decisions about their care.

As related in the Institute of Medicine's report (4) "To Err Is Human," the airline industry achieved significant safety gains by aggressively promoting the empowerment of each team member on an airplane to question each others actions. Airline policy included the requirement for every member of the team to speak up, even to the captain, if they thought a decision did not make sense. This notion of empowerment is closely related to collaboration and may help to explain the benefits of collaboration to patients. Both "To Err Is Human" and the IOMs more recent report "Crossing the Quality Chasm" (5) illustrate in frightening detail the safety and quality problems that are endemic in our health care system. They argue that an interdisciplinary, collaborative, patient-focused approach to patient management will result in safer, higher quality care.

THE ROLE OF THE NURSE

The definition of nursing is the diagnosis and treatment of human responses to actual or potential health problems. This definition implies that the nurse is focused on the whole person, not on the clinical pathology. Nurses care about the patient's emotional, psychological, and social response to illness, as well as the physiologic response. Given the nature of critical care, the SICU nurse places greater emphasis on monitoring the patient's physiologic response to illness and treatment, and on providing for the physical needs that a critically ill patient cannot manage.

As the member of the health care team who is at the bedside around the clock, the nurse plays a key role in communicating with the patient and family. Unlike in the past, patients and families now expect to be part of the health care team and to have an active role in making treatment decisions. Critical care nurses need to understand the diagnosis, prognosis, and treatment plan to better interpret them to the patient and the family. Surgeons are not always available to talk with multiple family members, and family members often do not fully understand the full context of discussion until the information has been repeated several times in different ways. Patients and families develop trust in the health care team when every member appears to understand and reinforce the treatment plan. For patients who develop complications and require complex care for an extended period of time, consistent communication from all members of the health care team is especially important. Periodic family conferences that include several members of the team are invaluable in allaying anxiety, ascertaining the wishes of the patient, and communicating a clear vision of the patient's current clinical course and the expected benefits of the treatment plan.

AIRWAY AND VENTILATOR MANAGEMENT
Routine SICU Care

All SICU patients require respiratory monitoring, and most require respiratory support ranging from supplemental oxygen to full ventilator support. Many surgical patients have underlying respiratory disease. They may have an abdominal or thoracic incision, which discourages them from coughing and deep breathing. Postoperatively, usually patients receive opiates, a further respiratory depressant, for pain relief. This combination of factors makes assessment and monitoring of respiratory status, with interventions as indicated, one of the major responsibilities of the SICU nurse. Assessment and monitoring include continuous or intermittent measurements of oxygen saturation, auscultation of lung sounds, observation of skin color and use of accessory muscles, and assessment of frequency and quality of respirations. In addition, experienced critical care nurses have learned that patients with respiratory insufficiency are also anxious and fearful.

Routinely, the SICU nurse encourages the patient to cough and deep breathe and assists the patients to change position every 2 h. In addition, the nurse assesses the patient's pain every 2 h or as indicated, and administers sufficient analgesia such that the patient is able to tolerate coughing, changing position, and early ambulation. Consensus exists that early ambulation for all but the most unstable patients is beneficial in preventing pulmonary complications. Coronary artery bypass (CAB) patients in particular have been well studied regarding repositioning and exercise tolerance. Goodwin et al. (6) described the early extubation and early ambulation protocol for CAB patients.

Nursing Considerations

They found that most patients were able to dangle at the bedside within 6 h of surgery and could get up to the chair within 8–12 h of surgery.

Even unstable patients can tolerate turning and repositioning. In a comprehensive review, Wheeler (7) concluded that, except for those patients with very low cardiac output, most patients tolerated turning with no lasting hemodynamic consequences. In addition, except for patients with unilateral lung disease, no single position promoted optimal oxygenation. For those with unilateral lung disease, oxygenation is maximized with the better lung positioned down.

Suctioning of Patients on Mechanical Ventilation

Nurses and respiratory therapists usually share the responsibility of suctioning and endotracheal tube care. Over the past 25 years, indications for suctioning, recommended frequency of suctioning, and optimal techniques for maximizing the benefits and minimizing the complications of suctioning have been controversial. A set of clinical practice guidelines for suctioning was published in 2001 by Brooks et al. (8). An interdisciplinary team performed an electronic literature search and reviewed 162 articles related to suctioning and, on the basis of this review, made several recommendations. Because only one article addressed the indications for suctioning, a recommendation was not made on that subject. The following summarizes their recommendations:

- Mechanically ventilated patients should receive additional oxygenation before and after suctioning.
- For mechanically ventilated cardiac, chronic obstructive pulmonary disease (COPD), and trauma patients, hyperoxygenation should be used during suctioning to maintain arterial oxygen saturation.
- The value of hyperinflation prior to suctioning was unclear. However, hyperinflation should not be performed before, during, and/or after suctioning of severely head injured patients in whom intracraneal pressure (ICP) is a concern. Minute ventilation should be increased by adjusting the rate but not the volume to minimize sudden increases in ICP during suctioning. Hyperinflation also is not recommended for patients after CAB and should be used with caution for other unstable patients, as it may be associated with increases in blood pressure.
- Hyperoxygenation is more effective via the ventilator than a manual resuscitation bag.
- Suctioning through an adapter while maintaining the patient on the ventilator may be as effective as hyperoxygenating before and after the procedure as a means of preserving oxygenation.
- Some evidence supports the use of a modified double-lumen endotracheal tube with capabilities for continuous or intermittent suctioning of subglottic secretions as a means of preventing subglottic aspiration.
- Insufficient evidence was found to recommend instillation of saline to loosen secretions. Most of the recent nursing literature discourages this practice.

Even though definitive research is lacking, studies (9–12) indicate that suctioning based on the assessed need is more appropriate than that using a fixed time schedule. In addition, the duration of suctioning should be limited to 15 s, suction should not be applied until the catheter is in place, the catheter should be rotated while being withdrawn, intermittent suction should be applied, and sufficient time should be allowed between passes to allow the patient to reoxygenate.

Until recently, it was the practice in many ICUs to routinely restrain all intubated patients. However, we have found that restraints are not necessary for patients who are alert and cooperative.

Care of Patients with Acute Respiratory Distress Syndrome

Acute respiratory distress syndrome (ARDS) patients present a unique critical care nursing challenge. In addition to their respiratory problems, ARDS patients also present challenges in regard to nutritional support, prevention of skin breakdown, and the need for emotional and psychological support. Prolonged mechanical ventilation imposes significant barriers to communication with the team. The nurse has an important role in assuring that the alert patient has a means to communicate, such as writing notes or using an alphabet or phrase board.

Many of the treatment strategies that may be tried for ARDS are frightening and uncomfortable to the patient, such as use of muscle relaxants, prone positioning, continuous lateral rotation, lung-protective ventilation techniques, and inhaled nitric oxide. The nurse has an important role in providing comfort and support by speaking to the patient, explaining procedures, being visible and available, and applying therapeutic touch. An essential role for the nurse is ensuring that the patient is adequately medicated to control anxiety, relieve discomfort, and promote rest.

Various specialty beds and positioning techniques have been tried since the late 1980s with the goals of improving oxygenation, preventing pulmonary complications, reducing ventilator time, and reducing length of ICU stay. Continuous lateral rotation, first on the Roto-rest bed, then with various models of continuous low air loss rotating beds, has been used. Several studies of the efficacy of these beds for various subgroups of patients have been published and report conflicting results. In those studies reporting positive results, patients have been put on the bed early in the course of hospitalization. Keeping a patient on the bed longer than 2 weeks has not been shown to improve outcomes. As the beds are expensive to rent, a protocol that helps the clinicians decide which patients may benefit and defines time limits for using the bed is desirable.

Prone positioning is another technique employed to improve the oxygenation of ARDS patients. Several studies have demonstrated improved oxygenation as a result of prone positioning. A study led by Gattinoni et al. (13), published in 2001, concluded that although prone positioning improves oxygenation, it does not improve survival. Safe prone positioning requires the participation of several members of the nursing staff. Development of a detailed procedure and appropriate staff training such that all individuals know their roles are essential. In particular, someone must be designated to stabilize the endotracheal tube and ventilator connection in order to prevent accidental extubation, which could be fatal. Attention also must be paid to appropriate cushioning and pressure reduction techniques, especially for facial prominences like the chin and forehead.

WOUND MANAGEMENT AND PRESSURE ULCER PREVENTION

Wound management has become a very complex field in the past 20 years. Consultation and collaboration with certified enterostomal (ET) nurses when treating complex wounds or pressure ulcers is beneficial for patients. ET nurses are specially trained in wound management and are experts in selecting the appropriate type of dressing for each patient. The ET nurse prescribes a treatment plan using the best dressing for that patient and collaborates with the ICU nurse in implementing the plan.

The purpose of dressings is to create the optimal environment for wound healing (14). They should be easy to apply, painless on removal, and require the fewest number of changes to save nursing time. Knowledge of the physiology of wound healing is helpful to nurses and all practitioners involved in managing wounds. We now know that most wounds heal best in a moist environment. Table 1 provides guidelines for suitable dressings for different types of wounds.

Several adjunctive therapies are currently being used for the treatment of complex acute and chronic wounds. These adjunctive therapies include electrical stimulation, topical oxygen, ultrasound, warmth therapy, and vacuum-assisted closure (VAC). The evidence for these therapies is limited but growing. In particular, the VAC system has been shown to enhance granulation tissue formation and to increase the blood flow and tissue oxygenation (15). Each clinician will need to periodically review the literature on these modalities in order to know which ones prove to be efficacious.

Approximately 40% of critically ill patients will develop pressure ulcers. In the author's experience, virtually 100% of long-term critically ill patients will develop a pressure ulcer unless aggressive steps are taken to prevent them. These steps include the performance by the nurse of a pressure ulcer risk assessment on admission to the unit and at predefined intervals. Then, on the basis of the assessed risk, specific interventions are implemented. High risk patients should have daily skin assessments, which are documented in the record. High risk patients should also be placed on low air loss beds or overlays, unless the unit is equipped with mattresses that provide effective pressure relief. The presence of a pressure ulcer adds significantly to the cost of care. A 1988 study estimated that the development of a stage III or IV ulcer added at least $25,000 to the cost of the hospital stay; in today's dollars the cost would be considerably increased (16,17).

The primary cause of pressure ulcers is tissue ischemia that occurs when external pressure exceeds the tissue capillary pressure. Shearing forces generated by sliding the patient up in bed or raising the head of the bed also contribute to ischemia and ulcer formation. Critically ill patients are often severely edematous and may have marginal tissue perfusion. These factors increase the likelihood that tissue ischemia will occur with any prolonged pressure. Frequent position changes and pressure relief are essential for these patients.

Common sites of pressure ulcers are the coccyx and heels. One reason that these sites are common is that ICU patients must be returned to the supine position frequently

Table 1 Selection of an Appropriate Wound Dressing

Type of wound	Suitable dressing
Closed wound healing by primary intention	Gauze dressing/adhesive film
Superficial partial thickness	Adhesive film/foam
Mild to moderate exudate	Hydrocolloid/hydrofiber/hydrogel
Contaminated, moderate to heavy exudate	Alginate/hydrofiber
Heavy exudate	Foam/hydrofiber/hydrocolloid
Dry necrotic	Hydrogel/hydrocolloid

in order to accurately measure pulmonary artery pressures. Decreasing the frequency of these measurements as soon as the patient becomes more stable may be helpful.

MANAGEMENT OF DIARRHEA

Management of enteral feeding–associated diarrhea is a significant critical care nursing problem. Diarrhea is a contributing factor to perineal skin excoriation and pressure ulcer development. The frequent bathing and bed changes required are also embarrassing and uncomfortable to the patient and very labor-intensive for the nursing staff.

The cause of diarrhea in patients receiving enteral feedings is not well understood. It has been attributed to hypoalbuminemia, bacterial contamination of formula, characteristics of particular tube feeding formulas, and concomitant drug therapy (18,19). Hypoalbuminemia leads to edema of the intestinal mucosa, which compromises absorption and disrupts the intravascular osmotic forces responsible for drawing substrates across the intestinal epithelial cells. Microbial contamination of enteral feeding during administration appears to play a significant role in the etiology of diarrhea (20). In terms of the characteristics of enteral feeding formulas that may affect the development of diarrhea, both the osmolality and fiber content of the formula have been implicated, although additional study is needed.

Another factor that may contribute to the development of diarrhea is medications that are given through the feeding tube. Some elixirs and suspensions are hyperosmolar or are dissolved in a hyperosmolar agent, such as sorbitol. Antacids containing magnesium hydroxide are also associated with diarrhea. Antibiotics may contribute to diarrhea, either by direct irritation of the intestinal mucosa or by causing a decrease in the normal gut flora, resulting in an overgrowth of toxin-producing bacteria, such as *Clostridium difficile*.

Several approaches can be taken to reduce the volume of diarrhea or to manage it. Medications that are being delivered via the feeding tube should be scrutinized to determine if those in hyperosmolar suspensions can be eliminated or given by another route. Once *C. difficile* has been excluded or treated, medications can be administered to reduce bowel motility. Care should be taken to maintain the tube feeding system as a closed system, such that bacteria are not introduced. Manufacturer's recommendations or unit policies regarding enteral feeding hang times should be followed closely. Skin excoriation and frequent clean-ups can be reduced through the use of fecal collection bags and membrane dressings that are applied to the skin for protection.

MANAGEMENT OF DELIRIUM

Delirium is a common occurrence in the ICU. The estimated prevalence ranges from 15% to 50%. Two recent prospective studies reported that 81% (21) and 83% (22), respectively, of the subjects developed delirium. Delirium is associated with poor outcomes, for example, increased length of stay, higher mortality rates, and the need for subsequent institutionalization (22,23). Ely et al. found in a 2001 study that the presence of delirium was the strongest independent predictor of hospital length of stay (21). The incidence of delirium increases with age and is especially common in mechanically ventilated patients. Delirium significantly increases nursing care requirements, especially in the hyperactive variation of the syndrome. Sometimes 1 : 1 observation is required to safely manage the patient and to prevent the patient from self-extubating or falling out of bed.

Nursing Considerations

To diagnose delirium, the following symptoms must exist:

- Global cerebral dysfunction involving the impairment of the ability to focus, sustain, or shift attention.
- Impairment of cognition, sometimes including illusions, delusions, or hallucinations.
- Onset over a short period of time.
- Presence of an underlying medical condition.

Delirium may take a hypoactive or hyperactive form. In the hypoactive form the patient is sluggish and lethargic. In the hyperactive form the patient is agitated, restless, and even combative.

The etiology of delirium is not well understood. Anticholinergic medications are a likely contributing factor. Other physiologic factors may include dementia, metabolic derangements, infections, multisystem failure, and hypoxia. Hospital-related factors may include immobility and physical restraint, sleep impairment from frequent assessments and interventions, and environmental factors such as the presence of around the clock light and noise in the ICU. Delirium frequently fails to be recognized in the ICU. The use of a delirium assessment tool, such as the confusion assessment method for the intensive care unit (CAM-ICU) (22,24), facilitates diagnosis and early treatment.

Multiple treatment options should be pursued when delirium is diagnosed. If the patient is reasonably stable, the nurse should try to batch assessments and cares during the night to allow periods of uninterrupted sleep. They should be sensitive to controlling noise and light during the night to promote sleep. Appropriate pain management and sedation also will promote sleep. As immobility appears to contribute to the development of delirium, restraints should be avoided and efforts made to get the patient out of bed during the day. The patient's medications should be reviewed, and anticholinergics eliminated when possible.

Medical treatment of delirium often requires the use of pharmacologic agents. The two main classes of drugs used to treat delirium are neuroleptics and benzodiazepines, although benzodiazepines themselves are associated with the development of delirium. Intravenous haloperidol is most commonly used. It may be titrated to effect with dosages as high as 10 mg every 15 min during acute episodes of agitation (25). When behavior is under control, the patient can be maintained on a routine dose of haloperidol until the delirium clears. Small doses of benzodiazepines may be used to decrease the amount of haloperidol needed. Patients on high doses of haloperidol or other neuroleptic agents should be monitored for the development of extrapyramidal symptoms, Q–T interval prolongation, torsades de pointes, and neuroleptic malignant syndrome.

SUMMARY

- Close collaboration between physicians and nurses in planning and providing care for the complex critically ill patient produces better outcomes.
- The whole patient is the focus of the nurse. In addition to monitoring physical response and providing for physical needs, nurses play a vital role in communication with patients and their families.
- An important part of critical care nursing is monitoring and supporting respiratory function. ICU nurses can identify impending respiratory failure early, position patients for improved respiratory function, and maintain patent airways.

- Guidelines for suctioning airways include: supplementary oxygen before suctioning, supplementary oxygen during suctioning for many patients, and avoiding hyperinflation in patients with severe head injury or after CAB. Suctioning through an adapter while the patient receives support from the ventilator may be of benefit.
- Airway suctioning should be performed as needed, rather than on a fixed schedule.
- Nurses are vital in assisting communication, allaying fears, and providing adequate analgesia and anxiolysis in patients requiring long-term mechanical ventilation.
- Pressure ulcers develop in ~40% of critically ill patients unless nurses identify high risk patients, place high risk patients on appropriate low air loss beds, and relieve pressure areas, especially the coccyx and heels.
- Diarrhea in the critically ill patient can be reduced by closed enteral feeding systems, limiting administration of hyperosmolar medications via the feeding tube, and identifying and treating antibiotic associated diarrhea. Fecal collection bags and membrane dressings can reduce excoriation.
- Components of delirium include: global cerebral dysfunction, impairment of cognition, rapid onset, and an underlying medical condition. Use of a delirium assessment tool can aid early diagnosis. Limiting assessments, controlling noise and light, and administering analgesics and sedatives are helpful. Neuroleptic agents and benzodiazepines are often used.

REFERENCES

1. Baggs JG, Schmitt MH, Mushlin AI, Mitchell PH, Eldredge DH, Oakes D, Hutson AD. Association between nurse–physician collaboration and patient outcomes in three intensive care units. Crit Care Med 1999; 27(9):1991–1998.
2. Baggs JG, Ryan SA, Phelps CE, Richeson JF, Johnson JE. The association between interdisciplinary collaboration and patient outcomes in a medical intensive care unit. Heart Lung 1992; 21(1):18–23.
3. Knaus WA, Zimmerman JE, Wagner DP. APACHE-acute physiology and chronic health evaluation: a physiologically based classification system. Crit Care Med 1982; 9:591–597.
4. Kohn L, Corrigan J, Donaldson M, eds. To Err is Human: Building a Safer Health System. Committee on Quality of Health Care in America, Institute of Medicine. Washington DC: National Academy Press, 1999.
5. Committee on Quality of Health Care in America. Crossing the Quality Chasm: A New Health System for the 21st Century. Institute of Medicine, 2001.
6. Goodwin MJ, Bissett L, Mason P, Kates R, Weber J. Early extubation and early activity after heart surgery. Crit Care Nurse 1999; 19(5):18–26.
7. Wheeler H. Positioning: one good turn after another? Nurs Crit Care 1997; 2(3):129–131.
8. Brooks D, Anderson CM, Carter MA, Downes LA, Keenan SP, Kelsey CJ, Lacy JB. Clinical practice guidelines for suctioning the airway of the intubated and nonintubated patient. Can Resp J 2001; 8(3):163–180.
9. Celik SS, Elbas NO. The standard of suction for patients undergoing endotracheal intubation. Intens Crit Care Nurs 2000; 16:191–198.
10. Wainwright SP, Gould D. Endotracheal suctioning: an example of the problems of relevance and rigour in clinical research. J Clin Nurs 1996; 5:389–398.
11. Wood CJ. Can nurses safely assess the need for endotracheal suction in short-term ventilated patients, instead of using routine techniques? Intens Crit Care Nurs 1998; 14:170–178.

12. AARC clinical practice guideline. Endotracheal suctioning of mechanically ventilated adults and children with artificial airways. American Association for Respiratory Care. Resp Care 1993; 38(5):500–504.
13. Gattinoni L, Tognoni G, Pesenti A, Taccone P, Mascheroni D, Labarta V, Malacrida R, Di Giulio P, Fumagalli R, Pelosi P, Brazzi L, Latini R. Effect of prone positioning on the survival of patients with acute respiratory failure. New Engl J Med 2001; 345(8):568–573.
14. Foster L, Moore P. Acute surgical wound care 3: fitting the dressing to the wound. Br J Nurs 1999; 8(4):200–206.
15. Krasner DL, Sibbald RG. Nursing management of chronic wounds: best practices across the continuum of care. Nurs Clin N Am 1999; 34(4):933–953.
16. Hadcock J. The development of a standardized approach to wound care in ICU. Br J Nurs 2000; 9(10):614–623.
17. Moody BL, Fanale JE, Thompson M. Impact of staff education on pressure sore development in elderly hospitalized patients. Arch Intern Med 1988; 148:2241–2243.
18. Burns PE, Jairath N. Diarrhea and the patient receiving enteral feedings: a multifactorial problem. J Wound Ostomy Continence Nurs Society 1994; 21:257–263.
19. Mobarhan S, DeMeo M. Diarrhea induced by enteral feeding. Nutr Rev 1995; 53(3):67–70.
20. Okuma T, Nakamura M, Totake H, Fukunaga Y. Microbial contamination of enteral feeding formulas and diarrhea. Nutrition 2000; 16(9):719–722.
21. Ely EW, Gautam S, Margolin R, Francis J, May L, Speroff T, Truman B, Dittus R, Bernard R, Inouye SK. The impact of delirium in the intensive care unit on hospital length of stay. Intens Care Med 2001; 27(12):1892–1900.
22. Ely EW, Inouye SK, Bernard GB, Gordon S, Francis J, May L, Truman B, Speroff T, Gautam S, Margolin R, Hart RP, Dittus R. Delirium in mechanically ventilated patients: validity and reliability of the confusion and assessment method for the intensive care unit (CAM-ICU). J Am Med Assoc 2001; 286(21):2703–2709.
23. Roberts BL. Managing delirium in adult intensive care patients. Crit Care Nurse 2001; 21(1):48–55.
24. Fraser GL, Riker RR. Monitoring sedation, agitation, analgesia and delirium in critically ill adult patients. Crit Care Clin 2001; 17(4):967–987.
25. Justic M. Does ICU psychosis really exist? Crit Care Nurse 2000; 20(3):28–37.

Part III
Pathophysiologic Conditions

C. Central Nervous System Function

15
Coma

Frederick Langendorf
Hennepin County Medical Center, Minneapolis, Minnesota, USA

INTRODUCTION

Coma sits at the end of a continuum of decreased levels of consciousness. It represents the brain's ultimate response to insult or injury. Coma can be an ominous medical emergency.

Coma is an eyes-closed, sleep-like, unarousable, unconscious state. The patient demonstrates no meaningful interaction with the environment and no awareness. Spontaneous respirations, various reflexes, and simple motor responses to noxious stimuli may or may not be present. The terms lethargy, obtundation, and stupor imply a higher level of consciousness than coma. As ambiguity surrounds these labels, describing the patient is more informative.

Whether a patient is arousable may be directly tested. Whether a patient is conscious is a matter of inference and even philosophy. Nevertheless, much is known about the anatomical substrate of consciousness.

ANATOMY AND PHYSIOLOGY

Two structures are necessary for our normal awake, aroused, aware, alert state. At least one cerebral hemisphere must be intact. The dispensability of one hemisphere (where consciousness is concerned) is demonstrated by the recovery of consciousness after hemispherectomy, a procedure still occasionally indicated for intractable epilepsy. Also required for consciousness is the ascending reticular activating system (ARAS). The ARAS is a series of neurons in the upper brainstem with bodies not discretely aggregated into a nucleus. The ARAS receives input from multiple sensory systems and projects to thalamus and cerebral cortex. Projections are principally cholinergic. The ARAS produces arousal, manifest as an eyes-open, wakeful-appearing state. Coupled to a functioning hemisphere, this arousal will generate consciousness. But without functioning hemispheres, the ARAS will produce an arousal-without-consciousness condition known as the vegetative state. The ARAS is transiently shut down during sleep by brain stem serotonergic systems. Consequently, destruction or inhibition of the ARAS or of both hemispheres will produce coma.

Severe bihemispheral dysfunction leading to coma can be caused by diminished cerebral blood flow (CBF) (Table 1). CBF depends on cerebral perfusion pressure

Table 1 Cerebral Blood Flow

	CBF (mL/100 g of brain per min)
Normal	50–55
Required for consciousness	25–30
Required for EEG activity (produced by post-synaptic potentials)	15–20
Required for cellular homeostasis	10–15

(CPP). Autoregulation ensures normal CBF through a range of CPPs from 60 to 160 mmHg by altering cerebral vascular persistance. Once CPP falls below 60 mmHg CBF will diminish. CPP, in turn, is the difference between the mean arterial pressure and the intracranial pressure. Both diminished blood pressure and increased intracranial pressure may diminish CBF to levels associated with coma (<25–30 mL/100 g of brain tissue/min). Diffuse metabolic or toxic injury to the brain also can cause bihemispheral dysfunction.

Structural abnormalities may cause coma by impingement on the ARAS. A mass lesion above the tentorium (the meningeal infolding that separates the cerebral hemispheres from the posterior fossa) may distort the ARAS through lateral displacement of the ARAS ("midline shift") or through transtentorial herniation. In transtentorial herniation, the medial temporal lobe moves across the edge of the tentorium and down along the brainstem. Bilateral mass effect in the hemispheres, for example from hydrocephalus, can produce central herniation through the tentorial opening containing the brainstem with resulting ARAS failure. The ARAS may be more directly affected by structural abnormalities below the tentorium, including brainstem lesions involving the ARAS and cerebellar lesions producing mass effect on the brainstem and ARAS.

DIFFERENTIAL DIAGNOSIS

Approach to Diagnosis

Almost any category of disease may produce coma. The crucial diagnostic challenge is distinguishing structural from nonstructural causes of coma. Suspicion of a structural problem mandates emergency cerebral imaging, which, in turn, can provide the anatomical mechanism of coma and a highly specific diagnosis. The discovery of a structural cause of coma may lead to life-saving surgery or other procedures.

Abrupt onset of coma suggests an intracranial structural catastrophe, although some nonstructural processes, such as anoxia, may exhibit sudden onset as well. Certain focal findings on neurological examination can suggest structural abnormality. These sets of findings can be diagnostic of a supratentorial mass lesion with transtentorial herniation or of an infratentorial mass lesion. A nonfocal examination does not rule out structural abnormality.

Major causes of coma and some diagnostic aids are listed in Tables 2 and 3.

Vascular Disease

Stroke usually does not disturb the level of consciousness. Nonetheless, a number of vascular pathologies can lead to coma principally by infarcting or compressing the

Table 2 Causes of Coma

Structural	Nonstructural
Vascular	Anoxia
Pontine hemorrhage	Shock
Brainstem infarction (basilar artery thrombosis)	Hypercapnea
	Temperature dysregulation
Cerebellar infarction or hemorrhage with brainstem compression	Hypothermia
	Heat stroke
Cerebral infarction or hemorrhage with herniation	Toxic
	Alcohol, methanol
Cerebral hemorrhage with intraventricular hemorrhage	Barbiturates
	Benzodiazepines
Subarachnoid hemorrhage	Opiates
Venous sinus thrombosis	Carbon monoxide
Hypertensive encephalopathy	Psychotropic drugs, including lithium and MAO inhibitors
Traumatic	
Penetrating injury	Anticholinergics
Diffuse axonal injury	Metabolic
Cerebral contusion or hematoma	Hyper- and hypoglycemia
Subdural or epidural hematoma	Acidosis
Cerebral fat embolism	Electrolyte disturbance: hyper- and hyponatremia; hyper- and hypocalcemia; hypomagnesemia
Neoplastic	
Tumor with herniation or brainstem compression	
	Endocrine disturbance: hypothyroidism, Addison disease
Multiple tumors	
Carcinomatous meningitis	Organ failure: hepatic encephalopathy, uremia
Infectious	Vitamin deficiency: Wernicke encephalopathy (thiamine deficiency)
Encephalitis	
Meningitis	Seizure-related
Sepsis	Status epilepticus, convulsive or non-convulsive
Abscess with herniation or brainstem compression	Post-ictal state
Demyelinating	
Acute disseminated encephalomyelitis	
Other	
Hydrocephalus	

ARAS. The pons is one of the typical sites for hypertensive hemorrhage and may involve the ARAS. Brainstem infarction also may impair the ARAS. These infarcts can occur with thrombosis or thromboembolism of the basilar artery. Cerebellar hemorrhage and infarction can compress the ARAS. Subarachnoid hemorrhage can cause coma through increased intracranial pressure, with or without hydrocephalus, and through processes not entirely understood. Thalamic hemorrhage, another typical hypertensive hemorrhage, can extend into the ventricular system to produce hydrocephalus and coma. Large supratentorial hemorrhages and infarcts may cause increased intracranial pressure, midline shift, or transtentorial herniation. Vascular events occur abruptly, although potentially coma-producing sequelae such as increased intracranial pressure, hydrocephalus, or transtentorial herniation may take time to evolve. Maximum mass effect from large

Table 3 Aids to the Differential Diagnosis of Coma

Coma presenting abruptly
  Anoxia
  Shock
  Trauma: contusion, diffuse axonal injury
  Vascular: pontine hemorrhage, subarachnoid hemorrhage
  Seizure-related
  Intoxication
Coma with focality on neurologic examination
  Vascular: infarction or hemorrhage
  Neoplastic: tumor, carcinomatous meningitis
  Traumatic: subdural or epidural hematoma, cerebral contusion
  Infection: abscess, herpes simplex encephalitis
  Hypoglycemia
  Post-ictal state
  Wernicke encephalopathy
Coma that resolves without specific treatment
  Intoxication
  Concussion
  Syncope
  Post-ictal state

infarcts with edema generally is reached 1–2 days after the stroke. Focal findings on neurological examination is the rule with vascular disease, although subarachnoid hemorrhage and venous sinus thrombosis are often nonfocal.

Some vascular causes of coma are neurosurgical emergencies, including cerebellar infarct or hemorrhage, intraventricular hemorrhage with hydrocephalus, and subarachnoid hemorrhage.

Trauma

Blunt injury may produce cerebral contusions or hematomas, which lead to increased intracranial pressure, midline shift, or herniation. Widespread shear injury that produces diffuse axonal injury (DAI) may be sufficient to cause coma. Subdural and epidural hematomas may produce mass effect, with resultant midline shift or transtentorial herniation. These types of brain injury may coexist.

Since the injury is usually severe and the coma immediate, trauma as the cause of coma is usually apparent. But some caveats are in order. Even with obvious head injury, some other problem, such as anoxia, seizure, or intoxication may have caused the injury or the ensuing coma. Apparently mild injuries sometimes may produce severe sequelae, especially when the patient is anticoagulated. Patients with subdural or epidural hematomas and little injury to underlying brain initially may appear intact. As the hematoma enlarges, the level of consciousness declines and focal signs appear. This phenomenon is the "talk and deteriorate" syndrome. Significant lesions, for example, bilateral frontal lobe or subdural hematomas, potentially requiring surgery, may produce a nonfocal examination. Cerebral imaging is usually diagnostic in trauma severe enough to produce coma. Sometimes, a severe degree of diffuse axonal injury may occur with little in the way of contusion or hematoma apparent on computed tomography (CT). Magnetic resonance imaging (MRI), with gradient echo sequences, is highly sensitive for the micro-hemorrhages associated with shear injuries.

Other Structural Pathologies

As with other structural abnormalities, tumors and focal infections can produce increased intracranial pressure or involve the ARAS. Neoplasms and focal infections generally produce progressive symptoms. Coma develops usually after the diagnosis is clear. In some exceptional circumstances, these pathologies can produce abrupt symptoms and mimic stroke. Some primary brain tumors and brain metastases (notoriously melanoma and renal cell carcinoma) can hemorrhage. Tumors and abscesses may produce hydrocephalus. A brain abscess may rupture into the ventricular system. Although not truly abrupt in onset, bacterial meningitis may progress very rapidly to coma. Focal examinations are the rule with neoplasms sizable enough to cause coma. Multiple tumors, such as metastases, may produce a nonfocal examination. Aside from abscess and herpes simplex encephalitis, the neurologic examination associated with infectious causes of coma is often nonfocal.

Nonstructural Pathologies

The entities listed in Table 2 affect the brain through many pathways. The precise mechanism of coma is unknown for many metabolic encephalopathies. These abnormalities are usually nonfocal, although hypoglycemia is a notorious exception. Anoxic coma typically occurs in the context of resuscitated cardiac arrest but may result from respiratory arrest or profound hypotension. Hypothermia below 32 °C may produce coma and even simulate brain death. Most metabolic encephalopathies will be evident on laboratory evaluation. Seizures responsible for coma may not be apparent clinically. Ongoing seizures, where the seizures cloud consciousness but do not cause convulsive movements, are called nonconvulsive status epilepticus. Alternatively, a post-ictal phase can account for coma; sometimes the preceding seizure is missed. Convulsive or nonconvulsive seizures may originate from an underlying cause, structural or nonstructural, that is by itself sufficient to cause coma.

APPROACH TO THE PATIENT WITH COMA

Given the life-threatening nature of many causes of coma, evaluation and management proceed rapidly and concurrently. The neurologic examination, despite its dependence on complicated anatomy and reflex arcs, has the simple purpose of separating structural from nonstructural causes of coma.

History

In the cases of trauma or cardiac arrest, history may be unavailable. When it is possible to obtain a history, the clinician should attempt to learn about the time course of onset, since some causes produce coma abruptly (Table 3). The history also should be directed to underlying medical conditions, medications, and any substance abuse. Preceding symptoms may suggest specific diagnoses: neurologic complaints such as lateralized weakness, numbness, or diplopia suggest structural abnormality. Headache suggests structural abnormality or infection. Fever may indicate infection. A history of epilepsy raises the question of seizures. Carbon monoxide poisoning is suggested by occupational exposure, headache, and multiple encephalopathic patients from the same location. With Wernicke encephalopathy, associated with acute thiamine deficiency, symptoms prior to coma include confusion, gait disorder, and diplopia. Findings indicating carbon monoxide poisoning or acute thiamine deficiency are not part of the usual laboratory evaluation of patients in coma. Clinical suspicion is of great importance in correctly diagnosing these conditions.

Examination

Vital Signs

Respirations should be carefully observed. Highly irregular patterns of respiration are associated with lower brainstem dysfunction. Rapid breathing can be a sign of hypoxia, acidosis, sepsis, hepatic encephalopathy, and some toxic overdoses. Hypotension suggests cardiovascular problems, internal hemorrhage, sepsis, endocrinopathy, or intoxication. Fever suggests infection but also may be seen with subarachnoid hemorrhage, pontine hemorrhage, and thyrotoxicosis. Hypothermia suggests intoxication, endocrinopathy, and Wernicke encephalopathy. Extreme dysregulation of body temperature either above or below normal is sufficient to cause coma.

General Examination

A careful inspection for signs of trauma will include an otoscopic examination for hemotympanum. Ophthalmoscopy may show papilledema, indicative of increased intracranial pressure; pre-retinal (also known as subhyaloid) hemorrhages, indicative of subarachnoid hemorrhage; or retinal hemorrhages and exudates suggestive of hypertensive encephalopathy. Nuchal rigidity, a sign of meningitis, should be tested, if no indication of trauma is present. An examination of the skin should not be overlooked. Important skin findings include a cherry-red appearance, suggestive of carbon monoxide poisoning; a petechial rash, suggestive of meningococcal meningitis or a bleeding disorder; dry, hot skin suggestive of heat stroke; jaundice, suggestive of hepatic encephalopathy or coagulopathy; or cyanosis. Examinations of the heart, lung, and abdomen are detailed in the following sections.

Mental Status Examination

Mental status examination establishes the level of alertness. It should be performed *and recorded* in sufficient detail that the next examiner can tell if the patient is better, worse, or the same. Stimuli should be delivered in order from least to most noxious, as needed to produce a response: normal voice, loud voice, touch, more aggressive tactile stimulus such as tapping on forehead or shaking limbs, and, finally, painful stimulus. Painful stimulus should be applied in the midline (brows, sternum) to assess general level of alertness, and then should be applied to each limb (pressure on an interphalangeal joint) to further assess symmetry.

From the mental status examination, a Glasgow Coma Score (GCS) can be determined (Table 4). This score is useful for comparing serial exams, for prognosticating outcome from head injury, and for giving other caregivers a fairly good idea of a patient's mental status in a few syllables. It is not a substitute for other parts of the examination, nor does it suffice to record a GCS without recording the specific findings.

Table 4 Glasgow Coma Scale

Best motor response	
Obeys commands	6
Localizes	5
Withdraws	4
Abnormal flexion	3
Abnormal extension	2
None	1
Verbal response	
Oriented	5
Confused	4
Inappropriate words	3
Incomprehensible	2
None	1
Eye opening	
Spontaneous	4
To voice	3
To pain	2
None	1

Cranial Nerve Examination

Examination of the *pupils* is critical. The efferent arm of the pupillary light reflex is mediated by parasympathetic fibers traveling on the outside of the third cranial nerve. Cranial nerve III travels just under the edge of the tentorium. Consequently, asymmetric or asymmetrically reactive pupils are signs of transtentorial herniation until proven otherwise. Ocular trauma, ophthalmic surgery, or eye drops can also produce pupillary asymmetry. Symmetrical but unreactive pupils imply bilateral midbrain dysfunction, often from more advanced herniation. Very small but reactive pupils are seen with pontine hemorrhage and narcotic overdose. Usually, ambient light in an emergency department is high intensity. Because of the critical nature of the pupillary examination, a very bright light source should be used and, if possible, the ambient light should be briefly dimmed.

Eye movements allow assessment of the cranial nerves III and VI, the midbrain, and the pons, and facilitate detection and localization of a structural process. The position of the eyes should be observed. The examiner should open the lids if necessary. Roving, conjugate, lateral eye movements are nonspecific, but persistent conjugate eye deviation suggests structural abnormality in either the hemisphere toward which the eyes are deviated or the pons on the opposite side. Nystagmoid jerks suggest seizures. Dysconjugate position of the eyes can be due to third nerve/midbrain dysfunction on the side of a laterally deviated eye or due to sixth nerve/pontine dysfunction on the side of a medially deviated eye. Vertical dysconjugacy suggests intrinsic brainstem dysfunction. If trauma has been excluded, eye movements can be induced by head turning. This maneuver stimulates a reflex originating from the vestibular system. The eyes move conjugately in the direction opposite to the head turn, when the brainstem and cranial nerves are intact. Asymmetric responses again indicate focal dysfunction of third nerve/midbrain or sixth nerve/pons. This reflex may be lost entirely in severe toxic, metabolic, or anoxic coma. A stronger stimulus for this reflex would be caloric testing (instilling cold water into the ear; eyes deviate conjugately toward the cold water). This examination is usually too time-consuming for use in the urgent evaluation of a comatose patient.

Corneal reflexes are mediated by cranial nerve V (afferent limb) and VII (efferent limb). Asymmetric responses indicate dysfunction at the level of the pons. Symmetric loss may again represent a nonstructural process. This reflex is tested by lightly touching the cornea (not the sclera) with tissue or cotton. As with examining pupils, the response on *both* sides must be noted when each side is stimulated.

Motor Examination

Spontaneous rhythmic, clonic movements suggest seizures. Irregular, twitchy, variably located movements represent myoclonus. Myoclonus typically is seen with anoxic encephalopathy, uremia, hepatic encephalopathy, and some intoxications. Persistently asymmetric spontaneous movements suggest a hemispheral or brainstem structural abnormality opposite the weak side. Noxious stimulation may produce movement where none was evident before. Asymmetric failure to move again suggests contralateral structural abnormality. Symmetrical extension of all four limbs, with internal rotation of the shoulders, represents extensor posturing. Arm flexion with leg extension represents flexor posturing. These findings suggest high brainstem dysfunction but can occur with nonstructural processes. Posturing also can occur spontaneously but is sufficiently stereotyped that the distinction from seizures should be obvious.

Interpretation of the Neurologic Examination

When brainstem function is intact and the physical examination is symmetric, bihemispheral dysfunction is the likely cause of coma. Often, a diffuse process is involved. Asymmetrical or focal findings suggest a structural lesion. In the comatose patient, focal findings on neurologic examination mandate an emergency cerebral imaging study to help determine the diagnosis. Nonstructural causes of focal examinations are uncommon but include hypoglycemia, Wernicke encephalopathy, post-ictal state and, rarely, hepatic encephalopathy. Conversely, some structural causes of coma may exhibit nonfocal examinations, including subarachnoid hemorrhage, venous sinus thrombosis, hypertensive encephalopathy, trauma with diffuse axonal injury, and acute disseminated encephalomyelitis. Bilateral subdural hematomas, infarcts, or neoplasms also may produce nonfocal examination. Because they are diagnostic, two clinical presentations deserve emphasis.

Supratentorial Mass Lesion with Transtentorial Herniation This lesion produces a highly characteristic sequence of events. It begins with the manifestation of the mass lesion: decreased level of consciousness, hemiparesis, and sometimes gaze deviation. The first sign of herniation is the asymmetrically enlarged, "blown" pupil, ipsilateral to the lesion in more than 90% of cases, but occasionally contralateral, when midbrain shift occurs. Loss of medial eye movement on the side of the large pupil follows. As herniation progresses to involve the midbrain, bilaterally unreactive pupils are seen. Concomitant posturing often is observed. Progression to the level of the pons will produce asymmetric loss of corneal reflexes and lateral, as well as medial, eye movements.

Infratentorial Lesion When a lower brainstem reflex fails in the face of preserved higher brainstem function, an infratentorial structural lesion is likely. Asymmetric eye movements or corneal reflexes with symmetric, reactive pupils suggest an infratentorial localization. Transtentorial herniation cannot account for these findings, because loss of brainstem function in transtentorial herniation proceeds in a rostral–caudal fashion as herniation proceeds. The initial findings are pupillary asymmetry or unreactivity.

Laboratory Examination and Other Tests

Laboratory evaluation for the comatose patient should include those items listed in Table 5. Results of liver and thyroid tests generally are not immediately available. In appropriate circumstances, serum cortisol concentrations, carbon monoxide serum concentrations, and serum concentrations of substances discovered in the urine toxicology screen can be added.

In the case of trauma, or when a structural cause is suggested by the history or physical examination, emergency imaging is indicated. In addition, if a nonstructural cause of coma is not rapidly identified, imaging is indicated. The initial imaging test should be a cranial CT scan without contrast injection. (Contrast may make recognition of a subarachnoid hemorrhage difficult.) CT is fast and generally available but has limitations. Artifact typically is seen between the temporal bones, which can obscure the brainstem. Small brainstem hemorrhages or infarcts may be missed. Brain infarction takes some time to become visible on CT: even large middle cerebral artery infarcts may take several hours to become visible. Subdural hematomas become isodense with brain in ~1 week, and bilateral subdural hematomas at this stage may be missed. MRI has logistical drawbacks but some diagnostic advantages. Diffusion weighted sequences on MRI can show cerebral infarction within less than one hour. However, MRI may be less sensitive for blood early, and lesions that represent neurosurgical emergencies are generally well seen on head CT.

Lumbar puncture is essential to diagnose meningitis. In cases of coma, obtaining a CT scan before performing a lumbar puncture is advisable. When bacterial meningitis is suspected, treatment should begin immediately, and a CT scan, lumbar puncture, and blood cultures obtained without delay.

Electroencephalography may be necessary to detect nonconvulsive seizures. This test generally follows other investigations.

Table 5 Laboratory Evaluation of Coma

Glucose
Electrolytes: Na, K, Cl, Ca, and Mg
BUN, creatinine
CBC with platelets
PT/PTT
Serum osmolality
ABG
Blood alcohol concentration
Urine toxicology screen
Liver function tests; ammonia
Thyroid function tests
Creatine kinase

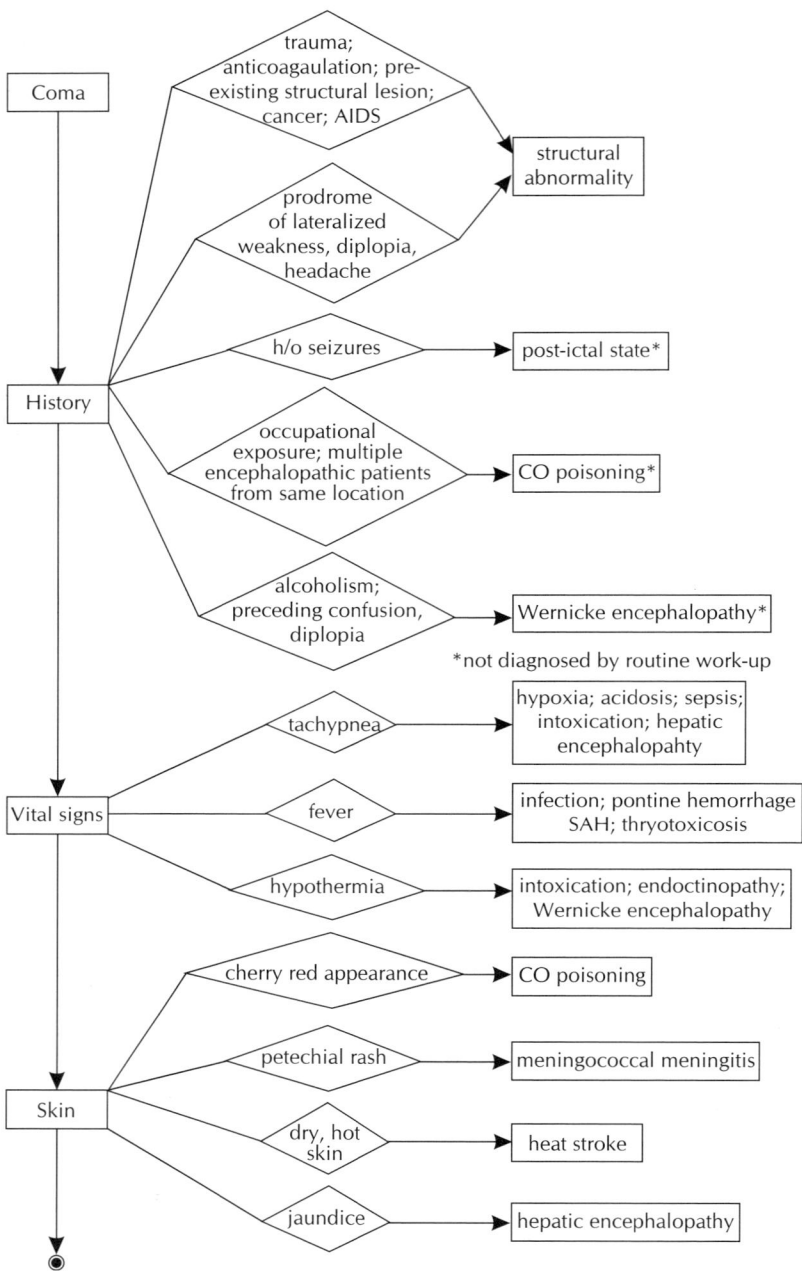

Figure 1 Approach to diagnosis and management of coma. (*Continued on next page.*)

Coma

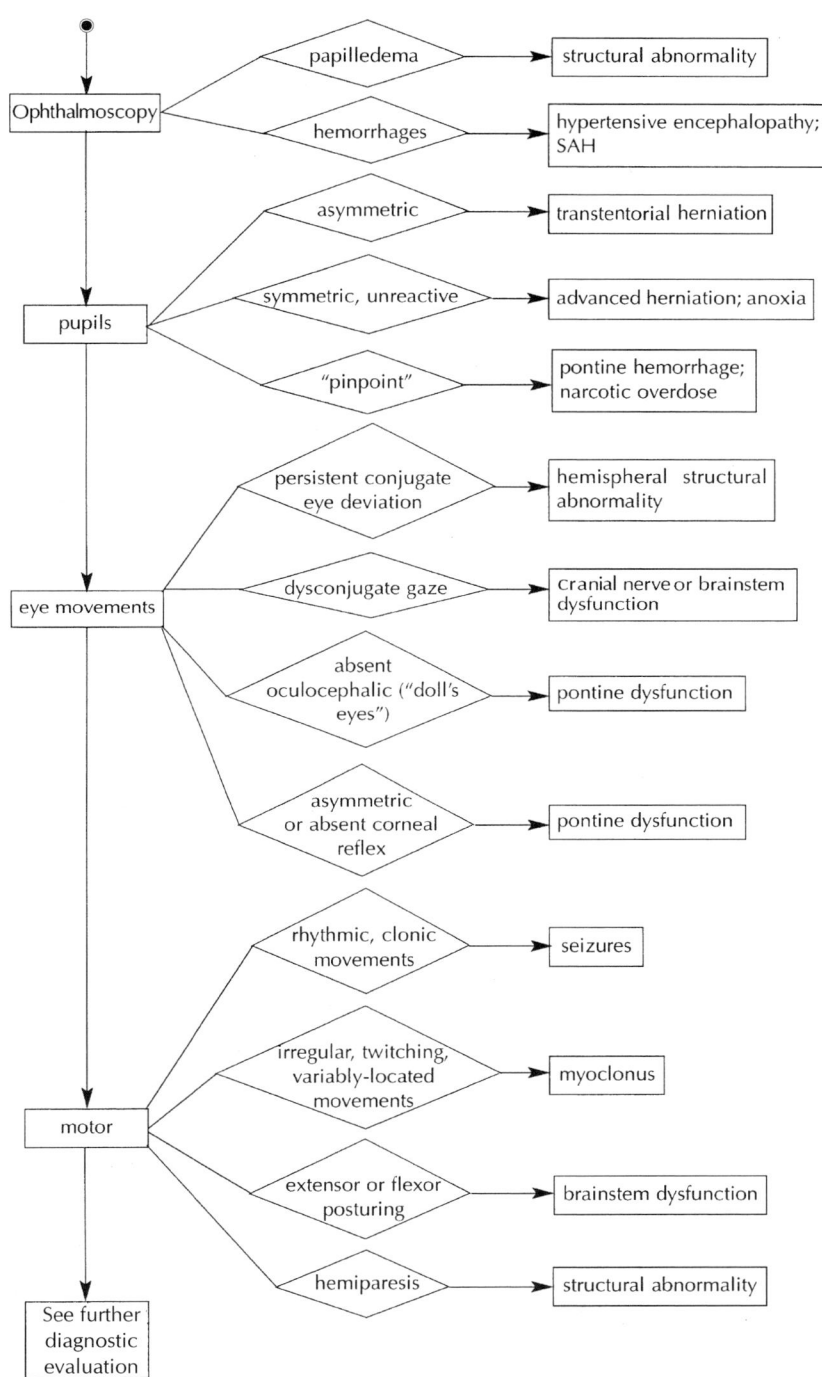

Figure 1 (*Continued on next page.*)

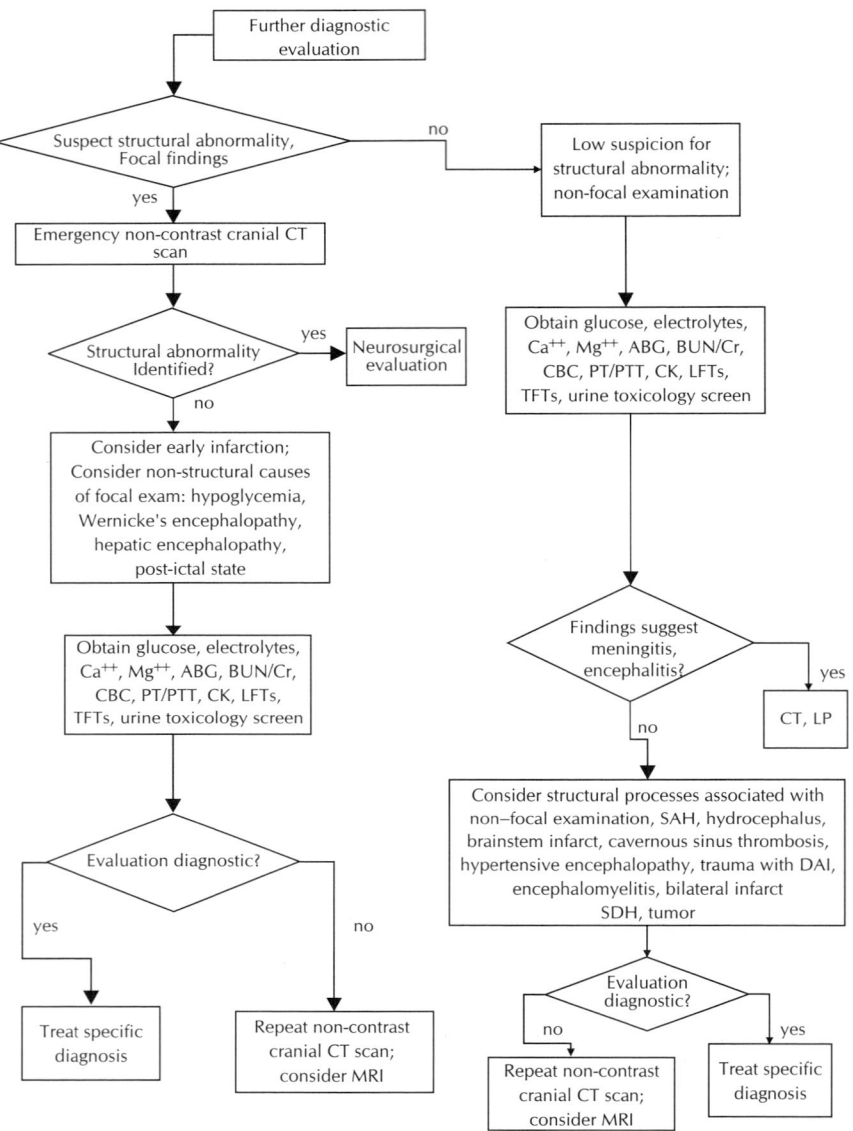

Figure 1 (*Continued*)

Emergency Management of Coma

Management strategies specific to the various causes of coma are beyond the scope of this chapter. A general approach to stabilizing the patient early will include addressing hypoventilation, hypoxia, hypotension, hypothermia, or marked hyperthermia. If intubation is required, care must be taken not to extend the neck of a patient in whom trauma has not been excluded. Intravenous lines must be established and blood for laboratory evaluation obtained. A glucose infusion should be given if any possibility of hypoglycemia exists. As glucose infusion can precipitate Wernicke's encephalopathy, 100 mg of thiamine should be administered concurrently. Naloxone can be administered for suspected narcotic overdose. Cervical spine films should be obtained if trauma cannot be excluded. A cranial CT scan should be obtained immediately if structural abnormalities are suspected.

PROGNOSIS

General Principles

Prognosis can be considered from two perspectives. *Given a comatose patient, what is the likely outcome?* The outcome is principally determined by the etiology of the coma. Provided that anoxia does not intervene, coma from intoxication usually results in a good outcome. Coma that is due to anoxic encephalopathy, subarachnoid hemorrhage, and severe head injury (with GCS <6) has a poor prognosis. Other causes occupy a middle ground (1). Outcome in coma often is described by the Glasgow Outcome Scale (GOS), initially developed for head injury (2) (Table 6). More information is obtained by answering the following question. *Given a diagnosis, what is the prognostic significance of coma?*

Determining prognosis presents a number of pitfalls. A strategy that may make a poor prognosis self-fulfilling is that treatment is often (and appropriately) limited when prognosis is thought to be poor. Data from a heterogeneous group of patients (e.g., with "nontraumatic coma") may not be highly predictive in the individual case. On the other hand, when homogeneous groups with regard to etiology, findings, and duration of coma are reported, the groups tend to be small. These constraints make confidence intervals large (3). Further, predictors of outcome often are based on a group of patients but not validated on a second group prospectively. Consequently, the positive and negative predictive value of these "predictors" is not known (4). These concerns surround the deeper question of how poor the prognosis needs to be to stop medical treatment. Decisions about limiting treatment need to be informed by as accurate a prognosis as possible. Treatment plans must be individualized with age, premorbid function, and, above all, the patient's wishes as determined from advance directives and surrogate decision makers included in the decision-making process.

Anoxic Encephalopathy

Among patients with anoxic coma for at least 6 h, only 13% recover to independence within 1 year (GOS 4–5), and 10% recover consciousness but are severely disabled (GOS 3) (5). Those destined to make a good recovery do so relatively quickly; about three quarters of the GOS 4–5 patients regain consciousness within 3 days. Investigators continue to search for ways to predict poor outcome with a high degree of certainty. Some

Table 6 Glasgow Outcome Scale

1	Death
2	Persistent vegetative state
3	Severe disability (disabled; dependent for activities of daily living)
4	Moderate disability (disabled but independent)
5	Good recovery (mild residual deficits)

examination findings are clearly helpful. The appearance of continuous myoclonus (irregular, synchronous or asynchronous limb and face twitching) is a negative prognostic factor and is associated with uniformly poor outcome (GOS 1–3) in two studies of anoxic coma (6,7). Absence of pupillary light reflexes on day 1, or absence of localized withdrawal to pain on day 3, also uniformly led to poor outcome (5). Several electroencephalographic patterns, including isoelectric ("flat") or discontinuous (burst-suppression) EEGs, and absent median nerve somatosensory evoked potentials predict poor outcome. These findings appear to add reliability when compared with predictions on the basis of physical examination alone (8). Whether they increase prognostic accuracy enough to significantly influence treatment decisions (specifically the decision to withdraw treatment) is debatable. These tests can support the decision-making process when some support is desired, either by physicians or family. Various MRI patterns may appear following anoxic injury that indicate widespread cerebral infarction, cortical infarction (laminar necrosis), or infarction of vulnerable subcortical structures, principally the basal ganglia. Whether any of these MRI patterns add prognostic information beyond what is obtainable from the physical examination is not known.

Traumatic Coma

Head injury may be closed (usually falls, motor vehicle accidents, and nonfirearm assaults) or penetrating (usually gunshot wounds). Prognostic information is different for the two injury types. Although data exist that correlate prognosis in head injury to GCS on presentation, certain cautions deserve emphasis. The GCS encompasses examinations possibly in keeping with brain death (GCS 3), with coma in the strict sense, and with a variety of lesser deficits. Some GCS scores may not meet a strict definition of coma. Consequently, prognosis of traumatic coma, compared to that of anoxic coma, is more difficult to assess. For patients with very low GCSs, outcome is clearly poor. Penetrating injury with a GCS of 3–5 (implying coma) is associated with 94% mortality and poor outcome among survivors (9). With closed head injuries, a GCS of 3–5 is associated with 81% mortality and improvement beyond vegetative state in only 12.5% (10). This figure is comparable to the dismal outcome from anoxic coma. In the GCS 3 subgroup, rare improvements were observed only in the group of patients under 40 years of age. Duration of traumatic coma correlates negatively with outcome (11).

As with anoxia, other predictors have been sought, particularly predictors of poor outcome reliable enough to justify stopping treatment. A "prediction tree" was developed on the basis of the pupillary reflex and motor response parts of the physical examination (prognostically helpful in anoxia). In addition, it incorporates age and the presence of an intracerebral lesion. Despite using these variables, the worst outcome group included a few patients who did well (12). A large number of additional factors, including systemic and intracranial pressure and findings on cerebral imaging studies, influence outcome. In this context, as in others, decisions about stopping treatment have to be individualized.

Subarachnoid Hemorrhage and Other Vascular Disease

About 10% of subarachnoid hemorrhage patients die before reaching the hospital. Of those who survive to hospital admission, about one-third will die and another third will be disabled. Patients comatose on admission have a still poorer prognosis. Seventy-two percent die, and 17% are disabled. Only 11% experience good recovery (13). Coma or near-coma at presentation does not appear to have a significant impact on surgical complications (14).

Coma at presentation is associated with poor outcome from intracerebral hemorrhage (15) and pontine hemorrhage.

Infection

A variety of infections (including infections remote from the nervous system) may be responsible for coma. With infection, coma generally takes hours to days to develop. Pneumococcal meningitis has neurologic sequelae in about one-third of children and a larger proportion of adults. In children with this illness, coma is a predictor of death and of neurologic sequelae, although some normal recoveries in children who have been comatose occur (16,17). Herpes simplex encephalitis causes death or severe disability in about one-third of patients. The development of coma or near-coma prior to initiating treatment is associated with poor outcome. Again, some patients demonstrate good recovery (18).

RELATIVES OF COMA

Locked-In State

A patient unable to move, including face movements, eye movements, and speech, may appear to be comatose while having entirely normal consciousness. This condition is known as the locked-in state. It can be produced by neuromuscular blockers, by Guillain–Barré syndrome (also known as acute inflammatory demyelinating polyradiculoneuropathy), and by myasthenia gravis. These conditions do not affect the central nervous system (and so leave consciousness unimpaired), but they render the CNS de-efferented. They are reversible. A bilateral ventral pontine infarct may produce a near locked-in state by eliminating lateral eye movements, facial movements, and limb movements. The more posteriorly and rostrally located ARAS is spared. This pathology may be irreversible. In all these cases, an EEG will show normal or near-normal function of cerebral cortex. Usually, hints of a locked-in state may be obtained from the physical examination. Some blinking or eye movement appropriate to context may be observed. Of note, loss of all cranial nerve reflexes (simulating brain death) has been seen in Guillain–Barré patients who ultimately recover (19).

Brain Death

Brain death is defined as the irreversible cessation of all cerebral hemisphere and brainstem function. This state is the creation of medical technology, specifically the mechanical ventilator. Once complete cessation of brain function (including the brainstem, which drives respirations) occurs, apnea follows. Apnea will rapidly lead to cardiac asystole. A ventilator will enable the heart to be oxygenated (and thus continue to beat, for which no brain input is required) after cessation of brain function. Published criteria for determining brain death may be found in the literature (20–23) (Table 7).

To satisfy the requirement of irreversibility, the underlying pathology must be known, and any possibility of recovery excluded. Eliminating potentially reversible causes of an unresponsive state simulating brain death, such as hypothermia, shock, intoxication, and metabolic encephalopathy, is mandatory. In addition, the duration of the brain death findings (not the underlying condition) should exceed 6 h. When the condition is known with certainty (for example, intracerebral mass lesion with herniation, as seen on cerebral imaging studies), 6 h is reasonable; with anoxia, a 24 h interval is recommended. A shorter interval for anoxia is permissible with confirmatory tests such as EEG and blood flow studies (22).

Table 7 Determination of Brain Death

1. Known, irreversible cause
      Clinical or imaging demonstration of process that accounts for findings
      Process is irreversible
      Exclusion of confounding medical condition, intoxication, or hypothermia
      Duration of findings in support of brain death >6 h
2. Absence of function of cerebral hemispheres and brainstem
      Coma/complete unresponsiveness, except for spinally mediated reflexes
      Absent brainstem reflexes
         Pupillary light, corneal, oculocephalic, oculovestibular, and
            oropharyngeal
         Apnea

Cessation of brain function implies unreceptivity and unresponsiveness (except for reflex movements mediated by the spinal cord), absent brainstem reflexes, and apnea. Unresponsiveness is shown by lack of response to visual, auditory, and noxious stimuli. Brainstem reflexes include pupillary, corneal, oculocephalic, oculovestibular, and gag reflexes. The oculovestibular reflex is tested by calorics (instilling cold water into the external auditory canal). Apnea testing is performed by removing the patient from the ventilator and providing 100% O_2 through a cannula inserted into the endotrachial tube. An ABG determination (typically drawn at 10 min) can demonstrate significant respiratory acidosis ($PCO_2 > 60$ torr), a finding that implies absence of respiratory drive (23). Confirmatory tests are not required if no doubt exists about the cause and irreversibility of the condition and the reliability of the examination. When confirmation of the clinical diagnosis of brain death is desired, a blood flow study can show absent CBF, from which irreversible cessation of brain function can be deduced. A conventional (catheter) angiogram is most reliable, but requires transportation of the patient to the angiography suite. Other tests are easier but have limitations. Transcranial Doppler may be unable to demonstrate blood flow in a small number of normal patients. A technetium-99m brain scan may miss blood flow to the brainstem. Where EEG confirmation is desired as another marker of absent cerebral function, special recording techniques are used which are aimed at maximizing the chance of detecting any cerebrally generated electrical potentials. Specialized EEGs can demonstrate false positives and negatives. The EEG may be isoelectric in such reversible settings as hypothermia and intoxication, and EEGs have appeared to demonstrate cerebral electrical activity in children with absent CBF on angiography (24).

That brain death is equivalent to cardiac death is now widely accepted and is made explicit by either statute or case law in all 50 states. The determination of brain death is required for harvesting of organs for transplant. Progression to brain death is certainly not required for stopping supportive medical treatments, including mechanical ventilation and intravenous hydration. Such treatments should be and usually are stopped when the prognosis is hopeless or when continued treatment would not be in keeping with the patient's wishes.

Persistent Vegetative State

Duration of coma longer than about 2 weeks is unusual. Patients usually recover ARAS function. If recovery of cerebral hemispheres also occurs, then consciousness will be regained. The recovery of the ARAS alone produces a condition known as the vegetative state. This state usually is seen as a residual of anoxia or trauma or as the end-stage of a degenerative or metabolic disorder. Patients in a vegetative state will exhibit sleep–wake cycles, some primitive orienting responses to stimuli, and other evidence of brainstem function such as roving eye movements, swallowing, grimacing, and spontaneous respirations. Cortically mediated responses, such as visually tracking a face, will be absent, and no evidence of consciousness will be elicited.

The vegetative state may be succeeded by the regaining of consciousness if the patient improves, but patients may linger in the vegetative state for years or even decades. The term "vegetative state," implying this set of examination findings, is often concatenated with "persistent," implying duration or prognosis. A multi-society task force reviewed data on the vegetative state, which included case reports of unusually late recoveries (25,26). Among patients in a vegetative state for 1 month (defined by the task force as persistent vegetative state, PVS), the outcome at 1 year was better for trauma than for nontraumatic causes but remained dismal. Among adults with traumatic PVS, 76% had an outcome of death, PVS, or severe disability (GOS 1–3). Only 7% made a good recovery. With nontraumatic PVS, 96% had an outcome of GOS 1–3, and only 1% made a good recovery. Outcome for children was only slightly better. This task force stated that a vegetative state was certain to be permanent if duration was >12 months for traumatic PVS, and if duration was >3 months for nontraumatic PVS.

The ethical and legal status of PVS patients has been a contentious matter. Although some argue that no permanently vegetative patients should receive supportive treatment because treatment is medically futile, others contend that all such patients should be supported because their lives are intrinsically valuable. In practice, the patient's treatment preferences (as determined by advance directive, or by family or other surrogate decision makers) should prevail in this context.

SUMMARY

- At least one cerebral hemisphere and the ARAS must be intact for consciousness to be present.
- Structural abnormalities may cause coma by impingement on the ARAS.
- The clinician must attempt to distinguish structural from nonstructural causes of coma.
- Suspicion of a structural problem mandates emergency imaging.
- Abrupt onset of coma suggests an intracranial structural catastrophe.
- Stroke usually does not disturb the level of consciousness. Vascular lesions that may produce coma include pontine hemorrhage, brainstem infarction, cerebellar hemorrhage, subarachnoid hemorrhage, and thalamic hemorrhage.
- Cerebellar infarction or hemorrhage, intraventricular hemorrhage with hydrocephalus, and subarachnoid hemorrhage are neurosurgical emergencies.
- Even with obvious head injury, causes such as anoxia, seizures, or intoxication may have preceded trauma or be responsible for coma.
- The "talk and deteriorate" syndrome may indicate epidural or subdural hematoma.
- Neoplasms and infections usually produced progressive symptoms. Coma is usually late.

- Hypothermia <32°C may cause coma and simulate brain death.
- History should include time and course of onset, underlying medical conditions, medications, and substance abuse. Preceding symptoms of lateralized weakness, numbness, diplopia, headache, previous seizures, and occupational exposure should be sought.
- Highly irregular breathing patterns suggest lower brainstem dysfunction. Rapid breathing is associated with hypoxia, sepsis, hepatic encephalopathy, and toxic overdoses.
- Hypothermia is associated with intoxication, endocrinopathy, and Wernicke encephalopathy.
- Inspect the patient for signs of trauma, including hemotympanum.
- Ophthalmoscopy should include examination for papilledema, pre-retinal hemorrhage, and retinal hemorrhage.
- Test for nuchal rigidity, if trauma is excluded.
- Examine skin for jaundice, petechial rash, cherry-red appearance, or hot dry appearance.
- Mental status examination should be performed and recorded in detail. GCS is useful for comparing serial examinations.
- Examination of the pupil is critical. Asymmetric or asymmetrically reactive pupils are signs of transtentorial herniation.
- Eye movements allow assessment of cranial nerves III and VI, the midbrain, and the pons and facilitate localization of a structural process.
- Asymmetric corneal reflexes may indicate pontine dysfunction.
- Motor examination should evaluate presence of spontaneous, rhythmic, clonic movements (seizures) and irregular twitching variably located movements (myoclonus).
- Bihemispheral dysfunction is the likely cause of coma when brainstem function is intact and physical examination is symmetric.
- Asymmetric or focal findings suggest a structural lesion. In a comatose patient, emergency cerebral imaging is indicated.
- When a lower brainstem reflex fails while higher brainstem function is preserved, an infratentorial structural abnormality is likely.
- Laboratory evaluation of the comatose patient should include those items listed in Table 5.
- In trauma, or when a structural cause is suspected, obtain emergency noncontrast head CT. Lesions that are neurosurgical emergencies are usually seen on CT scan.
- In patients with coma, obtaining a CT scan before lumbar puncture is advisable.
- In the emergency management of coma, glucose, thiamine, and naloxone should be administered.
- Coma from intoxication usually has a good prognosis, if anoxia is avoided.
- Coma from anoxic encephalopathy, subarachnoid hemorrhage, and severe head injury usually has a bad prognosis.
- The locked-in state (paralysis of eye movements, face, speech, and limbs with preserved consciousness) can simulate coma. This state can be produced by neuromuscular blockers, Guillain–Barré syndrome, myasthenia gravis, and brainstem infarction.

- Brain death is defined as the irreversible cessation of all cerebral hemisphere and brainstem function.
- See Table 7 for criteria of brain death.
- Recovery of ARAS without recovery of cerebral hemispheres produces the vegetative state.

REFERENCES

1. Levy DE, Bates D, Caronna JJ, Cartlidge NEF, Knill-Jones RP, Lapinski RH, Singer BH, Shaw DA, Plum F. Prognosis in nontraumatic coma. Ann Int Med 1981; 94:293–301.
2. Jennett B, Bond M. Assessment of outcome after severe brain damage: a practical scale. Lancet 1975; 7905:480–484.
3. Shewmon DA, DeGiorgio CM. Early prognosis in anoxic coma: Reliability and rationale. Neurol Clin 1989; 7:823–843.
4. Brody BA. Ethical issues raised by the clinical use of prognostic information. In: Evans RW, Baskin DS, Yatsu FM, eds. Prognosis of Neurological Disorders, 2d ed. New York: Oxford University Press, 2003:3–10.
5. Levy DE, Caronna JJ, Singer BH, Lapinski RH, Frydman H, Plum F. Predicting outcome form hypoxic–ischemic coma. J Am Med Assoc 1985; 253:1420–1426.
6. Krumholz A, Stern BJ, Weiss HD. Outcome from coma after cardiopulmonary resuscitation: relation to seizures and myoclonus. Neurology 1988; 38:401–405.
7. Wijdicks EFM, Parisi JE, Sharbrough FW. Prognostic value of myoclonic status in comatose survivors of cardiac arrest. Ann Neurol 1994; 35:239–243.
8. Basseti C, Bomio F, Mathis J, Hess CW. Early prognosis in coma after cardiac arrest: a prospective clinical, electrophysiological, and biochemical study of 60 patients. J Neurol Neurosurg Psychiat 1996; 61:610–615.
9. Aldrich EF, Eisenberg HM, Saydjari C, Foulkes MA, Jane JA, Marshall LF, Young H, Marmarou A. Predictors of mortality in severely head-injured patients with civilian gunshot wounds: a report from the NIH traumatic coma data bank. Surg Neurol 1992; 38:418–423.
10. Quigley MR, Vidovich D, Cantella D, Wilberger JE, Maroon JC, Diamond D. Defining the limits of survivorship after very severe head injury. J Trauma 1997; 42:7–10.
11. Katz DI, Alexander MP. Traumatic brain injury: predicting course of recovery and outcome for patients admitted to rehabilitation. Arch Neurol 1994; 51:661–670.
12. Choi SC, Muizelaar JP, Barnes TY, Marmarou A, Brooks DM, Young HF. Prediction tree for severely head-injured patients. J Neurosurg 1991; 75:251–255.
13. Kassell NF, Torner JC, Haley EC Jr, Jane JA, Adams HP, Kongable GL. The international cooperative study on the timing of aneurysm surgery. Part I: overall management results. J Neurosurg 1990; 73:18–36.
14. LeRoux PD, Elliott JP, Newell DW, Grady MS, Winn HR. The incidence of surgical complications is similar in good and poor grade patients undergoing repair of ruptured anterior circulation aneurysms: a retrospective review of 355 patients. Neurosurgery 1996; 38:887–895.
15. Lisk DR, Pasteur W, Rhoades H, Putnam RD, Grotta JC. Early presentation of hemispheric intracerebral hemorrhage: prediction of outcome and guidelines for treatment allocation. Neurology 1994; 44:133–139.
16. Kornelisse RF, Westerbeek CML, Spoor AB, van der Heijde B, Spanjaard L, Neijens HJ, de Groot R. Pneumococcal meningitis in children: prognostic indicators and outcome. Clin Infect Dis 1995; 21:1390–1397.
17. Pikis A, Kavaliotis J, Tsikoulas J, Andrianopoulos P, Venzon D, Manios S. Long-tern sequelae of pneumococcal meningitis in children. Clin Pediatr 1996; 35:72–78.

18. McGrath N, Anderson NE, Croxson MC, Powell KF. Herpes simplex encephalitis treated with acyclovir: diagnosis and long term outcome. J Neurol Neurosurg Psychiat 1997; 63:321–326.
19. Drury I, Westmoreland BF, Sharbrough FW. Fulminant demyelinating polyradiculoneuropathy resembling brain death. Electroencephalogr Clin Neurophysiol 1987; 67:42–43.
20. A definition of irreversible come: report of the *ad hoc* committee on the Harvard Medical School to examine the definition of brain death. J Am Med Assoc 1968; 205:337–340.
21. Diagnosis of brain death: statement issued by the honorary secretary of the Conference of Medical Royal Colleges and their faculties in the United Kingdom on 11 October 1976. Br Med J 1976; 2:1187–1188.
22. Guidelines for the determination of death: report of the medical consultants on the diagnosis of death to the President's Commission for the Study of Ethical Problems in Medicine and Biomedical and Behavioral Research. J Am Med Assoc 1981; 246:2184–2186.
23. Practice parameters for determining brain death in adults (summary statement): report of the Quality Standards Subcommittee of the American Academy of Neurology. Neurology 1995; 45:1012–1014.
24. Ashwal S, Schneider S. Failure of electroencephalography to diagnose brain death in comatose children. Ann Neurol 1979; 6:512–517.
25. The multi-society task force on PVS. Medical aspects of the persistent vegetative state (part 1). N Engl J Med 1994; 330:1499–1508.
26. The multi-society task force on PVS. Medical aspects of the persistent vegetative state (part 2). N Engl J Med 1994; 330:1572–1579.

16
Seizures

Frederick Langendorf
Hennepin County Medical Center, Minneapolis, Minnesota, USA

INTRODUCTION

The brain has a limited repertoire of responses to injury. Most of these responses are characterized by inhibition; for example, depressed level of consciousness, cognitive impairment, or focal deficits, such as hemiparesis. In contrast, seizures represent an excitatory response to brain insult or injury. Seizures may complicate trauma, medical illness, or almost any brain disorder. They may also occur in the absence of any discernable brain insult or abnormality (aside from the presence of the seizures themselves). Seizures range from violent convulsions to clinically enigmatic behavioral changes, diagnosed as seizures only by electroencephalography. The life-time probability of having a seizure is 5–10%. The prevalence of epilepsy is 0.5–1% (1). Seizures are relatively common occurrences in acutely ill patients and occur in 3.4% of patients admitted to a medical ICU for nonneurologic reasons (2).

This chapter will emphasize aspects frequently encountered in the ICU: new-onset seizure, post-traumatic seizures, and status epilepticus. Epilepsy syndromes and long-term management receive much less discussion, and pathophysiologic mechanisms of epilepsy are not mentioned.

A FRAMEWORK FOR CONSIDERING SEIZURES BY CAUSE
Definitions

Seizures may represent a response to acute brain injury or insult. Such seizures are said to be provoked or *acute symptomatic*. Alternatively, seizures may occur without any immediate antecedent insult to the brain. Such seizures are said to be unprovoked. When no underlying cause for unprovoked seizures is identified, they are *idiopathic* (or *cryptogenic*). When an underlying cause exists, seizures are *remote symptomatic*. Unlike acute symptomatic seizures, remote symptomatic seizures have an underlying cause, but, at a given time, no immediate antecedent insult is present. For example, a seizure associated with a brain tumor would usually be remote symptomatic; a seizure associated with hypoglycemia would be acute symptomatic. Some problems may lead to either acute symptomatic or remote symptomatic seizures. Early (first week) post-traumatic seizures are acute symptomatic; late post-traumatic seizures are remote symptomatic. This distinction is not merely academic: these two types of post-traumatic seizure have different pathogenesis, management, and prognosis.

Epilepsy is defined as recurrent (two or more) idiopathic or remote symptomatic seizures. Even multiple acute symptomatic seizures, for example, multiple febrile seizures, do not count as epilepsy. The presumption is that, between provocations, the brain returns to normal without a heightened tendency toward seizures. These distinctions drive the evaluation and management of seizures.

Acute Symptomatic Seizures

A wide variety of acute insults may lead to seizures (Table 1). The usual seizure type in these cases is convulsive (or generalized tonic–clonic). Although some of these conditions may recur or become chronic, they generally appear acutely.

Remote Symptomatic Seizures

A number of conditions can lurk about for some time before causing seizures. The seizures that ensue are remote symptomatic by definition (Table 2). Note that some conditions with abrupt onset may produce both acute and remote symptomatic seizures. The mechanism is likely to be different. For example, some long-term remodeling with gradual loss of inhibitory mechanisms in the brain takes place following head injury. This process would be a factor in only remote symptomatic seizures.

Among causes of remote symptomatic seizures, neoplastic, infectious, vascular, and inflammatory structural abnormalities of the brain are particularly important.

Table 1 Common Causes of Acute Symptomatic Seizures

Infection
  Meningitis
  Encephalitis
  Pyogenic abscess
Toxic
  Medications: antibiotics, antipsychotics, antidepressants
  Illicit drugs: cocaine, amphetamine
  Withdrawal: alcohol, benzodiazepines, barbiturates
Metabolic
  Hyper- and hypoglycemia
  Electrolyte disturbance: Na^+, Ca^{++}, Mg^{++}
  Organ failure: uremia and dialysis disequilibrium, hepatic encephalopathy
  Endocrine disturbance: thyrotoxicosis
Acute trauma
  Cerebral contusion
  Subdural hematoma
  Diffuse axonal injury
Acute stroke
  Intracerebral hemorrhage
  Subarachnoid hemorrhage
  Cerebral infarction
Anoxia
Hypertensive encephalopathy; eclampsia
Febrile seizures

Table 2 Common Causes of Remote Symptomatic Seizures

Neoplasm
   Primary or metastatic brain tumor
   Carcinomatous meningitis
   Paraneoplastic syndrome
Infection
   Cysticercosis
   HIV
Remote head injury
Remote stroke
Cerebral arterio-venous malformation
Vasculitis
   Primary (granulomatous) angiitis of the brain
   Systemic lupus erythematosis
Other inflammatory cause
   Sarcoidosis
Developmental disorder
   Tuberous sclerosis
   Focal cortical dysplasia
Inborn errors of metabolism
Other neurologic disorder
   Degenerative disorder: Alzheimer disease
   Multiple sclerosis
Alcoholism

Idiopathic Seizures and Epilepsy Syndromes

Isolated seizures, whether single or multiple, may have no discernable underlying cause. In some cases, multiple idiopathic seizures can coalesce into a specific epilepsy syndrome. An epilepsy syndrome, like any disease, will have a typical age of onset, specific symptoms (specific seizure type or types), specific test findings [electroencephalogram (EEG) patterns and imaging abnormalities] specific treatment, and prognosis. Idiopathic epilepsies may be *primary generalized* (with abnormal electrical activity widespread in the brain) or *localization related* (with abnormal electrical activity originating from one area of the brain).

Epilepsy syndromes present great variety. Some selected syndromes are listed in Table 3, which tabulates findings that set idiopathic epilepsies apart from acute and remote symptomatic seizures.

SEIZURE TYPES

Convulsive Seizures (Generalized Tonic–Clonic Seizures, Grand Mal Seizures)

Convulsive seizures are the most commonly encountered seizure type in hospitalized patients. These seizures may begin with a premonition or with a partial type of seizure that progresses. A tonic phase, with axial and limb stiffening, may or may not occur.

Table 3 Selected Epilepsy Syndromes

	Age at onset	Seizure type(s)	Treatment	Prognosis
Primary generalized				
Childhood absence epilepsy	3–10	Absence	Ethosuximide	Fairly good
Juvenile myoclonic epilepsy	8–30	Convulsive Absence Myoclonic	Valproate	Good, for control; poor, for remission
Localization-related				
Benign Rolandic epilepsy	3–13	Convulsive Simple partial	Most AEDs	Remits by age 20
Mesial temporal lobe epilepsy	6–15	Complex partial	Temporal lobectomy	Poor, without surgery

This phase can be associated with expiration against a closed larynx that produces a grunt and with tongue biting. Clonic movements are characterized by vigorous, synchronous, rhythmic limb movements of no more than 1–2 min duration. A postictal phase almost invariably occurs and lasts minutes, hours or, rarely, days. At the beginning of this interval, the patient may be incontinent. Consciousness gradually returns, and confusion, somnolence, or agitation may be experienced with restoration of consciousness.

Convulsive seizures are associated with increased heart rate and blood pressure. Lactic acidosis and transiently elevated serum prolactin concentrations may be found. Elevation of the serum prolactin is useful when excluding psychogenic seizures, seizure-like behavior from a conversion disorder, or malingering (3). Complications include tongue and mouth lacerations, shoulder subluxation, and aspiration. The abrupt loss of consciousness may cause falls and motor vehicle accidents.

Acute symptomatic seizures are usually convulsive in type. Disorders of glucose constitute a notorious exception: both hypo- and hyperglycemic seizures may be simple partial.

Remote symptomatic seizures may also be convulsive in type, and convulsive seizures can be seen with either generalized or localization-related idiopathic epilepsy. Consequently, the appearance of a convulsive (or generalized tonic–clonic) seizure does not identify the underlying process. In particular, "generalized" in the name of this type of *seizure* does not necessarily imply a primary generalized type of *epilepsy*.

Absence Seizures

Absence seizures are brief episodes of impaired consciousness which generally last less than a minute and have no prodrome and no postictal phase. The motor accompaniment, if any, is modest and may include eye flutter, facial movements, or some myoclonus. During this type of seizure, purposeful movement ceases. The patient may be unaware of the episode.

Absence seizures are seen with idiopathic generalized epilepsies. Unlike convulsive symptomatic seizures, they are not seen as an acute response to brain injury or insult. This seizure type does not generally respond to phenytoin or carbamazepine.

Myoclonic Seizures

Myoclonic seizures are rapid twitches or jerks. A single limb or a larger area of the body may be affected. Myoclonic seizures are seen with idiopathic generalized epilepsies.

As with absence seizures, they do not respond to phenytoin or carbamazepine, which can make them worse (4). Myoclonus can also be seen with many acute insults, including metabolic encephalopathy, intoxication, and, prominently, cerebral anoxia, where the continuous presence of myoclonus is associated with poor outcome (5). The boundary between myoclonus and seizure can be hard to define.

Complex Partial Seizures

Complex partial seizures, with their variability, bedevil epileptologists and nonspecialists alike. By definition, impairment of consciousness occurs but may be incomplete. In this type of seizure some interaction during the seizure and some memory of the event are possible. During this type of seizure, postures, such as head turning, or automatisms, such as picking at clothes, may be observed. Tone is generally preserved, but increase or decrease of tone may lead to falls. Auras and a postictal phase are common but not invariable.

Complex partial seizures are very common. Most are temporal lobe in origin, but they may arise from any lobe. They may be seen with remote symptomatic epilepsy or idiopathic localization-related epilepsy but are much less often acute symptomatic. Complex partial seizures are underdiagnosed. They should be considered in patients who have relatively brief, stereotyped episodes of altered mental status, especially those who have head injury or underlying cerebral structural abnormality.

Simple Partial Seizures

Simple partial seizures, by definition, do not compromise consciousness. But like complex partial seizures, they vary in manifestation according to the part of the brain from which they arise. They may involve motor movements (typically lateralized), sensory symptoms, special sensory symptoms (hallucinations), autonomic dysfunction, experiential phenomena such as fearfulness or a sense of familiarity. These seizures may progress ("secondarily generalize") into a convulsion. This seizure type may be seen with remote symptomatic epilepsy or idiopathic localization-related epilepsy and as an acute symptomatic seizure with hyper- and hypoglycemia.

DIFFERENTIAL DIAGNOSIS (Table 4)

An approach to differential diagnosis of possible seizures is shown in Figure 1.

Syncope

Global cerebral hypoperfusion (syncope) usually can be separated from seizures. A clinical context, such as dehydration or new medications predisposing to orthostatic hypotension, may favor syncope. Activities, including standing up quickly, prolonged singing, coughing, or micturition may provoke syncope. The prodrome of syncope, when present, is quite characteristic and includes lightheadedness, visual dimming, yawning, sweating, or nausea. (Patients may say that they felt as if about to faint.) Incontinence, injury, and tongue biting are uncommon, and an almost immediate return of normal mentation is typical. This absence of a postictal phase of gradual recovery is most helpful in separating seizure from syncope.

Table 4 Differential Diagnosis of Seizures—With Emphasis on Diagnostically Problematic Variants of Other Episodic Processes

Syncope
   Convulsive syncope
   Arrhythmias (may lack prodrome)
Transient ischemic attack (TIA)
   Sensory symptoms
   Aphasia
   Confusion (e.g., nondominant parietal lobe)
Migraine
   Atypical symptoms: numbness, dysarthria, vertigo
Psychiatric
   Fugue states
   Panic attacks
   Hyperventilation
Pseudoseizures
Sleep disorders
   Cataplexy
   Parasomnias
Movement disorders
   Dystonia (may be paroxysmal)
   Tics
Myoclonus unrelated to seizures
Transient global amnesia

When the diagnosis of syncope is clear, an EEG is of little value and is not recommended (6). Syncopal events from arrhythmias may occur without some provocative maneuver or context. Some myoclonus or stiffening is very common with syncope (7), and convulsive movements can occur (convulsive syncope). Complex partial seizures of frontal lobe origin may lead to falls and often are very short-lived with little postictal state. They can be mistaken for syncopal events.

Transient Ischemic Attacks

Focal cerebral hypoperfusion can cause a wide variety of different clinical syndromes. A transient ischemic attack (TIA) should be suspected when loss of neurologic function is related to a single vascular territory in the brain, including the optic nerve. Examples include hemiparesis, aphasia, and monocular blindness. Excitatory manifestations, such as involuntary movements, would not be expected with TIAs. Complex, nonlocalizing phenomena, such as confusion or automatisms, are not typical. The patient profile may favor a diagnosis of TIA. An older patient with vascular risk factors is likely to experience a TIA; whereas, a patient with an intracranial mass or severe head injury is more likely to have seizures.

Again, the distinction of TIA from seizure can be problematic. Numbness and tingling on one side can be a manifestation of an excitatory process (seizure) or an inhibitory process (TIA). Other focal loss of function, such as hemiparesis characteristically seen with TIA, may occur in the postictal phase of a seizure. Confusion (suggesting seizure) and aphasia (suggesting TIA) may be hard to distinguish.

Migraine

Migraine typically does not present a picture likely to be mistaken for seizure, but migraine can feature excitatory phenomena, such as visual changes or numbness, that may be separate from headache.

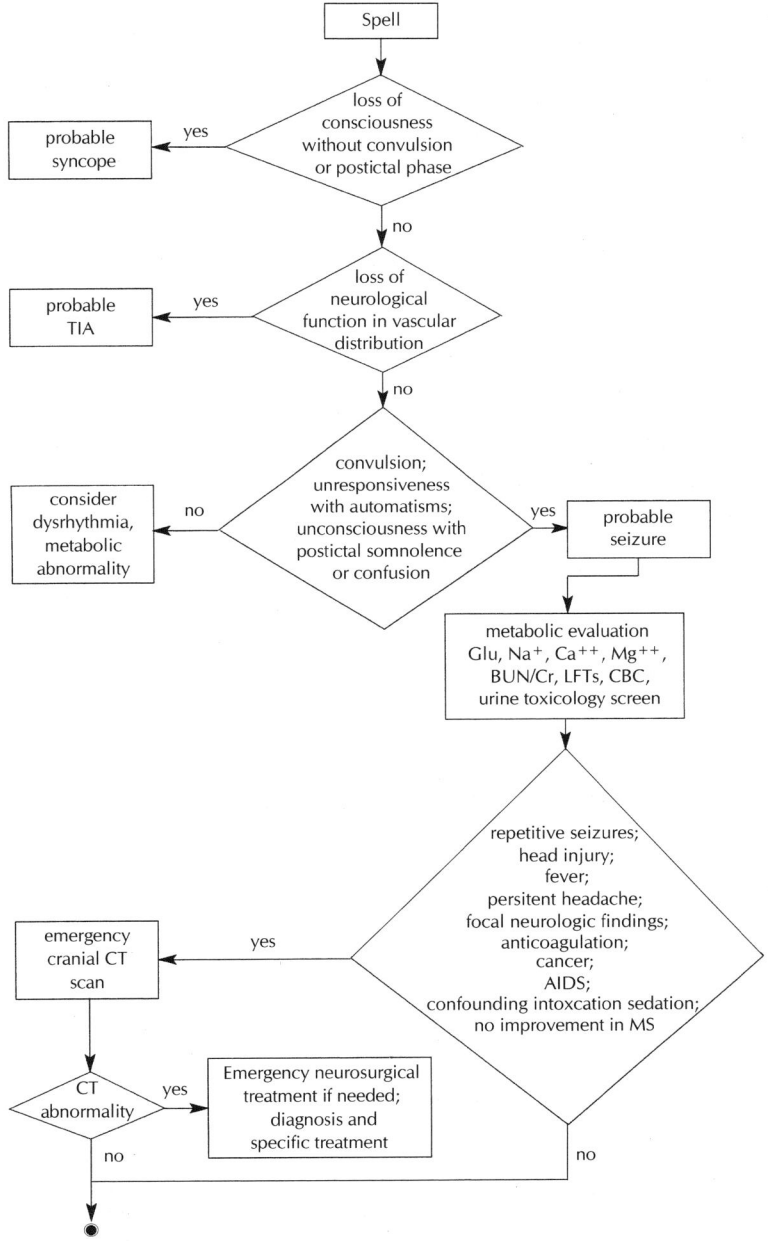

Figure 1 Approach to differencital diagnosis of possible seizures. (*Continued next page.*)

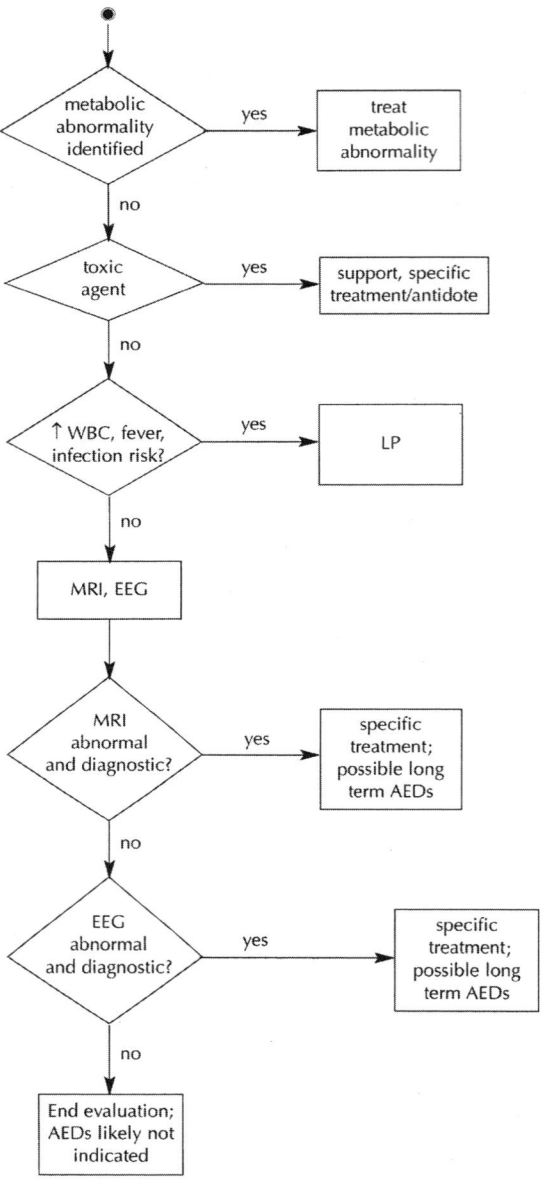

Figure 1 *Continued.*

Psychiatric Disorders

Prolonged episodes, for which the patient is later amnestic, are unlikely to be seizures if the patient was interacting normally at the time. Spells resembling seizures, called pseudoseizures or non-epileptic seizures, may be due to conversion disorder or malingering. When in doubt, the distinction between seizures and pseudoseizures can be made with EEG and concurrent video monitoring.

TREATMENT

Acute Symptomatic Seizures

The initial priority for acute symptomatic seizures is treatment of the underlying cause when possible and may include correcting a metabolic abnormality, withdrawing an offending medication, or treating an infection. When seizures are self-limited, antiepileptic drugs (AEDs) may not be needed. When seizures recur, or can be expected to recur, phenytoin may be inferior to other acute treatments. Long-term treatment with AEDs usually is not indicated.

Hyperglycemic seizures are best treated by correction of the hyperglycemia; phenytoin may be ineffective and impairs insulin secretion, a property that may exacerbate non-ketotic hyperglycemia (8,9). Hyponatremic seizures are treated with hypertonic saline. Care must be exercised to avoid overly rapid correction of hyponatremia with resultant central pontine myelinolysis. If antiepileptic medications are used for uremic seizures or seizures complicating hepatic encephalopathy, serum concentrations of these agents must be followed, particularly unbound (or "free") fractions of highly protein-bound drugs such as phenytoin. Drug metabolism and protein binding may be altered in these conditions.

Alcohol withdrawal seizures often occur in clusters. As with other alcohol withdrawal phenomena, withdrawal seizures are best treated with benzodiazepines, such as lorazepam (10); phenytoin is not effective (11). Seizures from tricyclic antidepressant overdose also are treated with benzodiazepines. Seizures complicating isoniazid overdose respond to pyridoxine.

Eclamptic seizures are effectively treated with magnesium sulfate. Phenytoin is less effective (12). Prolonged or repetitive febrile seizures are treated with benzodiazepines. Some causes of acute symptomatic seizures may predispose the patient to seizures at a later time (remote symptomatic seizures). Head injury, stroke, and some intracranial infections are some risk factors for remote symptomatic seizures. In these cases, a short course of an AED, for example phenytoin, is appropriate, if a seizure has intervened in the acute phase. Long-term treatment beyond several weeks to months is generally pursued only in the event of a seizure that occurs beyond the acute phase.

Remote Symptomatic Seizures

With remote symptomatic seizures, the discovery of an underlying cause is not easily translated into a treatment. Some causes are inherited or developmental. Potentially epileptogenic brain lesions from stroke, head injury, or infection (e.g., calcified cysticercosis lesions) may be permanent. Tumors and vascular malformations usually are not treated acutely. Consequently, patients with these pathologies may continue to experience seizures. Indeed, the recurrence rate for a single unprovoked seizure is significantly higher when the seizure was remote symptomatic and not idiopathic (13). Long-term antiepileptic therapy may be appropriate after a single remote symptomatic seizure. The decision about long-term treatment should include consideration of the EEG (which may help in the estimation of risk of recurrence), concurrent medical problems and medications, driving, employment, lifestyle, and patient preference.

Idiopathic Seizures

The decision about starting AEDs after the first idiopathic seizure generally is not made in the context of administering critical care. In most cases, long-term treatment with AEDs is not indicated.

ANTIEPILEPTIC DRUGS

AEDs in the Acute Setting

A number of AEDs may be administered in loading doses or rapidly acting regimens (see Table 5). These agents are used for status epilepticus (discussed subsequently), for acute repetitive seizures, or where rapid achievement of high blood concentration is desirable. Frequent settings requiring treatment include a single seizure when the risk of early recurrence is high, seizure prophylaxis in severe head injury (discussed subsequently), or augmentation of low AED serum concentration for patients with active chronic epilepsy.

Selection among these agents depends on the context. Specific treatment for acute symptomatic seizures (when any treatment beyond correcting the underlying cause is needed) has been discussed. Remote symptomatic seizures from structural brain abnormality can be expected to respond to either phenytoin or valproate. When administering loading doses of AEDs to patients with chronic epilepsy and low serum concentrations, matching the medication to the patient is essential. For patients with idiopathic epilepsy, identification of the underlying epilepsy syndrome is important. For example, phenytoin will often be ineffective for primary generalized epilepsy, whereas valproate may be successful. A review of the patient's AED regimens in the past and present, with attention to effectiveness, side effects, and toxicity, will usually lead to the right selection of AED. In the event of seizures from noncompliance, reinstating the patient's current regimen may be more beneficial than administering a loading dose of phenytoin or valproate, even if the current AED therapy does not permit loading.

Pharmacologic Considerations

Phenytoin is 90% protein-bound in most patients, but the unbound (or "free") fraction may be much higher than 10% in critically ill patients (14), pregnant patients, patients with renal failure or hypoalbuminemia, and patients receiving other highly protein-bound drugs. Consequently, "free" phenytoin serum concentrations are more informative than total serum concentrations and should be followed in critically ill patients. The half-life of

Table 5 Some AEDs for Acute Use

	Dose	Indication
Rectal diazepam (Diastat)	5–20 mg PR	Acute repetitive seizures
Lorazepam (Ativan)	0.1 mg/kg	Status epilepticus; alcohol withdrawal seizures
Phenytoin (Dilantin) or	20 mg[a]/kg	Status epilepticus
fosphenytoin (Cerebyx)	15 mg[a]/kg	Other settings for loading
Valproate sodium	20 mg/kg	Status epilepticus
(Depacon)	10–20 mg/kg	Other settings for loading
Propofol (Diprivan)	1–2 mg/kg over 5 min, then 2–4 mg/kg/h	Refractory status epilepticus
Midazolam (Versed)	0.2 mg/kg bolus, then 0.02–0.05 mg/kg/h	Refractory status epilepticus

Note: All delivered IV unless otherwise specified.
[a]Fosphenytoin ordered as 20 (or 15) mg phenytoin equivalents/kg.

phenytoin is ~24 h for most patients with serum concentrations in the conventional therapeutic range. The half-life may be shorter for some critically ill patients, including those patients with head injury (15). Twice a day dosing may be optimal. Owing to phenytoin's nonlinear kinetics, toxic serum concentrations may decline slowly. Phenytoin is an inducer of the cytochrome P450 system. Other medications metabolized by this pathway, especially warfarin, may need to be adjusted after co-administration of phenytoin.

Phenytoin is not water-soluble. The vehicle for IV phenytoin is propylene glycol, highly alkaline, which can cause tissue necrosis if extravasated. When IV phenytoin is desired and no central line is available, fosphenytoin is preferred. This phenytoin prodrug is water-soluble and rapidly converted to phenytoin. It is ordered in "milligram phenytoin equivalents" of the desired phenytoin dose.

Blood concentrations of phenytoin should be checked 2 h after administering a loading dose of either phenytoin or fosphenytoin. Steady state should be achieved 5 days after maintenance dosing is begun. The conventional therapeutic range for total phenytoin serum concentration is 10–20 µg/mL. The therapeutic range for free phenytoin is 1.0–2.0 µg/mL.

Valproate is also 80–90% protein-bound. High serum concentrations of this agent are generally better tolerated than those of phenytoin. Valproate pharmacokinetics are approximately linear. These features make following free valproate concentrations, a test not widely available, less important. The half-life of valproate is 8–15 h. Three times per day dosing in the critically ill patient is optimal. Valproate is an inhibitor of the cytochrome P450 system. Doses of warfarin and other drugs metabolized by this system may need to be adjusted when valproate is administered.

Valproate serum concentrations should be checked 2 h after administering a loading dose. Steady state is usually achieved 3 days after maintenance dosing is begun. The conventional therapeutic range for valproate is 50–100 µg/mL. Free concentrations of up to 20 µg/mL are generally well tolerated.

Long-Term Management

Most long-term AED considerations are beyond the scope of critical care management. Commonly used AEDs are listed in Table 6. All agents with the exception of levetiracetam are available in liquid, chewable, or sprinkle form compatible with tube-feeding.

Table 6 Some AEDs for Long-Term Management of Epilepsy

	Typical doses	Metabolism	Spectrum
Carbamazepine[a]	0.3–0.6 mg BID	CP450 inducer; autoinduces	LR
Lamotrigine	100–400 mg BID	Metabolized by CP450 system	LR,PG
Levetiracetam	500–1500 mg BID	Renally excreted unchanged	LR,PG
Phenytoin	3–5 mg/kg/day[b]	CP450 inducer; highly protein-bound	LR
Topiramate	100–200 mg BID	Renally excreted	LR,PG
Valproate[c]	1–3 g per day	CP450 inhibitor; highly protein-bound	LR,PG

Note: LR, localization-related epilepsy; PG, primary generalized epilepsy.
[a]Available as an extended release preparation (Tegretol XR or Carbatrol).
[b]3 mg/kg for elderly.
[c]Available as an extended release preparation (Depakote ER).

EVALUATION OF A FIRST SEIZURE

The principal goals in evaluation of a first seizure are adequate definition of the event, finding or excluding an acute or remote cause, and initiating appropriate treatment (Fig. 1).

History

The history should make every attempt to characterize the episode and consider context. Triggering events, any aura, the ictus, and the postictal phase should be sought in the history. When available, a description of the event from witnesses is of great importance. Previous episodes should be inquired about; significant medical problems and medications should be reviewed. For younger patients, a family history of epilepsy needs to be investigated. In the ill, hospitalized patient, a review of medications, previously obtained laboratory values, and any cerebral imaging studies is essential.

Laboratory Evaluation

A number of metabolic abnormalities make seizures more likely. Important parts of the metabolic evaluation include serum concentrations of glucose, sodium, calcium, magnesium, BUN, and creatinine. Liver function tests have implications for treatment, as well as for diagnosis. A CBC should be obtained. Urine toxicology screen may be appropriate. Lumbar puncture is indicated, if infection is part of the differential diagnosis.

Imaging

A seizure can be the manifestation of an intracranial catastrophe that requires emergency neurosurgical therapy. Emergency cerebral imaging is indicated for certain patients with new-onset seizure and high risk for intracranial structural pathology, with abnormal neurologic examinations, or with repetitive seizures. Guidelines for emergency imaging of seizure patients have been published (16) and are listed in Table 7. In these cases, a noncontrast CT scan is the initial examination. If a patient is alert, has no focal findings, and does not have a high risk for intracranial structural abnormality, and a magnetic resonance imaging (MRI) scan is available in $\sim$24 h, delaying imaging until MRI can be obtained is usually appropriate.

Table 7 Indications for Emergency CT Scanning in Patients with First-Time Seizure

---

Status epilepticus or acute repetitive seizures
Head injury
Fever
Persistent headache
Poor progression of mental status or confounding intoxication or sedation
Focal neurologic examination
Anticoagulation
History of cancer
History of AIDS

In most cases, the new onset of seizures should be evaluated with MRI, with imaging protocols appropriate to the detection of various developmental and acquired lesions related to epilepsy. Use of MRI is recommended, even if a CT scan were done as part of the emergency evaluation, unless CT findings were entirely explanatory (e.g., an acute intracranial hemorrhage) or a compelling metabolic cause were found (e.g., hypoglycemia). CT scans are less sensitive than MRI for a number of causes of remote symptomatic seizures (17). Although some metabolic and toxic problems potentiate seizure, a metabolic abnormality may not be the clear cause of the seizure. For example, a dialysis patient, at risk for seizures from metabolic encephalopathy, also is at risk for subdural hematoma. In such cases, obtaining MRI is reasonable.

Seizures can produce some acute MRI changes that mimic stroke. The MRI abnormalities presumably reflect transient edema, hyperemia, and blood–brain barrier alterations associated with seizures (18). Seizure-related MRI changes typically reverse.

Electroencephalogram (EEG)

The EEG may help answer several questions. *Was it a seizure?* In the event of spells of uncertain diagnosis, an EEG with typical seizure patterns ("spikes") makes seizure a more likely diagnosis. Spikes are seen in 2–4% of normal individuals; therefore, the EEG has a high positive predictive value for seizures only when high prevalence of seizure disorder in the study population is present. EEGs may be normal in patients with epilepsy. *What type of epilepsy?* Some EEG patterns are characteristic of specific epilepsy syndromes. *Are seizures likely to recur?* EEGs with spikes correlate with seizure recurrence (13). This finding can influence decisions about starting and stopping antiepileptic medications. *Are subclinical seizures occurring?* This question refers to seizures that are not apparent at the bedside. *Are pseudoseizures occurring?* For these last two questions, an answer may require long-term EEG with concurrent video monitoring. The use of EEG in status epilepticus is discussed.

POSTTRAUMATIC SEIZURES

Epidemiology and Definitions

The association between head injury and epilepsy was known to Hippocrates. Head injury increases the likelihood of developing epilepsy three-fold. As a risk factor for epilepsy, head injury is comparable to bacterial meningitis, heroin abuse, or a family history of seizures (19,20). Approximately 250,000 head injuries annually in the USA are serious enough to require admission to a hospital (21). Consequently, posttraumatic seizures represent a problem of considerable magnitude.

Head injuries can be categorized as penetrating (or missile) injuries on the one hand (mostly gunshot wounds), and closed (or blunt) injuries on the other (mostly falls, motor vehicle accidents, and non-firearm assaults). The designation as mild injury excludes skull fracture, intracranial structural abnormality, or a neurological deficit beyond brief unconsciousness or amnesia. Moderate injury includes intermediate-duration unconsciousness or amnesia, typically 30 min to 24 h, or skull fracture. In moderate injury, no intracranial contusion or hematoma is observed. Severe head injury often is defined by loss of consciousness or amnesia lasting more than 24 h, intracranial contusion, or hematoma.

Seizures have traditionally been divided into early (within 1 week of injury; acute symptomatic) and late (after 1 week; remote symptomatic). Treatment considerations are different for early and late posttraumatic seizures. Antiepileptic drugs may be beneficial in head injury patients with no seizures (seizure prophylaxis).

Risk

Acute symptomatic (early) seizures appear in 2–5% of patients with head injuries. Children are at greater risk for early seizures than adults. After severe head injury, the risk of early seizures rises to 10–15% for adults and 30–35% for children (22–25). Early seizures are followed by late seizures in 25–35% of adults with severe injury but are not predictive of late seizures in adults with mild injury or in children (22). Like other acute symptomatic seizures, early posttraumatic seizures tend to be convulsive (generalized tonic–clonic) in type. Apparent convulsions occurring within seconds of head injury may represent a more benign variant that bears little association with later seizures or structural brain abnormality. Some consider them similar to convulsive syncope (26). However, it is unlikely that an ictal EEG, which would settle the issue, will ever be recorded.

In a 50-year study of all Olmsted County, Minnesota patients treated for head injury, the incidence of remote symptomatic (late) seizures in the head-injured patient was compared with the incidence of unprovoked seizures in the general population (20,22). Late seizures were seen in 7.4% of children and 13.3% of adults with severe injury. Even mild head injury elevates the risk for late seizures.

Penetrating head injury carries a greater risk for seizure complications than closed head injury. In the Vietnam Head Injury Study, 53% of veterans who suffered a missile injury eventually experienced at least one late seizure. Multiple seizures occurred in the great majority of these cases. The first seizure occurred within 1 year of injury in about half of these patients, but the relative risk of a first seizure was significantly elevated even 10 years after injury (27).

Risk factors for seizures, both early and late, include structural abnormalities such as depressed skull fracture, subdural hematoma, and intracerebral hematoma (20,28,29). Blood in the brain is potentially epileptogenic in head injury as well as stroke. A high degree of global encephalopathy (confusion and depressed level of consciousness) is also a risk factor for seizures (30).

Diagnosis

Early seizures in the context of head injury mandate a noncontrast head CT, even if the injury otherwise seemed too insignificant to require imaging (31). Further information can be obtained from gradient echo MRI sequence, which can demonstrate small areas of intracerebral blood from shear injuries—a finding presumably correlating with diffuse axonal injury. Like first seizures for which no acute cause is known, late seizures should be evaluated with imaging, generally MRI.

EEG has a modest role to play. It is primarily helpful, usually in the context of long-term EEG monitoring when it captures a seizure episode that suggests the diagnosis of partial complex seizures or nonconvulsive status epilepeticus. If convulsive behavior is accompanied by a normal EEG, this finding can establish a diagnosis of pseudoseizures, which can occur in the context of head injury (32).

Posttraumatic seizures may be due to some other problem, such as alcohol withdrawal, or some other consequence of head injury, such as hyponatremia. Review of medications, laboratory studies, and evaluation for infection are important components of the diagnostic evaluation.

Treatment

Early seizures can create metabolic acidosis, hypertension, increased cerebral blood flow, and respiratory compromise in a head injury patient who is already unstable. Late seizures can disrupt and demoralize the recovering trauma victim. Yet, the head injured patient is particularly vulnerable to the cognitive side effects of antiepileptic medications (33,34). Treatment decisions must be made carefully.

Whether to use antiepileptic medications for seizure prophylaxis (i.e., in the absence of seizures) has been, until recently, a bedeviling question in head injury. Randomized, controlled studies of both phenytoin and valproate for patients with severe head injury have been reported. Phenytoin was effective in preventing early seizures; however, at 2 years postinjury, the cumulative probability of a seizure was similar in the treated and untreated groups (24). Valproate was as effective as phenytoin in the short-term, but a trend to more deaths in the valproate group was identified for unclear reasons. Valproate also does not prevent late seizures (35). Professional societies representing neurologists, neurosurgeons, and physiatrists have issued guidelines on seizure prophylaxis for severely head injured patients, that recommend antiepileptic medication for 1 week and no longer (36–38). Phenytoin may be preferable.

Decisions about starting antiepileptic medication after a single seizure are based on the anticipated rate of recurrence. For adults (but not for children), an early seizure will lead to a late seizure in less than one-third of patients with severe injury. The use of AEDs beyond a few weeks to months is not indicated. A late seizure, however, will lead to subsequent late seizures in a majority of cases (20,27), a finding consistent with the ominous prognosis of the first remote symptomatic seizure in other settings. Long-term antiepileptic therapy is recommended after a single late posttraumatic seizure. When compared with side effects of phenytoin, the neuropsychological profile of valproate is benign. Valproate may have advantages for long-term use (39). Head-injury patients are treated in the same way as other patients with multiple seizures and status epilepticus.

STATUS EPILEPTICUS

Definition and Epidemiology

Prolonged or recurrent seizures are a medical emergency. Status epilepticus (SE) is defined as a single continuous seizure or recurrent seizures with incomplete recovery of consciousness between seizure episodes that lasts at least 30 minutes. Thirty minutes is part of the definition of SE, because a 30 minutes interval is potentially associated with lasting brain damage. Another approach to defining SE identifies seizure patterns that are unlikely to be self-limited. Each of the following usually predicts further seizure activity if not treated: (1) 5 minutes of continuous seizure or (2) any two discrete seizures with incomplete recovery of consciousness in between. If not treated, SE likely will ensue. Beginning aggressive treatment in these cases, without waiting 30 minutes, is recommended (40).

Any type of seizure may be sufficiently prolonged or recurrent to constitute SE. When SE consists of seizures convulsive in type (generalized convulsive SE), the situation is most ominous and urgent. Other seizure types producing altered level of consciousness—absence and complex partial—pose diagnostic as well as management problems when they progress to SE.

The frequency of SE is high in children <1 year old and in the elderly. Acute symptomatic causes account for slightly more than half the cases (41). Virtually all of the causes, acute and remote, of a single symptomatic seizure can precipitate SE. SE also may occur in idiopathic epilepsy, especially when antiepileptic drug serum concentrations are low or as a first idiopathic seizure episode. SE can lead to neuronal damage and result in cognitive deficits (42). Mortality of SE is determined largely by underlying cause: mortality is higher for ominous precipitants such as stroke and anoxia, less for metabolic or toxic abnormalities, and least for the epilepsy patient with nontherapeutic amounts of medication.

Clinical Features of Generalized Convulsive Status Epilepticus

Early in the course of generalized convulsive status epilepticus (GCSE), discrete, typical convulsive seizures, featuring unconsciousness with tonic–clonic or clonic movements lasting 1–2 min, usually are observed. Before the patient can recover, another convulsion ensues. The recurrence of seizure activity before the patient has recovered from the previous one augments the deleterious systemic effects seen with convulsive seizures (43). These effects include catecholamine release, lactic acidosis, and hyperpyrexia. Catecholamine release may lead to arrhythmias, hypertension, and pulmonary edema. Rhabdomyolysis, with subsequent acute tubular necrosis and renal failure, can occur.

Early in its course, diagnosis of GCSE is not difficult. If seizures persist for a prolonged period of time, their morphology evolves. The seizures become less discrete, and the movements are less rhythmic and vigorous. In time, continuous irregular myoclonic movements, facial twitching, nystagmoid eye movements, or no movements at all may be the only observable signs. At this point, an EEG is needed for diagnosis, though even the EEG will evolve toward a less distinctive pattern. This evolution of uncontrolled GCSE probably represents the brain's reaction to failing support systems. As the seizures continue, blood pressure and cerebral perfusion eventually drop and serum glucose may decline, while the still-seizing brain continues to have high metabolic demands (44). The potential for brain damage persists until the abnormal electrical activity of the brain is treated.

Evaluation and Management of GCSE

Because GCSE frequently has an acute symptomatic cause, a "first seizure work-up" is indicated. Blood should be analyzed for glucose, sodium, calcium, magnesium, BUN, creatinine, liver function tests, and CBC. A urine toxicology screen should be obtained. Emergency CT imaging usually is indicated once the patient is stabilized. Lumbar puncture should be considered when meningitis or encephalitis is a consideration, though fever and leukocytosis are commonly seen with SE when no infection is present. Multiple arterial blood gas determinations usually are necessary. Antiepileptic drug serum concentrators will help identify the treated epileptic patient and suggest management strategies. An EEG is not needed to begin treatment unless the diagnosis is in considerable doubt. An EEG is required to manage refractory GCSE, because a prolonged course may lead to subclinical seizure activity. An EEG also is necessary for patients who cannot be followed clinically because they require therapy with muscle relaxants. AEDs are titrated to the EEG in these cases.

As with any unconscious and potentially unstable patient, an airway must be secured, vital signs monitored, and venous access achieved. Thiamine and glucose should be administered unless the serum glucose is known to be normal. Significant hyperpyrexia requires cooling. Metabolic acidosis often is self-limited but may require treatment if extreme. Consensus guidelines on treatment of GCSE may be found in Ref. (45). When identified, an underlying acute symptomatic cause should be treated.

The recommended first-line antiepileptic agent is lorazepam (0.1 mg/kg IV, no faster than 2 mg/min). Lorazepam is as immediately efficacious as diazepam (46) but has a longer duration of action. Lorazepam is more effective than phenytoin alone (47) and much easier to use than phenobarbital. Lorazepam can be used safely and effectively by paramedics for out-of-hospital SE (48). Phenytoin (20 mg/kg IV, no faster than 50 mg/min) or fosphenytoin (20 mg phenytoin equivalents/kg, up to 150 mg PE/min) should be added if lorazepam fails, or if seizure prevention beyond several hours is needed. Second-line drugs include additional phenytoin or fosphenytoin (5–10 mg/kg) and phenobarbital (20 mg/kg). Valproate (20–30 mg/kg) may be an option, especially if the patient has primary generalized epilepsy. Seizures refractory to these measures are treated with continuous infusion of propofol, midazolam, or pentobarbital. EEG monitoring is necessary when continuous infusions are employed. Refractory SE is best treated in collaboration with a neurologist or neuro-intensivist familiar with management of this challenging and life-threatening disorder.

Nonconvulsive Status Epilepticus

A plethora of diagnostic terms denote prolonged seizures with altered mental status but no convulsive movements and include epileptic encephalopathy, spike-wave stupor, and subtle SE. We prefer nonconvulsive status epilepticus (NCSE). Preferable is a name according to seizure type (e.g., complex partial SE); however, it is often hard in practice to deduce the underlying seizure type, even with EEG, if the seizures are prolonged or repetitive. In one study, NCSE was seen in 8% of patients with persistent coma but no clinical signs of seizure activity (49).

With NCSE, preceding discrete (and more readily recognizable) seizures may or may not occur. A waxing and waning pattern representing cycling through seizures and postictal states may or may not be present. The level of consciousness may be decreased, normal, or agitated. The content of consciousness is by definition abnormal, but may range from minimal confusion or speech hesitancy to bizarre behavior or mutism. There are some potential clues to this condition (Table 8), but the diagnostic difficulties are

Table 8 Some Clues to Nonconvulsive Status Epilepticus

Fluctuating mental status
Subtle motor signs: myoclonus, blinking, nystagmus
Mutism, verbal hesitancy, or perseveration
History of epilepsy
Low antiepileptic drug serum concentrations
Prior NCSE

always present. In the absence of a high degree of suspicion for NCSE, other causes of acutely altered mental status should be considered first. When the usual culprits—infection, intoxication, metabolic derangement, and structural abnormality—have been eliminated, NCSE should be considered. The EEG is critical for diagnosis. An infusion of a benzodiazepine may be given, if the EEG suggests on-going seizures. A benzodiazepine may restore both the patient's mental status and the EEG to normal, and provide diagnostic as well as therapeutic benefit.

NCSE is not associated with the systemic changes of GCSE (e.g., acidosis and hyperpyrexia), but adverse neurologic outcomes can occur. When compared with GCSE, treatment is less urgent and almost inevitably is delayed by diagnostic pitfalls and the need for EEG. Treatment usually starts with lorazepam. A second drug such as phenytoin or valproate, especially if an underlying primary generalized epilepsy is suspected, is needed if lorazepam is ineffective or if seizures recur. Refractory cases sometimes require similar treatment to refractory GCSE.

SUMMARY

- Acute symptomatic seizures are a response to brain injury or insult.
- Remote symptomatic seizures have an underlying cause, but, at a given time, no immediate antecedent insult is identified.
- Idiopathic seizures are unprovoked and have no underlying cause identified.
- Two or more idiopathic or remote symptomatic seizures are defined as epilepsy.
- Acute symptomatic seizures are usually convulsive.
- Although hyperglycemia or hypoglycemia can produce acute symptomatic seizures, they are frequently not of the convulsive type.
- Convulsive (or generalized tonic–clonic) seizures may begin with an aura or a partial type of seizure. They are followed by postictal somnolence, confusion, or agitation. They may be associated with hypertension, tachycardia, lactic acidosis, and elevated prolactin serum concentrations.
- Absence seizures are brief episodes of impaired consciousness with no prodrome and no postictal phase.
- Myoclonic seizures are rapid twitches and jerks and can be seen with metabolic encephalopathy, intoxication, and cerebral anoxia.
- Complex partial seizures are variable. Although consciousness is impaired, interaction during the seizure and memory of the event may occur. Automatisms are common.
- Simple partial seizures do not compromise consciousness. They involve stereotyped motor, sensory, autonomic, or experiential symptoms.
- Syncope may be distinguished from seizures by preceding activities including standing quickly and by the prodrome of lightheadedness, visual dimming, yawning, sweating, or nausea. Incontinence and tongue biting are uncommon. Absence of a postictal phase helps distinguish syncope from seizures.
- A transient ischemic attack (TIA) should be suspected when loss of neurologic function is related to a single vascular territory.

Seizures

- Treat the underlying cause whenever possible in acute symptomatic seizures. Hyperglycemia, hypoglycemia, hyponatremia, uremia, hepatic failure, alcohol withdrawal, tricyclic antidepressants, and isoniazid can cause seizures. Please see text for treatment.
- Eclamptic seizures are treated with magnesium sulfate.
- Long-term antiepileptic therapy may be appropriate after a single remote symptomatic seizure. Consider the EEG, concomitant medical problems, medications, employment, driving, lifestyle, and patient preferences.
- Frequent diagnoses requiring acute treatment include seizures in which the risk of early recurrence is high, seizure prophylaxis in severe head injury, and augmentation of deficient serum concentrations of antiepileptic medications.
- Phenytoin is 90% protein-bound in most patients, but the unbound fraction in critically ill patients may be higher than 10%. Follow unbound (free) phenytoin serum concentrations in the critically ill patient.
- Valproate is highly protein-bound. Unbound serum concentrations generally are not available and typically are not followed. Usual dose schedule is tid in critically patients.
- Warfarin dose may require adjustment with concomitant phenytoin or valproate therapy.
- Use fosphenytoin for intravenous administration when central venous access is not available.
- See flow chart (p. 213) for evaluation of first seizure.
- Indications for emergency CT scan include status epilepticus, acute repetitive seizures, head injury, fever, persistent headache, poor progression of mental status, focal neurologic examination, anticoagulation, cancer, and AIDS.
- Risks for both early and late posttraumatic seizures include depressed skull fracture, subdural hematoma, and intracerebral hematoma. Penetrating head injury confers higher risk than closed head injury.
- Severe head injury has a 10–15% risk for early acute symptomatic seizure in adults and 30–35% risk in children.
- Mild or severe head injury increases the risk for late remote symptomatic seizures.
- Noncontrast head CT is indicated for seizures associated with head injury, even when the injury otherwise seems mild enough to forego cranial imaging.
- One week of phenytoin therapy is recommended for seizure prophylaxis in severe head injury.
- Status epilepticus is defined as a single continuous seizure or recurrent seizures with incomplete recovery of consciousness between seizure episodes that last at least 30 min.
- Airway has the highest priority in the treatment of generalized convulsive status epilepticus (GCSE).
- Status epilepticus is an emergency. Five minutes of seizure or two discrete seizures with incomplete recovery warrant therapy.
- Perform a "first seizure work-up" for the patient with GCSE.
- Lorazepam is recommended for GCSE.
- Suspect nonconvulsive status epilepticus in patients with fluctuating mental status, myoclonus, blinking, nystagmus, mutism, verbal hesitancy, perseveration, history of epilepsy, inadequate doses of antiepileptic drugs, and prior nonconvulsive status epilepticus.

REFERENCES

1. Hauser WA, Hesdorffer DC. Epilepsy: Frequency, Causes and Consequences. New York: Demos, 1990.
2. Bleck TP, Smith MC, Pierre-Louis SJ-C, Jares JJ, Murray J, Hansen CA. Neurologic complications of critical medical illnesses. Crit Care Med 1993; 21:98–103.
3. Yerby MS, van Belle G, Friel PN, Wilensky AJ. Serum prolactins in the diagnosis of epilepsy: sensitivity, specificity, and predictive value. Neurology 1987; 37:1224–1226.
4. Genton P, Gelisse P, Thomas P, Dravet C. Do carbamazepine and phenytoin aggravate juvenile myoclonic epilepsy? Neurology 2000; 55:1106–1109.
5. Krumholz A, Stern BJ, Weiss HD. Outcome from coma after cardiopulmonary resuscitation: relation to seizures and myoclonus. Neurology 1988; 38:401–405.
6. Linzer M, Yang EH, Estes NAM III, Wang P, Vorperian VR, Kapoor WN for the Clinical Efficacy Assessment Project of the American College of Physicians. Diagnosing syncope. Part I: Value of history, physical examination, and electrocardiography. Ann Intern Med 1997; 126:989–996.
7. Lempert T, Bauer M, Schmidt D. Syncope: A videometric analysis of 56 episodes of transient cerebral hypoxia. Ann Neurol 1994; 36:233–237.
8. Harden CL, Rosenbaum DH, Daras M. Hyperglycemia presenting with occipital seizures. Epilepsia 1991; 32:215–220.
9. Malherbe C, Burrill KC, Levin SR, Karam JH, Forsham PH. Effect of diphenylhydantoin on insulin secretion in man. N Engl J Med 1972; 286:339–342.
10. D'Onofrio G, Rathlev NK, Ulrich AS, Fish SS, Freedlang ES. Lorazepam for the prevention of recurrent seizures related to alcohol. N Engl J Med 1999; 340:915–919.
11. Rathlev NK, D'Onofrio G, Fish SS, Harrison PM, Bernstein E, Hossack RW, Pickens L. The lack of efficacy of phenytoin in the prevention of recurrent alcohol-related seizures. Ann Emerg Med 1994; 23:513–518.
12. The Eclampsia Trial Collaborative Group. Which anticonvulsant for women with eclampsia? Evidence from the Collaborative Eclampsia Trial. Lancet 1995; 345:1455–1463.
13. Berg AT, Shinnar S. The risk of seizure recurrence following a first unprovoked seizure: a quantitative review. Neurology 1991; 41:965–972.
14. Zielmann S, Mielck F, Kahl R, Kazmaier S, Sydow M, Kolk J, Burchardi H. A rational basis for the measurement of free phenytoin concentration in critically ill trauma patients. Ther Drug Monit 1994; 16:139–144.
15. Boucher BA, Kuhl DA, Fabian TC, Robertson JT. Pharmacokinetics and drug disposition. Effect of neurotrauma on hepatic drug clearance. Clin Pharmacol Ther 1991; 50:487–497.
16. Greenberg MK, Barsan WG, Starkman S. Neuroimaging in the emergency patient presenting with seizure. Neurology 1996; 47:26–32.
17. Kilpatrick CJ, Tress BM, O'Donnell C, Rossiter SC, Hopper JL. Magnetic resonance imaging and late-onset epilepsy. Epilepsia 1991; 32:358–364.
18. Lansberg MG, O'Brien MW, Norbash AM, Moseley ME, Morrell M, Albers GW. MRI abnormalities associated with partial status epilepticus. Neurology 1999; 52:1021–1027.
19. Hauser WA, Annegers JF. Risk factors for epilepsy. In: Anderson VE, Hauser WA, Leppik IE, Noebels JL, Rich SS, eds. Genetic Strategies in Epilepsy Research. The Netherlands: Elsevier Science Publishers BV, 1991:45–52.
20. Annegers JF, Hauser WA, Coan SP, Rocca WA. A population-based study of seizures after traumatic brain injuries. N Engl J Med 1998; 338:20–24.
21. Thurman D, Guerrero J. Trends in hospitalization associated with traumatic brain injury. J Am Med Assoc 1999; 282:954–957.
22. Annegers JF, Grabow JD, Groover RV, Laws ER Jr, Elveback LR, Kurland LT. Seizures after head trauma: a population study. Neurology 1980; 30:683–689.
23. Desai BT, Whitman S, Coonley-Hoganson R, Coleman TE, Gabriel G, Dell J. Seizures and civilian head injuries. Epilepsia 1983; 24:289–296.

24. Temkin NR, Dikmen SS, Wilensky AJ, Keihm J, Chabal S, Winn HR. A randomized, double-blind study of phenytoin for the prevention of post-traumatic seizures. N Engl J Med 1990; 323:497–502.
25. Hahn YS, Fuchs S, Flannery AM, Barthel MJ, McLone DG. Factors influencing posttraumatic seizures in children. Neurosurgery 1988; 22:864–867.
26. McCrory PR, Bladin PF, Berkovic SF. Retrospective study of concussive convusions in elite Australian rules and rugby league footballers: phenomenology, aetiology, and outcome. Br Med J 1997; 314:171–174.
27. Salazar AM, Jabbari B, Vance SC, Grafman J, Amin D, Dillon JD. Epilepsy after penetrating head injury. I. Clinical correlates: a report of the Vietnam Head Injury Study. Neurology 1985; 35:1406–1414.
28. Jennett B. Epilepsy after non-missile head injuries. 2nd ed. Chicago, IL: William Heinemann, 1975.
29. D'Alessandro R, Ferrara R, Benassi G, Lenzi PL, Sabattini L. Computed tomographic scans in posttraumatic epilepsy. Arch Neurol 1988; 45:42–43.
30. Lewis RJ, Yee L, Inkelis SH, Gilmore D. Clinical predictors of post-traumatic seizures in children with head trauma. Ann Emerg Med 1993; 22:1114–1118.
31. Lee S-T, Lui T-N. Early seizures after mild closed head injury. J Neurosurg 1992; 76:435–439.
32. Barry E, Krumholz A, Bergey GK, Chatha H, Alemayehu S, Grattan L. Nonepileptic posttraumatic seizures. Epilepsia 1998; 39:427–431.
33. Dikmen SS, Temkin NR, Miller B, Machamer J, Winn HR. Neurobehavioral effects of phenytoin prophylaxis of posttraumatic seizures. J Am Med Assoc 1991; 265:1271–1277.
34. Smith KR, Goulding PM, Wilderman D, Goldfader PR, Holterman-Hommes P, Wei F. Neurobehavioral effects of phenytoin and carbamazepine in patients recovering from brain trauma: a comparative study. Arch Neurol 1994; 51:653–660.
35. Temkin NR, Dikman SS, Anderson GD, Wilensky AJ, Holmes MD, Cohen W, Newell DW, Nelson P, Awan A, Winn HR. Valproate therapy for prevention of posttraumatic seizures: a randomized trial. J Neurosurg 1999; 91:593–600.
36. Chang BS, Lowenstein DH. Practice parameter: antiepileptic drug prophylaxis in severe traumatic brain injury. Report of the Quality Standards Subcommittee of the American Academy of Neurology. Neurology 2003; 60:10–16.
37. Role of antiseizure prophylaxis following head injury. J Neurotrauma 2000; 17:549–553.
38. Brain Injury Special Interest Group of the American Academy of Physical Medicine and Rehabilitation. Practice parameter: antiepileptic drug treatment of posttraumatic seizures. Arch Phys Med Rehabil 1998; 79:594–597.
39. Dikmen SS, Machamer JE, Winn HR, Anderson GD, Temkin NR. Neuropsychological effects of valproate in traumatic brain injury. A randomized trial. Neurology 2000; 54:895–902.
40. Lowenstein DH, Alldredge BK. Status epilepticus. N Engl J Med 1998; 338:970–976.
41. Hesdorffer DC, Logroscino G, Cascino G, Annegers JF, Hauser WA. Incidence of status epilepticus in Rochester, Minnesota, 1965–1984. Neurology 1998; 50:735–741.
42. Dodrill CB, Wilensky AJ. Intellectual impairment as an outcome of status epilepticus. Neurology 1990; 40(suppl 2):23–27.
43. Walton NY. Systemic effects of generalized convulsive status epilepticus. Epilepsia 1993; 34(suppl 1):S54–S58.
44. Fountain NB, Lothman EW. Pathophysiology of status epilepticus. J Clin Neurophysiol 1995; 12:326–342.
45. Working Group on Status Epilepticus. Treatment of convulsive status epilepticus. Recommendations of the Epilepsy Foundation of America's working group on status epilepticus. J Am Med Assoc 1993; 270:854–859.
46. Leppik IE, Derivan AT, Homan RW, Walker J, Ramsay RE, Patrick B. Double-blind study of lorazepam and diazepam in status epilepticus. J Am Med Assoc 1983; 249:1452–1454.

47. Treiman DM, Meyers PD, Walton NY, Collins JF, Colling C, Rowan AJ, Handforth A, Faught E, Calabrese VP, Uthman BM, Ramsay RE, Mamdani MB, for the Veterans Affairs Status Epilepticus Cooperative Study Group. A comparison of four treatments for generalized convulsive status epilepticus. N Engl J Med 1998; 339:792–798.
48. Alldredge BK, Gelb AM, Isaacs SM, Corry MD, Allen F, Ulrich SK, Gottwald MD, O'Neil N, Neuhaus JM, Segal MR, Lowenstein DH. A comparison of lorazepam, diazepam, and placebo for the treatment of out-of-hospital status epilepticus. N Engl J Med 2001; 345:631–637.
49. Towne AR, Waterhouse EJ, Boggs JG, Garnett LK, Brown AJ, Smith JR Jr, DeLorenzo RJ. Prevalence of nonconvulsive status epilepticus in comatose patients. Neurology 2000; 54:340–345.

17
Head Injury

Anthony Bottini
Centracare Clinic—Neurosurgery, St. Cloud, Minnesota, USA

BASIC CONCEPTS

Head injury is one of the most common life-threatening conditions encountered in critical care. Approximately 50% of all deaths from trauma are associated with a significant head injury, and over 60% of deaths from motor vehicle accidents are caused by head injury. In the USA, a patient dies of a head injury every 12 minutes.

The optimal care of patients with head injury is constantly evolving. Since the brain does not respond well to injury, prevention of CNS injury, rather than attempts at repair, is imperative. The damage that occurs at the time of the patient's brain injury is largely irremediable. The focus of all therapeutic efforts subsequent to brain injury is prevention of secondary insults that will limit survival or increase the neurological deficits incurred from the primary injury. Efficient, accurate assessment and appropriate, timely intervention are essential in caring for patients with head injury. The Glasgow Coma Score should serve as the fundamental measure of injury at presentation and as the standard for serial comparison throughout the acute clinical course (Box 1).

The neuroanatomic substrate for consciousness resides primarily in the reticular activating system (RAS). RAS is diffusely distributed throughout the posterior portion of the brainstem and extends from the superior pons to the thalamus and the hypothalamus. Injury to this area through direct impact, concussion, or distortion by an intracranial mass will produce coma. Discrete injuries elsewhere in the cerebrum also will cause coma, although these areas are less commonly responsible for loss of consciousness following trauma (Box 2).

A more in-depth neurologic examination is done to assess those systems that may have localized pathologic intracranial conditions. These systems include the pupillary light reflex, motor system, and respiratory pattern. The pathway for the pupillary light reflex originates at the retina. The afferent limb includes the optic nerve and the dorsal midbrain. The efferent parasympathetic reflex arc, which acts to constrict the pupil, originates in the Edinger–Westphal nucleus of the midbrain, proceeds with the third cranial nerve to the ciliary ganglion, and finally passes through the short ciliary nerve to the iris. The efferent sympathetic supply, which dilates the pupil, passes from the hypothalamus downward through the lateral tegmentum of the brainstem to synapse in the interomediolateral cell column of the spinal cord from C8 to T2 and then returns upward through the sympathetic chain to the stellate ganglion. Sympathetic fibers travel with

Box 1 Glasgow Coma Scale

Eye opening (E)	
Spontaneous	4
To speech	3
To pain	2
None	1
Best motor response (M)	
Obeys commands	6
Localizes pain	5
Withdraws	4
Abnormal flexion	3
Extensor response	2
None	1
Best verbal response (V)	
Oriented	5
Confused conversation	4
Inappropriate words	3
Incomprehensible sounds	2
None	1
TOTAL (E + M + V) = 3–15	

Note: From Teasdale B, Jennett B. Assessment and prognosis of coma after head injury. Acta Neurochir (Wien) 1976; 34:45–55.

the carotid artery to the orbit and then pass through the long ciliary nerve to innervate the pupillodilatory mechanism of the iris.

In uncal herniation following head injury, the uncus of the temporal lobe is forced into the tentorial incisura and compresses the ipsilateral third cranial nerve. The parasympathetic supply to the pupil is interrupted, and the unbalanced sympathetic tone produces dilation of the ipsilateral pupil. Conversely, although far less commonly, trauma to the region of the cervical stellate ganglion or the carotid sheath may interrupt the sympathetic supply to the pupil and produce unbalanced parasympathetic tone. Pupillary constriction and ipsilateral miosis then occur. In this situation, the resulting anisocoria may be misinterpreted as contralateral pupillary dilation.

Box 2 Anatomic Substrates of Alertness

Reticular activating system (RAS): extends from superior half of pons through midbrain to hypothalamus and thalamus
Bilateral cerebral hemispheric lesions: produce transient unresponsiveness, especially if lesion involves mesial frontal region
Large unilateral lesions of dominant hemisphere: occasionally cause transient unresponsiveness
Posterior hypothalamic lesions: produce prolonged hypersomnia
Paraventricular thalamic nuclei: acute bilateral lesions that produce transient unresponsiveness and permanent severe amnestic dementia

Head Injury

Motor control originates in the primary motor cortex in the posterior frontal region, condenses into the internal capsule, and forms the corticospinal tract, which subsequently decussates in the lower medulla. This pathway, within the pyramidal tract, is found laterally at the level of the midbrain. In this area, the tract is susceptible to compression by either the herniating uncus of the temporal lobe or the free edge of the tentorium contralateral to the intracranial mass (Fig. 1). In the case of direct uncal compression of the pyramidal tract, the motor deficit is found contralateral to the intracranial mass. When the motor pathways are compressed by the free edge of the tentorium, hemiparesis is found ipsilateral to the mass lesion (Fig. 2). This false lateralizing finding, or Kernohan's notch phenomenon, is found in ~15% of patients with an asymmetric motor examination following closed head injury.

In comparison with the pupillary light reflex, motor findings following head injury are less reliable as a lateralizing sign. The clinician should remember that the mass lesion is usually on the side of the pupillary abnormality. Respiratory irregularities also have some value for localizing injury in the setting of progressive rostral-to-caudal brainstem herniation (Table 1).

SKULL FRACTURES

Skull fractures are a common finding after a severe head injury. In isolation they are infrequently a mechanism for neurologic injury. The search for a skull fracture should never become a primary objective in evaluation of the patient and should certainly never delay appropriate initial management of a patient with evidence of neurologic deterioration.

Linear Nondisplaced Skull Fractures

A linear, nondisplaced fracture is a stellate-appearing break of the cranial vault seen on plain radiographs of the skull. It is a direct effect of physical contact with the skull and

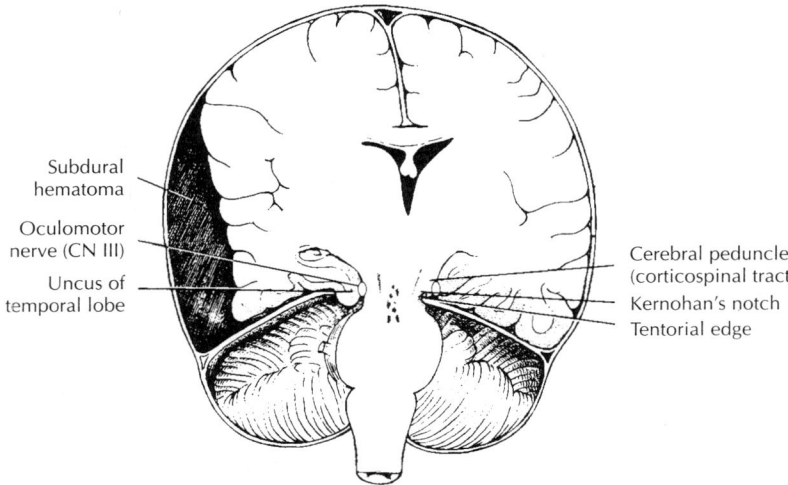

Figure 1 Uncal herniation in a coronal plane.

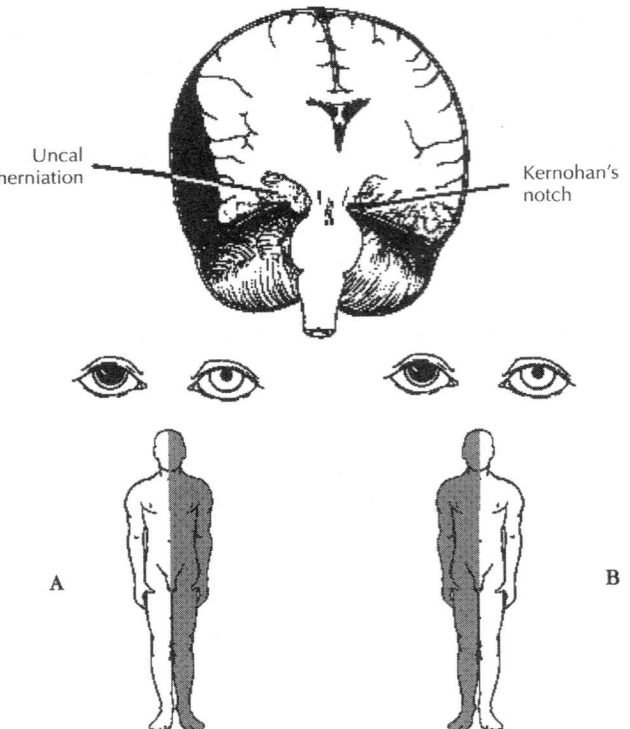

Figure 2 Lateralizing signs in uncal herniation. (A) Expected signs and (B) Kernohan's notch phenomenon.

Table 1 Respiratory Patterns in Coma

Pattern	Possible cause
Cheyne–Stokes respiration	Brief hyperpnea alternating with even shorter periods of apnea; represents loss of forebrain "smoothing" of respiratory response to PCO_2; found with bilateral thalamic lesions or lesions from cerebral hemispheres down to upper pons; also found with uremia or diffuse anoxia
Sustained regular hyperventilation	Lesions of midbrain or pons may produce rapid hyperpnea
Apneustic respiration	Lesions in lateral tegmentum of caudal pons may result in long periods of inspiration with breathholding followed by expiration
Cluster respiration	Lesions in lower pons or upper medulla may produce irregular pattern of clusters of respiration
Ataxic respiration	Damage to dorsomedial medulla may produce a completely irregular pattern of gasps and episodes of tachypnea; found in agonal patients as precursor to complete respiratory failure

reflects the amount of energy the skull has absorbed in the traumatic event. Patients with skull fractures commonly demonstrate little or no underlying neurologic injury because the energy of the impact has been expended in fracturing the skull; therefore, accelerational injury imparted to the underlying brain is minimized.

The most worrisome part of a linear skull fracture is that disruption of the inner table of the skull also may lacerate dural vascular structures. The most important of these structures, and the one most frequently injured, is the middle meningeal artery. This vessel is a branch of the external carotid artery that enters the skull under the temporal lobe through the foramen spinosum. The artery is contained intracranially within a shallow bone channel on the inner surface of the skull, which runs laterally and anteriorly from the foramen spinosum. Although the vessel is located within this channel, it is highly susceptible to injury when the skull is fractured. Near the lateral termination of the greater wing of the sphenoid bone, just anterior to and above the ear, the vessel leaves the bony channel to run between the leaves of the dura and branches widely to supply the lateral expanse of the supratentorial dura. Other vascular structures that may be imperiled by a linear skull fracture are the sagittal sinus and the lateral or sigmoid sinuses. Disruption of either a dural artery or vein may produce an epidural hematoma (EDH). A linear skull fracture in a conscious patient increases the risk of intracranial hematoma by a factor of 400 and increases the probability that the patient will require a craniotomy by a factor of 20 (1,2).

Identifying patients with linear fractures also specifies a patient population at greater risk for a major intracranial disaster. As a general principle, all patients with skull fractures should undergo CT scanning and close observation.

Depressed Skull Fractures

A depressed skull fracture occurs when a skull fragment is displaced one bone width below the surrounding skull. Such fractures are more common after severe or focal cranial impact than after the type of impact that produces linear fractures. In general, depressed fractures result from direct blows to the head, frequently those with small impact areas, and are more commonly associated with underlying brain and vascular injuries than are linear skull fractures.

An open, depressed skull fracture always requires surgical management. This type of injury represents a potential for bacterial contamination of the CSF pathways and the brain. It requires prompt and meticulous debridement, repair of any dural lacerations, and removal of contaminated skull fragments. Depending on the location, underlying structures, and depth of the depressed fragments, closed depressed skull fractures may be treated conservatively. Some neurosurgeons strongly argue that a depressed skull fracture represents a powerful predisposition to a posttraumatic seizure disorder and that elevation of these fractures is always indicated. Others have advocated a more conservative approach to the majority of these injuries (3,4). A depressed skull fracture, whether open or closed, necessitates neurosurgical consultation.

Basilar Skull Fractures

A basilar skull fracture is generally a clinical diagnosis rather than a radiographic one. Occasionally, a basilar fracture may be identified on a CT scan, but such a fracture is most commonly diagnosed through physical findings [e.g., hemotympanum, ecchymosis in mastoid region (Battle's sign), periorbital ecchymoses ("raccoon eyes"), or a CSF leak from ear or nose]. Fractures that cross the cribriform plate, paranasal sinuses, or mastoid cells of the petrous temporal bone and that breach the underlying dura may produce CSF leaks. Patients with suspected basilar skull fracture should be questioned closely for signs or symptoms of CSF otorrhea or rhinorrhea and examined serially to detect a leak or facial nerve paralysis. In patients who develop a CSF fistula following a closed head injury, ~85% will have cessation of leakage with a week of expectant treatment alone. During this time, the patient should remain in an upright position as much as possible because the pressure of the brain over the area of dural disruption may help to seal the fistula. Consideration also may be given to lumbar drainage of CSF to permit closure of the basilar CSF fistula. A persistent CSF leak disposes the patient to late infectious complications, such as meningitis or brain abscess, and surgery may be necessary if leakage has not stopped after 1 week. The use of prophylactic antibiotics in patients with basilar skull fractures, with or without evidence of a CSF leak, is controversial. Little clear, objective evidence exists to show that prophylactic antibiotics are effective, but data are available that demonstrate prophylactic antibiotics may change the nasopharyngeal flora to more pathogenic organisms, principally gram-negative enteric bacteria (5,6). Nasotracheal or nasogastric tubes should be used with great caution in patients with clinical signs of a basilar skull fracture, because they may penetrate the fracture and pass into the intracranial cavity. These patients should not have cotton swabs or other instrumentation placed in their external acoustic meatus.

Cranial nerve dysfunction, especially of the facial nerve, may result from a basilar skull fracture. Fractures that are transverse to the long axis of the petrous portion of the temporal bone are associated with a higher risk of facial nerve palsy, because they cross the path of the facial nerve in a transverse direction. Facial nerve palsies that are present immediately following trauma have a poorer prognosis than those that occur as a delayed complication, because an immediate facial palsy may indicate that the facial nerve was transected when the temporal bone was fractured. A delayed facial weakness, caused by nerve edema or the presence of a hematoma within the facial canal, has important implications for management. The paresis may be improved with surgical decompression of the facial nerve. This consideration emphasizes the need for close and careful observation of facial nerve function in a patient suspected of sustaining a basilar skull fracture.

HEMATOMAS

Epidural Hematoma

An EDH represents the greatest threat and the greatest challenge to clinicians who care for patients with brain injury. This type of hematoma most commonly results when the middle meningeal artery is lacerated along its course from its entrance into the intracranial cavity through the foramen spinosum to its eventual distribution and ramifications over the broad expanse of the supratentorial dura. The epidural space, usually only a potential space, is very distensible and is limited only by the attachment of the dura along the suture lines. Because the injury is arterial and the clot dissects the dura from the inner surface of the brain, the resulting lesion appears convex on axial imaging studies. EDHs are uncommon in elderly patients because the dura is often strongly adherent to the underlying surface of the skull. In the elderly, the epidural space may not exist.

The challenge involved in treating patients with EDH is early recognition. Most patients who suffer from an EDH have sustained little or no brain injury at the time of the trauma. The expanding hematoma in the epidural space represents a secondary injury that quickly may prove fatal. No one should ever die of an EDH. Because the neurologic prognosis is good in this group of patients, needless tragedy—irreversible brain injury or death—will occur as a result of a delay in recognizing this type of lesion. EDHs are most commonly found in a patient population younger than 40 years of age. Thus, this potentially fatal but easily treatable condition is an affliction of people who are in the prime of their lives.

A common clinical presentation for the patient with an EDH is a brief loss of consciousness in an accident, recovery of consciousness at the scene, and a near-normal neurologic examination on initial presentation to the paramedics or the emergency room. The patient subsequently undergoes a delayed, and sometimes rapidly progressive, neurologic deterioration. The pathophysiologic reason for this clinical course is that, although the patient suffers a minor cerebral contusion at the time of impact, the impact also produces a skull fracture and vascular laceration. Consciousness is soon regained, because the cerebral contusion is minimal. Consciousness deteriorates when hematoma within the epidural space begins to expand.

Initially, the brain shifts toward midline to accommodate this new intracranial mass, and CSF is displaced from the ventricles into the lumbar thecal sac to accommodate the growing extra-axial mass. As the dura is stretched, the patient complains of headache; as the mass out-grows the brain's ability to accommodate it, intracranial pressure (ICP) begins to rise, and the midline structures become distorted. The patient becomes less responsive, increasingly somnolent, and, finally, comatose. This clinical presentation of EDH is often described as the "lucid interval." Relatively early in this progression, the ipsilateral third cranial nerve may be compressed and initially may produce an oval pupil ipsilateral to the EDH. With further expansion of the hematoma, a widely fixed and dilated ipsilateral pupil occurs. (Patients who have a dilated, nonreactive pupil because of uncal herniation have always lost consciousness first.) With continued brainstem compression, the herniation syndrome becomes complete and the patient may develop bilateral pupillary abnormalities. Incomplete expressions of this syndrome may occur. The clinical findings may progress more slowly or to a lesser degree, and the predominant clinical complaint is increasing headache. Any patient with a linear skull fracture or with the progression of symptoms described above should be suspected of having an EDH or another type of space-occupying intracranial mass until proven otherwise.

The treatment of EDH usually demands immediate surgical management. Definitive treatment consists of a limited craniotomy with evacuation of the clot and control of the bleeding source. The presence of an EDH in a patient with signs of neurologic compromise is the paramount neurosurgical emergency. Some authors have advocated nonoperative management of small EDHs in patients who have no or minimal symptoms. The decision not to operate may initiate a precarious clinical course, and such a decision should be made only by a neurosurgeon.

Acute Subdural Hematoma

An acute subdural hematoma (ASDH) is the most commonly occurring intracranial mass lesion in patients who present to the emergency department with severe head injury. It is also the most common injury that produces a fatal outcome following trauma. Although

EDHs usually are not associated with underlying brain injury, ASDHs are usually a reflection of the amount of injury the brain has sustained. In severe injury, the brain suffers serious contusion, multiple small cortical veins are ruptured, and an ASDH is usually formed by venous bleeding from the cortical surface. Subdural hematomas form in the subdural space, the space between the brain or arachnoid membrane and the dura. Unlike the situation with EDH, the subdural space is not limited by suture lines. For this reason, subdural hematomas tend to spread widely over the convexity of the brain and form a concave appearance on axial imaging. The mortality rate from ASDHs ranges from 40% to 90%, and the outcome is related to two factors: the speed with which the clot is removed in a patient who is deteriorating and the extent of associated underlying brain injury. In a classic clinical study of patients with ASDH, severe morbidity and mortality were three times greater in patients who had an ASDH removed more than 4 h following trauma compared with those patients who were operated on within 4 h (7). Although subsequent clinical series have disputed these findings, the balance of available clinical literature suggests that speed is of the essence in diagnosing and treating ASDHs (8–11). The controversy in the literature may indicate that the extent of intrinsic cerebral injury likely has far more influence on outcome than the timing of surgery.

Clinical findings in a patient with an ASDH range from a patient who is deeply comatose from the time of injury to one who experiences a lucid interval comparable with that described with EDHs. A lucid interval at presentation is common among patients with EDH and less common for patients with subdural hematomas. Because ASDHs have a much higher incidence than EDHs, the majority of patients with a lucid interval will suffer from a subdural hematoma. Because both the EDH and the ASDH tend to occur over the lateral, frontal, or temporal regions, the mass effect from these lesions tends to be directed toward the midline. The ASDH produces a midline shift of the frontal and temporal lobes and, if not controlled, leads to uncal herniation by forcing the medial portion of the temporal lobe into the incisura. The surgical treatment of ASDH is similar to that of EDH. In both, a temporal trauma flap is fashioned, and a free bone flap is elevated over the frontal and temporal regions. For treatment of an ASDH, the dura must be opened before the hematoma can be removed. An ASDH is usually several centimeters thick, spreads out over the entire convexity of the brain, and is clotted and semifirm rather than liquid. The ASDH must be removed with a combination of suction and irrigation. The usual source of subdural bleeding is the small venules over the surface of the brain. It is unusual to find a discreet or major bleeding source when a subdural hematoma is removed. A major exception is the removal of a subdural clot produced by injury to a major venous structure such as the sagittal or lateral sinus.

Following the successful removal of an ASDH, the dura is closed, the bone flap is replaced, and an ICP monitor is customarily placed to aid in the management of intracranial hypertension as cerebral edema develops.

Traumatic Intracerebral Hematoma

A hematoma may form within the brain parenchyma itself as a result of trauma. Such hematomas are relatively uncommon and have an incidence ranging from 4% to 12% in patients who suffer severe closed head injury. Intracerebral hematomas are far less common than subdural hematomas; they occur with a frequency approximately equal to that of EDHs. Intracerebral hematomas result from severe disruption of the deep white matter and may occur at the time of injury. Alternatively, they may represent a coalescence of multiple smaller contusions contained within an injured lobe. Characteristically, these contusions, and thus the eventual hematoma, are found as a contrecoup accompaniment to trauma. Therefore, frontal intracerebral hematomas are most commonly found in patients who fall and strike the occipital region. These hematomas are expansile masses surrounded by edematous brain. They may elevate ICP and distort adjacent brain tissue sufficiently to mandate surgical removal. Most patients with large intracerebral hematomas resulting from trauma will have a profoundly altered state of consciousness and must be managed with close monitoring of ICP and neurologic status. Hematomas in proximity to the tentorial incisura (for example, those in the posterior frontal or anterior temporal lobes) are particularly dangerous. They may produce uncal herniation and brainstem injury with only a minimum of warning. Some neurosurgeons remove such hematomas prophylactically (12).

Delayed Traumatic Intracerebral Hematoma

A delayed traumatic intracerebral hematoma (DTICH) is found in patients with head trauma, CT scanning of whom showed no evidence of such a blood clot on admission. This type of hematoma develops hours to days following head injury and is more common in older patients (13). Following the removal of an extra-axial mass lesion such as a subdural hematoma, the brain underlying the hematoma re-expands. This portion of the brain has been severely traumatized by a combination of concussion and compression. Cerebral contusions frequently appear in the white matter upon re-expansion and then may coalesce to form a DTICH. Those patients who develop disseminated intravascular coagulopathy and fibrinolysis following a head injury may be at increased risk of developing a delayed intracerebral hematoma.

The clinical presentation of DTICH is neurologic deterioration in a patient who has been stable or who has shown improvement following the initial phases of head injury. DTICH may be heralded by an unexpected rise in the patient's ICP. Such deterioration should always prompt a search for a surgical intracranial lesion. A repeat CT scan is the most efficient means of diagnosing these hematomas. In patients who develop evidence of coagulopathy following head injury, serial CT scans may allow the early detection of a DTICH. As a matter of practice, CT scans of patients with severe head injury should be repeated routinely on postinjury days 1 and 3. The yield on these "routine" studies is high and helps to lessen the possibility of an unwelcome surprise later in the clinical course.

PATHOPHYSIOLOGY

Trauma produces a wide variation in the type of injury that the brain and its surrounding structures sustain. All of these injuries, edema, contusions, and hematomas, can be discussed in the context of the Monro–Kellie doctrine. This doctrine states that the intracranial capacity is a fixed volume occupied by brain, blood, CSF, and any other masses that may develop within this closed space. Because the space cannot expand, the amount of compliance available to buffer increased pressure is limited before pressure begins to elevate dramatically in response to an increasing mass. The intracranial mass that follows a head injury may be comprised of cerebral edema, hyperemia, an extra-axial or intra-axial hematoma, air, a penetrating object, or any combination of these elements.

The initial response of the system in terms of compliance is to displace CSF from the ventricles into the spinal thecal sac. This mechanism provides ~50–70 cc of additional intracranial volume to accommodate the mass. Venous capacitance vessels, providing an additional mechanism of compensation, collapse in response to rising ICP. When compliance is exhausted, the system's response to the addition of any further intracranial mass is rapidly increasing ICP. The management goal for head-injured patients is to preserve cerebral blood flow, minimize the formation of cerebral edema, and control ICP. Cerebral blood flow cannot be measured in most ICUs but must be inferred from a measurement of cerebral perfusion pressure (CPP), defined clinically as the difference between mean arterial pressure (MAP) and ICP. The formula to determine CPP is:

$$CPP = MAP - ICP$$

Under most circumstances, the cerebral blood flow will remain fairly constant within the limits of autoregulation (CPP = 60–150 mm Hg). Autoregulation is a physiologic accommodation that maintains near-constant cerebral blood flow over a wide range of perfusion pressures. Within the limits of cerebral autoregulation, cerebral ischemia will not occur. This mechanism is operant only in intact brain and is largely disrupted in edematous, traumatized, or ischemic brain where cerebral blood flow will vary directly with changes in CPP.

As ICP rises, CPP generally falls. If CPP falls below the lower limits of cerebral autoregulation, the traumatized brain becomes ischemic. This ischemia produces a secondary and sometimes devastating insult to vulnerable traumatized neural tissue. The actual incidence and relative contribution of cerebral ischemia that follows closed head injury has been vigorously debated by authorities in the field. Cerebral ischemia may affect only a minority of patients with severe head injury, although these patients tend to be more severely injured and have a worse prognosis (14). The more common response of cerebral blood flow to severe head injury is moderate to severe hyperemia, possibly to a greater extent in children and young adults. Such a finding probably reflects a failure of autoregulation and makes the cerebral capillary system vulnerable to hemorrhage or transudation of edema fluid into the interstitium.

MANAGEMENT OF ICP

A plan to manage intracranial hypertension, based on the Monro–Kellie doctrine, attempts to favorably affect each of the components that occupy intracranial volume (Fig. 3). The first line of defense is to remove those masses—epidural, subdural, or intracerebral hematomas—that are present when the patient arrives at the hospital. Usually, surgery for this indication has been performed before the patient arrives in the ICU, and the responsibility of the ICU physician is to monitor the patient carefully to detect the late development or recurrence of such a mass. At least 15% of patients who have undergone surgical removal of an intracranial hematoma will develop a delayed or recurrent hematoma after arriving in the ICU. The detection of such a lesion is the primary objective of all neurological and clinical monitoring. Any unexplained deterioration in the patient's neurologic status or an abrupt rise in ICP must alert the clinician to the possibility of the delayed development of a mass lesion. A corollary to this principle is that an unexplained rise in blood pressure may be a physiologic response to narrowed CPP as the

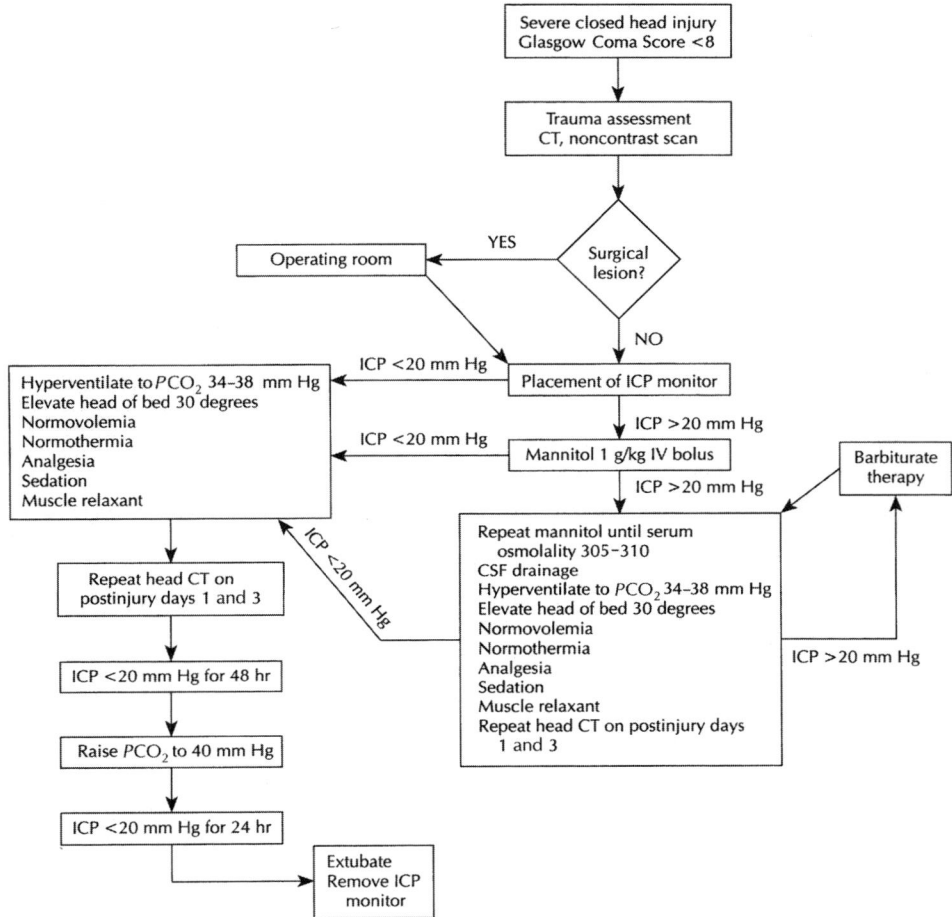

Figure 3 Management of intracranial pressure.

brain struggles to maintain adequate cerebral blood flow. The possibility of a delayed mass lesion always should be considered when systolic hypertension occurs in patients with head injury, especially in those patients who do not have ICP monitoring.

In those patients who have continuing ICP elevations following the evacuation of all surgical lesions, management is directed at increasing the compliance of the system through one of several manipulations. First and most effective is hyperventilation, which serves to constrict venous capacitance and to decrease the amount of intracranial volume taken by systemic blood. Hyperventilation also decreases the hyperemia that commonly follows head injury and has a direct and profound effect on ICP. The target PCO_2 is 34–38 mm Hg. End-tidal CO_2 measurements should be correlated with PCO_2 from arterial blood gas measurements and then followed closely. Excessive or inappropriate hyperventilation may worsen neurological outcome by increasing posttraumatic cerebral ischemia (15,16). The effect of hyperventilation on increased ICP may be temporary, and reduction in effect may be noted after 72–96 h (17,18). Positive end expiratory pressure may be used in patients with head injury at levels of 5–10 cm H$_2$O without significantly affecting ICP.

A second strategy for decreasing ICP is to treat the patient with a hyperosmotic agent, which decreases the amount of cerebral interstitial volume and cerebral edema. Mannitol is the drug of choice in most centers and is administered in a dose of 0.5–1 g/kg as a bolus injection over several minutes. Mannitol is most effective in decreasing ICP when given as a bolus, although some physicians use this agent in a drip form to maximize serum osmolarity. Mannitol may be infused until the serum osmolarity is in the range of 305–310. Increasing the osmolarity beyond this point does not significantly affect intracranial edema and potentiates serious electrolyte imbalances. The goal of mannitol therapy is to render the patient hyperosmotic but not hypovolemic. Hypovolemia may compromise the cerebral perfusion, and in patients with multiple trauma, such manipulation may limit the chance of survival. Nonosmotic diuretics also may be used to assist in the control of intracranial hypertension. Furosemide is the drug that has been used most often for this indication, and clinical evidence indicates that it acts synergistically with mannitol (19,20). The clinician should use caution, because combined therapy may produce profound dehydration much faster than either agent does alone and may lead to circulatory collapse. In its effect on ICP, furosemide appears to be less reliable as a sole agent than mannitol.

The next portion of the Monro–Kellie doctrine that can be manipulated is the intracranial volume occupied by CSF. Production of CSF will continue in the ventricles until very high ICP is reached. The development of posttraumatic hydrocephalus can be a terminal event. Compliance in the system may be increased by providing an alternative outlet for CSF drainage through placement of a ventriculostomy catheter, which can serve the dual role of providing ICP monitoring and an outlet for CSF flow.

In patients who are intubated, muscle relaxants used in conjunction with analgesics and/or sedatives are another useful adjunct for lowering ICP. These agents should be used with extreme caution in patients without ICP monitoring, because they have profound effects on neurological observation. Doses of these agents should be reduced or interrupted on a regular basis every few hours to permit monitoring of neurologic function. In those patients with continuous ICP monitoring, sedatives and muscle relaxants can be used with slightly more confidence, but intermittent neurological examination remains a priority. Elevation of the head of the patient's bed to control ICP is controversial in the literature, although in practice it is a nearly universal management technique. Typically, the patient's head is elevated ∼30 degrees to facilitate venous drainage and to diminish the formation of cerebral edema.

High-dose barbiturate therapy also has been used as a management option in patients with increased ICP (21–23). Most centers reserve this type of therapy for those patients who are hemodynamically stable and have intracranial hypertension that has proved refractory to conventional management. High-dose barbiturate therapy has the dual purpose of protecting the brain metabolically while decreasing cerebral blood flow and volume. The initiation and maintenance of pentobarbital coma is complex and dangerous (24). Its use should be considered only in patients who are not neurologically devastated, are young and not volume depleted, and have arterial pressure monitoring and Swan–Ganz monitoring catheters in place. The greatest risk with the initiation of barbiturate therapy is profound and refractory hypotension that makes hemodynamic monitoring and optimization necessary. Pentobarbital loading should be performed with a dose of 10 mg/kg over 30 min followed by a maintenance dose of 5 mg/kg/h for the next 3 h.

Long-term maintenance is then begun at 1–2 mg/kg/h and titrated to achieve ICP control. If ICP is not controlled, additional boluses of pentobarbital (100–200 mg) should be administered intravenously at a slow rate. Serum pentobarbital concentrations should be checked every 12 h for 48 h and subsequently at least every 24 h. Serum concentrations should be maintained at 3–4 mg/dL. The endpoint for pentobarbital therapy is ICP control. Pentobarbital is frequently a therapy of last resort. Once initiated, the drug should be used aggressively until ICP is controlled, or the patient displays signs of significant drug toxicity, such as refractory hypotension.

The use of steroids in patients with severe head injury is also controversial. Despite numerous clinical studies, not a single controlled study has shown evidence that administration of steroids improves patient outcome following severe head injury. New agents are under development and may be more effective in reducing cerebral edema and less likely to produce side effects. Presently, no indication for the use of steroids in head injury exists (25). Table 2 summarizes the pharmacologic control of ICP.

POSTTRAUMATIC SEIZURES

Posttraumatic seizures are relatively common among patients with severe head injury and have an estimated incidence of 20–50%. Higher rates are found in patients with depressed skull fractures or penetrating brain injuries and in children with severe head injuries. Seizures are most common from several hours to several days following severe head injury. Termed "early" seizures, they are a direct reflection of the injury to the brain. Although not considered epileptic, early seizures are a predisposing factor to the development of late seizures or posttraumatic epilepsy. However, the occurrence of early seizures following trauma does not mean that posttraumatic epilepsy is inevitable. The rationale for the use of anticonvulsants for early seizure prophylaxis is to decrease the incidence of these seizures, reduce the likelihood of late seizures, prevent acute complications of ictal events, and avoid further brain injury secondary to epileptiform discharge. In multiple

Table 2 Pharmacologic Control of ICP

Drug	Administration	Notes
Mannitol (osmotic diuretic)	Bolus IV dose: 1 g/kg	Effective until serum osmolality 305–310
Furosemide (loop diuretic)	Bolus IV dose: 10–20 mg (adult)	Less effective than mannitol; may potentiate electrolyte abnormalities if used in conjunction with osmotic diuretics
Vecuronium (paralyzing agent)	0.1 mg/kg IV dose or 1 μg/kg/min continuous IV infusion	Must be used in conjunction with a sedative
Lorazepam (sedative)	1–4 mg IV dose	Effect lasts 6–8 h, includes both sedation and relative amnesia
Pentobarbital (cerebral protective agent)	Loading dose: 10 mg/kg over 30 min Maintenance dose: 1–2 mg/kg/h	Hypotension is a common complication; drug is used until ICP is controlled or patient becomes refractorily hypotensive

double-blinded controlled studies, the most commonly used prophylactic anticonvulsant, phenytoin, has been shown to have an effect on the frequency of early seizures but no effect on that of late seizures. The use of phenytoin for patients with head injury is somewhat controversial (26). A conservative recommendation is that phenytoin be used as prophylaxis in all patients with acute severe head injury characterized by intracranial hematoma, contusion, depressed skull fracture, or open or penetrating injury. Anticonvulsants should be administered routinely to those patients who have suffered an early seizure.

If anticonvulsants are used, they must be administered in adequate dosage. Patients with head injury are hypermetabolic, and serum phenytoin concentrations are almost always subtherapeutic in the acute stage of management. Phenytoin is the drug of choice in this clinical setting, because it can be administered parenterally and has a relatively short half-life. When phenytoin is used in a critical care setting for a patient with head injury, serum drug concentrations should be followed at least daily to ensure that adequate blood concentrations are attained. Those patients who develop early seizures should be treated as though they were in status epilepticus with the intravenous administration of diazepam or lorazepam (Table 2).

SUMMARY

- All therapeutic efforts following brain injury attempt to prevent or reduce additional brain injury.
- Early, accurate diagnosis and therapy are essential to decrease morbidity and mortality.
- Initial assessment of patients with head injury must include Glasgow Coma Scale, pupillary light reflex, motor system evaluation, and respiratory pattern.
- A linear, nondisplaced skull fracture indicates increased risk for development of intracranial hematoma.
- An open depressed skull fracture requires surgical management. Any depressed skull fracture mandates neurosurgical consultation. Basilar skull fractures are diagnosed clinically. Prophylactic antibiotic therapy for basilar skull fracture is controversial.
- EDHs are common in young patients, usually following injury to a branch of the middle meningeal artery, and require emergency surgical evaluation. A lucid interval is characteristic of the patient's history.
- ASDHs are lesions most commonly associated with severe head injury. Rapid evacuation can decrease morbidity and mortality. ASDHs also may be characterized by a lucid interval. Development of systolic hypertension following head injury may indicate development of a new intracranial mass lesion.
- Management of increased ICP attempts to remove space-occupying masses, improve compliance with hyperventilation or mannitol, or decrease the volume of CSF with a ventriculostomy catheter.

REFERENCES

1. Dacey R, Alves W, Rimel R, Winn NR, Jane JA. Neurosurgical complications after apparently minor head injury; assessment of risk in a series of 610 patients. J Neurosurg 1986; 65:203–210.

2. Jennett B, Teasdale G. Early assessment of the head injured patient. In: Management of Head Injuries. Philadelphia: FA Davis, 1981.
3. Brackman R. Survey and follow-up of 225 consecutive patients with a depressed skull fracture. J Neurol Neurosurg Psychiatry 1971; 34:106.
4. Van den Heever H, Van der Merwe J. Management of depressed skull fractures. Selective conservative management of nonmissile injuries. J Neurosurg 1989; 71:186–190.
5. Hoff J, Brewin A. Antibiotics for basilar skull fractures. J Neurosurg 1976; 44:649.
6. Ignelzi R, VanderArk G. Analysis of the treatment of basilar skull fractures with and without antibiotics. J Neurosurg 1975; 43:721–726.
7. Seelig J, Becker D, Miller J, et al. Traumatic acute subdural hematoma. Major morbidity reduction in comatose patients treated within four hours. N Engl J Med 1981; 304:511–518.
8. Chiles BI, Cooper P. Extra-axial hematomas. In: Loftus C, ed. Neurosurgical Emergencies. Vol. 1. Park Ridge, IL: AANS, 1994:73–100.
9. Haselberger K, Pucher R, Auer L. Prognosis after acute subdural or epidural hemorrhage. Acta Neurochir (Wien) 1992; 90:111–116.
10. Stone J, Rifai M, Sugar O, et al. Subdural hematomas. I: acute subdural hematomas: progress in definition, clinical pathology and therapy. Surg Neurol 1983; 19:216–231.
11. Wilberger JJ, Harris M, Diamond D. Acute subdural hematoma: morbidity, mortality, and operative timing. J Neurosurg 1991; 74:212–218.
12. Andrews B, Chiles BW, Olsen W, Pihs LH. The effect of intracerebral hematoma location on the risk of brain-stem compression and on clinical outcome. J Neurosurg 1988; 69:518–522.
13. Fukamachi A, Kohno K, Nagaseki Y, et al. The incidence of delayed traumatic intracerebral hematoma with extradural hemorrhages. J Trauma 1985; 25:145–149.
14. Robertson C, Grossman R, Goodman J, Narayan RK. The predictive value of cerebral anaerobic metabolism with cerebral infarction after head injury. J Neurosurg 1987; 67:361–368.
15. Bouma G, Muizelaar J. Cerebral blood flow, cerebral blood volume, and cerebrovascular reactivity after severe head injury. J Neurotrauma 1992; 1:S333–S348.
16. Muizelaar J, Marmarou A, Ward J, et al. Adverse effects of prolonged hyperventilation in patients with severe head injury: a randomized clinical trial. J Neurosurg 1991; 75:731–739.
17. Havill J. Prolonged hyperventilation and intracranial pressure. Crit Care Med 1984; 12:72–74.
18. Van der Poel H. Cerebral vasoconstriction is not maintained with prolonged hyperventilation. In: Hoff J, Betz A, eds. Intracranial Pressure VII. Berlin: Springer-Verlag, 1989:899–903.
19. Pollay M, Fullenwider C, Roberts P, Stevens PA. Effect of mannitol and furosemide on blood–brain osmotic gradient and intracranial pressure. J Neurosurg 1983; 59:945–950.
20. Roberts P, Pollay M, Engles C, et al. Effect on intracranial pressure of furosemide combined with varying doses and administration of mannitol. J Neurosurg 1987; 66:440–446.
21. Eisenberg H, Frankowski R, Contant C, et al. High-dose barbiturate control of elevated intra-cranial pressure in patients with severe head injury. J Neurosurg 1988; 69:15–23.
22. Rea G, Rockswold G. Barbiturate therapy in un-controlled intracranial hypertension. Neurosurgery 1983; 12:401–404.
23. Rockoff M, Marshall L, Shapiro M. High-dose barbiturate therapy in humans: a clinical review of 60 patients. Ann Neurol 1979; 6:194–199.
24. Schalen W, Messeter K, Nordstrom C. Complications and side effects during thiopentone therapy in patients with severe head injuries. Acta Anaesthesiol Scand 1992; 36:369–377.
25. Marion D, Ward J. Steroids in closed-head injury. Perspect Crit Care 1990; 3:19.
26. Temkin N, Dikrnen S, Winn H. Posttraumatic seizures. Neurosurg Clin North Am 1991; 2:425–435.

18
Spinal Cord Injury

Anthony Bottini
Centracare Clinic—Neurosurgery, St. Cloud, Minnesota, USA

Critical care of patients with spinal cord injuries is a unique clinical challenge. These patients are usually young, recently healthy adults who have suffered a devastating injury that has dramatically altered their physiology, function, independence, and self-image. They are vulnerable to a variety of physiologic insults and complications that may contribute to serious, lifelong disability. Optimal management requires the physician to accurately assess and stabilize the cervical spinal injury, carefully monitor neurologic function, support the patient's homeostatic and recuperative mechanisms, and initiate physical and psychological rehabilitation.

CLINICAL ASSESSMENT

Assessment begins with a clear and detailed history of the patient's trauma and subsequent prehospital course. Important details include the mechanism of injury (e.g., flexion, extension, and rotation), the patient's realization of his/her deficit, and some understanding of the evolution of the neurologic deficit since the time of injury. The examiner should know whether the injury was initially complete or incomplete with subsequent progression. Details of the patient's extrication and transport to a hospital are also significant. Precautions undertaken to protect the patient's neurologic function during transport should be detailed, and a description of the patient's positioning, level of neurologic function, and immobilization measures in use at the time of unit admission should be documented.

The key element in assessment is a precise, complete, and carefully documented neurologic examination (1). Neurologic examination on admission is critical to establish the baseline with which subsequent physicians may compare their evaluations and determine the patient's neurologic course.

The patient's head and neck should be immobilized. Any cervical orthosis obscuring the clinician's view should be removed, and the neck examined. Obvious signs of injury to the neck should be noted, and carotid palpation and auscultation should be performed. Superficial temporal pulses also should be palpated, and any signs of trauma representing a threat to the airway noted. Careful palpation over the spinous processes also may enable the clinician to narrow his/her search for evidence of injury on a plain radiograph. The patient's head and neck should be maintained in a neutral position during the examination and not manipulated in any fashion. Typically, patients with spinal cord injuries do not have observable surface deformities, with the exception of those who have suffered a unilaterally locked facet with forced rotation of the head to one side. The Philadelphia collar or other stabilizing orthosis should be replaced after examination of the patient's neck.

Motor Examination

The motor examination is of primary importance. All major muscle groups in each of the four extremities should be serially examined, and the strength of muscle contraction carefully documented. A grading system, such as the one suggested in Box 1, is objective and allows different clinicians to make meaningful comparisons. A standard motor examination in spinal cord injured patients should test those muscle groups listed in Table 1. The reader is referred elsewhere for a description of the techniques for performing this examination (2). Special care should be taken to determine whether the muscles examined have any contractile function, including that which does not exceed the threshold for movement.

Sensory Examination

The sensory examination, performed next, should be a careful, systematic examination with a variety of modalities, including nociception, light touch, and proprioception. Multimodality testing is essential, because the structures within the spinal cord that conduct sensation decussate at different levels in the central nervous system and travel in different quadrants of the spinal cord (Fig. 1). Incomplete spinal cord lesions may produce a combination of sensory findings that depend on the tracts involved. Below the level of a complete lesion, all sensory modalities will be absent. Radicular pain or paresthesias may be present at the level of the injury and may have localizing value.

Pain sensation (nociception), as tested by a pinprick, is primarily mediated in the lateral spinothalamic tract. This modality is tested with a disposable pin proceeding in a systematic fashion from the lower extremities up the trunk to the upper extremities. Left and right extremities always should be examined in a serial fashion and compared. The chest and abdomen also should be examined over both the anterior surfaces and as far posteriorly as possible.

Light touch, carried through the spinal cord's posterior columns, may be tested either with manual touch, with a tissue, or with some other minimal stimulus. To further refine this examination, two point discrimination should be tested to detect more subtle loss of

Box 1 Grading System for Motor Examination of Patient with Spinal Cord Injury

---
5 Contraction against powerful resistance (normal power) = 100%
4 Contraction against gravity and some resistance = 75%
3 Contraction against gravity only = 50%
2 Movement possible only with gravity eliminated = 25%
1 Flicker of contraction but no movement = 10%
0 Complete paralysis = 0%

Source: From Clain A, ed. Hamilton Bailey's Demonstrations of Physical Signs in Clinical Surgery. Bristol: John Wright & Sons, 1980, p. 402. With permission of Butterworth-Heinemann Ltd.

Table 1 Testing of Muscle Groups in Standard Motor Examination of Patient with Spinal Cord Injury

Action	Muscle(s)	Root(s)	Peripheral nerve
Upper extremities			
1. Abduct (initial) arm and extend rotation of arm	Supraspinatous, infraspinatous	C5, C6	Suprascapular
2. Abduct arm (hold at 90 degrees against resistance)	Deltoid	C5	Axilliary
3. Flex arm (hand supine)	Biceps	C5, C6	Musculocutaneous
4. Flex arm (hand midway between supine and prone)	Brachioradialis	C5, C6	Radial
5. Extend arm	Triceps	C7	Radial
6. Extension of wrist			
a. Hand abducted (toward thumb)	Extensor carpi radialis longus	C5, C6	Radial
b. Hand adducted (toward fifth finger)	Extensor carpi ulnaris	C7, C8	Posterior interosseous
7. Flexion of wrist	Flexor carpi radialis	C6, C7	Median
8. Flexion of fingers	Flexor digitorium superficialis (proximal)	C7, C8, T1	Median
	Flexor digitorum profundus (distal)		
	a. First and second digits	C7, C8	Anterior interosseous
	b. Third and fourth digits	C7, C8	Ulnar
9. Palmar abduction of thumb	Abductor pollicis brevis	C8, T1	Median
10. Opposing thumb to base of fifth finger	Opponens pollicis	C8, T1	Median
11. Spreading and adducting fingers	Interossei	C8, T1	Ulnar
Lower extremities			
1. Flexion of hip	Iliopsoas	L1, L2, L3	Direct branches from root
2. Extension of hip	Gluteus maximus	L5, S1	Inferior gluteal
3. Adduction of thigh	Adductors	L2, L3, L4	Obturator
4. Extension of leg (lower)	Quadriceps femoris	L2, L3, L4	Femoral
5. Flexion of knee	Hamstrings	L5, S1, S2	Sciatic
6. Plantar flexion of foot	Gastrocnemius and soleus	S1, S2	Tibial
7. Dorsiflexion of foot	Anterior tibial	L4, L5	Deep peroneal
8. Inversion of foot	Posterior tibial	L4, L5	Tibial
9. Extension of toes	Extensor digitorum longus and extensor hallucis longus	L5, S1	Deep peroneal
10. Eversion of foot	Peroneal longus and brevis	L5, S1	Sciatic

Note: Underscoring indicates principal spinal nerve supply.
Source: Reprinted with permission from Weisberg L, Strub RL, Garcia CA. Essentials of Clinical Neurology, 2nd ed. Rockville, Md.: Aspen Publishers, 1989:12–13.

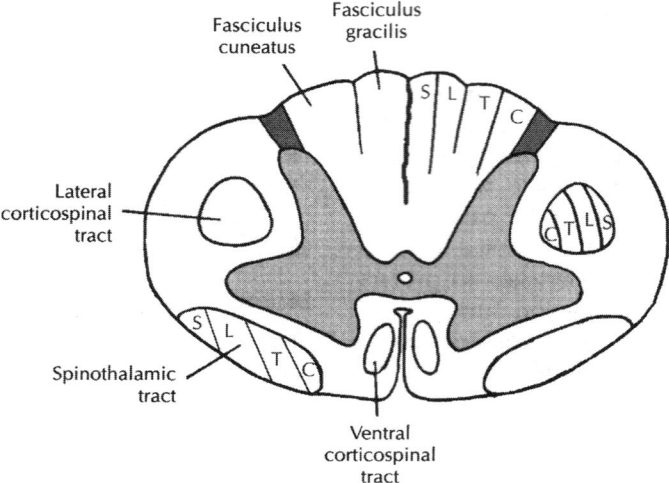

Figure 1 Cervical spinal cord anatomy. S, sacral; L, lumbar; T, thoracic; C, cervical.

sensation. A dermatomal diagram, in which the upper cervical dermatomes drape over the base of the neck and shoulders in a cape-like fashion, is shown in Fig. 2. These dermatomal distributions should be remembered in interpreting both the nociceptive and light touch portion of the sensory examination; sensation in this cape-like distribution may be misinterpreted as a preserved sensory level below an observed cervical motor level. In a patient with a high cervical motor level, preservation of sensation over the clavicular regions should not be misinterpreted as evidence of an incomplete cervical spinal cord injury.

Proprioception should be tested carefully over the patient's upper and lower extremities. In performing this examination, the examiner's thumb and forefinger are best positioned on the lateral aspects of the digit being tested. This position removes the additional pressure or light touch sensation differential that may result when the digit is alternatively deflected upward or downward. The examiner should take care to ensure that the patient is not able to see the direction of digit deflection. Both light touch and proprioception are mediated primarily through the posterior sensory columns.

Deep tendon reflexes should be tested over the biceps, triceps, brachioradialis, patellar, and Achilles' tendons. This examination should then be recorded in the medical record for later comparison. In addition to deep tendon reflexes, other reflexes should be tested in patients suspected of having a spinal cord injury, including the abdominal, cremastereric, bulbocavernosus, anal wink, and crossed adductor reflexes.

A rectal examination should always be performed in a patient with suspected spinal cord injury. Preservation of perirectal sensation is an important finding in a patient who appears to have an otherwise complete spinal cord injury. This so-called sacral sparing of sensation is a consequence of the onion skin-like lamination of fibers within the spinothalamic tract. Sacral fibers thst run in the ventrolateral portion of the tracts may be spared, even when deep intraparenchymal lesions occur. The distinction between an incomplete and complete cord syndrome has great significance for further diagnostics, therapeutics, and prognostication for the patient and family. The patient should be carefully examined for sphincter tone and anal reflexes for these same reasons.

Spinal Cord Injury

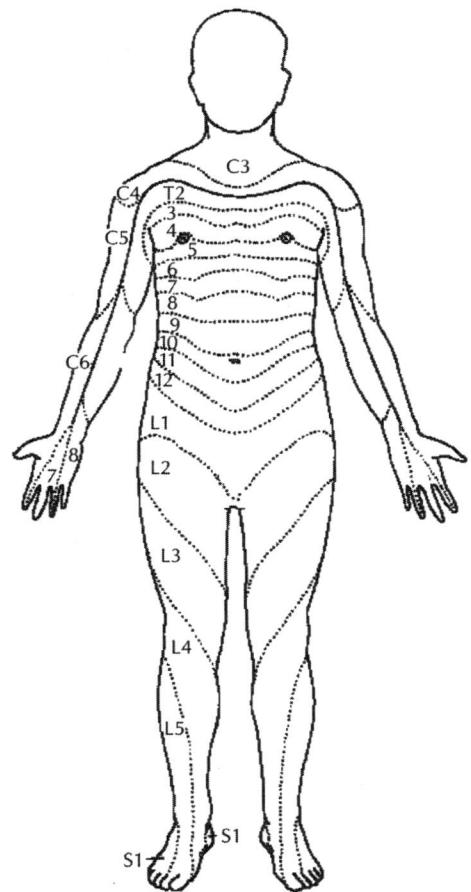

Figure 2 Dermatomal diagram for examination of patient with spinal cord injury.

RADIOGRAPHIC ASSESSMENT

The sensitivity and specificity of radiographic evaluation of intensive care unit patients with suspected spinal injuries has been the subject of a number of studies and reviews over the past decade (3). The minimal evaluation for patients in this category include a three-view cervical spine series with CT scanning supplementation in areas which are difficult to visualize, such as C6–T1 and the craniospinal junction. Any suspicious areas seen on plain films should be studied further with CT scanning through that area. The combination of normal plain films and normal CT scanning through the areas described earlier has a negative predictive value for significant spinal injury between 99% and 100% (4–8).

Awake, coherent patients may be studied further with dynamic flexion/extension views to search for ligamentous instability or other occult spinal injury. The combination of a normal three-view plain cervical spine series and a normal flexion/extension series also has a >99% sensitivity in the search for significant spinal injury (9). In patients who are obtunded or comatose, a spinal MRI study within the first 48 h following injury may eliminate the possibility of an undiagnosed clinically significant spinal ligamentous injury. MRI examination of the trauma patient is sometimes problematic because of limited scanner availability, the difficulty of patient transport, the presence or possibility of contained metal fragments, inadequate bone detail, the inability of trauma patients to cooperate with a prolonged study in the small confines of the gantry, and the large number of false positive examinations. A false positive examination may result in a prolonged, unnecessary immobilization of an obtunded patient (3,5,10–13).

Radiographic evaluation of a spinal cord injury always must begin with plain cervical spine films. The single most useful view is a lateral radiograph, which includes at least C1–C7 and, preferably, T1, as well. The examiner must develop and consistently use a systematized approach in studying cervical spine films. The most practical way to review cervical spine radiographs is to work from one direction to another. For example, the clinician can review findings from anterior to posterior, then cephalad to caudal. The clinician should initially study the retropharyngeal soft tissue to determine whether a hematoma, swelling, or other soft tissue sign provides a clue to the existence of a cervical spine injury. The examiner should study the anterior vertebral line to be certain that each of the vertebral bodies is properly aligned in a normal cervical lordotic configuration. Additionally, the examiner should look for avulsion fractures from the anterior end plates of these bodies, a finding that might indicate that the patient has suffered an unstable hyperextension injury. The vertebral bodies are next examined and counted. A cervical spine film that does not include C7 is judged inadequate and should be repeated. The heights of the vertebral bodies are studied for evidence of compression fractures, and their posterior margins are evaluated for a normal cervical lordotic configuration. Any subluxation or abrupt displacement of bone or vertebral bodies into the spinal canal should be noted. The spinal canal itself can be visualized as existing between the posterior margin of the vertebral bodies and the anterior margin of the spinous process. The normal diameter of an adult spinal cord is ~11 mm. Any lesser distance suggests cervical spinal canal stenosis of critical magnitude. The spinous processes should be examined for fractures or spacing irregularities. A flexion injury that disrupts the interspinous ligament is frequently noted by an increase in the interspinous distance between the two levels involved in the injury. This "fanning" of the spinous processes may be the only radiographic indication of a potentially unstable flexion injury.

The next area of study should be the C1–C2 complex. The base of the odontoid process should be carefully studied for evidence of fracture, angulation, or displacement, either anteriorly or posteriorly. Additionally, the preodontoid space, that is, the space between the posterior aspect of the anterior arch of C1 and the anterior portion of the odontiod process, should be <3 mm in adults. A widened preodontoid space suggests atlantoaxial instability. The relationship of the occiput and the foramen magnum to the odontoid process and C1 should be noted. In severe trauma, craniospinal dislocation may occur. Its presence carries a grim prognosis for the patient.

An anteroposterior cervical spine radiograph has limited utility in cervical spinal trauma. Careful inspection of the spinous processes on this view may disclose abnormal rotation between two levels. With forward displacement and locking of the superior facet, the spinous process of the vertebra cephalad to the dislocated level rotates toward the affected facet. This finding is pathognomonic for a unilaterally locked facet. An anteroposterior projection also may show irregular spacing of the spinous processes following a flexion injury or disruption of lateral border of the column of facets following a rotational injury.

Other radiographic projections add further dimensions to the radiographic examination. In a cooperative patient, an open mouth odontoid view is useful in studying the atlantoaxial complex and searching for a fracture (Jefferson fracture) of C1. Oblique views show the neural foramen and facet joints well and are useful in searching for locked facets. Flexion and extension lateral cervical spine films are invaluable in determining spinal stability, but they should never be obtained in patients who are intoxicated, have a diminished level of consciousness, or any evidence of neurological impairment. CT scanning of the cervical spine without intrathecal contrast enhancement is useful in studying Jefferson fractures or any vertebral body fracture or dislocation, particularly with sagittal and coronal reconstructions. Once they are stabilized, all patients with spinal cord injury should undergo either MRI or myelography to ensure that the spinal cord is not suffering continued compression by disc material, bone fragments, or extra-axial hematomas. See Fig. 3 for an approach to the patient with spinal cord injury.

NEUROLOGICAL SYNDROMES FOLLOWING SPINAL CORD INJURY

Patterns of spinal cord injury may be divided into complete and incomplete syndromes. With complete spinal cord injury, no motor or sensory function is detectable below the affected level. Before designating a lesion as complete, the patient should be examined carefully for evidence of preserved perianal sensation or sphincter tone. All sensory modalities, including pain, light touch, proprioception, and vibration should be tested before determining that a patient has a complete spinal cord injury. In acute spinal cord lesions, the muscles innervated below the level of a complete injury are flaccid and areflexic. In male patients, priapism accompanies spinal cord injury. With more chronic spinal cord injury, muscle tone is increased or spastic below the injury level. Hyperreflexia and up-going toes with plantar stimulation are found on examination. Common radiographic correlates of complete spinal cord injury are bilaterally locked facets or compression fractures of cervical vertebrae suffered in flexion or axial loading injuries.

Incomplete spinal cord injuries require a greater understanding of spinal cord anatomy. Three incomplete cord injury syndromes deserve special attention. Rarely are these syndromes present in the pure form; more commonly, an incomplete spinal cord injury shares elements of these syndromes (Fig. 4).

Brown–Sequard Syndrome

The Brown–Sequard syndrome follows hemisection of the spinal cord. Because of the different levels of decussation of the anterior spinothalamic tract and the posterior sensory columns, dissociation is noted between the sides of the sensory impairment occurring after this unilateral cord lesion. The lateral spinothalamic tract, which conveys pinprick and temperature sensation, enters the spinal cord through the dorsal roots and ascends one or two levels in the substantia gelatinosa before crossing through the ventral commissure to the opposite side of the spinal cord. In contradistinction, the posterior columns continue ipsilaterally until they decussate at the brain stem. If half of the cord is disrupted, loss of pain and temperature sensation begins approximately two dermatomal segments below and contralateral to the side of the lesion and extends caudally.

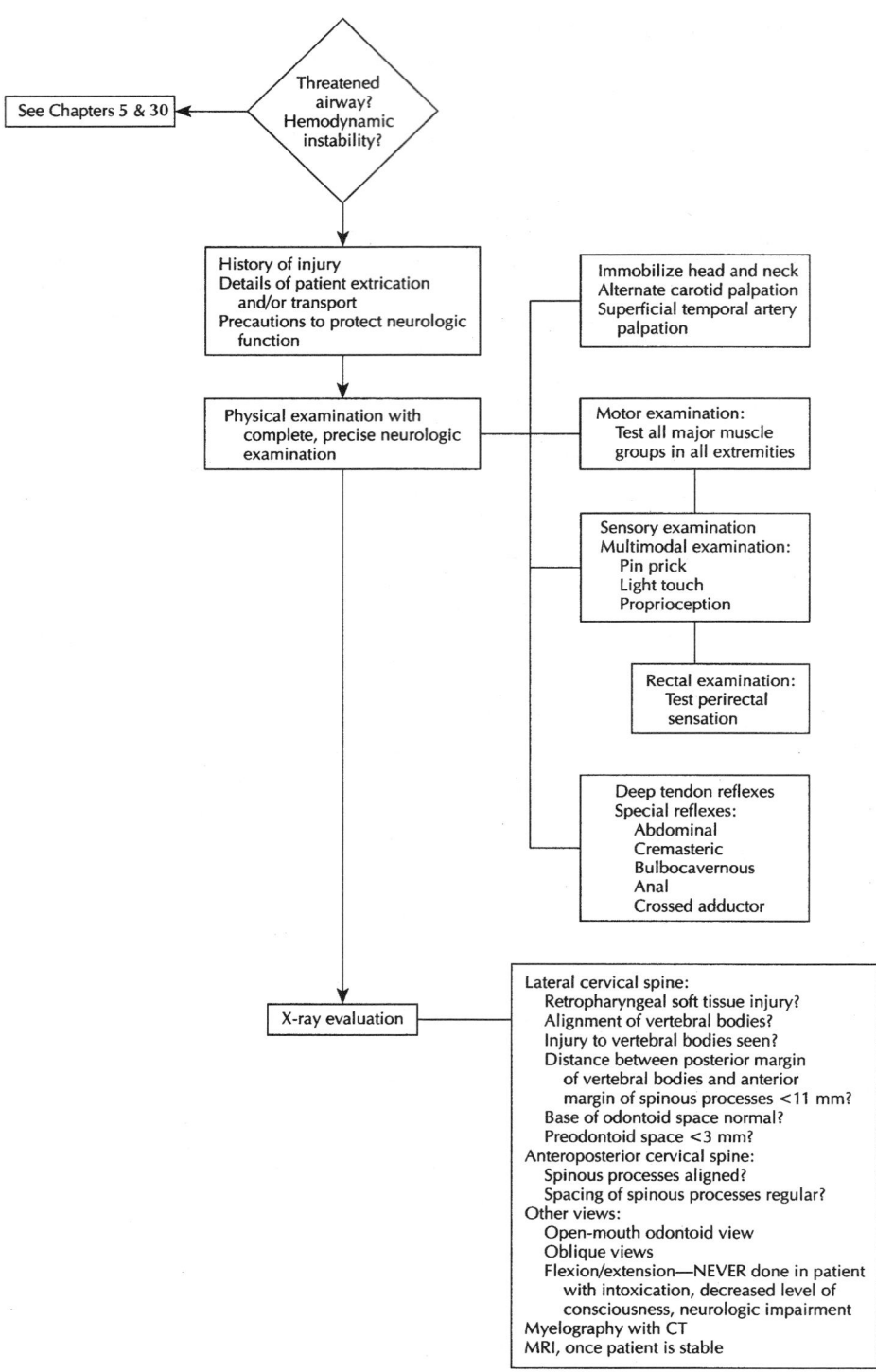

Figure 3 Approach to patient with spinal cord injury.

Spinal Cord Injury

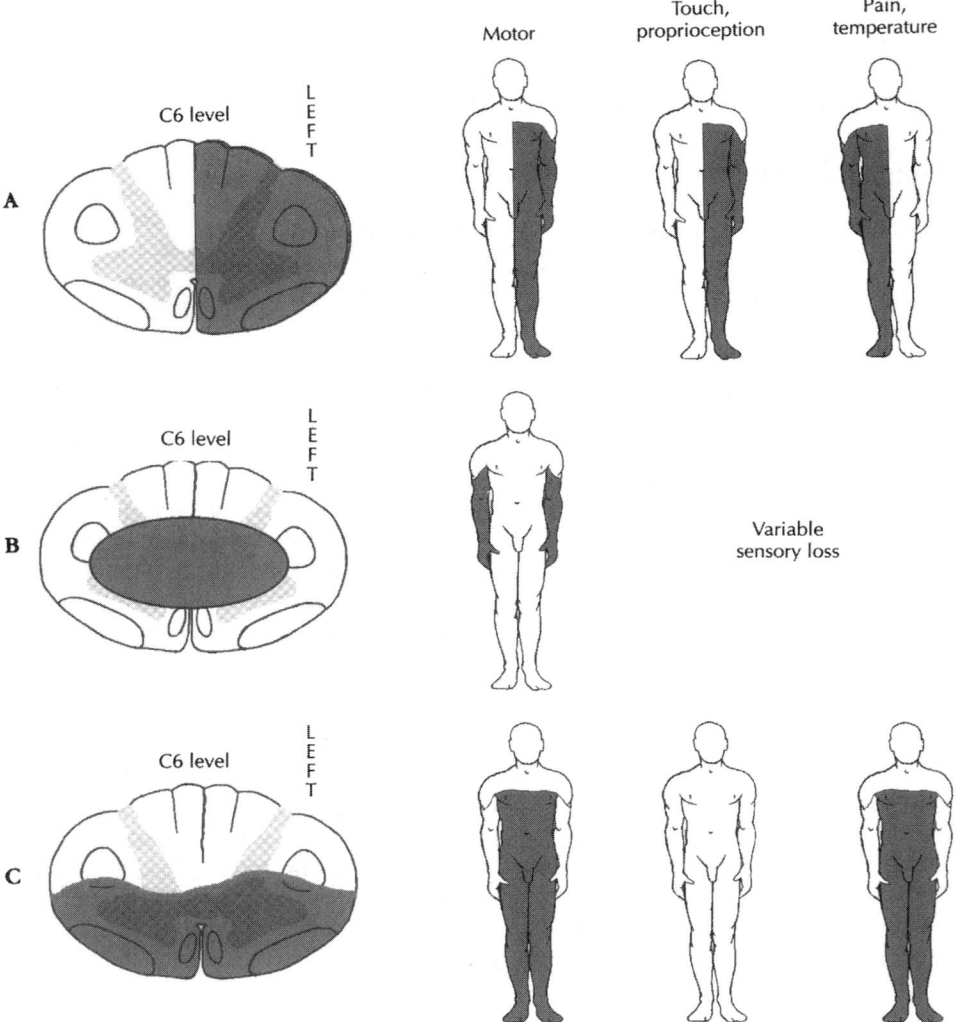

Figure 4 Incomplete lesions of spinal cord. (A) Brown–Sequard syndrome, characterized by: (1) contralateral loss of pain and temperature sensation, (2) ipsilateral loss of proprioceptive sensation and variable degrees of loss of light touch sensation, and (3) ipsilateral loss of motor function. (B) Central cord syndrome. Predominant weakness of arms is characteristic of central cord injury. (C) Anterior cord syndrome, characterized by: (1) loss of motor function below level of lesion, (2) loss of pain and temperature sensation, and (3) relative preservation of proprioception and light touch.

Beginning at the dermatome segment just below and ipsilateral to the level of the injury, proprioception and light touch are lost. Corticospinal tracts decussate at the level of the pyramids in the medulla and continue ipsilateral to the muscle groups they supply throughout the length of the spinal cord. Motor loss is, therefore, ipsilateral to the side of the hemisection. At the level of the lesion, segmental lower motor neuron findings and sensory loss may be found ipsilaterally, a consequence of damage to the anterior horn cells and roots. A pure Brown–Sequard syndrome after trauma is rare. More commonly, a partial Brown–Sequard pattern is noted with ipsilateral weakness and loss of light touch sensation and contralateral loss of pain and temperature sensation.

Central Cord Syndrome

A central cord syndrome is produced when the deepest regions of the cervical spinal cord are injured. Characteristically, distal weakness or paralysis of the upper extremities with relative sparing of motor function in the lower extremities is observed. The neuron cell bodies that control the upper extremities are located within the center of the cervical spinal cord at the level of the cervical enlargement. These cells are susceptible to posttraumatic ischemia as a consequence of their relatively higher metabolic rate and their increased distance from spinal cord blood supply. Variable sensory and bladder findings also may be present. This syndrome is most commonly seen following extension injuries when the gray matter of the cervical spinal cord is damaged. Complete recovery is possible; significant recovery is common.

Anterior Cord Syndrome

An anterior cord syndrome may occur after trauma when disc or bone fragments are driven into the spinal canal and compress the ventral spinal cord. On examination, these patients have suffered profound motor loss, as well as loss of pain and temperature sensation below the affected level (ventral spinothalamic tracts). Only posterior column function, light touch, and proprioceptive sensation may remain intact. Patients who suffer an anterior cord syndrome should be examined carefully for the presence of a ventral, extra-axial mass, such as a large disk herniation. Establishing the presence or absence of such a mass is necessary, if the deficit persists after realignment of the cervical spine. An anterior cord syndrome is not common after trauma; more commonly, it is produced by anterior spinal artery infarct. The possibility of a major thoracic vascular injury also should be considered in patients with evidence of thoracic spinal cord dysfunction.

STABILIZATION AND PROTECTION OF THE INJURED SPINE

All patients with known or suspected spinal injury require stabilization. A wide range of ancillary orthotics may be used in a critical care setting to immobilize an injured spinal column. These devices range from soft or semi-soft cervical collars such as a foam collar or the Philadelphia collar, to more reliable and complicated orthoses such as Gardener–Wells tongs, halo vests, and thoracolumbosacral braces (TLSO).

A cervical foam collar does not provide any measure of immobilization or security for patients with known or suspected spinal cord injury. They should never be used in an ICU. A Philadelphia collar, if properly applied, is more effective, particularly in preventing extremes of flexion and extension. However, this collar is difficult to tolerate over extended periods, becomes progressively less effective with use, and cannot be used to place traction or other distracting forces on the cervical spine.

The standard for acute immobilization of the unstable cervical spine remains the Gardener–Wells tongs. After shaving and anesthetizing an area immediately superior

Spinal Cord Injury

to the external acoustic meatus and slightly below the superior temporal line, these tongs are placed in the temporal region. Patient anxiety may be reduced during application, if the practitioner takes several minutes to explain the procedure to the patient and use analgesic and/or anxiolytic agents for premedication. The patient should be reassured that although initial placement of the tongs may cause discomfort, pain at the pin sites is short-lived and a significant decrease in neck pain occurs after traction is applied. Proper application of these tongs places the pins in a direct axial line above the external acoustic meatus and $\sim 0.5-1.0$ cm below the superior temporal line. Application in this area avoids the thin temporosquamosal skull and minimizes painful trauma to the temporalis muscle. Insertion of the tongs through the bulk of the temporalis muscle produces significant discomfort for the patient both at rest and upon opening the mouth to talk or to chew. Of importance, the points should not be placed at or above the superior temporal line: in this position they may slip during traction and produce a scalp laceration. The tong points may be placed either more anterior or posterior than the direct axial line above the external acoustic meatus if the practitioner wishes to place the patient's cervical spine in either extension or flexion. However, the indications for such a maneuver are uncommon.

An alternative to rigid skull fixation and traction is a halo ring placed early in the patient's hospital course. A halo system may be used as either an acute or long-term orthosis for an unstable cervical spine. Generally, halo immobilization is used as a long-term measure in those patients who have a vertebral fracture that does not require surgical stabilization. Initial placement of a halo ring as a means of providing skeletal traction, rather than Gardner–Wells tongs, may save the patient a second application of skeletal fixation, if any consideration is given to treating the injury with long-term immobilization. A halo ring is applied in much the same fashion as Gardner–Wells tongs. After shaving the scalp and injecting a local anesthetic, four pins are placed, two over the sides of the forehead and two over the parieto-occipital region. The remainder of the halo vest may or may not be initially connected to the halo ring. The ring alone may be used as a fixation device for axial skeletal traction. In the event that a satisfactory alignment is produced with distraction, the remainder of the vest and halo system may then be applied and normal anatomic alignment preserved while the patient heals.

Every ICU physician should be aware of halo vests, since their use may produce special problems in airway management or during resuscitation efforts. Intubation of a patient immobilized in a halo vest requires extra skill and some prior planning. Whenever possible, this intubation should be attempted only by or in the presence of someone with demonstrated expertise in intubation and only when other alternative measures such as fiber-optic laryngoscopy, bronchoscopy, or cricothyroidotomy are available. Electively, fiber-optic intubation is the procedure of choice. In a true emergency, when such a device is unavailable, blind nasal intubation should be attempted. Cricothyroidotomy should follow, if intubation attempts are unsuccessful. Loosening of the halo device to permit cervical extension is a distant third option. Such a maneuver might be considered in a life-or-death situation in a patient with a complete spinal cord injury.

Intensive care practitioners should inspect the patient's halo system upon admission to the ICU to determine how to remove the chest component quickly in the event that CPR is required. The majority of systems have hinges built into the sternal portion of the vest, which allow the practitioner to swing the anterior part of the vest away from the remainder of the halo device after disconnecting the abdominal straps. The vertical uprights remain in place such that cervical traction and stabilization may be maintained throughout resuscitation. For some older vest types, loosening the vertical upright supporting the head ring may be necessary. Because manipulation or removal of a halo orthosis may be unavoidable in an emergency, each patient immobilized in a halo apparatus must have a wrench that fits his/her hardware immediately available. This wrench should always be taped to the halo and should accompany the patient during any transport.

MEDICAL MANAGEMENT

Monitoring

Careful, detailed, serial neurological examinations at regular intervals are absolutely essential. These examinations are invaluable in monitoring the course of the patient's injuries, in detecting on-going injury to the spinal cord, and in formulating a rational treatment plan. The clinician's findings and the time of examination should be legibly and accurately recorded on the chart. The need for careful documentation of care and patient condition cannot be overemphasized.

Nursing orders also should include frequent neurologic checks. Initially these should be performed every hour in a patient with acute spinal cord injury and no less than twice in an 8 h period in any patient with spinal cord compromise. Patients who are in cervical traction or those patients with a known unstable spinal fracture or dislocation should have daily lateral cervical spine films to detect changes in alignment. Additionally, plain films should be repeated after any major event in the patient's hospital care, for example, an extended transport elsewhere in the hospital, a change in traction alignment or weights, placement in a halo vest, or adjustment of any orthotic device. Patients with spinal cord injury also should be routinely monitored with oxygen saturation monitors, careful fluid balance measurements, and daily weighs. In the acute setting, all patients with spinal cord injury should have a nasogastric tube placed at low continuous suction, and gastric aspirate should be monitored for pH levels. EKG monitoring, arterial pressure monitoring, and Swan–Ganz catheterization also may be indicated.

Steroids

The benefit of methylprednisolone therapy on neurologic recovery following acute spinal cord injury remains controversial. A single multicenter trial in 1985 reported that the administration of methylprednisolone within 8 h following acute spinal cord injury was associated with a significant improvement in motor function and sensation at a 6 month follow-up interval in comparison with control groups receiving either naloxone or placebo (14,15). This effect was observed in patients with both incomplete and complete spinal cord injuries. Methylprednisolone was administered as an initial intravenous bolus dose of 30 mg/kg, followed by a maintenance dose of 5.4 mg/kg/h for a total of 24 h of treatment. In this study, patients who were treated >8 h after injury with methylprednisolone experienced less recovery of motor function compared with placebo-treated patients. The authors of this study subsequently reported that the use of high-dose steroids was not associated with a statistically significant increase in treatment complications. They did report an increased incidence of infection and gastrointestinal bleeding among corticosteroid-treated patients that did not achieve statistical significance (16). The study concluded that methylprednisolone therapy was indicated for acute spinal cord-injured patients who could be treated within 8 h following injury. The authors recommended that this therapy not be initiated >8 h following injury (15).

Another multicenter trial of the use of methylprednisolone was subsequently performed and compared clinical results between patients who received steroid therapy for 24 h and a study group treated for 48 h. A placebo control group was not included in this study. The administration of methylprednisolone for 24 h following spinal cord injury was associated with an increase in serious medical complications. Complications increased with 48 h of steroid use.

Several additional studies sought to replicate the results of the initial multicenter trial. These investigators did not find the same improvement in neurologic outcome in spinal cord-injured patients treated with methylprednisolone. Multiple subsequent reviews of the use of methylprednisolone in the treatment of acute spinal cord injury have suggested that the available clinical evidence does not support the use of methylprednisolone for this indication. Several additional reviews supporting the use of methylprednisolone after acute spinal cord injury, including a Cochrane database of systemic reviews, have also been published.

Three North American multicenter randomized trials have been performed over the past 15 years in an attempt to address the issue of high dose corticosteriod treatment of acute spinal cord injured patients (3,11,13–17). The interested reader is referred to the wealth of clinical literature regarding this treatment (3, pp. S1–S199; 8,11, 13–17, 28–30,36,38,46,49).

The clinical literature in this area remains complex and results of studies are conflicting. The strongest conclusion possible from a review of available data is the administration of methylprednisolone within 8 h of acute spinal cord injury may produce some improvement in neurologic recovery (17). Current guidelines suggest that the use of methylprednisolone in the treatment of acute spinal cord injury should be regarded as an option and undertaken only with the knowledge that the possibility of serious side effects may outweigh the possibility of neurologic improvement as a result of this treatment.

Hemodynamics

A patient with cervical or thoracic spinal cord injury suffers a loss of sympathetic outflow with preservation of vagal afferents and efferents. Sympathetic supply originates in the hypothalamus and travels through the periaqueductal gray matter, pons, and posterolateral medulla to synapse within the interomediolateral cell column of the thoracic spinal cord. A complete spinal cord injury in the cervical region effectively removes all preganglionic sympathetic fibers. In contrast, the parasympathetic system retains input and output through the vagus nerve. In the acute phase, patients with spinal cord injury have unbalanced parasympathetic action, because they lose sympathetic mediated reflexes. A patient with an acute injury usually is brought to the emergency room with moderate hypotension and bradycardia. In the absence of associated injuries, these patients are not hypotensive as a result of hypovolemia. The loss of sympathetic tone may cause mean arterial pressures in the range of 70–80 mm Hg to persist even after administration of 4–6 L of resuscitation fluid. Invasive cardiac monitoring in young quadriplegic patients has demonstrated that they have an acutely elevated cardiac index; loss of sympathetic tone results in low systemic vascular resistance (18). Loss of peripheral vasoconstriction produces hypoperfusion of the renal and splanchnic beds by shunting blood flow to skin and skeletal muscle beds. Heat dissipation increases, and shivering occurs. Oliguria is commonly found in patients with acute spinal cord injury and, like hypotension, may be refractory to continued fluid administration. When pulmonary artery occlusion pressures exceed 18, administration of further volume may result in pulmonary edema or congestive heart failure. A patient with marginal pulmonary reserve may then require intubation and ventilatory support.

Investigators have extrapolated from traumatic brain injury studies that hypotension may increase morbidity and mortality in spinal cord-injured patients. Correction of systemic hypotension is desirable following spinal cord injury, although no direct evidence exists that moderate hypotension following spinal cord injury results in a worsened neurologic outcome. Clearly, in the care of a general trauma patient, systemic hypotension has been associated with poor outcome and must be corrected. However, clinical judgment suggests that in a young spinal cord-injured patient without other significant systemic trauma, modest hypotension (mean arterial pressures between 70 and 80) does not likely correlate with diminished neurologic outcome. Generally, systolic blood pressure less than 90 mm Hg should be avoided if possible. Volume replacement is the primary treatment. In selected patients, treatment with vasopressors or inotropic agents may be indicated. The goal of this therapy should be to increase mean arterial pressure to a range of at least 85–90 mm Hg for at least 7 days following acute spinal cord injury. Such therapy appears to be safe and may ultimately improve spinal cord perfusion and possibly neurologic outcome (3).

In the past, many clinicians commonly used alpha-agonists, such as phenylephrine or norepinephrine, to treat hypotension after spinal cord injury. Although these agents are effective in producing vasoconstriction in the periphery, they may decrease renal blood flow. Use of these agents also may elevate systemic blood pressure sufficiently to produce a reflex bradycardia. Most young patients with spinal cord injury have some degree of hypotension, but it rarely becomes symptomatic or requires treatment with alpha-agents. In the young oliguric patient, a better drug choice might be dopamine in renal dose (less than 5 $\mu g/kg/min$). The clearest indications for treatment of moderate hypotension are changes in mentation, evidence of myocardial ischemia, or urine output less than 0.5 mL/kg/h.

Hemodynamic management is far more difficult when the quadriplegic patient is elderly or has preexisting coronary disease. In these patients, symptomatic bradyarrhythmias are common and may be severe enough to produce profound hypotension or asystole. The treatment of choice is an anticholinergic drug such as atropine. Dopamine also may be used for its beneficial chronotropic effect. If bradycardia persists or has profound consequences, transvenous pacing may be necessary. In elderly patients or in patients experiencing congestive heart failure, pulmonary artery catheterization may be necessary to direct hemodynamic management. Clinicians also should recognize that many patients with spinal cord injury arrive in the ICU following vigorous fluid resuscitation both in the field and during the initial stage of evaluation and resuscitation in the emergency room. A great imbalance in intake compared to output during the initial hospitalization generally leads to fluid mobilization several days after admission. The failure to recognize and manage this expected diuresis may compromise patients with marginal respiratory function.

Respiratory System

The phrenic nerve arises from the C3 through the C5 level of the cervical spinal cord and innervates the diaphragmatic muscles. The intercostal nerves and accessory muscles of respiration also take their origin from the low cervical and thoracic spinal cord. Therefore, a lesion above C4 disrupts the diaphragm, as well as the accessory muscles of respiration. A lower cervical spinal cord lesion leaves the diaphragmatic function intact, while taking accessory muscle function away. Patients without phrenic nerve function cannot survive without ventilatory support. Those patients who sustain an injury above the C4 level require intubation in the field or they will not survive to reach the hospital. The great majority of these patients remain ventilator dependent for the remainder of their lives. The larger group of patients, those with injuries at C5 or below, who have lost their accessory muscles of respiration and intercostal muscles but have preserved phrenic muscle supply, are the focus of this discussion.

The inability to fix the thoracic cage during inspiration and to forcibly diminish its capacity during expiration through the use of intercostal muscles greatly diminishes the efficiency of the respiratory effort. Patients with acute spinal cord injury have flaccid accessory muscles and a compliant thoracic cage. This combination produces a functional flail chest. With time, the intercostal muscles redevelop tone and, although they may not regain innervation, they will contribute to the efficiency of respiration by producing a more rigid chest wall. Acutely, respiratory function is poor. If respiratory indicators are measured, they commonly fall below those levels that would prompt elective intubation in other patients. Of primary importance, the patient's tidal volume is notably reduced, a consequence of the loss of the intercostal muscles. Atelectasis is the immediate result of this inefficient respiratory mechanism and is exacerbated by the lack of deep breathing or an effective cough. Initially, these atelectatic changes may not be audible on auscultation or visible on chest radiographs. The first indication of the process may be a subtle decrease in lung compliance. Decreasing compliance increases ventilatory dead space, further reduces the efficiency of respiration, and increases atelectasis in an accelerating downward spiral. Respiratory failure in these patients is usually heralded by tachypnea; blood gas measurements may appear relatively normal until late stages of respiratory decompensation. Then, hypocapnea is supplanted by hypoxia as the patient progresses to respiratory arrest. Providing supplementary oxygen as the patient becomes hypoxic may, paradoxically, hasten respiratory failure by producing "absorption atelectasis." This phenomenon occurs when the gas mixture within the alveoli is composed of a high proportion of oxygen. In high concentrations, oxygen, which is rapidly absorbed from the alveoli, displaces nitrogen, which is not absorbed. Alveolar volume becomes proportionately less, and atelectasis increases (19).

Patients with spinal cord injuries may suffer other injury-associated pulmonary problems such as aspiration, near drowning, pulmonary edema, pulmonary contusion, and hemopneumothorax. Any or all of these problems may progress to adult respiratory distress syndrome (ARDS). The morbidity and mortality of ARDS is extremely high. At best, the progression of a quadriplegic patient to ARDS greatly prolongs the period of mechanical ventilation and hospitalization. Diminished pulmonary reserve substantially delays rehabilitation and impedes neurologic recovery. Preventing ARDS is clearly a high priority in the initial care of these patients. Most interventions consist of maintaining the patient's functional residual capacity. Cough and deep breathing instruction ("quad coughing") may be used, although the patient's functional limitations may minimize the efficacy of these interventions in the acute setting. Intermittent use of a continuous positive airway pressure (CPAP) mask may be the single most effective intervention in nonintubated quadriplegic patients. Continuously oscillating beds also have been shown to decrease the incidence of pulmonary complications in this patient group by diminishing atelectasis, minimizing the ventilation/perfusion mismatches, and draining secretions. Pulmonary secretions should be managed using orotracheal, nasotracheal, or endotracheal suctioning. Control of airway humidity with warm mist nebulizers facilitates mobilization of secretions and should not be neglected. Bronchodilator therapy also may be helpful.

Spinal cord-injured patients should be observed closely for evidence of pulmonary infection. Daily chest radiographs and frequent chest auscultation should be routine for these patients. Appropriate antibiotics should be administered immediately, if clinical or radiographic evidence of an incipient pneumonia is observed. Antibiotic therapy should start while cultures are pending. The decision to continue these agents should be based on the nature of the organisms cultured, sputum characteristics, chest films, and the clinical picture. Colonization of the tracheobronchial tree is an inevitable occurrence in these patients and a distinction must be drawn between colonization and pneumonia. Prophylactic antibiotics are not indicated.

Finally, endotracheal intubation should not be delayed in those patients who show signs of respiratory failure. Timely intubation may prevent unnecessary pulmonary or neurologic complications. Elective intubation in these patients with difficult airways is always preferred to an unplanned emergency intubation. Patients who have been intubated and have failed extubation trials, or patients who have marginal weaning ability should be considered for tracheostomy. Tracheostomy may provide improved respiratory efficiency, allow a ventilator-dependent patient to become independent, provide improved airway access for pulmonary toilet, allow more effective use of intermittent CPAP masks to minimize atelectasis, and provide ready airway control in the event of respiratory failure.

Deep Venous Thrombosis and Pulmonary Emboli

Pulmonary embolism is one of the most feared complications of spinal cord injury. Although low dose heparin therapy has been demonstrated as an effective prophylactic measure for thromboembolism, more recent studies have shown that better treatment alternatives exist. These treatments include the use of low molecular weight heparin, adjusted dose heparin, or anticoagulation used concurrently with pneumatic compression devices or electrical stimulation. Interventions that are at least partially effective include hydration, antiplatelet therapy with aspirin, continuously oscillating beds, and vena cava filters (20–22). These measures should be used in the order listed. Sequential compression stockings must be used continuously, even while transporting the patient or in the operating room, to be effective. The use of a mechanical inferior vena cava filter as a prophylactic measure for deep venous thrombosis should be reserved for those patients who have suffered either thromboembolic events despite adequate anticoagulation or have contraindications to the use of pneumatic compression devices or anticoagulation therapy (3,5,9,11,28,29).

The risk of increased thromboembolic events appears to diminish within 3 months following acute spinal cord injury; therefore, prophylactic therapy for this indication should be limited to the initial 3 months following injury (23–25). In patients with preservation of lower extremity motor function, thromboembolic prophylaxis may be terminated sooner.

Diagnosis of deep venous thrombosis may be performed with the use of duplex Doppler ultrasound with reported sensitivities in the 90% range. Fibrinogen scanning and D-dimer measurements are more sensitive but considerably less specific than noninvasive blood flow studies for the diagnosis of deep venous thrombosis (26). No specific test for deep venous thrombosis is entirely sensitive, specific, and reliable. When noninvasive studies are negative but a high degree of clinical suspicion remains, venography also may be considered as a diagnostic alternative. Of note, many patients with pulmonary embolism have negative venograms of their lower extremities (27).

Autonomic Dysreflexia

Autonomic dysreflexia refers to an exaggerated sympathetic response to afferent stimulation that results in hypertension, reflex bradycardia, sweating, cutaneous flushing above the level of the neurologic injury, and headaches. This condition follows resolution of spinal shock in ~70% of patients with spinal cord injuries above the T6 level and is usually triggered by visceral stimulation (28). The classic cause of this response is bladder distention, although skin stimulation and bowel distention also produce the syndrome. This problem also has been described as a response to endoscopic and urodynamic studies.

Autonomic dysreflexia may cause hypertension severe enough to produce myocardial infarction and subarachnoid or intracerebral hemorrhage. Emergency temporary blood pressure control may be achieved by using nifedipine 10 mg sublingually or phentolamine 5 mg intravenously. The clinician also should immediately determine and eliminate the source of the dysreflexic response. Patients undergoing endoscopic or urodynamic procedures should be premedicated with 10 mg of oral nifedipine just before the procedure to diminish the risk of this phenomenon. Stool softeners also should be routinely used to prevent constipation, rectal distention, or fecal impaction that may precipitate this dysreflexia.

GASTROINTESTINAL MANAGEMENT

Gastric atony and ileus of both the small and large bowel are almost an invariable consequence of spinal cord injury. This complication usually takes several days to develop following injury, and continuous nasogastric drainage is necessary to minimize the possibility of aspiration of stomach contents. Gastric atony with dilation also may compromise respiration as a result of subdiaphragmatic pressure. Ileus may persist for days or weeks and delay enteral nutrition for some patients for extended periods. In patients who require prolonged nasogastric suction, or in those who have copious gastric secretions, metabolic alkalosis may develop.

Stress ulceration may occur in these patients unless preventive measures are taken (see Chapter 37). H2 blockers or antacids should be administered by protocol to keep the gastric pH greater than 4.5. In those patients who develop gastric ulceration (or any other intra-abdominal complication), the usual clinical symptoms and signs may be obscured by the patient's spinal cord injury. A high index of suspicion of intra-abdominal pathology should be maintained in the presence of persistent fevers, unexplained sepsis, unstable hemoglobin concentration, or recurrent autonomic dysreflexia.

Nutritional Support Following Acute Spinal Cord Injury

Multiple clinical studies have addressed nutritional support following spinal cord injury over the past several decades. The marked hypermetabolic response commonly observed following acute traumatic brain injury does not occur following isolated acute spinal cord injury. Resting energy expenditure (REE) in spinal cord-injured patients is diminished, likely as a result of the flaccidity of musculature distal to the spinal cord transection or injury. Derived estimates of REE for these patients are usually inaccurate; therefore, indirect calorimetry is the best means to measure the energy expenditure in either the acute or chronic settings. The marked loss of lean body mass secondary to muscular atrophy following acute spinal cord injury is inevitable in the absence of neurologic recovery and is marked by a prolonged negative nitrogen balance, as well as rapid weight loss. Therefore, nutritional support of the acutely spinal cord-injured patient should be directed at satisfying caloric and nitrogen needs rather than achieving nitrogen balance (3, pp. S81–S89; 4,14,19,21).

Poikilothermia

Patients with a cervical or high thoracic injury suffer a functional sympathectomy and temporarily lose the capacity for peripheral vasoconstriction below the involved level. Because of their decreased ability to preserve heat, they shiver as a means of producing heat. These patients are not able to regulate body temperature effectively, are thoroughly dependent on their environment (poikilothermic), and are easily chilled. They may become hypothermic in an ICU unless appropriate care is provided.

Skin Breakdown

Patients who are immobile as a consequence of their neurologic deficit, cervical traction, pain, or spinal instability are at high risk of developing decubitus ulcers. In the spinal cord-injured patient the usual sites of breakdown are the sacral region and posterior aspects of the heels. An established decubitus ulcer can be a source of significant morbidity, delayed rehabilitation, prolonged hospitalization, and, occasionally, death. Prevention of this complication is a high priority in the nursing care of these patients.

In the acute care setting, continuously oscillating beds are the best methods of prevention. These devices allow greater patient motion than even the most conscientiously applied program of logrolling and repositioning, provide safety while the patient is stabilized with traction, and add pulmonary benefits as well. Air cushion beds also may be used with stable patients to minimize skin breakdown. Special care should be taken to ensure that the patient's heels do not rest on the mattress for prolonged periods. Small soft rolls under the calves can elevate the heels and prevent ulceration.

URINARY TRACT MANAGEMENT

Following an acute spinal cord injury, the urinary bladder is flaccid, and normal detrussor reflexes are abolished. The initial goals in management are to prevent distention and to monitor urinary output. Initially these goals are best accomplished with a continuous indwelling urinary catheter. A secondary goal should be to remove this catheter as soon as possible and use intermittent bladder catheterization. With the intermittent technique, urinary bladder volumes should not be allowed to exceed 400–500 mL. Routine urinalysis should be monitored and cultures obtained if evidence of urinary tract infection exists. The use of prophylactic antibiotics is controversial. We do not recommend such prophylaxis (29,30).

In the chronic phase of spinal cord injury, the bladder becomes hypertonic and spastic. Autonomic reflexes are reestablished, and bladder distention may trigger autonomic dysreflexia. Meticulous bladder management is necessary to prevent autonomic dysreflexia and to minimize the incidence of infection, vesico-ureteral reflux, hydronephrosis, calculi, and renal dysfunction in this patient population.

PREPARATION FOR REHABILITATION

Physical therapy should be initiated as soon as the patient is medically stable. Early goals are passive range-of-motion exercises, avoiding contractures and establishing a relationship with the providers who may be responsible for later substantive rehabilitation. The psychological effects of this therapy are of great benefit to the patient.

Psychological Factors

For many patients, quadriplegia is feared more than death and is without equal in psychological stress for the affected family, individual patient, and friends. Acceptance of quadriplegia is achieved only after terrible suffering, a profound sense of loss, and grieving for that loss. Just as every individual expresses any profound emotion differently, just as every family communicates and copes in its special manner, so do individuals and families differ in their responses, adjustment, and management of quadriplegia. The profundity of the loss and the wide range of responses, more than anything, must be remembered by the clinician caring for the quadriplegic patient and family. Psychological support and effective communication frequently become the greatest challenge for health care providers after the initial days of hospitalization.

The initial frenetic pace of care after a spinal cord injury serves the dual psychological purpose of convincing the patient and family that something is being "done" and allows them to concentrate on procedures, tests, and technology. This phase of care initiates the model response to the injury. Denial may last hours to days, or longer. Patients may make tentative, limited exploration of the prognosis attendant to their injury but generally are reluctant to ask "the question" directly. Occasionally, "the question" becomes almost palpable, underling every turn of conversation with care providers. The physician should be sensitive to the patient's readiness and desire to turn to this most serious issue. Timing is important, and a discussion of prognosis should not be forced on the patient. Conscious quadriplegics are acutely aware of their level of dysfunction and many have already assumed the worst. The patient may wait to choose the setting, company, and health care provider before opening the discussion. This communication is critical to the patient and should be conducted as an unhurried private conversation, in which the patient is free to assume control. On the basis of the facts, the clinician should determine the essential information to impart and then make certain that it is communicated effectively to the patient and family. They will remember little beyond the physician's estimate of the chances of recovery; further information should be provided as the patient directs. The patient should be advised frankly of the uncertainty of any clinical estimation regarding outcome, particularly in the complex setting of an incomplete spinal cord injury. The patient should be assured of receiving complete, honest answers to questions. A degree of denial has its merits early in the patient's clinical course, and no attempt should be made to force the patient to accept "the truth." Physicians should not allow their own emotional concerns about quadriplegia to become an added burden to the patient. Be cautious not to remove all hope, even if the situation appears hopeless. Allow the patient to cling to whatever level of denial they choose early in the clinical course. The skilled clinician's task is to allow the patient to replace denial with determined rehabilitation and a realistic view of what is possible, rather than what is impossible. This transition is more easily accomplished when the patient has rehabilitation and functional goals to concentrate on, not when they are lying immobile in the ICU.

As the patient's denial begins to falter, frustration, anger, and then depression often supervene. During these phases, the patient requires continued emotional support, communication, and understanding. In some communities, rehabilitated quadriplegic patients may be helpful as a source of support and can be helpful after the patient has progressed at least through the phases of denial and anger. Acceptance usually occurs during the rehabilitation process, long after the patient has left the critical care setting.

Family communication is another matter of great importance. Family members almost always ask the physician to estimate the chances of neurologic recovery early in the hospital course and commonly wish to withhold the full import of the injury from the patient. Be as open, forthcoming, and complete as possible in communicating with the family. Communication can be a complicated process in a critical care unit, and family members tend to compare statements made by different staff members. They become disconcerted by discrepancies, real or imagined. Understanding may be facilitated early in the clinical course by clearly identifying the principal provider and arranging periodic meetings to convey clinical information and to resolve uncertainties or conflicts. The process of grieving for the patient, accepting disability, and identifying realistic options must be accelerated for family and friends, if they are to be available as a source of support.

Families cope in a variety of ways. Initially, they tend to focus on the details of the injury or on the patient's care. This effort also may be a form of denial and lasts until it is displaced by a second phase, anger and frustration. Usually, the anger is directed at a specific target, commonly the nursing or medical staff. The family may insist that an individual or individuals not participate in the care of the patient. The inciting event for this anger is usually trivial, but the emotion is real and may lead to strained relations, a hospital transfer, or litigation if not dealt with effectively. Rarely does this hostility extend to include the primary physician and, frequently, that physician is in the best position to diffuse the situation. When these situations arise, as they almost inevitably do with every quadriplegic patient, the solution is usually to narrow the circle of staff members providing information, not to enlarge it.

SUMMARY

- Optimal management of patients with spinal cord injury requires immediate stabilization of the unstable spinal segment; accurate, well-documented neurologic assessment; and timely recognition and management of medical complications that may limit the patient's recovery.
- Careful motor examination must include all major muscle groups in each of the four extremities.
- Sensory examination should include nociception, light touch, and proprioception.
- Deep tendon reflexes should be carefully recorded for later comparison.

Spinal Cord Injury

- Preservation of perirectal sensation, sphincter tone, and anal reflexes may help distinguish incomplete from complete spinal cord injuries.
- Three-view cervical spine series with CT supplementation is indicated in initial evaluation. Dynamic flexion/extension views may be indicated in awake, coherent patients.
- In acute spinal cord lesions, muscles innervated below the level of complete injury are flaccid and without reflexes.
- Incomplete spinal cord syndromes include Brown–Sequard syndrome, central cord syndrome, and anterior cord syndrome. Incomplete spinal cord injury may contain elements of all three.
- All patients with known or suspected spinal cord injury require stabilization. Philadelphia collar, Gardener–Wells tongs, halo vests, and thoracolumbosacral braces are commonly used. A cervical foam collar does not provide immobilization and should not be used.
- For the patient in a halo vest requiring intubation, fiberoptic intubation is preferred. Blind nasal intubation is a second choice. Cricothyroidotomy is indicated if intubation via these means fails.
- On admission to the ICU, determine how to remove the chest component of the halo vest to perform CPR, should CPR become necessary. A wrench fitting the halo should be taped to the halo for emergencies.
- Administration of methylprednisolone to the patient with spinal cord injuries is controversial.
- Loss of sympathetic tone may produce hypotension despite intravenous fluid replacement. In a young patient with spinal cord injury, modest hypotension usually is well tolerated. Generally, systolic blood pressures <90 mmHg should be treated.
- A spinal cord injury above C4 disrupts function of the diaphragm and of the accessory muscles of respiration.
- Patients with lesions at C5 or below, who have lost accessory and intercostal muscles, have a functional flail chest.
- Patients with compromised respiratory function require close monitoring and timely endotracheal intubation with mechanical ventilatory support for respiratory failure.
- Low molecular weight heparin, adjusted dose heparin, and pneumatic compression devices are effective prophylaxis for pulmonary embolism. Prophylaxis is recommended for 3 months.
- Autonomic dysreflexia may be precipitated by bladder distention, skin stimulation, or bowel distention.
- Gastric atony and ileus are common. pH prophylaxis is recommended.
- Metabolic support should satisfy caloric and nitrogen needs but not aim at achieving nitrogen balance.
- Environmental temperature is important to prevent loss of heat.
- Pressure ulcers in the sacral region and posterior heels are common. Oscillating beds and elevating the heels can reduce these complications.
- Initially, indwelling urinary catheters are recommended. When intermittent catheterization is feasible, urinary bladder volumes should not exceed 400–500 mL.
- For many patients, the psychological stress of quadriplegia is without equal and may be feared worse than death. Sensitivity to the needs of patients and families is of great importance.

REFERENCES

1. Brazis P, Biller J. The localization of lesions affecting the spinal cord. In: Brazis P, Masden J, Biller J, eds. Localization in Clinical Neurology. Little, Boston, MA: Brown and Co., 1985.
2. Riddoch G. Aids to the Examination of the Peripheral Nervous System. London: Bailliere-Tindall. 1986.
3. Hadley M, et al. Guidelines for the management of acute cervical spine and spinal cord injuries: radiographic spinal assessment in symptomatic trauma patients. Neurosurgery 2002; 50(3 suppl):S36.
4. Borock E, et al. A prospective analysis of a two-year experience using computed tomography as an adjunct for cervical spine clearance. J Trauma 1991; 31:1001.
5. Brohi K, Wilson-Macdonald J. Evaluation of unstable cervical spine injury: a six year experience. J Trauma 2000; 49:76.
6. Freemyer B, et al. Comparison of five-view and three-view cervical spine series in the evaluation of patients with cervical trauma. Ann Emerg Med 1989; 18:818.
7. Tan E, et al. Is computed tomography of nonvisualized C7-T1 cost effective? J Spinal Disord 1999; 12:472.
8. Tehranzadeh J, Bonk R, Ansari A. Efficacy of limited CT for nonvisualized lower cervical spine in patients with blunt trauma. Skeletal Radiol 1994; 23:349.
9. Lewis L, et al. Flexion-extension views in the evaluation of cervical spine injuries. Ann Emerg Med 1991; 20:117.
10. Benzel E, et al. Magnetic resonance imaging for the evaluation of patients with occult spine injury. J Neurosurg 1996; 85:824.
11. D'Alise M, Benzel E, Hart B. Magnetic resonance imaging of the cervical spine in the comatose or obtunded trauma patient. J Neurosurg 1999; 91(suppl 1):54.
12. Emery S, et al. Magnetic resonance imaging of posttraumatic spinal ligament injury. J Spinal Disord 1989; 2:229.
13. Hall A, et al. Magnetic resonance imaging in cervical spine trauma. J Trauma 1993; 34:21.
14. Bracken M, et al. Efficacy of methylprednisolone in acute spinal cord injury. J Am Med Assoc 1984; 251:45.
15. Bracken M, et al. Methyprednisolone and neurological function 1 year after spinal cord injury: results of the National Acute Spinal Cord Injury Study (NASCIS-2). J Neurosurg 1985; 63:704.
16. Bracken M, et al. Methylprednisolone or naloxone treatment after spinal cord injury: 1 year follow-up data—results of the second national acute spinal cord injury study. J Neurosurg 1992; 76:23.
17. Bracken M, et al. A randomized, controlled trial of methylprednisolone or naloxone in the treatment of acute spinal-cord injury. Results of the Second National Spinal Cord Injury Study. N Engl J Med 1990; 322:1405–1411.
18. Mackenzie C, et al. Assessment of cardiac and respiratory function during surgery on patients with acute quadriplegia. J Neurosurg 1985; 62:843–849.
19. Rosner M. Medical management of spinal cord injury. In: Pitts LH, Wagner FC, eds. Craniospinal Trauma. New York: Thieme Medical Publishers, 1990.
20. Casa E, et al. Prophylaxis of venous thrombosis and pulmonary embolism in patients with acute traumatic spinal cord lesions. Paraplegia 1976; 14:178.
21. Becker D, et al. Prevention of deep venous thrombosis in acute spinal cord injury: use of rotating table. In: Green BA, Summer WR, eds. Continuous Oscillation Therapy: Research and Practical Applications. Miami: University of Miami Press, 1986.
22. Brackett T, Cordon N. Comparison of the wedge turning frame and kinetic treatment table in the acute care of spinal cord injury patients. Surg Neurol 1984; 22:53.
23. Naso F. Pulmonary embolism in acute spinal cord injury. Arch Phys Med Rehabil 1972; 55:275.

24. Lamb G, et al. Is chronic spinal cord injury associated with increased risk of venous thromboembolism? J Am Paraplegia Soc 1993; 16:153.
25. Perkash A, Prakash V, Perkash I. Experience with the management of thromboembolism in patients with spinal cord injury: Part I—Incidence, diagnosis and the role of some risk factors. Paraplegia 1978; 16(322).
26. Roussi J, et al. Contribution of D-dimer determination in the exclusion of deep venous thrombosis in spinal cord injury patients. Spinal Cord 1999; 37:548.
27. Geerts W, et al. A prospective study of venous thromboembolism after major trauma. N Engl J Med 1994; 331:1601.
28. Kurnick N. Autonomic dysreflexia and its control in patients with spinal cord lesions. Ann Intern Med 1956; 44:678.
29. Stover S, Lloyd L, Waites K, et al. Urinary tract infection in spinal cord injury. Arch Phys Med Rehabil 1989; 70:47.
30. Stickler D, Chawla J. An appraisal of antibiotic policies for urinary tract infection in patients with spinal cord injuries undergoing long-term intermittent catheterization. Paraplegia 1988; 26:215.

19
Stroke: Diagnosis and Management

Sabrina Walski-Easton and Edward Rustamzadeh
University of Minnesota, Minneapolis, Minnesota, USA

INTRODUCTION

Stroke ranks as the third leading cause of death in most industrialized nations and is the leading cause of long-term disability. The American Heart Association estimated the cost of stoke to be approximately 50 billion dollars in 2001 (1). Advances in the diagnosis of stroke, treatment options, intensive care management, and rehabilitation services have improved the prognosis for many patients with cerebrovascular accidents (2,3).

EPIDEMIOLOGY

The annual incidence of stroke is 200 per 100,000 (4) and after the age of 45, it is estimated that one out of four men and one out of five women will suffer a stroke. The National Institute of Neurological Disorders applies the term *stroke* to a group of disorders encompassing cerebral infarction, intracerebral hemorrhage, or subarachnoid hemorrhage resulting in neurological deficit (5). Roughly 70% of strokes are due to cerebral ischemia, another 27% are due to cerebral hemorrhage, and 3% are of undetermined cause (6). Ischemic strokes are a result of atherothromboembolism (50%), intracranial small vessel disease (25%), cardiac embolism (20%), and other etiologies (5%) (7). Overall, the 30-day mortality rate of ischemic stroke is significant (20–30%) (8,9). Deaths occurring within the first week of the stroke are often directly related to cerebral insult; whereas, late deaths are usually associated with complications such as deep venous thrombosis, pneumonia, and cardiac arrhythmias (9–12).

After 1 year, 20% of people with a first-time stroke will be completely dependent on others for care, and only 50% will be self-sufficient (13). The risk of a subsequent stroke within the first year is 10–16% and decreases to ∼5% per year thereafter (14). The prevalence of stroke, after adjusting for age, sex, and race, increased from 1.4% during the period of 1971–1975 to 1.9% during the period of 1988–1994 (15). The number of stroke-related deaths over the same period of time declined from 106/100,000 to 61/100,000 (16).

The risk factors associated with stroke can be divided into two groups: unmodifiable and modifiable.

Unmodifiable Risk Factors

In the first group are those factors that are not modifiable. These factors include age, gender, ethnicity, family history, and genetic disorders. Stroke is an age-dependent event. During the third and fourth decades, the incidence of stroke is 3/100,000; however, by the eighth to ninth decades, the incidence rises to 3/100 (8). For every successive 10 years after the age of 55, the risk of stroke doubles in both men and women (17). In general, men have a 30% higher risk of stroke than women, but because the life expectancy of women is longer, this risk reverses in the elderly (18). African American men have 104.1% higher stroke mortality rate than Caucasians (19). Furthermore, African Americans have a disproportionately younger age of onset for stroke. Hispanics have a similar risk of stroke as Caucasians, and the incidence of stroke in Asians lies between that of African Americans and Caucasians (20). The Framingham study revealed an increased risk of stroke in offspring with either a paternal or maternal history of stroke (21).

Homocystinuria, Fabry's disease, fibromuscular dysplasia, sickle cell disease, factor V Leiden mutation, anticardiolipin antibodies, and deficiencies in antithrombin III, factor XII, protein C and S, plasminogen, and plasminogen activator are all associated with an increased risk of stroke (22).

Modifiable Risk Factors

The second group comprises modifiable risk factors, which include hypertension, smoking, diabetes, atrial fibrillation, hyperlipidemia, and oral contraceptive use, particularly when combined with smoking.

Hypertension

Numerous studies have indicated that hypertension is a strong risk factor for all subtypes of stroke in both men and women and in all age groups (23). Both diastolic and systolic blood pressure have been shown to affect the incidence of stroke (23). A meta-analysis of prospective, randomized, and controlled trials revealed a 42% reduction in stroke risk, if diastolic blood pressure were lowered by 5–6 mm Hg (24). The Systolic Hypertension in the Elderly Program and the Multiple Risk Factor Intervention Trial showed that lowering systolic blood pressure below 140 mm Hg could reduce the risk of stroke by 36–40% (25).

Smoking

Smoking is another modifiable risk. Smoking is believed to induce atherogenesis and cause both ischemic and hemorrhagic stroke (26,27). A meta-analysis of 32 studies concerning the association of smoking and stroke revealed a relative risk factor of 1.5 for smokers (28). In white males 16,000 strokes per year are due to cigarette smoking (29). Furthermore, a body mass index (BMI) of ≥ 24 kg/m^2 combined with smoking is associated with 60% of strokes in men younger than 65 years of age (30).

Diabetes

Diabetes has been shown to have a relative risk ranging from 1.8 to 3.0 for ischemic stroke (17).

Cardiac Risk Factors

Atrial fibrillation alone has an annual risk for stroke of <3%. When combined with mitral stenosis, the risk of stroke increases 17-fold (31). The association of hyperlipidemia and stroke is not as well documented as the relation of stroke to coronary artery disease. One randomized, double-blinded study, investigating the effects of pravastatin (an HMG-CoA reductase inhibitor) in patients with previous myocardial infarctions and cholesterol levels ≤240 mg/dL, demonstrated a 31% reduction in the incidence of stroke in the experimental group when compared with the placebo group (32). The LIPID study found a 19% reduction in stroke incidence in patients receiving pravastatin with coronary artery disease and cholesterol serum concentrations between 155 and 271 mg/dL when compared with patients in the control group (33). The beneficial effects of statins are thought to include atherosclerotic plaque stabilization, improvement in endothelial plaque function, and beneficial effects on clotting, in addition to lowering serum cholesterol concentrations (34,35). Although the aforementioned data demonstrate a correlation between high serum cholesterol concentrations and ischemic stroke, low serum cholesterol concentration is related to a higher incidence of hemorrhagic type stroke (36).

Oral Contraceptives

The use of oral contraceptives (especially if the daily dosage is >50 μg of estrogen) has an increased risk of all stroke types with an odds ratio of 1.5. The odds ratio for a fatal event is 2.3 (37). Smoking increases this risk. Former users of oral contraceptives have an increased risk for stroke only if they continue smoking.

PATHOPHYSIOLOGY

Thrombosis, embolism, hemorrhage, and hypoperfusion are recognized causes of stroke. Table 1 lists common etiologies and rates from the National Institute of Neurological

Table 1 NINCDS Data Bank

NINCDS Data Bank	$N = 1805$
Cerebral ischemia	70%
Large artery stenosis	6%
Tandem arterial lesions	4%
Lacunae	19%
Cardioembolism	14%
Infarct of undetermined cause	27%
Cerebral hemorrhage	27%
Parenchymatous	13.5%
Subarachnoid	13.5%
Other	3%

Note: NINCDS, National Institute of Neurological and Communicative Disorders and Stroke.
Source: From Ref. (6).

Table 2 Sources of Cerebral Ischemia

Atherosclerosis	Complications of arteriography
Thrombus	Vasculitis
Stenosis	Infectious
Embolus, artery-to-artery	Pyogenic
Cardiogenic	Fungal
Myocardial infarction	Parasitic
Cardiac aneurysm	Viral
Arrhythmia	Inflammatory
Cardiomyopathy	Lupus erythematosus
Septal/foraminal defects	Polyarteritis nodosa
Valvular cardiac disease	Rheumatoid arthritis
Congenital	Giant cell arteritis
Rheumatic	Takayasu's disease
Prosthetic	Granulomatous angiitis
Bacterial endocarditis	Miscellaneous
Marantic endocarditis	Elevated intracranial pressure
Cardiac diagnostic procedures or surgery	Trauma
Atrial myxoma	Mass lesion
Hematological disorders	Large vessel disorders
Polycythemia	Aortic, vertebral artery, carotid
Thrombocytosis	
Sickle cell disease	Artery dissection
Thrombotic thrombocytopenic purpura	Traumatic
Disseminated intravascular coagulation	Atraumatic
Coagulation factor abnormalities	Direct vessel compromise
Other	Steal syndromes
Shock	Miscellaneous vasculopathy
Volume loss	Moyamoya
Sepsis	Fibromuscular dysplasia
Cardiogenic	Lipohyalinosis
Vasospasm	Radiation-induced
Migraine	Drug-related
Subarachnoid hemorrhage	Inherited disorders
	Other

Source: Adapted from Kiefer SP, Selman WR, Ratcheson RA. Clinical syndromes in cerebral ischemia. In: Tindall GT, Barrow DL, Cooper PR, eds. The Practice of Neurosurgery. Baltimore, MD: Williams & Wilkins, 1995.

and Communicative Disorders and Stroke. Table 2 lists common sources of cerebral ischemia.

Physiology of Ischemia

Although the brain comprises only 2% of the body's weight (1500 g), it consumes 20% of the body's oxygen and receives 17% of the cardiac output. Anaerobic glycolysis does not occur in neurons, and they have small glycogen and oxygen reserves. Consequently, neurons require a continuous supply of oxygen and glucose. The cerebral metabolic rate of oxygen consumption (CMrO$_2$) is 3.0–3.8 mL/100 g per min. This rate can increase up to 5% with focal cortical activity and can be decreased by drugs that reduce neuronal activity, such as pentobarbital. Oxygen availability is dependent on the cerebral blood flow (CBF), hemoglobin concentration, and arterial oxygen saturation, as shown in the relation:

$$O_2 \text{ availability} = \text{CBF} \times \text{arterial oxygen saturation} \times [\text{Hgb}] \times 1.39 \qquad (1)$$

To improve oxygen delivery to ischemic brain tissue, CBF may be augmented by increasing arterial blood pressure, perfusing collateral circulation, or by reperfusing ischemic areas. Maintenance of arterial oxygen saturations above 95% and hemoglobin concentrations above 10 g/dL increases oxygen availability to the ischemic penumbra.

Cerebral Blood Flow

Average normal CBF is 45–65 mL/100 g tissue/min. CBF in white matter is 20–30 mL/100 g/min, while CBF in gray matter is 75–80 mL/100 g/min. Loss of consciousness occurs when blood flow to the brain falls to <30 mL/100 g/min or ceases for 5–10 s. At a CBF of <25 mL/100 g/min, the EEG signals flatten, and neuronal dysfunction occurs. At levels <8–10 mL/100 g/min, ionic pump failure ensues and cell death occurs. The ischemic penumbra is observed with blood flow in the range of 10–25 mL/100 g/min. At this flow rate, neurons remain viable but are nonfunctional. These cells can be salvaged with return of blood flow. Depending on local conditions, such as glucose concentrations, temperature, and metabolic rate, neurons can survive indefinitely with a blood flow of ~18 mL/100 g/min (38).

Cerebral Autoregulation

To maintain constant CBF, the brain relies upon cerebral autoregulation. Autoregulation maintains CBF over a range of arterial pressures (usually 50–150 mm Hg) by varying cerebral pressure and vascular resistance.

CBF is defined by the equation:

$$\text{CBF} = \frac{\text{CPP}}{\text{CVR}} \qquad (2)$$

where CPP is cerebral perfusion pressure and CVR is cerebral vascular resistance.

$$\text{CPP} = \text{MAP} - \text{ICP} \qquad (3)$$

where MAP is mean arterial pressure and ICP is intracranial pressure.

CPP is affected by venous resistance. It is reduced in conditions such as cavernous sinus thrombosis in which venous resistance is elevated. Elevation of the head of the bed to 30 degrees can overcome the effects of increased venous resistance. CVR is linearly related to PCO_2 in the range of 20–80 mm Hg (38,39). CPP varies directly with MAP.

Autoregulation is altered in patients with untreated hypertension, such that the lower blood pressure limit of autoregulation is higher than normal (Fig. 1) (38,40). In areas of cerebral infarction and in the penumbral area, higher perfusion pressures are needed to

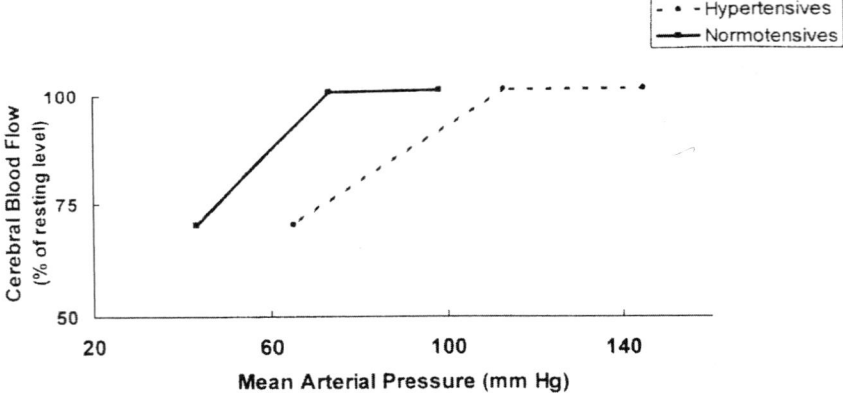

Figure 1 Cerebral autoregulation of blood flow in normotensive subjects and in hypertensive patients. CBF is maintained at a constant level between MAP 70 and 90 mm Hg and in hypertensive patients between 110 and 150 mm Hg. Neurologic symptoms occur at higher MAP in hypertensive patients.

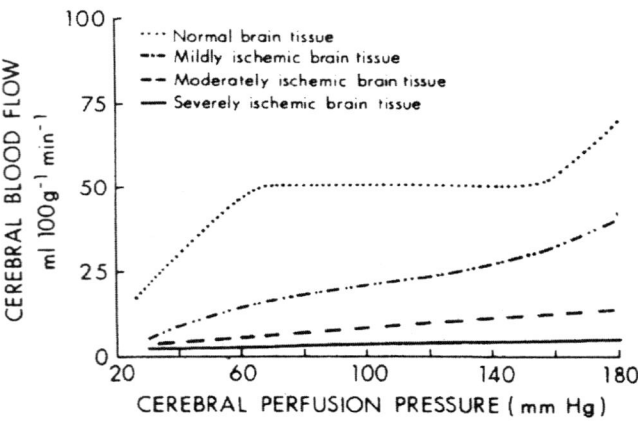

Figure 2 Cerebral autoregulation is impaired during focal ischemia and infarction. [From Ref. (16).]

maintain adequate blood flow (Fig. 2) (41). Therefore, systemic hypotension should be avoided in stroke patients to avoid increased neuronal damage.

DIAGNOSIS

Clinical Diagnosis

The clinical diagnosis of stroke depends on the time course of events and the resulting neurological deficits. Unlike brain tumors or intracranial infections, the onset of symptoms usually occurs rapidly, over several minutes to an hour, and symptoms may fluctuate

Stroke Diagnosis and Management

in severity. To diagnose a stroke correctly, the treating physician must be familiar with the various presentations of stroke that result from the different underlying pathophysiologies, including lacunar infarcts, major vessel thrombosis, posterior fossa infarcts, and watershed infarcts.

Lacunar Infarction

Lacunar infarcts occur deep in brain tissue areas that are perfused by perforating arteries that arise at right angles from major vessels. The affected area is <1.5 cm by definition (3,42). These infarcts occur mainly in hypertensive and diabetic patients and are primarily the result of lipohyalin degeneration of perforating arteries or from embolic microvascular occlusion (43,44). The commonly affected regions are the pons, internal capsule, thalamus, caudate, and the cerebral white matter. Clinically, lacunar infarcts produce a syndrome consisting of pure motor deficit, pure sensory deficit, dysarthria-clumsy hand, or ataxic-hemiparesis (Table 3) (42). As lacunar infarcts involve deeper regions of the brain, symptoms of aphasia, apraxia, and visual deficits should prompt a search for a different diagnosis.

Major Vessel Thrombosis

Unlike lacunar infarcts, major vessel occlusion involving the internal carotid, middle cerebral, anterior cerebral, or vertebrobasilar arteries often result in large territories of ischemia. Depending on location, supratentorial strokes result in contralateral weakness, facial palsy, contralateral neglect, or ipsilateral eye deviation. Expressive aphasia, in which the patient can comprehend verbal and written language but is unable to articulate the information, occurs with dominant frontal lobe strokes. Lesions involving the dominant superior temporal lobe result in receptive aphasia. The patient speaks fluently but nonsensically. Dominant parietal lobe strokes result in Gerstman's syndrome, in which the patient is unable to identify right vs. left, name individual fingers, and has difficulty calculating and writing. Nondominant parietal insults result in dressing apraxia, difficulty copying geometrical patterns, and loss of geographical memory. Patients with large ischemic cortical infarcts are at risk of developing malignant cerebral edema.

Table 3 Lacunar Syndromes

Syndrome	Lesion site	Clinical manifestation
Pure motor	Posterior limb of internal capsule, lower basis of pons, midportion of cerebral peduncle	Weakness of the face, arm, and leg
Pure sensory	Posterior ventral thalamus	Complete or partial sensory loss involving the face, arm, and leg
Dysarthria-clumsy hand	Basis pontis, genu of the internal capsule	Dysarthria, dysphagia, facial weakness, clumsiness of the hand
Ataxic-hemiparesis	Basis pontis, superior limb of the internal capsule	Hemiplegia, cerebellar dysmetria, and toppling

Posterior Fossa Infarctions

Infratentorial lesions may involve the corticospinal tracts and produce ipsilateral weakness if the lesion is below the decussation of the corticospinal tracts, or contralateral weakness if the lesion is above the decussation. Cerebellar infarctions are associated with vertigo, nausea, vomiting, dysmetria, intention tremor, and tendency to fall ipsilateral to the lesion. In proximity to the brainstem, these infarctions can lead to rapid deterioration and death if swelling, hemorrhagic conversion, or obstructive hydrocephalus occur. Cerebellar infarcts and hematomas are considered a neurosurgical emergency, and patients should be monitored closely in the intensive care unit for signs of deterioration. Brainstem infarctions result in cranial nerve palsies and can lead to deep coma if the reticular activating system is affected. Table 4 contains typical syndromes associated with brainstem strokes. Vertebrobasilar occlusion commonly occurs in stepwise fashion (45), and up to 50% of patients are comatose from ischemia of the reticular activating system (46,47).

Watershed Infarcts

Watershed infarcts result from hypoperfusion of anatomically vulnerable border zone regions, including medial frontal lobes, inferior lateral temporal lobes, posterior occipital lobes, basal ganglia, and cerebellum. These areas receive blood supply from end arteries of either the anterior cerebral artery and middle cerebral artery, or between the middle cerebral artery and the posterior cerebral artery. Watershed infarcts involving the basal ganglia can produce hemibalismus and Parkinson-like symptoms with myoclonus. Hippocampal infarcts can result in memory loss. Bilateral border zone infarcts, involving the territory of the middle cerebral artery and the anterior cerebral artery, can result in bilateral upper extremity weakness. The proximal muscles of shoulder and limb are affected although hand function is preserved. These findings are collectively known as the "man-in-the-barrel" syndrome. Bilateral border zone infarction of the posterior cerebral artery and the middle cerebral artery can result in cortical blindness of visual anosognosia (Anton syndrome).

Table 4 Brainstem Syndromes

Syndrome	Lesion site	Clinical manifestations
Weber	Midbrain	Ipsilateral cranial nerve 3 palsy, contralateral hemiplegia
Benedickt	Midbrain	Ipsilateral cranial nerve 3 palsy, contralateral tremor
Claude	Midbrain	Ipsilateral cranial nerve 3 palsy, contralateral ataxia
Millard–Gubler	Pons	Ipsilateral cranial nerves 6 and 7 palsy, contralateral hemiplegia
Foville	Pons	Ipsilateral facial palsy, contralateral hemiplegia
Locked-in	Pons	Preservation of consciousness with ocular communications, quadriplegia, and mutism
Wallenberg	Medulla	Ipsilateral facial sensory loss, ipsilateral Horner's, contralateral loss of temperature and pain

Radiological/Laboratory Diagnosis

Once the clinical diagnosis of stroke is suspected, prompt evaluation and treatment may improve outcome. Diagnoses mimicking stroke, such as hypoglycemia, migraine, or Todd's paralysis following seizures, should be excluded, and a CT scan should be obtained immediately to identify hemorrhage or early radiological signs of infarction. Early signs of infarct found with conventional CT include a dense middle cerebral artery sign (48), an obscure lentiform nucleus, loss of the insular ribbon, loss of gray and white differentiation, and gyriform contrast enhancement (49). If the patient's hemoglobin is ≤8 gm/dL, hematoma may be indistinguishable from normal brain (50). With diffusion-weighted imaging, magnetic resonance studies can verify ischemic areas of the brain where CT scanning may be inadequate. Diffusion-weighted imaging is useful up to 14 days following the onset of ischemia. Magnetic resonance angiography can detect flow voids in vessels occluded with thrombus. Figure 3 shows a diagnostic algorithm for stroke evaluation. Details of the NIH Stroke Scale may be found in the appendix to this chapter.

In addition to routine laboratory examination, and especially in patients with intracerebral hemorrhage, coagulation studies, including INR, PTT, PT, and fibrinogen

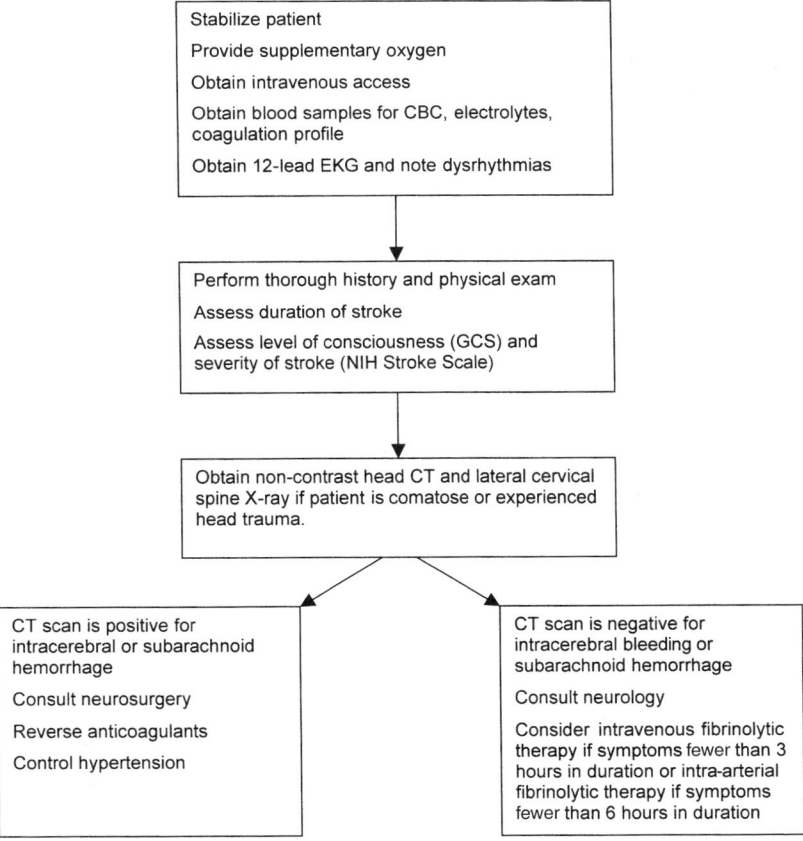

Figure 3 Approach to patient with suspected stroke.

levels, should be obtained. As acute stroke often precipitates a hypercoaguable state, in-depth laboratory testing for hypercoagulopathy should be delayed for several weeks.

MEDICAL THERAPY

A treatment plan must consider the patient's age, co-morbid conditions, advance directives, and prognostic factors.

Intensive Care Therapy

Intensive care units that have developed specialized stroke and nursing care protocols have been shown to reduce mortality rates and allow more patients to return to independent living after a stroke (2,3,51). In the first 24 h after an acute stroke, continuous monitoring of physiologic variables should be performed in an intensive care or stroke unit. Neurological examination should be performed every 1–2 h to detect progression of deficits or deterioration that require medical or surgical intervention. Sedatives and pain medications should be minimized to facilitate examination.

Cardiac

Patients with acute stroke may have concomitant cardiac disease and should be monitored for myocardial infarction, dysrhythmia, and congestive failure. Continuous EKG monitoring can be used to identify cardiac dysrhythmias, infarctions, or ischemia that require treatment. Monitoring is helpful in identifying dysrhythmias associated with embolic events, such as intermittent atrial fibrillation. Serial troponin determinations are useful in acute stroke to identify concomitant myocardial infarction.

Pulmonary

Respiratory status must be monitored carefully in stroke patients. These patients may have decreased level of consciousness and oropharyngeal dysfunction that increase the risk of hypoventilation, aspiration, and pneumonia. Prompt implementation of supplemental oxygen, suctioning of secretions, and endotracheal intubation should be performed when necessary. Treatment goals are a $PO_2 > 80$ mm Hg (95% saturation) and PCO_2 between 35 and 45 mm Hg. If endotracheal intubation is necessary, etomidate or thiopental will help prevent an increase in ICP. Administration of lidocaine will suppress coughing. Hypotension commonly occurs after endotracheal intubation and institution of positive pressure ventilation and may be minimized by intravenous volume replacement.

Fever

The risk of poor outcome after stroke has been shown to double for each 1°C increase in body temperature (39). Therefore, if fever is present, a complete evaluation for its source is mandatory.

Especially for patients with indwelling urinary catheters, a common fever source is infection of the urinary tract. Pulmonary sources of fever may be due to hypoventilation, poor clearing of secretions, or aspiration. Empiric antibiotic therapy should be initiated when fever is detected. If a pathogen is identified, antibiotic therapy may then be tailored to its sensitivities.

Returning body temperature to normal can be achieved with antipyretic medications, cooling mats, or wet towels. Although temperature reduction decreases neuronal metabolic rates by ~5% per degree, currently no evidence supports hypothermic therapy for acute stroke.

Electrolytes/Laboratory Examination

Frequent laboratory examinations are indicated to maintain normal serum glucose and electrolyte concentrations. Following stroke, glucose serum concentrations may be acutely elevated in patients without diabetes. Hyperglycemia may contribute to neuronal cell death and cerebral edema (38). Hyponatremia may potentiate cerebral edema and seizures. Patients receiving anticoagulation or thrombolytic therapy are at risk for systemic as well as intracranial bleeding complications, which require prompt recognition and treatment. Hemoglobin concentrations should be maintained at 10 g/dL to provide adequate oxygen carrying capacity to brain tissue.

Nutrition/Speech

Formal swallowing evaluations should be obtained for patients with hemispheric strokes, bulbar or pseudobulbar dysfunction, or language deficits. Oropharyngeal dysfunction often mandates restricted oral intake in stroke patients. Placement of nasojejuenal feeding tubes beyond the pylorus, to reduce the risk of aspiration, may be necessary for temporary enteral feedings, until oral feedings can be resumed.

Rehabilitation

Early mobilization and rehabilitation can help decrease the rate of complications from deep vein thrombosis, pulmonary embolism, decubitus ulcers, and contractures. Early mobilization is associated with improved recovery. To reduce the possibility of pulmonary embolism in high risk patients, we obtain duplex ultrasound examinations of the lower extremities in patients confined to bed rest for ≥3 days, or for those patients with limb paralysis, before they are mobilized or begin physical therapy.

Hemodynamic Optimization

Augmentation of blood flow may improve collateral circulation to ischemic areas or areas with tenuous blood flow. Intravenous volume replacement increases cardiac output and MAP. Maintaining the head level or with slight elevation (30 degrees) and midline improves CBF and facilitates venous drainage. To prevent obstruction of venous outflow, circumferential endotracheal tube dressings should be avoided. Maintenance of hemoglobin concentrations at 10 g/dL improves oxygen carrying capacity and rheologic properties of blood.

Blood Pressure

Hypertension pressure occurs in >80% of patients following acute CVA and usually returns to prestroke levels within 1 week. Compared with patients without hypertension, patients with pre-existing hypertension experience higher blood pressure elevations (52). In addition, autoregulation is altered in patients with untreated hypertension. The lower limit of regulation is higher than that found in nonhypertensive patients.

Significant elevations in blood pressure increase the risk of hemorrhage, recurrent hemorrhage, elevated ICP, and cerebral edema. However, adequate perfusion to vulnerable tissues may require an elevation in MAP. On the basis of the observation that the lower limit of autoregulation is 25% of the resting MAP in both normal and uncomplicated hypertensive patients, past treatment of stroke included the idea that arterial blood pressure can be safely lowered by 25%. Recently, randomized clinical trials indicate that antihypertensive treatment during acute stroke not only provides no benefit but also may worsen clinical outcome (52). This finding may be a consequence of altered cerebral autoregulation in the region of the stroke and the area of penumbra supplied by collateral circulation. These areas may require higher arterial pressure to allow adequate perfusion of viable brain tissue around the infarct.

No definitive study has identified the optimum blood pressure target in the treatment of acute stroke. A recent analysis of data from the International Stroke Trial demonstrated that both low blood pressure and high blood pressure were adversely associated with death or dependency (53). Early death increased by 17.9% for every 10 mm Hg the systolic blood pressure was below 150 mm Hg and by 3.8% for every 10 mm Hg the systolic rose above 150 mm Hg. The risk of recurrent stroke within 14 days was increased by 4.2% per 10 mm Hg rise in systolic blood pressure; whereas, cardiac deaths and stroke severity were associated with low systolic blood pressure. Patients with systolic blood pressures >200 mm Hg had a >50% increased risk of recurrence when compared with a patient with a systolic blood pressure of 130 mm Hg. No relationship was found between initial systolic blood pressure and intracranial hemorrhage. This study is limited in that only initial systolic blood pressure was analyzed. Optimum blood pressure treatments were not defined.

Because of the risk of worsening neurologic deficits with low blood pressure and the relatively low risk of mild or moderate hypertension in ischemic stroke, patients with acute stroke usually are not treated with antihypertensive medications unless systolic blood pressures ≥200 mm Hg or diastolic blood pressues >110 mm Hg are sustained (38,51). When treatment is indicated, short-acting antihypertensives should be used to provide slow reduction of blood pressure, avoid hypotension, and allow rapid reversal, if necessary.

For patients with intracerebral hemorrhage, a balance must be obtained between maintaining adequate cerebral perfusion and lowering blood pressure to reduce the risk of rebleeding. A goal of blood pressure reduction to prehemorrhage levels or by 20% appears to be reasonable, as autoregulation is maintained but shifted to the right with intracerebral hemorrhage. Autoregulation in this class of patients is similar to that of hypertensive patients (38).

Vasospasm-related cerebral ischemia has been successfully treated with hypertensive therapy. This finding raises the question of whether hypertensive therapy might also prove useful in ischemic stroke. A retrospective study reviewed patients with acute stroke and cerebral ischemia from large artery stenosis, sepsis, or neurological deterioration from hypotension who were treated with phenylephrine to increase blood pressure. Neurological improvement was demonstrated in one-third of patients, and no adverse effects were observed (54). For a select group of patients with vascular stenosis or large vessel occlusion, induced hypertension may be useful. For patients with sepsis, avoidance of hypotension may reduce further neurological deterioration. Hypotension during intubation, procedures, or from sedatives should be avoided.

Once the acute stroke has resolved, treatment of even mild hypertension can reduce the risk of recurrent stroke. Angiotensin converting enzyme (ACE) inhibitors, with or without diuretics, have been shown to reduce the risk of first stroke, recurrent stroke, and major vascular events in the HOPE and Progress trials (55). The benefits of

ACE inhibitor therapy may extend beyond lowering the blood pressure: both normotensive and hypertensive patients benefit from ACE inhibitor therapy. ACE inhibitor therapy should be instituted for all stroke patients prior to discharge, unless contraindications exist.

Neuroprotection

Agents designed to minimize infarct size and improve survival of cells in ischemic or hypoperfused areas have been the subject of much interest. Currently, no medications or treatment strategies have been shown to improve outcome (54).

Systemic Thrombolytic Therapy

Intravenous recombinant tissue plasminogen activator (IV rtPA) given within 3 h of onset of ischemic stroke in selected patients has been shown in the NINDS study to improve outcomes by 31% (absolute benefit, 11–15%) at 3 months (56,57). No statistically significant difference in mortality was demonstrated between rtPA and control groups, but the risk of symptomatic intracerebral hemorrhage increased from 0.6% in controls to 6% in treated patients. The risk-benefit ratio decreases significantly after a 3 h time interval (58–60). rtPA appears to be effective for all stroke subtypes, including strokes from small vessel disease, atherosclerosis, and embolic disease (61). Fibrinolytic therapy is recommended for patients with no evidence of intracerebral or subarachnoid hemorrhage on CT scan, if fibrinolytic therapy can be initiated within 3 h of the onset of symptoms and if no contraindications to fibrinolytic therapy are present (Table 5).

Table 5 Patient Eligibility Criteria for Systemic rtPA

Age ≥ 18 years

Diagnosis of ischemic stroke causing a potentially disabling neurological deficit. Reliable onset of symptoms <3 h prior to IV administration of rtPA. Initial CT brain imaging showing no signs of recent ischemia or early infarct signs no larger than one-third of the middle cerebral artery territory. No rapidly improving neurological deficits

No seizures at onset of stroke. No stroke or serious head injury in the previous 3 months. No major surgical procedure within the preceding 14 days

No gastrointestinal or urinary bleeding within the preceding 21 days. No recent myocardial infarction

No history or current signs of intracranial hemorrhage

Pretreatment blood pressure: systolic ≤ 185 mm Hg, diastolic ≤ 110 mm Hg[a]

Normal coagulation profile: INR ≤ 1.7, PTT in normal range, platelet count $\geq 100,000/mm^3$, blood glucose ≥ 50 and ≤ 400 mg/dL

Emergent ancillary care and facilities available during patient monitoring[b] to handle possible bleeding complication[c]

Potential treatment risk and benefit discussed with patient and/or family

[a]Recommended management: IV labetalol (10 mg over 1–2 min repeated every 10 min up to total dose of 150 mg); IV sodium nitroprusside (0.5–10 μg/kg per min).
[b]Monitoring in a dedicated stroke care facility (stroke unit) or intensive care unit recommended. Avoid placement of indwelling bladder catheter until 30 min after drug infusion. Avoid administration of antithrombotic or antiplatelet aggregating drugs, nasogastric tube, central venous access, and arterial punctures during the first 24 h.
[c]Bleeding should be considered as the likely cause of neurological worsening until CT is obtained. If signs of life-threatening bleeding occur, discontinue ongoing rtPA infusion; obtain blood sample for coagulation tests (hematocrit, hemoglobin, PTT, INR, platelet count, fibrinogen); obtain surgical consultation as necessary; consider transfusion, cryoprecipitate, fresh frozen plasma, donor platelets.

Because a significant number of patients are initially evaluated outside the 3 h treatment window, therapy is appropriate for a limited group.

Ancrod, a form of Malaysian pit viper venom, also has been shown in a randomized controlled trial to improve outcome by 22.7% (absolute benefit, 7.8%) without a statistically significant increase in symptomatic intracranial hemorrhage or mortality when given within 3 h of symptom onset (62). The venom decreases fibrinogen serum concentrations and stimulates the release of plasminogen activator from the endothelium. These effects improve blood rheology in the microcirculation and prevent further thrombosis. It is not yet approved in the USA by the FDA for use in ischemic stoke.

Neurointerventional Therapy

Intra-arterial Thrombolysis

Patients with acute ischemic middle cerebral artery (MCA) occlusion may be candidates for intra-arterial rtPA, if therapy is begun within 6 h of symptom onset. In contrast to systemic thrombolytic therapy, the window for beginning intra-arterial therapy is 3 h longer. The PROACT II study revealed significant improvement in outcome in patients treated with intra-arterial prourokinase and heparin when compared with heparin alone. Whereas 25% of control patients experienced significant neurologic disability, 40% of treated patients had no or minor neurological disability (62).

Angioplasty and Stenting

Percutaneous transluminal angioplasty and stenting offer promising alternatives for acute stroke treatment. The Carotid and Vertebral Artery Transluminal Angioplasty Study (CAVATAS) found that stenting and carotid endarterectomy are equally effective for up to 3 years (62). Stenting is currently performed in patients with contraindications to surgical therapy, including tumor induced stenosis, restenosis, radiation induced stenosis, and high risk co-morbid conditions. Intracranial angioplasty, with or without stenting, is feasible for the intracranial carotid artery, the MCA stem, and the basilar and vertebral arteries. It is particularly useful for stroke from arterial dissection and may obviate the need for anticoagulation. Interventional technologies such as catheters, baskets to prevent emboli, and stents continue to improve. Further studies are needed to better delineate risks and benefits and identify appropriate candidates for each procedure.

Anticoagulation

The International Stroke Trial and Chinese Acute Stroke Trial found a reduction of death and recurrent stroke with the administration of 160–300 mg of aspirin within 48 h of acute ischemic stroke (63). All patients without contraindications to aspirin therapy should receive aspirin immediately upon diagnosis (61). Other antiplatelet agents currently available include clopidogrel and dipyridamole. Clopidogrel can be administered to patients with gastrointestinal or respiratory contraindications to aspirin and has been shown to produce a similar reduction in the risk of ischemic stroke as aspirin (61). For secondary prevention of stroke, dipyridamole and aspirin combination is superior to aspirin alone (61) but confers a slightly higher bleeding risk.

In recent studies, intravenous anticoagulation with heparin or heparin-like agents (e.g., tinzaparin) have not been demonstrated to prevent early recurrent stroke or reduce the rate of neurological deterioration (22,61). Heparin has been administered in certain cases. Patients with crescendo TIAs often are treated with IV heparin until emergency surgical or interventional therapy is available. Heparin has been used in the treatment of arterial dissection and, controversially, in high grade carotid stenosis. New onset atrial fibrillation, intermittent atrial fibrillation, or atrial fibrillation with visible clot on ultrasound should prompt use of heparin anticoagulation. Stroke attributable to a cardiac embolic source, such as myocardial infarction with significant wall motion abnormality, dilated cardiomyopathy, or prosthetic valve, should prompt consideration for low dose IV anticoagulation therapy (PTT 50–60 s) and subsequent conversion to oral anticoagulation. Patients should be monitored for the development of heparin induced thrombocytopenia during therapy.

Oral anticoagulation with coumadin is instituted in patients at high risk for cardiac embolism. Again, atrial fibrillation and prosthetic heart valves constitute the most common reasons for therapy. Other indications include patent foramen ovale or hypercoagulable state. In patients with atrial fibrillation, 15–20% of ischemic cerebrovascular accidents are due to documented cardioembolic sources. The incidence ranges from 3% to 5% per year in patients greater than 60 years old with atrial fibrillation (51). The embolism rate for patients with mechanical valve replacement and therapeutic anticoagulation is $\sim$3% per year for mitral valves and 1.5% per year for aortic valves. Bioprosthetic valves have a 2–4% per year stroke risk without anticoagulation (38). Stroke patients often are at risk for injuries from falling and have increased risk for intracerebral hemorrhage when the patient is anticoagulated and a head injury occurs. This increased risk should be considered before beginning therapy.

Because acute stroke patients have a hypercoagulable state, are frequently bed ridden, and may have limb paralysis, they are at high risk for the development of deep venous thrombosis (DVT) or pulmonary embolus. In these patients, prophylactic treatment with subcutaneous heparin or low molecular weight heparin is indicated in the first 48–72 h after infarction, if risk factors for hemorrhagic complications are acceptable.

Hemorrhagic Complications

Anticoagulation and thrombolytic therapy increase risk of serious neurological or systemic bleeding complications. Hemorrhagic transformation of ischemic stroke can be a devastating event. The risk of hemorrhagic conversion of an ischemic infarction is 2–5% without thrombolytics or anticoagulation (38). Large infarct volume is associated with a higher risk of hemorrhagic transformation, and bolus dosing of IV heparin is associated with a higher rate of bleeding complications (22). The risk of bleeding complications must be balanced against the potential benefits of anticoagulation or thrombolytic therapy.

The bleeding risk for thrombolytic therapy is 6–10%. Coumadin therapy for atrial fibrillation is associated with a 10% per year risk of bleeding complications and a 0.3–2% risk of intracerebral hemorrhage. Antiplatelet therapy has a bleeding complication risk of 1–2% (22,38).

Strict monitoring of anticoagulation is essential to decrease the risk of bleeding complications. Many drug interactions increase or decrease the effect of anticoagulant therapy. Medications such as antibiotics and antiepileptic drugs may require adjustments in the doses of anticoagulants.

If hemorrhage occurs, coagulopathy should be corrected immediately. An advantage of both heparin and coumadin is the ability to be reversed in the event of bleeding.

Antiplatelet agents usually cannot be reversed. Platelet transfusions may improve clotting in severe cases. Bleeding with low molecular weight heparin therapy may be improved with administration of protamine. In rare cases, thrombotic agents can be considered with severe bleeding.

Management of Cerebral Edema

CPP should be maintained above 70 mm Hg. As cerebral edema increases, ICP rises, and CPP decreases [Eq. (3)]. Large hemispheric infarctions, especially in younger patients, may result in significant edema. Cerebral edema may precipitate cerebral herniation supratentorially or obstructive hydrocephalus and brainstem compression with cerebellar infarction. Neurological deterioration in a stroke patient should prompt emergency evaluation for hemorrhage by CT scan. If no hemorrhage is identified, cerebral edema (or rarely seizure activity) is the likely cause. Shift of the brain or frank edema may be seen on CT. Initial management should include securing the airway, oxygenating the patient, and maintaining adequate blood pressure. Adjunctive measures may then be implemented.

Hyperventilation

Mild hyperventilation (PCO_2 30–35 mm Hg) in intubated patients is a rapid method for reducing elevated ICP. Hypocarbia is postulated to induce vasoconstriction. The subsequent reduced blood flow leads to a reduction in ICP. Because of the reduction of CBF, the ischemic insult may be worsened. Hyperventilation, at best, is a temporary measure.

Osmotic Therapy

With neurologic deterioration, osmotic therapy with mannitol or glycerol should be instituted. An initial dose of 1 g/kg should be administered over 5–10 min. Longer administration times decrease effectiveness. Additional doses of 0.25–0.5 g/kg can be repeated every 6 h. Serum sodium concentration and osmolarity should be monitored before each additional dose. Therapeutic goals are sodium concentrations of 145–150 mEq/L and osmolarity of 310 mosm. The diuresis associated with osmotic therapy may cause hypokalemia and volume depletion. The osmotic gradient produced by these agents is thought to reduce blood viscosity and increase CSF absorption. Furosemide may increase the effect of osmotic therapy. Caution should be used in patients with heart failure or renal dysfunction, as intravascular volume rapidly increases temporarily with mannitol administration. Other complications include pulmonary edema, electrolyte abnormalities, renal failure (osmolarity >320), hemolysis, or hypersensitivity reaction. Although mannitol therapy is associated with a reduction in ICP, improvement in clinical outcome has not been demonstrated (64).

Steroids

Steroid therapy is indicated for the treatment of vasogenic edema. The edema in acute infarction is primarily cytotoxic and not responsive to steroid therapy. Patients with vasculitis-induced strokes should be treated with steroids. Cerebral edema may occur 2–5 days following onset of intracerebral hemorrhage. Steroids may be beneficial during this period.

Hypertonic Saline

Hyponatremia is a cause of cerebral edema. In recent years 3% or 5% hypertonic saline has been used to treat cerebral edema from trauma, tumor, or infarction. It is used primarily to keep serum sodium concentrations in the high normal range. Hyonatremia should be avoided, but hypernatremia is not recommended.

Barbiturate Coma

Failure of osmotic therapy for the treatment of cerebral edema often prompts consideration for induction of barbiturate coma. It has been used successfully for the treatment of elevated ICP in head injury. The mechanisms of action include reduction of cerebral metabolism with concomitant reduction in CBF, free radical scavenging, reduction of intracellular calcium, lysosomal stabilization, and vasoconstriction in normal brain tissue. Vasoconstriction in normal brain tissue may lead to shunting of blood flow to ischemic tissue. Initial treatment is a bolus dose of pentobarbital of 5 mg/kg IV over 30 min followed by 5 mg/kg every hour for 3 h. Maintenance dose is 1.0–1.5 mg/kg/h. Burst suppression on EEG indicates adequate therapy. A serum concentration of 3.5–5.0 mg% 1 h after loading dose is the clinical target, but clinical correlation is necessary. Invasive ICP monitoring should be performed. Thiopental also may be used. Thiopental is initiated with a 5 mg/kg bolus and 2.5–5 mg/kg/h maintenance dose. Occasional additional boluses may be required. High dose barbiturate therapy is associated with hypotension in up to 50% of cases, and pulmonary artery catheterization is recommended during therapy to monitor cardiac output (64). Adequate intravascular volume and vasoactive drugs such as dopamine are often necessary to maintain CPP (64).

A study of barbiturate coma in 60 patients with malignant cerebral edema secondary to MCA infarction revealed poor control of ICP without improvement in clinical outcome. Thiopental bolus doses did temporarily reduce ICP, and barbiturate therapy in stroke may be an effective temporizing option until definitive therapy can be instituted.

Failure of osmotic therapy and barbiturate therapy generally indicates a poor prognosis for stroke patients. Patients with nondominant infarctions are candidates for surgical decompressive craniectomy, a procedure that has a better outcome when performed early.

Seizure Prophylaxis

Stroke is the most common cause of epilepsy in adults over the age of 35 (65). Seizures after stroke occur in 5–20% of stroke patients, and 2.5% of patients develop recurrent seizures. Intracerebral hemorrhage has the highest seizure risk, estimated at 15.4%. Seizure risk for subarachnoid hemorrhage is 8.5%, for cortical infarction is 6.5%, and for TIA is 3.7% (66). Seizures as the presenting symptom occurred in 30% of patients with intracerebral hemorrhage and in 18% of subarachnoid hemorrhage patients (67,68).

The mechanisms for the development of poststroke seizures are not completely understood. They may occur from local ionic shifts that produce accumulation of intracellular calcium and sodium, which cause neuronal depolarization. Alternative mechanisms include hypoxia-induced release of excitatory neurotransmitters, electrical irritability of the ischemic penumbra, and replacement of normal tissue by neuroglia, immune cells, and gliotic scar.

Poststroke seizures are usually focal (61%) or focal with secondary generalization (28%) (69,70). They can generally be classified as early onset, late onset, episodic, recurrent (epilepsy), or status epilepticus. Early seizures are defined as occurring within the first 2 weeks following the initial stroke (70,71). Early seizures generally occur within the first 24–48 h, and 43–90% are reported to occur in the first day (69,72,73). Late onset seizures, those occurring more than 2 weeks after the initial stroke, are a risk factor for the development of recurrent seizures. These patients are more likely to have a permanent underlying lesion, such as scar tissue. For both ischemic and hemorrhagic strokes ~90% of patients with late onset seizures develop epilepsy; whereas, only 30–35% of patients with early onset seizures have recurrent seizures (67,74). If seizures recur, they usually appear within the first year (18). Status epilepticus is an uncommon event and occurs in ~9% of those patients who develop poststroke seizures (76).

Risk factors for the development of seizures include cortical location, large size, lobar or multilobar hemorrhage, venous infarction or sinus thrombosis, and severity of the initial clinical neurologic deficit when it reflects cortical infarct size (71,77–79). EEG findings can be helpful in predicting seizures. Periodic lateralizing epileptiform discharges (PLEDs) and focal spikes are associated with >75% risk of developing seizures; whereas, focal slowing, diffuse slowing, and a normal EEG are associated with risks of 20%, 10%, and 5%, respectively. EEG also is helpful in identifying nonconvulsive status epilepticus in patients with decreased mental status or unexplained neurologic deficits.

The treatment of seizures in the stroke patient follows the usual guidelines for other focal onset seizures, and these seizures usually respond well to single agent therapy (75). A loading dose for some anticonvulsants can be given to produce therapeutic concentrations rapidly. IV administration of a first line agent is often preferable in the stroke patient, because it allows rapid loading to achieve therapeutic drug concentrations and avoids the oral route in patients who may have a depressed level of consciousness or swallowing difficulties. Typical agents include short-acting benzodiazepines, phenytoin, IV phosphenytoin carbamazepine, and valproate. When administered intravenously, phosphenytoin produces less cardiac depression and less hypotension than phenytoin. Valproate may be used for focal onset or generalized seizures. Barbiturates or propofol may be needed for treatment of status epilepticus. Medication choice should be individualized to the patient's needs, and drug interactions must be recognized when prescribing anticonvulsants. For example, concurrent warfarin and phenytoin therapy can cause elevation of the INR. Drug serum concentrations should be monitored frequently to avoid subtherapeutic levels or toxicity. Frequent monitoring is particularly important in elderly patients who may have higher free drug concentrations from decreased protein binding and who are more susceptible to the sedative effects of anticonvulsants. Electrolyte abnormalities, such as hyponatremia, hypocalcemia, and hypomagnesemia, which can potentiate seizures, need to be avoided.

Prophylaxis is a controversial area in the treatment of poststroke seizures. Risks associated with seizures include aspiration, elevation of cerebral metabolic rate, increased ICP, and possible rebleeding. The Stroke Council of the American Heart Association recommends uniform seizure prophylaxis for patients with subarachnoid and intracerebral hemorrhage for approximately 1 month. If no seizures occur during the treatment period, seizure medications can be weaned (80,81). Patients who develop late onset seizures or seizures during the treatment period may require long-term seizure prophylaxis. No evidence for prophylactic anticonvulsant use in ischemic stroke without evidence of seizure activity exists (75).

SURGICAL MANAGEMENT

Supratentorial Infarcts

Approximately 10% of stroke patients develop malignant cerebral artery territory infarction. In this condition, the severe edema from the ischemia that leads to a stroke produces herniation. The mortality approaches 80% (82,83). Mori et al. (84) used decompressive craniectomy with or without resection of nonviable brain tissue in 19 patients with malignant infarction. Fifteen patients with similar symptoms received non-operative therapy. Mortality in the non-operative group was 67%; whereas, in the group treated surgically, mortality was 16%. Rieke et al. (85) found a mortality of 34% in 32 patients with large infarcts treated with decompressive craniectomy compared with a 76% mortality in 21 patients with similar massive infarcts treated without surgery. Of the patients treated surgically, 19% had an outcome rated as good at the time of discharge compared with 0% in the nonoperative group. Other studies advocate resection of infarcted tissue with possible temporal lobectomy for a herniating uncus (86,87). To be considered for surgical decompression, non-operative measures including hyperventilation, mannitol, hypernatremia, and barbiturate administration (88) must have been tried and failed. Decompression should be performed preferentially on nondominant hemisphere strokes to increase the chance of reasonable neurologic recovery (89).

Infratentorial Infarcts

Posterior fossa infarcts can rapidly deteriorate to a poor outcome without close monitoring. The lack of volume for brain expansion makes postinfarct swelling more likely to cause brainstem compression and herniation. Early surgical decompression in patients with evidence of neurologic deterioration can both prevent death and allow moderate to good functional outcomes. Treatment of large cerebellar infarcts with either ventriculostomy or decompressive craniectomy produces better results than medical management. Chen et al. (90) reported that 8 of 11 patients treated surgically for a cerebellar infarct survived and were able to function independently. Surgical decompression can be beneficial in comatose patients: relieving pressure on the brainstem can reverse coma (91,92). As the prognosis is poor, patients with brainstem infarcts should not be considered for surgical decompression.

Hemorrhage into the basal ganglia does not require surgical decompression. Ventriculostomy may be indicated. As the hemorrhages are deep in cerebral tissue, surgical decompression has dismal outcomes. For patients demonstrating herniation despite treatment with non-operative therapy, surgical decompression might be considered for salvage.

SUMMARY

- The term stroke is used to describe cerebral infarction, intracerebral hemorrhage, or subarachnoid hemorrhage that produces neurologic deficits.
- Modifiable risk factors include hypertension, smoking, diabetes, atrial fibrillation, hyperlipidemia, and oral contraceptive use.

- Nonmodifiable factors include age, gender, ethnicity, family history, and genetic disorders.
- Stoke symptoms usually develop rapidly over several minutes to 1 h and may fluctuate in severity.
- Lacunar infarcts typically occur in diabetic and hypertensive patients. Initial symptoms may be pure motor deficit, pure sensory deficit, dysarthria-clumsy hand, or ataxia-hemiparesis (see Table 3).
- Major vessel occlusion often produces large infarcts. Symptoms may include contralateral weakness, facial palsy, contralateral neglect, or ipsilateral eye deviation. Expressive aphasia is associated with frontal lobe strokes. Receptive aphasia is associated with temporal lobe strokes. Dominant parietal lobe strokes produce Gerstman's syndrome. Nondominant parietal lobe strokes produce dressing apraxia, difficulty copying geometrical patterns, and loss of geographic memory.
- Cerebellar infarcts are associated with vertigo, nausea, vomiting, dysmetria, intention tremor, and tendency for falling to the ipsilateral side.
- Cerebellar infarcts and hematomas are neurosurgical emergencies.
- Brainstem infarcts can produce cranial nerve palsies and lead to deep coma. See Table 4 for typical syndromes.
- Watershed infarcts occur in the vulnerable zones between anterior cerebral and middle cerebral arteries or between middle and posterior cerebral arteries.
- Suspect stroke in patients with slurred speech, upper extremity weakness, and facial droop.
- Immediately assess ABCs:
  A. Provide supplementary oxygen
  B. Obtain IV access
  C. Obtain blood samples for glucose, CBC, electrolytes with BUN and creatinine, and coagulation studies
  D. Obtain 12-lead electrocardiogram and note dysrhythmias
- Perform immediate neurologic assessment.
  Note whether onset of symptoms were within 3 h of evaluation
  Physical examination
  Neurologic examination—note level of consciousness (Glasgow coma scale) and level of stroke severity (NIH stroke scale)
- Obtain noncontrast CT scan of the head.
- Obtain lateral cervical spine X-rays if the patient is comatose or experienced trauma.
- If CT scan shows intracerebral or subarachnoid hemorrhage:
  Consult neurosurgery
  Reverse anticoagulants
  Treat bleeding disorders
  Control hypertension in the awake patient
- If CT scan shows no intracerebral or subarachnoid hemorrhage:
  patient probably has acute ischemic stroke and is a candidate for fibrinolytic therapy if:
  – No CT exclusions are observed
  – Neurologic deficits are not variable or rapidly improving
  – No contraindications to fibrinolytic therapy are present
  – Symptoms appeared <3 h before evaluation

- If CT scan shows no intracerebral or subarachnoid hemorrhage, but suspicion of subarachnoid hemorrhage is high, perform lumbar puncture, if no contraindications to lumbar puncture are present. Fibrinolytic therapy is contraindicated following lumbar puncture.
- Poor outcome for stroke is directly related to fever. Causes of fever should be diligently sought and treated.
- Hypertension in stroke patients is usually treated only if the systolic blood pressure is sustained at a level >200 mm Hg and the diastolic blood pressure is sustained at a level >110 mm Hg.
- Intravenous rtPA administered within 3 h of the onset of ischemic stroke improves outcomes (see Table 6).
- All patients without a contraindication to aspirin therapy should receive aspirin upon diagnosis of stroke. Clopidogrel can be administered to patients who cannot receive aspirin.
- Warfarin therapy is instituted for patients at risk for cardioembolism. These patients include individuals with mechanical prosthetic heart valves and those with atrial fibrillation.
- CPP = MAP − ICP should be maintained above 70 mm Hg. Measures to reduce ICP when it is elevated include mild hyperventilation for temporary control, mannitol, steroid therapy for vasculitic stroke, and correction of hyponatremia. If cerebral edema persists, barbiturate coma should be considered.
- Seizures in the stroke patient usually respond to single agent therapy.
- Seizure prophylaxis is recommended for patients suffering subarachnoid or intracerebral hemorrhage for ~1 month. Seizure prophylaxis is not recommended for ischemic stroke.
- Decompressive craniectomy may improve outcomes in malignant infarction and in posterior fossa infarcts in patients who demonstrate deterioration.

REFERENCES

1. American Heart Association. 2001. 2001 Heart and Stroke Statistical Update. http://www.americanheart.org/statistics/stroke.html.
2. Stroke Unit Trialists' Collaboration. Collaborative systematic review of the randomized trials of organized in-patient (stroke unit) care after stroke. BMJ 1997; 314:1151–1159.
3. Diez-Tajedor E, Fuentes B. Acute care in stroke: do stroke units make the difference? Cerebravasc Dis 2001; 11 (suppl 1):31–39.
4. Sudlow C, Warlow C. Comparing stroke incidence worldwide. What makes studies comparable? Stroke 1996; 27:550–558.
5. Ad Hoc Committee on Cerebrovascular Diseases. A classification and outline of cerebrovascular diseases III. Stroke 1990; 21:637–676.
6. Foulkes MA, Wolf PA, Price TR, et al. The Stroke Data Bank: Design, methods, and baseline characteristics. Stroke 1988; 19:547–554.
7. Davenport R, Dennis M. Neurological emergencies: acute stroke. J Neurol Neurosurg Psychiatry 200; 68:277–288.
8. Bonita R. Epidemiology of stroke. Lancet 1992; 339:342–344.
9. Dennis MS, Burn JP, Sandercock P, et al. Long-term survival after first-ever stroke: the Oxfordshire community stroke project. Stroke 1993; 24:796–800.

10. Bamford J, Dennis M, Sandercock P, et al. The frequency, causes and timing of death within 30 days of a first stroke: the Oxfordshire community stroke project. J Neurol Neurosurg Psychiatry 1990; 53:824–829.
11. Bounds JV, Wiebers DO, Whisnant JP, et al. Mechanisms and timing of deaths from cerebral infarction. Stroke 1981; 12:474–477.
12. Silver FL, Norris JW, Lewis AJ, et al. Early mortality following stroke: a prospective review. Stroke 1984; 15:492–496.
13. A practical approach to the management of stroke patients. In: Warlow CP, Dennis MS, Van Gijn, et al. Stroke: A practical guide to management. Oxford: Blackwell, 1996; 360–384.
14. Burn J, Dennis M, Bamford J, et al. Long-term risk of recurrence stroke after a first-ever stroke: the Oxfordshire community stroke project. Stroke 1994; 25:333–337.
15. Mayberg MR, Winn HR. Endarterectomy for asymptomatic carotid artery stenosis, resolving the controversy (Editorial). J Am Med Assoc 1995; 273:1459–61.
16. Mohr JP, Thompson JLP, Lazar RM. A Comparison of Warfarin and Aspirin for the Prevention of Recurrent Ischemic Stroke. N Engl J Med 2001; 345:1444–1451.
17. Sacco RL, Benjamin EJ, Broderick JP, et al. American Heart Association Prevention Conference IV. Prevention and rehabilitation of stroke: risk factors. Stroke 1997; 28:1507–1517.
18. Thompson DW, Furlan AJ. Clinical epidemiology of stroke. Neurosurg Clin N Am 1997; 8:265–269.
19. Heart and Stroke Facts. 1995 Statistical Supplement. Dallas, TX: American Heart Association. 1995; pp.11–12.
20. Howard G, Anderson R, Sorlie P, et al. Ethnic differences in stroke mortality between non-Hispanic Whites, Hispanic Whites, and Blacks: the national longitudinal mortality study. Stroke 1994; 25:2120–2125.
21. Kiely DK, Wolf PA, Cupples LA, et al. Familial aggregation of stroke. The Framingham study. Stroke 1993; 24:1366–1371.
22. Tegos TJ, Kalodiki E, Daskalopoulou S, Nicolaides AN. Stroke: epidemiology, clinical picture, and risk factors (I of III). Angiology 2000; 51:793–808.
23. Marmot MG, Poulter NR. Primary prevention of stroke. Lancet 1992; 339:344–347.
24. Collins R, Peto R, MacMahon S, et al. Blood pressure, stroke, and coronary heart disease. Part 2. Short-term reductions in blood pressure: overview of randomized drug trials in their epidemiological context. Lancet 1990; 335:827–838.
25. Prevention of stroke by antihypertensive drug treatment in older persons with isolated systolic hypertension. Final results of the systolic hypertension in the elderly program (SHEP). SHEP cooperative research group. J Am Med Assoc 1991; 265:3255–3264.
26. Kubota K, Yamaguchi T, Abe Y, et al. Effects of smoking on regional cerebral blood flow in neurologically normal subjects. Stroke 1983; 14:720–724.
27. Howard G, Wagenknecht LE, Burke GL, et al. Cigarette smoking and progression of atherosclerosis: The atherosclerosis risk in communities (ARIC) Study. J Am Med Assoc 1998; 279:119–124.
28. Shinton R, Beevers G. Meta-analysis of relation between cigarette smoking and stroke. Br Med J 1989; 25:789–794.
29. Klag MJ, Whelton PK. Risk of stroke in male cigarette smokers. N Engl J Med 1987; 316:628–629.
30. Fitzgerald AP, Jarret RJ. Body weight and coronary heart disease mortality an analysis in relation to age and smoking habit. 15 years follow-up data from the Whitehall study. Int J Obes Relat Metab Disord 1992; 16:119–123.
31. Halperin JL, Hart RG. Atrial fibrillation and stroke: new ideas, persisting dilemmas. Stroke 1988; 19:937–941.
32. Sacks FM, Pffefer MA, Moye LA, et al. For the Cholesterol and Recurrent Events Trial Investigators. The effect of pravastatin on coronary events after myocardial infarction in patients with average cholesterol levels. N Engl J Med 1996; 335:1001–1009.

33. Lipid study Group. Design Features and baseline characteristics of the LIPID (long-term intervention with pravastatin in ischemic disease) study: a randomized trial in patients with previous acute myocardial infarction and/or unstable angina pectoris. Am J Cardiol 1995; 76:474–479.
34. Vaughn CJ, Murphy MB, Buckley BM. Statins do more than just lower cholesterol. Lancet 1996; 348:1079–1082.
35. Rosenson RS, Tangney CC. Antiatherothrombotic properties of statins: Implications for cardiovascular event reduction. J Am Med Assoc 1998; 279:1643–1650.
36. Iso H, Jacobs DR Jr, Wentworth D, et al. Serum cholesterol levels and six-year mortality from stroke in 350,977 men screened for the multiple risk factor intervention trial. N Engl J Med 1989; 320:904–910.
37. Hannaford PC, Croft PR, Kay CR. Oral contraception and stroke. Evidence from the Royal College of General Practioners' Oral Contraception Study. Stroke 1994; 25:935–942.
38. Greenberg MS. "Handbook of Neurosurgery, 5th ed. Chapter 26: Cerebrovascular accidents." New York: Theime, 2001; pp. 736–745.
39. Caplan LR. Treatment of patients with stroke (Editorial). Arch Neurol 2002; 59:703–707.
40. Strandgaard S. Autoregulation of cerebral blood flow in hypertensive patients: the modifying influence of prolonged antihypertensive treatment on the tolerance to acute, drug-induced hypotension. Circulation. 1976; 53:720–727.
41. Powers W. Acute hypertension after stroke: the scientific basis for treatment decisions. Neurology. 1993; 43:61–67.
42. Fischer CM. Lacunar strokes and infarcts. Neurology 1982; 32:871–877.
43. Gorelick PB. Cerebrovascular disease, pathophysiology and diagnosis. Nurs Clin N Am 1986; 21:275–288.
44. Fischer CM. The anatomy and pathology of the cerebral vasculature. In: Meyer, JS (ed): Modern Concepts Cerebrovascular Disease. New York: Spectrum Publications, 1975.
45. Becker KJ. Vertebrobasilar Ischemia. New Horizons 1997; 5:305–312.
46. Kubik S, Adams RA. Occlusion of the basilar artery: a clinical and pathological study. Brain 1946; 69:6–121.
47. McDowell F, Potes J, Groch S. The natural history of internal carotid and vertebral-basilar artery occlusion. Neurology 1961; 11:153–157.
48. Leys D, Pruvo JP, Godefroy O, et al. Prevalance and significance of hyperdense middle cerebral artery in acute stroke. Stroke 1992; 23:317–324.
49. Jäger HR. Diagnosis of stroke with advanced CT and MR imaging. Br Med Bull 2000; 56:318–333.
50. Culebras A, Kase CS, Masdeu JC. Practice guidelines for the use of imaging in transient ischemic attacks and acute stroke: a report of the Stroke Council, American Heart Association. Stroke 1997; 28:1480–1497.
51. Treib J, Grauer MT, Woessner R, Morgenthaler M. Treatment of stroke in an intensive stroke unit: a novel concept. Intensive Care Med 2002; 26:1598–1611.
52. Blumenfeld JD, Laragh JH. Management of hypertensive crises: the scientific basis for treatment decisions. Am J Hypertension 2001; 14:1154–1167.
53. Leonardi-Bee J, Bath PMW, Phillips SJ, Sandercock PAG. Blood pressure and clinical outcome in the International Stroke Trial. Stroke 2002; 33:1315–1320.
54. Berenstein RA, Hemphill JC. Critical care of acute ischemic stroke. Curr Neurol Neurosci Rep 2001; 1:587–592.
55. Gorelick PB. Stroke prevention therapy beyond antithrombotics: unifying mechanisms in ischemic stroke pathogenesis and implications for therapy. Stroke 2002; 33:862–875.
56. The National Institute of Neurological Disorders and Stroke rtPA Stroke Study Group. Tissue plasminogen activator for acute ischemic stroke. N Engl J Med 1995; 333:1581–1587.
57. Albers GW, Bates VE, Clark WM, et al. Intravenous tissue type plasminogen activator for treatment of acute stroke: the standard treatment with alteplase to reverse stoke (STARS) study. J Am Med Assoc 2000; 283:1145–1150.

58. Hacke W, Caste M, Fieschi C, et al. Randomized double blind placebo-controlled trial of thrombolytic therapy with intravenous alteplase in acute ischemic stroke (ECASS II). Lancet 1998; 352:1245–1251.
59. Clark WM, Wissman S, Albers GW, et al. Recombinant tissue-type plasminogen activator (alteplase) for ischemic stroke 3 to 5 hours after symptom onset. J Am Med Assoc 1999; 282:2019–2026.
60. Hacke W, Kaste M, Fieschi C, et al. The ECASS study group. Intravenous thrombolysis with recombinant tissue plasminogen activator for acute hemispheric stroke. J Am Med Assoc 1995; 274:1017–1025.
61. Stapf C, Mohr JP. Ischemic stroke therapy. Annu Rev Med 2002; 53:453–475.
62. Sherman DG, Atkinson RP, Chippendale T, et al. Intravenous Ancrod for treatment of acute ischemic stroke. J Am Med Assoc 2000; 283:2395–2403.
63. International Stroke Trial Collaborative Group. 1997. The International Stroke Trialr (IST: a randomized trial of aspirin, subcutaneous heparin, both, or neither among 10435 patients with acute ischemic stroke. Lancet 349:1569–1581.
64. CAST (Chinese Acute Stroke Trial) Collaborative Group. 1997. CAST: randomized placebo-controlled trial of early aspirin use in 20000 patients with acute stroke. Lancet 349:1641–1649.
65. Hauser W, Annegers J, Kurland L. Incidence of epilepsy and unprovoked seizures in Rochester, Minnesota: 1935–1984. Epilepsia 1993; 34:453–468.
66. Kilpatrick C, Davis S, Tress B, et al. Epileptic seizures after stroke. Arch Neurol 1990; 47:157–169.
67. Sung C, Chu N. Epileptic seizures in intracerebral hemorrhage. J Neurosurg Psychiatr 1989; 52:1273–1276.
68. Rhoney D, Tipps L, Murray K, et al. Anticonvulsant prophylaxis and timing of seizures after aneurysmal subarachnoid hemorrhage. Neurology 2000; 55:258–265.
69. Gupta S, Naheedy M, Elias D, Rubino F. Postinfarction seizures: a clinical study. Stroke 1988; 19:1477–1481.
70. Davalos A, de Cendra E, Molins A, et al. Epileptic seizures at the onset of stroke. Cerebrovasc Dis 1992; 2:327–331.
71. Bladin C, Alexandrov A, Bellavance A, et al. Seizures after stroke: a prospective multicenter study. Arch Neurol 2000; 57:1617–1622.
72. Jennet B. Early traumatic epilepsy. Arch Neurol. 1974; 30:394–398.
73. Berger A, Lipton R Lesser M, et al. Early seizures following intracerebral hemorrhage: implications for therapy. Neurology. 1988; 38:1363–1365.
74. Sung C, Chu N. Epileptic seizures in thrombotic stroke. J Neurol 1990; 237:166–170.
75. Silverman IE, Restrepo L, Mathews GC. Poststroke Seizures. Arch Neurol 2002; 59:195–201.
76. Veioglu S, Ozmenoglu M, Boz C, Alioglu Z. Status epilepticus after stroke. Stroke. 2001; 32:1169–1172.
77. Lancman M, Golinstok A, Horcini J, Granillo R. Risk factors for developing seizures after a stroke. Epilepsia. 1993; 34:141–143.
78. Faught E, Peters D, Bartolucci, et al. Seizures after primary intracerebral hemorrhage. Neurology. 1989; 39:1089–1093.
79. Reith J, Jorgensen HS, Nakayama H, et al. Seizures in acute stroke. Stroke. 1997; 28:1585–1589.
80. Broderick J, Adams H Jr, Barsan W, et al. Guidelines for the management of spontaneous intracerebral hemorrhage: a statement for the healthcare professionals from a special writing group of the Stroke Council, American Heart Association. Stroke. 1999; 30:905–915.
81. Mayberg M, Batjer, Dacey R, et al. Guidelines for the management of aneurysmal subarachnoid hemorrhage: a statement for healthcare professionals from a special writing group of the Stroke Council, American Heart Association. Circulation. 1994; 90:2592–2605.
82. Moulin DE, Lo R, Chiang J, et al. Prognosis in middle cerebral artery occlusion. Stroke 1985; 16:282–284.

83. Hacke W, Schwab S, Horn M, et al. Malignant middle cerebral artery territory infarction: clinical course and prognostic signs. Arch Neurol 1996; 53:309–315.
84. Mori K, Aoki A, Yamamoto T, et al. Aggressive decompressive surgery in patients with massive hemispheric embolic cerebral infarction associated with severe brain swelling. Acta Neurochir 2001; 143:483–492.
85. Rieke K, Schwab S, Krieger D, et al. Decompressive surgery in space-occupying hemispheric infarction: results of an open, prospective trial. Crit Care Med 1995; 23 (9):1576–1587.
86. Ivamoto HS, Numoto M, Donaghy RMP. Surgical decompression for cerebral and cerebellar infarcts. Stroke 1974; 5:365–370.
87. Young PH, Smith KR Jr, Dunn RC. Surgical decompression after cerebral hemispheric stroke: indications and patient selection. South Med J 1982; 75:473–475.
88. Rengachary SS, Batnitzky S, Morantz RA, et al. Hemicraniectomy for acute massive cerebral infarction. Neurosurgery 1981; 8:321–328.
89. Loftus CM. Emergency surgery for stroke. In: Loftus CM, ed. Neurosurgical Emergencies: I. Chicago, Il: Am Assoc Neurologic Surg 1994.
90. Chen HJ, Lee TC, Wei CP. Treatment of cerebellar infarction by decompressive suboccipital craniectomy. Stroke 1992; 23:957–961.
91. Heros RC. Surgical treatment of cerebellar infarction. Stroke 1992; 23:937–938.
92. Laun A, Busse O, Calatayud V, et al. Cerebellar infarcts in the area of the supply of the PICA and their surgical treatment. Acta Neurochir. (Wien) 1984; 71:295–306.

APPENDIX

NIH Stroke Scale (Range 0–42; Score >22 Indicates Severe Neurologic Deficit)

1A. *Level of consciousness*
    0 Alert, keenly responsive
    1 Not alert, but arousable by minor stimulation to obey, answer, or respond
    2 Not alert, requires repeated stimulation to attend, or is obtunded and requires strong painful stimulation to make movements (not stereotyped)
    3 Comatose: responds only with reflex motor or (posturing) autonomic effects, or totally unresponsive, flaccid, and areflexic

1B. *Level of consciousness questions*
Patient is asked the month and his/her age
    0 Answers both questions correctly: must be correct (no credit for being close)
    1 Answers one question correctly, or cannot answer because of ET tube, orotracheal trauma, severe dysarthria, language barrier, or any other problem not secondary to aphasia
    2 Answers neither question correctly, or is aphasic, stuporous, or does not comprehend the questions

1C. *Level of consciousness commands*
Patient is asked to open and close the eyes, and then to grip and release the nonparetic hand. Substitute another one-step command if both hands cannot be used. Credit is given for unequivocal attempt even if it cannot be completed owing to weakness. If there is no response to commands, demonstrate (pantomime) the task. Record only the first attempt.
    0 Performs both tasks correctly
    1 Performs one task correctly
    2 Performs neither task correctly

2. *Best gaze*

   Test only horizontal eye movement. Use motion to attract attention in aphasic patients.

   0 Normal

   1 Partial gaze palsy (gaze abnormal in one or both eyes, but forced deviation or total gaze paresis is not present) or patient has an isolated cranial nerve 3, 4, or 6 paresis

   2 Forced deviation or total gaze paresis not overcome by oculocephalic (doll's eyes) maneuver (do not do caloric testing)

3. *Visual*

   Visual fields (upper and lower quadrants) are tested by confrontation. May be scored as normal if patient looks at side of finger movement. Use ocular threat where consciousness or comprehension limits testing. Then test with double-sided simultaneous stimulation (DSSS).

   0 No visual loss

   1 Partial hemianopia (clear cut asymmetry), or extinction to DSSS

   2 Complete hemianopia

   3 Bilateral hemianopia (blind, including cortical blindness)

4. *Facial palsy*

   Ask the patient (or pantomime) to show their teeth, or raise eyebrows and close close eyes. Use painful stimulus and grade grimace response in poorly responsive or noncomprehending patients

   0 Normal symmetrical movement

   1 Minor paralysis (flattened nasolabial fold, asymmetry on smiling)

   2 Partial paralysis (total or near total paralysis of lower face)

   3 Complete paralysis of one or both sides (absent facial movement in upper and lower face)

5. *Motor arm*

   Instruct the patient to hold the arms out-stretched, palms down (at 90 degrees if sitting, or 45 degrees if supine). If consciousness or comprehension impaired, cue patient by actively lifting arms into position while verbally instructing patient to maintain position

   0 No drift (holds arm at 90 degrees or 45 degrees for full 10 seconds)

   1 Drift (holds limbs at 90 degrees or 45 degrees position, but drifts before 10 full seconds but does not hit bed or other support)

   2 Some effort against gravity (cannot get to or hold initial position, drifts down to bed)

   3 No effort against gravity, limb falls

   4 No movement

   9 Amputation or joint fusion: explain

6. *Motor leg*

   While supine, instruct patient to maintain the nonparetic leg at 30 degrees. If consciousness or comprehension is impaired, cue patient by actively lifting leg into position while verbally instructing patient to maintain position. Then repeat in the paretic leg.

   0 No drift (holds leg at 30 degrees full 5 seconds)

   1 Drift (leg falls before 5 seconds, but does not hit bed)

   2 Some effort against gravity (leg falls to bed by 5 seconds)

   3 No effort against gravity (leg falls to bed immediately)

   4 No movement

   9 Amputation or joint fusion: explain

7. *Limb ataxia*
   (Looking for unilateral cerebellar lesion). Finger-to-nose-finger and heel–knee–shin tests are performed on both sides. Ataxia is scored only if clearly out of proportion to weakness. Ataxia is absent in the patient who cannot comprehend or is paralyzed.
   0 Absent
   1 Present in one limb
   2 Present in two limbs
   9 Amputation or joint fusion: explain
8. *Sensory*
   Test with pin. When consciousness or comprehension is impaired, score sensation normal unless deficit clearly recognized (e.g., clear-cut asymmetry of grimace or withdrawal). Only hemisensory losses attributed to stroke are counted abnormal.
   0 Normal, no sensory loss
   1 Mild to moderate sensory loss (pin-prick dull or less sharp on the affected side, or loss of superficial pain to pinprick but patient aware of being touched)
   2 Severe to total (patient unaware of being touched in the face, arm, and leg)
9. *Best language*
   In addition to judging comprehension of commands in the preceeding neurologic exam, the patient is asked to describe a standard picture, to name common items, and to read and interpret the standard text in the following box. The intubated patient should be asked to write.

   > You know how.
   > Down to earth.
   > I got home from work.
   > Near the table in the dining room.
   > They heard him speak on the radio last night.

   0 Normal, no aphasia
   1 Mild to moderate aphasia (some loss of fluency, word finding errors, naming errors, paraphasias, and/or impairment of communication by either comprehension or expression disability)
   2 Severe aphasia (great need for inference, questioning and guessing by listener, limited range of information can be exchanged)
   3 Mute or global aphasia (no usable speech or auditory comprehension) or patient in coma
10. *Dysarthria*
    Patient may be graded based on information already gleaned during evaluation. If patient is thought to be normal, have the patient read (or repeat) the standard text shown in the following box.

    > Mama
    > Tip-top
    > Fifty-fifty
    > Thanks
    > Huckleberry
    > Baseball player
    > Caterpillar

    0 Normal speech
    1 Mild to moderate (slurs some words, can be understood with some difficulty)
    2 Severe (unintelligible slurred speech in the absence of, or out of proportion to, any dysphasia or is mute/anarthric)
    3 Intubated or other physical barrier

11. *Extinction and inattention*

    Sufficient information to identify neglect may already be gleaned during evaluation. If the patient has severe visual loss preventing visual DSSS and the cutaneous stimuli are normal, the score is normal. Scored as abnormal only if present.

    0 Normal, no sensory loss
    1 Visual, tactile, auditory, spatial or personal inattention or extinction to DSSS in one of the sensory modalities
    2 Profound hemi-attention or hemi-inattention to more than one modality. Does not recognize own hand or orients to only one side of space

20
Encephalopathy

Jodie Herk Taylor
*University of Minnesota, Minneapolis, Minnesota and
Hennepin County Medical Center, Minneapolis, Minnesota, USA*

Encephalopathy is a derangement in mental status or level of consciousness secondary to a disease process extrinsic to the brain (1). Patients in the intensive care unit (ICU) often become confused or combative during their stay. The study by Fraser et al. (2) reports that a percentage of ICU patients as high as 74% experience at least one episode of confusion or encephalopathy (2). These episodes can be frightening to the patient and their loved ones and frustrating to the caregivers. Defining the etiology of the confusion and differentiating between emergency and non-emergency causes are essential to appropriate, prompt, and possibly life-saving treatment of the patient.

Basic rules to follow when first evaluating any and every patient with mental status changes are:

1. ABCs! Any patient who is obtunded and unable to protect his/her airway should first be intubated and mechanically ventilated. Following the maintenance of airway and breathing, a thorough evaluation of the patient's decreased level of consciousness may resume.
2. Vital signs are vital! After securing the airway, the patient's blood pressure, heart rate, temperature, respiratory rate, and arterial saturation should be evaluated. Deviations from normal values should place the patient in a setting where careful monitoring is possible. A differential diagnosis of the causes of the abnormality should be developed.
3. Specific laboratory tests should be obtained on each patient with a change in mental status. Blood glucose concentration is a must. Other appropriate studies may include ABG, WBC, hemoglobin, electrolytes, and troponin. Additional laboratory studies should be obtained and tailored to the specific situation and patient.

After following the foregoing steps, a thorough, orderly examination of *every* patient with confusion or coma should be performed. A stepwise evaluation of the patient should be initiated by first ruling out the emergency causes of encephalopathy. If emergency causes are included, less urgent etiologies must be considered.

EMERGENCY CAUSES OF MENTAL STATUS CHANGE

Reassess the ABCs

Airway and Breathing

The individual caring for the patient must establish the presence or absence of hypoxia in every patient with confusion. The most dangerous possible cause of confusion is hypoxia (Table 1). Decreased oxygen delivery to the brain produces a depressed level of consciousness. *The patient's saturation monitor may not correlate* with the arterial partial pressure of oxygen. If confusion is present with high SaO_2 values as determined by a saturation meter, an arterial blood gas should be obtained. A change in mental status that results from hypoxia may indicate life-threatening causes such as a tension pneumothorax, pulmonary embolism, or acute airway obstruction. Chest radiography should be performed on any patient with hypoxia. A chest X-ray is frequently helpful in identifying a reason for hypoxia. An arterial blood gas may identify shunt. Alternatively, the saturation of arterial blood with oxygen may be adequate, but the patient may, in fact, be hypercarbic. The partial pressure of CO_2 (PCO_2) in the arterial blood will not cause a decrease in oxygen saturation until the PCO_2 is well above the minimum level required for mental status changes. For example, the saturation monitor may indicate a saturation greater than 92% while the patient is hypercarbic with a PCO_2 of 70 mm Hg. For this reason, an arterial blood gas should be obtained on every patient with a decreased level of consciousness, and the saturation monitor should not solely be relied on when confusion persists despite a saturation reading consistent with adequate oxygenation.

Circulation

Hypotension from shock or cardiac dysfunction from either myocardial infarction (MI) or arrhythmias may cause acute mental status changes. Again, the brain experiences decreased oxygen delivery. In these cases, improvement in oxygen delivery by appropriately increasing either hemoglobin concentration or cardiac output can be life saving. Patients who have altered mental status from a circulatory cause will not be able to communicate chest pain. An electrocardiogram (EKG) should be obtained to evaluate the possibility of MI or arrhythmia. Hypotensive or tachycardic trauma patients, postoperative patients, or any patient at risk for bleeding should have the hemoglobin concentration determined to evaluate possible hemorrhage.

Disability

In critically ill patients, a cerebrovascular accident (CVA) can cause an acute change in mental status. Focal neurologic signs are often present, but lack of focal findings does

Table 1 Emergency Causes of Encephalopathy (*Always* Rule These Out *First!*)

Hypoxia
Hypercarbia
Cardiac arrhythmias
Stroke
Hypoglycemia
Shock (hemorrhagic or septic)

not eliminate the possibility of a CVA. When stroke is suspected, the clinician should obtain an emergency head CT without contrast to determine the presence of an acute hemorrhagic CVA or other intracranial pathology. CT is limited in identifying an ischemic CVA. If this diagnosis strongly suspected and the head CT is negative, a brain MRI should be obtained.

Other Emergency Causes

Hypoglycemia can cause a profound decrease in mental status. Seizures and focal neurologic abnormalities can occur with low serum glucose concentrations. A blood glucose concentration should be obtained in all patients with an alteration in mental status and all patients who are not emerging from anesthesia or sedation as expected. If hypoglycemia is not recognized or treated in a timely manner, significant, preventable brain injury may result.

Sepsis can produce changes in mental status. In fact, one of the earliest signs of sepsis in a patient is encephalopathy. *Any patient who exhibits tachypnea, respiratory alkalosis, and mental status changes should be evaluated for sepsis.* These changes usually occur before fever, positive blood cultures, or hypotension.

After evaluating the patient for emergency causes of mental status changes, classification by systems is frequently helpful (Table 2). The following diagnoses should be made *only after* ruling out other, more urgent causes of disturbances in cerebral function.

Neurologic Causes of Mental Status Changes/Encephalopathy As described earlier, CVA can occur in ICU patients without a prior history of such an event. Patients with atrial fibrillation or other risk factors for clot formation are at higher risk. Surgical patients who have been immobile for a prolonged period of time may develop occult DVTs that can embolize through a patent foramen ovale and cause an ischemic stroke. If an ischemic stroke is confirmed, and the time from onset of symptoms to potential

Table 2 Other Causes of Encephalopathy (*Systems Approach*)

Neurologic	Meningitis, encephalitis
	Posttraumatic encephalopathy
Metabolic	Hypo/hypernatremia
	Hypo/hypercalcemia
	Hypo/hyperosmolar states
	Vitamin deficiency
Endocrine	Diabetes, hypothyroidism
	Hyperthyroidism, hyperparathyroidism
	Hypo/hyperadrenalism
Cardiovascular	Post-CABG encephalopathy
Iatrogenic	Sleep/wake cycle disturbances
	Sleep deprivation
	Drugs (narcotics, sedatives, steroids, etc.)
Hepatic	Hepatic encephalopathy
Infectious	Septic encephalopathy
Renal	Uremic encephalopathy, dialysis
	Disequilibrium syndrome
	Aluminum toxicity

treatment is <3 h, TPA may be appropriate treatment. A neurology consultation should be obtained.

If hemorrhagic stroke is identified, a neurosurgeon should be consulted. The PT/INR and PTT should be measured, and any anticoagulants or medications inhibiting platelet function should be discontinued.

Although meningitis occurs infrequently in the surgical ICU, it can cause a change in a patient's mental status. Patients at increased risk are those who have had a recent violation of the dura resulting from use of an epidural catheter, back or neck surgery, placement of a ventriculostomy catheter, or head trauma. Immunocompromised patients have increased risk of developing meningitis, and fungal meningitis should be considered. Lumbar puncture should be obtained, if the patient is suspected of having meningitis or encephalitis. Glucose, protein, cell count, Gram stain, and cultures of bacteria, viruses, and fungi in the spinal fluid should be obtained.

Special situations to consider: Patients with traumatic brain injuries often will have mental status abnormalities for several days to weeks following the trauma. These patients can be combative, agitated, and unable to follow commands. After evaluating them for other medical causes of mental status changes, a repeat head CT may be appropriate, especially early in the hospital stay. Such patients may develop extension of an existing contusion or hematoma, which may require intervention. Once progression of a brain injury has been ruled out, these patients may be monitored with serial examinations, and minimal sedation to allow administration of routine nursing and medical care. When used, sedation in these patients should be decreased enough to allow for a thorough neurologic examination *at least* once daily. Any deterioration in neurologic examination or focal findings on examination should prompt a repeat head CT. The typical course of traumatic brain injury in young patients is gradual improvement.

Metabolic/Electrolyte Causes of Mental Status Change: ICU patients typically receive fluids and nutrients intravenously or enterally. The normal regulatory mechanisms such as thirst are bypassed. Electrolyte abnormalities can easily occur. Hyponatremia, hypernatremia, hypercalcemia, and hypocalcemia can produce changes in mental status and are frequently encountered. Hyper- and hypo-osmolal states can also cause mental status changes.

Hyponatremia is the most common electrolyte abnormality in the ICU. It is associated with an increased mortality when compared with patients with normal serum sodium concentrations (3). The brain has great capacity to adapt to changes in serum electrolytes and serum osmolality. When a decrease in osmolality is sensed, the brain begins to lose electrolytes and organic solutes within minutes, a process that is complete within 48 h of sustained hyponatremia (4). As a result of this compensatory mechanism, brain water increases 3–6% when serum sodium decreases by 22–27% (4). Despite the efficacy of this adaptive mechanism, brain swelling may occur with profound acute hyponatremia. The neurologic consequences of hyponatremia depend on the rapidity of change in electrolyte concentration or osmolality rather than on the absolute value. For example, a serum sodium concentration of 130 mEq/L that rapidly falls from 145 may induce neurologic symptoms; whereas, a patient with a serum sodium concentration of 115 mEq/L may be asymptomatic, if the development of hyponatremia were gradual (5).

Acute hyponatremia (that develops in <48 h) is generally hospital-acquired and frequently occurs postoperatively, with excessive volume resuscitation or with diuretic use (6). Abrupt decreases in serum sodium concentration can cause mental status changes by increasing cerebral edema and causing subsequent intracranial hypertension.

Encephalopathy

Hypoxia, young age, and estrogens have been associated with a poorer tolerance to hyponatremia. One study demonstrated that permanent brain damage and death was 25 times greater in menstruant women than in men or in postmenopausal women (7). An alteration in mental status is the most common manifestation, but the symptoms can range from lethargy and confusion to coma. The severity of symptoms is increased with a more rapid fall in serum sodium concentration. Often, these symptoms are insidious in onset but can progress rapidly. Consequently, early recognition of minor symptoms is important. Seizures can occur in response to hyponatremia and require immediate control. The serum sodium concentration should be corrected to 120–125 mEq/L with use of a hypertonic (3%) saline solution (8). Correction beyond 120–125 mEq/L should *never* be accomplished quickly, because central pontine myelinolysis (CPM) may occur. With rapid correction of the serum sodium concentration, the serum is unable to rapidly re-establish the normal concentration of osmolytes and electrolytes that were lost during the previous adaptation to hyponatremia. The result of rapid sodium replacement is cerebral dehydration, which subsequently leads to the demyelination (8).

Patients with poor nutrition, patients with burns, and patients with liver disease are at increased risk for developing CPM. Of note, burned patients can develop CPM in the face of normal or near-normal serum sodium. This finding suggests that the osmotic shifts experienced by these patients can be enough to cause CPM. In general, correction of serum sodium concentration after acute hyponatremia confers a *lower risk* of CPM than does correction of the serum sodium concentration in patients with chronic hyponatremia.

- The accepted algorithm for correcting hyponatremia is to limit correction to <15 mEq/L per 24 h. If other risk factors for CPM are present, the correction should be limited to <10 mEq/L per 24 h.
- The postoperative period is a critical time during which hypotonic fluid should be avoided in order to prevent the development of hyponatremic encephalopathy and potentially permanent neurologic damage (8).

Special situations to consider: Hyponatremia frequently develops in patients who sustain a subarachnoid hemorrhage from aneurysm rupture. Occurrence of hyponatremia is attributed to a cerebral salt-wasting syndrome and is usually *not* a result of the syndrome of inappropriate antidiuretic hormone (SIADH) secretion. These patients often are treated with fluid restriction. Fluid restriction can exacerbate their hypovolemia and can increase the risk for vasospasm and subsequent cerebral infarction. Normal intravascular volemia should be maintained with normal saline. In some cases, hypertonic saline can be used.

Chronic hyponatremia is generally acquired as an outpatient and is usually better tolerated than acute hyponatremia. By itself, chronic hyponatremia has not been shown to cause permanent neurologic sequelae. However, patients with chronic hyponatremia can still develop neurologic symptoms, which are likely a result of cerebral solute losses (8). The symptoms are less obvious and can consist of headache, lethargy, weakness, or confusion. In patients who are able to maintain oral intake, restriction of free water intake to <1000 cc per day can help to improve symptoms and increase serum sodium. Remember that patients with chronic hyponatremia are at greater risk for development of CPM with correction of the serum sodium concentration than are patients with acute hyponatremia.

The CNS symptoms of *hypernatremia* are usually seen at concentrations >160 mEq/L or at osmolalities >320 mOsm/kg. This electrolyte disorder is common in patients with impaired ability to maintain hydration. In the SICU, hypernatremia is encountered in neurosurgical trauma patients who develop central diabetes insipidus from an intracranial injury, or in those patients treated with mannitol to decrease intracranial pressure. As with hyponatremia, symptoms can range from lethargy to seizures and coma. The symptoms are seen more often during rehydration and may result from cerebral edema during the rehydration process. Rehydration should be performed slowly (5). The patient's free water deficit should be calculated [Eq. (1)]. The rate of free water administration to correct the serum sodium concentration should not exceed at 0.7 mEq/L per h. A useful guideline is to administer half of the free water deficit to the patient over the first 24 h and administer the other half over the subsequent 48 h. Occasionally, vasopressin administration is required to prevent persistent free water loss. When vasopressin is used, the patient's serum sodium concentration should be carefully monitored to avoid water intoxication and hyponatremia.

$$\text{Free water deficit (L)} = \frac{\text{Patient's serum sodium} - 140}{140} \times \text{weight (kg)} \times 0.6 \quad (1)$$

Malignancy, hyperparathyroidism, and immobility are the main causes of *hypercalcemia*. The neurologic manifestations of hypercalcemia include lethargy, confusion, and ultimately coma. With hyperparathyroidism, seizures or internuclear ophthalmoplegia may occur. When symptoms occur in hypercalcemic patients, they are directly proportional to the degree of hypercalcemia and usually appear when serum calcium concentrations are >14 mg/dL. At any calcium level associated with neurologic symptoms, prompt emergency treatment is necessary. Corrections of volume deficits and forced diuresis are initiated. Further discussion may be found in Chapter 43.

Hypocalcemia in the SICU is most often encountered after multiple blood transfusions. The citrate in transfused blood products binds calcium. Other causes of hypocalcemia in the SICU include parathyroid injury, parathyroid surgery, or pancreatitis. The most common CNS manifestations are seizures, irritability, confusion, anxiety, delirium, hallucinations, and psychosis. Usually prior to CNS symptoms, patients with hypocalcemia will demonstrate perioral numbness or tingling in the fingertips. Treatment of symptomatic patients is calcium replacement. Of note, hypomagnesemia often accompanies hypocalcemia. The presence of hypomagnesemia decreases circulating parathyroid hormone levels (5). Therefore, magnesium should be given to hypocalcemic patients who fail to respond to calcium supplementation.

Osmolar abnormalities are common in critically ill patients. Most hypo-osmolar states are associated with hyponatremia. Hyperosmolar states can occur with or without hypertonicity. Solutes that freely cross the extracellular (ECF) and intracellular fluid (ICF) compartments are considered ineffective solutes. An increase in the concentration of these ineffective solutes can result in hyperosmolality. Solutes that are primarily located in the ECF compartment are effective solutes and increase the tonicity between the extracellular and intracellular compartments. Therefore, an increase in tonicity results in cellular dehydration as ICF volume shifts to the ECF compartment. The brain is particularly sensitive to cellular dehydration and, consequently, neurologic symptoms frequently occur in hyperosmolar states with hypertonicity. These conditions can occur as a result of pure water loss, hypotonic fluid loss, or effective solute gain. Hyperosmolar states can follow gastrointestinal or rental fluid losses. Symptoms include obtundation or other manifestations of CNS depression. In situations of hyperosmolar, nonhypertonic states, the CNS abnormalities are due to the solute toxicity itself (e.g., ethanol) and not by the change in ICF volume.

Thiamine deficiency is associated with Wernicke's encephalopathy. Although not commonly observed, Wernicke's encephalopathy has been reported to be evident in 2–3% of all brain pathology specimens (9). The classical triad of this disorder is confusion, impaired extraocular movements with nystagmus, and ataxia. The ocular symptoms do not have to be present in this diagnosis. Symptoms can occur abruptly or evolve gradually. In the SICU, thiamine deficiency can be seen in patients who are malnourished or who chronically consume alcohol. Alcohol is known to interfere with the gastrointestinal transport of thiamine, and patients who chronically consume excessive alcohol are known to have decreased thiamine stores (9). Patients admitted to the SICU with high blood alcohol concentration should be presumed to have thiamine deficiency. These patients should receive thiamine and folate supplementation. Administration of glucose without thiamine in deficient patients may exacerbate symptoms of Wernicke's encephalopathy.

Endocrine Causes of Mental Status Changes: In the SICU, the presence of *diabetes mellitus* in most patients is known. Surgical stress and infection may precipitate development of a hyperglycemic state with resulting, neurologic symptoms. Acute stroke, confusion, and aphasia have been reported (10). Cerebral infarction and degeneration of cortical neurons, which may be evident on a CT scan, occur with poor long-term glucose control. A recent trial reported decreased complications from surgical procedures with strict blood glucose control (11).

Central neurologic manifestations of *hypothyroidism* produce dementia, seizure, ataxia, and psychosis. These symptoms abate with thyroid hormone replacement. Autoimmune thyroiditis has been associated with neurologic symptoms that range from focal neurologic deficits to global confusion (12). The syndrome of "Hashimoto's encephalopathy" is rare. (Only approximately 30 cases are reported in the literature.) It can occur despite normal thyroid hormone serum concentration and is thought to result from an autoimmune process (12). The condition responds to steroid treatment. Thyrotoxicosis may produce psychosis or unmask a pre-existing psychiatric disorder. Seizures may occur in thyrotoxic patients and have been reported in 1–9% of these patients (10).

Up to 25% of patients with hyperparathyroidism exhibit a CNS disturbance, which can range from overt psychosis and confusion to subtle distractability. These psychiatric changes do not correlate well with calcium concentrations and may be a consequence of an increased parathyroid hormone level (10). Overall alertness decreases with serum calcium concentrations >14 mg/dL.

Cushing's syndrome and Addison's disease may produce mental status changes that are reversible with appropriate treatment.

Cardiovascular Causes of Mental Status Change: Myocardial infarction and dysrhythmias are important, and possibly life threatening, emergency causes of mental status changes. Other cardiovascular causes of encephalopathy exist. Patients who have undergone coronary artery bypass (CAB) or other cardiac surgery utilizing the heart–lung bypass machine may experience postoperative mental status changes. This phenomenon occurs in a high percentage of patients undergoing on-pump CAB and is seen more often in older patients and those individuals experiencing longer pump run times. The etiology of this disorder is not well understood. It may be a consequence of intraoperative cerebral hypoxia. The alteration in mental status can prolong the patient's time on the ventilator and ICU length of stay. Previous studies have shown that depression of neuropsychological status may persist for up to one year (13). However, a recent study observed a generalized improvement in cognitive function after an average of 9 days (14). Prior to improvement, these patients can become belligerent. Haloperidol may be appropriate treatment. Benzodiazepines can worsen the patient's confusion.

Iatrogenic Causes of Mental Status Change: The patient in the ICU is continuously awakened for nursing care, vital sign assessments, and examinations from various doctors. Lights are on during the night, and the patient's day/night cycles can become reversed. This atmosphere compromises adequate, restful sleep. Days to weeks of sleep deprivation can produce confusion. Older patients are especially sensitive to their environment and depend on environmental cues to keep their lives in order. Removing an elderly patient from a familiar setting can unmask underlying dementia. The lack of normal environmental cues coupled with administration of unusual medications and sleep deprivation, can lead to encephalopathy. Although a typical response is to further sedate the belligerent, confused patient, increasing environmental cues, such as turning off the lights at night, may help modify the patient's behavior. If necessary, small amounts of haloperidol may lessen agitation. Benzodiazepines should be avoided in this population. Later symptoms of withdrawal can occur and further cloud the patient's mental status.

Anesthetics, narcotics, and sedatives can compromise a patient's mental status. Despite their side effects, these drugs often are necessary to treat pain and to sedate patients requiring mechanical ventilation. Patients who receive narcotics or benzodiazepines for a prolonged period of time may experience withdrawal symptoms, if these medications are discontinued abruptly. Gradual weaning of those agents may obviate these withdrawal symptoms.

Steroids can cause an encephalopathy, with psychosis as the classic presentation. Overt steroid psychosis occurs in <1% of patients receiving steroids (15). The more common symptoms are tremulousness, inability to concentrate, and insomnia. Treatment is discontinuation of the steroids. Antipsychotics or mood stabilizers are used as necessary (15).

Hepatic Causes of Mental Status Changes: Patients with acute or chronic liver disease may display signs of hepatic encephalopathy (HE). Hepatic encephalopathy reflects a spectrum of neuropsychiatric abnormalities seen in patients with liver dysfunction after exclusion of other known brain disease (16). HE can be associated with acute liver failure, cirrhosis and portal hypertension, or portal-systemic bypass with or without intrinsic hepatocellular disease. This disturbance in cognition can range from a shortened attention span to coma and can have an abrupt or insidious onset. Focal findings are unusual. The mental status changes seen in HE are not pathognomonic, and other causes, such as structural or metabolic abnormalities, need to be eliminated.

The pathogenesis of hepatic encephalopathy is not fully defined. It is thought to be a result of CNS exposure to toxins that are not cleared by the liver. Bacterial breakdown of foodstuffs or blood in the intestine can produce these toxins. Although many agents, such as ammonia, short chain fatty acids, false neurotransmitters, and gamma-amino-butyric acid (GABA), have been investigated, multiple factors are the likely cause of HE (17). Although ammonia levels are often obtained in patients suspected of having HE, its plasma levels do not correlate with the severity of the encephalopathy (17). Glutamine concentrations in the CSF are elevated in patients with HE. This amino acid is a substrate for many neurotransmitters in the brain, and glutamine concentrations in the CSF *do* parallel the extent of encephalopathy. This assay requires lumbar puncture and may not be obtainable at all hospitals. A lumbar puncture may not be prudent on these patients, who often demonstrate severe coagulopathy. CT or MR neuroimaging techniques cannot be used to detect HE, which demonstrates no structural abnormality on these studies. PET scanning or labeled neurotransmitter scans may improve diagnostic ability in the future.

In patients with chronic liver disease, gastrointestinal bleeding, high-protein diet, infection, drugs, and electrolyte abnormalities can precipitate HE. For patients receiving tube feeds or hyperalimentation *and who have evidence of HE*, nutrition with high levels of branched chain amino acids (BCAAs) should be routine. This practice is derived from evidence that patients with hepatic failure have a decreased ability to metabolize aromatic amino acids and will preferentially utilize BCAAs for energy. With the subsequent decreased availability of BCAAs, fewer of these amino acids are available to the CNS to produce essential neurotransmitters. The patient will then utilize aromatic amino acids to produce false neurotransmitters, which have been implicated in the pathogenesis of HE. Increasing the availability of BCAAs theoretically will reduce encephalopathy.

Other aspects of treatment attempt to decrease bacterial count in the gastrointestinal tract to reduce bacterial substrates, and the resulting toxins affecting the brain. Lactulose is the mainstay of therapy for patients with HE. It is administered either orally or rectally. Lactulose is metabolized by intestinal bacteria to acidify the colonic environment. Increased acidity converts ammonia into an ionized form, which is less absorbable. The antibiotics neomycin and metronidazole have been used to decontaminate the colon and decrease HE. Administration of these antibiotics is generally reserved for those patients who are refractory to lactulose treatment.

Septic Encephalopathy: Septic encephalopathy is an acute change in mental status secondary to an infectious process extrinsic to the brain. Patients with sepsis can have a range of symptoms including lethargy, confusion, disorientation, agitation, stupor, and coma. *Changes in mental status, respiratory alkalosis, and tachypnnea are often the first signs of sepsis, and all patients with this constellation of symptoms should be presupposed to have sepsis, until it is excluded.* Septic encephalopathy reportedly develops in 9–71% of all septic patients (18), but since many of these patients are concomitantly treated with sedatives, paralytic agents, mechanical ventilation, and narcotics, the incidence of encephalopathy may be under reported. The wide variation of incidence in the literature reflects the various definitions of encephalopathy, most of which are subjective. A recent prospective study evaluated electroencephalograms (EEGs) of septic patients and found that impaired subcortical and cortical pathways occurred in 34% and 84%, respectively (19). The cortical impairment correlated with the severity of the illness, and generally reverses as the patient's condition improves (19). Another recent study, which utilized standardized methods for scoring encephalopathy, found the incidence of septic encephalopathy to be between 50% and 62%, with no differences noted among age, sex, and laboratory evaluation (20). When compared with patients without encephalopathy, those who exhibit septic encephalopathy demonstrated increased mortality (20); however, it is unclear whether the encephalopathy itself is concomitant with more severe disease.

The etiology of septic encephalopathy was initially thought to be the result of microabscesses in the brain or of microorganisms in the blood affecting brain function. This hypothesis was not supported by pathologic tissue examination or by blood cultures of septic patients. Also, the onset of encephalopathy frequently precedes any objective measurement of infection. More likely, the changes in mental status are multifactorial and may include the "action of inflammatory mediators on the brain or a cytotoxic response by brain cells to these mediators" (21). The pathophysiologic mechanism may additionally be explained by a cytokine-induced decrease in systemic vascular resistance, which overwhelms the body's compensatory mechanisms for maintaining cerebral perfusion. Another possibility is that cerebral edema occurs during sepsis, which decreases cerebral blood flow. This occurrence has been demonstrated in septic pigs (2,21).

Early diagnosis of septic encephalopathy can be life saving. If diagnosed promptly, appropriate therapy may be initiated. The mental status changes are reversible and resolve with resolution of the inflammatory process. Generally, these patients are somnolent and display decreased spontaneous activity; however, if agitation occurs, sedation is appropriate.

Uremic Encephalopathy: Patients with renal failure can develop neurologic manifestations that result from metabolic derangements. The symptoms of uremic encephalopathy are nonspecific and the *severity of symptoms does not correlate with laboratory evaluation.* Because of the similarity of signs and symptoms to other, more urgent causes of mental status change, uremic encephalopathy is a diagnosis of exclusion. Other causes should be excluded before establishing this diagnosis.

A classic, although nonspecific, sign is asterixis. Early CNS symptoms include impaired concentration, apathy, dysarthria, and insomnia (22). Late symptoms can range from hallucinations to convulsions and coma. Seizures develop more often in patients who have massive, rapid shifts in electrolytes or pH. Such shifts may be seen in acute renal failure. The etiologic agent or agents responsible for uremic encephalopathy are not well understood. Several agents have been studied, including creatinine and BUN. However, both humans and animals dialyzed against a high urea dialysate show dramatic improvement in neurologic symptoms despite high serum urea concentrations (23). Injection of creatinine or its metabolites has not induced neurologic symptoms. The only etiologic agent clearly involved in the pathogenesis of neurologic symptoms is parathyroid hormone (22). Its mechanism of neurotoxicity is controversial.

Neurodiagnostic testing may be abnormal in patients suspected of having uremic encephalopathy; however, these are not specific. EEG testing, also nonspecific, can be of some diagnostic value if serial examinations are performed (22).

The "dialysis disequilibrium syndrome" can occur during the initiation of dialysis in patients who are profoundly uremic. This syndrome is thought to result from brain swelling that occurs in response to a lag in osmolar and electrolyte shifts between the blood and brain in patients initiating dialysis. This syndrome should be considered in encephalopathic renal failure patients. The occurrence of mental status changes around the time of dialysis should distinguish this diagnosis from the more insidious changes characteristic of uremic encephalopathy (22).

Aluminum neurotoxicity also can be seen in renal failure patients. This progressive myoclonic dementia was initially induced by aluminum contamination of the dialysate; today, however, the aluminum content in this fluid is routinely tested. The disorder can still be seen in patients taking aluminum compounds for control of hyperphosphatemia. Patients initially present with stammering. Gradually, the syndrome leads to seizures and dementia. Aluminum deposition on tissue biopsy proves the diagnosis.

Improved understanding of the pathophysiologic mechanisms involved with uremic encephalopathy may lead to definitive treatment in the future.

SUMMARY

- When evaluating a patient for encephalopathy:
  1. Assess the airway as first priority; secure an airway as necessary.
  2. Monitor vital signs; do not forget the respiratory rate.
  3. Obtain a serum blood glucose concentration.
  4. Obtain an arterial blood gas to identify hypoxemia and associated acid–base disorders.
- Encephalopathy may be an early manifestation of septic shock or myocardial infarction.
- Thorough neurologic examination is vital. Head CT and MRI may be indicated.
- Meningitis should be considered in patients who have recently been treated with an epidural catheter or ventriculostomy catheter. It should also be considered in patients with head trauma, recent back surgery, or recent neck surgery.
- Hyponatremia is the most common electrolyte abnormality in the ICU and may cause mental status changes. Seizures caused by hyponatremia require expeditious correction of the serum sodium concentration to 120–125 mEq/L.
- Hypernatremia should be corrected gradually.
- Hypercalcemia may produce a range of neurologic abnormalities. Initial treatment is correction of volume deficits and forced diuresis.
- Hypocalcemia usually occurs after thyroid or parathyroid surgery. Asymptomatic patients generally do not require calcium replacement.
- Thiamine deficiency is a common contributor to encephalopathy in the chronically malnourished or alcoholic patient.
- Endocrine causes of mental status changes include: diabetes mellitus, hypothyroidism, hyperthyroidism, hyperparathyroidism, Cushing's syndrome, and Addison's disease.
- Treatment of hepatic encephalopathy includes metabolic support with branch chain amino acid formulations, lactulose, neomycin, and metronidazole.
- Etiology of uremic encephalopathy is poorly understood. Underlying renal failure should be treated. Aluminum toxicity may be a cause.

REFERENCES

1. Dorland's Illustrated Medical Dictionary. 26th ed. Philadelphia, PA: W.B. Saunders Co., 2000.
2. Fraser GL, Prato S, Riker RR, Berthiaume D, Wilkins ML. Evaluation of agitation in ICU patients: incidence, severity, and treatment in the young versus the elderly. Pharmacotherapy 2000; 20:75–82.
3. Decaux G, Musch W, Soupart A. Hyponatremia in the intensive care: from diagnosis to treatment. Acta Clin Belg 2000; 55:68–77.
4. Verbalis JG, Gullans SR. Hyponatremia causes large sustained reductions in brain content of multiple organic osmolytes in rats. Brain Res 1991; 567:274–282.
5. Riggs JE. Neurologic manifestations of fluid and electrolyte disturbances. Neurol Clin 1989; 7(3):509–523.
6. Soupart A, Decaux G. Therapeutic recommendations for management of severe hyponatremia: current concepts on pathogenesis and prevention of neurologic complications. Clin Nephrol 1996; 46(3):149–169.

7. Ayus JC, Wheeler JM, Arieff AI. Postoperative hyponatremic encephalopathy in menstruant women. Ann Intern Med 1992; 117:891–897.
8. Soupart A, Decaux G. Therapeutic recommendations for management of severe hyponatremia: current concepts on pathogenesis and prevention of neurologic complications. Clin Nephrol 1996; 46(3):149–169.
9. Albers JW, Nostrant TT, Rigs JE. Neurologic manifestations of gastrointestinal disease. Neurol Clin 1989; 7(3):525–548.
10. Kaminski HJ, Ruff RL. Neurologic complications of endocrine diseases. Neurol Clin 1989; 7(3):489–507.
11. Van den Berghe G, Wouters P, Weekers F, Verwaest C, Bruyninckx F, Schetz M, Vlasselaers D, Ferdinande P, Lauwers P, Bouillon R. Intensive insulin therapy in critically ill patients. N Engl J Med 2001; 345(19):1359–1367.
12. Chen HC, Masharani U. Hashimoto's encephalopathy. South Med J 2000; 93(5):504–506.
13. Hammeke TA, Hastings JE. Neuropsychologic alterations after cardiac operations. J Thoracic Cardiovasc Surg 1988; 96:326–331.
14. Mullges W, Berg D, Schmidtke A, Weinacker B, Toyka KV. Early natural course of transient encephalopathy after coronary artery bypass grafting. Crit Care Med 2000; 28(6):1808–1811.
15. Wada K, Yamada N, Sato T, Suzuki H, Miki M, Lee Y, Akiyama K, Kuroda S. Corticosteroid induced psychotic and mood disorders. Psychosomatics 2001; 42(6):461–466.
16. Ferenci P, Lockwood A, Mullen K, Tarter R, Weissenborn K, Blei AT. Hepatic Encephalopathy—Definition, nomenclature, diagnosis, and quantification: Final Report of the Working Party at the 11th World Congresses of Gastroenterology, Vienna, 1998. Hepatology 2002; 35:716–721.
17. Rothstein JD, Herlong HF. Neurologic manifestations of hepatic disease. Neurol Clin 1989; 7(3):563–569.
18. Sprung CL, Peduzzi PN, Shatney CH, Schein RMH, Wilson MF, Sjeagren JN, Hinshaw LB. The Veterans Administration Systemic Sepsis Cooperative Study Group. Impact of encephalopathy on mortality in the sepsis syndrome. Crit Care Med 1990; 18:801–806.
19. Zauner C, Gendo A, Kramer L, Funk GC, Bauer E, Schenk P, Ratheiser K, Madl C. Impaired subcortical and cortical sensory evoked potential pathways in septic patients. Crit Care Med 2002; 30(5):1136–1139.
20. Eidelman LA, Putterman D, Putterman C, Sprung CL. The spectrum of septic encephalopathy. J Am Med Assoc 1996; 275(6):470–473.
21. Papadopoulos MC, Davies DC, Moss RF, Tighe D, Bennett ED. Pathophysiology septic encephalopathy: a review. Crit Care Med 2000; 28(8):3019–3024.
22. Moe SM, Sprague SM. Uremic Encephalopathy. Clin Nephrol 1994; 42(4):251–256.
23. Merrill JP, Legrain M, Hoigne R. Observations on the role of urea in uremia. Am J Med 1953; 14:519–520.

D. Cardiovascular Function

21
Altered Cardiac Physiology

Vivian L. Clark
Henry Ford Hospital, Detroit, Michigan, USA

James A. Kruse
Detroit Receiving Hospital, Detroit, Michigan, USA

Richard W. Carlson
Maricopa Medical Center, Phoenix, Arizona, USA

Knowledge of the physiology and manifestations of altered cardiac function is essential for effective clinical management of critically ill patients. Equally important is clinician awareness of the potential effects of critical illness itself on cardiac physiology. Anticipation and recognition of these effects allow the rational selection and titration of therapy to optimize cardiac function, restore vital organ perfusion, and aid in preventing or minimizing organ system failure.

NORMAL PHYSIOLOGY

Cardiac performance and myocardial oxygen demand are dependent on four major factors: heart rate, preload, afterload, and contractility (1,2). As cardiac output (CO) is the product of heart rate and stroke volume, both bradydysrhythmias and tachydysrhythmias can adversely affect it.

Heart Rate

The ability to tolerate abnormal cardiac rhythms is largely dependent on the patient's underlying ventricular function. For example, an individual with chronic left ventricular dysfunction or marked left ventricular hypertrophy may tolerate atrial fibrillation poorly, even if it results in only a modest increase in heart rate. On the other hand, an otherwise normal individual at rest may tolerate rates of 200 min^{-1} or more without significant hemodynamic consequences. Treating dysrhythmias usually improves cardiac function in acutely ill patients. Most sustained dysrhythmias of ventricular origin will require pharmacologic or electrical conversion; whereas, the adverse effects of supraventricular dysrhythmias often respond to rate control measures alone. Sinus tachycardia never occurs as a primary dysrhythmia. Rather, this rhythm represents a compensatory response to either a physiologic or pathologic condition, such as exercise, fever, hypoxia, hypovolemia, anemia, heart failure, thyrotoxicosis, agitation, or pain. Certain drugs (e.g., β-adrenergic agonists) can produce sinus tachycardia. Therefore, a patient with sinus tachycardia requires a diligent search for an underlying cause. Efforts to slow this rhythm using digoxin or β-blockers are rarely appropriate; instead, treatment should focus on correcting the underlying cause.

Preload

Preload refers to ventricular end-diastolic volume and is a measure of myocardial fiber stretch just prior to contraction. The Frank–Starling principle expresses the relationship between preload and stroke volume generated during a subsequent systole. This relationship is depicted in Fig. 1. The point at which ventricular volume is maximal indicates end-diastolic myocardial fiber stretch. Although the Frank–Starling principle is based on myocardial fiber length or ventricular volume, for clinical purposes, preload is frequently estimated by ventricular filling pressure, because volume measurements are not readily obtainable at the bedside (2,3). The relationship between ventricular pressure and ventricular volume during diastole is termed *compliance* (also referred to by its reciprocal, stiffness). This stiffness can be represented graphically by the slope of the diastolic portion of the ventricular pressure–volume loop (Fig. 2). If chamber compliance is assumed to be constant, then changes in intracavitary pressure will be proportional to changes in chamber volume. However, myocardial compliance is altered in a number of disease states. For example, in a low-compliance (stiff) ventricle, such as that observed in a patient with myocardial hypertrophy, a given change in ventricular volume will result in a greater change in ventricular pressure compared with that seen in an individual with normal compliance (4,5). Certain drugs can also affect ventricular compliance. For example, β-adrenergic catecholamines decrease myocardial compliance; whereas, β-blockers and calcium-channel blockers produce the opposite effect.

In the absence of valvular stenosis, atrial pressure is in equilibrium with ventricular pressure at end-diastole. Right atrial pressure or central venous pressure (CVP), which is

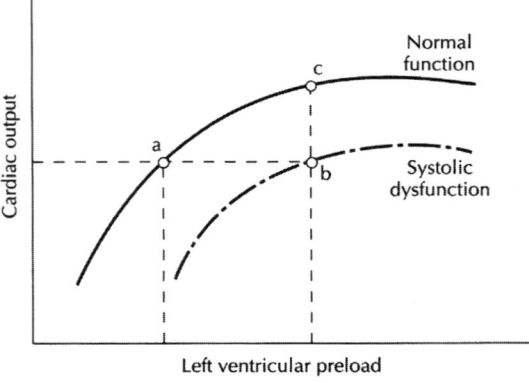

Figure 1 Relationship between preload and CO in normal cardiac function and systolic dysfunction. Normal heart (a) requires lower preload than heart with impaired systolic function (b) to maintain normal resting CO. A given preload level results in higher CO in normal heart (c) compared with heart with impaired systolic function (b).

Altered Cardiac Physiology

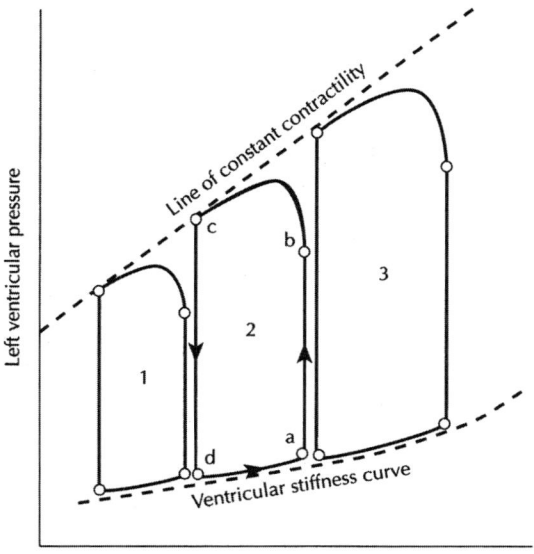

Figure 2 Left ventricular pressure–volume loops showing changes in preload and afterload. Loop 2 represents a normal cardiac cycle. During diastole (segment d–a), the ventricle fills and pressure increases until end-diastolic pressure and end-diastolic volume are attained (a), representing preload. The slope of curve (d–a) is a measure of ventricular stiffness. During isovolumic contraction (both valves closed), pressure rapidly increases whereas volume remains the same (segment a–b). When intraventricular pressure exceeds central aortic pressure, the aortic valve opens, and systole ensues (b). Point b represents afterload. As the ventricle empties, the ventricular pressure falls until it is below aortic pressure and the aortic valve then closes (c). Stroke volume is indicated by the distance between points b and c along the x-axis. During the isovolumic relaxation period (both valves closed), the ventricular pressure falls rapidly (segment c–d) until it is below left atrial pressure; the mitral valve then opens (point d), beginning a new cycle. Changes in preload and afterload are evident in loops 1 and 3. Note the point c of each loop falls along the line of constant contractility, indicating the same inotropic state for all three loops. Changes in contractility would be indicated by a deviation from this line.

nearly equivalent to right atrial pressure, is therefore commonly used as a surrogate for right ventricular filling pressure. Except in certain postcardiac surgery patients, left atrial pressure is not directly accessible to the clinician; however, the balloon-tipped pulmonary artery (PA) catheter allows left atrial pressure to be estimated (3,5). During balloon inflation, a continuous static column of fluid exists between the monitoring orifice at the tip of the catheter and the left atrium. Thus, pulmonary artery occlusion pressure (PAOP) and right atrial pressure serve as indirect estimates of left and right ventricular filling pressures, respectively (Fig. 3a).

According to the Frank–Starling relationship, inadequate preload, such as occurs with hypovolemia, results in decreased CO. If the degree of volume depletion is severe, it will result in hypotension and frank circulatory shock (6). Factors that can lead to increased preload include intravascular volume overload, systolic ventricular dysfunction, and diastolic ventricular dysfunction. Patients with abnormal ventricular function

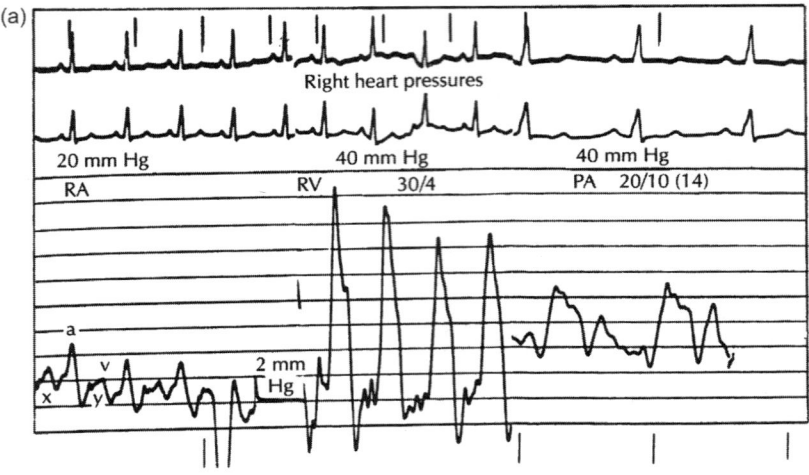

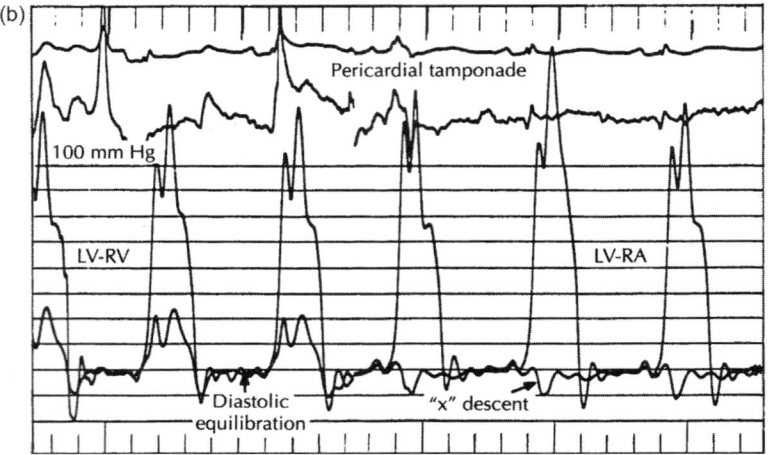

Figure 3 (a) Normal pressure sweep during right heart catheterization as the PA catheter is advanced from the right atrium (RA) to the right ventricle (RV), to the PA. Normal *a* and *v* waves are shown in RA and PAOP (wedge) waveforms. (b) Pressure sweep during right heart catheterization showing characteristic hemodynamic findings of pericardial tamponade: elevated filling pressures, decreased pulse pressures, and equalization of diastolic pressures. (Adapted from Kruse JA, Armendariz E. Hemodynamic monitoring. In: Carlson RW, Geheb MA, eds. Principles and Practice of Medical Intensive Care. Philadelphia: W.B. Saunders, 1993:1079–1103, and Clark VL. Pericardial tamponade. In: Kruse JA, Fink MP, Carlson RW, eds. Saunders Manual of Critical Care. Philadelphia: Elsevier, 2002, with permission.)

generally require higher filling pressures to maintain optimal CO (3). Increasing right- and left-sided preload can eventually lead to peripheral and pulmonary vascular congestion, respectively. Severe increases in left ventricular pressure can increase PAOP sufficiently to cause hydrostatic pulmonary edema with attendant hypoxemia and possibly respiratory failure.

Afterload

Afterload can be defined as overall resistance or impedance to ejection of blood by the ventricles (2). Blood pressure is the simplest measure of afterload. Systemic blood pressure can be used to estimate left ventricular afterload, and pulmonary arterial pressure can be used to estimate right ventricular afterload. Afterload also can be represented as the ventricular pressure at the end of isovolumic contraction (see Fig. 2). As this pressure increases, resistance to ventricular ejection rises and the ventricle must exert greater force during systole. Increases in afterload, therefore, are associated with increases in myocardial oxygen consumption (MvO_2). The added work imposed by an elevation in afterload can also precipitate heart failure in patients with underlying cardiac disease. Vascular resistance represents another way of quantifying afterload (2). Systemic vascular resistance (SVR) and pulmonary vascular resistance (PVR) can be calculated at the bedside using the CO obtained by the thermodilution PA catheter and the pressure gradient across the respective vascular beds (Table 1). Factors that lead to increased afterload include systemic hypertension (both essential and secondary varieties), use of vasoconstricting agents, and conditions resulting in obstruction to ventricular outflow such as aortic valvular stenosis. Positive pressure ventilation, use of positive end-expiratory pressure, pulmonary embolism, and pulmonary arterial hypertension (both primary and that secondary to left ventricular dysfunction or mitral valvular disease) increase right ventricular afterload. Left ventricular afterload is decreased by systemic vasodilation (which can occur spontaneously in sepsis and cirrhosis), arteriovenous shunting, and a variety of drugs, including nitroprusside and other vasodilating agents.

Table 1 Formulas and Normal Ranges for Common Hemodynamic Variables

Variable/formula	Range
Right atrial or central venous pressure (CVP)	2–8 mm Hg
Right ventricular pressure [s/d]	15–30/2–8 mm Hg
Pulmonary artery pressure (PAP) [s/d/$\bar{x}$]	15–30/4–8/12–15 mm Hg
Pulmonary artery occlusion pressure (PAOP)	5–12 mm Hg
Mean arterial pressure (MAP) [$=d + \{(s - d)/3\}$]	85–100 mm Hg
Cardiac output (CO)	4.5–6.0 L/min
Cardiac index (CI) [$=$CO/BSA]	2.6–3.8 L/min/m^2
Stroke volume (SV) [$=1000 \times$ CO/HR]	60–90 mL
Stroke index (SI) [$=1000 \times$ CO/(HR $\times$ BSA)]	35–50 mL/m^2
Right ventricular stroke work index (RVSWI) [$=$SI $\times$ ($\overline{\text{PAP}}$ − PAOP) $\times$ 0.0136]	8–12 g m/m^2
Left ventricular stroke work index (LVSWI) [$=$SI $\times$ (MAP − CVP) $\times$ 0.0136]	40–60 g m/m^2
Systemic vascular resistance index (SVRI) [$=$(MAP − CVP) $\times$ 80/CI]	1400–2100 dyne s/cm^5/m^2
Pulmonary vascular resistance index (PVRI) [$=$($\overline{\text{PAP}}$ − PAOP) $\times$ 80/CI]	180–400 dyne s/cm^5/m^2
Ejection fraction (EF) [$=100 \times$ SV/EDV]	55–75%

Note: s, systolic; d, diastolic; $\bar{x}$, mean; BSA, body surface area (m^2); EDV, ventricular end-diastolic volume (mL).

Contractility

Contractility refers to the intrinsic inotropic property of the myocardium that is independent of the effects of changes in preload, afterload, or heart rate. Although the position of the pressure–volume loop changes as preload, afterload, and ventricular stiffness are varied, the position of the end-systolic pressure–volume point (Fig. 2) is constrained to move along a given straight line as long as contractility is constant. An increase in contractility results in an increase in the slope of this line; whereas, a decrease in contractility results in a shallower slope. Clinically, ejection fraction (Table 1) is sometimes used to gauge contractility, although in reality this variable also is influenced to some degree by both preload and afterload (4). Contractility may be increased in hypertrophic cardiomyopathy, in some hypermetabolic states (e.g., thyrotoxicosis), and by inotropic agents such as β-adrenergic agonists, milrinone, and digoxin. Contractility is diminished in myocardial ischemia or infarction, in cardiomyopathic processes, in sepsis, and by a variety of drugs, including β-blockers and calcium-channel blockers.

The overall work performed by the ventricle is the product of pressure and volume, represented by the area within the pressure–volume loop. Calculated stroke work index thus can be used to assess the total contractile work generated by the left or right ventricle (see Table 1).

PATHOPHYSIOLOGY OF HEART FAILURE

Abnormal systolic function, one of the most frequently encountered cardiac disorders, is a common cause of postoperative complications. The most common causes are ischemic heart disease, hypertensive heart disease, valvular heart disease, and dilated cardiomyopathy. The hallmark of systolic dysfunction is impaired contractility, which is usually secondary to myocardial ischemia, necrosis, or fibrosis. In an effort to maintain adequate CO, several compensatory responses, including salt and water retention, that are due to activation of neurohormonal mechanisms, occur (2,4). Fluid retention leads to ventricular dilation, and as a consequence, preload is elevated. This increase in preload serves as a compensatory mechanism that helps maintain a normal level of cardiac work by way of the Frank–Starling relationship (see Fig. 1). The pressure–volume relationship in systolic dysfunction is depicted in Fig. 4 (loop 3). Stroke volume is impaired, but in mild cases near normal CO may be maintained by compensatory tachycardia.

The elevated filling pressures and low CO resulting from systolic dysfunction are associated with several clinical manifestations (Table 2). In addition to tachycardia, these include neck vein distention, peripheral edema, and the presence of rales (indicating pulmonary vascular congestion and pulmonary edema). If systolic function is severely impaired, hypotension and signs of diminished end-organ perfusion, such as oliguria and changes in mentation, may be observed. Many patients with systolic dysfunction are asymptomatic under normal conditions, but clinical symptoms may be precipitated by the stress of sepsis, trauma, or surgery. Two-dimensional echocardiography or multiple uptake-gated acquisition (MUGA) scanning usually demonstrate a reduced ejection fraction and increased ventricular volume.

Figure 1 demonstrates the relationship between filling pressure and CO in a normal heart and in a heart with abnormal systolic function. Patients with systolic dysfunction may be quite sensitive to changes in preload, and their clinical condition may deteriorate

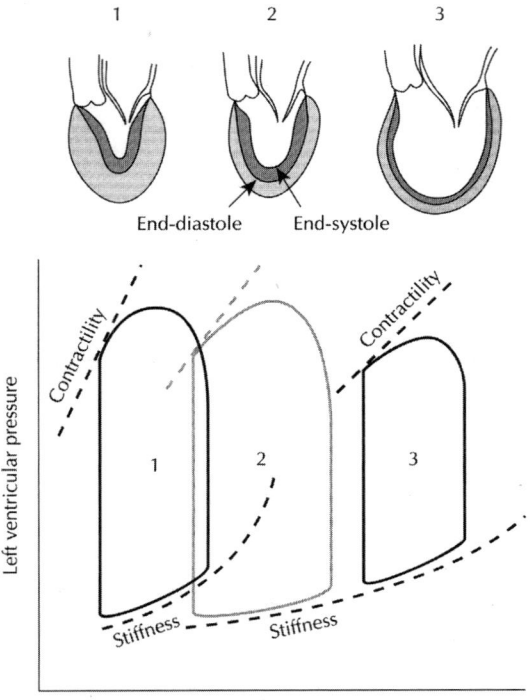

Figure 4 Left ventricular pressure–volume loops comparing normal ventricular function (loop 2) with pure diastolic dysfunction (loop 1) and pure systolic dysfunction (loop 3). Note that left ventricular volume is lower than normal in diastolic dysfunction but higher than normal in systolic dysfunction. End-diastolic pressure is increased and stroke volume may be decreased in both disorders. The increased slopes of the diastolic (bottom) portion of loop 1 indicates increased intrinsic stiffness (decreased compliance) characteristic of diastolic dysfunction. In systolic dysfunction, the ventricular stiffness curve is normal, but stiffness is increased because the ventricle is distended. The slope of the respective contractility lines demonstrates diminished contractility characteristic of systolic dysfunction and augmented contractility that may be seen in diastolic dysfunction.

when subjected to either hypovolemia or fluid overload. In addition, increased afterload may lead to clinical decompensation. This condition can occur as a result of increasing MvO_2 in the face of coronary artery disease or simply from the greater work load imposed on an already failing heart. Perioperative use of the balloon-tipped thermodilution PA catheter for hemodynamic monitoring in selected patients with known systolic dysfunction may allow early recognition and prevention of cardiac decompensation (3).

A number of pharmacologic agents are useful for treating systolic dysfunction (2,7). In cases where fluid overload, indicated by edema or pulmonary congestion, is present without compromise of CO, diuretics alone may be effective. Loop diuretics such as furosemide, bumetanide, or torsemide are the agents of choice. Nitrates, which also reduce preload, are a useful adjunct, particularly in patients with underlying coronary artery disease. Nitrates can be administered orally, topically, or by continuous intravenous infusion. If low CO accompanies congestion, then digoxin combined with diuretics may be of benefit. Digoxin is particularly useful in patients with atrial dysrhythmias, such as

Table 2 Clinical Features Frequently Present in Heart Failure

Mechanism	Finding
Elevated filling pressures	Rales, rhonchi
	Distended neck veins
	Hepatic congestion
	Pulmonary congestion
	Peripheral edema
	Hypoxemia
	Pleural effusions
	Ascites
Low cardiac output	Tachycardia
	Low pulse pressure
	Oliguria
	Altered sensorium
	Cold extremities
	Anorexia

atrial fibrillation or flutter, but has also been shown to be of value in individuals in sinus rhythm (7).

Afterload-reducing agents are now considered a standard treatment for patients with systolic dysfunction and low CO, and they have been shown in a number of clinical trials to improve survival in patients with heart failure (8). In emergency situations, nitroprusside can be useful because it is administered by intravenous infusion, has a short half-life, and can be titrated easily. However, nitroprusside use requires intra-arterial pressure monitoring. It can be used only for a short duration, because cyanide and thiocyanate toxicity may develop with high-dose or prolonged infusions, particularly in individuals with renal insufficiency. Nesiritide, a recombinant form of B-type natriuretic peptide, has recently been approved for acute cardiac decompensation in patients without hypotension. It has vasodilator properties, promotes diuresis, opposes the activity of the renin–angiotensin system, and has a better safety profile than nitroprusside. It is administered as an intravenous bolus followed by a continuous infusion given for up to 48 h. In general, it does not require the use of invasive hemodynamic monitoring (9). For long-term treatment, angiotensin-coverting enzyme (ACE) inhibitors are the agents of choice, but they too must be used with caution in patients with impaired renal function. A newer class of related agents, angiotensin receptor inhibitors, is a good alternative in patients intolerant of ACE inhibitor side effects. Other afterload-reducing agents that may be of value include hydralazine, prazosin, and high-dose intravenous nitroglycerin. β-Blockers have been shown to be beneficial in the treatment of chronic left ventricular dysfunction but generally have no role in the treatment of acutely decompensated heart failure.

Patients with severe compromise of systolic function, particularly when accompanied by hypotension, may require inotropic agents such as dobutamine, dopamine, or amrinone for short-term hemodynamic support (7). Dobutamine, a β-adrenergic catecholamine, usually increases CO without significantly increasing MvO_2, and it often lowers PAOP. Because dobutamine has peripheral vasodilating properties, it may not increase blood pressure and should not be given to patients with uncontrolled hypotension. Dopamine has both α- and β-adrenergic properties and may be effective in increasing both CO and blood pressure in hypotensive patients. The improvement in blood pressure, however, may occur at the expense of increasing both MvO_2 and PAOP. Dopamine also stimulates dopaminergic receptors in the splanchnic and renal vasculature. At low doses dopamine may augment renal perfusion and increase urine output, but it has not been shown to have renal protective effects or improve renal recovery in acute renal failure. Phosphodiesterase-III inhibitors, such as amrinone and milrinone, have both inotropic and vasodilating properties. Although they are not catecholamines, their effects are similar to dobutamine.

Diastolic dysfunction is increasingly recognized as an important cause of cardiac decompensation. Patients with this abnormality generally have reduced myocardial compliance or abnormal myocardial relaxation with impaired ventricular filling, while often demonstrating normal or even hypercontractile systolic function (10–12). The pressure–volume loops in Fig. 4 illustrate some of the physiologic characteristics of diastolic dysfunction compared with normal function and systolic dysfunction. Most notable are the increased stiffness of the ventricle, as shown by the steeper slope of the diastolic portion of the loop, and the relatively low ventricular volumes.

Diastolic dysfunction is seen most often in patients with severe left ventricular hypertrophy, which may be idiopathic, secondary to long-standing hypertension, or the result of outflow obstruction, such as that caused by aortic stenosis. It also can occur in ischemic heart disease, in which it is frequently combined with systolic dysfunction. Less commonly, diastolic dysfunction can be due to infiltrative cardiomyopathy, restrictive cardiac disease, or pericardial disease leading to inadequate ventricular filling. Hypertrophy and ischemia both impair myocardial relaxation and alter ventricular compliance (13). Increased cardiac chamber stiffness also results in elevation of filling pressure for any given level of ventricular volume or preload. This disturbance in the pressure–volume relationship in diastolic dysfunction can be seen in Fig. 4 (loop 1). The increase in venous pressure provides some degree of compensation by maintaining the driving pressure for diastolic filling, but high pulmonary and systemic venous pressures can lead to congestive manifestations. Left ventricular diastolic dysfunction thus produces clinical signs and symptoms of pulmonary congestion and the hemodynamic abnormality of an elevated PAOP.

Distinguishing diastolic heart failure from that due to systolic dysfunction has important management implications (Table 3) (13,14). Patients with diastolic dysfunction often have normal cardiac size on physical examination and chest roentgenography,

Table 3 Characteristics and Treatment of Systolic and Diastolic Dysfunction

	Systolic dysfunction	Diastolic dysfunction
Ventricular size	Dilated	Hypertrophied
Contractility	Decreased	Normal to increased
Cardiac output	Low	Low or normal
Clinical findings	Pulmonary congestion	Pulmonary congestion
	Peripheral congestion	Peripheral congestion
	S3 gallop rhythm	S4 gallop rhythm
Acute treatment	Diuresis	β-Adrenergic blockers
	Afterload reduction	Calcium-channel blockers
	Inotropic drugs	ACE inhibitors
	Intra-aortic balloon pump	

although signs of left ventricular hypertrophy such as a prominent, sustained point of maximal impulse are often present. Although a third heart sound is frequently present in patients with systolic dysfunction, those with diastolic dysfunction often have an S4 gallop rhythm. Both groups may have signs of pulmonary and peripheral congestion. Two-dimensional echocardiography with Doppler sonography can prove extremely useful in identifying patients with diastolic dysfunction. This imaging modality often will demonstrate significant left ventricular hypertrophy with normal ventricular size, along with normal or hyperdynamic systolic function in these patients. Doppler examination may reveal abnormal indices of diastolic function, such as altered mitral flow velocity patterns.

Appropriate treatment for patients with pure diastolic dysfunction may differ markedly from that of patients with pure systolic dysfunction. Inotropic agents such as β-agonists and digoxin can actually worsen cardiac failure that is due to purely diastolic dysfunction. This effect also may be true of preload- and afterload-reducing drugs such as diuretics, nitrates, and vasodilators, although some reduction in preload with diuretics may be necessary if significant edema or pulmonary vascular congestion is present. Patients frequently improve clinically with agents such as β-blockers and nondihydropyridine calcium-channel blockers, which improve myocardial relaxation and thereby enhance ventricular compliance (13,14). β-Blockers also may improve diastolic filling by slowing the heart rate. In addition these drugs can be used to treat associated hypertension, which often underlies diastolic dysfunction. ACE inhibitors have been shown to effectively lead to regression of myocardial hypertrophy and may be useful in some patients. In acute decompensation, short-term use of nesiritide, which improves myocardial relaxation, may be beneficial in patients who fail to respond to conventional therapy.

When hypotension occurs in patients with isolated diastolic dysfunction, the pure α-adrenergic agonist phenylephrine may be more effective than catecholamines that combine both α- and β-adrenergic effects. This agent is particularly important in those with diastolic dysfunction caused by hypertrophic obstructive cardiomyopathy. Patients having systolic dysfunction, in common with individuals with diastolic dysfunction, have high resting filling pressures and tend to be sensitive to changes in preload. Even relatively mild degrees of hypovolemia or hypervolemia should be avoided, since they may lead to marked clinical deterioration (14). Acutely decompensated patients and those at high risk for major shifts in intravascular volume may benefit from invasive hemodynamic monitoring with a balloon-tipped thermodilution PA catheter. Such monitoring allows for early detection of such volume shifts and assists with titration of intravenous fluids and diuretics.

Because individuals with diastolic dysfunction have abnormal diastolic filling, tachydysrhythmias, particularly atrial fibrillation and atrial flutter, are poorly tolerated and should be treated aggressively. Intravenous β-blockers or calcium-channel blockers, such as diltiazem, should be used for rate control. These drugs should be chosen over digoxin.

PERICARDIAL TAMPONADE

Pericardial tamponade is a clinical syndrome characterized by peripheral venous congestion and low CO that is due to impaired cardiac filling from accumulation of fluid in the pericardial sac. If severe, this condition can lead to extreme hemodynamic compromise and frank circulatory shock. Ventricular compliance is decreased in tamponade, not because of intrinsic myocardial stiffness, as occurs in ischemia or hypertrophy, but because of the constraint to normal diastolic filling imposed by the surrounding pericardial effusion (15,16). Thus, tamponade resembles a form of diastolic dysfunction. Its development and severity are dependent on both the volume of pericardial fluid and the rapidity with which it accumulates. For example, patients with end-stage renal disease may develop very large pericardial effusions over a long period without progressing to tamponade; whereas, a patient with a stab wound to the chest may develop tamponade with only 50 mL of fluid in the pericardial sac. This effect is due to the lack of distensibility of the pericardium unless tension is applied over a prolonged period of time.

Pericardial effusions can result from a number of causes. The most common are pericarditis (either idiopathic or secondary to infection), radiation therapy, collagen vascular disease, hypothyroidism, malignancy, uremia, and open heart surgery. Effusions associated with bacterial infections or malignancy are particularly likely to progress to tamponade. Hemopericardium is a common cause of tamponade in the surgical intensive care unit. It can occur as a consequence of blunt or penetrating thoracic trauma, aortic dissection, open heart operations, myocardial rupture, or iatrogenic myocardial perforation by vascular catheters or pacing wires. Hemopericardium also may be a complication of coronary perforation during percutaneous coronary interventions.

As fluid accumulates in the pericardial sac, right atrial pressure rises and limits venous return. This limitation results in peripheral venous congestion and decreased CO, which in turn leads to the typical signs and symptoms of tamponade. The patient usually will complain of dyspnea and chest discomfort, both of which are aggravated by assuming a supine position. Other common symptoms include nausea, anorexia, fatigue, and malaise. These symptoms may occur acutely or have an insidious onset. Important findings on physical examination include hypotension with pulsus paradoxus (an inspiratory drop in systolic pressure of at least 10 mm Hg), elevated jugular venous pressure, tachycardia, tachypnea, a quiet precordium on auscultation, and dullness to percussion of the posterior chest just below and medial to the left scapula (Ewart's sign). A pericardial friction rub may or may not be present. If the accumulation of fluid has occurred slowly, evidence of chronic venous congestion, including ascites and lower extremity edema, may be observed. The electrocardiogram commonly shows sinus tachycardia with reduced QRS voltage. Electrical alternans (beat-to-beat alternation in QRS amplitude) and diffuse ST-segment elevation characteristic of pericarditis also may be present. Chest radiography typically shows an enlarged cardiac silhouette with a globular shape but no evidence of associated pulmonary vascular congestion. The cardiac silhouette may be normal in those patients with small, but rapidly accumulating pericardial effusions.

Pericardial tamponade causing hypotension can be difficult to distinguish from other causes of shock. The finding of jugular venous distension is important and should alert one to the possibility of tamponade and helps to exclude hypovolemia. Central venous catheterization will reveal a correspondingly elevated right atrial pressure. PA catheterization will show equalization of diastolic pressures and reduced CO (Fig. 3b). Echocardiography can confirm or exclude the presence of pericardial fluid. In addition, the echocardiogram may reveal evidence of tamponade, such as inspiratory collapse of right heart chambers. Echocardiographic findings of tamponade may be present even before clinical findings become apparent (17).

Pericardial tamponade is a medical emergency and requires prompt intervention. Volume loading may be useful as a temporizing measure by increasing mean systemic pressure and thus improving right heart filling and CO. Definitive treatment includes needle or catheter pericardiocentesis or pericardial window placement. For medical causes of pericardial effusion, the latter has the advantage of providing tissue for diagnosis and also of preventing reaccumulation of fluid.

CARDIAC FUNCTION IN SEPSIS AND SEPTIC SHOCK

A distinct hemodynamic pattern occurs in patients with sepsis and septic shock. Characteristic findings include a low SVR, secondary to peripheral vasodilation, and, in many cases, increased CO (18,19). In addition, some patients experience a potentially reversible impairment in systolic function. This impairment is associated with acute left ventricular dilation, decreased contractility, and diminished ejection fraction. Decreased contractility in the face of increased CO may seem contradictory, but can occur because of marked decrease in afterload, increase in preload, and tachycardia, all of which serve to counter the negative inotropic effect. This abnormality affects approximately half of patients with septic shock and appears to be mediated by a circulating myocardial depressant factor. Patients who develop these changes appear to have a higher mortality rate compared with those who do not. For survivors, abnormalities in ventricular function gradually reverse as resolution of sepsis occurs.

The mainstays of treatment for severe sepsis include appropriate antibiotic therapy and drainage of closed space infections. In selected patients drotrecogin alfa (recombinant activated protein C) has been efficacious. Measures to maintain adequate perfusion and reverse the shock state are also important. Initial management should include fluid resuscitation to restore and optimize preload. Clinical investigations have shown that, in general, the optimal PAOP for patients with sepsis is ~12 mm Hg (19). This level is lower than the optimal PAOP for patients with cardiogenic shock from acute myocardial infarction; the difference probably relates to increased ventricular stiffness that occurs with myocardial ischemia. Frequently, patients with severe sepsis require several liters of isotonic fluid administered intravenously over only a few hours. Patients with severe sepsis are susceptible to pulmonary edema on the basis of several factors. The vigorous fluid resuscitation that is often required increases the risk of cardiogenic pulmonary edema. In addition, these patients are at high risk of developing acute lung injury and acute respiratory distress syndrome. PA catheterization can be helpful for titrating fluid therapy and assessing cardiac function in selected critically ill patients with severe sepsis and septic shock.

Along with optimization of preload, many patients will require administration of sympathomimetic agents (e.g., dopamine, norepinephrine, or both) to treat hypotension (20). These agents generally are employed only in patients who remain hypotensive or exhibit other signs of impaired organ perfusion despite optimization of left ventricular preload.

SUMMARY

- Cardiac performance and oxygen demand depend on heart rate, preload, afterload, and contractility.
- Sinus tachycardia is a compensatory response to either a physiologic or pathologic condition.

- Preload is the ventricular end-diastolic volume.
- Ventricular compliance is approximated by the reciprocal of the slope of the diastolic portion of the ventricular pressure–volume loop.
- PAOP and CVP are indirect estimates of left ventricular and right ventricular preload, respectively. An assumption about compliance is implicit when volume is inferred from pressure measurements.
- Patients with impaired ventricular function usually have higher filling pressures.
- Systemic and pulmonary arterial blood pressures provide simple estimates of left ventricular and right ventricular afterload, respectively.
- SVR and PVR are useful estimates to left and right ventricular afterload, respectively, when CO and pressure gradients across the systemic and pulmonary vascular beds are available.
- Clinically, ejection fraction provides an estimate of contractility, although ejection fraction is also affected by preload and afterload.
- Physical work performed by the heart is represented by the area contained within the ventricular pressure–volume loop.
- Impaired contractility is characteristic of systolic dysfunction.
- Patients with either systolic or diastolic dysfunction are sensitive to changes in preload.
- Consider the use of inotropic agents in patients with severely compromised systolic function.
- Diastolic dysfunction can be an important cause of cardiac decompensation (see Table 3).
- Use agents that improve myocardial compliance to treat diastolic dysfunction.
- Pericardial tamponade is a form of diastolic dysfunction that requires prompt recognition and emergency treatment.
- Sepsis is commonly associated with low SVR and high resting CO. Transient systolic dysfunction is common. Patients need fluid resuscitation to restore and optimize preload and may require sympathomimetic agents, if hypotension persists despite adequate volume expansion.

REFERENCES

1. Opie LH. Mechanisms of cardiac contraction and relaxation. In: Braunwald E, Zipes DP, Libby P, eds. Heart Disease. 6th ed. Philadelphia: W.B. Saunders, 2001:443–478.
2. Little RC, Little WC. Cardiac preload, afterload and heart failure. Arch Intern Med 1982; 142:819–822.
3. O'quin R, Marini JJ. Pulmonary artery occlusion pressure: clinical physiology, measurement and interpretation. Am Rev Resp Dis 1983; 128:319–326.
4. McElroy PA, Shroff SG, Weber KT. Pathophysiology of the failing heart. Cardiol Clin 1989; 7:25–37.
5. Wiedermann HP, Matthay MA, Matthay RA. Cardiovascular-pulmonary monitoring in the intensive care unit. Chest 1984; 85:537–549, 656–668.
6. Bressack MA, Raffin TA. Importance of venous return, venous resistance, and mean circulatory pressure in the physiology and management of shock. Chest 1987; 92:906–912.

7. Bristow MR, Port JD, Kelly RA. Treatment of heart failure: pharmacological methods. In: Braunwald E, Zipes DP, Libby P, eds. Heart Disease. 6th ed. Philadelphia: W.B. Saunders, 2001:562–599.
8. Flather MD, Torp-Pedersen C, Yusuf S, Ball S, Kober L, Pogue J, Pfeffer M, Moye L, Hall A, Braunwald E, Murray G, Long-term ACE-inhibitor therapy in patients with heart failure or left-ventricular dysfunction: a systematic overview of data from individual patients. ACE-Inhibitor Myocardial Infarction Collaborative Group. Lancet 2000; 355:1575–1581.
9. Hobbs RE, Mills RM, Young JB. An update on nesiritide for treatment of decompensated congestive heart failure. Expert Opin Investig Drugs 2001; 10:935–942.
10. Tresch DD. Clinical manifestations, diagonstic assessment, and etiology of heart failure in elderly patients. Clin Geriatr Med 2000; 16:445–456.
11. Cohen GI, Pietrolungo DO, Thomas JD, Klein AL. A practical guide to assessment of ventricular diastolic function using Doppler echocardiography. J Am Coll Cardiol 1996; 27:1753–1760.
12. Kitzman DW, Gardin JM, Gottdiener JS, Arnold A, Boineau R, Aurigremma G, Marino EK, Lyles M, Cushman M, Enright PL. Importance of heart failure with preserved systolic function in patients >65 years of age. Am J Cardiol 2001; 87:413–419.
13. Harizi RC, Blanco JA, Alpert JS. Diastolic function of the heart in clinical cardiology. Arch Intern Med 1988; 148:99–109.
14. Cody RJ. The treatment of diastolic heart failure. Cardiol Clin 2000; 18:589–596.
15. Ameli S, Shah PK. Cardiac tamponade: pathophysiology, diagnosis and management. Cardiol Clin 1991; 9:665–674.
16. Spodick DH. Pathophysiology of cardiac tamponade. Chest 1998; 113:1372–1379.
17. Tsang TS, Oh JK, Seward JB. Diagnosis and management of cardiac tamponade in the era of echocardiography. Clin Cardiol 1999; 22:446–452.
18. Vincent J-L. Cardiovascular alternations in septic shock. J Antimicrob Chemother 1998; 41(suppl A):9–15.
19. Kumar A, Haery C, Parillo JE. Myocardial dysfunction in septic shock. Crit Care Clin 2000; 16:251–287.
20. Task Force of the American College of Critical Care Medicine, Society of Critical Care Medicine. Practice parameters for hemodynamic support of sepsis in adult patients in sepsis. Crit Care Med 1999; 27:639–660.

22
Cardiac Arrhythmias and the Perioperative Period

Charles C. Gornick
Minneapolis Heart Institute, Minneapolis, Minnesota, USA

Arthur H. L. From
VA Medical Center, Minneapolis, Minnesota, USA

INTRODUCTION

Cardiac arrhythmias are common management problems. During the perioperative period cardiac arrhythmias can cause considerable morbidity, including myocardial ischemia, hemodynamic compromise, and stroke; these complications can be life threatening. Thus, recognizing and understanding the etiology and appropriate management of arrhythmias are critical components of perioperative care.

Among surgical patients, the diagnosis and treatment of cardiac arrhythmias must take into consideration the severity of any concomitant heart and lung disease. These diseases, along with the stress associated with surgery, are often causally related to the arrhythmia. Further, the presence of significant renal dysfunction may affect the pharmacologic approach selected. Clinical history can be quite variable. In some patients, a history of primary arrhythmias, or arrhythmias complicating long established heart disease, may be present. In other patients, a new arrhythmia may develop without clinically evident heart disease. Furthermore, arrhythmias may develop only during acute stress, such as that occurring during the perioperative period, or as result of peri- or postoperative complications such as myocardial infarction, pulmonary embolism, or serious infection. Last, as expected, the likelihood of arrhythmia development is greatest in patients with underlying cardiac or pulmonary disease or debilitation resulting from other chronic diseases. Following the onset of an arrhythmia, the physician should look carefully for immediate precipitating factors that may be readily correctable.

Factors that can precipitate arrhythmias include volume overload with congestive heart failure, myocardial ischemia, pulmonary embolism, acid/base abnormalities, electrolyte abnormalities, adverse drug effects, and sepsis. If present preoperatively, these abnormalities should be treated before surgery to decrease the likelihood of subsequent arrhythmias. Additionally, patients with heart disease often have an underlying arrhythmia substrate. The stress associated with the perioperative period can increase the frequency of premature atrial or ventricular beats. These ectopic beats can trigger supraventricular or ventricular arrhythmias. The importance of accurate diagnosis of cardiac arrhythmias cannot be overemphasized, because arrhythmia-specific treatment options are more likely to be effective.

BRADYARRHYTHMIAS (Fig. 1)

Sinus Node Dysfunction

Sinus node dysfunction is a common cause of bradyarrhythmia, the frequency of which increases with age (1–4). Sinus bradycardia may occur without symptoms, or hemodynamic consequences may result from the inappropriately slow heart rate. Generally, if the heart is otherwise normal, slow rates are well tolerated. In contrast, in patients with heart disease, a heart rate of 80–90 per min during the postoperative period may better maintain cardiac output than a rate of 50 per min. The diseased heart is often stroke volume limited as the result of systolic or diastolic dysfunction. Therefore, the ability to increase cardiac output is less dependent on the Starling mechanism and is more dependent on the ability to increase heart rate. Hence, in patients with heart disease, the lower cardiac output associated with slow and limited heart rate may induce or exacerbate signs of decreased perfusion. Near-syncope or syncope can result if sinus pauses are of long duration (5).

In other patients tachycardia can be precipitated by bradycardia-associated ectopy resulting in the so-called "tachycardia–bradycardia syndrome" (6) (Fig. 2). In this syndrome, symptoms relating to either bradycardia or tachycardia may predominate. The usual tachyarrhythmias are atrial fibrillation or atrial flutter. Other primary atrial or AV nodal reentrant tachycardias also may occur. Any of these arrhythmias may be symptomatic. With spontaneous or therapeutic interruption of the tachyarrhythmia, severe symptomatic bradycardia may supervene because of "overdrive" suppression of sinus node function. Also, pharmacologic treatment aimed at controlling the tachyarrhythmia, by further depressing sinus node function, may precipitate or accentuate bradycardia.

Etiology

The mechanisms underlying sinus node dysfunction are not well defined. Abnormalities have been classified as intrinsic, when apparent abnormality of the SA node or SA nodal exit block exist. Abnormalities are considered extrinsic when abnormal neural input to the node or drugs suppress nodal function (5). Examples of external neural input on sinus node function would include enhanced vagal tone precipitated by severe pain or stimulation of the tracheobronchial tree with suction of secretions.

Often overlooked causes of sinus node dysfunction are pharmacologic therapies for cardiovascular or general medical problems (7).

Treatment

Excessive vagal stimulation related to significant pain or to events such as tracheobronchial suctioning can be minimized by appropriate pain management or techniques limiting duration of tracheal stimulation. In extreme cases, during needed secretion suctioning, short-acting anticholinergic drugs (e.g., atropine) or sympathomimetic drugs present in inhalers can be used to prevent bradycardia.

Patients presenting with symptoms of sinus node dysfunction require careful scrutiny of their medications. β-Adrenergic blockers, Ca^{++} channel blockers, digoxin, sympatholytic antihypertensive agents, and antiarrhythmic agents are long-established causes of sinus node dysfunction. Symptoms may abate when treatment is stopped. Drugs less commonly

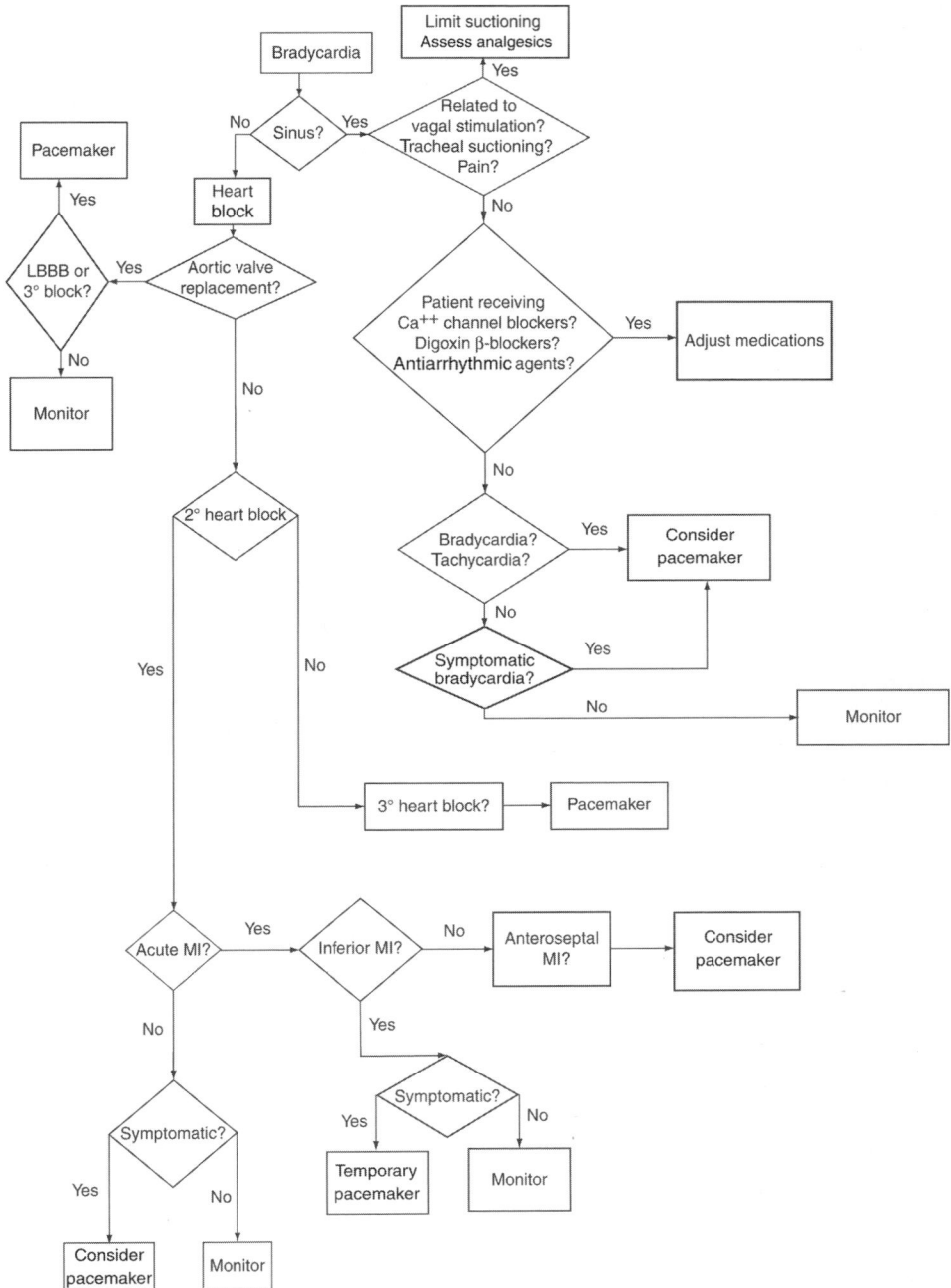

Figure 1 Approach to bradyarrhythmias.

associated with sinus node dysfunction include lithium carbonate, cimetidine, antidepressants such as amitriptyline, and phenothiazines (7). If sinus bradyarrhythmia is present, the patient's entire medication list needs to be reviewed. A pharmacology database should be queried for any unfamiliar agent. The results of a drug query can be both surprising and enlightening.

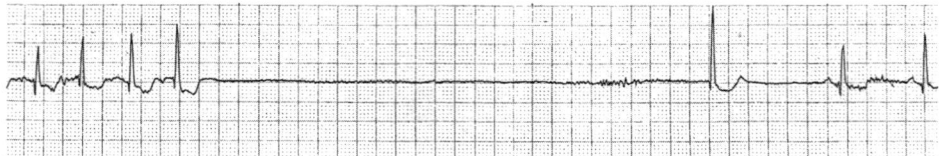

Figure 2 ECG lead II demonstrating conversion of atrial fibrillation (left side of tracing), resulting in prolonged asystole until interrupted by a junctional beat followed by sinus rhythm.

In patients with symptomatic sinus node dysfunction without an otherwise correctable cause, electrical pacing is standard therapy (8–10). If the need for pacing is estimated to be only short term, a temporary pacing system can be used for a few days. If the perioperative period has uncovered significant sinus node dysfunction that is expected to persist (including sinus bradycardia caused by necessary drugs) and be symptomatic following recovery from the surgical procedure, permanent pacing is indicated. Pacing is effective because, in patients with symptoms resulting from bradycardia, the resting heart rate is increased and, with rate responsive pacemakers, chronotropic incompetence can be alleviated. In patients with sinus bradycardia and predominantly tachycardia-related symptoms, chronic pacing may prevent recurrence or permit the use of suppressive antiarrhythmic therapy that would otherwise be limited by the underlying sinus node dysfunction. Pacing should be reserved for symptomatic patients. No evidence demonstrates that pacing improves longevity in asymptomatic patients either short or long term (11–13). A detailed discussion of appropriate pacemaker selection will be presented subsequently.

Abnormalities of AV Conduction

In the presence of intermittent or established complete heart block (Figs. 3 and 4), the severity of symptoms depends on the rate of the subsidiary pacemaker. An adequate heart rate is often maintained by a junctional pacemaker, usually originating in the His bundle. Under these circumstances, symptoms may be mild, and hemodynamic

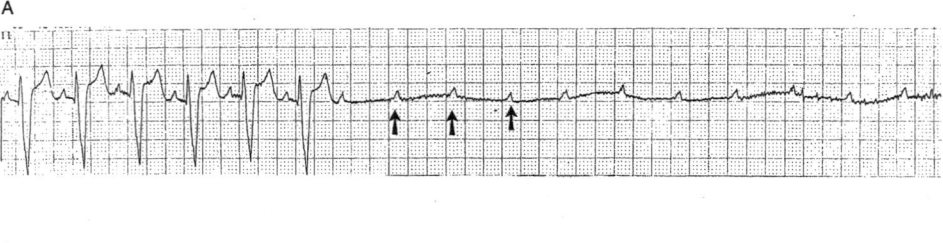

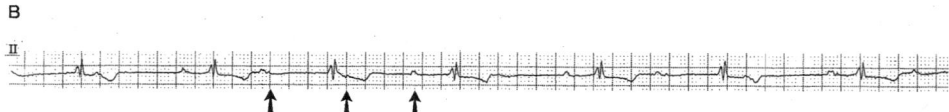

Figure 3 (A) ECG lead II demonstrating sinus rhythm with AV conduction interrupted by complete AV block. Nonconducted P waves indicated by arrows. (B) Incomplete AV block characterized by P waves (arrows) that conduct only intermittently to the ventricles. The irregularity of the QRS response supports some conduction from the atrium to the ventricles.

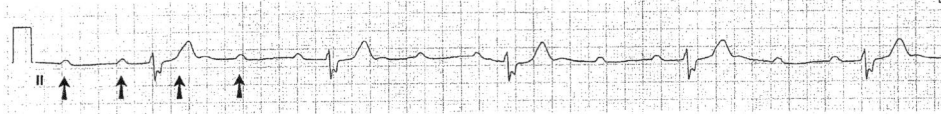

Figure 4 ECG lead II demonstrating compete AV block. Note the P waves indicated by arrows are completely disassociated from the QRS. The widened QRS suggests a low junctional or ventricular escape rhythm.

compromise is minimal. A lower, slower (and less reliable) ventricular escape rhythm, characterized by wide and aberrant QRS configuration, often results in significant hemodynamic compromise, including hypotension and congestive heart failure. Frank syncope occurs as a result of transient asystole or bursts of ventricular tachycardia associated with severe bradycardia (Stokes–Adams attacks) (14). Clinically significant AV conduction disturbances are usually readily diagnosed by ECG (Figs. 3 and 4). However, when symptoms are intermittent, continuous ECG monitoring is required.

Etiology

Ischemic heart disease is frequently thought to be the cause of AV conduction abnormalities. In fact, only ~20% of cases can be directly attributed to this cause by pathologic examination. Primary degeneration of the conduction system (Lev-Lenegre's disease) is more often the cause (15). Lev-Lenegre's disease may be inferred when a careful history and physical examination appear to exclude other causes. In the surgical patient, underlying conduction system disease may be uncovered by the stress and hemodynamic demands of the perioperative period.

AV block occurs in 5–8% of patients with acute myocardial infarction. Because myocardial infarction can occur in perioperative patients, it should be considered as a possible etiologic factor in patients exhibiting otherwise unexplained AV block during this period. Further, early diagnosis of postoperative acute myocardial infarction is important, because percutaneous angioplasty techniques can be employed, even though postprocedure anticoagulation may be limited as a consequence of the primary surgical procedure. During the surgical recovery period, wound pain and level of consciousness may mask symptoms, such as chest pain, that are typically seen with myocardial infarction. Although myocardial infarction more commonly complicates cardiac surgery or major vascular surgery, any surgical procedure can be associated with acute myocardial infarction. Despite efforts to diagnose, characterize, and optimally treat heart disease prior to elective surgery, myocardial infarction occurs in some patients. Further, in patients requiring emergency surgery, only limited preoperative risk assessment can be made.

With inferior myocardial infarction, partial (usually Möbitz Type I) or complete heart block may occur. Temporary pacing may be required in the presence of hemodynamic instability from severe bradycardia, marked left ventricular dysfunction, or clinically significant right ventricular infarction. In many patients, pacing is not required. The symptoms resulting from the heart block (which is usually associated with a stable junctional escape rhythm of 40–55 beats per minute) are minimal, and the prognosis for complete recovery of AV nodal function is excellent. Permanent pacing should be reserved for those with significant block persisting for at least 7–10 days (16–18).

In contrast, AV block associated with antero-septal myocardial infarction is usually a result of extensive myocardial damage, and the short- and long-term prognosis with or without pacing is poor (16–20). Temporary transvenous or transcutaneous pacing should be instituted or be available in all patients with secondary AV block or complete AV block associated with acute antero-septal infarction. In patients with antero-septal infarction complicated by a new left bundle branch block (or so-called bifascicular block comprising right bundle branch block associated with either left anterior or left posterior hemiblock), a stand-by transcutaneous pacing system should be placed while preparing for transvenous pacing. Complete heart block may develop in 20–30% of these patients (21). Alternatively, these patients can be monitored with a transcutaneous pacing system set on stand-by (after testing to assure reliable capture). The latter approach assumes that 24 h capability of placing a reliable, emergency transvenous temporary system is present.

Valvular heart disease, particularly calcific aortic stenosis, may be associated with impaired AV conduction (22). This abnormal condition results from extension of valvular calcification into the bundle of His or proximal bundle branches that traverse the ventricular septum. Additionally, surgical replacement of the aortic valve may result in heart block when sutures are placed too deeply in the ventricular septum. Therefore, new left bundle branch block or complete heart block following aortic valve surgery will require permanent dual chamber pacing. In such patients the long-term risk of recurrent AV block is high.

Temporary Pacing

When heart block is likely to be temporary and is not symptomatic (as in acute inferior myocardial infarction), treatment is not required. If the patient is symptomatic, treatment with atropine, isoproterenol, dopamine, or dobutamine may occasionally be successful. These drugs are less desirable than temporary pacing, because they have potentially adverse effects on the heart and peripheral vasculature. In asymptomatic patients, our practice is to place temporary transcutaneous pacing patches (23), ensure that they function properly, and leave them in standby mode. If transcutaneous pacing is subsequently required for more than a brief period, temporary transvenous ventricular pacing is instituted. Prolonged transcutaneous stimulation can be uncomfortable. In some patients with complete heart block, such as those with associated, severe right ventricular infarction, temporary dual chamber pacing may afford an additional hemodynamic advantage, because the atrial contribution to right ventricular filling and cardiac output may be considerable (30).

Although patients with AV block associated with acute antero-septal infarction may be temporarily stabilized with drugs or transcutaneous pacing, temporary transvenous pacing is the most reliable therapeutic modality. In the setting of acute antero-septal infarction, an apparently reliable or pharmacologically supported ventricular escape rhythm may rapidly deteriorate. A transcutaneous pacemaker can be used to support the patient, while preparations are made for placing a temporary transvenous pacing system. Similarly, a standby transcutaneous pacing system should be placed in patients with new, myocardial infarction-related bundle branch block, while preparing for transvenous pacing.

A previous point requires emphasis. In patients without acute antero-septal myocardial infarction, AV block must be establised as irreversible before placing a permanent pacemaker. For example, in the setting of drug induced or aggravated AV block, adequate time must be allowed for medications to "wash out."

Permanent Pacing

Progressive advances in technology have made a wide variety of reliable pacing systems available. Thus, once a patient has a definite indication for pacemaker implantation, the next important decision is the type of pacing system to use.

Pacemaker Code

Agreed-on symbols or codes to describe pacemakers are an indispensable means of communication. In 1974 The Inter-Society Commission on Heart Disease Resources (ICHD) recommended a three-position letter code to provide a simple way of describing pacing systems (24). As pacemakers have become more complicated, this system has been modified with additional letter positions (25). Table 1 summarizes the widely used positions in pacemaker coding system. Addition of an R to the three-position code indicates the pacemaker has an additional sensor that increases heart rate in response to exercise.

General Considerations

Pacemakers that utilize atrial sensing, maintain AV synchrony, and have rate responsiveness often improve cardiac function significantly. AV synchrony, with an appropriately timed PR interval, augments left ventricular filling when systolic contraction and/or diastolic relaxation abnormalities are present. Among older patients, decreased ventricular compliance is common, although often not recognized (26). This diastolic abnormality is more likely in the presence of hypertension with associated left ventricular hypertrophy (27).

In many patients with "sick sinus syndrome," AV conduction is intact. In such patients, VVI pacing can induce retrograde atrial activation during ventricular contraction and produce the "pacemaker syndrome" (28). This syndrome is characterized by symptoms induced by hypotension and a sensation of pulsation and fullness in the neck with symptoms occuring during intermittent periods of ventricular pacing.

Appropriate Pacemaker Selection

In most patients, dual chamber pacing is desirable. In some instances, atrial pacing decreases the frequency of atrial arrhythmias. Most current dual chamber pacing systems have a feature that recognizes rapid atrial arrhythmias. This capability prevents the ventricles from being paced at the elevated atrial rate. The device will transiently ignore or not track the atrium until the atrial rate is within a predetermined range. When the atrial arrhythmia terminates, the device will return to tracking the atrium and pacing the ventricle at an appropriate rate. Heart rate response to exercise is an important consideration in selected patients. If a patient has chronotropic competence of the SA node,

Table 1 Three-Position ICHD Code

Chamber(s) paced (I)	Chamber(s) sensed (II)	Mode of response(s) (III)
V = Ventricle	V = Ventricle	V = Ventricle
A = Atrium	A = Atrium	I = Inhibited
D = Double	D = Double	D = Double
	O = None	O = None

tracking the atrial response during exercise yields the most physiologic ventricular pacing rate. In ~25% of patients with complete AV block, the SA node does not respond with an appropriate rate increase with exercise. In such patients, a rate responsive pacing system, using a sensor incorporated into the pacing system, can improve exercise performance by permitting appropriate increases of heart rate and cardiac output.

In patients with chronic left ventricular dysfunction and dysynchrony of contraction (usually associated with a wide QRS), pacing systems utilizing an atrial, right ventricular, and left ventricular lead can be beneficial. This pacing mode can resynchronize contraction, improve hemodynamic performance, ameliorate congestive heart failure symptoms, and perhaps improve mortality (29,30). The left ventricular lead is placed either transvenously via the coronary sinus or on the left ventricular epicardium via a surgical approach.

In summary, current pacing systems involving multiple leads and complex programming are available. They provide reliable long-term pacing that may improve hemodynamic performance and symptoms when used appropriately.

TACHYARRHYTHMIAS—PRIMARY ATRIAL ARRHYTHMIAS (Figs. 5 and 6)

Atrial Fibrillation

Etiology

Preoperative chronic atrial fibrillation is commonly present in older patients (Fig. 7). In the general population, among individuals over age 70 years, the incidence of atrial fibrillation is ~9% (31). Further, among older patients, atrial fibrillation is usually associated with underlying cardiac diseases such as coronary artery diseases, hypertension, valvular heart diseases, or cardiomyopathy. Systemic disorders such as hyperthyroidism or amyloidosis are less-frequent causes. In such patients, previously well-tolerated chronic atrial fibrillation may be replaced by accelerated rates postoperatively, Hemodynamic consequences of the tachycardia may occur. Increased ventricular response rate may result from the stress of surgery or withdrawal of chronic medications during the perioperative period. Generally, the patient's history and physical examination, together with the ECG, chest X-ray, and/or echocardiogram, will identify the arrhythmia and reveal the presence and severity of the underlying cardiac disease.

Atrial fibrillation commonly occurs in response to the stress of surgery, with its attendant increase of sympathetic nervous system activity, or is associated with perioperative complications such as myocardial infarction, pulmonary embolism, or severe infection. When approaching a patient with new-onset postoperative atrial fibrillation, the physician should consider additional precipitating or exacerbating factors, such as acute bleeding, altered volume status, hypoxia, acid/base abnormalities, or electrolyte abnormalities, including reduced serum K^+ and Mg^{++}. In many patients with or without underlying cardiac disease, atrial fibrillation manifests itself only during the stress of surgery. In such patients, reversion to sinus rhythm occurs spontaneously during the postoperative recovery period.

The incidence of atrial fibrillation after cardiac surgery, either coronary artery bypass surgery or valve surgery, is as high as 30–50% and increases with the severity of ventricular dysfunction and the age of the patient. Other predisposing factors include

Perioperative Cardiac Arrhythmias

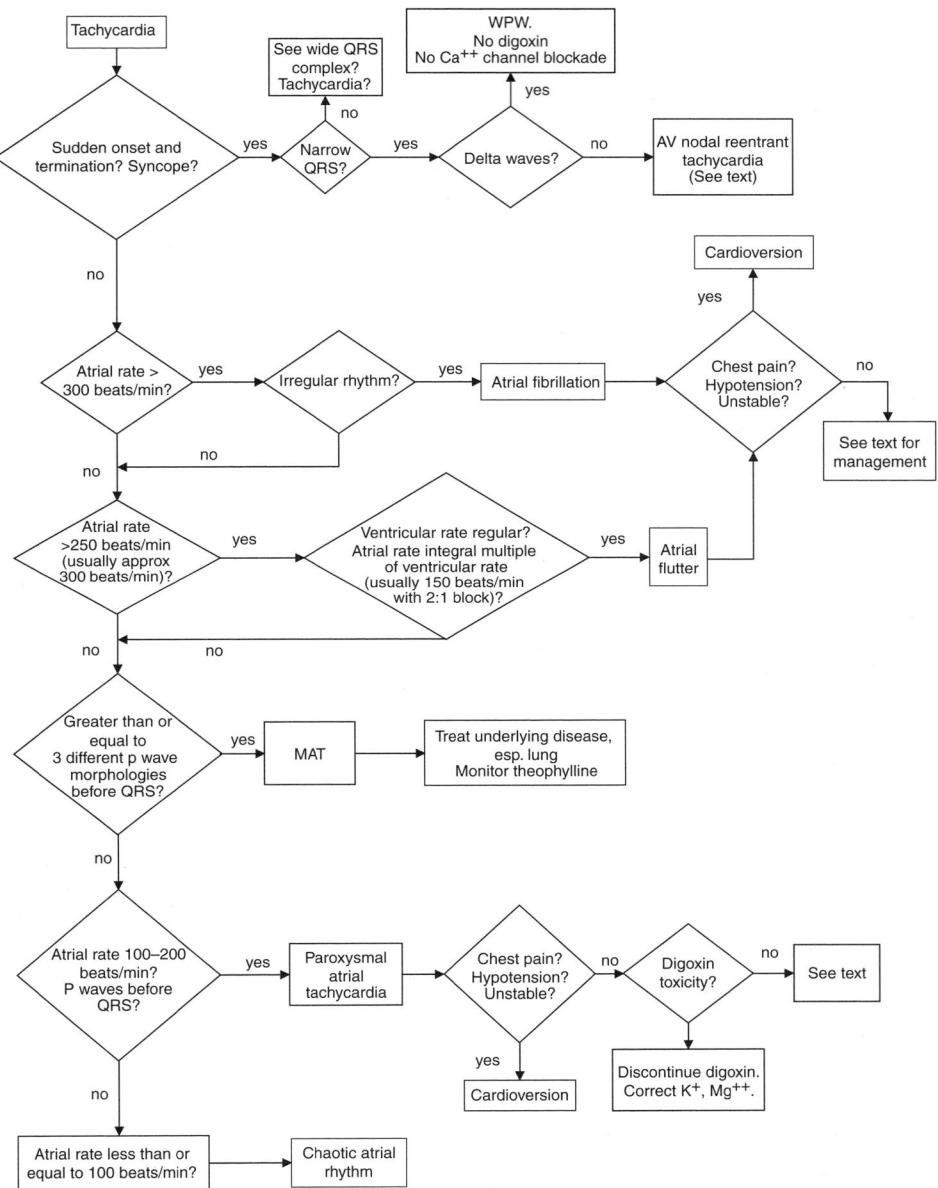

Figure 5 Approach to tachycardia.

previous history of atrial fibrillation and more complicated heart surgery, such as valve replacement. Typically, the peak occurrence of atrial fibrillation is between days 3 and 5 following cardiac surgery. Atrial fibrillation after cardiac surgery prolongs hospitalization and increases costs (32).

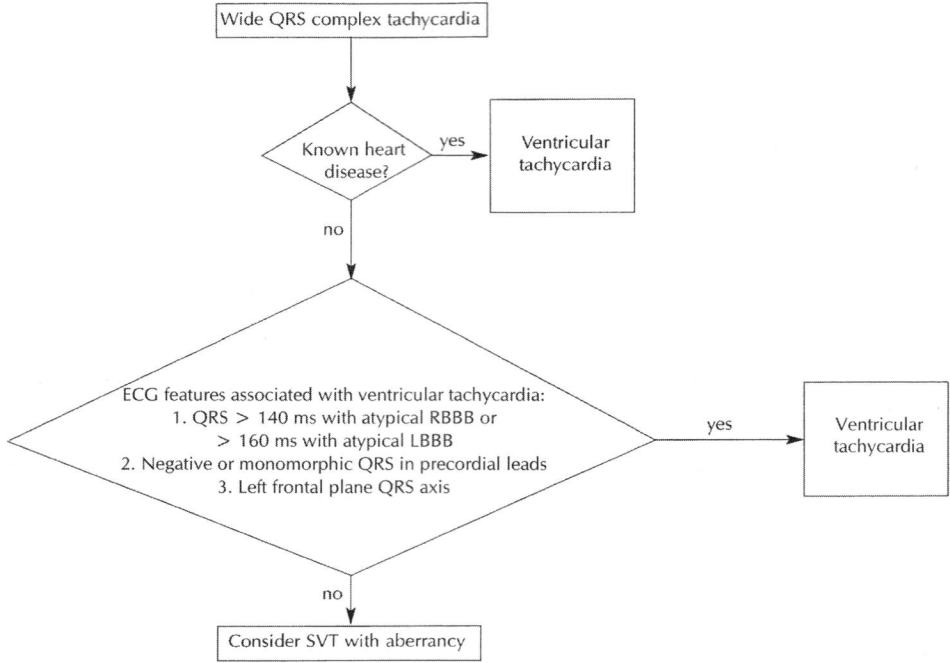

Figure 6 Approach to wide complex tachycardia

Pre- and postoperative use of β-adrenergic blocking drugs has been effective in reducing the incidence of atrial fibrillation complicating cardiac surgery. Generally, chronic β-adrenergic blocker therapy should not be stopped prior to surgery. Continuing β-blocker therapy in the case of cardiovascular surgery is especially important. Pretreatment with amiodarone for 1 week prior to cardiac surgery and a few days following surgery has been shown to reduce the incidence of atrial fibrillation from 53% to 25% (33).

Clinical Presentation

The clinical presentation of atrial fibrillation in postoperative patients depends on the ventricular response rate, on the severity of ventricular dysfunction, and on factors such as the presence of severe coronary obstruction or mitral stenosis (Fig. 8). In many patients with acute postoperative atrial fibrillation, symptoms may be absent or be experienced as merely a sensation of an irregular heart beat, despite the presence of a rapid ventricular response. Patients with significant left ventricular dysfunction, severe coronary artery disease, or severe left ventricular relaxation problems, resulting from hypertrophy, are generally less tolerant of the arrhythmia. These patients often have signs and symptoms of congestive heart failure, angina, or hemodynamic compromise.

Atrial fibrillation is easily diagnosed by ECG features that include absence of regular atrial activity, a fine or coarse undulating baseline, and irregularly irregular R–R intervals (Figs. 7 and 8). Occasionally, an especially coarse undulating baseline with so-called "fibrillatory" waves may be confused with other atrial arrhythmias such as atrial flutter or paroxysmal atrial tachycardia, both of which may also be associated

Perioperative Cardiac Arrhythmias 333

A

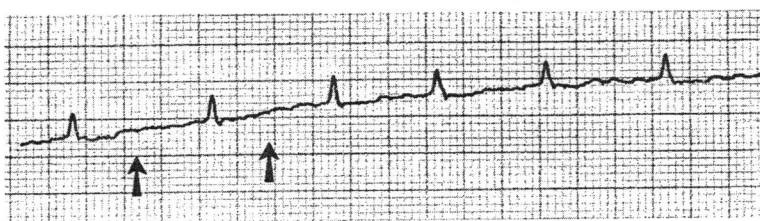

B

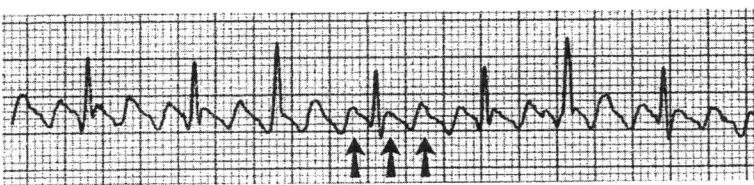

C

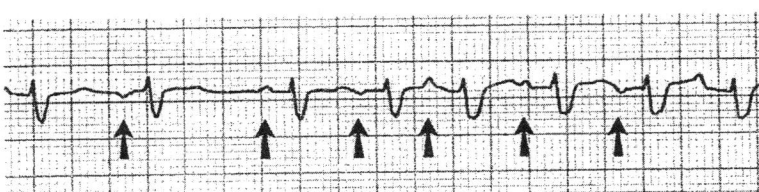

Figure 7 ECG lead II—(A) atrial fibrillation. Note the irregular ventricular response rate which is characteristic and fine undulation of the baseline produced by the fibrillating atrium. (B) Atrial flutter. Note the "saw tooth" appearance of the baseline produced by the fluttering atria. The ventricular response rate is always a multiple of the flutter rate (in this example 2 : 1 or 3 : 1). (C) Mutifocal atrial tachycardia (MAT). This rhythm is characterized by multiple different P wave morphologies indicated by arrows.

with variable AV conduction. This confusion often occurs when the ventricular response is not very irregular.

When the ventricular response without drug therapy is less than 80 beats per minute and increases only modestly in response to stress, associated disease of the AV node is present. In contrast, a resting ventricular response of 120–160 beats per minute suggests that AV nodal function is normal. If the resting ventricular response is more than 150 beats per minute, the sympathetic nervous system is activated by the postsurgical state, any associated complications, or the stress of the altered hemodynamic state created by atrial fibrillation. Resting ventricular rates of more than 200 beats per minute suggest the presence of enhanced AV nodal conduction or the presence of an accessory AV connection. Under the latter circumstances, the QRS morphology is aberrant ("pre-excited"), and the rhythm may be confused with ventricular tachycardia.

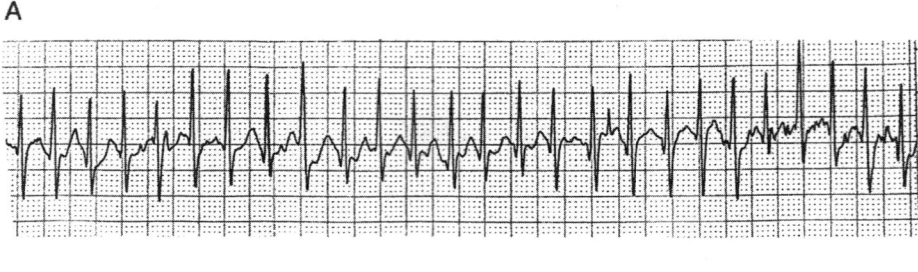
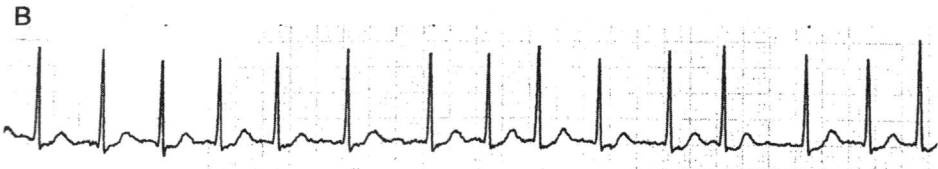

Figure 8 ECG lead II—(A) atrial fibrillation with a very rapid ventricular response and (B) atrial fibrillation in the same patient as (A), following pharmacologic slowing of the ventricular response rate.

In addition to its effect on cardiac performance, persistent atrial fibrillation increases the risk of stroke. This risk is further increased when fibrillation is accompanied by risk factors including hypertension, diabetes, prior stroke, or preexisting heart disease. In contrast, younger patients with so called "lone" atrial fibrillation, defined by the absence of the above risk factors, have an extremely low risk for embolism (50).

Treatment

With acute onset of atrial fibrillation or with rate acceleration early after operation in patients with chronic atrial fibrillation, severe symptoms, including hypotension, pulmonary edema, and new, or worsening, angina can occur. Under these circumstances the arrhythmia must be rapidly controlled or corrected. The most efficacious treatment for new-onset atrial fibrillation is electrical cardioversion under sedation. Synchronized DC cardioversion, with a biphasic discharge waveform, improves the immediate rate of success and should be used.

If the atrial fibrillation is chronic or recurs following cardioversion, then intravenous β-adrenergic blocking drugs such as esmolol (34), or Ca^{++} channel antagonists such as diltiazem (35), and digoxin can be used to slow the ventricular rate. In patients with significant left ventricular dysfunction, both β-adrenergic blocking agents and Ca^{++} channel blockers must be used with caution, because administration of these agents increases the risk of inducing severe hypotension or worsening of congestive heart failure. Adjunctive therapy to control congestive failure, hypotension, and angina must also be employed to stabilize the patient. Drug dosages should be adjusted, if diminished renal and hepatic function are present.

In patients with atrial fibrillation and a rapid ventricular response but without significant symptoms, the initial goal is control of ventricular rate. In the absence of specific contraindications to β-adrenergic blocking drugs, an intravenous preparation with a short half-life, such as esmolol, is the initial drug of choice in most postoperative patients (36,37).

In situations when β-adrenergic blocking drugs are relatively contraindicated, intravenous diltiazem can be used. Diltiazem may be useful for patients with severe left ventricular dysfunction, requring catecholamine support to maintain hemodynamic stability, or with significant lung disease, particularly bronchospasm (38). The dose of intravenous diltiazem can be gradually increased to control ventricular rate without precipitating severe hypotension or worsening of congestive heart failure in many, but not all, patients.

Patients without underlying heart disease, who develop atrial fibrillation and experience few or no symptoms, present a lower level of risk. In this group of patients, attention to rate control is recommended. Long periods of increased heart rate can, over time, lead to progressive symptoms, because tachycardia-related cardiomyopathy may develop (39).

Infrequently, patients with atrial fibrillation exhibit a ventricular rate greater than 200 beats per minute (Fig. 8). If the QRS complexes are wide and bizarre (normal QRS complexes may be interspersed), conduction through an accessory AV connection, such as seen with the Wolff–Parkinson–White Syndrome (WPW), should be considered. In treating atrial fibrillation with a very rapid response from antegrade conduction though an accessory pathway, digoxin and verapamil are contraindicated, as they may further accelerate conduction through the accessory connection, increase the ventricular rate excessively, and, induce ventricular fibrillation. Indeed, rapid rate induced ventricular fibrillation is thought to be the mechanism for the rare instances of sudden death that occur in patients with accessory AV connections.

The most appropriate initial therapy in these patients is cardioversion followed by treatment with a type I (see Table 2) antiarrhythmic and β-adrenergic blocking drug. Both drugs decrease conduction velocity through the accessory connection and the AV node. Pharmacological therapy should be attempted only if immediate cardioversion is not possible. In the hemodynamically unstable patient, an intravenous bolus of lidocaine

Table 2 Classification of Antiarrhythmic Agents

Type IA	Quinidine
	Procainamide
	Disopyramide
Type IB	Lidocaine
	Mexiletine
Type IC	Flecanide
	Propafenone
Type II	Beta-blockers
Type III	Amiodarone
	Sotalol
Type IV	Diltiazem
	Verapamil
Others	Digoxin
	Adenosine
	Ibutilide
	Dofetilide

followed by a continuous infusion, if there is a reduction of ventricular rate following the bolus infusion, may be the safest initial therapeutic choice. This agent slows accessory pathway conduction velocity in some patients and is less likely than other antiarrhythmic agents to worsen hypotension. If lidocaine fails, an intravenous infusion of procainamide, given slowly to avoid inducing or worsening hypotension, will often slow conduction in the accessory connection enough to reduce the ventricular rate to more tolerable levels or to convert the arrhythmias to sinus rhythm. Even if initially successful, drug treatment is most often a temporary expedient. If the atrial fibrillation is not converted by drug therapy, DC cardioversion will be required.

In patients with acute onset atrial fibrillation, including that occurring in the postoperative period, the risk of systemic embolization becomes significant after 24–48 h. In the absence of contraindications, an anticoagulation strategy with heparin or warfarin should be considered, if the atrial fibrillation persists for a longer period. In these patients rate control is of paramount importance, if cardioversion is to be deferred. Because the anticoagulation protects patients from systemic embolization, they can be observed safely for a few weeks. Postoperative (particularly after cardiac surgery) patients will often spontaneously convert to sinus rhythm during the observation period. If atrial fibrillation persists, then elective cardioversion can be performed with a great likelihood of success. Following elective cardioversion, the decision to administer temporary or chronic suppressive antiarrhythmic drug therapy is based on the clinical estimation of the probability of recurrence.

Chronic Therapy

In patients with stress-induced atrial fibrillation following coronary artery bypass, noncardiac surgery, or an acute medical illness, chronic treatment is often unnecessary. Therapy may be terminated after resolution of the precipitating event and reinstituted only if atrial fibrillation recurs. In practice, most patients in this category have their antiarrhythmic medication discontinued during the hospitalization or at the first postoperative clinic visit. In postoperative patients in whom atrial fibrillation has been a chronic or recurrent problem preoperatively, permanent therapy will be required if arrhythmia suppression (as opposed to rate control) is chosen.

Electrical cardioversion of patients with atrial fibrillation has an initial success rate of ≥90% (40). Factors associated with a higher initial success rate include younger age and shorter duration of arrhythmia (41). The major problem in treating chronic or recurrent atrial fibrillation is maintenance of sinus rhythm after cardioversion. With chronic or recurrent fibrillation, a recurrence rate of 80% at 1 year should be expected following cardioversion, unless antiarrhythmic pharmacologic agents are administered (42).

The recently completed Atrial Fibrillation Follow-up Investigation of Rhythm Management (AFFIRM) trial was performed in older patients with persistent atrial fibrillation who were relatively asymptomatic. This study demonstrated that, when rate control (accompanied by anticoagulation with warfarin) was compared with sinus rhythm maintainence (these patients also received warfarin), no real differences in outcome with regard to mortality or quality of life were observed (43,44).

In patients who use antiarrhythmic drugs to maintain sinus rhythm, the choice of drug is largely empiric. Individual drug toxicities, side effects, and proarrhythmic responses, as well as the nature and severity of the underlying heart disease, should be taken into account. Table 3 summarizes the commonly used antiarrhythmic medications that have been used to control recurrences of atrial fibrillation.

Table 3 Antiarrhythmic Drugs

Drug	Oral dose (mg)	Therapeutic level (µg/mL)	Major elimination route	Primary side effects
Quinidine	300–600 q.6h	3–6	Liver	Diarrhea, GI upset, cinchonism
Procainamide	750–1250 q.6h	4–10	Kidneys	Lupus syndrome GI upset
Disopyramide	100–400 q.6–8h	2–5	Kidneys	Urinary retention, dry mouth, congestive failure
Flecainide	100–200 q.12h	0.2–1.0	Liver	Proarrhythmia, CNS symptoms
Propafenone	150–300 q.8–12h	0.2–3.0	Liver	Unusual taste, GI upset, conduction disturbances
Amiodarone	200–400 q.d.	0.5–1.5	Kidneys	Photosensivity, liver/lung toxicity, thyroid abnormalities
Ethmozine	200–300 q.8h	—	Liver	CNS sympotoms, GI upset, conduction disturbances
Mexiletine	150–300 q.8h	0.75–2	Liver	CNS symptoms, GI upset
Sotalol	80–160 q.12h	—	Liver	CNS symptoms, conduction disturbances, proarrhythmia
Dofetilide	0.25–0.50 q.12h	—	Kidneys	QT prolongation with *torsades de pointes*

Patients should be monitored in the hospital during initial treatment with many antiarrhythmic drugs. Close monitoring will facilitate the early detection of marked QT prolongation and/or frank arrhythmia in a safe environment and ensure medication is otherwise well tolerated before discharge. Electrolyte abnormalities must be corrected before drug therapy, and potential adverse interactions of the antiarrhythmic agent with other drugs such as digoxin, warfarin, and cimetidine must be recognized. Drug administration, metabolism and excretion are important considerations. For example, procainamide is hazardous in patients with significant renal dysfunction, because clearance of this drug occurs via renal excretion. In contrast, quinidine, now a less frequently used agent, is metabolized by the liver before excretion; hence, this agent is hazardous in patients with significant hepatic disease. These factors should be considered before selecting any drug for use in any patient.

Propafenone and sotalol (45,46), both of which combine β-adrenergic blocking properties with antiarrhythmic properties, have been reported to be successful in maintaining sinus rhythm for 1 year in 40–67% of cases (46,47). Amiodarone, has been successful in restoring and maintaining sinus rhythm for 1 year in up to 79% of patients in whom other antiarrhythmic agents have failed (48). Results of the AFFIRM trial indicated that amiodarone was the most effective agent in maintaining sinus rhythm when compared with other agents, including sotalol. Newer agents such as dofetilide were not included in the AFFIRM trial. Agents such as procainamide and moricizine have been used successfully to prevent recurrent atrial fibrillation. Their success rates are lower than that of amiodarone and those recently reported for dofetilide.

The American College of Cardiology (ACC) and the American Heart Association (AHA) have published guidelines in the selection of antiarrhythmic agents used to suppress atrial fibrillation (49). In general, class IC agents should be avoided if any prior history of heart disease, particularly ischemic heart disease, is elicited. Depending on the antiarrhythmic agent chosen, digitalis (or alternatively β-adrenergic blockers or Ca^{++} channel antagonists) are given in conjunction to provide AV slowing, should atrial fibrillation recur. In patients receiving sotalol, a powerful β-adrenergic blocker, additional β-blockade is unnecessary.

For the patient who requires maintenance of sinus rhythm, especially when other drugs have failed, or if the patient has severe underlying heart disease which increases the likelihood of recurrence, we use amiodarone or dofetilide (48). Amiodarone has the additional benefit of slowing conduction through the AV node, should atrial fibrillation recur. After a loading dose of amiodarone is administered, doses of ≤ 200 mg/day may be effective (50). Proarrhythmia is less of a problem with amiodarone than with other antiarrhythmic medications, and LV function is not significantly depressed by orally administered amiodarone. Amiodarone is likely the most efficacious drug; however, amiodarone-associated noncardiac organ system toxicity, especially thyroid, hepatic and pulmonary, is always a concern. The use of chronic amiodarone therapy commits the physician to an organized follow-up plan to detect toxic effects on the thyroid, lung, and liver. Amiodarone is one of the few agents that can be started in an out-patient setting (200 mg/day) with out-patient follow-up.

Dofetilide effectively prevents the recurrence of atrial fibrillation. Further, use of the drug appears to be safe in patients with underlying heart disease, including congestive heart failure, so long as specific administration precautions are taken (50,51). Initiation of dofetilide requires hospitalization to monitor QT interval. Renal function is critical for clearance of dofetilide, and dose adjustments must be made in patients with reduced renal function. Additionally, care needs to be taken to avoid medications that affect dofetilide metabolism or affect the QT interval. With careful monitoring, the incidence of *torsades de pointes* has been kept low. Before being certified to prescribe this drug, each physician and the supplying pharmacy must undergo formal training from the sponsoring pharmaceutical corporation.

Prediction of long-term maintenance of sinus rhythm, with or without suppressive drug treatment, has been correlated with younger age, shorter duration of atrial fibrillation, a low New York Heart Association functional class, and absence of rheumatic heart disease (52).

Chronic atrial pacing has been demonstrated to reduce the occurrence rate of atrial fibrillation in patients with sinus node dysfunction and consequent sinus bradycardia (53). Recently, dual site atrial pacing (simultaneous pacing of high and low right atrium) (54) and Bachmann's bundle pacing (85) have demonstrated some success in reducing the incidence of recurrent atrial fibrillation.

Surgical and, in some cases, catheter-based ablation procedures have been used with success in preventing recurrence of atrial fibrillation in patients not satisfactorily controlled with medical therapies. The different types of surgical procedures employed have been recently reviewed (55). The atrial maze operation utilizes multiple incisions made in both atria. The subsequent incisional scars limit the amount of myocardium that could potentially participate in sustaining the multiple reentry loops, the basis of the arrhythmia. Reported results indicate that postoperative left atrial transport function returns in many patients. However, some patients need chronic pacing to maintain heart rate, probably a result of co-existing intrinsic sinus node dysfunction. Generally the maze procedure is combined with other cardiac surgery, such as mitral valve replacement. Recently, a limited maze procedure has been devised. This procedure uses surgically placed microwave or radiofrequency lesions in various patterns in the left atrium alone. Reported success rates are as high as 70%. The latter procedure can be performed much more quickly and is increasing in popularity as a result.

Catheter-based ablation procedures for atrial fibrillation also have been reviewed recently (56). These procedures have success (60–80%) in selected patients with atrial fibrillation of the paroxysmal type and otherwise normal hearts. These procedures involve electrical isolation of the pulmonary veins with radiofrequency or other forms of energy. Unfortunately, serious complications including symptomatic pulmonary vein stenosis can occur. The results of catheter-based maze-like techniques for the control of chronic atrial fibrillation, especially in abnormal hearts, have been disappointing.

If the ventricular response rate to atrial fibrillation cannot be controlled with drug therapy, radiofrequency ablation of the AV node is an excellent option (57). AV node ablation is combined with ventricular pacing (VVI or VVIR) to produce a controlled regular ventricular rate that markedly decreases patient symptoms and prevents the development of a tachycardia associated myocardiopathy.

Atrial fibrillation and anticoagulation

In patients with rate controlled chronic atrial fibrillation in whom symptoms are absent or mild, studies have demonstrated that low-intensity warfarin therapy (INR 2–3) decreases the risk for stroke to rates close to that of age-matched controls and is safe even in elderly patients (58–61). Evidence that aspirin may reduce the risk of stroke exists (59). Our current practice is to treat all older patients with chronic atrial fibrillation with low-intensity warfarin, unless major contraindications are present. Aspirin is used for patients who are not considered eligible for warfarin therapy.

To summarize, the results of the AFFIRM study, combined with data supporting the safety of carefully monitored low-intensity anticoagulation, indicate that repeated attempts to maintain sinus rhythm in otherwise asymptomatic or mildly symptomatic patients are no longer appropriate, because the risk of proarrhythmia may outweigh the benefits of sinus rhythm.

The role of warfarin in preventing stroke may be more than just prevention of embolization from left atrial thrombi. An echocardiographic study suggested that other mechanisms, including mitral valve disease, patent foramen ovale, regional ventricular wall motion abnormalities, atrial septal aneurysm, carotid atherosclerotic disease, and ascending aortic and aortic arch athero-thrombotic lesions, may also be responsible (62).

Others have cited the low incidence of embolism in patients with "lone atrial fibrillation" and believe that this finding supports the concept that embolism associated with atrial fibrillation results from coexisting cardiovascular disease (63).

Elective Cardioversion

There are several caveats that apply to elective cardioversion. A major concern is the possibility of embolism associated with the procedure. Although the risk for stroke is low (64), in patients in whom atrial fibrillation has been present for >48 h, standard practice is anticoagulation with warfarin for 3–4 weeks before and 3–4 months following cardioversion. The rationale for continuing anticoagulation following successful cardioversion is the known delay in return of atrial mechanical function in some patients (65) and the high rate of recurrent atrial fibrillation.

Approximately 10–20% of patients receiving Class I antiarrhythmic therapy will convert to sinus rhythm prior to cardioversion (66). Additionally, ~30% of patients with atrial fibrillation can be converted with ibutilide, an intravenous Class III agent (67,68). The drug is most effective when atrial fibrillation or flutter is of recent onset (i.e., <30 days). We have occasionally used ibutilide for cardioversion, when avoiding the brief general anesthesia required for electrical cardioversion is necessary. In patients who have failed electrical cardioversion, ibutilide administered 20–30 min prior to a repeat attempt with electrical cardioversion has substantially improved the success rate (69). *Ibutilide must be used very cautiously if the patient has recently received other antiarrhythmic drugs.* When ibutilide is used, the patient must be NPO and carefully monitored for a few hours after drug administration; the incidence of polymorphic ventricular tachycardia following ibutilide has been reported to be as high as 8.3% (67). Dofetilide, which is used for chronic therapy, can result in an ~40% conversion rate during the initial dosing phase. During this time, the patient must be monitored in the hospital. Conversion usually occurs after the third or fourth dose, and, if it does not occur, elective cardioversion can be performed prior to discharge. Postconversion, warfarin is recommended for at least a few weeks in patients with a low likelihood of recurrence and 3–6 months with a higher likelihood of recurrence. Transesophageal echocardiography has been used to identify left atrial thrombus prior to cardioversion. Absence of left atrial thrombus lessens the need for anticoagulation prior to, *but not following, cardioversion*, unless a major contraindication to anticoagulation exists (70).

In patients with atrial fibrillation of short duration (i.e., <48 h), the role of anticoagulation with warfarin after cardioversion is unclear. We recommend initial heparinization on admission, if cardioversion is to be delayed. For postoperative patients with atrial fibrillation that requires cardioversion and who also have risk factors for embolization, anticoagulation may be prudent, until the risk of an early recurrence is past.

Atrial Flutter

Etiology

Atrial flutter occurs more frequently in older than in younger patients. It is uncommon in the absence of underlying heart or advanced pulmonary disease. Typical atrial flutter is a reentrant rhythm that uses the isthmus between the tricuspid valve and inferior vena cava as the reentrant pathway. In atypical atrial flutter, the reentrant pathway is present in other areas of the right or left atrium.

Clinical Presentation

In typical atrial flutter, the flutter rate its ~300 beats/min with a 2:1 AV block. The resulting ventricular rate is 150 beats/min. In the absence of ventricular ectopy or varying AV conduction, the rate is regular. As in patients with atrial fibrillation, symptoms from atrial flutter are dependent on the ventricular rate and the presence of underlying heart or lung disease. Typical atrial flutter is characterized by predominantly negative flutter waves, described as "saw tooth" in appearance (Figs. 7 and 9). The flutter waves most often are seen in inferior leads II, III, and AVF on the surface ECG. This pattern may be obscured by the QRST complex. Occasionally, flutter waves are best seen in lead VI. In atypical flutter, other patterns of regular rapid atrial activation are seen that depend on the location of the underlying re-entry circuit. The atrial flutter rate is typically 250–340 beats/min with 2:1 AV block. Less frequently, a greater degree of AV block is present. In these patients the ventricular response rate is usually greater than or less than 150 beats/min. Rarely, 1:1 conduction occurs, unless accelerated AV nodal conduction or an accessory AV connection is present (Fig. 9). In patients who initially have 2:1 AV block, 1:1 AV conduction can occur, if the atrial flutter rate is slowed with antiarrhythmic drugs. For example, if the atrial rate slows from 300 (where there is 2:1 conduction) to 200 (where there is 1:1 conduction), the ventricular rate will increase from 150 to 200 beats/min. Among patients with primary abnormalities of AV nodal function, or those receiving drugs that depress AV nodal conduction, AV block may be greater than 2:1 (Fig. 7). The ventricular rate is always an integral multiple of the atrial flutter rate, unless complete heart block with a junctional or ventricular escape rhythm develops. Atrial flutter is distinguished from other tachycardias originating in the atrium primarily by rate. With atrial flutter, the atrial rate in the absence of antiarrhythmic drug effect, is generally >250 beats/min. The atrial rate in primary atrial tachycardias is usually lower.

Because an atrial flutter rate of 300 beats/min is usually accompanied by 2:1 AV block, atrial flutter should be suspected in every regular supraventricular tachycardia with a ventricular rate of ~150 beats/min, even if flutter waves are not readily visible on ECG. If the patient is stable, maneuvers that transiently increase AV block, such as carotid massage or administration of adenosine (6–12 mg, IV bolus), can be used to unmask flutter waves (Fig. 10). If conversion to sinus rhythm occurs with these maneuvers, then AV nodal or AV re-entrant rhythm (rather than atrial flutter) is the likely diagnosis (Fig. 10). An atrial electrogram obtained from an intra-atrial or an esophageal electrode can also be helpful in making an accurate diagnosis. In postoperative cardiac

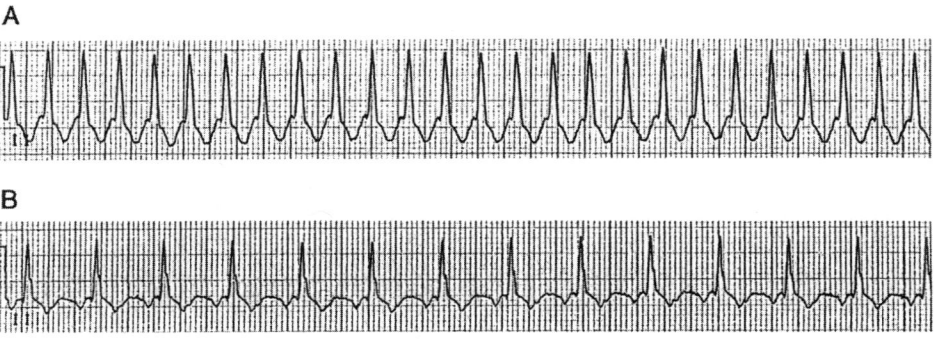

Figure 9 ECG lead II—(A) atrial flutter with 1:1 ventricular response rate. The QRS makes interpretation of the rhythm difficult because the flutter waves are obscured. (B) Atrial flutter from the same patient after pharmacologic slowing of AV conduction. The flutter waves are now visible as an undulating baseline.

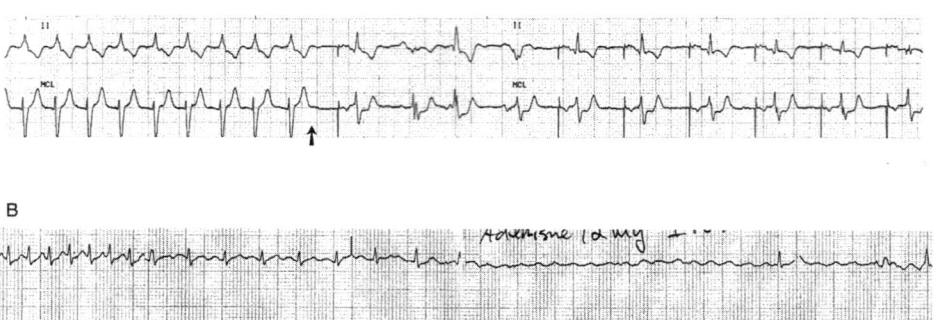

Figure 10 ECG leads II and MCL—(A) adenosine termination of a somewhat wide complex arrhythmia indicated by the arrow. The rhythm converts to an AV paced rhythm indicating that interruption of conduction through the AV junction was important in maintaining the tachycardia. (B) Adenosine induced AV block in a patient with atrial flutter. Note on the left very rapid AV conduction or 1 : 1 followed by slowing of AV conduction 2 : 1, followed by complete AV block with flutter waves not conducted to the ventricles leading to transient asystole. In this case the nature of the underlying atrial arrhythmia is unmasked by the use of pharmacologic AV block induction with adenosine.

surgery patients, if temporary atrial wires are placed for postoperative pacing, the diagnosis of atrial flutter can be made readily by recording from the leads. Further, rapid pacing techniques using the atrial leads often can terminate the arrhythmia.

The reported incidence of systemic embolism complicating atrial flutter is lower than that seen in atrial fibrillation. This finding may be related to the mechanical activity of the atria during flutter. Atrial activity, in atrial flutter, is more coordinated than that of atrial fibrillation, and less stagnation of blood in the atrium results. Recently, echocardiographic studies of patients with atrial flutter have demonstrated a surprisingly high incidence of thrombus in the left atrial appendage and/or evidence of blood stasis ("smoke") (71). Hence, although the embolic risk with flutter is undoubtedly lower than that incurred with atrial fibrillation, anticoagulation of postoperative patients with prolonged atrial flutter is prudent, because systemic embolism can occur (72–74).

Acute Therapy

Patients with atrial flutter and rapid ventricular response (≥ 150 beats/min) may present with no, mild, or severe symptoms. If symptoms are severe, the treatment of choice is QRS synchronized DC cardioversion or atrial overdrive pacing. The latter is particularly useful following cardiac operations when a temporary atrial lead is in place (75). In patients with severe chronic lung disease, in whom even a brief period of general anesthesia may be undesirable, overdrive pacing can be done after the percutaneous placement of a right atrial electrode catheter (76). The advantages of DC cardioversion are that it is generally available, highly effective, and can be used in anticoagulated patients.

In patients with acute atrial flutter with less severe or no symptoms, the usual ventricular response is ≤ 150 beats/min. Early cardioversion by QRS synchronized DC cardioversion or overdrive pacing remains the most efficient treatment. Initial therapy with digoxin and procainamide results in conversion in 10–20% of cases. Up to 50% of patients with acute atrial flutter associated with surgery or stress convert to sinus rhythm with intravenous esmolol therapy. This drug should be considered if the patient has no major contraindications. Esmolol may increase the degree of AV block and reduce the ventricular response rate (36,37). However, in some patients with good AV nodal function, the dose of esmolol required may cause significant hypotension. In the absence of contraindications, such as recent therapy with an antiarrhythmic agent, ibutilide can be used for cardioversion as described for atrial fibrillation. The expected success rate is 40–60%. Conversion usually occurs within 30 min following the end of the infusion. The patient monitored for polymorphous ventricular tachycardia for a few hours following ibutilide infusion (67).

Some patients with atrial flutter demonstrate a degree of AV block greater than 2:1 without prior drug therapy. These patients often have a slow flutter rate (between 180 and 220 beats/min). The ventricular rate in these patients is usually between 60 and 100 beats/min. This presentation is more common in patients with severe underlying heart disease associated with abnormalities of the sino-atrial node, intra-atrial conduction system, and AV node. A strong case can be made for simply anticoagulating these patients, if the ventricular response rates at rest and with stress are acceptable. The presence of significant AV node disease substantially increases the hazards of rate control and antiarrhythmic suppressive therapy. If the patient is cardioverted to sinus rhythm, bradycardia may worsen, because rate control or suppressive therapy may cause additional sinus node suppression. Antiarrhythmic drugs also may cause or increase AV block. Hence, this approach is feasible only with backup permanent pacing. The mode of pacing should be DDD or DDDR pacing, if the patient is in sinus rhythm, or VVI or VVIR, if the patient remains in flutter. Backup pacing should be available if cardioversion is attempted, because successful conversion may unmask severe sinus node dysfunction.

When in atrial flutter, a small number of patients exhibit 1:1 AV conduction and very rapid ventricular rates. Like atrial fibrillation, this rapid response suggests that accelerated AV nodal conduction or an accessory AV connection is present. The latter is suggested by abnormal QRS morphology compatible with preexcitation. This ECG pattern may be confused with ventricular tachycardia, especially in the absence of variable AV block. Even if the diagnosis is uncertain, the rapid heart rate itself poses a major threat to the patient and urgent cardioversion or rate slowing is indicated.

Chronic Therapy

After acute atrial flutter has been converted, the duration of drug therapy is variable and largely determined by the cause of the flutter. In patients with acute stress-induced atrial flutter following cardiac surgery, therapy may be terminated after a few days to weeks and reinstituted only if flutter recurs. In patients with chronic atrial flutter, pharmacologic control of ventricular rate, particularly during exercise, is often difficult or impossible to achieve, if the patient has normal AV nodal function. Thus, cardioversion and suppressive drug therapy, rather than rate control, is the therapeutic goal. The long-term suppressive strategies available are the same as those described for atrial fibrillation. Additionally, dofetilide, by slowing atrial conduction velocity, can be quite effective in chronically suppressing atrial flutter, both typical and atypical.

Catheter ablation of the flutter "circuit" with radiofrequency energy has been used to treat chronic or recurrent atrial flutter (77). Ablation of the isthmus between the tricuspid valve and inferior vena cava can be curative in a substantial number of patients with typical atrial flutter. In atypical atrial flutter, ablation success can be achieved with careful mapping of the reentrant pathway of the arrhythmia. Unfortunately, up to 30% of patients subsequently develop atrial fibrillation, which, in some cases, can be suppressed with antiarrhythmic therapy (78). If drug regimens or flutter ablation therapies fail, catheter ablation of the AV node followed by VVI or VVIR pacemaker implantation is the therapy of choice.

Available data indicate anticoagulation for chronic atrial flutter or for cardioversion of patients with atrial flutter of >48 h is beneficial. With contraindications to anticoagulation, a transesophageal echocardiogram should be obtained. In the presence of clot or "smoke" in the left atrial appendage, cardioversion will have a higher risk of thromboembolic complications, and short-term anticoagulation should be reconsidered. If cardioverted (with or without anticoagulation), these patients always should be placed on suppressive antiarrhythmic therapy for several months, if the risk for recurrence is minimal, or permanently, if the risk of recurrence is high. If suppressive therapy is considered unsafe, cardioversion should not be attempted, because the likelihood of recurrence is high.

Multifocal Atrial Tachycardia

Etiology

Multifocal atrial tachycardia (MAT) is a common arrhythmia that is almost never primary (79) (Fig. 7). It is most frequently encountered in the medical or surgical intensive care unit in patients with severe cardiac or pulmonary disease, particularly those with exacerbations of chronic obstructive lung disease. It may result from a stress precipitated surge in plasma catecholamine levels combined with atrial abnormalities such as acute stretch. Patients receiving theophylline, agents related to theophylline, or catecholamine containing bronchodilators are particularly susceptible to MAT. The theophylline serum concentration should be determined in any patient with MAT who receives or is suspected of receiving this drug. Of note, MAT is not a manifestation of digitalis toxicity, but digitalis toxicity may supervene when that agent is used in a vain attempt to control the ventricular rate response.

Clinical Presentation

The characteristic ECG pattern is a rapid, irregular ventricular rhythm with each QRS complex preceded by P waves of varying morphology (Fig. 7). Nonconducted premature P waves are also frequent. The typical heart rate is 100–130 beats/min. Faster rates may occur and be complicated by aberrant ventricular conduction (80). MAT may be associated with intermittent atrial flutter or fibrillation. Usually, three or more different P wave morphologies are required for diagnosis (81). If the ECG pattern is similar, but the atrial rate is ≤100 beats/min, the term "chaotic atrial rhythm" is sometimes used. If the ventricular rate is more than ∼130 beats/min, MAT may worsen ischemia or compromise hemodynamic status in patients who are already quite ill. In clinically stable patients, the rhythm generally poses no threat, unless the ventricular response becomes very rapid (∼150 beats/min).

Acute Therapy

The primary intent of therapy is treatment of the underlying disease and elimination of other precipitating causes of MAT, such as theophylline toxicity. The major indication for treating MAT is a ventricular rate that is not tolerated by the patient. β-Adrenergic blocking drugs or Ca^{++} channel antagonists may be useful to control the ventricular rate (82). The role of β-adrenergic blockers is limited by the severity of the coexisting lung disease, although low dose esmolol therapy is often effective and well tolerated in such patients. If these drugs fail, a standard antiarrhythmic agent can be added in an attempt to slow the atrial rate (79). Digoxin is usually ineffective, and, if vigorously administered, may induce digitalis toxicity. In refractory cases of more chronic MAT, we have had some success with amiodarone therapy. Amiodarone not only slows atrial rate, but also slows AV conduction; both effects result in slower ventricular rates.

Other Primary Atrial Tachycardias

Etiology

Sustained paroxysms of atrial tachycardia (AT) are relatively uncommon when compared with atrial fibrillation and flutter. However, short asymptomatic bursts often are detected during ECG monitoring (Holter or in-hospital monitoring). AT has several intra-atrial electrophysiological mechanisms and is usually associated with underlying cardiac disease (83). A relatively small number of cases of AT with variable atrioventricular nodal block are a result of digitalis toxicity, although this arrhythmia is considered characteristic of digitalis toxicity (84).

Clinical Presentation

As in other atrial tachyarrhythmias, heart rate and underlying severity of heart or lung disease determine whether the patient experiences significant symptoms. When AT is a consequence of digitalis toxicity, patients may have other symptoms such as nausea, vomiting, confusion, and rarely, yellow vision.

The atrial rates can vary widely from just over 100 to over 200 beats/min. P waves are present before each QRS complex, unless AV block is present (Fig. 11). The P wave may have a normal axis, a finding that suggests an origin in the high right atrium. Alternatively, P waves may have a superiorly directed axis with negative P waves in inferior leads, a combination consistent with a low atrial origin, so-called "inferior atrial rhythm." Atrial flutter and AT usually are distinguished by the atrial rate. Carotid sinus massage or intravenous adenosine (6–12 mg, IV bolus) may induce AV block in AT with 1:1 conduction. This response identifies the atrium as the source of the arrhythmia. If either carotid sinus massage or adenosine terminates the arrhythmia, AV nodal re-entry or re-entry using an accessory connection should be considered.

Acute and Chronic Therapy

Therapy is determined by clinical urgency and etiology of the arrhythmia. AT with AV block suggests digitalis toxicity. When digitalis toxicity is suspected, the drug should be withheld and hypomagnesemia and hypokalemia, if present, should be corrected. Digoxin antibody administration usually is not required unless AT is rapid or the patient experiences adverse symptoms. A substantially elevated serum digoxin concentration (>3 ng/mL) supports a diagnosis of digoxin toxicity. Unstable patients with frank digitalis toxicity should not be cardioverted, because cardioversion confers substantial danger of post-cardioversion ventricular arrhythmias. Antibody administration is the preferred treatment.

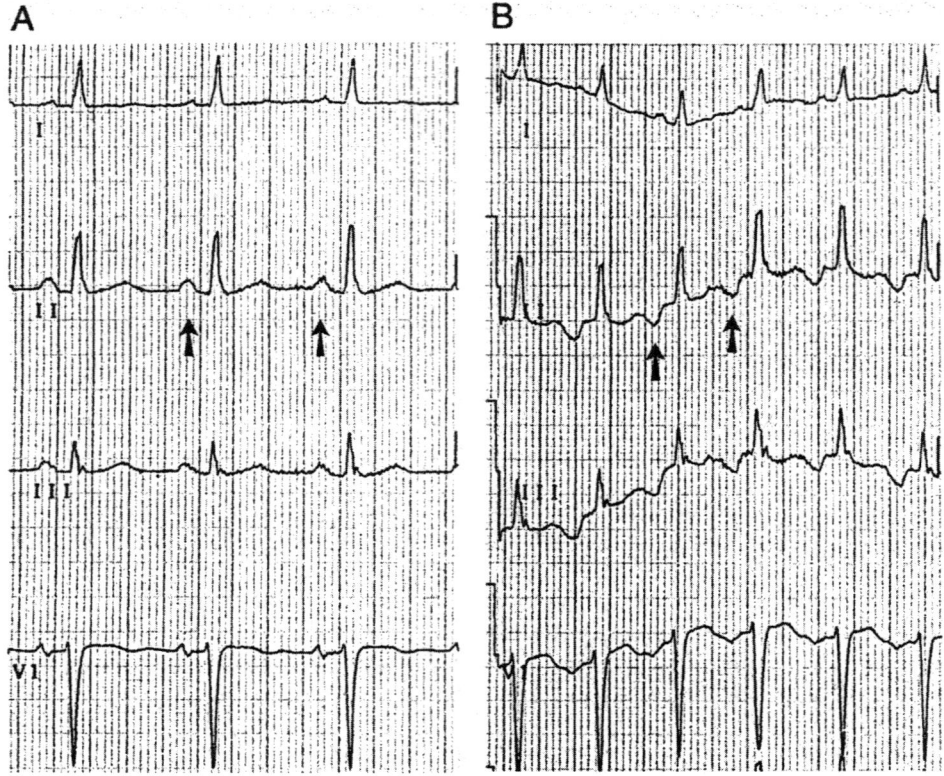

Figure 11 ECG in (A) demonstrates normal sinus rhythm with P waves indicated with arrows. (B) ECG is taken from the same patient during his atrial tachycardia. Note the different heart rate and P wave (arrows) morphology.

If digoxin is not the cause of AT, the usual case, and the patient is clinically unstable, cardioversion should be performed. In patients with an intra-atrial, reentrant tachycardia, conversion to sinus rhythm may occur. Various antiarrhythmic drugs used for suppression of atrial fibrillation and flutter may be effective in suppressing recurrent AT. If the arrhythmia is automatic in origin, stimulants such as theophylline and caffeine should be avoided, and a trial of β-adrenergic blocker therapy may be warranted. Treatment with Ca^{++} channel blockers also can be effective. In patients with recurrent drug resistant AT, an electrophysiological study may be useful in clarifying the nature of the arrhythmia. Surgical or catheter ablation of an atrial focus has been successful in selected cases (106). AV nodal ablation combined with ventricular or dual chamber pacing is reserved for refractory cases.

Nonparoxysmal Junctional Tachycardia

Etiology

Nonparoxysmal junctional tachycardia (NPJT) is an accelerated junctional rhythm with ventricular rate between 70 and 140 beats/min (85). It may be caused by digitalis toxicity (84) or be associated with cardiac surgery, acute myocardial infarction, pulmonary embolization, sepsis, or other severe illnesses that elevate serum catecholamine concentrations. It should not be confused with a junctional escape rhythm that occurs in the presence of physiological or pathological sinus bradycardia, because the junctional escape rate is usually less than <80 beats/min even during periods of increased sympathetic activity.

Clinical Presentation

The patient may be asymptomatic or have symptoms and signs of the underlying disease. AV dissociation may produce "cannon A waves" in the jugular venous pulse. The intensity of the first heart sound varies for the same reason. The junctional rate exceeds that of the sinus node. The ventricular rate is generally somewhat irregular as a consequence of intermittent sinus capture beats and periodic resetting of the sinus node by retrograde atrial activation. Loss of the atrial contribution to ventricular filling may precipitate or aggravate heart failure. Episodes of more rapid NPJT may be confused with slow ventricular tachycardia when aberrant intraventricular conduction is present.

Acute Therapy

When NPJT is a manifestation of digitalis toxicity, and the patient is hemodynamically stable, withholding digoxin and correcting hypomagnesemia and hypokalemia are appropriate. If the patient is unstable, and the arrhythmia is thought to be contributory, digitalis antibody can be administered.

In the absence of digitalis toxicity, nothing need be done beyond treating the underlying problem in a stable patient. If lack of atrial "kick" is associated with hemodynamic instability, atrial pacing may be used to overdrive the junctional pacemaker and restore a normal sequence of contraction. If the heart rate is excessive, a short-acting β-adrenergic blocking drug, such as esmolol, may be administered cautiously to slow the rate. However, this strategy is unlikely to correct the arrhythmia. As this tachyarrhythmia is transient during acute illness or perioperative stress, no chrornic therapy is recommended.

AV NODAL AND AV REENTRANT ARRHYTHMIAS

In the absence of a prior history of tachycardia, the initial appearance of these arrhythmias in the perioperative period is uncommon, but not rare.

AV Nodal Reentry

Etiology

AV nodal reentry tachycardia is usually precipitated by a premature atrial impulse that is conducted slowly through the AV nodal region in the antegrade direction, re-enters a fast conduction pathway, and propagates in the retrograde direction (Fig. 12). This pattern of slow antegrade conduction with fast retrograde conduction (slow–fast AV nodal reentry) can continue as a circus movement tachycardia, until the circuit destabilizes spontaneously or a therapeutic maneuver or drug treatment terminates it. A much less common form (fast–slow AV nodal reentry) results from antegrade conduction

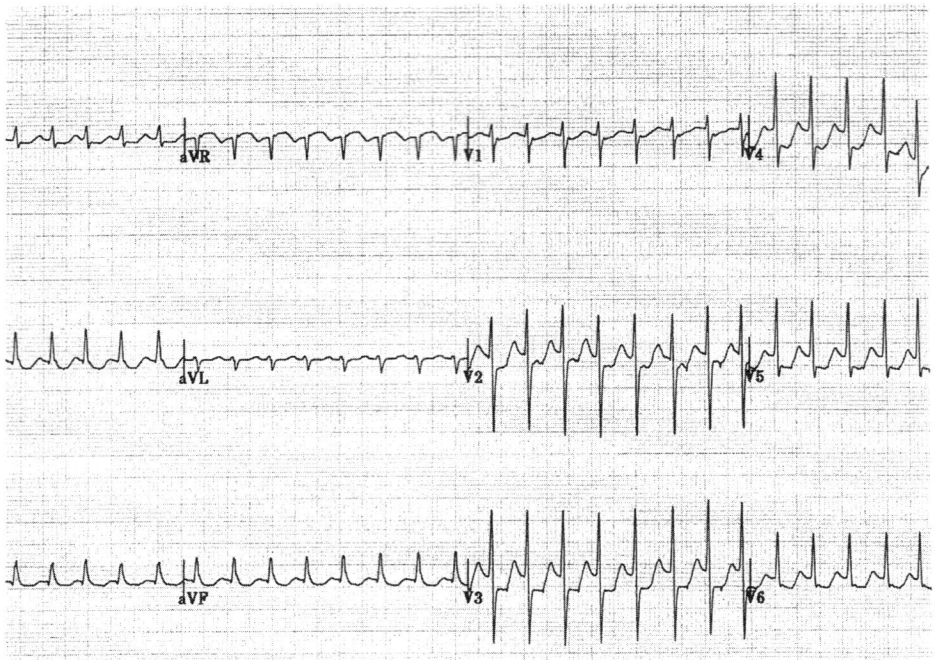

Figure 12 12 Lead ECG in patient with AV node reentry. Note the absence of visible P waves (see text).

down a fast pathway and retrograde conduction via the slow pathway. In most patients, only one form of the tachycardia is observed. However, intermediate forms with variable conduction times in either antegrade or retrograde direction may occur.

Clinical Presentation

Typically, attacks of tachycardia begin and end suddenly. Generally, the heart rate is in the range of 160–180 beats/min but faster rates may occur and occasionally result in syncope. Syncope may result, in part, from the hemodynamic consequences of simultaneous contraction of the atria and ventricles, the rapid rate itself, or other neurally mediated causes (86).

The ECG during tachycardia usually has a narrow QRS complex or a QRS morphology similar to that present when the patient is in sinus rhythm. Typical right or left bundle branch block conduction pattern may also occur. In the common slow–fast tachycardia, the atria and ventricles are activated nearly simultaneously. Consequently, the P wave is buried in the QRS complex (Fig. 12). An esophageal or atrial electrode can be used at the bedside to document simultaneous activation of the atria and ventricles. In the uncommon form of AV node reentry (fast–slow), a retrograde P wave may be visible during tachycardia, and the distance from the preceding R wave to the P is longer than the subsequent PR interval. During sinus rhythm, patients with AV nodal reentry tachycardia do not have delta waves to suggest ventricular preexcitation. Although a probable diagnosis of AV nodal reentry can often be made from clinical and ECG features, an invasive electrophysiological study is needed to confirm the diagnosis.

Acute Therapy

Before receiving medical attention, patients already may have discovered that certain maneuvers, such as breath holding, Valsalva maneuver, or carotid massage, can interrupt the tachycardia (87). When these maneuvers are successful, termination of tachycardia is the rule in contrast to the transient increase in AV block seen in patients with primary atrial tachycardias. If vagal maneuvers fail, intravenous adenosine or a Ca^{++} channel blockers, such as verapamil, are usually successful. Adenosine (6–12 mg, IV bolus) is preferable, because the rapid onset and termination of action limits the duration of any side effects. Intravenous verapamil (5–15 mg, IV over a few minutes) is also quite effective, but can result in significant hypotension, particularly if rapid conversion to sinus rhythm does not occur. Pretreatment with intravenously administered Ca^{++} has been shown to prevent or attenuate the hypotension without affecting the AV nodal blocking effect (105). DC cardioversion is rarely necessary.

Chronic Therapy

Patients with infrequent, brief, well-tolerated episodes of AV nodal reentrant tachycardia that are self terminating may require no therapy. If drug therapy is necessary, β-adrenergic blockers, Ca^{++} channel blockers, and antiarrhythmic drugs have been used with varying degrees of success.

Catheter modification of the AV node has been found to be extremely effective in treating both "slow" and "fast" pathway tachycardias in >95% of patients (88,89). Selective AV nodal modification is occasionally complicated by complete AV block, a complication more common when ablation of a "fast" pathway is attempted (89). Catheter ablation has become the primary therapy in many patients with frequent symptomatic episodes of AV nodal reentry tachycardia, because the success rate is high and pharmacological agents offer only moderate efficacy. Further, every antiarrhythmic agent has the potential to cause proarrhythmia and other side effects.

AV Reentry Tachycardia and the WPW Syndrome

Etiology

AV reentry tachycardia uses an accessory pathway and the normal specialized AV conduction system as a macro-reentry tachycardia loop (90). The arrhythmia is precipitated by premature atrial or ventricular impulses that are conducted at differing velocities through the normal AV specialized conduction system and the accessory connection.

Clinical Presentation

Similar to AV nodal reentry tachycardia, episodes of AV reentry tachycardia start and end abruptly. Tachycardia rates are comparable to those seen with AV nodal reentry. The ECG in sinus rhythm may demonstrate evidence of ventricular preexcitation in the form of delta waves (90) (Fig. 13). The presence of delta waves depends on the location of the connection, its ability to conduct in an antegrade fashion, and the conduction properties of the AV node. If the connection does not conduct in an antegrade direction, it is called "concealed".

Orthodromic reciprocating tachycardia (ORT) (Fig. 14), the most common form of AV reentrant tachycardia, utilizes the normal AV node and His conduction system in an antegrade direction and the accessory connection in a retrograde direction to complete the reentry loop. Hence, delta waves, if present during sinus rhythm, disappear during

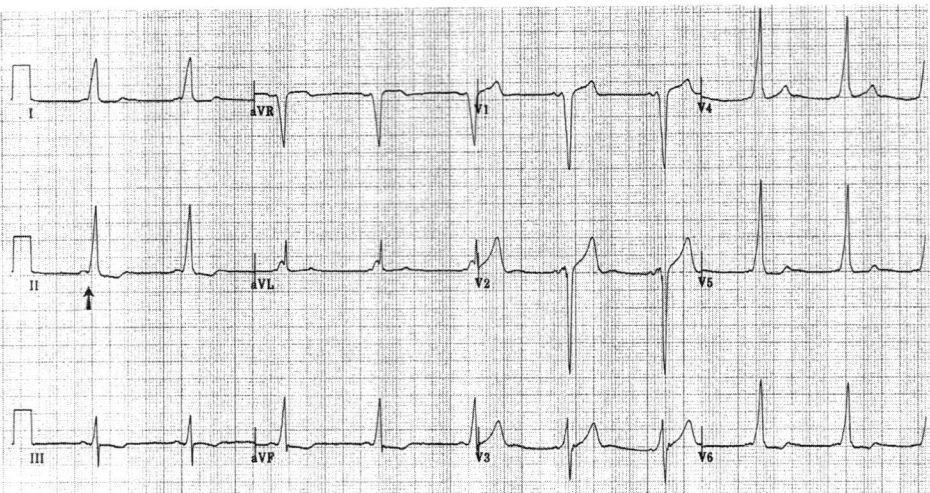

Figure 13 12 Lead ECG demonstrating ventricular pre-excitation. Note the short PR (arrow) with slurred (delta wave) upstroke of the QRS indicating early activation of the ventricles via an accessory AV connection.

the tachycardia (Fig. 14). The ventricular rate during ORT is frequently in the range of 180–200 beats/min, although faster rates (200–240 beats/min) are occasionally encountered. Unlike AV node reentry, careful examination of the ECG during ORT often will reveal a distinct retrograde P wave following the QRS (Fig. 14). The timing

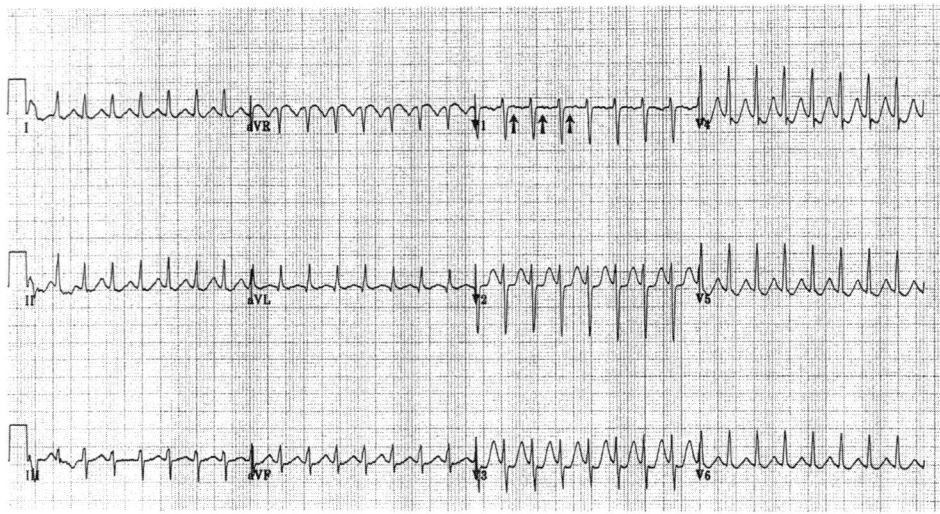

Figure 14 12 Lead ECG demonstrating tachycardia consistent with antegrade conduction down the AV node (normal QRS) and retrograde conduction via an accessory connection. Retrograde P waves are indicated with arrows.

of the P waves is such that the R–P interval is usually less than the subsequent P–R interval. During ORT, the QRS is typically narrow, but right or left bundle branch block may occur.

Antidromic reciprocating tachycardia (ART) is much less common and involves antegrade conduction through the accessory connection with retrograde conduction via the His bundle and AV nodal conduction system (90). In ART, the QRS is wide and bizarre, because abnormal ventricular activation spreads away from the ventricular insertion of the accessory connection.

Patients with accessory connections may experience severe symptoms, usually the result of the especially fast ventricular rates in response to atrial fibrillation or flutter. Fast ventricular rates occur when the accessory pathway has a rapid antegrade conduction velocity and a short refractory period. Under these conditions, the QRS is wide and bizarre.

Other accessory AV connections exist that are variants of preexcitation, but are less common. One example is an atriofasicular connection that arises in the right atrium and inserts in the region of the right bundle branch. Others are nodofasicular and nodoventricular connections that may arise in the AV node and insert in the vicinity of the right bundle branch or right ventricle (91).

Acute Therapy

As in AV nodal reentry tachycardia, patients may use the Valsalva maneuver or carotid massage to interrupt episodes of tachycardia. These maneuvers can be successful, because AV nodal conduction is slowed by vagal (cholinergic) stimulation, and the AV node is always a component of the re-entry pathway. If vagal maneuvers fail, and QRS morphology is normal, or if the QRS morphology is a typical right or left bundle branch block, then adenosine (6–12 mg, IV bolus) or verapamil (5–15 mg, IV over a few minutes) can be used to terminate orthodromic tachycardia. Whether vagal maneuvers, adenosine, or verapamil are used, termination nearly always occurs with inscription of a P wave, because block occurs in the AV node. Synchronized DC cardioversion can be employed, if the drug therapy fails.

If antidromic tachycardia with either antegrade conduction through an accessory connection and retrograde conduction through the normal conduction system or atrial fibrillation or flutter with rapid antegrade conduction through an accessory pathway is suspected, prompt cardioversion is the safest and most expeditious therapy and will likely be successful. If the wide complex tachycardia is well tolerated, slow IV infusion of procainamide (10–15 mg/kg) given at a rate of no greater than 25 mg/min, with careful monitoring for hypotension, may be successful. *Digoxin and Ca^{++} channel blockers (classically verapamil) should be avoided in treatment of these tachycardias. These drugs may facilitate conduction through the accessory connection and further accelerate heart rate.*

Chronic Therapy

As in AV nodal reentry, no treatment may be necessary in patients with infrequent, well-tolerated, and self terminating episodes of orthodromic AV reentry tachycardia. In patients with ORT requiring treatment, drugs that slow AV nodal conduction such as digoxin and Ca^{++} channel blockers may be effective. However, these drugs can potentially increase the frequency of tachycardia by providing the critical AV nodal delay required for an impulse to reenter the accessory connection. Drugs that slow accessory pathway conduction such as β-adrenergic blockers and most antiarrhythmic drugs can be used successfully (92).

In patients with antidromic tachycardia or rapid ventricular response to atrial fibrillation, antiarrhythmic drugs are especially important. Amiodarone has been found to be particularly effective in the management of some refractory tachycardias.

Catheter ablation is a relatively safe and effective curative therapy (>90%) for patients with accessory connections and frequent tachycardia (93,94). The high success rate coupled with the low complication rate makes catheter ablation the preferred treatment in most patients with accessory connections who are symptomatic. Catheter ablation is especially useful in patients with atrial fibrillation or flutter and rapid conduction through an accessory pathway.

Although the patient may have few symptoms related to the arrhythmia, the medical approach commits these often young patients to a lifetime of dependence on antiarrhythmic drugs and with their attendant side effects and toxicities.

VENTRICULAR ARRHYTHMIAS

Premature Ventricular Contractions and Nonsustained Ventricular Tachycardia (NSVT)

Etiology

Premature ventricular contractions (PVCs) and runs of nonsustained ventricular tachycardia (NSVT) are common, especially in older patients. PVC frequency also increases with the presence of heart disease. PVCs may be encountered in the absence of clinically evident heart disease, but most often, they complicate ischemic or other causes of heart disease. Frequently, ECG monitoring, including perioperative monitoring, detects these frequently asymptomatic arrhythmias.

Clinical Presentation

Many patients are unaware of the arrhythmia. The palpitations or sensations of throbbing in the neck are presumably caused by "cannon A waves." Anxiety may result from awareness of an irregular heart rhythm. Clinical observation indicates that most PVCs are asymptomatic, even in patients who complain of symptoms. Perception of PVCs is more likely to occur when the patient is at rest, especially before sleep when external stimuli are minimal.

On the ECG, PVCs are usually easily recognized by their QRS patterns of atypical LBBB or RBBB, or of greater degrees of aberration. A full compensatory pause usually occurs, because block of the next sinus beat results from retrograde conduction and penetration of the sinus node by the PVC. Usually, the coupling interval between the PVC and the preceding normal QRS complex is fixed, and the mechanism is considered re-entry or triggered via a pathway within a ventricle. If retrograde conduction is absent, as with closely coupled PVCs, and the subsequent sinus P wave is conducted, the PVC is said to be interpolated. When the coupling interval is variable but the interval between PVCs is constant, or a multiple of a constant interval, ventricular parasystole is present. Parasystole is thought to derive from a competing ventricular pacemaker. NSVT has ECG features comparable to those described subsequently for sustained ventricular tachycardia.

Acute and Chronic Therapy

Evidence exists that frequent PVCs, PVCs in pairs, short PVC runs of <5 beats, and NSVT of <20–30 s duration are independent markers for sudden death *in the presence* of significant underlying heart disease (95–97). However, no data indicate that treatment with antiarrhythmic drugs, with the possible exception of amiodarone, improves prognosis of this group (98). Amiodarone therapy produces mixed results, when used in patients with cardiomyopathy at high risk after myocardial infarction. The lesson of the Cardiac Arrhythmia Suppression Study (CAST) study is that certain antiarrhythmic drugs actually increase mortality after myocardial infarction, despite their efficacy in controlling ventricular ectopy (99). Whether these data apply to other antiarrhythmic drugs or other cardiac diseases remains to be determined. Effective treatment of the high risk patient group with ectopy and decreased LV function involves placement of implantable cardiac defibrillators, a topic that will subsequently be discussed.

Symptomatic patients with no, or modest, heart disease should be reassured that PVCs are not dangerous. Reassurance often will reduce anxiety and make sensed PVCs tolerable. β-adrenergic blockers may be used for their anxiolytic effect, in the absence of contraindications; however, control of PVCs is often ineffective. Therapy with antiarrhythmic drugs in this group should be reserved for the very few patients with intractable and distressing symptoms willing to accept risks inherent in such therapy. Table 3 summarizes the drugs commonly used in the treatment of ventricular arrhythmias.

Similar considerations apply to NSVT in asymptomatic patients who have relatively well preserved left ventricular function. In patients with an ejection fraction of <30–35%, complex ventricular ectopy identifies a group of patients at high risk for sudden death (95–97). The MADITT trial using ambulatory monitoring evaluated post-MI patients with ejection fractions <35% and NSVT (>3 beats) (100). Patients were subjected to electrophysiological testing. If inducible ventricular tachycardia were present and not suppressible with antiarrhythmic drugs, the patients were randomized to receive conventional therapy or an implantable defibrillator (ICD). A significant reduction in arrhythmic death was demonstrated in the ICD group.

In contrast, in a group of patients referred for coronary artery bypass with ejection fractions <35% and an abnormal signal averaged ECG, implantation of a defibrillator at the time of surgery did not have a survival benefit (101). This lack of improvement may have resulted from favorable effects of revascularization on the survival of patients with significant left ventricular dysfunction.

In the second MADITT trial, ICD implantation in patients with ischemic heart disease and an ejection fraction of $\leq$30%, and who did not receive electrophysiological evaluation, produced a survival benefit. Thus, ICD therapy is becoming standard in patients with ischemic heart disease with low ejection fractions. Survival benefit also has been demonstrated in hypertrophic cardiomyopathy patients. Additional studies are ongoing in patients with other forms of cardiomyopathy to assess the role of ICD use. Patients considered for the prophylactic use of ICDs should not be at high risk of death from other causes and should have a reasonable cardiovascular prognosis, if the fatal ventricular arrhythmia is prevented.

Sustained Ventricular Tachycardia and Ventricular Fibrillation

Etiology

Chronic ischemic heart disease with myocardial scarring and left ventricular dysfunction is by far the most common substrate for recurrent ventricular tachycardia, ventricular fibrillation, and sudden death (Fig. 15). Acute myocardial ischemia/infarction can be

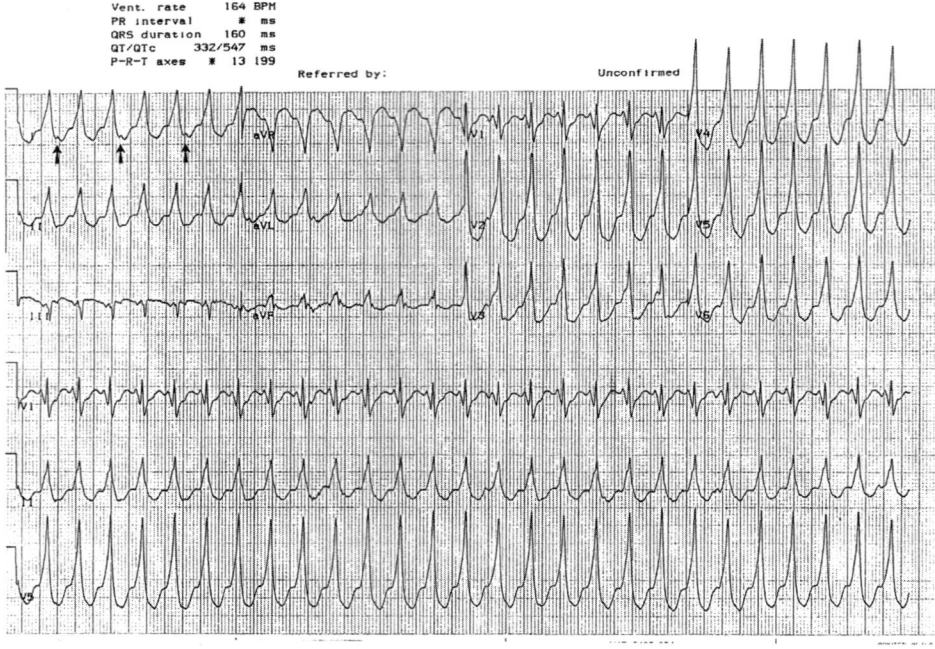

Figure 15 12 Lead ECG demonstrating ventricular tachycardia. Note the wide bizarre QRS with an atypical bundle branch block appearance. Note also ventricular atrial dissociation. Retrograde P waves are indicated with arrows.

complicated by significant ventricular arrhythmias. The stress of surgery, including the hypercoaguable state that exists perioperatively, can precipitate acute myocardial ischemia.

The next most common cause of nonischemic ventricular arrhythmias is nonischemic myocardiopathy with left ventricular dysfunction. Common causes of left ventricular dysfunction include valvular disease, long-standing hypertension, idiopathic cardiomyopathy and, chronic alcohol abuse.

Drug-induced ventricular arrhythmias, including those associated with QT prolongation (*torsades de pointes*) (102) (Fig. 16) and digitalis toxicity (84), must also be considered. Drugs associated with QT prolongation and *torsades de pointes* include most standard antiarrhythmic drugs such as quinidine, procainamide, disopyramide, propafenone, sotalol, and dofetilide. In contrast, amiodarone is an uncommon cause of this

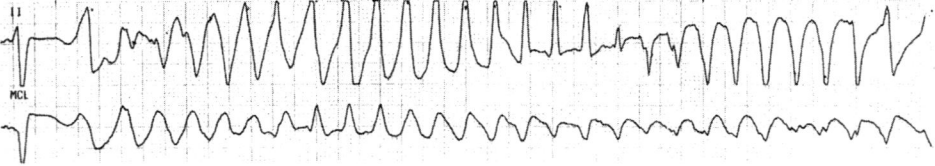

Figure 16 ECG lead II and MCL demonstrating *torsades de pointes*. Note the almost undulating changing polarity QRS characteristic of this tachycardia.

arrhythmia, despite the usual presence of QT prolongation (102). Psychotropic drugs, such as amitryptyline and phenothiazines, also may result in QT prolongation and torsades (102). Antibiotics, such as IV erythromycin and other drugs known to prolong the QT interval, have also been implicated (102). Other abnormalities associated with the long QT syndrome include hypokalemia, hypomagnesemia, lithium therapy, and severe bradyarrhythmias, such as sinus node dysfunction or complete heart block (14,102). Heritable cardiac ion channel abnormalities are associated with QT prolongation, ventricular arrhythmias, and premature death (103–106). Further, increasing evidence suggests that people with excessive QT lengthening, in excess of the expected dose related response, and ventricular arrhythmia in response to these drugs and electrolyte abnormalities, may have mild versions of the cardiac channel disease. The precipitating agent may worsen the channel problem to the degree that it becomes clinically significant (106). A detailed discussion of these entities is beyond the scope of this chapter.

Clinical Presentation

Although most patients with severe ventricular arrhythmias have significant cardiac disease, in some individuals the arrhythmia may be the first manifestation of the disease. Even among patients with a known history of heart disease, the clinical course may have been quite stable until onset of the arrhythmia.

Initial symptoms often include palpitation, weakness, dizziness, angina, or symptoms of heart failure. More dramatic presentations are syncope or cardiac arrest. The presenting symptoms and signs are generally proportional to the rate of tachycardia and severity of cardiac disease. If the ventricular tachycardia rate is slow and underlying heart disease is mild, few symptoms may be experienced. Acute myocardial ischemia/infarction should always be considered as a possible cause.

Physical findings relatively specific for ventricular tachycardia include intermittent cannon A waves in the jugular venous pulse and variation in intensity of the first heart sound. Both findings occur as a result of AV dissociation. In contrast, if retrograde AV conduction is present, these findings are absent, and the jugular venous pulse demonstrates continuous cannon A waves.

In severely ill patients, ventricular fibrillation is a terminal, secondary event. Patients already hospitalized for advanced illness consistently have low success when presentation for ventricular fibrillation is attempted. This category includes postoperative patients, with severe complications that are not responding to treatment. Thus, defining the resuscitation status of all patients with severe illnesses is essential. This decision should include a detailed evaluation of long-term prognosis and should incorporate the views of the patient and family. Prior determination of resuscitation status can prevent tragic, futile efforts that deny the patient and family the comfort and dignity of a peaceful death.

Ventricular tachycardia is characterized by abnormal QRS morphology and duration and is one of the causes of "wide QRS complex tachycardia" (Fig. 15). Other causes include: (i) supraventricular tachycardias with RBBB, LBBB, or nonspecific intraventricular conduction delay and (ii) tachycardias involving ventricular activation via an accessory pathway, such as the WPW syndrome (107). Physicians are generally eternal optimists and prefer to make the most benign diagnosis in the face of a wide QRS complex tachycardia. If the tachycardia is well tolerated, absence of alarm is the rule. The responsible physician should understand that, in patients with underlying heart disease, *most wide QRS complex tachycardias are ventricular tachycardia* (107).

A number of criteria have been proposed for analysis of wide complex QRS tachycardias (108), including:

1. AV dissociation (present in ~50% of ventricular tachycardias) should be carefully sought by looking for P waves independent of QRS complexes in the 12 lead ECG (Fig. 15).
2. The presence of occasional fusion or normal QRS beats strongly supports AV dissociation.
3. Unless typical RBBB or LBBB is present, a diagnosis of ventricular tachycardia is strongly favored, especially if an earlier ECG with sinus rhythm does not show comparable QRS morphology.
4. Ventricular tachycardia is usually monomorphic (Fig. 15).
5. QRS duration >140 ms with atypical RBBB or 160 ms with atypical LBBB (Fig. 15) favors ventricular tachycardia.
6. A negative, monomorphic QRS complex in all precordial leads is nearly always ventricular tachycardia.
7. A markedly leftward frontal plane QRS axis is highly suggestive of ventricular tachycardia, unless this left axis deviation pre-exists.

Even with these useful guidelines and a strong probability that a wide QRS tachycardia is ventricular tachycardia, electrophysiological study may be required to define the true nature of a tachycardia.

Torsades de pointes (Fig. 16) is the type of ventricular tachycardia most often associated with QT prolongation, although monomorphic ventricular tachycardia may also occur with QT prolongation. *Torsades de pointes* is characterized by rapid rate and marked variations of QRS morphology (i.e., rapid changes of the QRS from positive to negative) over short periods of time. Persistent torsades may result in cardiovascular collapse and deteriorate into ventricular fibrillation. Torsades often is initiated by a long–short sequence of R–R intervals. For example, a sinus beat followed by a PVC generates a compensatory pause, and the next sinus beat has marked prolongation of the QT interval with a significant after potential that can trigger the arrhythmia (102).

Digitalis associated ventricular tachycardia or fibrillation may occur in the patient with severe heart disease, even if digoxin serum concentrations are not markedly elevated. Hypokalemia and hypomagnesemia can potentiate this arrhythima (84). In patients with less severe disease, ventricular arrhythmias may occur with higher digoxin concentrations. The classical, but uncommon, digitalis induced bidirectional ventricular tachycardia is thought to result from alternation of intra-ventricular conduction pathways (84).

Ventricular fibrillation is characterized by chaotic variations in the ECG baseline that may be coarse in amplitude or quite fine. The term ventricular flutter has been used to designate regular sinusoidal oscillations of moderate amplitude, with the rates varying from 175 to 300 cycles/min.

Acute Therapy

Acute therapy is dictated by the clinical presentation. If the patient with ventricular tachycardia is stable enough to tolerate a brief delay in cardioversion, a 12 lead ECG should be obtained. A standard ECG will aid initial diagnosis and, most importantly, will be useful for reference in those patients undergoing subsequent electrophysiological study. In the unstable patient with ventricular tachycardia, a monitor strip may be all that is obtainable. Immediate synchronized DC cardioversion is indicated following adequate sedation.

Patients who are stable can be treated with lidocaine, procainamide, or amiodarone. If tachycardia persists, DC cardioversion can be performed under brief general anesthesia. In patients with acute, recurring ventricular tachycardia or fibrillation, intravenous amiodarone is often effective when other agents have failed and should be considered early, if lidocaine fails.

For patients with ventricular fibrillation, the American Heart Association Advanced Cardiac Life Support (ACLS) guidelines for emergency therapy should be followed (109). In all patients with ventricular arrhythmias, particular attention should be paid to identifying underlying myocardial infarction, ischemia, heart failure, pulmonary embolus, electrolyte disturbunces, acid/base abnormalities, arterial blood gas abnormalities, and possible drug toxicity. Correction of such abnormalities facilitates resuscitation. If acute myocardial ischemia is thought to be a possible cause, emergency coronary angiography with acute coronary intervention should be considered after resuscitation. Even in the postoperative period, when use of anticoagulation is of increased risk, acute coronary intervention can be performed and may be lifesaving.

Chronic Therapy

Long-term therapeutic goals and approach to treatment are determined by severity of the arrhythmia and associated cardiac and noncardiac diseases. The primary determinants of subsequent untoward events are the severity of left ventricular dysfunction and the presence of myocardial ischemia.

We perform angiography to assess severity of underlying coronary disease and to assess left ventricular function in patients with acute ventricular arrhythmias, with or without myocardial infarction, unless age or debility is a contraindication. In the presence of severe coronary disease we recommend revascularization without further evaluation of the arrhythmia. After optimal management of the coronary artery disease, the patient then undergoes an electrophysiological study to determine whether an inducible ventricular arrhythmia is present. In patients without critical coronary disease, we perform electrophysiological testing following angiography. In the setting of nonacute ischemic heart disease, electrophysiological testing results in arrhythmia induction in ∼80–90% of cases in patients with a clinical history of ventricular tachycardia. In nonischemic cardiomyapathy, the yield is ∼50% or less (110).

Currently, the most successful therapy for patients with symptomatic life threatening ventricular arrhythmias, in whom a clear reversible precipitating factor is not present, is the implantable cardioverter-defibrillator (ICD). Mortality rates as low as 7% over the first year following implantation have been reported along with an arrhythmic death rate over 5 years of follow-up of <5% (93). The Antiarrhythmic vs. Implantable Defibrillators Trial found a significant benefit with the device when compared with pharmacologic therapy (111). In our experience, adjunctive drug therapy, usually amiodarone, and radiofrequency catheter ablation of the site of origin of the tachycardia may reduce frequency of ICD discharges in patients, when the electrical discharges compromise quality of life. Fortunately, with modern devices capable of rapid pacing conversion of ventricular tachycardia, the frequency of uncomfortable shocks is usually low.

Unfortunately, many patients who have suffered significant ventricular arrhythmias are poor candidates for aggressive therapy with implanted devices. Included in this group are patients with severe intractable heart failure and those with significant multisystem diseases. Additionally, some elderly patients are quite averse to this form of treatment. In such patients, we have used amiodarone empirically. This therapy has been well tolerated, even in the presence of severe left ventricular dysfunction. Concerns about long-term complications, including serious hepatic and pulmonary toxicity, need to be balanced against potential benefit of the drug. We regularly monitor thyroid and liver function and obtain pulmonary function testing and chest X-rays.

In addition to amiodarone, sotalol (a type 3 antiarrhythmic agent with β-adrenergic blocking properties) also has been reported to be effective in treating ventricular tachyarrhythmias. It can be used if the ejection fraction is not severely depressed and no other contraindications to β-adrenergic blockade exist (47,112).

Therapy for Long QT Associated Ventricular Tachycardia

Temporary ventricular pacing or acceleration of heart rate with infusion of isoproterenol or dobutamine are frequently successful in shortening the Q–T interval and abolishing torsades (102). Withdrawal of the offending drug and correction of hypokalemia and hypomagnesemia are important treatments in this disorder. Intravenous magnesium infusion is often effective in controlling torsades, even in patients without magnesium deficiency. Magnesium infusion is *now first line therapy* (102). If persistent, marked bradycardia is the inciting factor, then permanent pacing will be required (VVIR or DDDR as appropriate).

Therapy for Digitalis Toxic Ventricular Tachycardia

If the patient is not compromised by a relatively slow tachycardia, withholding digitalis, correcting electrolyte deficiencies, and careful monitoring are appropriate. If major toxicity, characterized by elevation of serum potassium concentrations, severe tachy- or bradyarrhythmias, and hemodynamic instability is present, digoxin antibody (FAB) is the most effective treatment.

ANTITACHYCARDIA AND DEFIBRILLATOR DEVICES

As pointed out earlier, ICDs are highly effective in preventing recurrent ventricular arrhythmic or sudden arrhythmic cardiac death in appropriate patients (113). A consideration that deserves emphasis is that such therapy is "after-the-fact." Recurrence of arrhythmia is common, and, in many patients, ancillary treatment with drugs or catheter ablation is required. Despite the need for adjunctive antiarrhythmic therapy, this new treatment with an ICD is a welcome addition to current options, because drugs have a high failure rate.

Recently, combining ICD therapy with biventricular pacing has shown some promise in improving heart failure symptoms and perhaps mortality. The decision to implant a defibrillator in a younger individual with an episode of sudden cardiac death is relatively easy, but the decision is more difficult in the elderly patient, particularly those patients with complex, multisystem diseases.

The success of ICD devices in prolonging life has generated another social issue: When can such patients be permitted to drive their automobiles? Physicians should consult the detailed recommendations included in the AHA/NASPE Medical/Scientific Statement 135 and relevant state regulations.

ACKNOWLEDGMENTS

The authors thank Margaret Fashinbauer for her assistance in preparation of the figures and manuscript and the personnel in the Cardiac electrophysiology sections at the Mpls VAMC, and Mpls Heart institute for their assistance in caring for our patients.

SUMMARY

- Cardiac arrhythmias are common problems. Diagnosis and treatment must recognize concomitant heart and lung disease. Accurate diagnosis is imperative.
- Precipitating causes of arrhythmias include: volume overload, myocardial ischemia, pulmonary embolism, acid/base disorders, electrolyte abnormalities, adverse drug effects, and sepsis.
- Sinus node dysfunction is a common cause of bradyarrhythmias.
- The diseased heart is often stroke volume limited, and a heart rate of 80–90 beats/min may be needed to maintain cardiac output in the postoperative period.
- Pain control and careful techniques for tracheobronchial suctioning can limit vagal stimulation.
- Medications including beta blockers, calcium channel blockers, digoxin, antihypertensive agents, and antiarrhythmic drugs are associated with sinus node dysfunction.
- Patients with symptomatic sinus node dysfunction with no identifiable reversible cause should be treated with a pacemaker.
- Clinically significant heart block is usually identified with a standard ECG.
- With intermittent or established complete heart block, severity of symptoms depends on the subsidiary pacemaker rate.
- In patients with inferior myocardial infarction, pacing is not required unless bradycardia is severe, LV dysfunction is marked, or RV infarction is present.
- Temporary transvenous pacing is the most reliable therapy in all patients with second degree or third degree AV node block associated with acute anteroseptal myocardial infarction.
- When indicated, pacemakers with atrial sensing, which can maintain AV synchrony and respond to rate, can improve cardiac function significantly. In most patients, dual chamber pacing is desirable.
- Atrial fibrillation may occur in response to surgical stress, perioperative myocardial infarction, pulmonary embolus, or severe sepsis. Other potential causes are acute hemorrhage, hypoxia, acid/base abnormalities, hypokalemia, and hypomagnesemia.
- Pre- and postoperative beta blockers reduce incidence of atrial fibrillation after cardiac surgery.
- Atrial fibrillation is diagnosed by ECG features including: irregular atrial activity, fine or coarse undulating baseline, and irregular R–R intervals.
- In atrial fibrillation, a ventricular rate of ≤ 80 beats/min suggests disease of the AV node. A rate of 120–160 suggests a normal AV node. A rate >150 suggests increased sympathetic tone, and a rate >200 suggests enhanced AV nodal conduction or an accessory AV connection.
- Synchronized DC cardioversion under sedation is the most efficacious therapy for patients with atrial fibrillation associated with hypotension, pulmonary edema, or angina.
- Ventricular rate can be controlled with beta blockers, calcium channel blockers, or digoxin. Diltiazem may be useful for patients with severe LV dysfunction, with a need for catecholamine support, or with severe bronchospasm.
- Patients with atrial fibrillation of >48 h duration should be anticoagulated, if no contraindication is present.

- In chronic rate controlled atrial fibrillation, low-intensity warfarin therapy decreases the risk for stroke.
- In patients with chronic atrial fibrillation who are candidates for cardioversion, anticoagulation with warfarin for 3–4 weeks before and 3–4 months after cardioversion is standard practice to reduce the possibility of embolism.
- In typical atrial flutter, the atrial rate is ~300 beats/min, and the ventricular rate is usually 150 beats/min. The ventricular rate is usually regular. Atrial flutter should be suspected in every regular supraventricular tachycardia with a ventricular rate of 150 beats/min.
- Atrial flutter is distinguished from other atrial tachycardias by atrial rate. With atrial flutter, the atrial rate is usually ≥250 beats/min. In primary atrial tachycardias, it is usually lower.
- The incidence of systemic embolism in atrial flutter is lower than that of atrial fibrillation.
- For atrial flutter with severe symptoms, QRS synchronized DC cardioversion is the treatment of choice.
- Multifocal atrial tachycardia is a complication of severe cardiac or pulmonary disease and is associated with exacerbation of chronic obstructive lung disease.
- Multifocal atrial tachycardia may be a complication of digoxin therapy.
- Primary therapy of multifocal atrial tachycardia is treatment of the underlying disease or elimination of the precipitating causes, such as theophylline toxicity.
- Paroxysmal atrial tachycardias have atrial rates of 100–200 beats/min. P waves are present before each QRS complex, unless A–V block is present.
- Cardioversion is contraindicated for digoxin toxicity.
- AV nodal and AV reentrant arrhythmias are uncommon in the perioperative period in those patient with no previous history of tachycardia.
- AV nodal tachycardia usually begins and ends suddenly. The ventricular rate is usually 160–180 beats/min. QRS morphology is usually narrow. Commonly, the P wave is buried in the QRS complex.
- Acute therapy for AV nodal tachycardia includes vagal maneuvers, adenosine, or verapamil.
- AV reentrant tachycardia starts and ends suddenly. Sinus rhythm ECG may demonstrate delta waves. In orthodromic reciprocating tachycardia, delta waves disappear during the tachycardia. Ventricular rate is usually 180–200 beats/min. A retrograde P wave frequently follows a narrow complex QRS.
- Acute therapy for orthodromic AV reentrant tachycardia includes vagal maneuvers, adenosine, or verapamil. Cardioversion may be indicated if these measures fail.
- Digoxin and verapamil should be avoided in wide complex antidromic tachycardia.
- PVCs are usually asymptomatic. The QRS may demonstrate atypical LBBB or RBBB. A full compensatory pause occurs.
- Therapy of PVCs with antiarrhythmic drugs should be reserved for patients with intractable symptoms who are willing to accept the risks of therapy.
- ICD therapy is of benefit in patients with ischemic heart disease and low ejection fractions.
- Drugs associated with prolongation of the QT interval can produce ventricular tachycardias. Many antiarrhythmic drugs and digoxin are associated with QT prolongation.
- In severely ill patients, ventricular fibrillation is a terminal, secondary event. Defining resuscitation status in severely ill patients is essential.

- Most wide complex tachycardias are ventricular tachycardia. Immediate synchronized DC cardioversion is indicated in the unstable patient after sedation is accomplished.
- Stable patients can be treated with lidocaine, procainamide, or amiodarone.
- Follow ACLS guidelines for ventricular fibrillation.
- The implantable cardioverter-defibrillator is the most successful therapy for life threatening ventricular arrhythmias.
- Isoproterenol or dobutamine may be useful for long QT associated ventricular tachycardia.
- Intravenous magnesium is the first line therapy for *torsades de pointes*.
- Digoxin antibody should be administered for severe digoxin toxicity. Indications include severe tachy- or bradyarrhythmias, hemodynamic instability, or hyperkalemia.

REFERENCES

1. Rokseth R, Hatle L. Prospective study on the occurrence and management of chronic sinoatrial disease, with follow-up study. Am Heart J 1985; 109:513–522.
2. Hartel G, Talvensaari T. Treatment of sinoatrial syndrome with permanent cardiac pacing in 90 patients. Acta Med Scand 1975; 198:341–347.
3. Jordan J, Yamaguchi I, Mandel M. Function and dysfunction of the sinus node: clinical studies in the evaluation of sinus node function. In: Bonke F, ed. The Sinus Node: Structure, Function, and Clinical Relevance. The Hague: Martinus Nijhoff, 1978:3–22.
4. Rickards A, Donaldson R. Rate responsive pacing. Clin Prog Pacing Eletrophysiol 1983; 1:21–29.
5. Benditt D, Milstein S, Goldstein M, Reyes W, Gornick C. Sinus node dysfunction: pathophysiology, clinical features, evaluation and treatment. In: Zipes D, Jalife J, eds. Cardiac Electrophysiology: From Cell to Bedside. Philadelphia, PA: WB Saunders, 1990:708–734.
6. Short D. The syndrome of alternating bradycardia and tachycardia. Br Heart J 1954; 16:208–214.
7. Benditt D, Sakaguchi S, Goldstein M, Lurie K, Gornick C, Adler S, eds. Sinus node dysfunction: pathophysiology, clinical features, evaluation and treatment. 2d ed. Philadelphia, PA: W.B. Saunders Company, 1995.
8. Skagen K, Hansen J. The long-term prognosis for patients with sinoatrial block treated with permanent pacemaker. Acta Med Scand 1975; 199:13–15.
9. Sasaki S, Takeuchi A, Ohzeki M, et al. Long-term follow-up of paced patients with sick sinus syndrome. In: Steinbach K, Glogar D, Laszkovics A, et al., eds. Cardiac Pacing. Proceedings of the VIIth World Symposium on Cardiac Pacing, Darmstadt, Steinkopff Verlag, 1983:85–90.
10. Conde C, Leppo J, Lipski J, et al. Effectiveness of pacemaker treatment in the bradycardia–tachycardia syndrome. Am J Cardiol 1973; 32:209–214.
11. Alt E, Volker R, Wirtzfeld A, et al. Survival and follow-up after pacemaker implantation: a comparison of patients with sick sinus syndrome, complete heart block and atrial fibrillation. PACE 1985; 8:849–855.
12. Wohl A, Laborde J, Atkins JM et al. Prognosis of patients permanently paced for sick sinus syndrome. Arch Intern Med 1976; 136:406–408.
13. Lichstein E, Aithal H, Jonas S, et al. Natural history of severe sinus bradycardia discovered by 24 hour Holter monitoring. PACE 1982; 5:185–189.
14. Parkinson J, Papp C, Evans W. The electrocardiogram of the stokes–adams attack. Br Heart J 1941; 3:171–199.

15. Davies M, Anderson R, Becker A. The Conduction System of the Heart. London: Butterworth & Co., 1983.
16. Rotman M, Wagner G, Wallace A. Bradyarrhythmias in acute myocardial infarction. Circulation 1972; 45:703.
17. Norris R, Mercer C. Significance of idioventricular rhythms in acute myocardial infarction. Prog. Cardiovasc. Dis. 1974; 16:455.
18. Norris R. Heart block in posterior and anterior myocardial infarction. Br Heart J 1969; 31:352.
19. Mavric Z, Zaputovic L, Matana A, et al. Complete heart block associated with acute myocardial infarction. Am Heart J 1990; 119:823.
20. Kostuk W, Beanlands D. Complete heart block associated with acute myocardial infarction. Am J Cardiol 1970; 26:380.
21. Lamas G, Muller J, Turi Z, Stone P, Rutherford J, Jaffe A, et al. A simplified method to predict occurrence of complete heart block during acute myocardial infarction. Am J Cardiol 1986; 57:1213–1219.
22. Waller B. Clinicopathological correlations of the human cardiac conduction system. In: Zipes D, Jalife J, eds. Cardiac Electrophysiology: From Cell to Bedside. Philadelphia, PA: W.B. Saunders, 1990:249–269.
23. Madsen J, Meibom J, Videbach R. Transcutaneous pacing: experience with the Zoll noninvasive temporary pacemaker. Am Heart J 1988; 116:7–10.
24. Parsonnet V, Furman S, Smyth N. Implantable cardiac pacemakers: status report and resource guidelines. Circulation 1974; 50:A21.
25. Parsonnet V, Furman S, Smyth N. Revised code for pacemaker identification. PACE 1981; 4:400.
26. Lakatta E, Mitchell J, Pomerance A, Rowe G. Human aging: changes in structure and function. J Am Coll Cardiol 1987; 10:42A–47A.
27. Lakatta E. Do hypertension and aging have a similar effect on the myocardium? Circulation 1987; 75:169–177.
28. Barold S, Zipes D. Cardiac pacemakers and antiarrhythmic devices. In: Braunwald E, ed. Heart Disease: A Textbook of Cardiovascular Medicine. Philadelphia, PA: W.B. Saunders, 1992:726–755.
29. Ukkonen H, Beanlands RS, Burwash IG, de Kemp RA, Nahmias C, Fallen E, et al. Effect of cardiac resynchronization on myocardial efficiency and regional oxidative metabolism. Circulation 2003; 107(1):28–31.
30. Bradley DJ, Bradley EA, Baughman KL, Berger RD, Calkins H, Goodman SN, et al. Cardiac resynchronization and death from progressive heart failure: a meta-analysis of randomized controlled trials. J Am Med Assoc 2003; 289(6):730–740.
31. Kannel W, Abbott R, Savage D, McNamara P. Epidemiologic features of chronic atrial fibrillation. N Engl J Med 1982; 306:1018–1022.
32. Aranki S, Shaw D, Adams D, Rizzo R, Couper G, VanderVliet M, et al. Predictors of atrial fibrillation after coronary artery surgery. Circulation 1996; 94:390–397.
33. Daoud E, Strickberger S, Man C, Goval R, Deeb G, Boiling S, et al. Preoperative Amiodarone as prophylaxis against atrial fibrillation after heart surgery. New Engl J Med 1997; 337:1785–1791.
34. The Esmolol vs Placebo Multicenter Study Group, Anderson S, Blanski L, Byrd R, Das G, Engler R, et al. Comparison of the efficacy and safety of esmolol, a shortacting beta blocker, with placebo in the treatment of supraventricular tachyarrhythmias. Am Heart J 1986; 111:42–48.
35. Salerno D, Dias V, Kleiger R, Tschida V, Sung R, Sami M, et al. Efficacy and safety of intravenous diltiazem for treatment of atrial fibrillation and atrial flutter. Am J Cardiol 1989; 63:1046–1051.
36. Gray R, Bateman T, Czer L, Conklin C, Matloff J. Esmolol: a new ultrashort-acting beta-adrenergic blocking agent for rapid control of heart rate in postoperative supraventricular tachyarrhythmias. J Am Coll Cardiol 1985; 5:1451–1456.

37. Platia E, Michelson E, Porterfield J, Das G. Esmolol versus verapamil in the acute treatment of atrial fibrillation or atrial flutter. Am J Cardiol 1989; 63:925–929.
38. Kopecky S, Gergh B, McGoon M, Whisnant J, Holmes D, Ilstrup D, et al. The natural history of lone atrial fibrillation. N Engl J Med 1987; 317:669–674.
39. Umana E, Solares CA, Alpert MA. Tachycardia-induced cardiomyopathy. Am J Med 2003; 114(1):51–55.
40. Lown B, Perlroth M, Kaidbey S, Abe Y, Harken D. Cardioversion of atrial fibrillation. N Engl J Med 1963; 269:325–331.
41. Kreiner G, Heinz G, Siostrzonek P, Gossinger H. Effect of slow pathway ablation on ventricular rate during atrial fibrillation, Dependence on electrophysiological properties of the fast pathway. Circulation 1996; 93:277–283.
42. Lundstrom T, Ryden L. Chronic atrial fibrillation: longterm results of direct current conversion. Acta Med Scand 1988; 223:53–59.
43. Wyse DG. The AFFIRM trial: main trial and substudies-what can we expect? J Interv Card Electrophysiol 2000; 4(suppl 1):171–176.
44. Wyse DG, Waldo AL, DiMarco JP, Domanski MJ, Rosenberg Y, Schron EB, et al. A comparison of rate control and rhythm control in patients with atrial fibrillation. N Engl J Med 2002; 347(23):1825–1833.
45. Antman E, Beamer A, Cantillon C, McGowan N, Friedman P. Therapy of refractory symptomatic atrial fibrillation and atrial flutter: A staged care approach with new antiarrhythmic drugs. J Am Coll Cardiol 1990; 15:698–707.
46. Juul-Moller S, Edvardsson N, Rehnqvist-Ahlberg N. Sotalol versus quinidine for the maintenance of sinus rhythm after direct current conversion of atrial fibrillation. Circulation 1990; 82:1932–1939.
47. Haverkamp W, Martinez-Rubio A, Hief C, Lammers A, Muhlenkamp S, Wichter T, et al. Efficacy and safety of D,L-sotalol in patients with ventricular tachycardia and in survivors of cardiac arrest. J Am Coll Cardiol 1997; 30:487–495.
48. Gold R, Haffajee C, Charos G, Sloan K, Baker S, Alpert J. Amiodarone for refractory atrial fibrillation. Am J Cardiol 1986; 57:124–127.
49. Fuster V, Ryden LE, Asinger RW, Cannom DS, Crijns HJ, Frye RL, et al. ACC/AHA/ESC Guidelines for the Management of Patients With Atrial Fibrillation: Executive Summary. A Report of the American College of Cardiology/American Heart Association Task Force on Practice Guidelines and the European Society of Cardiology Committee for Practice Guidelines and Policy Conferences (Committee to Develop Guidelines for the Management of Patients With Atrial Fibrillation) Developed in Collaboration With the North American Society of Pacing and Electrophysiology. Circulation 2001; 104(17):2118–2150.
50. Middlekauff H, Wiener I, Saxon L, Stevenson W. Low-dose amiodarone for atrial fibrillation: time for a prospective study? Ann Intern Med 1992; 116:1017–1020.
51. Saliba WI. Dofetilide (Tikosyn): a new drug to control atrial fibrillation. Cleve Clin J Med 2001; 68(4):353–363.
52. Van Gelder I, Crijns H, Van Gilst W, Verwer R, Lie K. Prediction of uneventful cardioversion and maintenance of sinus rhyhtm from direct-current electrical cardioversion of chronic atrial fibrillation and flutter. Am J Cardiol 1991; 68:41–46.
53. Andersen H, Thuesen L, Bagger J, Vesterlund T, Thomsen P. Prospective randomised trial of atrial versus ventricular pacing in sick-sinus syndrome. Lancet 1994; 344:1523–1528.
54. Prakash A, Saksena S, Hill M, Krol R, Munsif A, Giorgberidze I, et al. Acute effects of dual-site right atrial pacing in patients with spontaneous and inducible atrial flutter and fibrillation. J Am Coll Cardiol 1997; 29:1007–1014.
55. Gillinov AM, Blackstone EH, McCarthy PM. Atrial fibrillation: current surgical options and their assessment. Ann Thorac Surg 2002; 74(6):2210–2217.
56. Saad EB, Marrouche NF, Natale A. Ablation of atrial fibrillation. Curr Cardiol Rep 2002; 4(5):379–387.

57. Touboul P. Atrioventricular nodal ablation and pacemaker implantation in patients with atrial fibrillation. Am J Cardiol 1999; 83(5B):241D–245D.
58. Ezekowitz M, Bridgers S, James K, Carliner N, Colling C, Gornick C, et al. Warfarin in the prevention of stroke associated with nonrheumatic atrial fibrillation. N Engl J Med 1992; 327:1406–1412.
59. Stroke Prevention in Atrial Fibrillation Investigators. Stroke prevention in atrial fibrillation study: final results. Circulation 1991; 84:527–539.
60. The Boston Area Anticoagulation Trial for Atrial Fibrillation Investigators. The effect of low-dose warfarin on the risk of stroke in patients with non-rheumatic atrial fibrillation. N Engl J Med 1990; 323:1505–1511.
61. Petersen P, Boysen G, Godtfredsen J, Andersen E, Andersen B Placebo-controlled, randomised trial of warfarin and aspirin for prevention of thromboembolic complications in chronic atrial fibrillation: the Copenhagen AFASAK study. Lancet 1989; 1:538–545.
62. Archer SL, James KE, Kvemen L, Cohen IS, Ezekowitz MO, Gornick CC. Role of transesophageal echocardiography in the detector of left atrial thrombus in patients with chronic non-rheumatic atrial fibrillation. Am Heart J 1995; 130:287–295.
63. Chesebro J, Fuster V, Halperin J. Atrial fibrillation—risk marker for stroke. N Engl J Med 1990; 323:1556–1558.
64. Arnold A, Mick M, Mazurek R, Loop F, Trohman R. Role of prophylactic anticoagulation for direct current cardioversion in patients with atrial fibrillation or atrial flutter. J Am Coll Cardiol 1992; 19:851–855.
65. Manning W, Leeman D, Gotch P, Come P. Pulsed Doppler evaluation of atrial mechanical function after electrical cardioversion of atrial fibrillation. J Am Coll Cardiol 1989; 13: 617–623.
66. Fenster P, Comess K, Marsh R, Katzenberg C, Hager W. Conversion of atrial fibrillation to sinus rhythm by acute intravenous procainamide infusion. Am Heart J 1983; 106:501–504.
67. Stambler B, Wood M, Ellenbogen K, Perry K, Wakefield L, VanderLugt J, et al. Efficacy and safety of repeated intravenous doses of ibutilide for rapid conversion of atrial flutter or fibrillation. Circulation 1996; 94:1613–1621.
68. Kowey P, VanderLust J, Luderer J. Analysis of safety and risk/benefit of ibutilide for conversion of atrial fibrillation/flutter. Am J Cardiol 1996; 78(8A):46–52.
69. Khoury DS, Assar MD, Sun H. Pharmacologic enhancement of atrial electrical defibrillation efficacy: role of ibutilide. J Interv Card Electrophysiol 1997; 1(4):291–298.
70. Manning W, Silverman D, Gordon S, Krumholz H, Douglas P. Cardioversion from atrial fibrillation without prolonged anticoagulation with use of transesophageal echocardiography to exclude the presence of atrial thrombi. N Engl J Med 1993; 328:750–755.
71. Irani W, Grayburn P, Afridi I. Prevalence of thrombus, spontaneous echo contrast, and atrial stunning in patients undergoing cardioversion of atrial flutter. A prospective study using transesophageal echocardiography. Circulation 1997; 95:962–966.
72. Diner BM. Evidence-based emergency medicine. Anticoagulation or antiplatelet therapy for non-rheumatic atrial fibrillation and flutter. Ann Emerg Med 2003; 41(1):141–143.
73. Segal JB, McNamara RL, Miller MR, Powe NR, Goodman SN, Robinson KA, et al. Anticoagulants or antiplatelet therapy for non-rheumatic atrial fibrillation and flutter. Cochrane Database Syst Rev 2001(1):CD001938.
74. Mehta D, Baruch L. Thromboembolism following cardioversion of "common" atrial flutter. Risk factors and limitations of transesophageal echocardiography. Chest 1996; 110:1001–1003.
75. Wells J Jr, MacLean W, James T, Waldo A. Characterization of atrial flutter—studies in man after open heart surgery using fixed atrial electrodes. Circulation 1979; 60:665–673.
76. Sowton E, Holt P. Strategies for the management of tachyarrhythmias. Pacing Clin Electrophysiol 1986; 9(6 Pt 2):1304–1308.
77. Feld G, Fleck R, Chen P, Boyce K, Bahnson T, Stein J, et al. Radiofrequency catheter ablation for the treatment of human type 1 atrial flutter. Circulation 1992; 86:1233–1240.

78. Poty H, Saoudi N, Nair M, Anselme F, Letac B. Radiofrequency catheter ablation of atrial flutter. Circulation 1996; 94:3204–3213.
79. Benditt D, Benson D Jr, Dunnigan A, Gornick C, Anderson R. Atrial flutter, atrial fibrillation, and other primary atrial tachycardias. Med Clin N Am 1984; 68:895–918.
80. Chung E. Manual of Cardiac Arrhythmias. Stoneham, MA: Butterworth, 1986.
81. Shine K, Kastor J, Yurchak P. Multifocal atrial tachycardia: Clinical and electrocardiographic features. N Engl J Med 1968; 279:344–349.
82. Salerno D, Anderson B, Sharkey P, Iber C. Intravenous verapamil for treatment of multifocal atrial tachycardia, with and without calcium pretreatment. Ann Intem Med 1987; 107:623–628.
83. Swerdlow C, Liem L. Atrial and junctional tachycardias: Clinical presentation, Course, and therapy. In: Zipes D, Jalife J, eds. Cardiac Electrophysiology: From Cell to Bedside. Philadelphia, PA: W.B. Saunders, 1990:742–755.
84. Fisch C. Digitalis induced tachycardias. In: Surawicz B, Reddy C, Prystowsky E, eds. Tachycardias. Boston, MA: Martinus Nijhoff, 1984:399–406.
85. Wantanabe Y, Nishimura M, Noda T, Habuchi Y, Tanaka H, Homma N. Atrioventricular junctional tachycardias. In: Zipes D, Jalife J, eds. Cardiac Electrophysiology: From Cell to Bedside. Philadelphia, PA: W.B. Saunders, 1990:564–570.
86. Leitch J, Klein G, Yee R, Leather R, Kim Y. Syncope associated with supraventricular tachycardia: an expression of tachycardia rate or vasomotor response? Circulation 1992; 85:1064–1071.
87. Waxman M, Wald R, Sharma A, Huerta F, Cameron D. Vagal techniques for termination of paroxysmal supraventricular tachycardia. Am J Cardiol 1980; 46:655.
88. Jackman W, Beckman K, McClelland J, Wang X, Friday K, Roman C, et al. Treatment of supraventricular tachycardia due to atrioventricular nodal reentry by radiofrequency catheter ablation of slow-pathway conduction. N Engl J Med 1992; 327:313–318.
89. Lee M, Morady F, Kadish A, Schamp D, Chin M, Scheinman M, et al. Catheter modification of the atrioventricular junction with radiofrequency energy for control of atrioventricular nodal reentry tachycardia. Circulation 1991; 83:827–835.
90. Gornick C, Benson D. Electrocardiographic aspects of the preexcitation syndromes. In: Benditt D, Benson D, eds. Cardiac Preexcitation Syndromes: Origins, Evaluation, and Treatment. Boston, MA: Martinus Nijhoff, 1986:43–73.
91. Gallagher J, Selle J, Sealy W, Colavita P, Fedor J, Littmann L, et al. Variants of pre-excitation: update 1989. In: Zipes D, Jalife J, eds. Cardiac Electrophysiology: From Cell to Bedside. Philadelphia, PA: W.B. Saunders, 1990:480–502.
92. Wellens H, Brugada P, Penn O, Gorgels A, Smeets J. Pre-excitation syndromes. In: Zipes D, Jalife J, eds. Cardiac Electrophysiology: From Cell to Bedside. Philadelphia, PA: W.B. Saunders, 1990:691–702.
93. Schluter M, Geiger M, Siebels J, Duckeck W, Kuck K-H. Catheter ablation using radiofrequency current to cure symptomatic patients with tachyarrhythmias related to an accessory atrioventricular pathway. Circulation 1991; 84:1644–1661.
94. Lesh M, Van Hare G, Schamp D, Chien W, Lee M, Griffin J, et al. Curative percutaneous catheter ablation using radiofrequency energy for accessory pathways in all locations: results in 100 consecutive patients. J Am Coll Cardiol 1992; 19:1303–1309.
95. Gradman A, Deedwania P, Cody R, Massie B, Packer M, Pitt B, et al. Predictors of total mortality and sudden death in mild to moderate heart failure. J Am Coll Cardiol 1989; 14:564–590.
96. Mukharji J, Rude P, Poole K, Gustafson, N, Thomas L, Strauss H, et al. Risk factors and sudden death following acute myocardial infarction: two year follow-up. Am J Cardiol 1984; 54:31–36.
97. Bigger J, Fleiss J, Kleiger R, Miller J, Rolnitsky L, Group tMPI. The relationship between ventricular arrhythmias, left ventricular dysfunction and mortality in the two years after myocardial infarction. Circulation 1984; 69:250–258.

98. Investigators ATM-A. Effect of prophylactic amiodarone on mortality after acute myocardial infarction and in congestive heart failure: meta-analysis of individual data from 6500 patients in randomised trials. Lancet 1997; 350:1417–1424.
99. The Cardiac Arrhythmia Supression Trial (CAST) Investigators. Preliminary report: effect of encainide and flecainide on mortality in a randomized trial of arrhythmia supression after myocardial infarction. N Engl J Med 1989; 321:406–412.
100. Moss A, Hall J, Cannom D, Daubert J, Higgins S, Klein H, et al. Improve survival with an implanted defibrillator in patients with coronary disease at high risk for ventricular arrhythmia. New Engl J Med 1996; 335:1933–1940.
101. Bigger J, Investigators CABGCPT. Prophylactic use of implanted cardiac defibrillators in patients at high risk for ventricular arrhythmias after coronary artery bypass graft surgery. New Engl J Med 1997; 337:1569–1575.
102. Jackman W, Friday K, Anderson J, Aliot E, Clark M, Lazzara R. The long QT syndromes: a critical review, new clinical observations and a unifying hypothesis. Prog Cardiovasc Dis 1988; 31:115–172.
103. Wickenden A. K(+) channels as therapeutic drug targets. Pharmacol Ther 2002; 94(1–2):157–182.
104. Wall TS, Freedman RA. Ventricular tachycardia in structurally normal hearts. Curr Cardiol Rep 2002; 4(5):388–395.
105. Ikeda T. Brugada syndrome: current clinical aspects and risk stratification. Ann Noninvasive Electrocardiol 2002; 7(3):251–262.
106. Priori SG, Napolitano C. Genetic defects of cardiac ion channels. The hidden substrate for torsades de pointes. Cardiovasc Drugs Ther 2002; 16(2):89–92.
107. Akhtar M, Shenasa M, Mohammand J, Caceres J, Tchou P. Wide QRS complex tachycardia: reappraisal of a common clinical problem. Ann Intern Med 1988; 109:905–912.
108. Wellens H, Conover M. The ECG in Emergency Decision Making. Philadelphia, PA: W.B. Saunders, 1992.
109. Dummy UR. Guidelines for cardiopulmonary resuscitation emergency cardiovascular care. Circulation 2000; 102(suppl I):I-1-I-384.
110. Naccarelli G, Prystowsky E, Jackman W, Heger J, Rahilly G, Zipes D. Role of electrophysiologic testing in managing patients who have ventricular tachycardia unrelated to coronary artery disease. Am J Cardiol 1982; 50:165–171.
111. Investigators TAvIDA. A comparison of antiarrhythmic-drug therapy with implantable defibrillators in patients resuscitated from near-fatal ventricular arrhythmias. N Engl J Med 1997; 337:1576–1583.
112. Mason J, Investigators Esvem. A comparison of electrophysiologic testing with Holter monitoring to predict antiarrhythmic drug efficacy for ventricular tachyarrhythmias. N Engl J Med 1993; 329:445–451.
113. Winkle R, Mead R, Ruder M, Gaudiani V, Smith N, Buch W, et al. Long term outcome with the implantable cardioverter-defibrillator. J Am Coll Cardiol 1989; 13:1353–1361.

23
Myocardial Infarction

Steven M. Hollenberg
Cooper University Hospital, Camden, New Jersey, USA

Sandeep Nathan
Rush–Presbyterian–St. Luke's Medical Center, Chicago, Illinois, USA

ANATOMY OF ACUTE INFARCTION
Definitions

Ischemic heart disease results from an inadequate level of coronary blood flow to meet myocardial oxygen demand. Since the heart extracts oxygen nearly maximally at baseline, increases in myocardial oxygen demand must be met by commensurate increases in coronary blood flow. Myocardial infarction occurs when prolonged occlusion of coronary flow results in myocardial necrosis. Acute coronary syndromes are a family of disorders that share similar pathogenic mechanisms and represent different points along a continuum. They include unstable angina pectoris, non-ST-segment elevation myocardial infarction (NSTEMI), ST-segment elevation myocardial infarction (STEMI), and sudden cardiac death (SCD).

Myocardial ischemia or infarction is associated almost immediately with reduction in segmental contraction. Although sequential contraction abnormalities can result in part from myocardial necrosis, areas of nonfunctional but viable myocardium can also cause or contribute to the development of systolic dysfunction. Reversibly dysfunctional myocardium is classified into two main categories: stunned and hibernating. Myocardium reperfused after ischemia initially may exhibit profound contractile dysfunction despite restoration of normal blood flow. Eventually, recovery of contractile function may occur. This transient postischemic dysfunction is termed "stunning." Hibernating myocardium is in a state of persistently impaired myocardial function at rest as a consequence of severely reduced coronary blood flow. The reduced myocardial contractile function in an area of hypoperfusion can be viewed as a response to restore equilibrium between flow and function. Decreased function in response to decreased flow minimizes the potential for ischemia or necrosis. Both stunned and hibernating myocardium possess contractile reserve, and function of both may improve with time or revascularization.

Pathogenesis

The common link between the various acute coronary syndromes is the rupture of a vulnerable, but previously quiescent, coronary atherosclerotic plaque. Exposure of plaque contents to the circulating blood pool triggers the release of vasoactive amines, activation of platelets, and the coagulation cascade. The extent of resultant platelet aggregation, thrombosis, vasoconstriction, and microembolization dictates the clinical manifestations of the syndrome. The relative fibrin and platelet content of these lesions varies. Unstable angina/ NSTEMI is associated more often with platelet-rich lesions; whereas, STEMI is associated with fibrin-rich clot. It should be noted that all lesions contain some degree of both components. These observations form the scientific rationale for the use of fibrinolytic ("thrombolytic") agents in STEMI and the use of platelet inhibitors in unstable angina/NSTEMI.

Classification of infarctions into "transmural" and "nontransmural" largely has been abandoned with the recognition that electrocardiographic criteria are neither sensitive nor specific to make this distinction. Similarly, the previously used designations of Q-wave and non-Q-wave infarctions have been replaced by STEMI and NSTEMI infarctions, respectively. These newer categories provide descriptive accuracy and shift the focus to the treatment window during which time myocardium may yet be salvageable. This classification is clinically important; patients with STEMI are eligible for fibrinolytic therapy; whereas, patients with NSTEMI are not. STEMI is usually transmural and results most often from total coronary occlusion; whereas, NSTEMI is usually subendocardial and results from subtotal coronary occlusion. Unstable angina may clinically mimic myocardial infarction. The detection of elevated cardiac enzyme serum concentrations signifying recent or ongoing myocyte necrosis is a key feature separating unstable angina from NSTEMI. Although treatment for these latter two syndromes are fairly similar, STEMI presents important differences in prognosis and treatment. These differences are briefly summarized below; however, the primary focus of this chapter remains STEMI.

Distributions of the Major Coronary Arteries

The left anterior descending coronary artery (LAD) supplies the anterior left ventricle, anterior septum, and, usually, the left ventricular apex; the LAD has septal and diagonal branches. Evidence for anterior infarction is seen in electrocardiographic (EKG) leads V_1-V_5. The right coronary artery (RCA) supplies the inferior left ventricular wall, usually the inferior septum, most of the right ventricle, and the sinus node. The RCA is dominant (i.e., it gives rise to a posterior descending artery which supplies left ventricular myocardium in the inferior septal region) in 80% of patients. Signs of inferior infarction are seen in EKG leads II, III, and aVF. The circumflex coronary artery runs in the atrioventricular (A–V) groove; obtuse marginal (OM) branches supply the lateral and posterolateral left ventricle. Findings of lateral infarction are seen in EKG leads I, aVL, V_5, and V_6.

DIAGNOSIS OF ACUTE INFARCTION

The diagnosis of acute myocardial infarction is made on the basis of a compatible clinical presentation, electrocardiographic changes, and a rise and fall in enzymes indicative of myocardial damage. The differential diagnosis of acute infarction includes dissecting aortic aneurysm, pericarditis, pulmonary embolism, pneumonia, and pneumothorax. Gastrointestinal disorders such as esophageal inflammation, peptic ulcer disease, and cholecystitis may mimic acute myocardial infarction. Costochondritis can provide acute chest pain. The presentation of myocardial infarction in surgical patients may be subtle. Postoperative effects of surgery and analgesics used for postoperative pain can mimic or mask the classic features of myocardial infarction, including substernal chest pain with radiation to the arm, neck, or jaw; dyspnea; nausea; and diaphoresis. The vigilant clinician must maintain a high index of suspicion and a low threshold for obtaining a 12-lead ECG.

The classic electrocardiographic feature of acute infarction is ST-segment elevation, followed by T-wave inversion, and ultimate development of Q-waves. The presence of pre-existing left bundle-branch block (LBBB) or a permanent pacemaker can mask the classic electrocardiographic findings. Nonetheless, new LBBB with a compatible clinical presentation should be considered acute myocardial infarction and treated accordingly. Indeed, recent data suggest that patients with STEMI and new LBBB may gain greater benefit from reperfusion strategies than those with ST elevation and preserved ventricular conduction. True posterior myocardial infarction, which usually accompanies inferior infarction, can be subtle; hallmarks include prominent R-waves, tall upright T-waves, and depressed ST segments in leads V_1 and V_2. The clinician also must recognize electrocardiographic "imposters" of acute infarction, which include pericarditis, J-point elevation, Wolff–Parkinson–White syndrome, and hypertrophic cardiomyopathy.

The classic biochemical marker of acute myocardial infarction is elevation of creatine phosphokinase (CPK) serum concentration. The CPK-MB isoenzyme is found primarily in cardiac muscle, and only small amounts are present in skeletal muscle and the brain. CPK serum concentration peaks during the first 24 h following myocardial infarction and then decreases rapidly. Lactate dehydrogenase (LDH) serum concentration peaks at 72–96 h and may be used to detect recent infarction, which is associated with an increase in the LDH_1, isoenzyme.

Elevations in troponin T and troponin I are more specific biochemical markers of cardiac muscle damage. Their use is becoming more widespread and has replaced the use of CPK-MB in many settings. Rapid point-of-care troponin assays, which have become available in the past few years, have further extended the clinical use of this marker. Troponins are more sensitive and specific for the detection of myocardial damage, and troponin elevation in patients without ST elevation (or, in fact, without elevation of CPK-MB) identifies a subpopulation at increased risk for complications. Troponins may not be elevated until 6 h after an acute event. Once elevated, they remain high for days to weeks, limiting their utility to detect late reinfarction.

THROMBOLYTIC THERAPY FOR ACUTE MYOCARDIAL INFARCTION

Early reperfusion of an occluded coronary artery is indicated for all eligible candidates. Thrombolytic therapy has been proven to decrease mortality in patients with ST-segment elevation. Patients treated early derive the most benefit. Indications and contraindications for thrombolytic therapy are listed in Table 1. Contraindications can be regarded as absolute or relative. In the surgical patient, thrombolysis may pose a prohibitive risk. Emergency coronary angiography (with percutaneous coronary intervention as clinically indicated) may be preferable, if facilities are readily available. In contrast to the treatment of STEMI, thrombolytics have shown no benefit (with an increased risk of adverse events in some trials) when used for the treatment of unstable angina/NSTEMI.

Table 1 Indications and Contraindications for Thrombolytic Therapy in Myocardial Infarction

Indications
   Symptoms consistent with acute myocardial infarction
   EKG showing 1 mm (0.1 mV) ST elevation in at least two contiguous leads or new LBBB
   Presentation within 12 h of symptom onset
   Absence of contraindications
Contraindications
   Absolute
     Active internal bleeding
     Intracranial neoplasm, aneurysm, or A–V malformation
     Stroke or neurosurgery within 6 weeks
     Trauma or major surgery within 2 weeks which could be a potential source of serious rebleeding
     Aortic dissection
   Relative
     Prolonged (>10 min) or clearly traumatic cardiopulmonary resuscitation[a]
     Severe uncontrolled hypertension (>200/110 mm Hg)[a]
     Trauma or major surgery within 6 weeks (but >2 weeks)
     Pre-existing coagulopathy
     Active peptic ulcer
     Infective endocarditis
     Pregnancy
     Chronic severe hypertension

[a]Could be an absolute contraindication in low-risk patients with myocardial infarction.

Thrombolytic Agents

Streptokinase

Streptokinase (SK) is a single-chain protein produced by α-hemolytic streptococci, which produces a systemic lytic state for ~24 h. SK is given as a 1.5-million-unit IV infusion over 1 h. Hypotension with infusion usually reverses with administration of IV fluids and a decreased infusion rate, but allergic reactions are possible. Hemorrhagic complications are the most feared side effect. The rate of intracranial hemorrhage is ~0.5%.

Tissue Plasminogen Activator

Tissue plasminogen activator (t-PA) is a recombinant protein that is more fibrin-selective than streptokinase and produces a higher early coronary patency rate. On the basis of the favorable results of the Global Utilization of Streptokinase and Tissue Plasminogen Activator for Occluded Coronary Arteries (GUSTO) trial, t-PA usually is administered in divided doses: 15 mg bolus, 50 mg IV over the initial 30 min, and 35 mg over the next 60 min. This dosing scheme is known as an accelerated regimen. Adjustment for weight is preferred for patients <67 kg. Allergic reactions do not occur, because t-PA is not antigenic. The rate of intracranial hemorrhage may be slightly higher than that with SK and is estimated to be 0.7%.

Reteplase

Reteplase (r-PA) is a deletion mutant of t-PA with an extended half-life. It is administered as two 10 mg boluses 30 min apart. r-PA originally was evaluated in angiographic trials which demonstrated improved coronary flow at 90 min when compared with t-PA. Subsequent trials demonstrate similar 30-day mortality rates. The reason enhanced patency with r-PA did not translate into lower mortality is uncertain.

Tenecteplase

Tenecteplase (TNK-t-PA) is a genetically engineered t-PA mutant with amino acid substitutions that result in prolonged half-life, resistance to plaminogen-activator inhibitor-1 (PAI-1), and increased fibrin specificity. TNK-t-PA is given as a single bolus, adjusted for weight. A single bolus of TNK-t-PA has been shown to produce coronary flow rates identical to those seen with accelerated t-PA and to yield equivalent 30-day mortality and bleeding rates. On the basis of these results, single-bolus TNK-t-PA is an acceptable alternative to t-PA.

Other new thrombolytics include lanoteplase (n-PA), a deletion mutant of t-PA with a prolonged half-life that is given as a single bolus (120,000 U/kg). Angiographic studies demonstrated increased normalization of coronary blood flow (TIMI grade 3) with n-PA when compared with t-PA, an equivalent 30-day mortality rate, but a higher rate of bleeding. Staphylokinase, a plasminogen activator produced by certain strains of *Staphylococcus aureus*, is as potent as t-PA and significantly more fibrin-specific. Disadvantages of staphylokinase include a short half-life, antigenicity, and induction of antibodies. Site-directed mutagenesis, as well as conjugation with polyethylene glycol, are being investigated in an attempt to reduce the immunogenicity of staphylokinase and to increase its plasma half-life.

The ideal thrombolytic agent has not yet been developed. Newer recombinant agents with greater fibrin specificity, slower clearance from the circulation, and more resistance to plasma protease inhibitors are being studied.

Combination Fibrinolytic and Anti-Platelet Therapy in Acute STEMI

Thrombolytic monotherapy for acute STEMI is successful in achieving normal (TIMI grade 3) flow in only ~50–60% of patients enrolled in large thrombolytic trials. Although the newer fibrinolytic agents have demonstrated somewhat higher rates of TIMI grade 3 flow when compared with accelerated-dose t-PA, associated improvement in mortality rates has not been observed. Platelet-rich thrombi may be responsible for a substantial proportion of thrombolytic failures. Furthermore, fibrinolysis is known to activate platelets and release PAI-1, which may interfere with the thrombolytic effect of fibrin-specific agents such as t-PA, r-PA, and TNK. These events may result in further thrombus formation, subsequent reocclusion, and reinfarction in a significant number of patients.

Researchers have proposed that the combination of a glycoprotein IIb/IIIa inhibitor with a reduced dose of fibrinolytics would maximize inhibition of platelet aggregation without increasing serious bleeding complications. Although early studies showed improved patency demonstrated by a larger percentage of patients with TIMI 3 flow, this approach has not improved clinical outcomes. In the GUSTO V trial, which enrolled over 16,000 patients presenting with STEMI, reduced-dose r-PA plus abciximab, reduced the 30-day occurrence of secondary endpoints such as reinfarction and ventricular dysrhythmias compared with standard dose reteplase. In this large trial, no difference in 30-day or 1-year mortality between the groups was observed. Glycoprotein IIb/IIIa inhibitors are currently not recommended either alone or in combination with thrombolytics as pharmacologic reperfusion therapy. These agents have shown substantial benefit as adjunctive pharmacotherapy in primary percutaneous coronary intervention (PCI) in STEMI as discussed below.

The glycoprotein IIb/IIIa inhibitors also play a pivotal role in the medical and mechanical management of unstable coronary syndromes and NSTEMI. Significant differences in structure, half-life, and receptor affinity exist among the three commercially available glycoprotein agents and are summarized below. Reduced rates of death and MI have been demonstrated with all three agents. Even greater benefit is realized when they are combined with percutaneous revascularization. These agents are best utilized in patients with high-risk characteristics (dynamic ECG changes, cardiac enzyme elevation, or persistent anginal symptoms despite institution of standard antiplatelet/antithrombotic therapies). Preferably, those patients should be considered for early invasive therapy. The importance of careful patient selection was emphasized by the negative results of the GUSTO IV trial; a trend towards higher mortality was seen in relatively low-risk patients receiving prolonged (24–48 h) infusions of abciximab with the minority of patients proceeding to PCI.

"Facilitated" early PCI refers to planned PCI after reduced dose pharmacological reperfusion therapy. This strategy has been shown to be feasible and safe. Studies are currently underway to determine whether this approach, utilizing either glycoprotein IIb/IIIa agents alone or in combination with reduced-dose thrombolytics, could provide the optimal reperfusion strategy.

Glycoprotein IIb/IIIa Receptor Antagonists

Abciximab (ReoPro)

Abciximab is a chimeric murine–human monoclonal antibody Fab fragment that binds with relatively high affinity to platelet receptors. The plasma half-life of this large-molecule agent is short (10–30 min), but the duration of biologic action is longer than that seen with either of the two other small molecule agents. Its prolonged effect is a consequence of the strength of the bond formed with the surface of the activated platelet. Since a relatively low ratio of abciximab molecules to platelets exists (i.e., limited plasma pool of unbound drug), platelet transfusions may be helpful in the event of a major bleeding complication. Abciximab is currently approved for elective PCI or unstable coronary syndromes with planned PCI.

Tirofiban (Aggrastat)

Tirofiban is a relatively small molecular weight, synthetic, nonpeptide agent with a half-life of ~2.5 h. It has a lower receptor affinity than abciximab. This agent is approved for the medical management of unstable angina/NSTEMI with or without planned PCI. Given the large drug to platelet ratio (i.e., large plasma pool of free drug) seen with this agent as well as with eptifibitide, platelet transfusions are generally not as helpful in the event of a major bleed. If hemorrhage occurs, the drug simply should be stopped and supportive therapy instituted during the relatively short period of biologic activity.

Eptifibatide (Integrilin)

Eptifibatide is a small molecular weight, cyclic heptapeptide with a 2 h half-life. Like tirofiban, it is approved for the medical management of unstable angina with or without subsequent PCI. It may also be used as adjunctive therapy in elective PCI.

PRIMARY PCI IN ACUTE MYOCARDIAL INFARCTION

Rapid restoration of coronary blood flow is the initial goal of therapy for acute myocardial infarction. As many as one-half to two-thirds of patients presenting with acute myocardial infarction may be ineligible for thrombolytic therapy, and these patients should be considered for primary PCI. Primary PCI can achieve reperfusion of the infarct vessel

Myocardial Infarction

without the risk of bleeding associated with thrombolytic therapy. In experienced hands, initial success rates exceed 90%. Complications include reinfarction in 2–4% (a rate lower than with thrombolytics), distal embolization of thrombus, ventricular arrhythmias, and transient, but severe, hypotension associated with the Bezold–Jarisch reflex, which is more common with reperfusion of the RCA.

The major advantages of primary PCI over thrombolytic therapy include a higher rate of TIMI trial grade 3 (normal) flow, lower risk of intracranial hemorrhage, and the ability to stratify risk based on the severity and distribution of coronary artery disease. Several randomized trials have suggested that PCI is preferable to thrombolytic therapy for AMI patients at higher risk, including those >75 years of age, those with anterior infarctions, and those with hemodynamic instability. The largest of these trials is the GUSTO-IIb Angioplasty substudy, which randomized 1138 patients. At 30 days, a clinical benefit was observed in the combined primary endpoints of death, nonfatal reinfarction, and nonfatal disabling stroke in the patients treated with PTCA when compared with t-PA. No difference was seen in the "hard" endpoints of death and myocardial infarction at 30 days.

Of note, these trials were performed in institutions in which a team skilled in primary angioplasty for acute myocardial infarction was immediately available with standby surgical backup, allowing for prompt reperfusion of the infarct-related artery. More important than the method of revascularization is the time to revascularization. If primary PCI can be performed in a timely manner (ideally within 60 min) by highly experienced personnel, PCI may be the preferred method of revascularization. Advantages of PCI include more complete revascularization with improved restoration of normal coronary blood flow and detailed information about coronary anatomy. Historically, it has been felt that PCI requires a substantial time delay, and therefore thrombolytic therapy may be preferable, but new data have called for a reevaluation of this widely held viewpoint. Three recent studies (PRAGUE-2, DANAMI-2, and Air-PAMI) have investigated the often difficult decision between in-house thrombolysis vs. hospital transfer for PCI. In PRAGUE-2, no difference in mortality between patients treated within 3 h either with thrombolysis using streptokinase or off-site PCI was found. Interestingly, in patients treated between 3 and 12 h, transfer for PCI conferred significant mortality benefit, despite increasing the time to treatment. Similar results were found in DANAMI-2. Referral for primary PCI reduced the occurrence of a composite endpoint of death, reinfarction, or stroke when compared with thrombolysis using t-PA. While these data are intriguing, the importance of procedural volume and experience in producing these results has been underscored by retrospective studies. Those studies suggest that in the community setting (as opposed to PCI performed as part of a controlled clinical trial), mortality rates after myocardial infarction with routine primary PCI and thrombolytic therapy are currently equivalent. More controversial is the issue of performing PCI at centers without onsite surgical backup. While emerging data suggest that this practice is not only feasible but also safe, further large-scale investigations will be necessary to clarify this issue. In certain subpopulations primary PCI is clearly preferred. These subsets are listed in Table 2.

Coronary Stenting and Glycoprotein IIb/IIIa Antagonists

Primary angioplasty for acute myocardial infarction results in a significant reduction in mortality but is limited by the possibility of abrupt vessel closure, recurrent in-hospital ischemia, reocclusion of the infarct-related artery, and restenosis. The PAMI Stent trial was designed to test the hypothesis that routine implantation of an intracoronary stent

Table 2 Percutaneous Intervention vs. Thrombolytic Therapy for Acute Myocardical Infarction

Situations in which PCI is clearly preferable to thrombolytics in acute myocardial infarction
    Contraindications to thrombolytic therapy
    Cardiogenic shock
    Patients in whom uncertain diagnosis prompted cardiac catheterization, which revealed coronary occlusion
Situations in which PCI *may be* preferable to thrombolytics in acute myocardial infarction
    Elderly patients (>75 years)
    Hemodynamic instability
    Large anterior infarction
    Patients with a prior myocardial infarction or prior coronary artery bypass grafting

would reduce angiographic restenosis and improve clinical outcomes compared to primary balloon angioplasty alone. This large, randomized, multicenter trial involving 900 patients did not show a difference in mortality at 6 months but did show improvement in ischemia-driven target vessel revascularization and less angina in the stented patients when compared with PTCA alone.

Glycoprotein IIb/IIIa receptor antagonists inhibit the final common pathway of platelet aggregation by binding platelet membrane glycoprotein IIb/IIIa receptors, which are responsible for binding of circulating von Willebrand factor and fibrinogen with resultant crosslinking of activated platelets. Their use in percutaneous intervention has become routine. In the context of emergency infarct PCI, they have demonstrated particular benefit. The ReoPro and Primary PTCA Organization Randomized Trial (RAPPORT) compared the glycoprotein IIb/IIIa inhibitor abciximab to placebo in 483 patients with acute STEMI undergoing primary PTCA. The trial showed no difference in the primary endpoint of death, nonfatal MI, or any repeat revascularization procedure at 6 months, but the incidence of death, reinfarction, or urgent revascularization was lower with abciximab vs. placebo at day 7. Bleeding complications, which occurred mostly at arterial access sites, were more common with abciximab. The ADMIRAL trial (Abciximab Before Direct Angioplasty and Stenting in MI Regarding Acute and Long Term Follow Up) was the first placebo-controlled study to evaluate abciximab as an adjunct to primary PTCA and stenting in acute myocardial infarction patients. Abciximab used before stenting improved coronary patency and resulted in a nearly 50% relative risk reduction in the incidence of death, recurrent MI, and urgent revascularization at 30 days. The abciximab group experienced increased incidence of minor bleeding.

The Controlled Abciximab and Device Investigation to Lower Late Angioplasty Complications (CADILLAC) trial randomized 2082 patients to either angioplasty alone, angioplasty plus abciximab, stenting alone, or stenting plus abciximab. The composite endpoint of death, reinfarction, disabling stroke, and repeat revascularization was reduced from 20.0% with PTCA alone to 16.5% with PTCA and abciximab, and from 11.5% with stent alone to 10.2% with stent and abciximab. These findings achieved statistical significance. This study has led to the recent FDA approval of stents (with or without abciximab) for use in infarct PCI.

Other Indications for Angioplasty in Acute Myocardial Infarction

In patients who fail thrombolytic therapy, salvage PTCA is indicated. Although the initial success rate is lower than that of primary angioplasty, reocclusion is more common, and mortality is higher. The RESCUE trial focused on a subset of acute myocardial infarction patients with anterior infarction and demonstrated a reduction in the combined endpoint of death or congestive heart failure at 30 days in the group receiving salvage PTCA.

There is no convincing evidence to support empirical delayed PTCA in patients without evidence of recurrent or provokable ischemia after thrombolytic therapy. The TIMI IIB trial and other studies suggest that a strategy of "watchful waiting" allows identification of patients who will benefit from revascularization.

MEDICAL THERAPY FOR MYOCARDIAL INFARCTION

Aspirin

Unless contraindicated, all patients with a suspected acute coronary syndrome (STEMI, NSTEMI, and unstable angina) should be given aspirin, 160–325 mg, within the first 10 min of hospital evaluation. The aspirin must be chewed to accelerate absorption. Aspirin has been shown to reduce mortality in acute infarction to the same degree as thrombolytic therapy, and its effects are additive to thrombolytics. In addition, aspirin reduces the risk of reinfarction.

Once begun, aspirin probably should be continued indefinitely. Aspirin irreversibly inactivates platelet cyclooxygenase, inhibits platelet aggregation, and reduces the release of platelet-derived vasoconstrictors such as serotonin and thromboxane A_2. Recent data suggest that the anti-inflammatory effects of aspirin may play a role in inhibiting plaque rupture as well. Toxicity with aspirin is mostly gastrointestinal; enteric-coated preparations may minimize these side effects.

Thienopyridines

Ticlopidine and clopidogrel are the two currently available thienopyridine antiplatelet agents. The latter compound is the newer and more potent of the two and, in combination with aspirin, is a key component of the medical regimen poststent deployment, as well as following intravascular brachytherapy for the treatment of in-stent restenosis. These agents exert their antiplatelet effect through irreversible binding of platelet membrane adenosine diphosphate receptors, which mediate platelet aggregation. The side effect of neutropenia is less often associated with clopidogrel than with ticlopidine, a finding that makes clopidogrel the preferred agent at present. Although the use of clopidogrel in acute myocardial infarction (STEMI) has not been investigated directly on a large scale, it may be considered as an alternative antiplatelet agent in patients with true aspirin allergy (bronchospasm, anaphylaxis, etc.). An oral loading dose of 300 mg of clopidogrel may be administered to achieve rapid antiplatelet effect. Continuing therapy is daily administration of 75 mg. In contrast to STEMI, for the treatment of unstable angina, clopidogrel has clearly demonstrated incremental benefit when used with aspirin. In the Clopidogrel in Unstable Angina to prevent Recurrent Events (CURE) trial, 12,562 patients were randomized to receive clopidogrel or placebo in addition to standard therapy with aspirin within 24 h of unstable angina symptoms. Clopidogrel significantly reduced the risk of myocardial infarction, stroke, or cardiovascular death from 11.4% to 9.3%, a finding that achieved statistical significance. It should be noted that this benefit came with a 1% absolute increase in major, non-life threatening bleeds ($p = 0.001$) as well as a 2.8% absolute increase in major, life-threatening bleeds associated with CABG within 5 days ($p = 0.07$). These data have raised concerns about giving clopidogrel prior to knowledge of the coronary anatomy.

Heparin

Administration of full-dose heparin after thrombolytic therapy with t-PA is essential to diminish reocclusion after successful reperfusion. Dosing should be adjusted to weight, using a bolus of 80 U/kg and an initial infusion rate of 18 U/kg/h, with adjustment to keep the partial thromboplastin time (PTT) between 50 and 70 s. Heparin should be continued for 24–48 h.

Low molecular weight heparins (LMWH) have several theoretical advantages over unfractionated heparin. Because of a higher resistance to inactivation by platelet factor 4 and a lower affinity for heparin-binding proteins, LMWHs have a more predictable pharmacokinetic profile, greater bioavailability, and longer plasma half-life, all of which result in more predictable and reliable anticoagulant effects. LMWHs may be given once or twice daily as subcutaneous injections at fixed or weight-adjusted doses, a schedule that simplifies administration and eliminates the need for laboratory monitoring and dose adjustment.

LMWHs have been studied in several large randomized trials in patients with unstable angina or NSTEMI. In both the Efficacy and Safety of Subcutaneous Enoxaparin in Non-Q-Wave Coronary Events (ESSENCE) study and the TIMI IIB trial, the combined endpoint of death, myocardial infarction, or recurrent ischemia at 14 days was significantly reduced (15% relative risk reduction) with enoxaparin therapy when compared with unfractionated heparin. The data regarding other LMWHs have not been as positive as the enoxaparin data. When investigated, no significant benefit from dalteparin treatment in patients already on aspirin was observed. LMWH has reduced clearance in renal insufficiency and should be used with caution in such patients. A commercially available test to measure its anticoagulant effect is not available. Trials of LMWH are underway to evaluate the safety and efficacy of combination therapy with thrombolytic agents in treatment of STEMI.

Nitrates

Nitrates have a number of beneficial effects in acute myocardial infarction. They reduce myocardial oxygen demand by decreasing preload and afterload and also may improve myocardial oxygen supply by increasing subendocardial perfusion and collateral blood flow to the ischemic region. Occasional patients with ST elevation from occlusive coronary artery spasm may have dramatic resolution of ischemia with nitrates. In addition to their hemodynamic effects, nitrates also reduce platelet aggregation. Despite these benefits, the recently reported GISSI-3 and ISIS-4 trials failed to show a significant reduction in mortality from routine acute and chronic nitrate therapy. Nitrates remain first-line agents for the symptomatic relief of angina pectoris and for myocardial infarction complicated by congestive heart failure.

Our practice is administration of sublingual nitroglycerin to all patients presenting with chest pain, unless the systolic blood pressure is <100 mm Hg or evidence of right ventricular infarction is present. For patients with persistent chest pain, intravenous nitroglycerin is infused at 10 μg/min and increased in increments of 5–10 μg/min every 5 min until the pain resolves.

The major adverse effects of nitrates are hypotension and headache. Nitrates should be used with great caution in patients with right ventricular infarction who may not tolerate decreases in filling pressure. Similarly, precipitous decreases in blood pressure in patients presenting with inferior myocardial infarction should raise the suspicion of right ventricular involvement. Nitrate-induced hypotension usually is caused by vasodilation and is treated with rapid bolus infusion of intravenous fluids.

β-Blockers

The β-blockers are beneficial both in the early management of myocardial infarction and as long-term therapy. In the prethrombolytic era, early intravenous atenolol was shown to significantly reduce reinfarction, cardiac arrest, cardiac rupture, and death. For patients receiving t-PA, immediate β-blockade with metoprolol resulted in a significant reduction in recurrent ischemia and reinfarction.

Administration of intravenous β-blockers should be strongly considered for patients with acute myocardial infarction, especially those with continued ischemic pain and sympathetically mediated hypertension or tachycardia. Therapy should be avoided in patients with moderate or severe heart failure, hypotension, severe bradycardia or heart block, and severe bronchospastic disease. Metoprolol can be given as a 5 mg IV bolus, repeated every 5 min for a total of three doses. Because of its brief half-life, esmolol may be advantageous in situations requiring control of heart rate when rapid drug withdrawal may be needed if adverse effects occur.

Oral β-blockade should be initiated in all patients who can tolerate it, even if they have not been treated with intravenous β-blockers. The major side effects include exacerbation of heart failure, hypotension, conduction abnormalities, and bronchospasm.

Angiotensin-Converting Enzyme Inhibitors

Angiotensin-converting enzyme (ACE) inhibitors are known to reduce mortality and improve symptoms in patients with symptomatic left ventricular dysfunction from a variety of causes and to prevent progression to symptomatic heart failure in patients with asymptomatic left ventricular dysfunction. Several large randomized trials, most recently the Heart Outcomes Prevention Evaluation (HOPE) study, have demonstrated that ACE inhibitors decrease mortality after myocardial infarction. This improved survival is additive to the benefits of aspirin and β-blockers. The mechanisms responsible probably include limitation in the progressive left ventricular dysfunction and enlargement (remodeling) that often occur after infarction. A reduction in ischemic events was seen as well. Recent studies have suggested that ACE inhibitors can ameliorate endothelial dysfunction in atherosclerosis.

Although the trials have demonstrated a benefit with ACE inhibitors for all patients postinfarction, patients with significant left ventricular dysfunction (ejection fraction <40%) have the most to gain. ACE inhibitors should be started early, preferably within the first 24 h after infarction. Immediate intravenous ACE inhibitor administration with enalaprilat has not been shown to be beneficial. Patients should be started on low doses of oral agents (captopril 6.25 mg three times daily). The dose should be increased rapidly to the range demonstrated beneficial in clinical trials (captopril 50 mg three times daily, enalapril 10–20 mg twice daily, lisinopril 10–20 mg once daily, or ramipril 10 mg once daily).

Calcium Antagonists

Randomized clinical trials have not demonstrated a mortality benefit for calcium-channel blockers for routine use after myocardial infarction. Meta-analyses suggest that high doses of the short-acting dihydropyridine, nifedipine, increase mortality in myocardial infarction. Adverse effects of calcium channel blockers include bradycardia, atrioventricular block, and exacerbation of heart failure. Patients with NSTEMI who are not in congestive heart failure, however, appear to have a significant reduction in reinfarction and recurrent ischemia when treated with diltiazem.

Although routine administration of calcium blockers in acute myocardial infarction is not indicated, these agents are useful for patients whose postinfarction course is complicated by recurrent angina, because these agents not only reduce myocardial oxygen demand but also inhibit coronary vasoconstriction. For hemodynamically stable patients, diltiazem can be administered. A typical starting dose is 60–90 mg orally every 6–8 h. In patients with severe left ventricular dysfunction, long-acting dihydropyridines without prominent negative inotropic effects, such as amlodipine, nicardipine, or the long-acting preparation of nifedipine, may be preferable; increased mortality with these agents has not been demonstrated.

Antiarrhythmics

Routine prophylactic administration of lidocaine is no longer recommended. Even though lidocaine decreases the frequency of premature ventricular contractions and early ventricular fibrillation, overall mortality is not decreased. Meta-analyses of pooled data have demonstrated *increased* mortality from the routine use of lidocaine.

Lidocaine infusion is clearly indicated after an episode of sustained ventricular tachycardia or ventricular fibrillation and should be considered in patients with nonsustained ventricular tachycardia. Lidocaine is administered as a bolus of 1 mg/kg (not to exceed 100 mg), followed by a second bolus of 0.5 mg/kg 10 min later, followed by infusion at 1–3 mg/min. Lidocaine is metabolized by the liver. In patients with liver disease, the elderly, and patients who have congestive heart failure severe enough to compromise hepatic perfusion, lower doses should be used. Toxic manifestations primarily involve the central nervous system and can include confusion, lethargy, slurred speech, and seizures. Because the risk of malignant ventricular arrhythmias decreases after 24 h, lidocaine is usually discontinued after this point. For prolonged infusions, monitoring of lidocaine serum concentrations (therapeutic between 1.5 and 5 micrograms/mL) is sometimes useful.

Intravenous amiodarone is an alternative to lidocaine for ventricular arrhythmias. Amiodarone is given as a 150 mg IV bolus over 10 min, followed by 1 mg/min for 6 h, then 0.5 mg/min for 18 h.

Perhaps the most important point in the prevention and management of arrhythmias after acute myocardial infarction is maintaining normal serum potassium and magnesium serum concentrations. Serum electrolytes should be followed closely, particularly after diuretic therapy. Routine administration of magnesium has not been shown to reduce mortality after acute myocardial infarction, but empiric administration of 2 g of intravenous magnesium in patients with early ventricular ectopy is often probably a good idea.

COMPLICATIONS OF ACUTE MYOCARDIAL INFARCTION

Postinfarction Angina and Infarct Extension

Causes of ischemia after infarction include decreased myocardial oxygen supply from coronary reocclusion or spasm, mechanical problems that increase myocardial oxygen demand, and extracardiac factors such as hypertension, anemia, hypotension, or hypermetabolic states. Nonischemic causes of chest pain, such as postinfarction pericarditis and acute pulmonary embolism, should also be considered.

Immediate management includes aspirin, β-blockade, IV nitroglycerin, heparin, consideration of calcium-channel blockers, and diagnostic coronary angiography. Postinfarction angina is an indication for revascularization. PTCA can be performed if the culprit lesion is suitable, but the clinician must recognize that acute outcomes and long-term patency may not be as good as those achieved with elective angioplasty. CABG should be considered for patients with left main disease, three vessel disease, and those unsuitable for PTCA. If the angina cannot be controlled medically, or is accompanied by hemodynamic instability, an intra-aortic balloon pump should be inserted.

Ventricular Free Wall Rupture

Ventricular free wall rupture typically occurs during the first week after infarction. The classic patient is elderly, female, and hypertensive. Free wall rupture is a catastrophic event with shock and electromechanical dissociation. Salvage is possible with prompt recognition, pericardiocentesis, and thoracotomy. Emergency echocardiography or pulmonary artery catheterization can aid diagnosis.

Ventricular Septal Rupture

When septal rupture occurs, signs include severe heart failure or cardiogenic shock, a pansystolic murmur, and parasternal thrill. The hallmark finding is a left-to-right intracardiac shunt ("step-up" in oxygen saturation from right atrium to right ventricle). Distinguishing septal rupture from mitral regurgitation with a pulmonary artery catheter tracing can be difficult. Both can produce dramatic "v" waves in the pulmonary artery occlusion pressure (PAOP) tracing. Echocardiography can be diagnostic. Surgical repair is required.

Acute Mitral Regurgitation

Papillary muscle *dysfunction* is common after inferior myocardial infarction but is rarely important hemodynamically. The characteristic holosystolic apical murmur of mitral regurgitation is typically present. Papillary muscle *rupture*, in contrast, produces pulmonary edema and shock. A murmur may not be present if cardiac output is sufficiently decreased. Acute treatment includes afterload reduction with nitroprusside and intra-aortic balloon pumping as temporizing measures. Definitive therapy is surgical valve repair or replacement.

Right Ventricular Infarction

Right ventricular infarction occurs in as many as 30% of patients with inferior infarction and is clinically significant in 10%. Signs include hypotension, elevated neck veins, and clear lung fields. Although these patients appear to be in cardiogenic shock, right ventricular infarction confers a better prognosis.

The diagnosis of right ventricular infarction is made by identifying ST elevation in right precordial leads, or by characteristic hemodynamic findings on right heart catheterization (elevated right atrial and right ventricular end-diastolic pressures with normal to low PAOP and low cardiac output). Echocardiography can demonstrate depressed right ventricular contractility and can help differentiate right ventricular infarction from tamponade, which may produce similar clinical and hemodynamic findings.

Treatment, in addition to rapid reperfusion of the occluded coronary artery, if necessary, includes fluid resuscitation with normal saline boluses to increase left ventricular filling pressure and inotropic therapy with dobutamine or possibly amrinone to stimulate RV contractility. Patients who do not rapidly improve with fluids need hemodynamic monitoring to guide therapy. For continued hemodynamic instability, an intra-aortic balloon pumping may be useful. An intra-aortic balloon pump can counteract elevated right ventricular pressures and volumes, which increase wall stress and oxygen consumption and decrease right coronary perfusion pressure, factors that exacerbate right ventricular ischemia. Nitrates, which may reduce right ventricular preload, and consequently decrease cardiac output, should be avoided.

Cardiogenic Shock

Cardiogenic shock as a complication of acute myocardial infarction is associated with a high mortality rate. In some series, mortality approaches 60–90%. Hemodynamically, cardiogenic shock is defined as a cardiac index <1.8 L/min per m^2 with an elevated PAOP, generally >18 mm Hg. Prompt reperfusion of the occluded coronary artery is the only way to reduce the mortality associated with cardiogenic shock. Because thrombolytic therapy alone does not appear to be very effective in cardiogenic shock, primary PCI is recommended. An intraaortic balloon pump should be placed before the PCI to stabilize the patient, to enhance coronary blood flow, and to reduce myocardial oxygen demand. Urgent coronary artery bypass surgery may be an alternative, if prompt angioplasty is not feasible.

SUMMARY

- Acute coronary syndromes include unstable angina pectoris, non-ST-segment elevation myocardial infarction (NSTEMI), ST-segment elevation myocardial infarction (STEMI), and sudden cardiac death.
- Myocardial ischemia or infarction is associated with reduction of segmental contraction.
- Stunning is defined as transient contractile dysfunction despite restoration of coronary blood flow.
- Hibernating myocardium is defined as a state of persistently impaired myocardial function at rest, which results from impaired coronary blood flow.
- STEMI is associated with fibrin rich clot; hence, fibrinolytic therapy is indicated.
- NSTEMI is associated with platelet rich lesions; hence, platelet inhibitors are indicated.

- STEMI usually results from total coronary artery occlusion.
- NSTEMI is usually subendocardial and results from subtotal coronary occlusion.
- Diagnosis of acute myocardial infarction is based on clinical presentation, ECG changes, and a rise and fall of enzymes indicating myocardial damage. In the postoperative patient, typical symptoms may be masked. Obtain a 12-lead ECG whenever myocardial ischemia or infarction is suspected.
- ECG findings of acute infarction are typically ST-segment elevation followed by T-wave inversion and subsequent appearance of Q-waves. New LBBB with appropriate clinical presentation should be considered acute infarction.
- Troponins are specific biochemical markers of myocardial damage. Typically, increase of serum troponin concentration occurs 6 h after acute infarction. Troponins may remain elevated for days to weeks.
- Thrombolytic therapy decreases mortality in patients with STEMI. Early treatment produces the best outcomes.
- Thrombolytic therapy is not indicated for NSTEMI.
- Glycoprotein IIb/IIIa inhibitors are important in treatment of unstable angina, NSTEMI, and after percutaneous revascularization.
- PCI should be considered as primary therapy for patients who are not eligible for fibrinolytic therapy.
- More important than the method of revascularization is the time to revascularization. Ideally revascularization can be performed within 60 min of onset of infarction.
- Salvage PCI is indicated for patients who fail thrombolytic therapy.
- All patients with a suspected coronary syndrome should receive aspirin, unless aspirin is contraindicated. Aspirin must be chewed and preferably should be administered within 10 min of beginning evaluation.
- Clopidogrel is used after coronary stenting and after brachytherapy for stent restenosis.
- Heparin therapy after thrombolytic therapy is indicated. Low molecular weight heparin has benefit over unfractionated heparin.
- Nitrates reduce myocardial oxygen demand by decreasing preload and afterload. They may improve myocardial oxygen supply by increasing subendocardial perfusion and collateral blood flow. Nitrates should be considered for patients with chest pain, unless systolic blood pressure <100 mm Hg or right ventricular infarction is present.
- β-Blockers should be administered to patients with acute myocardial infarction unless they demonstrate heart failure, hypertension, severe bradycardia, heart block, or bronchospastic disease.
- ACE inhibitors have demonstrated additive benefit to aspirin and β-blockade after myocardial infarction.
- Calcium channel blockers are not routinely indicated in acute myocardial infarction, but are useful for patients with recurrent angina after infarction.
- Maintenance of normal serum potassium and magnesium concentrations is important for preventing dysrhythmias after myocardial infarction.
- Complications of acute myocardial infarction include postinfarction angina and infarct extension, ventricular free wall rupture, ventricular septal rupture, acute mitral regurgitation, right ventricular infarction, and cardiogenic shock.

SUGGESTED READING

β-Blocker Heart Attack Trial Research Group: A randomized trial of propranolol in patients with acute myocardial infarction. I. Mortality results. J Am Assoc Med 1982; 247:1707–1714.

CAPTURE Investigators. Randomised placebo-controlled trial of abciximab before and during coronary intervention in refractory unstable angina: the CAPTURE Study. Lancet 1997; 349:1429–1435.

Cohen M, Demers C, Gurfinkel EP, et al. A comparison of low-molecular-weight heparin with unfractionated heparin for unstable coronary artery disease. Efficacy and safety of subcutaneous enoxaparin in non-Q-wave coronary events study group. N Engl J Med 1997; 337:447–452.

Fibrinolytic Therapy Trialists' (FTT) Collaborative Group. Indications for fibrinolytic therapy in suspected acute myocardial infarction: collaborative overview of early mortality and major morbidity results from all randomised trials of more than 1000 patients. Lancet 1994; 343:311–322.

Grines CL, Browne KF, Marco J, et al. A comparison of immediate angioplasty with thrombolytic therapy for acute myocardial infarction. N Engl J Med 1993; 328:673–679.

Gruppo Italiano per lo Studio della Sopravvinza nell'Infarto Miocardico (GISSI). Effectiveness of intravenous thrombolytic treatment in acute myocardial infarction. Lancet 1986; 2:397–402.

GUSTO Investigators. An international randomized trial comparing four thrombolytic strategies for acute myocardial infarction. N Engl J Med 1993; 329:673–682.

GUSTO Angiographic Investigators. The effects of tissue plasminogen activator, streptokinase, or both on coronary-artery patency, ventricular function, and survival after acute myocardial infarction. N Engl J Med 1993; 329:1615–1622.

Gutstein DE, Fuster V. Pathophysiology and clinical significance of atherosclerotic plaque rupture. Cardiovasc Res 1999; 41:323–333.

Hochman JS, Sleeper LA, Webb JG, et al. Early revascularization in acute myocardial infarction complicated by cardiogenic shock. N Engl J Med 1999; 341:625–634.

ISIS-2 Collaborative Group. Randomised trial of intravenous streptokinase, oral aspirin, both, or neither among 17 187 cases of suspected acute myocardial infarction: ISIS-2. Lancet 1988; 2:349–360.

ISIS-4 (Fourth International Study of Infarct Survival) Study Group: ISIS-4. A randomised factorial trial assessing early oral captopril, oral mononitrate, and intravenous magnesium sulphate in 58,050 patients with suspected acute myocardial infarction. Lancet 1995; 345:669–685.

LATE Study Group. Late assessment of thrombolytic efficacy (LATE) study with alteplase 6-24 hours after onset of acute myocardial infarction. Lancet 1993; 342:759–766.

Libby P. Current concepts of the pathogenesis of the acute coronary syndromes. Circulation 2001; 104:365–372.

Montalescot G, Barragan P, Wittenberg O, et al. Platelet glycoprotein IIb/IIIa inhibition with coronary stenting for acute myocardial infarction. N Engl J Med 2001; 344:1895–1903.

Ohman EM, Armstrong PW, Christenson RH, et al. Cardiac troponin T levels for risk stratification in acute myocardial ischemia. N Engl J Med 1996; 335:133–1341.

Pfeffer MA, Braunwald E, Moye LA, et al. Effect of captopril on mortality and morbidity in patients with left ventricular dysfunction after myocardial infarction. Results of the Survival and Ventricular Enlargement Trial. N Engl J Med 1992; 327:669–677

Rogers WJ, Canto JG, Lambrew CT, et al. Temporal trends in the treatment of over 1.5 million patients with myocardial infarction in the United States from 1990 to 1999. J Am Coll Cardiol 2000; 36:2056–2063.

Ryan TJ, Anderson JL, Antman EM, et al. American College of Cardiology/American Heart Association guidelines for the management of patients with acute myocardial infarction. 1999 Update. A report of the American College of Cardiology/American Heart Association Task Force on Practice Guidelines. J Am Coll Cardiol 1999; 34:890–911.

Scandinavian Simvastatin Survival Study Group. Randomised trial of cholesterol lowering in 4444 patients with coronary heart disease: The Scandinavian Simvastatin Survival Study (4S). Lancet 1994; 344:1383–1389.

Yusuf S, Sleight P, Pogue J, et al. Effects of an angiotensin-converting-enzyme inhibitor, ramipril, on cardiovascular events in high-risk patients. N Engl J Med 2000; 342:145–153.

24
Hypertensive Emergencies

Rakesh Gupta and John W. Hoyt
St. Francis Medical Center, Pittsburgh, Pennsylvania, USA

A common description of a patient having a hypertensive emergency includes markedly elevated blood pressure (systolic pressure 200–240 mm Hg/diastolic pressure 120–140 mm Hg) with evidence of end organ damage, such as hypertensive encephalopathy, intracranial hemorrhage, aortic dissection, pulmonary edema, or myocardial ischemia. Even though the incidence of hypertensive emergencies has been declining, in part because of better pharmacologic treatment, a significant number of patients develop dangerously elevated blood pressure in the operating room, recovery room, SICU, emergency room, and the hospital ward on a daily basis. These elevations of blood pressure may or may not be associated with symptoms but, depending on past medical history, may put the patient at increased risk for cardiovascular and CNS complications. The physician evaluating a patient with acutely elevated blood pressure often feels compelled to "do something" to correct the problem. This chapter discusses the physiologic reasons for initiating treatment and provides guidelines on when to treat, how to treat, and how to monitor treatment.

Common causes of hypertensive crises include sudden reduction or withdrawal of antihypertensive medications; ingestion of substances (legal and illicit) that will increase blood pressure, such as sympathomimetic drugs, cocaine, and PCP; perioperative hypertension; secondary hypertension, such as pheochromocytoma or renovascular hypertension; and hypertension associated with pregnancy (preeclampsia/eclampsia). Hospitalized patients are at risk for episodes of hypertension and tachycardia when facing the anxiety and stress of invasive procedures and surgery. Patients with a history of hypertension are particularly at risk to develop substantial elevations of blood pressure and heart rate in the hospital. These abnormalities can occur even if their blood pressure has been well controlled as outpatients. Stress and anxiety before surgery, and pain and fear after surgery, can trigger a hypertensive crisis.

TYPES OF HYPERTENSIVE CRISES

Hypertensive crises are commonly subdivided into hypertensive emergency and hypertensive urgency, depending on whether there is evidence of end organ damage. As stated earlier, hypertensive crisis can be seen with systolic blood pressure of 200–240 mm Hg or diastolic pressures of 120–140 mm Hg. In hypertensive emergency, one sees signs and symptoms of damage to target organs in conjuction with the elevated blood pressure. Organs commonly affected in hypertensive emergencies include the brain (encephalopathy, intracranial hemorrhage, subarachnoid hemorrhage, or thrombotic stroke), heart (myocardial ischemia, acute pulmonary edema secondary to left ventricular failure, or aortic dissection), and kidneys (acute renal failure). In hypertensive urgency, there is no evidence of acute end organ damage. Table 1 lists potential causes of hypertensive crisis.

Differentiating between hypertensive emergency and hypertensive urgency is important in selecting appropriate therapy and monitoring. The level of blood pressure alone is not diagnostic of an emergency. A pregnant female with eclampsia can have complications and evidence of end organ damage with a blood pressure of 180/110 mm Hg, whereas a chronic noncompliant hypertensive patient can have a blood pressure >220/130 mm Hg with no acute target organ damage. Patients with hypertensive emergencies need immediate reduction of blood pressure, usually with parenteral medications, and require close observation in intensive care units. Patients with hypertensive urgencies can be treated with oral medications to achieve a gradual reduction in blood pressure over 24 h. Patients with hypertensive urgencies require close monitoring; however, they do not necessarily need to be monitored in an intensive care unit.

INITIAL EVALUATION

When evaluating a patient with severely elevated blood pressure, the physician must rapidly identify evidence of acute target organ damage that would require rapid and emergent treatment. A brief but focused history and physical examination and selected laboratory tests can help differentiate between hypertensive emergency and hypertensive urgency. When obtaining the history, the physician should focus on the onset of symptoms (acute vs. several days). Is there evidence of target organ damage (does the patient complain of a headache, blurred vision, chest pain, or shortness of breath)? Have there been

Table 1 Causes of Hypertensive Crisis

Neurologic
   Intracranial hemorrhage
   Subarachnoid hemorrhage
   Acute head trauma/injury
Vascular
   Recent vascular surgery
Cathacholamine excess states
   Pheochromocytoma
   Withdrawal of centrally acting alpha-2 agonist (clonidine/methyldopa)
   Sympathomimetic agents (over-the-counter cold medications)
   Illicit drug use (phencyclidine/LSD/cocaine)
Miscellaneous
   Perioperative hypertension secondary to pain/anxiety
   Renovascular hypertension
   Preeclampsia/eclampsia
   Severe burns

recent changes in medications [did the patient decrease or stop their antihypertensive medications, is the patient taking any over-the-counter cold medications (sympathomimetic agents)]? Does the patient have a history of illicit drug use, such as cocaine or LSD? Anxiety and pain are commonly overlooked provocative factors, especially in hospitalized and postoperative patients. The initial physical examination should be brief but thorough and focus on finding evidence of target organ damage. With a rapid neurologic examination, a physician should ascertain whether the patient is oriented to person, place, and time and determine whether the patient has a new focal deficit. Are the pupils equal or unequal? Are retinal hemorrhages present? Evidence of an S-3 gallop or rales on auscultation of the heart and lungs indicate acute left ventricular dysfunction. Unequal pulses in the arm or the presence of an abdominal bruit should make one suspicious of an aortic dissection. Laboratory data also can assist in the diagnosis and treatment of hypertensive crisis. An EKG and cardiac enzymes can help evaluate a patient for cardiac ischemia. A chest X-ray will assess the pulmonary vasculature and the diameter of the aorta. Urinalysis and serum BUN/creatinine can help evaluate renal function. However, since even the quickest of "STAT" labs in the hospital can take some time, a physician should not delay therapy while waiting for laboratory results, if the patient exhibits evidence of a hypertensive emergency by history and physical examination alone (see Table 2).

Table 2 Intial Evaluation

History
    Recently changed/stopped antihypertensive therapy?
    Are the symptoms sudden or gradual?
    Are CNS symptoms present (headache, visual changes, nausea, vomiting)?
    Is there any chest pain or dyspnea?
    Has the patient had recent vascular surgery (lower extremity bypass, CABG)?
    Is the patient pregnant?
    Does the patient have any pain?
    Is the patient taking any cold medications?
    Does the patient use any illicit drugs?
Physical examination
    New focal neurologic deficits
    Orientation to person, place, and time
    Stiff neck
    Unequal pupils
    Retinal hemorrhages
    Unequal pulses in arms
    Abdominal bruits
    S-3 gallop
    Rales
Laboratory tests
    EKG
    Cardiac enzymes
    Chest X-ray
    Urinalysis
    Serum BUN/creatinine
    Urine and plasma cathecholamines (if pheochromocytoma is suspected)

MANAGEMENT OF HYPERTENSIVE CRISIS

Evaluating the hospitalized patient with an acute elevation of blood pressure and deciding to treat with an appropriate antihypertensive agent is difficult and many times arbitrary. A person with normal cardiac and CNS function can tolerate substantial elevations of blood pressure without risk. On the other hand, the patient with a history of cardiac ischemia or previous myocardial infarction is at significant risk, if systolic blood pressure is >200 mm Hg, diastolic blood pressure is >110 mm Hg, and heart rate is >100. Ideally, this type of patient should receive antihypertensive therapy before symptoms develop. On most occasions, the physician will be notified by the nurse that blood pressure is elevated. On further evaluation, the patient is free of symptoms. A decision to treat must be based on a knowledge of the patient's history, particularly of the heart and CNS, and a knowledge of the physiologic impact of hypertension with or without tachycardia on important body systems.

Rapid treatment becomes essential, if patient evaluation identifies complications of the acutely elevated blood pressure. Chest pain consistent with angina may be present, but many times is a poor indicator of significant ischemia. Diabetic patients, in particular, are known to develop prominent ischemia by various indicators and yet be free of chest pain. New ST depression or T-wave inversion is a good indicator of cardiac complications of hypertension. The absence of these findings, however, does not mean the absence of ischemia. Left ventricular wall motion abnormalities demonstrated by transesophageal echocardiography are earlier indicators of ischemia, but this study is impractical for the usual patient with hypertension. Other findings, such as a new cardiac gallop or pulmonary rales, likely indicate a decompensating hypertensive state that must be treated immediately. On many occasions, beginning treatment in the absence of signs and symptoms is appropriate to prevent known cardiac and CNS complications of hypertension.

The initial treatment goal in hypertensive emergencies is reduction of blood pressure, not to normal levels, but to one that is lowered sufficiently to allow autoregulation to be restored. If blood pressure is dropped further, the resulting hypoperfusion may worsen organ damage. In most instances, blood pressure should be lowered ~25% from the hypertensive emergency levels. Patients with neurologic signs and symptoms require blood pressure reduction over 1–2 h, whereas those exhibiting cardiovascular complications need a decrease in blood pressure in a matter of a few minutes. After blood pressure is controlled for a suitable period of time to allow autoregulation to be reestablished (12–24 h), oral medications can be started and parenteral antihypertensive agents can be withdrawn gradually. Patients with hypertensive urgency require a gradual decrease in blood pressure over several hours to one day. Oral medications usually suffice in the treatment of hypertensive urgency. For the management of hypertensive complications, see sections on Cardiac/Vascular and CNS Complications.

ANTIHYPERTENSIVE AGENTS

Anxiety and pain are frequently under diagnosed and under treated causes of malignant hypertension in hospitalized patients. When pain or anxiety are the causes, short-acting analgesics such as fentanyl, administered intravenously in doses of 50–100 µg, and anxiolytics such as midazolam, given parenterally in doses of 1–2 mg, frequently will resolve the hypertensive crisis. No other treatment is needed, except for instituting a better program of pharmacologic pain and anxiety management. For patients who fail to improve with sedation and analgesia, this therapy should not be continued to the point that level of consciousness is altered just to lower blood pressure. An antihypertensive agent must be selected, if concern about cardiac or CNS complications of the elevated blood pressure is present.

Numerous options exist for the medical treatment of hypertensive crisis. In general, a patient with true hypertensive emergency should be treated with intravenous medications, either by continuous infusion or by intermittent bolus. Those with hypertensive urgency can be treated with oral medications and close follow-up. However, chronically hypertensive patients may not tolerate oral medications immediately following abdominal surgery: they require parenteral antihypertensive medications for control of high blood pressure (Table 3).

Sodium nitroprusside has been a first-line agent for treatment of hypertensive emergencies for many years. Nitroprusside, a direct vasodilator, has the benefit of having a very quick onset of action (<1 min) and a quick cessation of effect (<5 min) after discontinuation of the medication, a combination that allows nitroprusside to be titrated easily and helps avoid prolonged hypotension. The usual dose ranges from 0.5 to 10 μg/kg/min. Doses at the maximal range should be used for <10 min to minimize potential cyanide toxicity. Sulfhydryl groups in erythrocytes release cyanide ions from nitroprusside. Liver disease, lack of sulfhydryl groups, or renal disease affect the metabolism of nitroprusside. Evidence of cyanide toxicity includes tachyphylaxis, headaches, confusion, air hunger, normal PaO_2 with decreased oxyhemoglobin saturation on arterial blood gas analysis, and metabolic acidosis. Treatment involves the use of nitrite (sodium nitrite or inhaled amyl nitrite), which oxidizes normal ferrous hemoglobin to ferric hemoglobin (methemoglobin), which in turn binds cyanide to form stable cyanomethemoglobin. Thiosulfate is then administered, and cyanide is transferred from cyanomethemoglobin to thiosulfate in the liver by the enzyme rhodanase to form thiocyanate. Thiocyanate ions are subsequently excreted by the kidneys. Thiocyanate toxicity occurs with serum concentrations >10 mg/dL. Thiocyanate toxicity may be seen in patients with decreased renal function, high infusion rates, and prolonged (>3 day) infusions. Clinical signs and symptoms include tinnitus, blurred vision, headaches, nausea and vomiting, restlessness, delerium, and seizures. Thiocyanate toxicity is reversible when the medication is stopped. Thiocyanate can be cleared by hemodialysis, if needed.

Approved by the FDA in 1998 for the short-term (<48 h) management of severe hypertension, fenoldopam is a relatively new medication for the treatment of hypertensive emergencies. A selective dopamine-1 agonist, fenoldopam is a vasodilator with specific actions on renal, splanchnic, and coronary circulations. It lacks dopamine-2, alpha-adrenergic, or beta-adrenergic activity; therefore, its dose can be titrated upwards until vasodilatation and subsequent decrease in blood pressure occurs. During infusion, it has shown some benefit in patients with renal impairment by improving natuiresis, diuresis, and creatinine clearance. Another benefit of fenoldopam is that it lacks a toxic metabolite and therefore avoids the cyanide and thiocyanate toxicity seen with nitroprusside. It has a serum half-life of 7–9 min and is available only in the intravenous form. Side effects include headache, dizziness, flushing, reflex tachycardia, excessive hypotension, and brisk diuresis.

Table 3 Parenteral Medications for Treatment of Hypertensive Emergencies

Drug	Dosage	Onset	Duration of action	Comments
Sodium nitroprusside	0.5–10 μg/kg/min	Immediate	2–3 min	Inexpensive; quickest onset and cessation; risk of thiocyanate/cyanide toxicity; levels should be monitored; must shield from light
Fenoldopam	0.01–1.6 μg/kg/min	Rapid (<15 min)	10 min	Lacks toxic metabolites seen with nitroprusside; dose should be adjusted according to response of blood pressure
Labetolol	20 mg over 1–2 min Repeat every 15 min or 2 mg/min to max dose of 300 mg, then maintenance rate of 2–4 mg/h	5–10 min	3–6 h	Can cause significant bronchoconstriction; avoid in patients with heart block or severe LV dysfunction
Esmolol	500 μg/kg bolus then 50–300 μg/kg/min	5–10 min	18–30 min	Same as labetolol
Nicardipine	5–15 mg/h	15 min	2–4 h	Commonly used in postvascular and cardiac surgical patients; can cause phlebitis if infused peripherally for >24 h
Nitroglycerin	5–300 μg/min	1–2 min	3–5 min	Reduces preload and, to a lesser extent, afterload; tolerance may develop with prolonged use; can cause severe headaches
Hydralazine	5–20 mg bolus	10–20 min	3–6 h	Preferred agent for eclampsia
Enalaprilat	0.625–5 mg bolus	15 min	6–12 h	Can cause angioedema
Phentolamine	5–15 mg bolus every 10 min	1–2 min	3–10 min	Use restricted for catecholamine crisis; see profound decrease in BP if volume depleted

Labetolol and esmolol are two beta-blockers commonly used in the treatment of hypertensive emergency. Labetolol has mixed beta- and alpha-blocking activity. It can be given as an intermittent bolus (20 mg) over 1–2 min or a continuous infusion (2 mg/min up to a total of 300 mg). It has been used frequently for patients with aortic dissection and hypertensive encephalopathy, as well as postoperative patients and patients with pheochromocytoma. Labetolol acts quickly (5–10 min) and its effect will last 3–6 h. Esmolol is commonly used in patients with cardiac disease who have hypertensive emergencies. Esmolol is a short-acting selective beta-1 blocking agent. It is given as a 500 µg/kg bolus over 1 min and then started at 50 µg/kg/min. Esmolol is subsequently titrated by 50 µg/kg/min increments every 5 min to a maximum of 300 µg/kg/min. Esmolol also has the advantage of having a very quick onset of action (5–10 min) and short duration of action (half-life 7 min). Both labetolol and esmolol can cause bronchoconstriction, heart block, and left ventricular dysfunction. These complications of beta-blockade are contraindications to the use of these agents when a patient has wheezing, history of significant reactive airway disease, low cardiac output syndrome, or heart block.

Nicardipine, an intravenous dihydropyridine calcium channel antagonist, is longer acting than either nitroprusside or fenoldopam. Generally, it does not depress cardiac conduction and does not decrease left ventricular function. It is commonly used both for patients with coronary artery disease and after cardiac surgery, because it causes coronary artery dilation. Usual doses range from 5 to 15 mg/h.

Intravenous nitroglycerin is commonly used for hypertensive emergencies in settings of coronary insufficiency such as unstable angina, myocardial infarction, or left ventricular failure. It is frequently administered after coronary artery bypass surgery. Nitroglycerine dilates coronary arteries and promotes blood flow to ischemic areas. At low doses, it is a venodilator and, consequently, decreases preload. At higher doses it causes arterial dilation and can decrease blood pressure. Doses range from 5 to 300 µg/min. It has a quick onset of action and short duration of action.

Hydralazine has a long history of safety and efficacy. Onset of action of a starting IV dose of 5 mg is within 10 min, and the duration of action is 3–8 h. After the initial dose has been administered and the patient's response assessed, subsequent doses of 10–20 mg can be administered every 15–30 min until the desired lowering of blood pressure is achieved. Hydralazine has become the drug of choice in the treatment of hypertension associated with eclampsia. Hydralazine acts as a direct arteriolar vasodilator and is associated with reflex tachycardia. It should be avoided in patients with myocardial ischemia or aortic dissection.

Enalaprilat is the only intravenous angiotensin converting enzyme inhibitor available. Initial dose is 0.625 mg and additional doses of 0.625 mg may be given to a maximum of 5 mg every 6 h. Onset of action is within 15 min, and its effect usually lasts 6 h, but can last up to 12 h.

Phentolamine mesylate is a pure nonselective alpha blocking agent that has a quick onset of action (within 1–2 min). Phentolamine's use is limited to cathecholamine crises, such as a drug overdose (cocaine, amphetamines), clonidine withdrawal, or pheochromocytoma. Doses range from 5 to 15 mg every 15 min as needed.

Several oral agents are available for the treatment of hypertensive urgencies. These include captopril, clonidine, labetolol, nifedipine, and nimodipine. Patients being treated for hypertensive urgencies can be safely watched on the regular hospital ward with frequent serial examinations and monitoring by an automated noninvasive blood pressure cuff.

CARDIAC/VASCULAR COMPLICATIONS AND THEIR MANAGEMENT

Cardiovascular complications represent the greatest concern for patients in hypertensive crisis. Hypertension increases cardiac risk by increasing myocardial oxygen demand and altering its balance work supply. The determinants of myocardial oxygen demand include systolic blood pressure, heart rate, and cardiac wall tension. Myocardial oxygen supply is governed by hemoglobin concentrations, oxygen saturation of hemoglobin, and flow of blood through the coronary arteries. Unlike most organs in the body, blood flow to the heart does not occur during systole. When the heart is in systole, high chamber and muscle pressures preclude blood flow. As a result, blood flow to the myocardium must occur during diastole. Diastolic blood pressure and diastolic time become essential determinants of myocardial oxygen supply. The primary determinant of diastolic time is heart rate. When heart rate increases, systole stays essentially the same, but diastole progressively shortens. At a heart rate of 60, more time is spent in diastole than in systole, and the mycocardium is well perfused, if adequate diastolic pressure and minimal coronary occlusion are present. At a heart rate of 90, systolic and diastolic times are approximately equal. At a heart rate of 120, significant compromise of diastolic time has occurred. At some point in the elevation of heart rate, the balance of myocardial oxygen supply and demand will fail, and ischemia may result. If the ischemia persists, muscle will die, and usually a subendocardial myocardial infarction will occur. This sequence of events prompts most physicians to act to lower the blood pressure for the hospitalized patient with a hypertensive crisis.

The importance of heart rate must be emphasized. The patient with a normal heart rate and elevated blood pressure has increased myocardial oxygen demand and is at risk for ischemia. If tachycardia is added to hypertension, the problem is worsened, since tachycardia increases myocardial oxygen demand and decreases myocardial oxygen supply, as well, by reducing diastolic time. The tachycardia may reflect the endogenous state of the patient, or it may be created by the pharmacologic choice of the physician, since many antihypertensive agents are associated with reflex tachycardia. Independent of the cause of tachycardia, gains made in reducing myocardial oxygen demand by lowering systolic blood pressure may be offset by the deleterious effects of tachycardia. Intravenous nitroglycerin and β-blockers (in the absence of severe heart failure) are usually the drugs of choice to decrease blood pressure and heart rate to produce the beneficial effects of decreasing myocardial oxygen demand and increasing myocardial oxygen supply.

Severe left ventricular dysfunction leading to acute pulmonary edema can result from both myocardial ischemia and the increase in afterload associated with hypertensive crisis. Increase in afterload, with its attendant increase in impedance to ejection of the stroke volume, may lead to an acute decrease in cardiac output. A depressed cardiac output may occur, especially in patients who have valvular heart disease, such as mitral regurgitation. Decreasing blood pressure greatly decreases the workload on a failing left ventricle. Treatment of acute pulmonary edema includes preload reduction with an intravenous diuretic, such as furosemide, and afterload reduction with an appropriate antihypertensive. The target reduction in blood pressure should be one that improves cardiac perfusion and relieves symptoms.

Patients with hypertensive emergencies associated with aortic dissection are treated more aggressively than those with other types of hypertensive emergencies. Most hypertensive emergencies require a 20–25% reduction in blood pressure in a matter of minutes to several hours. An aortic dissection, however, requires an immediate decrease in blood pressure to a systolic pressure of <120 mm Hg. Usually, an intravenous β-blocker, which will decrease aortic shear stress through its negative-chronotropic and ionotropic effects, is given along with a vasodilator, such as nitroprusside, to rapidly decrease the blood pressure. Aortic dissections involving the ascending aorta and aortic arch are surgical emergencies, and pharmacologic treatment is only a temporary adjunct to definitive surgical repair. Dissection may occur distal to the left subclavian artery and involve the descending aorta. In the absence of renal artery compromise, mesenteric ischemia, or impending rupture, this type of dissection can be treated medically with strict control of blood pressure.

Coronary artery bypass surgery, operations that require cross clamping of the aorta, such as repair of aortic aneurysms and renal revascularization, and operations on carotid arteries are sometimes followed by severe hypertension. Patients who have had recent vascular surgery require immediate lowering of blood pressure. Elevated shear stress from even moderate elevation in blood pressure can threaten suture lines after recent vascular surgery. Hypotension should be avoided to lessen the danger of thrombosis. Most surgeons prefer to use short-acting agents, such as nitroprusside or fenoldopam, to avoid the risk of prolonged hypotension. Intravenous nitroglycerin is used commonly for treatment of hypertension in postoperative coronary artery bypass patients.

CNS COMPLICATIONS AND THEIR MANAGEMENT

The potential for CNS complications mandates urgent lowering of blood pressure in a hypertensive crisis. Blood flow to the brain is autoregulated: between mean blood pressures of 50 and 150 mm Hg, CNS blood flow remains nearly constant. With pathologic alterations to the brain, such as head trauma, surgery, and encephalopathy, a loss of autoregulation may occur. Brain tissue may experience substantial increases in blood flow (hyperperfusion) with subsequent worsening cerebral edema and increasing intracranial pressure. Patients with elevated intracranial pressure commonly develop petechial hemorrhages and microinfarcts.

Patients with papilledema or new retinal hemorrhages or exudates have hypertensive emergencies and often have some degree of hypertensive encephalopathy. Common signs and symptoms of CNS dysfunction secondary to hypertensive emergencies include headache, nausea, vomiting, visual disturbance, focal neurologic deficit or weakness, and varying degrees of obtundation.

Nitroprusside, with its rapid onset of action, is the drug of choice for blood pressure reduction for most hypertensive emergencies with neurologic complications. Labetolol is frequently used. Antihypertensive agents that can impair mental status, such as clonidine and methyldopa, should be avoided. Generally, the goal is reduction of blood pressure by 25% over 2–3 h. The clinician should avoid decreasing the blood pressure by more than 25% to prevent cerebral hypoperfusion and ischemia. In patients with intracranial hemorrhage or new thrombotic stroke, reduction of blood pressure remains controversial.

SUMMARY

- Hypertensive crises are associated with sudden reduction or withdrawal of antihypertensive medications, ingestion of sympathomimetics and other legal or illicit substances that increase blood pressure, perioperative hypertension, pheochromocytoma, renovascular hypertension, pre-eclampsia, and eclampsia.

- Hypertensive emergency is associated with end organ damage, including encephalopathy, intracranial hemorrhage, subarachnoid hemorrhage, stroke, myocardial ischemia, left ventricular failure, aortic dissection, and acute renal failure.
- Hypertensive urgency is not associated with end organ damage.
- Systolic blood pressures in the range of 200–240 mm Hg and diastolic pressures in the range of 120–140 mm Hg are associated with hypertensive crisis. Level of blood pressure alone is not diagnostic of an emergency. Hypertensive emergencies can occur at lower blood pressures in certain individuals.
- Initial evaluation should focus on identifying the presence of acute end organ damage, including acute onset of headache, blurred vision, chest pain, shortness of breath, or focal neurologic deficit.
- Important parts of the initial evaluation include changes in antihypertensive medication, use of over-the-counter medications (sympathomimetic agents), and pain and anxiety.
- The initial goal of treatment is reduction of blood pressure to a level that allows autoregulation to be restored.
- Agents available for treatment of hypertensive crises include sodium nitroprusside, fenoldopam, labetolol, esmolol, nicardipine, hydralazine, and enaliprilat.
- Hypertension increases cardiac risk. The patient with elevated blood pressure has increased myocardial oxygen demand. Tachycardia further increases myocardial oxygen demand, while potentially reducing myocardial oxygen supply.
- Decreasing blood pressure decreases the workload on a failing left ventricle.
- Aortic dissection requires immediate reduction of blood pressure to a systolic pressure below 120 mm Hg. Intravenous beta-blockers are usually used.
- Sodium nitroprusside is the usual drug of choice for hypertensive emergencies with neurologic complications.

BIBLIOGRAPHY

1. Calhoun DA, Oparil S. Treatment of hypertensive crisis. N Engl J Med 1990; 323:1177–1183.
2. Smith CB, Flower LW, Reinhardt CE. Control of hypertensive emergencies. Hypertens Emerg 1991; 89:111–119.
3. Rahn KH. How should we treat a hypertensive emergency? Am J Cardiol 1989; 63:48C–50C.
4. Ferguson RK, Vlasses PH. Hypertensive emergencies and urgencies. J Am Med Assoc 1986; 255:1607–1613.
5. Koch-Weser J. Drug therapy: hydralazine. N Engl J Med 1976; 295(suppl 6):320.
6. Murphy C. Hypertensive emergencies. Emerg Med Clin North Am 1995; 13:973–1007.
7. Vaughan CJ, Delanty N. Hypertensive emergencies. Lancet 2000; 356:411–417.
8. Gifford RW. Management of hypertensive crisis. J Am Med Assoc 1991; 266:829–835.
9. Prisant M, Carr AA, Hawkins DW. Treating hypertensive emergencies. Postgrad Med 1993; 93:92–110.
10. Townsend R. Hypertensive crisis. In: Lanken PN, Hanson CW, Manaker S, eds. The Intensive Care Unit Manual. Philadelphia, PA: W.B. Saunders Company, 2001:603–614.
11. Elliot WJ. Hypertensive emergencies. Crit Care Clin 2001; 17 435–451.
12. Ram CVS. Management of hypertensive emergencies: changing therapeutic options. Am Heart J 1991; 122:356–363.

25
Cardiopulmonary Interactions

Michael R. Pinsky
University of Pittsburgh Medical Center, Pittsburgh, Pennsylvania, USA

The primary goal of the cardiorespiratory system is to continually deliver adequate amounts of O_2 to meet the metabolic demands of the tissues. Oxygen delivery (DO_2) is a function of arterial O_2 content and cardiac output. Alterations in both arterial O_2 content and cardiac output occur routinely during spontaneous ventilation and can be quite abnormal and life-threatening in patients with either cardiovascular instability or respiratory insufficiency. Furthermore, artificial ventilation and ventilatory maneuvers (such as bag sigh/suctioning) can profoundly alter not only gas exchange (arterial O_2 content) but cardiac output as well. With an understanding of these interactions during both spontaneous and artificial ventilation, the physician can comprehend the impact that application and withdrawal of ventilatory therapies will have on the patient's overall cardiovascular homeostasis. Ventilation alters cardiovascular function in four primary ways (see Table 1).

CARDIOPULMONARY INTERACTIONS
Intrapulmonary Gas Exchange and Work of Breathing

First, determination of intrapulmonary gas exchange and the work-cost of breathing shows that ventilation modulates the levels of CO_2 and O_2 in the blood. Although mild hypoxemia and hypercarbia stimulate sympathetic tone, which increases blood pressure and cardiac output (1,2), profound hypoxemia ($PaO_2 < 35$ torr) and hypercarbia (if associated with acidemia, pH < 7.25) blunt the vascular response to sympathetic stimulation (2). In patients with markedly increased work-cost of breathing, even adequate intrapulmonary gas exchange does not decrease the metabolic load imposed by this increased energy expenditure (3). In some critically ill patients with limited cardiac reserve, the work-cost of breathing induces a marked increase in respiratory muscle O_2 demand that may result in a global O_2 demand in excess of the body's ability to deliver O_2 and still maintain its normal metabolic function (4). Ventilation also may alter the distribution of blood flow among organs.

Changes in Lung Volume

The lung is supplied with a large number of vagal and sympathetic afferent fibers. Normal ventilation is associated with an inspiration-induced tachycardia (respiratory sinus

Table 1 Effects of Ventilation on Cardiac Function

Intrapulmonary gas exchange and work of breathing
   Determines PaO_2 and $PaCO_2$ by altering VO_2, VCO_2, Qs/Qt, and Vd/Vt
Lung volume
   Alters pulmonary vascular resistance
Intrathoracic pressure
   Alters pressure gradients for venous return and LV ejection
Ventricular interdependence
   Alters LV diastolic compliance

arrhythmia) induced by transient withdrawal of parasympathetic tone (5–7). In contrast, large tidal volume ventilation induces cardio-depression by withdrawal of sympathetic tone (8,9). These interactions rarely impair cardiovascular function but may complicate the interpretation of cardiovascular function in critically ill patients.

As lung volume changes, so does pulmonary vascular resistance (PVR), and hence right ventricular (RV) ejection pressure load. Varying ejection pressure load can have a profound effect on RV performance, because the ability of the thinner-walled right ventricle to adapt to increasing loads is markedly limited when compared with that of the left ventricle. Under normal conditions, PVR is least at end-expiration, which at rest is defined as functional residual capacity (FRC). PVR increases as lung volume varies in either direction from FRC (10–12). As lung volume increases above FRC, alveolar vessels are compressed, and pulmonary vascular cross-sectional area decreases. The result is increased alveolar vessel resistance (10,13). As lung volume decreases below FRC, terminal airways collapse, and, by the process of hypoxic pulmonary vasoconstriction, pulmonary vasomotor tone increases. The result is again increased PVR (14,15).

FRC is very variable, even in normal humans. End-expiratory lung volume decreases with recumbency, muscle weakness, tense ascites, abdominal surgery and thoracic surgery, and in most patients with acute respiratory distress syndrome (ARDS). End-expiratory lung volume increases during acute hyperventilation associated with exercise, acute hyperinflation associated with exacerbations of chronic obstructive pulmonary disease (COPD, asthma), or inadequate expiratory time to allow for complete exhalation.

Positive end-expiratory pressure (PEEP) also increases end-expiratory lung volume. All the gas exchange and hemodynamic effects of PEEP therapy are related to the degree to which lung volumes are increased (16–24). When end-expiratory lung volume is below FRC and PEEP increases it back to normal, PVR should decrease as terminal airways reopen and alveolar gas is refreshed (16,17,19). If PEEP therapy over-distends lung units, either regionally or globally, then PVR will increase. With increased PVR, RV ejection is reduced, and cardiac output decreases (17). This over-distention-induced decrease in cardiac output is most pronounced in patients with acute hypovolemia (20) or exacerbations of obstructive lung disease. In the latter condition, the decrease in cardiac output is due to the combined effects of increased RV ejection pressure load and decreased RV distension mediated venous return.

In patients with normal cardiopulmonary function, positive-pressure ventilation decreases cardiac output by decreasing the pressure gradient for venous return to the heart; whereas, spontaneous ventilation increases cardiac output by increasing venous return above that of an apneic baseline (25–31) (Table 2). Spontaneous breathing increases cardiac output in individuals with normal cardiopulmonary function, because

Table 2 Hemodynamic Effects of Ventilation

Changes in lung volume
   Alters autonomic tone (respiratory sinus arrhythmia)
   Alters PVR
   Mechanical compression of the heart
Changes in ITP
   Alters the pressure gradient for venous return
   Alters the pressure gradient for LV ejection

they have a highly preload-sensitive heart, compliant lungs that transmit a majority of the increased airway pressure to the pleural surface, and a PVR that is very low. In contrast, most critically ill patients do not have normal cardiopulmonary function. Varying degrees of cardiac, systemic vascular, pulmonary vascular, pulmonary parenchymal, and effective circulating blood volume abnormalities exist in most critically ill patients, and all these factors are modified by ventilation. Both positive-pressure ventilation and PEEP have been documented to decrease splanchnic blood flow (32,33). Selective intestinal mucosal ischemia has been reported in both canine and human studies when high levels of PEEP have been used to support arterial oxygenation (34–36).

Changes in Intrathoracic Pressure

Gas moves between the lungs and the airway opening in response to pressure gradients between these two regions. Since the heart is in the chest, while the rest of the body and cardiovascular system is not, changes in intrathoracic pressure (ITP) will alter the pressure gradients for both venous return to the heart and left ventricular (LV) ejection from the heart. These responses are independent of the heart itself.

As lung volume increases above FRC, the heart is compressed within the cardiac fossa. Since RV volume and diastolic compliance is greater than LV volume and diastolic compliance, the initial effects of increasing lung volume will be to decrease RV end-diastolic volumes (37). Eventually, biventricular diastolic compliance will decrease if lung volume increases sufficiently.

All forms of ventilation phasically increase lung volume, although spontaneous and positive-pressure ventilation have the exact opposite effects on ITP. Spontaneous inspiration decreases ITP through the actions of respiratory muscle effort, lung compliance, and airway resistance. Thus, vigorous spontaneous inspiratory effort against an inspiratory load (bronchospasm, vocal cord paralysis, upper airway obstruction, and excessive inspiratory resistance in a CPAP system) markedly decreases ITP. In contrast, positive-pressure inspiration increases ITP as a function of tidal volume delivered and thoracopulmonary compliance. Accordingly, large tidal volume (>15 mL/kg) positive-pressure breathing, "normal" tidal volume (<10 mL/kg) positive-pressure breathing in the presence of decreased thoracopulmonary compliance, or the use of excessive amounts of PEEP all markedly increase ITP (38).

Before addressing the effects of ITP on cardiac function, the relationship between airway pressure and ITP requires examination. Increases in airway pressure may not produce similar increases in ITP in all patients. Although approximately two-thirds of the increase in airway pressure is transmitted to the pleural space in patients with normal lungs and normal tidal volumes, this relationship does not always apply to patients with lung disease (1,22,26,39–41). Patients with acute lung injury have reduced lung compliance and may not transmit as much of the increase in airway pressure to the pleural surface as do patients with normal lung compliance. Patients with obstructive lung disease may transmit more of the airway pressure to the pleural surface than normal subjects. They also may manifest intrinsic hyperinflation (often referred to as auto-PEEP). Patients experiencing auto-PEEP have end-expiratory airway pressure equal to atmospheric pressure by convention referred to as zero, but their lung volume is increased as if an external amount of PEEP were present. Clinically, one can document whether a patient has auto-PEEP by a variety of methods. The easiest way is occluding the airway at end-expiration and immediately measuring the airway pressure. If auto-PEEP is present, airway pressure should rapidly rise to the least auto-PEEP level. Although it is difficult to measure the degree to which airway pressure is transmitted to the pleural surface, a pulmonary artery catheter may allow an estimation. One can examine the swings in diastolic pulmonary arterial pressure during ventilation. Changes in pulmonary arterial diastolic pressure should closely follow changes in ITP in most conditions not associated with pulmonary hypertension.

Venous return to the heart from the body is determined by the pressure gradient between the heart (right atrial pressure) and the large venous reservoirs (mean systemic pressure) (28). Mean systemic pressure (not to be confused with mean arterial pressure) is determined by the circulating blood volume, peripheral vasomotor tone, and blood flow distribution. Any process that increases right atrial pressure will decrease this pressure gradient, decrease venous return, and, ultimately, reduce cardiac output. Since the right ventricle is a highly compliant structure, changes in surrounding ITP are directly transmitted to right atrial pressure. Since ITP is normally sub-atmospheric at end-expiration and decreases further during spontaneous inspiration, right atrial pressure usually does not rise during spontaneous ventilation. When the pressure gradient for venous return is increased, as in recumbency and with fluid overload, spontaneous inspiration-induced decreases in right atrial pressure accelerate venous blood flow (27,29,42–44). This process is referred to as the thoracic pump.

Positive-pressure inspiration, on the other hand, increases right atrial pressure by increasing ITP. Consequently, venous return is impeded (26,28,29,45,46). This ITP-induced decrease in venous return is the primary hemodynamic effect of positive-pressure ventilation on the cardiovascular system under most conditions (22). In addition, in fluid resuscitated subjects with an intact abdomen, the usual diaphragmatic descent during positive-pressure inspiration pressurizes the abdominal compartment and increases inferior vena caval pressure. This mechanism has the effect of minimizing the decrease in the venous return pressure gradient, such that, under these conditions, venous return often is unaffected by small tidal volume positive-pressure ventilation (47–49).

The left ventricle ejects its blood into an extra-thoracic arterial circuit. The pressure required to accomplish this ejection is the pressure across the wall of the left ventricle, the transmural pressure (50). Assuming that pericardial pressure and ITP are similar and that no aortic outflow obstruction exists, then transmural LV ejection pressure can be defined by the following equation:

Transmural LV ejection pressure = Aortic pressure − ITP

For a constant aortic pressure, increasing ITP will decrease LV ejection pressure; whereas, decreasing ITP will increase LV ejection pressure. Thus, both increases and decreases in ITP will alter LV ejection pressure and LV afterload (50–52). Vigorous spontaneous inspiratory efforts against an inspiratory resistance (bronchospasm, stiff lungs, and airway obstruction) can profoundly decrease ITP, which, by simultaneously increasing LV ejection pressure and augmenting venous return, can precipitate acute LV failure and cardiogenic pulmonary edema (53). The initial hemodynamic improvement seen in patients with cardiogenic pulmonary edema, who are emergently intubated and ventilated (41,54), may result from removing these exaggerated negative swings in ITP by eliminating the inspiratory obstruction and spontaneous respiratory efforts against the obstruction to decrease LV afterload. On the other hand, in the hemodynamically unstable patient requiring mechanical ventilatory support, removing such support may increase afterload and metabolic stress to the extent that such patients may not only "fail" their weaning trial, but may develop worsening cardiovascular instability during the weaning process (55). Management of such a situation may require the temporary use of inotropic agents or adjustment of intravascular volume.

Positive swings in ITP, as occur during positive-pressure inspiration, not only will decrease LV afterload, but will also decrease venous return (52). Since the ability to increase ITP by mechanical means is usually associated with similar ITP-induced decreases in venous return, the beneficial effects of increasing ITP on cardiovascular function are limited (16,19). Clearly, the overall effect of increasing ITP is dependent on the degree to which cardiac output is responsive to changes in LV preload and afterload (52). In patients with LV failure and volume overload, increases in ITP increase cardiac output, because ITP-induced decreases in LV ejection pressure override the ITP-induced decreases in pressure gradient for venous return (16,19,38,41,56).

Ventricular Interdependence

Since the two ventricles share a common intraventricular septum, changes in RV volume, which shift the septum, can change LV diastolic compliance. Consequently, changes in lung volume and ITP alter LV diastolic compliance by altering RV end-diastolic volume (ventricular interdependence) (37,57,58). In the setting of acute RV failure from pressure overload (acute cor pulmonale), as may occur following either massive pulmonary embolism or hyperinflation with fluid resuscitation, LV end diastolic volume may be reduced despite a "normal" LV filling pressure. Accordingly, measures of LV filling pressure alone (pulmonary capillary occlusion pressure; Ppao) will not reflect actual LV volume status when ITP and RV volumes are changing. This concern is more of a problem with spontaneous inspiration, when RV volumes normally increase, than with positive-pressure inspiration, when RV volumes normally decrease. Ventilation-induced changes in RV volume, which reciprocally change LV diastolic compliance and, by inference, LV preload, are thought to be the major causes of pulsus paradoxus seen in patients with acute exacerbations of asthma and chronic obstructive lung disease (37,42,59,60). On the basis of the above discussion, one can predict which strategies will be effective in minimizing the detrimental effects of ventilation while optimizing the beneficial ones (Table 3).

CLINICAL APPLICATIONS OF CARDIOPULMONARY INTERACTIONS

The effect of ventilation on a patient will be dependent on the baseline level of cardiorespiratory function and the mode of ventilation used. In the spontaneously ventilating patient, concerns regarding ventilatory support, with or without endotracheal intubation,

Table 3 Physiologic Strategies to Minimize the Detrimental Effects of Mechanical Ventilation

Maximize venous return
Prevent right atrial pressure from increasing
   Keep ITP elevations small
      Small tidal volumes (<10 mL/kg)
      Brief inspiratory time
      Least amount of PEEP necessary to maintain arterial oxygenation
   Prevent hyperinflation-induced cor pulmonale
      Least amount of PEEP necessary to maintain arterial oxygenation
      Prolonged expiratory time
Maximize mean systemic pressure
   Maintain effective circulating blood volume
      Use least amount of sedation to facilitate synchrony with ventilation
      Fluid resuscitation as necessary to maintain LV filling
      Military anti-shock trousers (MAST)
      Avoid massive thoracentesis or paracentesis
   In the fluid-resuscitated subject with a persistently low right atrial pressure and cardiac output, vasopressor therapy to increase peripheral vasomotor tone

Minimize LV afterload
Abolish vigorous negative swings in ITP during spontaneous ventilation
   Remove impediments to spontaneous inspiratory efforts
      Intubation for upper airway obstruction
      Bronchodilator therapy for bronchospasm
      Paracentesis (to an abdominal pressure <12 mm Hg) for tense ascities
Minimize vigorous inspiratory efforts during positive-pressure ventilation
   In partial ventilatory assist modes (e.g., IMV, pressure support)
      Low resistance respiratory circuits
      High bias flows
      Extrinsic PEEP equal to or greater than intrinsic PEEP
      Patient-matched inspiratory flow rates (usually >60 L/min)
   In total ventilatory support (e.g., CMV, assist-control)
      Extrinsic PEEP equal to or greater than intrinisic PEEP
      Patient-matched inspiratory flow rates (usually >60 L/min)

should be directed at determining the primary factor(s) that may induce cardiovascular instability. Hypovolemia, if associated with hypoperfusion, can induce acute respiratory muscle failure and, if prolonged, death (3,20). Loss of vasomotor tone, as may occur in sepsis or anaphylactic shock, can have the same effects. Placing such patients on positive-pressure ventilation can induce acute circulatory collapse, if circulating blood volume and vasomotor tone are not sustained at normal levels.

Several cardiac factors appear to play major roles in determining the degree of ventilation-induced cardiovascular instability (61,62). Clearly, cardiovascular insufficiency will be exaggerated during weaning trials (discussed earlier), as the increased metabolic demand is coupled with increased afterload. Occult mesenteric ischemia, as assessed by tonometry (63), is a common finding in patients failing a weaning trial. Patients with chronic obstructive lung disease, who are able to wean from mechanical ventilatory support, increase their cardiac output during weaning but keep their arterio-venous O_2 content difference (DvO_2) constant. In contrast, those subjects unable to wean increase both their cardiac output and their DvO_2, a phenomenon consistent with worsening cardiovascular performance (64,65). Hyperinflation can induce tamponade-like physiology, with pulsus paradoxus and diastolic equilibration of intracardiac pressures (27).

Increased ITP can induce relative hypovolemia (discussed earlier), which may correct with fluid resuscitation (27,58). Both hyperinflation and pulmonary embolism can induce RV pressure overload (acute cor pulmonale), which will impair LV filling by the mechanism of ventricular interdependence. Appropriate therapy is reversal of the primary process (66). Finally, LV failure can occur if marked negative swings in ITP sufficiently increase LV ejection pressure (50,53). How then does one prevent or reverse these processes? Table 4 lists some general principles useful in minimizing the detrimental effects of mechanical ventilation. Useful principles for patients, including those breathing spontaneously, are:

1. Avoid large swings in ITP
2. Minimize the work-cost of breathing
3. Retune end-expiratory lung volume to FRC

Clearly, the degree to which adequate gas exchange may be compromised in order to keep the increases in lung volume and ITP small requires balance. New studies have suggested that permissive hypercarbia, if not associated with acidemia, can be well tolerated in the patient with severe reversible airflow obstruction. The benefits of permissive hypercarbia are less barotrauma and less hemodynamic instability.

In heart failure patients, the transition to positive-pressure ventilation often is associated with improved cardiovascular performance, rather than deterioration, as a consequence of the reduced preload and afterload (67,68). These effects can be so pronounced as to be identifiable during the inspiratory phase of ventilation (56,69).

Although these principles seem reasonable, no controlled clinical trial has proven their effectiveness in maintaining hemodynamic stability. Given the complex nature and unpredictable course of critically ill patients, such a clinical study may not be feasible. In practice, if these broad principles are used, the work-cost of breathing can be minimized, the metabolic load (O_2 demand) of the respiratory muscles decreased, and patient anxiety reduced (3). Since dynamic hyperinflation is commonly seen in patients with chronic obstructive lung disease, using enough externally applied PEEP to offset the patient's own auto-PEEP during spontaneous ventilation is rational. This additional PEEP can be provided with CPAP employing a bias flow circuit with or without the

Table 4 Clinical Strategies to Minimize the Detrimental Effects of Mechanical Ventilation

Allow the patient to breathe spontaneously
   Assist-control ventilation
   Partial ventilatory support
      Intermittent mandatory ventilation (IMV) with back-up pressure-support ventilation
      Pressure support ventilation
Avoid hyperinflation
   Prolonged expiratory time
   Bronchodilator therapy to relieve air trapping and minimize auto-PEEP
   Use least PEEP

application of positive-pressure breaths. If end-expiratory airway and alveolar pressure can be equalized by this method, then excess negative swings in ITP during spontaneous inspiration can be avoided. Please note that, like auto-PEEP, these large negative swings in ITP may not be appreciated from inspection of the airway pressure signal alone.

Since pressure support ventilation, of all the partial ventilatory support modes, is associated with the lowest magnitude swings in ITP during matched tidal breaths, it may be the optimal method of partial ventilatory support in the hemodynamically unstable patient requiring mechanical ventilatory support. Although clinical trials are (not?) available to support this concept, it may represent the least stressful method of weaning such patients if other methods, such as t-tube weaning and IMV withdrawal, are unsuccessful.

The practical goal of the physician caring for such patients is identifying the cardiopulmonary interactions that determine the cardiovascular status of the patient. The clinician must, therefore, work to optimize the beneficial aspects of these interactions without impairing gas exchange or venous return.

USING CARDIOPULMONARY INTERACTIONS TO DIAGNOSE CARDIOVASCULAR INSUFFICIENCY

Employing a different perspective, one can use the known hemodynamic effects of breathing in the diagnosis of preload-responsiveness. Since right atrial pressure (Pra) is the backpressure against venous return, if Pra should decrease during spontaneous inspiration, then venous return will transiently increase. Cardiac output will consequently increase. If, however, the right ventricle is unable to dilate further, then Pra will not decrease during inspiration, even though ITP decreases. At the extreme, spontaneous inspiration-associated increases in Pra reflect severe RV failure and are referred to as Kussmaul's sign.

Magder et al. (70) used the fall in Pra to predict which patients would increase their cardiac outputs in response to a defined fluid challenge. They found that if Pra decreased by >2 mm Hg during a spontaneous breath, then cardiac output increased in 16 of 19 patients in response to 250–500 mL saline bolus infusion. If Pra did not decrease, then cardiac output increased in only 1 of 14 patients. These data are important, because they focus on both RV function and spontaneous ventilation, two areas of study with few clinical trials. These workers recently documented that this approach can also be used to predict subsequent changes in cardiac output in response to increasing levels of PEEP in mechanically ventilated subjects (71). A potential limitation of these studies is reliance on RV performance as the signal transducer for blood flow. They do not address the issue of LV performance, which would need to be assessed separately.

Other studies have focused on the effects of positive-pressure ventilation on LV output. Positive-pressure ventilation induces cyclic changes in LV stroke volume through similar cyclic changes in venous return. The magnitude of these changes in stroke volume is a function of the tidal volume, the subsequent increase in ITP, and the extent of changes in LV output resulting from LV filling pressure. Beat-to-beat changes in LV stroke volume can be monitored easily as beat-to-beat changes in arterial pulse pressure, since the only other determinants of pulse pressure, arterial resistance, and compliance cannot change enough to alter pulse pressure during a single breath.

Based on this logic, Perel et al. (72) examined the systolic pressure variation (SPV) induced by a defined positive-pressure breath both in animals, made hypovolemic or in heart failure, and in humans. They demonstrated that a decrease in systolic pressure from an apneic baseline identified hemorrhage and was minimized by fluid resuscitation (72–74). The concept of SPV assumes that all the changes in systolic pressure can be explained by parallel changes in LV stroke volume (75). Unfortunately, Denault et al. (38) could not demonstrate any relation between LV stroke volume, estimated by transesophageal echocardiographic analysis, and SPV, a finding that suggests that factors other than LV stroke volume contribute to SPV. Michard et al. (76,77) reasoned that arterial pulse pressure variation (PPV) would more accurately reflect changes in LV stroke volume because, unlike SPV, PPV is not influenced by ITP changes. They compared SPV with PPV as predictors of the response of cardiac output to fluid loading in septic, ventilator-dependent patients. Their data convincingly demonstrated that both PPV and SPV of $\geq 15\%$ were far superior to measures of either Pra or pulmonary artery occlusion pressure in predicting an increase in cardiac output after volume loading. Furthermore, the greater the PPV or SPV, the greater was the increase in cardiac output. However, PPV was associated with greater precision and less bias than SPV (74). Subsequently, other investigators validated these findings in different patient populations (78,79).

Since PPV may reflect LV stroke volume changes, the finding that aortic flow variation, as measured by transesophageal 2D pulsed Doppler echocardiography, follows a similar response to fluid loading as does PPV is not surprising (80). The flow variation data are very important, because flow is the primary variable from which SPV and PPV derive their validity. Though less invasive than arterial pressure monitoring, echocardiographic analysis is far from ideal as a hemodynamic monitoring tool, because it requires the continuous presence of an experienced operator, as well as expensive and often scarce equipment. Minimally invasive esophageal pulsed Doppler techniques have recently been developed that continuously measure descending aortic flow on a beat-to-beat basis. To the extent that descending aortic flow varies proportionally with aortic outflow, these measures of descending aortic flow accurately asses stroke volume variation.

SUMMARY

- Spontaneous ventilation can increase oxygen consumption, venous return, and LV ejection pressure. If a critically ill patient can breathe spontaneously without increases in the work-cost of breathing, increasingly negative swings in ITP, or hyperinflation, spontaneous breathing is preferred.
- Positive-pressure ventilation attempts to decrease the work-cost of breathing while maintaining gas exchange.
- Positive-pressure ventilation increases ITP and decreases cardiac output by decreasing venous return.
- PVR increases as lung volume becomes either greater or less than functional residual capacity (FRC).
- PEEP increases end-expiratory lung volume. PVR will be minimized if PEEP brings lung volumes to normal FRC.
- Biventricular diastolic compliance will decrease if lung volumes increase.
- The right ventricle is a compliant structure, and increases in ITP are transmitted to the right ventricle and right atrium. Venous blood flow may decrease.
- Changes in ITP modulate LV ejection pressure.

- Increasing RV volume decreases LV compliance.
- To minimize detrimental effects of mechanical ventilation, avoid large swings in ITP, minimize the work-cost of breathing, and return end-expiratory lung volume to FRC.
- Successful weaning from mechanical ventilation will depend on the effect of resumption of spontaneous ventilation on cardiac function.

APPENDIX—CASE EXAMPLES

Case 1

A 34-year-old, 105 kg female underwent a routine cholecystectomy. She was extubated postoperatively and was returned to her ward bed. For the next two days the patient complained of vague abdominal pain, nausea, and mild dyspnea. D5NS was administered at the rate of 125 mL/h until she could start taking fluids p.o. On the second postoperative day she developed increasing epigastric pain, fever (39.5 °C), tachycardia (HR 125, regular), nausea, and respiratory distress. Arterial blood gas analysis revealed a PaO_2 of 55 torr, $PaCO_2$ of 30 torr, and pH of 7.48, while breathing 2 L O_2 nasal via a cannula. Chest roentgenogram revealed bilateral lower lobe atelectasis and pleural effusions. Blood chemistries revealed a leukocytosis with a left shift, hematocrit 34%, and a moderately elevated serum amylase. All other chemistries were normal.

The patient was given supplemental oxygen (40% by face mask), encouraged to deep breathe and cough, and transferred immediately to the intensive care unit. Blood cultures and a repeat arterial blood gas analysis demonstrated a PaO_2 of 42 torr, $PaCO_2$ of 45 torr, and a pH of 7.31. Respiratory rate was 32 breaths/min, temperature was 39.5 °C, blood pressure 98 by palpation, and pulse 125 beats/min. With increasing agitation, central cyanosis, and presumed impending respiratory arrest, an attempt at awake endotracheal intubation was performed but was unsuccessful. The patient was sedated with midazolam, easily intubated, and given positive-pressure ventilation with the following settings: tidal volume 1200 mL, frequency 15 per min, FiO_2 0.5, and 5 cm H_2O of PEEP.

Within minutes of the intubation the patient became less responsive and profoundly hypotensive. Blood pressure was 60 by palpation, and pulse was thready at a rate of 150 per min. Good breath sounds without wheezing were heard bilaterally. A portable chest roentgenogram demonstrated that the endotracheal tube was in proper position and that a significant amount of the atelectasis observed in the previous film had resolved. Repeat arterial blood gas analysis revealed a PaO_2 of 255 torr, $PaCO_2$ of 25 torr, and pH of 7.31. The tidal volume was reduced to 800 mL, a central venous catheter was placed, and rapid fluid resuscitation with NS in 250 mL boluses was performed. After approximately 1000 mL NS had been infused, the patient stabilized with a blood pressure of 135/75 and pulse 85 per min. The metabolic acidosis resolved within an hour. Follow-up blood culture was negative, and the patient was successfully extubated to a 24% FiO_2 face-mask on the following day.

Comment

The patient demonstrated most of the detrimental effects on venous return of positive-pressure ventilation. Her clinical course was one of postoperative atelectasis in a volume-depleted patient. These features were complicated by her obesity and the upper

Cardiopulmonary Interactions

abdominal incision. Her fluid requirements in the setting of recent abdominal surgery with third space fluid loss, fever, and no oral intake resulted in a hypovolemic state. Her thoracic compliance was decreased by obesity. Consequently, her ITP increased more in response to increased lung volume than would occur in a non-obese patient. Furthermore, as documented by the repeat arterial blood gas analysis, the initial tidal volume delivered was too high. The positive-pressure ventilation-induced rise in ITP was greater than that needed to sustain gas exchange. The choice of initial tidal volume settings, though based on actual body weight, should be referenced to ideal body weight, since the extra fat contributed little to metabolic demand. Furthermore, initial tidal volumes should be set more toward 6 mL/kg.

Appropriate treatment of such a patient may include tracheal intubation, if obtundation prevents the use of mask CPAP. Several clinical measures and the clinical context all suggest hypovolemia. Thus, rapid and aggressive fluid resuscitation may be necessary in such patients to prevent a hypotensive crisis.

Case 2

A 65-year-old, 65 kg male with a past history of severe COPD secondary to tobacco use (125 pack/year exposure) develops acute hemoptysis and syncope. By esophago-gastroendoscopy an arterial bleeding site is documented at the base of a duodenal ulcer. The patient underwent a routine vagotomy and pyloroplasty with over-sewing of the ulcer. He was returned to the intensive care unit intubated. Since the patient had a past history of severe COPD (FEV_1/FVC ratio = 0.25, FEV_1 = 900 mL) no attempt to wean the patient from mechanical ventilatory support was attempted on the first postoperative day. On the second postoperative day the patient was hemodynamically stable and afebrile. Arterial blood gas analysis revealed a PaO_2 of 120 torr, $PaCO_2$ of 35 torr, and pH of 7.44 on an FiO_2 of 0.4. The patient was ventillated with intermittent mandatory ventilation (IMV), a tidal volume of 700 mL, and a frequency of 20.

Weaning was attempted by progressively decreasing the IMV frequency in 5 breath increments every 4 h as tolerated. Although the patient appeared comfortable with a ventilatory frequency of 15 per min, when the rate was reduced further he became agitated, tachypneic (respiratory rate of 35 per min), tachycardic (pulse 125 sinus), and had diffuse wheezing. Pulmonary arterial and radial arterial catheters were inserted, and the following hemodynamic data were obtained during weaning trials:

	IMV ventilator rate		
Measurement	20	15	10
PaO_2	120	115	85
$PaCO_2$	35	37	67
pH	7.44	7.43	7.18
RR	20	25	35
HR	95	105	125
Pra	15	17	32
Ppa	35/18	36/20	56/35
$Ppao$	12	13	30
$Part$	110/75	112/80	75/45

The patient's IMV rate was returned to 20, and he was given inhalation bronchodilator therapy. He exhibited hemodynamic stabilization within 1 h. Afterward, the patient was placed on maintenance bronchodilator therapy, given supplemental levels of PEEP until Ppa diastolic pressure rose, and the tidal volume was decreased to 600 mL. These therapies resulted in arterial blood gas analysis of PaO_2 of 125 torr, $PaCO_2$ of 48 torr, and pH of 7.38. Repeat weaning from the lower tidal volume with 6 cm H_2O PEEP successfully allowed the patient to be extubated within 24 h.

Comment

Patients with severe COPD have an increased work-cost of breathing. Furthermore, their ability to exhale is time-limited. Air-trapping is a risk when ventilatory rates are high. This patient initially received an excessive minute ventilation, which resulted in a mild respiratory alkalosis. The patient was unable to maintain that excessively high level of minute ventilation during weaning for two reasons. First, the work-cost of breathing was too high. Second, air-trapping as a consequence of the high spontaneous ventilatory rate decreased respiratory muscle efficiency further and increased ITP. The increased ITP caused an increase in intrathoracic vascular pressure. Note the diastolic equilibration of pressures. Supplemental extrinsic PEEP to offset the auto-PEEP effect allowed spontaneous ventilatory efforts to occur without large swings in ITP, which increase the work-cost of breathing.

Therapies that limit hyperinflation will improve mechanical efficiency of the respiratory muscles and will prevent increases in end-expiratory ITP and large swings in ITP during ventilation. Bronchodilator therapy, permissive hypercarbia, and supplemental extrinsic PEEP all function to achieve this goal.

REFERENCES

1. Grenvik A. Respiratory, circulatory and metabolic effects of respiratory treatment. Acta Anaesth Scand (suppl) 1966.
2. Vatner SF, Rutherford JD. Control of the myocardial contractile state by carotid chemo- and baroreceptor and pulmonary inflation reflexes in conscious dogs. J Clin Invest 1978; 63:1593–1601.
3. Roussos C, Macklem PT. The respiratory muscles. N Engl J Med 1982; 307:786–797.
4. Aubier M, Vires N, Sillye G, Mozes R, Roussos C. Respiratory muscle contribution to lactic acidosis in low cardiac output. Am Rev Respir Dis 1982; 126:648–652.
5. Painal AS. Vegal sensory receptors and their reflex effects. Physiol Rev 1973; 53:59–88.
6. Shepherd JT. The lungs as receptor sites for cardiovascular regulation. Circulation 1981; 63:1–10.
7. Tang PC, Marie FW, Amassain VE. Respiratory influence on the vasomotor center. Am J Physiol 1957; 191:218–224.
8. Daly MB, Hazzledine JL, Ungar A. The reflex effects of alterations in lung volume on systemic vascular resistance in the dog. J Physiol (London) 1967; 188:331–351.
9. Glick G, Wechsler AS, Epstein DE. Reflex cardiovascular depression produced by stimulation of pulmonary stretch receptors in the dog. J Clin Invest 1969; 48:467–472.
10. Hakim TS, Michel RP, Chang HK. Effect of lung inflation on pulmonary vascular resistance by arterial and venous occlusion. J Appl Physiol 1982; 53:1110–1115.
11. West JB, Dollery CT, Naimark A. Distribution of blood flow in isolated lung; relation to vascular and alveolar pressure. J Appl Physiol 1964; 19:713–724.

12. Whittenberger JL, McGregor M, Berglund E, et al. Influence of state of inflation of the lung on pulmonary vascular resistance. J Appl Physiol 1960; 15:878–882.
13. Howell JBL, Permutt S, Proctor DF, et al. Effect of inflation of the lung on different parts of the pulmonary vascular bed. J Appl Physiol 1961; 16:71–76.
14. Brower RG, Gottlieb J, Wise RA, Permutt W, Sylvester JT. Locus of hypoxic vasoconstriction in isolated ferret lungs. J Appl Physiol 1987; 63:58–65.
15. Hakim TS, Michel RP, Minami H, Chang K. Site of pulmonary hypoxic vasoconstriction studied with arterial and venous occlusion. J Appl Physiol 1983; 54:1298–1302.
16. Calvin JE, Driedger AA, Sibbald WJ. Positive end-expiratory pressure (PEEP) does not depress left ventricular function in patients with pulmonary edema. Am Rev Resp Dis 1981; 124:121–128.
17. Canada E, Benumnof JL, Tousdale FR. Pulmonary vascular resistance correlated in intact normal and abnormal canine lungs. Crit Care Med 1982; 10:719–723.
18. Cassidy SS, Robertson CH, Pierce AK, et al. Cardiovascular effects of positive end-expiratory pressure in dogs. J Appl Physiol 1978; 44:743.
19. Grace MP, Greenbaum DM. Cardiac performance in response to PEEP in patients with cardiac dysfunction. Crit Care Med 1982; 20:358–360.
20. Harken AH, Brennan MF, Smith N, Barsamian EM. The hemodynamic response to positive end-expiratory ventilation in hypovolemic patients. Surgery 1974; 76:786–793.
21. Jardin F, Farcot JC, Boisante L, et al. Influence of positive end-expiratory pressure on left ventricular performance. N Engl J Med 1981; 304:387.
22. Luce JM. The cardiovascular effects of mechanical ventilation and positive end-expiratory pressure. J Am Med Assoc 1984; 252:807–811.
23. Marini JJ, Culver BN, Butler J. Mechanical effect of lung distension with positive pressure on cardiac funtion. Am Rev Resp Dis 1980; 124:382–386.
24. Pick RA, Handler JB, Murata GH, Friedman AS. The cardiovascular effects of positive end-expiratory pressure. Chest 1982; 82:345–350.
25. Brecher Ga, Hubay CA. Pulmonary blood flow and venous return during spontaneous respiration. Circ Res 1955; 3:40–214.
26. Cournaud A, Motley HL, Werko L, et al. Physiologic studies of the effect of intermittent positive pressure breathing on cardiac output in man. Am J Physiol 1948; 152:162–174.
27. Guntheroth WG, Morgan BC, Mullins GL. Effect of respiration on venous return and stroke volume in cardiac tamponade. Mechanism of pulsus paradoxus. Circ Res 1967; 20:381–390.
28. Guyton AC, Lindsey AW, Abernathy B, et al. Venous return at various right atrial pressures and the normal venous return curve. Am J Physiol 1957; 189:609–615.
29. Holt JP. The effect of positive and negative intrathoracic pressure on cardiac output and venous return in the dog. Am J Physiol 1944; 142:594–603.
30. Morgan BC, Martin WE, Hornbein TF, et al. Hemodynamic effects of intermittent positive pressure respiration. Anesthesiology 1960; 27:584–590.
31. Seely RD. Dynamic effects of inspiration on the simultaneous stroke volumes of the right and left ventricles. Am J Physiol 1948; 154:273–280.
32. Kiefer P, Nunes S, Kosonen P, Takala J. Effect of positive end-expiratory pressure on splanchnic perfusion in acute lung injury. Intensive Care Med 2000; 26:376–383.
33. Lefrant JY, Juan JM, Bruelle P, Demaria R, Cohendy R, Aya G, Oliva-Lauraire MC, Peray P, Robert E, de La Coussaye JE, Eledjam JJ, Dauzat M. Regional blood flows are affected differently by PEEP when the abdomen is open or closed: an experimental rabbit model. Can J Anaesth 2002; 49:302–308.
34. Fournell A, Scheeren TW, Schwarte LA. PEEP decreases oxygenation of the intestinal mucosa despite normalization of cardiac output. Adv Exp Med Biol 1998; 454:435–440.
35. Jedlinska B, Mellstrom A, Jonsson K, Hartmann M. Influence of positive end-expiratory pressure ventilation on peripheral tissue perfusion evaluated by measurements of tissue gases and pH. An experimental study in pigs with oleic acid lung injury. Eur Surg Res 2000; 32:228–235.

36. Lehtipalo S, Biber B, Frojse R, Arnerlov C, Johansson G, Winso O. Effects of positive end-expiratory pressure on intestinal circulation during graded mesenteric artery occlusion. Acta Anaesthesiol Scand 2001; 45:875–884.
37. Janicki JS, Weber KT. The pericardium and ventricular interaction, distensibility and function. Am J Physiol 1980; 238:H494–H503.
38. Denault AY, Gasior TA, Gorcsan J, Mandarino WA, Deneault LG, Pinsky MR. Determinants of aortic pressure variation during positive-pressure ventilation in man. Chest 1999; 116:176–186.
39. Conway CM. Hemodynamic effects of pulmonary ventilation. Br J Anaesth 1975; 47:761–766.
40. Goldberg HS, Rabson J. Control of cardiac output by systemic vessels: circulatory adjustments of acute and chronic respiratory failure and the effects of therapeutic interventions. Am J Cardiol 1981; 47:696.
41. Rasanen J, Nikki P, Heikkila J. Acute myocardial infarction complicated by respiratory failure. The effects of mechanical ventilation. Chest 1984; 85:21–28.
42. Bromberger-Barnea B. Mechanical effects of inspiration on heart functions: a review. Fed Proc 1981; 40:2172–2177.
43. Scharf SM, Brown R, Saunders N, et al. Effects of normal and loaded spontaneous inspiration on cardiovascular function. J Appl Physiol 1979; 47:582–590.
44. Wise RA, Robotham JL, Summer WR. Effects of spontaneous ventilation on the circulation. Lung 1981; 159:175–192.
45. Braunwald E, Binion JT, Morgan WL, Sarnoff SJ. Alterations in central blood volume and cardiac output induced by positive pressure breathing and counteracted by metraminol (Aramine). Circ Res 1957; 5:670–675.
46. Pinsky MR. Determinants of pulmonary arterial flow variation during respiration. J Appl Physiol 1984; 56:1237–1245.
47. Kitano Y, Takata M, Sasaki N, Zhang Q, Yamamoto S, Miyasaka K. Influence of increased abdominal pressure on steady-state cardiac performance. J Appl Physiol 1999; 86:1651–1656.
48. Kraut EJ, Anderson JT, Safwat A, Barbosa R, Wolfe BM. Impairment of cardiac performance by laparascopy in patients receiving positive end-expiratory pressure. Arch Surg 1999; 134:76–80.
49. Van den Berg PC, Jansen JR, Pinsky MR. Effect of positive pressure on venous return in volume-loaded cardiac surgical patients. J Appl Physiol 2002; 92:1223–1231.
50. Buda AJ, Pinsky MR, Ingels NB, Daughters GT, Alderman EL. Effect of intrathoracic pressure on left ventricular performance. N Engl J Med 1979; 301:453–459.
51. Peters J, Kindred MK, Robotham JL. Transient analysis of cardiopulmonary interactions II. Systolic events. J Appl Physiol 1988; 64:1518–1526.
52. Pinsky MR, Matuschak GM, Klain M. Determinants of cardiac augmentation by increases in intrathoracic pressure. J Appl Physiol 1985; 58:1189–1198.
53. Stalcup SA, Mellins RB. Mechanical forces producing pulmonary edema in acute asthma. N Engl J Med 1977; 297:592–596.
54. Rasanen J, Vaisanen IT, Heikkila J, et al. Acute myocardial infarction complicated by left ventricular dysfunction and respiratory failure. The effects of continuous positive airway pressure. Chest 1985; 87:158–162.
55. Beach T, Millen E, Grenvik. Hemodynamic response to discontiunance of mechanical ventilation. Crit Care Med 1973; 1:85–90.
56. Fellahi JL, Valtier B, Beauchet A, Bourdarias JP, Jardin F. Does positive end-expiratory pressure ventilation improve left ventricular function? A comparative study by transesophageal echocardiography in cardiac and noncardiac patients. Chest 1998; 114:556–562.
57. Olsen CO, Tyson GS, Maier GW, et al. Dynamic ventricular interaction in the conscious dog. Circ Res 1983; 52:85–104.
58. Taylor RR, Corell JW, Sonnenblick EH, Ross Jr J. Dependence of ventricular distensibility on filling the opposite ventricle. Am J Physiol 1967; 213:711–718.

59. Brinker JA, Weiss I, Lappe DL, et al. Leftward septal displacement during right ventricular loading in man. Circulation 1980; 61:626–633.
60. Ruskin J, Bache RJ, Rembert JC, Greenfield Jr. Pressure-flow studies in man: effect of respiration on left ventricular stroke volume. Circulation 1973; 48:79–85.
61. Frazier SK, Stone KS, Schertel ER, Moser DK, Pratt JW. A comparison of hemodynamic changes during the transition from mechanical ventilation to T-piece, pressure support, and continuous positive airway pressure in canines. Biol Res Nurs 2000; 1:253–264.
62. Pinsky MR. Breathing as exercise: the cardiovascular response to weaning from mechanical ventilation. Intensive Care Med 2000; 26:1164–1166.
63. Mohsenifar Z, Hay A, Hay J, Lewis MI, Koerner SK. Gastric intramural pH as a predictor of success or failure in weaning patients from mechanical ventilation. Ann Intern Med 1993; 119:794–798.
64. De Backer D, El Haddad P, Preiser JC, Vincent JL. Hemodynamic responses to successful weaning from mechanical ventilation after cardiovascular surgery. Intensive Care Med 2000; 26:1201–1206.
65. Jubran A, Mathru M, Dries D, Tobin MJ. Continuous recordings of mixed venous oxygen saturation during weaning from mechanical ventilation and the ramifications thereof. Am J Respir Crit Care Med 1998; 158:1763–1769.
66. Sibbald WJ, Driedger AA. Right ventricular function in disease states: pathophysiologic considerations. Crit Care Med 1983; 11:339–345.
67. Heney MF, Johansson G, Haggmark S, Biber B. Analysis of left ventricular systolic function during elevated external cardiac pressures: an examination of measured transmural left ventricular pressure during pressure-volume analysis. Acta Anaesthesiol Scand 2001; 45:868–874.
68. Kaplan LJ, Bailey H, Formosa V. Airway pressure release ventilation increases cardiac performance in patients with acute lung injury/adult respiratory distress syndrome. Crit Care 2001; 5:221–226.
69. Karlocai K, Jokkel G, Kollai M. Changes in left ventricular contractility with the phase of respiration. J Auton Nerv Syst 1998; 73:86–92.
70. Magder S, Georgiadis G, Cheong T. Respiratory variations in right atrial pressure predict the response to fluid challenge. J Crit Care 1992; 7:76–85.
71. Madger S, Lagonidis D, Erice F. The use of respiratory variations in right atrial pressure to predict the cardiac output response to PEEP. J Crit Care 2001; 16:108–114.
72. Perel A, Pizov R, Cotev S. Systolic blood pressure variation is a sensitive indicator of hypovolemia in ventilated dogs subjected to graded hemorrhage. Anesthesiology 1987; 67:498–502.
73. Szold A, Pizov R, Segal E, Perel A. The effect of tidal volume and intravascular volume state on systolic pressure variation in ventilated dogs. Intensive Care Med 1989; 15:368–371.
74. Tavernier B, Makhotine O, Lebuffe G, Dupont J, Scherpereel P. Systolic pressure variation as a guide to fluid therapy in patients with sepsis-induced hypotension. Anesthesiology 1998; 89:1313–1321.
75. Bennett-Guerrero E, Kahn RA, Moskowitz DM, Falcucci O, Bodian CA. Comparison of arterial systolic pressure variation with other clinical parameters to predict the response to fluid challenges during cardiac surgery. Mt Sinai J Med 2002; 69:96–100.
76. Michard F, Chemla D, Richard C, Wysocki M, Pinsky MR, Lecarpentier Y, Teboul JL. Clinical use of respiratory changes in arterial pulse pressure to monitor the hemodynamic effects of PEEP. Am J Respir Crit Care Med 1999; 159:935–939.
77. Michard F, Boussat S, Chemla D, Anguel N, Mercat A, Lecarpentier Y, Richard C, Pinsky MR, Teboul JL. Relation between respiratory changes in arterial pulse pressure and fluid responsiveness in septic patients with acute circulatory failure. Am J Respir Crit Care Med 2000; 162:134–138.

78. Berkenstadt H, Margalit N, Hadani M, Friedman Z, Segal E, Villa Y, Perel A. Stroke volume variation as a predictor of fluid responsiveness in patients undergoing brain surgery. Anesth Analg 2001; 92:984–989.
79. Reuter DA, Felbinger TW, Kilger E, Schmidt C, Lamm P, Goetz AE. Optimizing fluid therapy in mechanically ventilated patients after cardiac surgery by on-line monitoring of left ventricular stroke volume variations. Comparison with aortic systolic pressure variations. Br J Anaesth 2002; 88:124–126.
80. Feissel M, Michard F, Mangin I, Ruyer O, Faller JP, Teboul JL. Respiratory changes in aortic blood velocity as an indicator of fluid responsiveness in ventilated patients with septic shock. Chest 2001; 119:867–873.

26
Vascular Emergencies in the Surgical Intensive Care Unit

Alexandre d'Audiffret, Steven Santilli, and Connie Lindberg
VA Medical Center, Minneapolis, Minnesota, USA

INTRODUCTION

With advances in surgical and anesthesia techniques and the increasing complexity of surgical patients, the management of the intensive care unit (ICU) patient population frequently includes vascular injuries. As 20–30% of the population over the age of 60 suffers from peripheral arterial disease, a significant number of vascular problems can be expected during any ICU admission (1). In addition, complications may result from therapeutic vascular interventions or the placement of indwelling arterial catheters necessary to monitor and stabilize the critically ill patient.

ACUTE ARTERIAL INSUFFICIENCY

The etiology of acute arterial insufficiency may be divided into three main categories: thrombosis, thromboembolism, and non-occlusive ischemia. Regardless of the etiology, prompt diagnosis and intervention are essential to prevent limb loss. Several studies have demonstrated that irreversible peripheral nerve and muscle damages occur after 3–6 h of ischemia (2). Timely diagnosis of the threatened limb can be challenging and depends on the patient's degree of alertness, hemodynamic status, and known history of chronic arterial insufficiency. The five cardinal features of arterial insufficiency classically have been described as pain, paralysis, paresthesia, pallor, and pulselessness. A certain level of experience is necessary to determine the true severity of the ischemic event and the need for intervention before full development of these five signs.

Lower Extremity Ischemia
Clinical Presentation
The diagnosis and etiology of the threatened lower extremity begins with history and physical examination. Thorough historical and physical examination remain of primary importance and, combined with the use of a Doppler probe, allow stratification of the severity of the ischemia and the proper therapeutic intervention. The Society for Vascular

Surgery/International Society for Cardiovascular Surgery Committee on Reporting Standards has established three categories of ischemia (3):

1. *Viable*: Not immediately threatened, intact capillary return, no muscle weakness, no sensory loss, audible Doppler arterial signal with an ankle pressure >30 mm Hg, and audible venous signal.
2. *Threatened*: Salvageable limb with proper treatment, slow capillary refill, mild muscle weakness, mild sensory loss, inaudible arterial signal, and audible venous signal.
3. *Major tissue loss*: Amputation regardless of treatment, no capillary refill, profound paralysis, anesthesia, and no arterial or venous signal.

A complete physical examination should include assessing the presence or absence of all extremity pulses, timing of capillary refill, noting the level of skin temperature changes, status of venous filling, determining the presence of arterial and venous Doppler signals, and performing an ankle systolic pressure measurement.

Differential Diagnosis

Acute Arterial Thrombosis: Acute arterial thrombosis occurs most commonly in patients with known arterial occlusive disease or a history of claudication and may follow episodes of hypovolemia, hypotension, decreased cardiac output, or transient hypercoagulability. On physical examination, occlusive disease is often present in the contralateral limb. Of note, patients with pre-existing occlusive disease have well-developed collaterals and may often be better able to tolerate an ischemic insult than an individual with acute thrombosis and no collateral flow.

Arterial Thromboembolism: A history of recent myocardial infarction, mural thrombus, or atrial fibrillation should raise the suspicion of an embolic event. On examination, a simple pulse examination, as well as the presence of a clear demarcation in the skin temperature, easily determine the level of occlusion. In addition, the contralateral pulse examination is often normal.

Non-occlusive Ischemia: This term is commonly associated with mesenteric ischemia; however, in the critically ill patient on multiple vasopressors, peripheral vasoconstriction may be severe enough to abolish Doppler signals in both distal upper and lower extremities. On examination, a blue discoloration is present in all digits and toes; however, proximal pulses in the groin, popliteal fossa, and brachial artery are preserved. No intervention is necessary, because resolution is the rule with hemodynamic improvement.

Medical and Surgical Treatment

Assessment to measure the degree of ischemia is essential to determine the need for therapeutic intervention. A guiding principle is that the patient's life takes priority over limb. Independently of the severity of the ischemia, the patient's hemodynamic status will be the limiting factor in the decision about the feasibility and extent of intervention.

Protective measures include hemodynamic optimization, anticoagulation (if not contraindicated) to protect collateral vascular beds, and extremity skin protection to prevent pressure ulcers on the heels, malleoli, and toes.

Surgical revascularization is indicated only in hemodynamically stable patients. In the case of embolic disease of the lower extremity, a simple embolectomy often can be performed via a femoral approach under local anesthesia. In contrast, patients with thrombotic disease need to undergo diagnostic angiography. Finally, patients with non-salvageable limbs should undergo prompt amputation. The acidosis and other complications of myonecrosis may significantly worsen the prognosis.

Upper Extremity Ischemia

Clinical Presentation

The principles for lower extremity also apply to the upper extremity. In contrast to the lower extremity, the presence of multiple collaterals at the level of the shoulder and elbow account for the low incidence of critical upper extremity ischemia. Only 10–15% of acute occlusions of the subclavian or axillary artery and 3% of acute brachial artery occlusions result in a threatened limb (4). The physical examination should highlight the elements already mentioned for the examination of the lower extremity.

Differential Diagnosis

Arterial Thromboembolism: Approximately 15% of embolic events involve the upper extremities. Of the embolic sources, 80–90% are cardiac in origin (atrial fibrillation or myocardial infarction), 5–10% are noncardiac (aneurysmal aorta or axillary artery), and 5–10% are unknown (5). As in lower extremity ischemia, intervention is indicated only in cases of threatened limbs.

Acute Arterial Thrombosis: Upper extremity occlusive disease commonly involves the innominate artery and the subclavian arteries. An acutely threatened limb from chronic occlusive disease is a rare entity, because a well-developed collateral network is present. Symptomatic chronic arterial insufficiency may result from brachial arterial puncture. An estimated 45% of patients with an arterial injury after brachial puncture for vascular diagnostic or other interventional procedures will have chronic symptoms, and 20% will require surgical intervention (6). Intervention at the time of diagnosis is rarely needed and can be addressed once the patient has stabilized.

Vasospasm or Non-occlusive Ischemia: Arteries in the upper extremities, especially in younger patients, are extremely prone to vasospasm. As a result, ischemic changes in the hands and digits may result from shock, attempts at arterial cannulation, and from the use of vasopressors. As previously mentioned, critical upper limb ischemia is a rare entity and surgical treatment is seldom necessary. Complications associated with arterial cannulation will be discussed later.

Medical and Surgical Treatment

Chronic ischemia of the upper extremity does not necessitate any intervention while the patient is in the ICU. Follow-up in the vascular noninvasive laboratory and vascular surgery clinic is indicated. In the case of embolic disease, an embolectomy is indicated in all cases, unless precluded by the hemodynamic status of the patient. An embolectomy can be performed under local anesthesia via a brachial artery approach above the elbow, or in the antecubital fossa, to selectively thrombectomize the ulnar and radial arteries. These patients should be anticoagulated if possible at the time of diagnosis, and anticoagulation should be continued postoperatively. Non-occlusive ischemia is managed conservatively, as previously described for the lower extremity.

ACUTE MESENTERIC ISCHEMIA

The etiology of mesenteric ischemia can be divided into two main categories: arterial and venous. Arterial causes are more common and include superior mesenteric artery emboli, superior mesenteric artery thrombosis, and non-occlusive mesenteric ischemia. Mesenteric venous thrombosis accounts for <5% of all cases of acute mesenteric ischemia.

Clinical Presentation and Differential Diagnosis

The clinical presentation of acute mesenteric ischemia consists of acute nonspecific abdominal complaints. Only a high index of suspicion and careful attention to risk factors will lead to a timely diagnosis, the most important determinant of outcome. Superior mesenteric artery emboli should be suspected in patients with atrial fibrillation, a recent MI, evidence of synchronous emboli, or recent proximal aortic instrumentation. A history of chronic mesenteric ischemia and diffuse atherosclerosis, associated with an episode of hypotension or dehydration, should raise suspicion for superior mesenteric artery thrombosis. Patients receiving vasopressors, who have low cardiac output and hypotension, are at risk for non-occlusive mesenteric ischemia, which is essentially severe mesenteric vasospasm. Finally, mesenteric venous thrombosis is seen in patients with known hypercoagulabilty states, recurrent deep vein thromboses, and associated dehydration.

Medical and Surgical Management

The primary objective is to establish the diagnosis of mesenteric ischemia prior to the onset of small bowel infarction, which is associated with 90% mortality (7). Angiography remains the gold standard for the diagnosis of acute mesenteric ischemia. An angiogram will determine mesenteric flow, the presence of vasospasm, and the state of the collateral circulation proximal and distal to the occlusion. Placement of a catheter at the ostium of the superior mesenteric artery allows delivery of papaverine to manage vasospasm during the perioperative period. The majority of patients with mesenteric ischemia will require laparotomy to re-establish vascular flow, assess intestinal viability, and resect compromised bowel.

The diagnosis of mesenteric venous thrombosis is made with contrast-enhanced computed tomography. Once the diagnosis is confirmed, the patient should be anticoagulated. Surgical intervention is indicated if intestinal ischemia is suspected.

Two of the worst complications following mesenteric revascularization are rethrombosis (associated with 100% mortality) and failure to properly recognize the compromised bowel. As a result, patients should remain anticoagulated after thrombectomy, and a second-look procedure should be planned within 24–48 h of the first laparotomy.

PHLEGMASIA CERULEA DOLENS AND VENOUS GANGRENE

Advanced cases of iliofemoral deep venous thrombosis have been described as phlegmasia alba dolens and phlegmasia cerulea dolens. Phlegmasia alba dolens is defined as diffuse swelling and pallor of the involved extremity, with associated moderate pain as a consequence of iliofemoral venous thrombosis. In contrast, patients with phlegmasia cerulea dolens have a severely cyanotic limb. They complain of extreme pain and tenderness, petechiae are present, and pedal pulses are diminished or absent. Both the deep and superficial venous systems are completely thrombosed. Advanced cases may present with hemorrhagic bullae and distal gangrenous changes. Phlegmasia cerulea dolens may represent a progression of phlegmasia alba dolens or may occur *de novo*. Treatment involves anticoagulation and thrombectomy or thrombolysis. Anticoagulation is commonly successful in cases of phlegmasia without venous gangrene. Thrombectomy is performed if the patient's limb fails to improve after 12 h of anticoagulation, or if gangrenous changes occur in the limb. Fasciotomies offer mixed results and are not routinely recommended (8). Patients are often too ill to undergo general anesthesia. Mortality is estimated to be between 20% and 40%. Although the amputation rate is 20–60%, most amputations are minor (9).

COMPLICATIONS ASSOCIATED WITH INVASIVE MONITORING

Arterial complications associated with hemodynamic monitoring may be the result of indwelling arterial catheters or from an inadvertent arterial injury while placing central venous access.

Radial Artery Catheterization

The radial artery is the most commonly involved site, because ease of placement of a catheter makes it the primary choice for arterial catheterization. Up to 5% of patients have an incomplete palmar arch. An incomplete palmar arch without significant retrograde collateral circulation, such that the radial artery alone supplies blood to the hand, has been reported in 1.6% of patients. As a result, appropriate tests to perform are the Allen's test and the Doppler test, which assess digital and palmar flow with occlusion of the radial artery (10). Despite the high incidence of compromised flow in the radial artery, critical digital ischemia is an uncommon problem. If clinical ischemia is present, catheter removal is the first intervention. In some cases, embolectomy with radial reconstruction may be necessary. Up to 29% of patients develop radial artery thrombus distal to the catheter site after 4–10 days. In addition, 30% develop thrombi at the time of decannulation (11,12). However, nearly all patients recanalize the thrombosed segments and do not develop evidence of digital ischemia. The superficial arch is the principal source of flow to the digit and is primarily derived from the ulnar artery.

Brachial Artery Complications

Brachial artery complications occur in individuals with inadequate collateral circulation, such as patients with diabetes and peripheral vascular disease. Brachial artery occlusion, in the context of poor collateral circulation, produces a high incidence of critical ischemia, because it leads to loss of flow in both the ulnar and radial arteries. Despite the low incidence of these complications, the brachial artery should not be used as a site of arterial cannulation unless absolutely necessary.

Axillary Artery Catheterization

Complications associated with axillary artery catheterization are not only ischemic in nature but also neurologic, as hematoma within the arterial sheath leads to compression of the surrounding nerves. The incidence of complications associated with axillary catheters is estimated at 2.5% (13).

Access Complications

Finally, access complications occur. These complications are associated with central venous cannulation and involve subclavian and carotid puncture. Management depends on the coagulation status of the patient, the vessel involved, and the size of the arterial injury. For patients with ongoing hemorrhage or acute neurologic changes as a result of arterial thrombosis or expanding hematoma, emergency surgical consultation should be sought.

VASCULAR COMPLICATIONS ASSOCIATED WITH VASCULAR PROCEDURES

Aortic Procedures

Perioperative Bleeding

Bleeding after aortic aneurysm repair or aortic bypass procedure should be minimal. Should hemorrhage occur, knowledge of the location of the cross-clamp, especially whether it was above or below the celiac axis, will help predict the etiology of the hemorrhage. The crucial point is recognition of surgical bleeding. A useful guideline is: a patient with normal coagulation factors, whose aorta is clamped below the celiac axis, should not require more than 2 units of packed red blood cells during the subsequent 8 h to maintain a stable hemoglobin. Patients who require supraceliac clamping, or who have a thoraco-abdominal aortic aneurysm repair, could have a coagulopathy associated with transient liver ischemia. This coagulopathy needs to be recognized and corrected. A complication, often overlooked, is splenic laceration associated with thoraco-abdominal aneurysm repair or retroperitoneal aneurysm repair that requires supraceliac clamping. Splenic injury has been reported in up to 25% of these cases.

Colon Ischemia Following Abdominal Aneurysm Repair

Ischemic colitis is a serious complication following abdominal aortic aneurysm repair. It occurs in 1% of elective cases and in up to 5% of emergency cases for ruptured aneurysm. Persistent acidosis, excessive fluid requirement, and loose stools following aneurysm repair should prompt a diagnostic colonoscopy (14) (refer also to section on Acute Mesenteric Ischemia).

Lower Extremity Ischemia Following Aortic Procedures

Extremity pulses, including femoral pulses, should be carefully monitored following abdominal aortic procedures. The etiology of the ischemic limb after an aortic procedure is generally either technical or embolic. Prompt recognition is crucial to assure timely correction and limb salvage (refer also to section on Acute Arterial Insufficiency).

CAROTID ENDARTERECTOMY

Carotid endarterectomy is a safe and effective procedure with a low complication rate when performed by an experienced surgeon. Close monitoring for changes in hemodynamic status, development of hematoma, or hyperperfusion syndrome is required during the 6 h following carotid endarterectomy.

Hypotension/Hypertension

Alterations in blood pressure are common after carotid endarterectomy and are likely related to the sinus nerve of Hering, a branch of the glossopharyngeal nerve ending at the carotid bifurcation. A large body of literature associates blood pressure fluctuation with an increased incidence of perioperative stroke; therefore, pharmacological treatment is initiated for a systolic pressure <110 mm Hg and >170 mm Hg. Sodium nitroprusside or neosynephrine are commonly used.

Cervical Hematoma

Cervical hematoma may occur in up to 6.5% of patients; however, reintervention is necessary in <1.5% in our institution (15). The patient's neck should be monitored periodically at the time of neurologic evaluation. In cases of acute respiratory distress secondary to a cervical hematoma, the neck wound should be reopened and the hematoma evacuated prior to reintubation. The tracheal deviation is often too severe to permit safe reintubation.

Hyperperfusion Syndrome

Cerebral hemorrhage, or hyperperfusion syndrome, after carotid endarterectomy is a rare phenomenon associated with correction of a critical stenosis in the face of a contralateral occlusion, stroke, or severe postoperative hypertension. This phenomenon is thought to be associated with cerebral edema followed by hemorrhage and may occur immediately or up to 5 days postoperatively. The affected patient suffers form severe unilateral headaches and seizures. Treatment is aimed at limiting cerebral edema, controlling blood pressure, and preventing seizures.

SUMMARY

- Etiology of acute arterial insufficiency may be caused by thrombosis, thromboembolism, or non-occlusive ischemia.
- The five cardinal features of arterial insufficiency are pain, paralysis, paresthesia, pallor, and pulselessness.
- A guiding principle is that the patient's life takes precedence over limb.
- Many critically ill patients have chronic peripheral vascular disease and risk factors for acute vascular injury. The clinician must have a high index of suspicion for vascular injury and recognize limb or visceral ischemia early.
- Three categories of ischemia are viable, threatened, and major tissue loss. Careful history, physical examination, and Doppler evaluation can help to stratify the degree of injury.
- Physical examination of the lower extremity should include presence or absence of pulses, timing of capillary refill, level of skin temperature change, status of venous filling, presence of arterial and venous Doppler signals, and ankle systolic pressure measurements.

- Critical upper extremity ischemia is less common than critical lower extremity ischemia.
- Recent myocardial infarction, mural thrombus, or atrial fibrillation are associated with thromboembolism.
- Mesenteric ischemia may be arterial (95%) or venous (5%).
- Superior mesenteric artery emboli may occur in patients with atrial fibrillation, recent myocardial infarction, synchronous emboli, or recent aortic instrumentation who report abdominal pain.
- Angiography can determine mesenteric flow, the presence of vasospasm, and the state of collateral circulation.
- The majority of patients with mesenteric ischemia will require laparotomy.
- Patients receiving vasopressors are at risk for non-occlusive mesenteric ischemia.
- Phlegmasia alba dolens is a consequence of iliofemoral venous thrombosis. The lower extremity shows diffuse swelling and pallor. Pain is usually moderate.
- Phlegmasia cerulea dolens results from complete thrombosis of the superficial and deep venous systems. Findings include a severely cyanotic, painful limb with petechiae and hemorrhagic bullae. Early diagnosis and treatment with anticoagulation, thrombectomy, or thrombolysis may save life and limb.
- Arterial monitoring catheters may be associated with distal ischemia. The brachial artery should not be used unless absolutely necessary.
- Aortic reconstructive surgery may be associated with surgical bleeding, splenic injury, colon ischemia, and lower extremity ischemia.
- Carotid endarterectomy may be associated with altered blood pressure, cervical hematoma, or hyperperfusion syndrome.

REFERENCES

1. Hirsch A, et al. The Minnesota regional arterial disease screening program: towards a definition of community standards of care. Vasc Med 2001; 6(2):87–96.
2. Harman J. The significance of local vascular phenomena in the production of ischemic necrosis in skeletal muscle. Am J Pathol 1948; 25:625.
3. Rutherford R, et al. Suggested standards for reports dealing with lower extremity ischemia. J Vasc Surg 1986; 64:80.
4. Ricotta J, et al. Management of acute ischemia of upper extremity. Am J Surg 1983; 145(5):661–666.
5. Abbot W, et al. Arterial embolism: a 44 year perspective. Am J Surg 1982; 143:460–465.
6. Menzoian J, et al. Management of the upper extremity with absent pulses after cardiac catheterization. Am J Surg 1978; 135:484.
7. Geelkerken R, et al. Mesenteric vascular disease: a review of diagnostic methods and therapies. Cardiovasc Surg, 1995; 3(3):247–269.
8. Weaver F, et al. Phlegmasia cerulea dolens: therapeutic considerations. South Med J 1988; 81:306–312.
9. Perkins J, et al. Phlegmasia cerulea dolens and venous gangrene. Br J Surg 1996; 83(1):19–23.
10. Husum B, et al. Arterial dominance in the hand. Br J Anaesth 1978; 50:913–916.

11. Bedford R, et al. Complications of percutaneous radial artery cannulation: an objective prospective study in man. Anesthesiology 1973; 38:228–236.
12. Bedford R, et al. Radial artery function following percutaneous cannulation with 18 and 20 gauge catheters. Anesthesiology 1977; 47:37.
13. Bryan-Brown C, et al. The axillary artery catheter. Heart Lung 1983; 12:492–497.
14. Bast, Ischemic disease of the colon and rectum after surgery for abdominal aortic aneurysm: a prospective study of the incidence and risk. Eur J Vasc Surg 1990; 4:253.
15. Treiman R, et al. The influence of neutralizing heparin after carotid endarterectomy on postoperative stroke and wound hematoma. J Vasc Surg 1990; 11:252.

E. Pulmonary Function

27
Acute Lung Injury

Larry A. Woods, Alan J. Cropp, and Bhagwan Dass
St. Elizabeth Hospital Medical Center, Youngstown, Ohio, USA

INTRODUCTION

Acute lung injury (ALI), first described by Ashbaugh in 1967 (1), is a disorder with varying degrees of pulmonary cellular damage (parenchymal and vascular) that alters alveolar capillary membrane permeability, produces accumulation of noncardiogenic extravascular lung water, and results in hypoxic respiratory failure. Patients with this syndrome have dyspnea, refractory hypoxia, reduced lung compliance, and diffuse radiologic changes. Acute respiratory distress syndrome (ARDS) is a more severe subset of ALI characterized by dyspnea, refractory hypoxemia, decreased lung compliance, and diffuse radiologic changes that occur in the absence of cardiac failure or chronic lung disease. The American–European Consensus Conference on ARDS of 1994 defines ALI as "a syndrome of inflammation and increased permeability that is associated with a constellation of clinical, radiologic, and physiologic abnormalities that cannot be explained by, but may coexist with, left atrial or pulmonary capillary hypertension." It is associated most often with sepsis syndrome, aspiration, primary pneumonia, or multiple traumas. Much less common associations include cardiopulmonary bypass, multiple transfusions, fat embolism, and pancreatitis. ALI and ARDS are acute in onset and persistent, for example, lasting days to weeks; are associated with one or more known risk factors; are characterized by arterial hypoxemia resistant to oxygen therapy alone; and demonstrate diffuse radiologic infiltrates. Chronic lung diseases such as interstitial pulmonary fibrosis and sarcoidosis, which would technically meet the criteria for the chronicity, are excluded by this definition (2). The criteria recommended by this consensus committee are enumerated in Table 1. This definition emphasizes that ALI/ARDS is not the result of primary cardiac disease as the cause of the hypoxia and radiographic findings (2), although patients with this condition can become fluid overloaded or develop concurrent heart failure (3).

With improved ICU care and new treatment strategies, a gradual increase in the percentage of survivors of ALI has been observed. In the 1970s and 1980s, the mortality rate was ~60%. Currently, the average mortality rate is ~35%, and some centers report even lower mortality (4).

Table 1 Recommended Criteria for ALI and ARDS

	Timing	Oxygenation	Chest radiograph	Pulmonary artery wedge pressure
ALI	Acute onset	$PaO_2/FIO_2 < 300$ mm Hg (independent of level of PEEP)	Bilateral infiltrates seen on frontal CXR	<18 mm Hg when measured and no clinical evidence of left atrial hypertension
ARDS	Acute onset	$PaO_2/FIO_2 < 200$ mm Hg (independent of level of PEEP)	Bilateral infiltrates seen on frontal CXR	<18 mm Hg when measured and no clinical evidence of left atrial hypertension

INCIDENCE

ALI/ARDS affects ~150,000 persons annually in the United States alone (5). The annual incidence of ARDS in the United States was found to be 75 cases per 100,000 population in a study conducted by the National Institutes of Health (NIH) (6). A study from Utah reported an incidence of 4.8–8.3 per 100,000 population per year (7). Valta's European study found an incidence of 4.9 per 100,000 population per year for ARDS (8). In one of the first studies to use the definition of the consensus conference of 1994, the reported incidence of ALI and ARDS was found to be 17.9 per 100,000 and 13.5 per 100,000, respectively.

RISK FACTORS

Conditions associated with the development of ALI/ARDS include factors causing direct lung injury or systemic injury that affect the lungs (Table 2). ALI is usually an acute process developing within 24 h of the inciting incident. When ALI/ARDS develops 72 h or later after the inciting event, the respiratory failure usually is due to a delayed infectious process.

Overall, sepsis syndrome has the highest risk for the development of ALI/ARDS (10). Gastric aspiration and trauma are frequently associated with ALI. Pepe et al. (11) found the risk of developing ARDS doubles for each concurrent disorder present.

Factors demonstrated to increase the risk of ARDS in the presence of the foregoing conditions include age, female gender (trauma only), severity of illness [measured by APACHE II or lung injury severity score (ISS)], cigarette smoking, chronic alcohol abuse, or a combination of these factors (12).

MEDIATORS OF ALI

ALI/ARDS results from cascading inflammatory events thought to be responsible for the capillary membrane breakdown and vascular changes seen in this condition.

Acute Lung Injury

Table 2 Major Categories of ARDS Risk

Direct injury
  Aspiration
  Diffuse pulmonary infection (e.g., bacterial, viral, pneumocystis, etc.)
  Infection
  Near drowning
  Toxic inhalation
  Lung contusion
Indirect injury
  Sepsis syndrome with or without significant hypotension (e.g., systolic blood pressure ≤90 mm Hg) and with or without evidence of infection outside the lung. This syndrome can be described as having both signs of systemic inflammation (i.e., by abnormalities of body temperature, heart rate, respiratory rate, and white blood cell count) and signs of organ dysfunction, including, but not limited to, pulmonary, hepatic, renal, central nervous, and cardiovascular symptoms.
  Severe intrathoracic trauma as indicated by
    Clinical description
    Scoring systems such as the ISS or APACHE II/III
    Treatment interventions such as the treatment intervention scoring system
  Hypertransfusion for emergency resuscitation
  Cardiopulmonary bypass (rare)

A stimulus, such as trauma or sepsis, causes the release of inflammatory cytokines, including tumor necrosis factor (TNF), interleukin-1 (IL-1), interleukin-6 (IL-6), and interleukin-8 (IL-8). Although not specific markers for ALI/ARDS, both TNF and IL-1 concentrations are increased in bronchoalveolar lavage fluid of patients with this syndrome. TNF and IL-1 stimulate the production of IL-8, which is a strong chemoattractant for neutrophils and which triggers the acute inflammation within the lungs. In addition, concentrations of IL-8 are increased in the bronchoalveolar lavage and pulmonary edema fluid of patients who have developed ARDS. Higher concentrations of IL-8 in ARDS patients are associated with higher mortality, but no specific threshold of IL-8 is associated with death. Blood IL-6 concentrations have been found to be more predictive of patient outcome in this syndrome than those of IL-8. Concentrations of IL-6 are significantly higher and persist for a longer period of time in patients who do not survive (13–15).

The neutrophils that are attracted by IL-8 and other stimuli accumulate in the air spaces and interstitium of the lungs. When activated, they release toxic mediators, such as reactive oxygen species, platelet aggregation factor, metabolites of arachidonic acid, and proteases. These substances cause damage to the capillary endothelium and alveolar epithelium. As normal barriers are lost, protein escapes through the alveolar capillary membrane into the airspace of the lung. The resultant pulmonary edema causes surfactant dysfunction and necrosis of type I alveolar cells. Type II alveolar cells undergo hyperplasia. Damage to type I alveolar cells increases entry of fluid into the alveoli and decreases clearance of fluid from the alveoli. Damage to type II alveolar cells is associated with decreased production of surfactant with resultant decreased compliance and alveolar collapse. The result is diffuse alveolar damage, which is seen histologically during the early stages of ALI/ARDS.

PATHOPHYSIOLOGY

The pathologic progression of ALI/ARDS is consistent and does not depend on the underlying cause. The process follows three overlapping phases of injury and repair of both lung parenchyma and pulmonary vasculature.

Phase I, lasting 0–7 days, is the acute or exudative phase. Its hallmark is the breakdown of the pulmonary capillary–alveolar membrane with subsequent increase in vascular permeability. This injury results in interstitial–alveolar edema, often recognized on chest radiograph as pulmonary edema. Proteins and cellular debris form hyaline membranes. Multiple alveoli collapse. Intravascular platelet aggregation and fibrin deposition form microthrombi and perpetuate pulmonary hypertension.

During phase II, days 5–14, the first signs of repair appear. This interval is the subacute or proliferative phase. A hyperplastic response of type II alveolar epithelial cells is noted during this period. Fibroblasts begin the transformation of the intra-alveolar fluid into granulation tissue, a process that precedes the deposition of collagen in the third phase. This fibrotic phase may start as early as day 10 in some areas of the lung. This stage varies in duration, but typically lasts until the third week of the illness.

The fibrotic phase, or phase III, starts at approximately the third week. The result of this fibrotic process is loss of alveoli, thickened membranes, and a less distensible lung. The lung parenchyma becomes diffusely emphysematous as the third phase progresses. The pulmonary vasculature is not spared in the inflammatory process. The microthrombi seen in the acute phase persist and may obstruct larger arterioles. Thickening of vessel walls results from intimal and medial hypertrophy, which occurs in the subacute and fibrotic phases. Finally, the loss of pulmonary vasculature is proportional to the decrease in alveolar units. All of these events result in a continuation of the pulmonary hypertension seen at the onset of the acute stage (16).

Underlying changes in lung structure are accompanied by changes in lung function. Injury to the alveolar capillary membrane epithelium results in increased permeability. This increased permeability is both to fluids and to large-molecular-weight proteins. The disruption of the epithelial side of the membrane allows passage of an exudative fluid directly into the alveoli. The fluid found in patients with cardiogenic pulmonary edema caused by increased hydrostatic forces in the presence of an intact membrane is low in protein content, and alveolar edema is less pronounced. Worsened gas-exchange occurs as a result of ventilation–perfusion (V/Q) mismatch. In contrast, noncardiogenic lung water, high in protein, is caused by increased membrane permeability. Widespread alveolar flooding ensues, and large areas of unventilated lung are still perfused. This intrapulmonary shunt causes hypoxia, which characteristically is not responsive to supplemental levels of inspired oxygen. Also seen are under-perfused but well-ventilated areas of the lung, which result in increased dead space.

The decrease in compliance that occurs in the acute phase is not fully understood. It is thought to occur initially by quantitative and qualitative changes in surfactant produced by type II alveolar epithelial cells. The presence of leaking plasma proteins renders surfactant ineffective in reducing surface tension. Lung compliance is consequently decreased, and increased pressures are needed to expand the lungs.

Increased pulmonary vascular pressures without a concomitant increase in left ventricular filling pressures are thought to occur in the early phase of ARDS. Initially, pulmonary hypertension is caused by cell-injury mediators. The resulting vasoconstriction is followed and perpetuated by microthrombi and vascular collapse as extravascular lung

Acute Lung Injury

water increases. As the process continues into the second and third phases, the underlying causes of hypoxia, decreased compliance, and pulmonary hypertension become more complex. In the proliferative and fibrotic phases, causes of hypoxia include not only increased right to left intrapulmonary shunting but also newly developed areas of V/Q mismatch, as well as gas-diffusion abnormalities. This condition results from loss of alveolar units, loss of pulmonary vasculature, and the widened septal membranes seen with fibrosis. The proliferating type II alveolar epithelial cells replace surfactant. Lung compliance remains low and usually is decreased further by the large amount of collagen deposited in the repair phase. Obliteration of pulmonary vasculature and diffuse vessel wall hypertrophy sustain the previously increased pulmonary artery pressures.

CLINICAL COURSE

Despite multiple causes, the clinical presentation of ALI is quite uniform. After the initial insult, a latent period extends from a few hours to several days. As the cell-injury mediators are released and the capillary permeability increases, tachypnea appears. In the early stages of ALI, the precipitating injury usually is the primary focus of the physician's efforts. Pulmonary impairment usually appears within 48 h. During physical examination, the patient may appear agitated. Fever, dyspnea, tachypnea, and cough develop. Use of respiratory accessory muscles, sternal retractions, and paradoxic abdominal movements with respirations may signal impending respiratory collapse. On pulmonary examination, diffuse crackles in the chest can be auscultated. As this condition closely resembles cardiogenic pulmonary edema, careful attempts should be made to look for signs of congestive heart failure or fluid overload. ABG studies reveal hypoxemia with a widening alveolar–arterial gradient, a reflection of intrapulmonary shunting. Initially, respiratory alkalosis is usually present. The shunt fraction, Q_S/Q_T (i.e., the portion of non-ventilated blood flow divided by the total pulmonary blood flow), is increased and may be 30% or greater in patients with severe lung injury. Resulting hypoxemia is usually severe and frequently requires endotracheal intubation and mechanical ventilation. In addition, static lung compliance, measured by dividing the tidal volume by the plateau pressure minus the positive end expiratory pressure (PEEP), is decreased. The plateau pressure is obtained by occluding the exhalation circuit at end inspiration or by adding an inspiratory pause of 1–2 s. The decreased lung compliance can be less than 30 mL/cm H$_2$O in ARDS patients (normal is 80–100 mL/cm H$_2$O). Leukocytosis may be present and reflect the underlying cause or nonspecific inflammatory response of the lung.

Radiographic examination early in the course of ALI may reveal completely normal results. As the injury progresses, interstitial edema followed by bilateral fluffy infiltrates representing alveolar flooding occurs. Normal heart size and lack of pleural effusion may help to distinguish noncardiogenic pulmonary edema from cardiac-induced pulmonary edema. The institution of mechanical ventilation and PEEP may initially appear to cause clearing of the chest X ray (CXR) by hyperinflation, but results should not be confused with injury regression. The CXR eventually takes on the "ground-glass" appearance of interstitial fibrosis and may demonstrate hyperlucent zones representing lung remodeling and emphysematous changes. CT scans generally are not indicated for patients with ARDS. The risk of transport of a critically ill patient must be weighed against the benefit of identifying more subtle pulmonary interstitial changes, cavitations, pleural effusions, and pneumothorax.

The clinical course of ALI may take several paths and is dependent on a variety of factors (17). ALI with rapid reversal is seen in patients who are otherwise healthy and young and who develop the injury from a single cause (i.e., high-altitude sickness, drug ingestion, or fat embolism). Improvement may be as rapid as the onset, with little or no pulmonary sequelae. Patients who are older or develop ALI secondary to "high-risk" or multiple causes (e.g., sepsis) have a more protracted course and experience greater morbidity and mortality. Nonsurvivors with ALI/ARDS usually die during the first 2 weeks, frequently from the underlying disease, sepsis, or organ failure syndrome. Patient's surviving into phase III of the disease have a better prognosis, although recovery may take weeks or months.

Pulmonary sequelae in survivors of ALI vary and are related to both severity and duration of injury. Those patients with rapid disease reversal have little, if any, pulmonary abnormalities when compared with those with protracted courses. Improvement in lung function has been shown to occur through at least 6 months following extubation, but no further improvement has been shown at 1 year (18). Some patients have residual hyper-reactive airways; whereas, others may develop varying degrees of restrictive lung dysfunction and gas-exchange abnormalities (19,20). Despite improvement in lung function to near normal in many cases, those who survive ALI still have a decreased quality of life as measured by surveys comparing survivors with a control group (21).

MANAGEMENT

The management of ALI and ARDS is mainly supportive. Treatment of the underlying cause is the initial step in the management of this syndrome. At this time, no known treatment exists to reverse increased vascular permeability changes or fibrosis occurring with ALI.

The need to assess volume status and proceed with fluid resuscitation is an essential basic step in managing ARDS. Intravascular volume must be adequate to maintain gas exchange, oxygen delivery, and hemodynamic stability. Pulmonary artery catheter insertion may be essential in these assessments. Although volume–pressure relationships are variable, maintaining a pulmonary capillary wedge pressure between 12 and 15 mm Hg has been a useful clinical practice. Cardiac output may be negatively affected by the use of PEEP (see Chapter 25). Inotropic support may be needed if adequate intravascular volume has already been achieved. Controversy about the preference for crystalloid or colloid solutions persists. Maintaining adequate oxygen-carrying capacity provided by hemoglobin should not be neglected, and patients should be transfused when indicated to increase oxygen delivery to tissues (see Chapter 53).

Continued vigilance for signs of infection is necessary. Fastidious care should be given to all intravascular monitoring and other indwelling devices in accordance with the infection control policies of each institution. In cases in which fever and leukocytosis are present without an obvious source, fungal infection, sepsis from indwelling invasive lines, and sinus infection as a result of intubation should be considered. If fever and leukocytosis occur without an obvious source before lung injury, suspicion should be focused on the lower torso as the source of infection. If this phenomenon should occur after the establishment of ALI, a pulmonary source is likewise strongly suspected (22). Malnutrition compromises host defenses. Early and appropriate nutritional support is vital and is discussed in more detail in Chapter 3.

The treating physician must anticipate many of the general medical complications resulting from ALI, for example, aspiration, cardiac dysrhythmias, stress ulcers with Gl bleeding, and pulmonary embolism. Ventilator-associated complications may include barotrauma with mediastinal and retroperitoneal dissection of air, pneumothorax, subcutaneous emphysema without pneumothorax, nosocomial pneumonias, and sinusitis. Prophylactic measures (e.g., the use of sequential leg compression devices, stress ulcer prophylaxis, and careful attention to intravenous and arterial access catheters) may be beneficial in avoiding some of these complications.

HYPOXIA

By definition, patients with ALI/ARDS have severe hypoxia, for which a combination of high oxygen supplement and PEEP is the mainstay of treatment. Usually, the magnitude of respiratory failure mandates that the patient be intubated and, initially, 100% FIO_2 is used to ensure adequate oxygen saturation. Once satisfactory oxygen saturation is achieved, the FIO_2 should be decreased and titrated to maintain oxygen saturation >90%. An FIO_2 >50% appears to put the patient at risk from O_2 toxicity and absorption atelectasis; therefore, other measures to enhance oxygen saturation should be employed, if necessary (23,24). Usually, additional therapies include PEEP, often at levels >20 cm H_2O, to achieve adequate oxygenation with decreased FIO_2. Unfortunately, PEEP at high levels increases the probability of complications, including barotrauma, decreased cardiac output, and overdistension of normal alveoli. The treatment goal is the use of the least PEEP necessary to keep the oxygen saturation >90% at safe levels of FIO_2. Pulse oximetry can assist with rapid lowering of FIO_2 and reduce the need for serial arterial blood gases. For the critically ill patient, establishing a correlation between the saturation determined by the pulse oximeter and the saturation independently measured by the co-oximeter in an arterial blood gas study is necessary. As pulse oximetry has an error of approximately ~2%, a saturation measured at <92% may represent a dangerously low PaO_2 and requires further evaluation.

Other measures to improve oxygenation include diuresis and decreasing oxygen consumption. With diuresis, hypotension and reduced organ perfusion need to be avoided. Reducing oxygen consumption may require the use of antipyretic agents for those patients who are febrile and paralytic agents (along with sedatives) to eliminate respiratory muscle use. Oxygen delivery can be enhanced by transfusion of packed red blood cells. The benefits of transfusion to increase oxygen-carrying capacity must be balanced against the risks.

MECHANICAL VENTILATION

Almost all patients with ALI/ARDS will be managed with mechanical ventilation. Support strategies have undergone significant change over the past 5 years, and new ventilator strategies may be a factor in the improved mortality now being seen in this condition. In ALI, all alveoli are not affected to the same extent. Some alveoli collapse from debris or from loss of surfactant with subsequent microatelectasis. As the disease is heterogeneous, areas of normal lung, with normal lung compliance, are present. With tidal volumes of 10–15 cc/kg, these normal alveoli become over-distended.

Over-inflated alveoli in animal studies have been shown to develop pathological abnormalities similar to ALI/ARDS (25,26). In addition, excessive lung stretch has been associated with release of the inflammatory cytokines (27). This finding suggests that overdistension or stretch of normal lung units may worsen lung injury and should be avoided. Using lower tidal volumes (5–7 cc/kg) or decreasing PEEP can decrease the lung stretch. A recent study has shown a decrease in mortality rate with the use of decreased tidal volumes in these patients (28). With this strategy, a decrease in tidal volume may result in an increased PCO_2 and respiratory acidosis. In response to this potential result of low tidal volume therapy, permissive hypercapnia has been recommended in patients who require low tidal volumes to keep pulmonary plateau pressures <30 cm H_2O (28). Adverse effects of permissive hypercapnia include severe acidemia with subsequent circulatory failure, increased intracranial pressure, and muscle weakness. Some authors have advocated the use of sodium bicarbonate infusion to treat the acidemia. In addition, these patients may become agitated and frequently require sedatives.

ALTERNATIVE VENTILATOR STRATEGIES

Open-lung ventilation uses pressure-control mode. This mode of ventilation is based on the hypothesis that the lung can be protected by limiting distending volume and pressure by maintaining a level of PEEP that prevents the cyclical stretch of the majority of alveoli. This approach incorporates a smaller tidal volume (<6 cc/kg) and higher level of PEEP. The pressure limited ventilation strategy uses distending pressures of ≤ 20 cm H_2O, peak airway pressures of ≤ 40 cm H_2O, and sodium bicarbonate infusion to manage acidosis. In one report, the incidence of barotrauma and the time for weaning were reduced. Using this form of mechanical ventilation, a recent trial demonstrated a 28% mortality rate, significantly lower than that reported in other studies (4).

Prolonging the inspiratory time is an another strategy frequently employed to improve gas exchange in patients with severe ALI. Prolongation of inspiratory time is used to recruit more alveoli for gas exchange by providing the diseased lung units with time to open. In this mode of ventilatory support, the peak flow rate may be decreased, the decelerating waveform may be used, or end inspiratory pause may be employed. With inverse ratio ventilation, inspiratory time exceeds the exhalation time. Mean airway pressures are usually increased. Inverse-ratio ventilation is thought to induce intrinsic PEEP. Unpublished data demonstrate a shift in the V/Q distribution towards deadspace ventilation that is far in excess of that seen with comparable levels of PEEP (29). Unfortunately, this method of ventilation is poorly tolerated without heavy sedation and neuromuscular paralysis.

Tracheal gas insufflation (TGI) provides gas flow near the carina. This mode of ventilation is thought to enhance elimination of carbon dioxide by washing carbon dioxide out of large airways during exhalation. TGI has been used in conjunction with lung protective ventilation to limit hypercapnia. Adverse effects include increased airway pressure, barotrauma, and airway mucosal dryness. High-frequency ventilation (HFV) allows the use of small tidal volumes (1–5 mL/kg) at rates of 60–360 breaths per minute. It allows the use of higher end expiratory alveolar pressures and volumes to achieve high levels of lung recruitment. The roles of HFV in ARDS require further study.

Prone positioning as a method to increase oxygenation was first described in the early 1970s. It is postulated to improve V/Q mismatch, to decrease shunt flow, and to improve uniformity of ventilation by favorably altering the transpleural pressure gradient (30,31). The frequency with which patients in prone position need to return to supine position is unknown. Prone positioning is controversial at this time; complications such as facial compression and displacement of tubes and catheters limit its use. No studies establishing definite benefit of prone positioning on survival are available.

Extracorporeal support with veno-arterial extracorporeal membrane oxygenation (ECMO) or veno-venous low frequency positive pressure ventilation with extracorporeal carbon dioxide removal (LFPPV–ECCOR) may be used as an adjunct to manage severe ARDS. The risk of ventilator associated lung damage, risk of acidosis, and refractory hypoxemia theoretically support these modes of respiratory support. Perhaps to a greater degree than other modes of ventilatory support, these strategies allow the lungs to rest while the underlying lung injury reverses. Prospective randomized trials question survival benefit. Resources necessary for ECMO or LFPPV–ECCOR are extensive and not universally available (32,33). Extracorporeal support, at this time, is limited to specialized centers. Liquid ventilation using perfluorocarbons has been shown to improve lung compliance, shunt fraction, and gas exchange (34). Liquid ventilation may be more widely used in the future.

PHARMACOLOGIC THERAPIES

Several pharmacologic therapies are postulated to have beneficial effects in patients with ALI/ARDS. These treatments include surfactant, nitric oxide, antioxidants, prostaglandins, ketoconazole, and activated protein C. Steroids probably have been most extensively studied and may be indicated in the later stages of ALI/ARDS (35–37). Table 3 lists these agents, their mechanisms of action, and their methods of administration. Further study is necessary before recommending these therapies as standard care.

Table 3 Pharmacologic Therapies in ARDS/ALI

Drug	Mechanism of action	Method of administration
Surfactant therapy	Produced by type II alveolar cells; decreases surface tension at the air–fluid interface of the alveoli	Aerosolized
Nitric oxide	Selective pulmonary vasodilator	Inhalation
Steroids	Antifibrotic effect	Oral/IV/inhalation
Prostaglandins (PGE1)	Improvement in oxygenation and vasodilatation	IV liposomal
Ketoconazole	Antifungal; inhibits thromboxane, leukotriene, and tissue-factor	IV/oral
Lisofylline	Aminophylline derivative; adenosine receptor antagonist	IV
Activated protein C (drotrecogin alfa activated)	Endogenous protein; antithrombotic, anti-inflammatory, and profibrinolytic	IV
N-acetylcysteine	Antioxidant	Oral

SUMMARY

- ALI/ARDS is a severe respiratory failure with dyspnea, refractory hypoxemia, decreased lung compliance, and diffuse CXR changes in the absence of cardiac failure or chronic lung disease. ARDS is a more severe subset of ALI.
- Sepsis, gastric aspiration, and trauma are the most common causes of ALI/ARDS.
- Mediators of ALI include endotoxins, eicosanoid metabolites, and cytokines.
- ALI proceeds through an acute (exudative), subacute (proliferative), and chronic (fibrotic) phase. This process produces loss of alveoli, thickened membranes, and decreased compliance.
- Clinical presentation of ALI is stereotypic. After a latent interval, shunt fraction increases and hypoxemia usually requires aggressive support. CXR usually reveals a "ground-glass" appearance.
- Overall mortality remains high. Death usually results from organ-failure syndrome.
- Treatment of ALI and ARDS usually requires mechanical ventilation with PEEP, volume resuscitation to maintain oxygen transport and hemodynamic stability, inotropic support, and metabolic support.
- Newer strategies to support pulmonary gas exchange may improve mortality.

REFERENCES

1. Ashbaugh DG, Bigelow DB, Petty TL, Levine BE. Acute respiratory distress in adults. Lancet 1967; 2:319–323.
2. Bernard GR, Artigas A, Brigham KL, Carlet J, Falke K, Hudson L, Lamy M, Legall JR, Morris A, Spragg R. The American–European consensus conference on ARDS: definitions, mechanisms, relevant outcomes, and clinical trial coordination. Am J Respir Crit Care Med 1994; 149:818–824.
3. Zimmerman GA, Morris AH, Cengiz M. Cardiovascular alterations in acute respiratory distress syndrome. Am J Med 1982; 73:25–34.
4. Amato MB, Barbas CS, Mediros DM, Magaldi RB, Schettino GP, Lorenzi-Filho G, Kairalla RA, Deheinzelin D, Munoz C, Oliveria R, Takagaki TY, Carvalho CR. Effect of protective-ventilation strategy on mortality in the acute respiratory distress syndrome. N Engl J Med 1998; 338:347–354.
5. Ranieri VM, Suter PM, Tortorella C, De Tullio R, Dayer JM, Brienza A, Bruno F, Slutsky AS. Effect of mechanical ventilation on inflammatory mediators in patients with acute respiratory distress syndrome: a randomized controlled trial. JAMA 1999; 282(1):54–61.
6. National Heart and Lung Institute: Task Force on Problems, Research Approaches: The Lung Program. Washington DC: Department of Health, Education, and Welfare, 1972; 165–180 (Publication No. (N III) 73–432).
7. Thomsen GE, Morris AH. Incidence of adult respiratory distress syndrome in the state of Utah. Am J Respir Crit Care Med 1995; 152:965–971.
8. Valta P, Uusaro A, Nunes S, Ruononen E, Takala J. Acute respiratory distress syndrome: frequency, clinical course, and cost of care. Crit Care Med 1999; 27:2367–2374.
9. Luhr OR, Antonsen K, Karlsson M, Aardal S, Thorsteinsson A, Frostell CG, Bonde J. Incidence and mortality after acute respiratory failure and acute respiratory distress syndrome in Sweden, Denmark, and Iceland. Am J Respir Crit Care Med 1999; 159:1849–1861.

10. Hudson LD, Milberg JA, Anardi D, Maunder RJ. Clinical risks for development of the acute respiratory distress syndrome. Am J Respir Crit Care Med 1955; 151(2 Pt 1):293–301.
11. Pepe PE, Potkin RT, Reus DH, Hudson LD, Carrico CJ. Clinical predictors of the adult respiratory distress syndrome. Am J Surg 1982; 144(1):124–130.
12. Steinberg KP, Hudson LD. Acute lung injury and acute respiratory distress syndrome. The clinical syndrome. Clin Chest Med 2000; 21(3):401–417, vii (Review).
13. Hack CE, DeGroot ER, Felt-Bersma RJ, Nuijens JH, Strack Van Schijndel RJ, Eerenberg-Belmer AJ, Thijs LG, Aarden LA. Increased plasma levels of IL-6 in sepsis. Blood 1989; 74:1704–1710.
14. Goldie AS, Fearon KC, Ross JA, Barclay GR, Jackson RE, Grant IS, Ramsay G, Blyth AS, Howie JC. Natural cytokine antagonists and endogenous antiendotoxin core antibodies in sepsis syndrome. JAMA 1995; 274:172–177.
15. Pinsky MR, Vincent JL, Daviere J, Alegre M, Kahn RJ, Dupont E. Serum cytokine in human septic shock: relation to multiple system organ failure and mortality. Chest 1993; 103:565–575.
16. Tomashhefski JF Jr. Pulmonary pathology of adult respiratory distress syndrome. Clin Chest Med 1990; 11:593–619.
17. Hansen-Flaschen J, Fishman AP. Adult respiratory distress syndrome: clinical features and pathogenesis. In: Fishman AP, ed. Pulmonary Diseases and Disorders. Vol. 3. 2d ed. New York: McGraw-Hill, 1988:2201–2213.
18. McHugh LG, Milberg JA, Whitcomb ME, Schoene RB, Maunder RJ, Hudson LD. Recovery of function in survivors of the acute respiratory distress syndrome. Am J Respir Crit Care Med 1994; 150(1):90–94.
19. Elliott CG. Pulmonary sequelae in survivors of the adult respiratory distress syndrome. Clin Chest Med 1990; 11(4):789–800.
20. Elliott CG, Morris AH, Cengiz M. Pulmonary function and exercise gas exchange in survivors of adult respiratory distress syndrome. Am Rev Respir Dis 1981; 123(5):492–495.
21. Davidson TA, Caldwell ES, Curtis JR, Hudson LD, Steinberg KP. Reduced quality of life in survivors of acute respiratory distress syndrome compared with critically ill control patients. JAMA 1999; 281(4):354–360.
22. Montgomery AB, Stager MA, Carrico CJ, Hudson LD. Causes of mortality in patient with the adult respiratory distress syndrome. Am Rev Respir Dis 1985; 132:485–489.
23. Sackner MA, Landa J, Hirsh J, Zapata A. Pulmonary effects of oxygen breathing. Ann Intern Med 1975; 82:40–43.
24. Singer MM, Wright F, Stanley LK, Roe BB, Hamilton WK. Oxygen toxicity in man: a prospective study in patients after open-heart surgery. N Engl J Med 1970; 283:1473–1477.
25. Tsuno K, Prato P, Kolobow T. Acute lung injury from mechanical ventilation at moderately high airway pressures. J Appl Physiol 1990; 69:956–961.
26. Tsuno K, Miura K, Takeya M, Kolobow T, Morioka T. Histopathological pulmonary changes from mechanical ventilation at high peak airway pressures. Am Rev Respir Dis 1991; 143:1115–1120.
27. Chiumello D, Pristine G, Slutsky AS. Mechanical ventilation affects local and systemic cytokines in an animal model of acute respiratory distress syndrome. Am J Respir Crit Care Med 1999; 160(1):109–116.
28. Brower RG, Matthay MA, Morris A, Schoenfeld D, Thompson BT, Wheeler A. The Acute Respiratory Distress Syndrome Network. Ventilation with lower tidal volume as compared with traditional tidal volumes for acute lung injury and the acute respiratory distress syndrome. N Engl J Med 2000; 342:1301–1308.
29. Lim JP-K, Abrams JH. Ventilator pressure waveform affects V/Q distribution for comparable mean airway pressures. Presented at the Society of Critical Care Medicine's Educational and Scientific Symposium, January 31, 1994.

30. Mure M, Domino KB, Lindhal SG, Hlastala MP, Alterneier WA, Glenny RW. Regional ventilation–perfusion distribution is more uniform in the prone position. J Appl Physiol 2000; 88:1076–1083.
31. Amis TC, Jones HA, Hughes JM. Effect of posture on inter-regional distribution of pulmonary ventilation in man. Respir Physiol 1984; 56:145–167.
32. National Heart, Lung and Blood Institute. Extracorporeal support for respiratory insufficiency: a collaborative study in response to RFP-NHLI-73–20. Bethesda U.S. Department of Health, Education, and Welfare: National Institute of Health, 1979:247–264.
33. Zapol WM, Snider MT, Hill JD, Fallat RJ, Bartlett RH, Edmunds LH, Morris AH, Peirce EC II, Thomas AN, Proctor HJ, Drinker PA, Pratt PC, Bagniewski A, Miller RG Jr. Extracorporeal membrane oxygenation in severe acute respiratory failure. JAMA 1979; 242:2193–2196.
34. Mrozek JD, Smith KM, Bing DR, Meyers PA, Simonton SC, Connett JE, Mammel MC. Exogenous surfactant and partial liquid ventilation: physiologic and pathologic effects. Am J Respir Crit Care Med 1997; 156:1058–1065.
35. Meduri GU, Belenchia JM, Estes RJ, Wunderink RG, EL Torky M, Leeper KV Jr. Fibroproliferative phase of ARDS: clinical findings and effects of corticosteroids. Chest 1991; 100:943–952.
36. Meduri GU, Chinn AJ, Leeper KV, Wunderink RG, Tolley E, Winer-Muram HT, Khare V, EI Torky M. Corticosteroid rescue treatment of progressive fibroproliferation in late ARDS: patterns of response and predictors of outcome. Chest 1994; 105:1516–1527.
37. Meduri GU, Headley AS, Golden E, Carson SJ, Umberger RA, Kelso T, Tolley EA. Effect of prolonged methylprednisolone therapy in unresolving acute respiratory distress syndrome: a randomized controlled trial. JAMA 1998; 280:159–165.

28
Bronchospasm

Stephen Trzeciak and R. Phillip Dellinger
Cooper University Hospital, Camden, New Jersey, USA

The surgeon may be required to participate in the critical care management of the patient with bronchospasm during postoperative bronchospasm exacerbations and following trauma. Bronchospasm is defined as *reversible* obstructive airway disease. The hallmark of obstructive airway disease is airflow limitation with an impediment to expiration. Asthma is the prototype of bronchospasm, and this chapter is mainly devoted to the management of status asthmaticus. However, chronic obstructive pulmonary disease (COPD) patients also may have some component of reversible obstruction. The pharmacologic therapy of bronchospasm is similar for asthma and COPD. Although reversibility is anticipated in asthma, the degree of reversibility in COPD may vary from significant response to bronchodilator therapy to no response at all. Independent of the etiology (asthma or COPD), bronchospasm predisposes a patient to postoperative or post-traumatic pulmonary complications through an increased risk of atelectasis and the direct physiologic consequences of bronchospasm itself.

PATHOPHYSIOLOGY

Bronchospasm is the result of small airway smooth muscle contraction that produces airflow obstruction. The majority of patients with bronchospasm have significant chronic inflammation that initiates and perpetuates bronchospasm. This inflammation is characterized by infiltration of the bronchial wall with inflammatory cells, bronchial mucosal edema, mucous production, and smooth muscle hyperplasia. Treatment must be directed at both the bronchospasm (bronchodilator therapy) and the inflammation (anti-inflammatory therapy). Although bronchodilator therapy may be lifesaving, its benefits may be short lived. Anti-inflammatory therapy is essential to reverse the underlying inflammation.

Severe bronchospasm can produce mixed hypoxemic and hypercapnic respiratory failure, although the latter almost always predominates. Hypoxemia in severe bronchospasm is a result of decreased ventilation relative to perfusion (low V/Q areas). The reasons for ventilatory failure in severe bronchospasm are many. Acute airway edema and bronchospasm increase resistance to both inspiration and expiration. Expiratory obstruction increases the time necessary for complete emptying of the breath. When bronchospasm becomes severe, "air trapping" may occur as the need for increased expiratory time becomes greater and greater. When air trapping is evident, inspiration occurs before total emptying of the previous breath. Air trapping is associated with higher end-expiratory lung volumes (higher functional residual capacity). Worsened compliance is a consequence of the increase in functional residual capacity. An increase in the inspiratory work of breathing results from the worsened compliance. The diaphragm, which normally has optimal contractile force in its dome-shaped resting position, assumes a flattened position as hyperinflation worsens. Compromise of diaphragmatic function results. The combination of inspiratory resistance, air trapping, and diaphragm dysfunction increases the work of breathing and may result in ventilatory failure and progression to respiratory arrest.

CLINICAL FINDINGS AND PHYSICAL EXAMINATION

All wheezing is not bronchospasm. The differential diagnosis of wheezing and clues to diagnosis are shown in Box 1. The patient with severe bronchospasm is usually profoundly tachypneic and tachycardiac and may have difficulty in talking. Expiratory wheezing correlates with the degree of obstruction. Inspiratory wheezing also may be heard. The absence of wheezing in the severely bronchospastic patient is an ominous sign that indicates expiratory flow is too low for wheezing to be heard.

Accessory muscle use (such as sternocleidomastoid muscles) in acute bronchospasm indicates severe airway obstruction ($FEV_1 < 1.0$) (1). Another potential physical finding in severe airway obstruction is pulsus paradoxus, a decrease in systolic blood pressure of 15 mm Hg or more with inspiration. When increased inspiratory effort causes dramatic swings in intrathoracic pressure, pulsus paradoxus is a result of decreased cardiac output during inspiration. Paradoxical breathing is a physical finding seen in respiratory

Box 1 Differential Diagnosis of Wheezing and Clues to Diagnosis

---
Asthma
Chronic obstructive pulmonary disease (COPD)
Congestive heart failure
   Ischemic heart disease or pre-existing cardiomyopathy of any etiology
   Increased jugular venous pressure, presence of S_3, or rales on physical
     examination
   CXR findings of pulmonary edema or suggestive of heart failure
Upper airway obstruction (i.e., subglottic stenosis, vocal cord paralysis, etc.)
   Wheezing greatest over trachea, inspiratory stridor
   Relief of all airflow limitation after endotracheal intubation
Anaphylaxis
   Inciting event (i.e., insect sting, drug ingestion, etc.)
   +/− urticarial rash
Endobronchial obstruction
   Risk factors for lung cancer or foreign body aspiration
   Localized wheezing
Pulmonary embolus (*rarely* presents with severe bronchospasm)
   Risk factors for pulmonary embolism, pleuritic chest pain
Toxic fume exposure

failure. Normally, the diaphragm moves downward as it contracts, and the abdomen moves outward with inspiration. With diaphragmatic failure, the diaphragm moves upward, stabilizes the ribcage, and assists the intercostal muscles' inspiratory effort. As the diaphragm moves upward, the abdomen is observed moving inward with inspiration (2). Paradoxical breathing is an indicator of ventilatory failure and possible impending respiratory arrest (3). Prompt intubation should be considered.

Physicians are notoriously inaccurate in judging the severity of bronchospasm on physical examination and subjective patient assessment (4). Although routine spirometry (performed by first obtaining a full inspiration, followed by a maximal forced expiration) is the gold standard of measuring obstruction (forced expiratory volume in 1 s [FEV_1]), it is impractical in the patient in distress. A more practical test is peak expiratory flow rate (PEFR). This measurement can be done with a portable handheld spirometer. PEFR is reliable and requires less patient cooperation than full spirometry, because peak PEFRs occur early in the forced expiratory maneuver. Interpretation of PEFR assumes that the patient performed the test correctly with full and cooperative effort. PEFR is higher in younger adults, males, and taller individuals. A PEFR <125 L/min indicates severe and potentially life-threatening airflow obstruction.

Laboratory Data

Routine laboratory tests are of minimal value for the management of acute bronchospasm. White blood cell count may be mildly elevated as a consequence of stress or of the adrenergic agents used for treatment. Patients receiving albuterol therapy may have hypokalemia.

At the onset of bronchospasm, arterial blood gas analyses (ABGs) may be impressively abnormal, but the patient may still respond quickly and dramatically to vigorous bronchodilator therapy. Because most patients with asthma will respond to bronchodilator therapy, ABGs obtained at the onset of symptoms poorly predict outcome. The decision to intubate early in the course of bronchospasm is usually made on clinical evidence of impending respiratory failure rather than ABG data. Therefore, ABG values may contribute to decisions concerning intubation, but only after the patient has received significant bronchodilator therapy. A normal $PaCO_2$ in an asthmatic with respiratory distress is an ominous sign, because a tachypneic patient with preserved ventilatory capacity would be expected to have a low $PaCO_2$. In the case of a patient with severe bronchospasm refractory to beta-adrenergic therapy, a normal $PaCO_2$ may indicate respiratory fatigue, the onset of ventilatory failure, and an increased risk of respiratory arrest. The presence of lactic acidosis is also a significant concern for impending respiratory arrest. ABGs are important for ongoing management of severe bronchospasm in the intubated patient.

TRADITIONAL MEDICAL THERAPY

Bronchodilator Therapy

All initial bronchodilator regimens should be built around inhaled beta-2 selective agonists. Onset of effect is immediate, and the ratio of therapeutic efficacy to toxicity is optimal (5). Nebulized albuterol is recommended. Routes and dosages for adrenergic therapies are listed in Table 1. The frequency of inhaled therapy depends on the severity of the bronchospasm and risk for cardiac side effects. For severe asthma, initial therapy,

Table 1 Adrenergic Agonists for Acute Severe Bronchospasm

Agent	Route of administration	Duration (h)	Dosage
Albuterol	Aerosol, 0.5% solution	4–6	Adults: 2.5–5.0 mg (0.5–1.0 mL) in 5 mL of normal saline solution
Terbutaline	Parenteral, 0.1% solution (SC)	4–6	0.01 mL/kg; typical adult dose 0.25 mL
Epinephrine	Parenteral, 1:1000 dilution (SC)	1–2	0.01 mL/kg; maximum of 0.3–0.5 mL

recommended by the National Institute of Health [NIH] expert panel (6), is 2.5–5.0 mg of nebulized albuterol (0.5–1.0 mL of 0.5% solution in 5 mL of normal saline) every 20 min for three doses. In the young, previously healthy bronchospastic patient with life-threatening asthma, continuous nebulized albuterol therapy may have greater efficiency and has been shown to have a similar safety profile when compared with intermittent therapy (7–9). Because of the tachycardia that can be induced with beta-agonists, the frequency of bronchodilator therapy may have to be limited in patients with known or suspected ischemic heart disease. However, in young, otherwise healthy asthmatic patients with life-threatening bronchospasm, tachycardia is not an appropriate indicator for limiting therapy of inhaled beta-agonists. For these patients, chest pain or premature ventricular contractions believed related to adrenergic therapy are reasons to decrease the frequency of beta-agonist therapy.

Inhaled beta-2 selective agonists can be delivered successfully via metered dose inhaler (MDI) and spacer, rather than nebulizer. MDIs and nebulizers have been shown to be equally efficacious for acute severe bronchospasm (10,11). The requirement for less patient coordination and cooperation is the main reason to use nebulized bronchodilators instead of MDIs in the most severe cases of bronchospasm. The patient is essentially "taken out of the loop," and maximal delivery is ensured. In general, nebulization is preferred for severe bronchospasm and is readily adaptable for use with mechanical ventilation. The handheld nebulizer is preferred but requires lip-sealing around the mouthpiece. If a lip-seal cannot be maintained by the patient, delivery of nebulized therapy by a face mask is necessary. When bronchodilator therapy is administered in the intubated patient, the dose of aerosol medication should be doubled. Particle impact on the endotracheal tube may reduce effective medication delivery by 50% or more.

Patients with severe bronchospasm who are in need of endotracheal intubation and mechanical ventilation or are at imminent risk of respiratory arrest may benefit from subcutaneous beta-agonists in addition to aerosolized beta-2 selective agents (12). The cardiac side effects of subcutaneous epinephrine and subcutaneous terbutaline are equivalent (13), and neither agent has been proven to be more efficacious than the other. Terbutaline is the preferred agent in the pregnant patient; epinephrine would be contraindicated. The typical adult doses of epinephrine and terbutaline are provided in Table 1. Subcutaneous epinephrine may be repeated in the initial management of life-threatening bronchospasm as many as three times (every 15 min).

Subcutaneous epinephrine or terbutaline therapy confers more risk of toxicity than inhaled beta-2 selective agonists. Subcutaneous beta-adrenergic therapy should always be administered with caution and is contraindicated in patients with known or suspected ischemic heart disease. Beta-1 activity (tachycardia and increased myocardial oxygen demand) may precipitate an acute coronary event. The use of subcutaneous epinephrine or terbutaline for patients with asthma is indicated as follows:

- In patients who have not responded significantly to inhaled bronchodilator therapy
- In combination with inhaled therapy for patients in extreme respiratory distress and clinical findings of impending respiratory failure

Inhaled anticholinergic therapy is not as effective as inhaled beta-agonists for acute bronchospasm. It has an adjunctive therapeutic role. Although ipratropium has less peak bronchodilating effect and a less predictable clinical response when compared with beta-agonists, it likely provides additive effect to albuterol. Most studies in patients for both asthma and COPD demonstrate a benefit from adding ipratropium to beta-agonists in combination therapy for acute bronchospasm (14,15). The onset of action of anticholinergic therapy begins ~30 min after administration and peaks in ~2–3 h. The effect lasts 4–6 h. The recommended dose of ipratropium is 0.5 mg (nebulized) every 30 min for three doses and then every 2–4 h as needed (6).

Anti-inflammatory Therapy

Corticosteroids are a cornerstone of therapy for all patients with severe or persistent bronchospasm (16,17) and are indicated for acute exacerbations of COPD (18) and asthma. The major anti-inflammatory benefit from corticosteroids is probably delayed for ~6 h, although a partial response is achieved earlier in the course of therapy. Intravenous methylprednisolone, 120–180 mg/day divided q4–6 h, is recommended for the first 48 h of acute asthma exacerbation requiring hospitalization and for the onset of severe bronchospasm in a hospitalized patient (6). As the patient improves, the IV dose is tapered and replaced with an oral regimen.

OTHER MEDICAL THERAPIES

The use of methylxanthines (theophylline or intravenous aminophylline) for acute bronchospasm is controversial (19,20). Although methyxanthines are proven bronchodilators in comparison with placebo, additional clinical efficacy is questionable when added to a full therapeutic regimen of inhaled beta-2 selective agonists. Some prospective studies demonstrate a benefit with the addition of aminophylline to a beta-agonist regimen, although most studies do not confirm this finding. Meta-analysis has failed to demonstrate a statistically significant treatment effect, but reveals significant toxicity (21,22). Currently, the addition of theophylline or aminophylline to a full therapeutic regimen of conventional therapy for acute bronchospasm cannot be recommended. We prescribe theophylline as part of a regimen for acute bronchospasm only for the patient who takes theophylline chronically as an outpatient.

Intravenous magnesium, a long-known smooth muscle relaxer, has the potential to reverse bronchoconstriction through inhibition of the calcium channel and decreased acetylcholine release. Although study results are mixed, one recent, well-developed study supported benefit in patients with severe bronchospasm (23,24). Because of variability in trial results and the benign side effect profile, we sometimes add magnesium sulfate (2 g intravenously) to our therapeutic regimen for patients with refractory bronchospasm in dire circumstances.

An asthmatic patient who fails to improve with conventional therapy may be a candidate for heliox. Heliox is a blended mixture of helium and oxygen usually administered in mixtures of 60:40 or 70:30. Because helium is less dense than air, heliox decreases turbulent flow in the large airways and simultaneously decreases airway resistance. Heliox has been shown to decrease pulsus paradoxus and to increase peak expiratory flow (25). It may reduce the risk of respiratory muscle fatigue in the interval between initiating conventional therapy and achieving maximal bronchodilatory and anti-inflammatory effects. No large controlled studies have demonstrated an outcome benefit. Heliox administered as a 60:40 or 70:30 mixture corresponds to an FIO_2 of 40% or 30%, respectively. The inability to deliver high flow oxygen with heliox therapy may limit its use in a patient with significant hypoxemia. In the mechanically ventilated patient it is likely to reduce auto-PEEP.

IV fluid administration for the purpose of liquefying or loosening secretions has no role; however, repletion of decreased intravascular volume is clearly indicated. Antibiotics are not indicated for acute bronchospasm, unless pneumonia is present.

Considerations in the Intubated and Mechanically Ventilated Patient

The basis for the decision to intubate patients with status asthmaticus is most frequently clinical deterioration (26). Common indications for endotracheal intubation are listed in Box 2. Because the use of mechanical ventilation for severe bronchospasm has the potential for serious adverse consequences, mechanical ventilation should be performed with great caution. The pitfalls of ventilatory management of severe bronchospasm are usually related to air trapping and intrinsic positive end-expiratory pressure (intrinsic PEEP or auto-PEEP).

Intrinsic PEEP is present when the end-expiratory lung volume represents a volume at which air would continue to escape, if expiration were allowed to continue. Expiratory time is inadequate to allow full exhalation of a ventilator breath, and expiratory flow is still occurring when the next ventilator breath is delivered (Fig. 1). As the flow at end-expiration is not zero, a pressure gradient at end-expiration relative to atmospheric pressure (zero set PEEP) or extrinsic PEEP (ventilator set PEEP) persists (27). Therefore, PEEP exists, although it is not set on the ventilator, or is in excess of the PEEP that is set on the ventilator. As obstructive airway disease increases the need for expiratory time, mechanically ventilated patients with obstructive airway disease are at increased risk for intrinsic PEEP.

Box 2 Indications for Intubation of the Bronchospastic Patient

Apnea or near-apnea
Altered mental status (presumably related to either hypercapnia, hypoxemia, or both)
Central cyanosis
Severe respiratory distress not responding to aggressive bronchodilator therapy
Rising partial pressure of arterial carbon dioxide ($PaCO_2$) and pH falling to less than 7.25 despite aggressive bronchodilator therapy

Bronchospasm

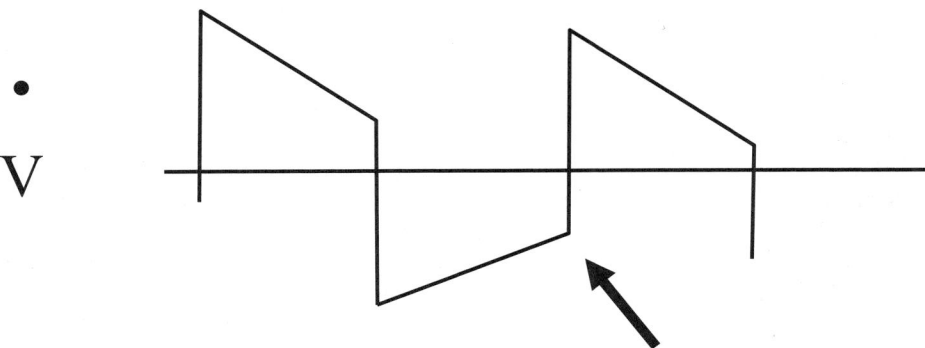

Figure 1 Intrinsic PEEP as demonstrated on a flow over time waveform.

The sequelae of intrinsic PEEP include barotrauma (discussed later in this section), impairment of gas exchange (inducing or severely worsening a respiratory acidosis), and hemodynamic compromise. Intrinsic PEEP may cause a hemodynamically significant elevation of intrathoracic pressure by decreasing venous return to the right side of the heart. This effect decreases left heart filling pressure and ultimately may reduce cardiac output. A patient with low intravascular volume is especially sensitive to the hemodynamic effects of intrinsic PEEP. Intrinsic PEEP must be suspected whenever an intubated patient with severe bronchospasm becomes hypotensive. The presence or absence of intrinsic PEEP may be confirmed at the bedside by checking graphic flow waveforms (Fig. 1) on the ventilator.

The best immediate intervention for the hemodynamic effects of intrinsic PEEP is disconnecting the patient from the ventilator for several seconds and allowing the patient to exhale completely. If hypotension immediately resolves, this maneuver is both diagnostic and therapeutic. Mechanical ventilation should then be reinstituted with a ventilator strategy to limit intrinsic PEEP by decreasing inspiratory time relative to expiratory time. This strategy is best accomplished by decreasing the respiratory rate to allow the patient more time to exhale between breaths. Decreasing the tidal volume will also reduce intrinsic PEEP, although to a lesser degree. With volume cycled ventilation, the inspiratory time is dependent on the peak inspiratory flow rate, an adjustable variable that determines how rapidly the breath will be delivered. The choice of inspiratory flow waveform also influences inspiratory to expiratory (I : E) ratio. When providing volume cycled ventilation in the presence of bronchospasm-induced intrinsic PEEP, the peak inspiratory flow rate should be set at 80–100 L/min with a square waveform to limit the inspiratory time and allow more time in the respiratory cycle for expiration. Note that the I : E ratio should not be the primary goal in managing intrinsic PEEP. Rather, the chief determinant of instrinsic PEEP is the *absolute* time of expiration for each breath. Decreasing the respiratory rate is the critical intervention. Patients with acute bronchospasm are at risk for barotrauma caused by air trapping, especially when mechanical ventilation is initiated. The risk of barotrauma correlates with peak alveolar pressure. Peak alveolar pressure is best estimated by inspiratory plateau pressure (IPP), rather than the peak airway pressure. An IPP greater than 35 mm Hg correlates with alveolar overdistension and an increased risk for barotrauma. Accurately measuring the IPP may require deep sedation and/or brief neuromuscular blockade. In order to decrease the IPP, the tidal volumes should be reduced, and intrinsic PEEP should be minimized as much as possible.

If hypotension occurs shortly after initiating mechanical ventilation, the possibility of tension pneumothorax should be considered immediately. A chest radiograph should not be required for this diagnosis. Tension pneumothorax is a clinical diagnosis identified by physical examination. It requires immediate evacuation by needle aspiration followed by chest tube insertion.

Using lower respiratory rates and tidal volumes to avoid adverse sequelae during mechanical ventilation of severe bronchospasm may induce a respiratory acidosis. Accepting this higher $PaCO_2$ and lower pH in order to avoid complications of intrinsic PEEP is called *permissive hypercapnia* (28,29). Permissive hypercapnia may be necessary to avoid intrinsic PEEP and barotrauma. This ventilator strategy is typically well tolerated, even at extremely high levels of $PaCO_2$ (30). If necessary, a bicarbonate infusion may be used to keep the pH at an acceptable level (typically $\geq 7.20-7.25$) (31).

Extrinsic PEEP (ventilator-set PEEP) is unnecessary in severe bronchospasm and should not be applied, with one exception. When intrinsic PEEP is present and cannot be eliminated, it may cause increased work of breathing for a patient who is triggering ventilator breaths spontaneously. To trigger the ventilator to deliver a breath in this circumstance, the patient must first generate an inspiratory effort large enough to overcome the level of intrinsic PEEP, before the sensitivity setting is overcome. This high inspiratory effort may be associated with inability to trigger and ventilatory "dysynchrony." Applying extrinsic PEEP at a level just below the intrinsic PEEP allows a patient to trigger the ventilator more easily. This application of PEEP decreases the effort required to initiate a breath, decreases dysynchrony in the awake patient, and may improve patient comfort. However, application of extrinsic PEEP in this situation must be done with great caution.

In the presence of severe intrinsic PEEP, some patients with severe bronchospasm may require the use of neuromuscular blockade to control respiratory rate early in the course of mechanical ventilation. However, neuromuscular blocking agents (NMBAs) should be administered with caution when necessary, and avoided if possible. The concomitant use of glucocorticoids in these patients increases the risk of having prolonged paralysis following discontinuation of NMBAs. Therefore, NMBAs should be discontinued as soon as possible. Propofol may offer an alternative to NMBAs in the hemodynamically stable patient.

SUMMARY

- Bronchospasm is a *reversible* obstructive airway disease and airflow limitation.
- All wheezing is not bronchospasm (see Box 1).
- Asthma is the prototype of bronchospasm; however, COPD patients may also have some component of reversible obstruction.
- Therapy should focus on treatment of bronchospasm (bronchodilator therapy) and inflammation (anti-inflammatory therapy).
- Use inhaled beta-2 selective agonists (i.e., albuterol) as the most essential component of initial therapy. Use subcutaneous epinephrine or terbutaline in combination with inhaled therapy in selected patients who are in extreme distress or those in whom inhalation therapy has failed.

- Use of theophylline or IV aminophilline in acute bronchospasm is controversial and, in general, cannot be recommended.
- Inhaled anticholinergic therapy (i.e., ipratropium) has an adjunctive role.
- Administer steroids to patients with severe or persistent bronchospasm.
- Mechanically ventilated patients with bronchospasm are at risk for barotrauma. First, suspect and rule out tension pneumothorax if hypotension occurs.
- Intrinsic PEEP increases intrathoracic pressure, which may impair venous return to the heart and cause hemodynamic compromise.
- Intrinsic PEEP in mechanically ventilated patients may be identified with flow graphic waveforms (see Fig. 1).
- Manipulate respiratory rate, tidal volume, and I : E ratio to limit intrinsic PEEP in mechanically ventilated patients.

REFERENCES

1. McFadden ER, Kiser R, DeGroot WJ. Acute bronchial asthma: relations between clinical and physiologic manifestations. N Engl J Med 1973; 288:221.
2. Tobin MJ, Perez W, Guenther SM, et al. Does rib cage-abdominal paradox signify respiratory muscle fatigue? J Appl Physiol 1987; 63:851.
3. Yanos J, Keamy MF, Leisk L. The mechanisms of respiratory arrest in inspiratory loading and hypoxemia. Am Rev Respir Dis 1990; 141:933.
4. Shim CS, Williams MH. Evaluation of the severity of asthma: patients versus physicians. Am J Med 1980; 68:11–13.
5. Stiell IG, Rivington RN. Adrenergic agents in acute asthma: valuable new alternatives. Ann Emerg Med 1983; 12:493–500.
6. U.S. Department of Health and Human Services, National Institutes of Health, National Heart, Lung, and Blood Institute. Expert panel report 2: guidelines for the diagnosis and management of asthma. NIH Publ No 97-4053, 1997.
7. Baker EK, Willsie SK, Marinac JS, et al. Continuously nebulized albuterol in severe exacerbations of asthma in adults: a case-controlled study. J Asthma 1997; 34:521.
8. Rudnitsky GS, Eberlein RS, Schoffstall JM, et al. Comparison of intermittent and continuously nebulized albuterol for treatment of asthma in an urban emergency department. Ann Emerg Med 1993; 22:1842.
9. Lin Y, Sauter D, Newman T, et al. Continuous versus intermittent albuterol nebulization in the treatment of acute asthma. Ann Emerg Med 1993; 22:1847.
10. Idris AH, McDermott MF, Raucci JC, et al. Emergency department treatment of severe asthma: metered dose inhaler plus holding chamber is equivalent in effectiveness to nebulizer. Chest 1993; 103:655.
11. Rodrigo C, Rodrigo G. Salbutamol treatment of acute severe asthma in the ED: MDI versus hand-held nebulizer, Am J Emerg Med 1998; 16:637.
12. Appel D, Karpel P, Sherman M. Epinephrine improves expiratory airflow rates in patients with asthma who do not respond to inhaled metaproterenol sulfate. J Allergy Clin Immunol 1989; 84:90.
13. Amory DW, Burnham SC, Cheney FW. Comparison of the cardiopulmonary effects of subcutaneously administered epinephrine and terbutaline in patients with reversible airway obstruction. Chest 1975; 67:279.
14. Karpel JP, Schacter EN, Fanta C, et al. A comparison of ipratropium and albuterol vs albuterol alone for the treatment of acute asthma. Chest 1996; 110:611.

15. Karpel JP. Bronchodilator responses to anticholinergic and beta-adrenergic agents in acute and stable COPD. Chest 1991; 99:871.
16. Haskell RJ, Wong BM, Hansen JE. A double-blind, randomized clinical trial of methylprednisolone in status asthmaticus. Arch Intern Med 1983; 143:1324–1325.
17. Jantz MA, Shan SA. Corticosteroids in acute respiratory failure. Am J Resp Crit Care Med 1999; 160:1079.
18. Niewoehner DE, Erbland ML, Deupree RH, et al. Effect of systemic glucocorticoids on exacerbations of chronic obstructive pulmonary disease. N Engl J Med 1999; 340:1941.
19. Newhouse MT. Is theophylline obsolete? Chest 1990; 98:1–4.
20. Niewoehner DE. Theophylline therapy-A continued dilemma. Chest 1990; 98:5.
21. Littenberg B. Aminophilline in severe acute asthma: a metaanalysis. J Am Med Assoc 1988; 259:1678.
22. Rodrigo C, Rodrigo G. Treatment of acute asthma: lack of a therapeutic benefit and increase of the toxicity from aminophylline given in addition to high doses of salbutamol delivered by metered-dose inhaler. Chest 1994; 106:1071.
23. Green SM, Rothcock SG. Intravenous magnesium for acute asthma: failure to decrease emergency treatment duration or need for hospitalization. Ann Emerg Med 1992; 21:260.
24. Silverman RA, Osborn H, Runge J, et al. Acute Asthma/Magnesium Study Group. IV magnesium sulfate in the treatment of acute severe asthma: a multicenter randomized controlled trial. Chest 2002; 122:489.
25. Manthous CA, Hall JB, Melmed A, et al. Heliox improves pulsus paradoxus and peak expiratory flow in nonintubated patients with severe asthma. Am J Respir Crit Care Med 1995; 151:310.
26. Zimmerman JL, Dellinger RP, Shah AN, et al. Endotracheal intubation and mechanical ventilation in severe asthma. Crit Care Med 1993; 21:1727.
27. Wiener C. Ventilatory management of respiratory failure in asthma. J Am Med Assoc 1993; 269(16):2128–2131.
28. Bidani A, Tzouanakis AE, Cardenas VJ, et al. Permissive hypercapnia in acute respiratory failure. J Am Med Assoc 1994; 272:957.
29. Tuxen DV. Permissive hypercapnia ventilation. Am J Respir Crit Care Med 1994; 150:870.
30. Adnet E, Plaisance P, Borron SW, et al. Prolonged severe hypercapnia complicating near fatal asthma in a 35-year-old woman. Intens Care Med 1998; 24:1335.
31. Menitove SM, Goldring RM. Combined ventilator and bicarbonate strategy in the management of status asthmaticus. Am J Med 1983; 74:898.

29
Venous Thromboembolism

Mark D. Cipolle
Lehigh Valley Hospital, Allentown, Pennsylvania, USA

Historically, the diagnosis and treatment of pulmonary embolism (PE) have presented challenges for clinicians (1). In the surgical intensive care unit (SICU), the diagnosis of PE is often complicated by superimposed lung injury, and treatment decisions are often affected by relative or absolute contraindications to anticoagulation or thrombolytic therapy. At some time, most critically ill patients manifest clinical findings that are consistent with PE, including dyspnea, chest pain, ventilation–perfusion (V/Q) mismatch, or elevated central venous pressure (CVP). A systematic approach to the diagnosis and treatment of PE is necessary to minimize the possibility of a missed diagnosis and to prevent the risk of unnecessary therapy.

INCIDENCE

PE is the third leading cause of death in the United States and the most common secondary diagnosis in patients who die on a medical service. The most common preventable cause of in-hospital mortality, it is the cause of death in 4–7% of emergency hip surgery patients, 0.34–1.7% of elective hip surgery patients, and 0.1–0.8% of general surgery patients (2–4). PE occurs in ~35–50% of patients with documented proximal deep venous thrombosis (DVT) (5,6). In total, 10% of PE victims die within 1 h of the event. Of the remaining 90%, only one-third will be correctly diagnosed: of these patients in whom therapy is instituted, 8% will die. In the larger group with undiagnosed PE, the mortality is ~30% (4). Consequently, correctly establishing the diagnosis of PE decreases mortality by three-to fourfold. Figure 1 outlines the scope of the problem of PE.

RISK FACTORS

Several well-documented risk factors for the development of venous thromboembolism (VTE) are shown in Box 1.

The incidence of DVT can be as high as 30% and 70% in major abdominal surgery and orthopedic surgery, respectively. The incidence of fatal PE is 1–2% in major abdominal surgery and 2–5% in orthopedic procedures. The contribution of a surgical procedure

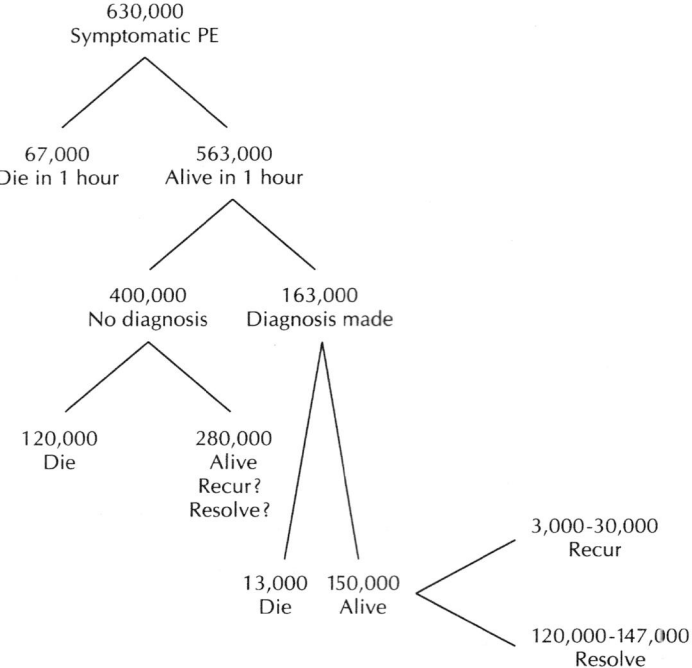

Figure 1 Scope of problem of pulmonary embolism.

to the risk of VTE is not easily separable from the risk associated with the underlying disease, age, and preoperative immobility. Of patients over the age of 40 who undergo major surgery, 15–50% develop DVT (4). Not all detectable DVT carry the same risk of embolism. Venous thrombi located in or above the popliteal vein are associated with a much higher risk of PE when compared with more distal thrombi (7).

PE is reported to occur in 0–22% of trauma patients. Despite prophylaxis, up to 24% of moderately to severely injured trauma patients have CT proven asymptomatic PE (8). The estimated mortality ranges from 8–35% (9,10). Trauma patients with moderate-to

Box 1 Risk Factors for VTE

Heart disease
Advanced age
Shock
Trauma
Obesity
Estrogen therapy, pregnancy
Malignancy
Surgery
Immobility, paralysis
Previous PE or DVT
Indwelling venous catheters
Antithrombin III deficiency
Other hypercoagulable disorders

severe injury have a 58% incidence of DVT without prophylaxis (11). In patients with head and chest trauma, the incidence is 40%; in those with femur fracture, the incidence approaches 80%. In lower extremity fractures, venous thrombi are often found bilaterally. All trauma patients, regardless of the site of injury or the patient's age, have increased risk of PE (4). A cumulative risk may be present when more than one risk factor is identified; therefore, the surgical intensivist must maintain a high index of suspicion for VTE in all patients admitted to the SICU or trauma unit. PE should be included in the differential diagnosis of shock. Subtle manifestations of PE include worsening hypoxemia and respiratory alkalosis in a ventilated patient; dyspnea that is unresponsive to bronchodilators in a patient with chronic obstructive pulmonary disease; unexplained fever, atelectasis, or peripheral infiltrate on chest radiograph; and sudden pulmonary hypertension or elevated CVP. These findings should increase the suspicion of PE. All SICU and trauma patients should have adequate VTE prophylaxis. If PE occurs, the diagnosis and treatment of VTE must be confirmed rapidly.

DIAGNOSIS

Correctly diagnosing PE and instituting appropriate therapy decreases the mortality from $\sim$30% to 8%. Diagnosis of PE can be difficult, because clinical findings and objective tests can lead to an outcome that neither confirms nor excludes PE. This difficulty is emphasized by Goldhaber and Henekens (12). Of 54 patients with massive PE, only 16 were correctly diagnosed before death. Furthermore, patients >70 years of age or patients with pneumonia had the correct antemortem diagnosis made only 10% and 21% of the time, respectively. The consequences of a missed diagnosis may be fatal; whereas, anticoagulation therapy, instituted in a patient who has been falsely diagnosed with PE, presents the potential for significant risk without any benefit. Clinical findings are unreliable, and objective tests, such as V/Q and helical CT scans, are frequently nondiagnostic. Consequently, the critical care physician is often confronted with difficult choices. Should a patient with a 20% probability of having PE, an estimate consistent with a low-probability V/Q scan, receive anticoagulation therapy if 10% of patients die within 1 h of sustaining a PE? Should a patient with risks for anticoagulation and diagnostic testing that is indeterminate, but suggests a risk for PE >20%, be treated with anticoagulation? Should pulmonary angiography, with its attendant discomfort, risk, and expense, be the standard for diagnosis in patients for whom long-term anticoagulation is of significant risk? Ideally, a diagnostic strategy would allow the clinician to make the appropriate choices rationally. Though difficult choices exist for certain patients, a practical plan for diagnosis is useful and incorporates both clinical findings and objective tests (13).

The signs and symptoms of PE are listed in Table 1. The classic clinical triad of PE—dyspnea, pleuritic chest pain, and hemoptysis—occurs in only 20% of patients with major PE (14). In SICU patients, concomitant cardiopulmonary disease or lung injury reduces the sensitivity and specificity of clinical signs and symptoms. Despite these limitations, clinical assessment remains valuable. In both the Prospective Investigation of Pulmonary Embolism Diagnosis (PIOPED) and McMaster studies of the accuracy of V/Q lung scanning, a pretest probability, on the basis of clinical findings, was assigned. Patients were categorized as low, intermediate, or high probability prior to obtaining a V/Q scan. In the PIOPED study, the prevalence of PE was 9% in the low pretest probability group, 30% in the intermediate group, and 68% in the high-probability group (15). In the McMaster study, comparable results of 15% in the low-probability

Table 1 Clinical Manifestations of PE

Sign/symptom	%Seen
Tachypnea	85
Pleuritic chest pain	73
Rales (localized)	60
Increased S_2	60
Apprehension	60
Cough	60
Tachycardia	40
Fever	45
Thrombophlebitis	40
Hemoptysis	34
Supraventricular tachycardia	15
Proximal DVT	70–90 (majority "silent")

group, 38% in the intermediate group, and 79% in the high-probability group were obtained (16). In these studies, no standardized protocol was used to establish clinical risk.

Assigning an accurate pretest probability clearly allows efficient use of other diagnostic tests. Wells et al. (13) developed a clinical model to stratify patients. Their initial model incorporated clinical findings and risk factors. The clinical findings included dyspnea or worsening of chronic dyspnea, pleuritic chest pain, chest pain that is not retrosternal and not pleuritic, an arterial saturation <92% while breathing room air that corrects with oxygen supplementation <40%, hemoptysis, and pleural rub. Risk factors included surgery within the previous 12 weeks, complete bed rest for 3 or more days in the 4 weeks before presentation, previous DVT or objectively diagnosed PE, fracture of a lower extremity and immobilization of the fracture within 12 weeks, strong family history of DVT or PE, cancer, postpartum state, and lower extremity paralysis. Another important feature of the stratification was the possibility of a diagnosis other than PE that was as likely, or more likely, to explain the clinical findings. Patients were then stratified into low, moderate, and high probability of having PE. When the pretest probability was combined with V/Q scanning and bilateral leg vein ultrasonography, PE was reliably diagnosed in 96% of patients. Their model was subsequently simplified. Using stepwise regression analysis, significant variables were identified and their respective weights were used to score patients (see Box 2).

Box 2

Clinical signs and symptoms of DVT (minimum of leg swelling and pain with palpation of the deep veins)	3.0 points
An alternative diagnosis is less likely than PE	3.0 points
Heart rate >100	1.5 points
Immobilization or surgery in the previous 4 weeks	1.5 points
Previous DVT/PE	1.5 points
Hemoptysis	1.0 points
Malignancy (receiving treatment, treated in the last 6 months, or palliative treatment)	1.0 points

Source: From Ref. (17).

Patients with a score of ≤2.0 were considered to have low probability for PE. Patients with scores of 2.0–6.0 were considered to have moderate probability, and patients with scores >6.0 had high probability. The prevalence of PE was 2% in the low-probability group, 19% in the moderate-probability group, and 50% in the high-probability group. These investigators used the pretest probability obtained by this simplified method combined with an assay for D-dimer to exclude PE in patients with a score of ≤4 and a negative assay for D-dimer.

These findings support the concept of obtaining a pretest probability by clinical assessment and combining it with results of objective tests to refine diagnosis. Several objective tests, in addition to D-dimer assay, are used to aid the diagnosis of PE.

Pulmonary Angiography

Pulmonary angiography is the accepted diagnostic reference standard for establishing the presence or absence of PE (18,19). Selective techniques and magnification have made this tool even more powerful in recent years.

A diagnosis of PE is confirmed when the angiogram demonstrates a constant intraluminal filling defect on multiple films, or when a sharp cutoff is consistently observed in multiple views in a vessel >2.5 mm in diameter. Abnormalities, such as oligemia, vessel pruning, and loss of filling of vessels, are nonspecific and may be the result of pneumonia, atelectasis, adult respiratory distress syndrome, pulmonary hypertension, chronic obstructive pulmonary disease, or carcinoma.

Clinically significant complications, including tachycardia, myocardial injury, cardiac perforation, cardiac arrest, and hypersensitivity reaction to contrast material, occur in 3–4% of patients. Hull et al. (5) observed that ~20% of patients with clinically suspected PE and abnormal perfusion lung scans had a severe enough primary illness that they could not undergo pulmonary angiography. The mortality associated with pulmonary angiography varies from 0.2% to 0.5%. Absolute contraindications to pulmonary angiography are allergy to contrast material and severe pulmonary hypertension (20). Concerns for morbidity and mortality, technical requirements, and inapplicability to some of the most critically ill patients have prompted investigation into other diagnostic tests.

V/Q Scanning

V/Q scanning has had an important role in the diagnosis of PE. Injection of technetium-99m-labeled microaggregated human albumin particles, 10–30 μm in diameter, temporarily occludes <0.5% of pulmonary capillary beds. Ventilation scanning has been added to perfusion scanning to differentiate embolic occlusions from perfusion defects from other causes, such as pneumonia or atelectasis. Ventilation scanning usually is performed with ^{133}Xe (20).

Prospective studies have compared the probability of PE, determined by detection of defects with various scanning procedures, with that determined by pulmonary angiography (5,15,16,21,22). V/Q scanning suffers from lack of specificity. Only a normal scan, which is found in 5–10% of scans, or a high-probability scan in a patient with a high prescan probability of PE, is useful as a diagnostic endpoint. The criteria used for classifying V/Q scans are not uniform. The greatest variability occurs in the intermediate-probability category (23). In general, the probability of PE increases with the size of the perfusion defect and the amount of V/Q mismatch. Two important prospective studies for determining the accuracy of V/Q scanning are those of Hull et al. (5,16) and the PIOPED study (15). Hull and his colleagues observed that patients with segmental or greater perfusion defects with V/Q mismatch (high probability) had an 86% probability of having a PE on pulmonary angiogram; however, 25–40% of patients with a low-probability scan had PE demonstrated by angiography. Hull and colleagues recommended not withholding anticoagulation therapy solely on the basis of a low-probability V/Q scan (5).

PIOPED was a multicenter trial that included 931 patients with clinically suspected PE. In total, 88% of patients with a high-probability scan had PE confirmed by angiography (102 of 116 patients). However, only 41% of patients with PE (102 of 251 patients) had a high-probability V/Q scan. Of 322 patients with intermediate-probability scans, 105 (33%) had PE. These investigators found a 12% frequency of PE in patients classified as low probability on the V/Q scan. Overall, the sensitivity of the V/Q scan was determined to be 98%. However, the overall specificity was only 10%. Although the specificity could be increased by making the criteria for PE more stringent, sensitivity was lost (15).

Helical Computed Tomography

The advent of helical computed tomography, or spiral volumetric tomography, allows images to be obtained from a patient holding inspiration for a single breath. Van Strijen et al. (24) evaluated the sensitivity and specificity of 258 helical CT scans for diagnosing PE. When compared with pulmonary angiography, helical CT scan had a sensitivity of 69% and a specificity of 86%. In a study of 299 patients with a positive test for D-dimer, sensitivity and specificity of helical CT scan were 69% and 91%, respectively. These authors concluded that helical CT scan should not be used as the sole test for diagnosing PE. Rather, when combined with lung scanning and ultrasound examination of the lower extremity, helical CT scanning may reduce the need for pulmonary angiography (25).

For subsegmental isolated PE, sensitivity is ~30%. As these isolated subsegmental emboli are associated with a significant risk of recurrence, diagnosis of these emboli is important (26). In his review of PE diagnosis, Kearon concluded that lobar or main pulmonary artery intraluminal filling defects have a positive predictive value of 85% and are equivalent to a high-probability V/Q scan. Segmental, and especially subsegmental, defects are nondiagnostic. In these cases, additional testing may be necessary. A normal helical CT scan is equivalent to a low-probability V/Q scan and does not exclude the diagnosis of PE (26).

Ultrasonographic Examination of the Lower Extremities for DVT

DVT of the leg is the origin of PE in most patients. Examination of the lower extremities for the presence of DVT is an indirect means of diagnosing PE (13,26). Hull and colleagues evaluated the role of noninvasive DVT testing in the diagnosis of PE (5,16,27). Several important observations were made in these studies. The frequency of proximal DVT was related to the likelihood of PE observed with V/Q scans: DVT was found in <1% of patients with normal lung scans; whereas, DVT was demonstrated in 49% of patients with large perfusion defects and V/Q mismatch. Patients with low- and intermediate-probability V/Q scans had a 15–27% rate of proximal DVT (16). These findings were interpreted to show that patients with clinically suspected PE and abnormal V/Q scans have a substantial frequency of proximal DVT.

Should a patient with a non-high-probability V/Q scan and a negative noninvasive examination be treated for DVT? In a study of 371 patients, those individuals with low- or intermediate-probability V/Q scans and normal serial impedance plethysmography (IPG) examinations (six times over a 2 week period) had a <3% chance of having DVT or PE in the 3 months following the index event that prompted evaluation for PE (27). Further, no patient died of VTE during this 3 month period. This study was limited to patients with good cardiopulmonary reserve. The authors concluded that withholding anticoagulation therapy is an acceptable strategy for managing patients with adequate cardiopulmonary reserve, nondiagnostic lung scan results, and negative serial IPGs. As duplex scanning of the lower extremities is more sensitive and specific than IPG, this strategy could also be followed in patients with a negative duplex scan for DVT.

D-Dimer Assay

D-dimer is derived from cross-linked fibrin that is lysed by plasmin. Although elevated serum concentrations of D-dimer have been observed in patients with PE, an increase in D-dimer is associated with many other conditions, including age, sex, smoking, body mass index, cholesterol, blood pressure, CRP, fibrinogen, von Willebrand factor, and plasmin–antiplasmin complex (28). D-dimer is frequently elevated in patients with recent surgery (29). A normal blood concentration of D-dimer is useful for excluding the possibility of PE (26). Assays for D-dimer are of two types: very highly sensitive and moderate-to-highly sensitive. Although their negative likelihood ratio is sufficient to exclude PE, many of the very highly sensitive assays are not practical for clinical diagnostic use. Moderate-to-highly sensitive assays do not have a high enough negative likelihood ratio to exclude PE and must be combined with another diagnostic test (26).

Combinations of Diagnostic Tests

Box 3 summarizes combinations of diagnostic tests for PE (26).

Box 3 Test Results That Confirm or Exclude the Presence of PE

Tests that confirm PE
    Pulmonary angiography: intraluminal filling defect
    Helical CT scan: intraluminal filling defect in a lobar or main pulmonary artery
    V/Q scan: high-probability scan and moderate/high clinical probability
Tests that exclude PE
    Pulmonary angiogram: normal
    Perfusion scan: normal
    D-dimer test: normal test that has sensitivity $\geq 85\%$ and specificity $\geq 70\%$ and
        (a) low clinical suspicion for PE
        or
        (b) normal alveolar dead space fraction, $VD/VT = (P_aCO_2 - P_eCO_2)/P_aCO_2$, where P_eCO_2 is the partial pressure of carbon dioxide in mixed expired gas
    Nondiagnostic V/Q scan or normal helical CT scan, and normal proximal venous ultrasound scans and
        (a) low clinical suspicion for PE
        or
        (b) normal D-dimer test that has sensitivity at least 85% and specificity at least 70%

Evidence of acute DVT with nondiagnostic V/Q scan or helical CT scan confirms the need for anticoagulation for treatment of the DVT. With acute PE, DVT is demonstrated in 75% of patients with venography and in 50% of patients with compression ultrasonography.

Noninvasive testing may be nondiagnostic in 30–60% of patients. Prevalence of PE in this group of patients is ~20%. As demonstrated in the PIOPED study, the majority of patients with PE had a low- or intermediate-probability V/Q scan. Pulmonary angiography should be considered to confirm the diagnosis in these patients. Alternatively, those patients with nondiagnostic noninvasive testing that includes ultrasonography of the proximal veins may be evaluated with serial ultrasound examinations of the proximal veins of the lower extremities. This recommendation is based on the observation that proximal vein thrombosis occurs before PE. Ultrasound examinations of such patients demonstrate abnormal findings in ~2% of patients. Those patients with normal serial testing have a low risk for developing PE (26). A single normal ultrasound examination is likely insufficient to withhold anticoagulation. Only 5 of 22 patients with PE, diagnosed by pulmonary angiography or high-probability V/Q scan, had a positive duplex examination the day before, the day of, or the day after diagnosis of PE (10).

See Figs. 2–4 for a diagnostic approach to hemodynamically stable patients.

PROPHYLAXIS

The key to reducing morbidity and mortality from VTE is prophylaxis. Although anticoagulation therapy is very effective in preventing death from this condition, the vast majority

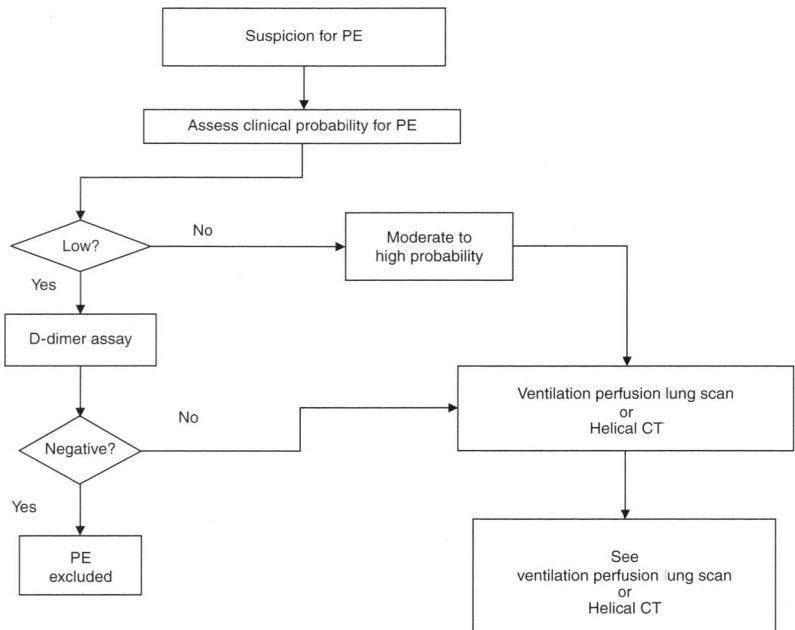

Figure 2 Approach to PE.

Venous Thromboembolism

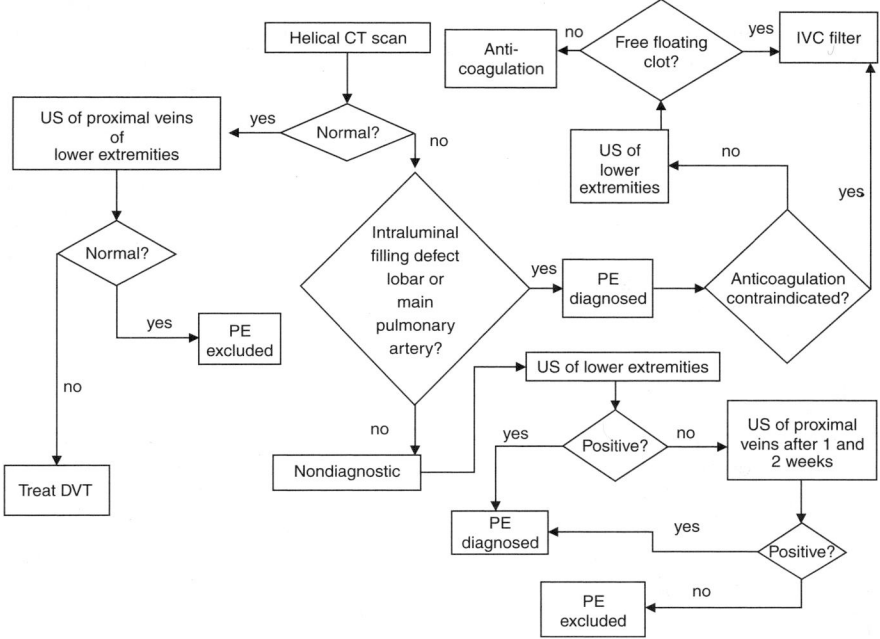

Figure 3 Use of helical CT in management of PE.

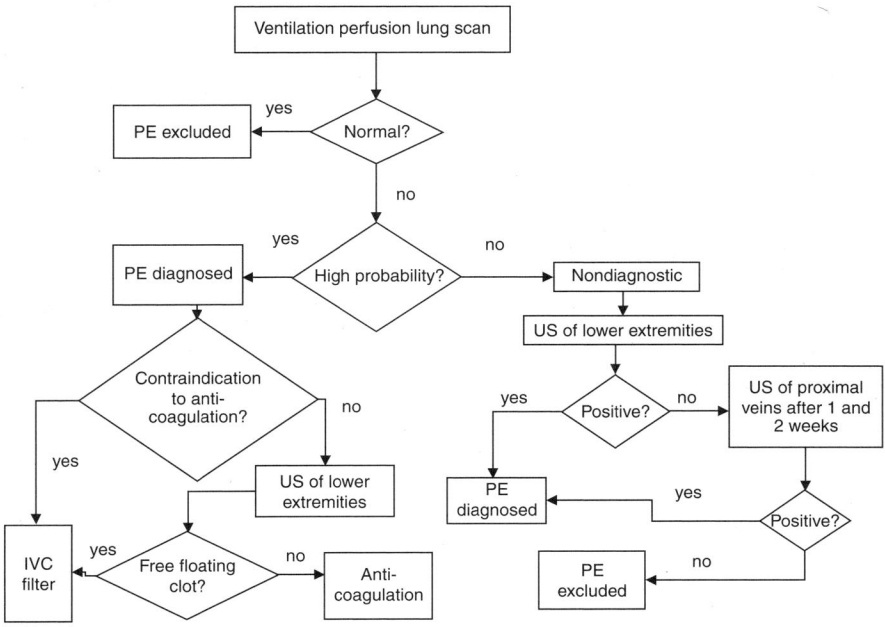

Figure 4 Use of ventilation perfusion lung scan in management of PE.

of patients die of PE either within the first hour of the event or without a diagnosis. Prophylaxis is much more effective for prevention of death and morbidity from PE when compared with anticoagulation for treatment of an established embolus. Routine use of effective prophylaxis in patients undergoing elective general surgery could prevent 4000–8000 postoperative deaths yearly in the United States (30). Studies proving the efficacy of VTE prophylaxis, particularly in surgical patients, have been well summarized (30–33). Subcutaneous low-dose heparin, low-molecular-weight heparin (LMWH), oral anticoagulation, pneumatic compression devices, and graduated compression stockings (GCS) are current means of providing prophylaxis. The form of prophylaxis used depends on the risk of VTE for the patient. Table 2 outlines the risk stratification of VTE for surgical patients.

Low-Dose Heparin

Low-dose heparin generally is given as a dose of 5000 units subcutaneously 2 h preoperatively and every 8–12 h postoperatively. Much lower doses of heparin are required to inhibit the initiation of blood coagulation than are needed for the treatment of established DVT or PE (31). A large multicenter international trial involving more than 4000 patients (32) and an analysis of 70 randomized trials that included more than 16,000 patients (31) have established the efficacy of low-dose heparin as a prophylactic agent for postoperative VTE.

Collins et al. (31) performed an exhaustive overview of 70 studies involving 16,000 patients in general, orthopedic, and urologic surgery. This study demonstrated a reduction in DVT from 22% to 9% with the use of subcutaneous heparin and found a significant

Table 2 Classification of Risk of Postoperative VTE

	Risk (%) related to		
Risk category	Calf vein thrombosis	Proximal vein thrombosis	Fatal pulmonary embolism
High risk	40–80	10–20	1–5
General, urologic surgery in patient >40 years with recent history of DVT or PE			
Extensive pelvic or abdominal surgery for malignant disease			
Major orthopedic surgery of lower limbs			
Moderate risk	10–40	2–10	0.1–0.7
General surgery in patients >40 years that lasts 30 min or more, in patients <40 years receiving oral contraceptives, and women >35 years having emergency cesarean section			
Low risk	<10	<1	<0.01
Minor surgery (<30 min) in patients >40 years with no additional risk factors			
Uncomplicated surgery in patients <40 years with no additional risk factors			

Source: Hull RD, Pineo GF. Prophylaxis of deep venous thrombosis and pulmonary embolism. Med Clin NA 1998; 82:477–493.

reduction in fatal PE in the patients treated with low-dose heparin. Low-dose heparin caused no apparent increase in deaths. Collins et al. estimated that using low-dose subcutaneous heparin decreased the odds of having proximal DVT by approximately two-thirds and of having postoperative PE by one-half.

In major orthopedic surgery, the administration of low-dose heparin reduced DVT by approximately two-thirds in elective surgery and trauma. In hip fracture patients, the use of low-dose heparin may be limited. Kakkar et al. (34) reported that 22 of 50 hip fracture patients still sustained a postoperative DVT despite receiving low-dose heparin therapy.

Data on increased bleeding associated with the use of low-dose heparin in postoperative patients have been incomplete and inadequate in many trials. In their overview of the randomized trials, Collins et al. (31) demonstrated that the absolute excess of bleeding attributable to low-dose heparin was ~2%. Although the multicenter trial showed a slight increase in bleeding morbidity in the low-dose heparin group (117 wound hematomas in control patients vs. 158 in heparin-treated patients), no difference between groups in deaths from hemorrhage was observed (32).

Low-Molecular-Weight Heparin (LMWH)

Another primary prophylactic agent is LMWH. LMWH, with molecular weights of 4000–6500 Da, has a longer half life than unfractionated heparin. It can be administered subcutaneously once or twice daily. When administered to healthy volunteers, subcutaneous LMWH produced peak plasma anti-Xa activities at least 6× greater than those obtained with conventional heparin given in the same dosage (35). LMWH has much greater bioavailability when compared with unfractionated heparin. As clearance is primarily renal, it should be used cautiously in patients with renal insufficiency and should not be used in patients in whom the creatinine clearance is <30 mL/min. LMWH has been shown to be effective in preventing postoperative thromboembolic complications in patients having elective hip surgery (36) and in general surgery patients (37,38). In a meta-analysis, LMWH and unfractionated heparin were compared. In surgical patients, LMWH provided superior protection (39). Bleeding complications appeared to be minimal with LMWH. LMWH is an efficacious prophylactic agent that may be safer than conventional heparin.

Many studies have demonstrated the superiority of LMWH over unfractionated heparin in the prevention of VTE in the high- and highest-risk surgical patients (see Table 2). Most patients admitted to an SICU fall into these categories. If the bleeding risk is acceptable, these patients should receive LMWH as the primary form of VTE prophylaxis, unless the creatinine clearance is <30 mL/min. In that case, they should receive unfractionated heparin, 5000 units every 8 h. The highest risk patients should have combination therapy that includes both compression devices and anticoagulation, if the bleeding risk is acceptable.

Oral Anticoagulants

Oral anticoagulation started in the immediate postoperative period is a very effective DVT prophylaxis in hip arthroplasty, knee arthroplasty, and hip fracture patients. Many studies have shown warfarin to be superior to unfractionated heparin. The warfarin dose should be adjusted to produce an INR of 2.0. Orthopedic patients should receive warfarin therapy for at least 7–10 days postoperatively. In high risk orthopedic patients, LMWH and oral anticoagulation appear to have similar efficacy and similar risk of bleeding (33).

Sequential Compression Devices

Sequential compression devices prevent venous thrombosis by enhancing blood flow in the deep veins of the legs. These devices have been shown to increase fibrinolytic activity systemically (40–42). In 15 of 22 studies, sequential compression has been demonstrated to significantly reduce the formation of postoperative thrombi. This type of prophylaxis is effective in moderate-risk general surgical patients and in patients undergoing minor surgery, major knee surgery, prostate surgery, and pelvic surgery. It is the method of choice for prophylaxis in patient groups in which anticoagulation is either contraindicated or ineffective (30). Sequential compression devices are virtually free of clinically important side effects and offer a valuable alternative in patients who have a high risk of bleeding.

Graduated Compression Stockings (GCSs)

GCSs reduce venous stasis by applying compression to the ankle and calf. Greater pressure is applied more distally. Although they have been shown to increase the velocity of venous blood flow, the mechanism by which they provide prophylaxis is unclear. Use of these stockings provides prophylaxis in low-risk general surgery patients (30). Efficacy in moderate- to high-risk patients has not been demonstrated (30). Our institution has abandoned the use of GCSs, because patients developed lower extremity ulcers or worsened pre-existing ulcers as a result of the GCSs. These stockings should not be used for prophylaxis in patients with peripheral vascular disease.

Vena Cava Interruption

Vena cava interruption initially required laparotomy for either suturing or clipping of the vena cava. These procedures were associated with a high mortality rate, recurrence of PE, and lower extremity edema (43). Simpler and safer procedures are now available. Inferior vena cava (IVC) filters or umbrellas may be inserted via a transvenous approach using local anesthesia. Recent reports recommend the use of removable IVC filters in high-risk trauma and general surgery patients (44).

The following are indications for the use of vena cava filters (45,46):

- Recurrent PE despite anticoagulation therapy
- PE or proximal DVT in patients with a contraindication to anticoagulation therapy
- Development of bleeding or thromboembolic complications secondary to anticoagulation therapy
- Progression or extension of an iliofemoral thrombus despite adequate anticoagulation therapy
- Demonstration of large, free-floating thrombi in iliac veins or the IVC
- Treatment following a single massive PE event when a recurrent embolus may prove fatal

Additional indications include:

- Need for prophylaxis in patients at very high risk for recurrent PE
- CNS bleeding and lower extremity fractures in patients with multiple trauma

Recommendations (33)

Choice of prophylaxis depends on the patient risk and the surgical procedure.

General Surgery

Low-Risk Patients: Early ambulation is recommended. Additional prophylaxis is not required.

Moderate-Risk Patients: Subcutaneous low-dose unfractionated heparin in a dose of 5000 units every 8–12 h or subcutaneous LMWH heparin is recommended for moderate-risk patients. Sequential compression devices may be used as an alternative and may be the initial choice for patients with a high bleeding risk.

Higher-Risk Patients: VTE prophylaxis with low-dose unfractionated heparin, LMWH, or pneumatic compression devices. Pneumatic compression devices are recommended for those higher-risk patients with a higher risk of bleeding.

Very High-Risk Patients: Pharmacologic prophylaxis with low-dose unfractionated heparin or LMWH should be combined with pneumatic compression devices. If risk is sufficiently high, perioperative LMWH or warfarin should be considered after discharge.

Gynecologic Surgery

Early mobilization is recommended for patients undergoing brief procedures for benign disease. For patients without risk factors undergoing major surgery for benign disease, low dose unfractionated heparin (LDUH) bid is recommended. LMWH or pneumatic compression devices, started before surgery and continued for several days postoperatively, are alternatives. For patients undergoing major surgery for malignancy, LDUH tid is recommended. Alternatives include LDUH combined with pneumatic compression devices or higher doses of LMWH.

Urologic Surgery

Early ambulation is recommended for patients undergoing low risk or transurethral procedures. LDUH, LMWH, or pneumatic compression devices are recommended for patients undergoing major open procedures. Combining LMWH or LDUH with pneumatic compression devices is recommended for the highest-risk patients.

Major Orthopedic Surgery

Elective Hip Replacement: LMWH, started 12 h before surgery, administered 12–24 h after surgery or 4–6 h after surgery at half the usual high-risk dose, and then continued at the high-risk dose on postoperative day 1 is recommended. Adjusted-dose warfarin administered to achieve a target INR of 2.5, with a range of 2.0–3.0, started preoperatively or immediately after surgery, is a recommended alternative. Adjusted-dose heparin therapy started preoperatively is acceptable. Pneumatic compression devices may provide additional benefit. LDUH, aspirin, dextran, and pneumatic compression devices alone are not recommended.

Elective Knee Replacement: LMWH or adjusted-dose warfarin is recommended. Pneumatic compression devices are an acceptable alternative. LDUH is not recommended.

Hip Fracture Surgery: LMWH or adjusted-dose warfarin is recommended. LDUH may be acceptable but has limited data to support its use. Aspirin alone is not recommended.

Other Orthopedic Considerations

Postoperative anticoagulation for 7–10 days is recommended, although the optimum duration of therapy is unknown. For high-risk patients, LMWH therapy in addition to the 7–10 days of postoperative therapy may be beneficial. Longer duration of therapy is recommended for high-risk patients. Routine duplex ultrasonography of the lower extremities is not recommended.

Neurosurgery

Pneumatic compression devices are recommended for patients undergoing intracranial procedures. LDUH or LMWH postoperatively are acceptable. A combination of LDUH or LMWH and pneumatic compression devices may be more effective than either form of prophylaxis alone.

Trauma

LMWH should be started as soon as possible in trauma patients with a risk factor for VTE. Initial prophylaxis with pneumatic compression devices should be started, if LMWH will be delayed or the patient's bleeding risk prohibits its use. For high-risk patients whose prophylaxis is less than ideal, duplex ultrasound examinations should be performed for screening. IVC filters are recommended, if DVT is identified and anticoagulation is contraindicated. IVC filters are not recommended for prophylaxis

Acute Spinal Cord Injury

LMWH is recommended for patients with acute spinal cord injury. LDUH and pneumatic compression devices are not recommended. Pneumatic compression devices may have benefit in combination with LDUH or LMWH. They may be used if patients cannot receive anticoagulant therapy after injury. LMWH or full-dose warfarin should be continued in the rehabilitation period.

Medical Conditions

Acute MI: LDUH or IV heparin should be administered to patients with acute MI.

Ischemic Stroke: Patients with ischemic stroke and limitations on mobility should receive prophylaxis with LDUH, LMWH, or danaparoid. Pneumatic compression devices should be used if anticoagulation is contraindicated.

General Medicine

LDUH or LMWH is recommended for patients with risk factors, including malignancy, heart failure, severe lung disease, and requirement for bed rest.

Special Conditions

Pregnancy (47): Subcutaneous low-dose heparin is recommended for high-risk patients. For patients undergoing planned cesarean section, especially if they have no risk factors, prophylaxis is of uncertain benefit. Prophylaxis with low-dose unfractionated heparin is recommended for patients requiring emergency cesarean section.

Cipolle et al. have demonstrated that adherence to an evidence-based protocol for prophylaxis in high-risk patients, including trauma patients, which used a combination of pneumatic compression devices and LMWH, produced excellent VTE prevention. Over a 6 year study period, ultrasound proven DVT had an incidence of 2.5%, of which 25% were symptomatic, and PE incidence was 0.3%. Even with reduced duplex ultrasound screening, the low incidence of PE was observed. The authors concluded that an evidence-based VTE prophylaxis protocol is of greater importance in preventing PE in trauma patients than is routine duplex ultrasound examination (10).

TREATMENT

Anticoagulation remains the mainstay of treatment for VTE. Thrombolysis has not yet gained wide acceptance as a first-line therapy. This limitation arises from bleeding risk. Lytic therapy has been reserved for use in unstable patients with massive PE or as part of a study protocol. Surgical thromoembolectomy is reserved for patients with postembolic systemic hypotension who have contraindications to, or have had, unsuccessful thrombolysis.

The ultimate goals of therapy are to prevent morbidity and mortality from PE and to prevent long-term complications of VTE. The optimum therapy depends on the patient's clinical status and cardiopulmonary reserve. Anticoagulation allows the fibrinolytic system to act unopposed and should limit the size of any embolic material that may be dislodged. In contrast, thrombolysis and embolectomy are therapies designed to actively remove PE.

Anticoagulation

Anticoagulation is the initial choice for therapy. Heparin does not lyse clots; rather, it prevents further clot formation. A randomized trial of heparin in the treatment of PE was discontinued after use in only 35 patients, because the investigators thought that withholding heparin in the control group was unethical (48). Continuous intravenous infusion of heparin is more effective than intermittent subcutaneous administration of heparin in preventing recurrent thromboembolism, a consequence of the delay in achieving anticoagulation when heparin is used subcutaneously. Hull et al. (49) reported that the relative risk of recurrent VTE was 15× higher in patients demonstrating inadequate anticoagulation therapy during the first 24 h, whether the heparin was given intravenously or subcutaneously.

Once the diagnosis of proximal DVT or PE has been confirmed, rapid anticoagulation is mandated. Therapy may be initiated with unfractionated heparin 5000–10,000 units/kg IV bolus followed by continuous infusion of 500–1500 units/h to maintain the PTT 1.5–2× the control value. The risk of major bleeding with full therapeutic doses of heparin ranges from 1% to 33%. Bleeding complications during heparin therapy do not correlate closely with elevated PTT (50,51). Most studies indicate a frequency of 5–10% (52,53). Continuous infusion results in fewer bleeding complications than intermittent injection (52).

LMWH has been used for treatment of both DVT and PE. It can be administered, using guidelines based on patient weight, as initial therapy. With dosing based on weight, dose adjustment and laboratory monitoring are not required. Outpatient therapy is possible. When compared with intravenous unfractionated heparin, therapy with LMWH is less costly. Several studies have evaluated long-term clinical outcomes with LMWH in comparison with unfractionated heparin (54–65).

Outcomes are comparable with the two approaches. Hull et al. (59) demonstrated lower rates of recurrence and bleeding with LMWH compared with unfractionated heparin. Two meta-analyses (66,67) suggest that LMWH is superior to unfractionated heparin with respect to recurrence and bleeding. Treatment of VTE with LMWH has advantages in patients without critical illness; whereas, problems arise in patients in the SICU. A major problem in the critically ill patient is the presence of renal failure, which contraindicates use of LMWH. Reversing subcutaneous LMWH is more difficult than discontinuing intravenous unfractionated heparin in patients who may be bleeding or who may require invasive procedures. Reduction in laboratory monitoring and early discharge are not easily demonstrated cost savings in the critically ill patient. As with all decisions in medicine, risks and benefits of LMWH therapy must be carefully considered.

The following factors have been associated with increased risk of bleeding during heparin therapy:

- Dose of heparin
- PTT >3× control
- Intermittent subcutaneous infusion > continuous infusion
- Thrombocytopenia
- Vitamin K deficiency
- Advanced age
- Underlying disease (e.g., malignancy, GI bleeding, renal or hepatic failure)
- Use of aspirin, NSAIDS, and lytic agents

Heparin-associated thrombocytopenia, an important drug reaction, is discussed in Chapter 52.

Early initiation of warfarin therapy shortens both the duration of heparin therapy (from 9.5 to 4.1 days) and the length of hospital stay by 4–5 days (68,69). In SICU patients, who frequently require surgical or other invasive procedures, early initiation of warfarin therapy may not always be feasible. If these procedures are required, the heparin dose can be decreased or stopped temporarily, and the effects will begin to reverse in 1–2 h. Anticoagulation with warfarin can be reversed by the addition of fresh frozen plasma, vitamin K, or both.

Initation of anticoagulation therapy with warfarin alone is not recommended. In addition to its well-known effect on coagulation factors, warfarin reduces blood concentrations of protein C, a naturally occurring antithrombin. Protein C has a half-life of 4–6 h and is depleted early with warfarin therapy. Such depletion creates the potential for a hypercoagulable state. Warfarin therapy must be initiated with simultaneous infusion of heparin to prevent hypercoagulability. Although the prothrombin time may be in the therapeutic range by the second or third day, the patient is not effectively anticoagulated until factors II, VII, IX, and X have been depleted. The half-life of factor X is about 4–5 days (52).

Generally, warfarin has been administered as a once-daily dose to maintain the prothrombin time at 1.5–2× that of control. Hull et al. (70) have shown that doses producing a lower PT are just as effective and result in fewer bleeding complications over a 3-month period. In their study, the conventional treatment group (average PT 19 s) and the study group (average PT 15 s) had an equal incident of recurrent DVT. The study group had only two patients with bleeding complications, and the conventional group had 11 bleeding complications.

For uncomplicated VTE, 3 months of oral anticoagulation therapy is recommended. Shorter duration of anticoagulation has resulted in excessively high recurrence rates of DVT (71,72). Reports by Hull and associates (73,74) have shown that providing a dose of warfarin to keep the PT between 1.5 and 2× that of control resulted in only a 2% recurrence of proximal DVT. In the subsequent 9 months, only 4% of patients experienced recurrence. Others have reported higher PE recurrences (17–23%) during anticoagulation therapy (75–77). As Hirsch and Hull (78) have suggested, the variability in these recurrence rates may be related to the delay in initiating therapeutic anticoagulation. They recommend that patients with a previous thromboembolic episode or those with persistent risk factors undergo anticoagulation therapy for at least 1 year. Patients who have had more than two thromboembolic episodes should be treated indefinitely.

Recently, the NIH-sponsored multicenter Prevention of Recurrent Venous Thromboembolism (PREVENT) trial demonstrated a 64% reduction in episode of recurrent VTE in patients receiving long-term warfarin therapy compared with a placebo control group. Of the 253 patients assigned to placebo, 37 patients experienced recurrence of VTE, whereas only 14 of 255 patients in the low-dose warfarin group had recurrence. Major bleeding and mortality were equivalent in both groups. In this trial, the initial VTE event was idiopathic in the sense that the VTE was not associated with recent surgery, trauma, or metastatic cancer. Patients in this study completed at least 3 months of uninterrupted full-dose warfarin therapy (79).

The most common complication of warfarin therapy is bleeding. In one report, major hemorrhage requiring transfusions or termination of oral anticoagulation therapy occurred in 2% of patients, and minor bleeding occurred in 4.8% (80). Skin necrosis is an important complication of warfarin therapy. Warfarin-induced skin necrosis begins as a painful erythematous patch of skin that rapidly progresses to a hemorrhagic area. Necrosis occurs and is followed by infection. More than 90% of patients affected are women, and necrosis generally begins between the second and fifth days of therapy (80). A postulated mechanism is microvascular thrombosis, secondary to depletion of protein C. Warfarin should be discontinued and heparin therapy begun as soon as this problem is recongnized.

The most important contraindication to warfarin therapy is pregnancy, because warfarin is associated with many fetal abnormalities. In a review of 418 pregnancies in which warfarin was administered, one-sixth of the pregnancies resulted in abnormal live-born infants and another one-sixth ended in abortion with stillbirths. Complications were seen most frequently when warfarin was used during the first trimester of pregnancy. Pregnant patients should be maintained on subcutaneous heparin or should be considered for vena cava interruption. Heparin is associated with a somewhat higher incidence of prematurity and stillbirths than is warfarin. The overall fetal mortality is ~20% in both groups. However, warfarin is associated with a 10-fold higher incidence of congenital abnormalities (81).

The following well-described conditions and drugs potentiate the effects of warfarin:

Conditions: alcoholism; cardiac, hepatic, or renal failure; cholestasis; hypoalbuminemia; fever; and malnutrition

Drugs: aspirin, NSAIDs, amiodarone, clofibrate, H_2-receptor blockers, sulfa drugs, danazol, disulfiram, glucagon, metronidazole, quinidine, tamoxifen, thyroxine

New Agents for Anticoagulation

The thrombin inhibitors hirudin, bivalirudin, and argatroban are FDA-approved drugs for intravenous use as an alternative to unfractionated heparin or LMWH in patients with heparin-induced thrombocytopenia. Ximelagatran, an oral agent that does not require monitoring, shows great promise as an alternative to warfarin for the prevention of VTE (82).

In contrast to heparin and LMWH, which blocks factor Xa in an antithrombin-dependent fashion, newer factor Xa inhibitors are also able to inactivate Xa bound to phospholipid surfaces, as well as free factor Xa (83,84). One of these synthetic pentasaccharides, fondaparinux, was found to be safe and equivalent to enoxaparin in the prevention of VTE after orthopedic surgery and has FDA approval for this use. It is administered subcutaneously once daily, does not require monitoring, and has been shown to be equivalent to adjusted-dose intravenous unfractionated heparin in the initial treatment of hemodynamically stable patients with PE (85–89). A new long-acting synthetic factor Xa inhibitor, idraparinux, with a half-life of 4 days, has shown great promise as an agent that can replace warfarin for long-term therapy for the prevention of recurrent VTE. This drug is administered subcutaneously once weekly and is currently in phase III trials (90).

Orally administered heparin is currently in phase III trials and has been an effective prophylaxis in patients undergoing hip or knee arthroplasty and for treatment of VTE. It may be an alternative to warfarin in patients with atrial fibrillation (91,92).

Thrombolytic Therapy

Advocates of lytic therapy observe that the case fatality rate of 15% for PE, which has not changed since the 1960s (93), is unacceptable but not surprising, as the usual treatment for PE continues to be anticoagulation therapy alone.

Thrombolytic therapy can accelerate clot lysis, improve pulmonary reperfusion, and rapidly reverse right heart failure, the usual immediate cause of death in PE (94). The high initial recurrence rates with the use of anticoagulation therapy alone, reported in some studies, may be a consequence of failure to lyse the embolic source from the pelvic or deep veins. Proponents of thrombolytic therapy maintain that recurrence could be averted by thrombolytic therapy. Although initial reports indicated no improved long-term survival or reduction in morbidity in PE patients treated with thrombolytic therapy, compared with those receiving conventional anticoagulation therapy (94–96), the Urokinase Pulmonary Embolism Trial (UPET) (97) demonstrated more complete resolution of PE in patients treated with lytic therapy. This result was documented by preservation of the normal pulmonary vascular response to exercise. Patients treated with heparin alone demonstrated a markedly abnormal rise in pulmonary artery pressure and pulmonary vascular resistance when undergoing bicycle exercise. In addition, the PE patients assigned to heparin only were in a more symptomatic functional class than those who had initially received thrombolytics followed by heparin.

Urokinase, streptokinase, and recombinant tissue plasminogen activator (rTPA) are approved for treatment of PE. rTPA provides clot specific lysis. It activates plasminogen without depleting fibrinogen. Thus, rTPA offers the potential of thrombolytic efficacy with fewer bleeding complications, when compared with streptokinase and urokinase (98). Trials by Goldhaber and colleagues (98–102) have shown that rTPA dissolved thrombi more rapidly and with fewer bleeding problems than did urokinase. In these studies, lysis was checked with a combination of a 2 h angiogram and a 24 h lung scan.

The risk of bleeding from lytic therapy is not precisely known, but is probably greater than the risk associated with conventional anticoagulation. In the UPET study (97), 10% of patients who received urokinase, as opposed to only 4% of patients treated with heparin, had bleeding of sufficient magnitude to require cessation of therapy or transfusion.

Controversy still persists concerning the role of thrombolytic agents in the primary treatment of VTE. In 1980, a consensus development conference of the National Institutes of Health suggested that thrombolytic therapy was not being used often enough. Their guidelines recommended the use of thrombolytic therapy for patients with obstruction of blood flow to a lobe or multiple pulmonary segments and for patients with hemodynamic compromise, regardless of the anatomic size of the embolus. A multicenter study in the United States recently carried out a 1-year survey in patients with PE diagnosed by high-probability lung scan or positive pulmonary angiogram. Of 2539 patients identified as having PE, 1345 (53%) would have been acceptable candidates for treatment with thrombolytic therapy (103).

Thrombolysis has the potential for widespread use as a therapeutic regimen among PE patients rather than being limited to use in patients with massive PE, who are hemodynamically unstable. Thrombolytic therapy should help advance the care of patients with VTE.

Pulmonary Embolectomy

Surgical embolectomy is reserved for patients with postembolic systemic hypotension who have an absolute contraindication to thrombolytic therapy or for those who deteriorate despite thrombolytic therapy. The outcome is dependent on surgical skill, interval to surgical intervention, and degree of cardiopulmonary disease. An emergency embolectomy is occasionally lifesaving (104).

Since the advent of cardiopulmonary bypass, the operative mortality for pulmonary embolectomy has steadily fallen from a rate of 60% to ~15%. The major sources of morbidity and mortality are severe hypoxia, prolonged hypoxia, acidosis, shock, and cardiopulmonary arrest prior to angiography or the induction of anesthesia. Patients in such moribund states should be placed on partial cardiopulmonary bypass prior to angiography or induction of anesthesia (105–107). A few patients have been saved through extracorporeal membrane oxygen support with or without pulmonary embolectomy (108,109). Most surgeons place a vena cava filter in patients who are undergoing pulmonary embolectomy. Complications of pulmonary embolectomy include hemorrhagic infarction and massive endobronchial hemorrhage after revascularization of ischemic lung tissue. Other complications, such as bleeding, right ventricular failure, cerebral anoxia, or cardiac arrest, are not necessarily a direct result of the procedure; they can be a result of massive PE or lytic therapy.

SUMMARY

- PE should be considered when (1) worsening hypoxemia and respiratory alkalosis occur in a patient being mechanically ventilated, (2) dyspnea in a patient with COPD does not improve with bronchodilator therapy, (3) a patient develops atelectasis or a peripheral infiltrate on CXR, (4) sudden onset of pulmonary hypertension or elevated CVP occurs, (5) pleuritic chest pain or chest pain that is not retrosternal and not pleuritic occurs (6) hemoptysis occurs, (7) a pleural rub is detected, and (8) an arterial saturation <92% while breathing room air that corrects with supplementary oxygen of <40% is observed.

- In addition to the risk factors listed, consider PE in patients with (1) surgery within the previous 12 weeks, (2) complete bed rest for 3 or more days in the 4 weeks before presentation, (3) fracture of a lower extremity and immobilization of the fracture within 12 weeks, and (4) postpartum state.
- Pulmonary angiography is the diagnostic standard. Absolute contraindications include allergy to radiocontrast agents and severe pulmonary hypertension.
- A normal V/Q scan excludes PE. Only 5–10% of V/Q scans are normal. A normal helical CT scan does not exclude a diagnosis of PE.
- Combinations of clinical findings and objective tests, outlined in Box 3, aid in the diagnosis of PE. For hemodynamically stable patients, see Figs. 1–3 for a diagnostic flow chart.
- For patients with a low clinical suspicion for PE, nondiagnostic testing for PE, and no evidence of DVT on evaluation of the lower extremities, serial evaluations of the lower extremities with ultrasound or impedance plethysmography may allow anticoagulation to be withheld, if DVT does not occur in the follow-up period.
- As mortality associated with PE occurs either in the first hour or before a diagnosis is established, prophylaxis, rather than treatment of an established embolus, reduces mortality more effectively.
- Effective prophylactic measures include low-dose heparin, LMWH, warfarin, and sequential compression devices. Choice of prophylaxis depends upon patient risk factors and planned surgical procedure.
- Anticoagulation with continuous intravenous heparin is the standard therapy for PE. Inadequate anticoagulation in the first 24 h is associated with increased recurrent thromboembolism. Administering warfarin early shortens duration of heparin therapy.
- Thrombolytic therapy can accelerate clot lysis, improve pulmonary reperfusion, and reverse right heart failure. Consider using thrombolytic therapy for patients with obstruction of blood flow to a lobe or to multiple segments.
- Vena cava filters can be used to reduce morbidity and mortality from PE in clinical conditions listed.

REFERENCES

1. Newman G. Pulmonary thromboembolism: a historical perspective. J Thorac Surg 1989; 4:1.
2. Kakkar VV, Flank C, Howe CT, et al. Natural history of postoperative deep vein thrombosis. Lancet 1969; 2:230.
3. Carter C, Gent M. The epidemiology of venous thrombosis. In: Hirsch J, Marder V, eds. Hemostasis and Thrombosis: Basic Principles and Practice. Philadelphia, PA: JB Lippincott, 1982:805.
4. Dalen JE, Paraskos Ja, Ockenc IS, et al. Venous thromboembolism. The scope of the problem. Chest 1986; 89(suppl):370S.
5. Hull RD, Hirsch J, Carter CJ, et al. Pulmonary angiography, ventilation scanning, and venography for clinically suspected pulmonary embolism with abnormal perfusion scan. Ann Intern Med 1983; 98:891.
6. Dorfman GS, Cronan JJ, Tuppu TB, et al. Occult pulmonary embolism: a common occurrence in deep vein thrombosis. Am J Roentgenol 1987; 148:263.
7. Moser KM, LeMoine JR. Is embolic risk conditioned by location of deep venous thrombosis? Ann Intern Med 1981; 94:439.

8. Schultz DJ Brasel KJ, Washington L, Goodman LR, Quickel RR, Lipchik RJ, Clever T, Weigelt J. Incidence of asymptomatic pulmonary embolism in moderately to severely injured trauma patients. J Trauma—Injury Infect Critic Care 2004; 56:727–733.
9. Kudsk KA, Fabian TC, Baurn S, et al. Silent deep vein thrombosis in immobilized multiple trauma patients. Am J Surg 1989; 158:515–519.
10. Cipolle MD, Wojcik R, Seislove E, et al. The role of surveillance duplex scanning in preventing venous thromboembolism in trauma patients. J Trauma 2002; 52:453–462.
11. Geerts WH, Code Kl, Jay RM, et al. A prospective study of VTE after major trauma. N Engl J Med 1994; 331:1601–1606.
12. Goldhaber SZ, Hennekens CH. Time trends in hospital mortality and diagnosis of pulmonary embolism. Am Heart J 1982; 104:305.
13. Wells PS, Ginsberg JS, Anderson DR, Kearon C, Gent M, Turpie AG, Bormanis J, Weitz J, Chamberlain M, Bowie D, Barnes D, Hirsh J. Use of a clinical model for safe management of patients with suspected pulmonary embolism. Ann Intern Med 1998; 129:997–1005.
14. Wenger NK, Stein PD, Willis PW. Massive acute pulmonary embolism. The deceptively nonspecific manifestations. J Am Med Assoc 1972; 220:843.
15. The PIOPED investigators. Value of the ventilation/perfusion scan in acute pulmonary embolism. Results of the prospective investigation of pulmonary embolism diagnosis (PIOPED). J Am Med Assoc 1990; 263:2753–2759.
16. Hull RD, Hirsh J, Carter CJ, Raskob GE, Gill GJ, Jay, RM, et al. Diagnostic value of ventilation—perfusion lung scanning in patients with suspected pulmonary embolism. Chest 1985; 88:819–828.
17. Wells PS, Anderson DR, Rodger M, Ginsberg JS, Kearon C, Gent M, Turpie AGG, Bormanis J, Weitz. J, Chamberlain M, Bowie D, Barnes D, Hirsh J. Derivation of a simple clinical model to categorize patients probability of pulmonary embolism: increasing the models utility with the SimpliRED D-dimer. Thromb Haemost 2000; 83:414–420.
18. Robin ED. Overdiagnosis and overtreatment of pulmonary embolism. The emperor may have no clothes. Ann Intern Med 1977; 87:775.
19. Hull RD, Raskob GE, Hirsch J. The diagnosis of clinically suspected pulmonary embolism, practical approaches. Chest 1986; 89(suppl):417S.
20. Spence TH. Pulmonary embolization syndrome. In: Civetta JM. Kirby RR. Taylor RW, eds. Critical Care. Philadelphia, PA: JB Lippincott, 1988:101.
21. Goldhaber SZ, ed. Strategies for diagnosis. Pulmonary Embolism and Deep Venous Thrombosis. Philadelphia, PA: WB Saunders, 1985:79.
22. Goldhaber SZ, Hennekens CH. Time trends in hospital mortality and diagnosis of pulmonary embolism. Am Heart J 1982; 104:305.
23. Webber MM, Gomes AS, Roe D, et al. Comparison of Biello, McNeil, and PIOPED criteria for the diagnosis of pulmonary emboli on lung scans. Am J Roentgenol 1990; 154:975.
24. van Strijen MJ, De Monye W, Kleft GJ, Bloem JL. Diagnosis of pulmonary embolism with spiral CT: a prospective cohort study in 617 patients. Radiology 1999; 213 S:127.
25. Perrier A, Howarth N, Didicr D, Loubeyre P, Unger PF, de Moerlosse P, Slosman D, Junod A, Bounameaux H. Performance of helical computed tomography in unselected outpatients with suspected pulmonary embolism. Ann Intern Med 2001; 135:88–97.
26. Kearon C. Diagnosis of pulmonary embolism. Can Med Assoc J 2003; 168:183–194.
27. Hull RD, Raskob GE, Coules G, et al. A new non-invasive management strategy for patients with suspected pulmonary embolism. Arch Intern Med 1989; 149:2549.
28. MacCallum PK, Cooper JA, Martin J, Howarth DJ, Meade TW, Miller GJ. Haemostatic and lipid determinants of prothrombin fragment F1.2 and D-dimer in plasma. Thromb Haemost 2000; 83:421.
29. Doukctis JD, McGinnis J, Ginsberg JS. The clinical utility of a rapid bedside D-dimer assay for screening deep vein thrombosis following orthopaedic surgery. Thromb Haemost 1997; 78:1300–1301.

30. Hull RD, Raskon GE, Hirsch J. Prophylaxis of venous thromboembolism: an overview. Chest 1986; 89(suppl):374S.
31. Collins R, Scrimgeour A, Yusuf S, et al. Reduction in fatal embolism and venous thrombosis by perioperative administration of subcutaneous heparin. N Engl J Med 1988; 318:1162.
32. An international multicenter trial: Prevention of fatal pulmonary embolism by low doses of heparin. Lancet 1975; 2:45.
33. Geerts WH, Heit JA, Clageet GP, Pineo GF, Colwell CW, Anderson FA, Wheeler HB. Prevention of venous thromboembolism, Chest 2001; 119:132S–175S.
34. Kakkar VV, Corrigan T, Spindler J. et al. Efficacy of low doses of heparin in prevention of deep vein thrombosis after major surgery. A double blind randomized trial. Lancet 1972; 2:101.
35. Bergqvist D, Hedman U, Sjorin E, Holmer E. Anticoagulant effects of two types of low molecular weight heparin administered subcutaneously. Thromb Res 1983; 32:381.
36. Turpie ACG. Low molecular weight heparins: deep vein thrombosis prophylaxis in elective hip surgery and thrombotic stroke. Acta Chir Scand 1988; 543(suppl):85.
37. Bergqvist D. Prophylaxis of postoperative deep vein thrombosis in general surgery: experience with fragmin. Acta Chir Scand 1988; 543(suppl):87.
38. Hauch O, Jorgensen LN, Kolle TR, et al. Low molecular weight heparin (Logiparin™) as thromboprophylaxis in elective abdominal surgery. Acta Chir Scand 1988; 543(suppl):90.
39. Jorgensen LN, Wille-Jorgensen P, Hauch O. Prophylaxis of postoperative thromboembolism with low-molecular-weight heparins. Br J Surg 1993; 80:689–704.
40. Allenby F, Pflug JJ, Boardman I, Clavin JS. Effects of external pneumatic compression on fibrinolysis in men. Lancet 1973; 2:1412.
41. Tarnaz TJ, Fohr PA, Davidson AG, et al. Pneumatic calf compression, fibrinolysis, and the prevention of deep venous thrombosis, Surgery 1980; 88:489.
42. Inada K. Lioke S, Shirai N, et al. Effects of intermittent pneumatic leg compression for prevention of postoperative deep venous thrombosis with special reference to fibrinolytic activity. Am J Surg 1988; 155:602.
43. Greenfield LJ. Evolution of venous interruption for pulmonary thromboembolism. Arch Surg 1992; 127:622–626.
44. Offner PJ, Hawkes A, Madayag R, Seale F, Maines C. The role of temporary inferior vena cava filters in critically ill surgical patients. Arch Surg 2003; 138:591–595.
45. Kempczinski RF. Surgical prophylaxis of pulmonary embolism. Chest 1986; 89(suppl):384S.
46. Greenfield LJ. Current indications for, and results of, Greenfield filter placement. J Vasc Surg 1984; 1:502.
47. Hull RD, Pineo GF. Prophylaxis of deep venous thrombosis and pulmonary embolism. Med Clinics N Am 1998; 82:447–493.
48. Barritt DW. Jordan SD. Anticoagulant drugs in the treatment of pulmonary embolism. A controlled trial. Lancet 1960; 1:1309.
49. Hull RD, Raskob GE, Hirsch J, et al. Continuous intravenous heparin compared with intermittent subcutaneous heparin in the initial treatment of proximal vein thrombosis. N Engl J Med 1986; 315:1109.
50. Basu D, Gallus A, Hirsch J, et al. A prospective study of the value of monitoring heparin treatment with the activated partial thromboplastin time. N Engl J Med 1972; 287:324.
51. Deykin D. Regulation of heparin therapy. N Engl J Med 1972; 287:355.
52. Stead R. Clinical pharmacology. In: Goldhaber SZ, ed. Pulmonary Embolism and Deep Vein Thrombosis. Philadelphia, PA: WB Saunders, 1985:99.
53. Kelton JG, Hirsch J. Bleeding associated with antithrombotic therapy. Semin Hematol 1980; 17:259.
54. Koopman MMW, Prandoni P, Piovella F, et al. Treatment of venous thrombosis with intravenous unfractionated heparin administered in the hospital as compared with subcutaneous low-molecular weight heparin administered at home. N Engl J Med 1996; 334:682–687.

55. The Columbus Investigators. Low-molecular-weight heparin in the treatment of patients with venous thromboembolism. N Engl J Med 1997; 337:657–662.
56. Simonneau G, Sors H, Charbonnier B, et al. A comparison of low-molecular-weight heparin with unfractionated heparin for acute pulmonary embolism. N Engl J Med 1997; 337:663–669.
57. Hull RD, Raskob GE, Brandt RF, et al. Low-molecular-weight heparin vs. heparin in the treatment of patients with pulmonary embolism. Arch Intern Med 2000; 160:229–236.
58. Prandoni P, Lensing AWA, Buller HR et al. Comparison of subcutaneous low molecular weight heparin with intravenous standard heparin in proximal vein thrombosis. Lancet 1992; 339:441–445.
59. Hull RD, Raskob GE, Pineo GF, et al. Subcutaneous low-molecular-weight heparin compared with continuous heparin in the initial treatment of proximal vein thrombosis. N Engl J Med 1992; 326:975–982.
60. Lindmarker P, Holmstrom M, Granqvist S, et al. Comparison of once-daily subcutaneous fragmin with continuous intravenous unfractionated heparin in the treatment of deep vein thrombosis. Thromb Haemost 1994; 72:186–190.
61. Fiessinger JN, Lopez-Fernandez M, Gatterer E, et al. Once daily subcutaneous dalteparin, a low molecular weight heparin, for the initial treatment of acute deep vein thrombosis. Thromb Haemost 1996; 76:195–199.
62. Luomanmaki K, Granqvist S, Hallert C, et al. A multicentre comparison of once-daily subcutaneous dalteparin (low molecular weight heparin) and continuous intravenous heparin in the treatment of deep vein thrombosis. J Intern Med 1996; 240:85–92.
63. Kirchmaier CM, Wolf H, Schaefer H, et al. Efficacy of a low molecular weight heparin administered intravenously or subcutaneously in comparison with intravenous unfractionated heparin in the treatment of deep venous thrombosis: Certoparin study group. Int Angiol 1998; 17:135–145.
64. Meyer G, Brenot F, Pacouret G, et al. Subcutaneous low-molecular-weight heparin fragmin versus intravenous unfractionated heparin in the treatment of acute non massive pulmonary embolism: an open randomized pilot study. Thromb Haemost 1995; 74:1432–1435.
65. Lopaciuk S, Meissner AJ, Filipecki S, et al. Subcutaneous low molecular weight heparin versus subcutaneous unfractionated heparin in the treatment of deep vein thrombosis: a Polish multicenter trial. Thromb Haemost 1992; 68:14–18.
66. Siragusa S, Cosmi B, Piovella F, et al. Low-molecular-weight heparins and unfractionated heparin in the treatment of patients with acute venous thromboembolism: results of a meta-analysis. Am J Med 1996; 100:269–277.
67. Gould MK, Dembitzer AD, Doyle RL, et al. Low-molecular-weight heparins compared with unfractionated heparin for treatment of acute deep venous thrombosis. Ann Intern Med 1999; 130:800–809.
68. Gallus A, Jackman J, Tillet J, et al. Safety and efficacy of warfarin started early after submassive venous thrombosis or pulmonary embolism. Lancet 1986; 2:1293.
69. Rosiello RA, Clan CK, Tencza F, et al. Timing of oral anticoagulation therapy in the treatment of angiographically proven acute pulmonary embolism. Arch Intern Med 1987; 147:1469.
70. Hull RD, Hirsch J, Jay R, et al. Different intensities of oral anticoagulation therapy in the treatment of proximal vein thrombosis. N Engl J Med 1982; 301:1076.
71. O'Sullivan EE. Duration of anticoagulant therapy in venous thromboembolism. Med J Aust 1972; 2:1104.
72. Holmgren K, Andersson G, Fagrelli B, et al. One-month versus six-month therapy and the probabilities of recurrent thromboembolism and hemorrhage. Am J Med 1986; 81:255.
73. Hull RD, Delmore T, Genton E, et al. Warfarin sodium versus low dose heparin in the long-term treatment of venous thrombosis. N Engl J Med 1979; 301:355.

74. Hull RD, Carter C, Hirsch J, et al. Adjusted subcutaneous heparin versus warfarin sodium on the long-term treatment of venous thrombosis. N Engl J Med 1982; 306:189.
75. Urokinase Pulmonary Embolism Trail: a national cooperative study. Circulation 1973; 47(suppl 2):1.
76. Wheeler AP, Jaquess RDB, Newman JH. Physician practices in the treatment of pulmonary embolism and deep venous thrombosis. Arch Int Med 1988; 148:132.
77. Monreal M, Ruiz J, Salvador, et al. Recurrent pulmonary embolism: a prospective study. Chest 1989; 95:976.
78. Hirsch J, Hull RD. Treatment of venous thromboembolism. Chest 1986; 89(Suppl):426S.
79. Ridker PM, Goldhaber SZ, Danielson E, Rosenberg Y, Eby CS, Deitcher SR, Cushaman M, Moll S, Kessler CM, Elliott CG, Paulson R, Wong T, Baucr KA, Schwartz BA, Miletich JP, Bounameaux H, Glynn RJ. PREVENT investigators. Long-term, low intensity warfarin therapy for the prevention of recurrent venous thromboembolism. N Engl J Med 2003; 348:1425–1434.
80. Peterson CE, Kwaan HC. Current concepts of warfarin therapy. Arch Int Med 1986; 146:581.
81. Hall JG, Pauli RM, Wilson KM. Maternal and fetal sequelae of anticoagulation during pregnancy. Am J Med 1980; 68:122.
82. Francis CW, Berkowitz SD, Comp PC, Lieberman JR, Ginsberg JS, Paiement G, Peters GR, Roth AW, McElhattan J, Colwell CW, EXULT study group. Comparison of ximelagatran with warfarin for the prevention of venous thromboembolism after total knee replacement. N Engl J Med 2003; 349:1703–1712.
83. Vlasuk GP. Structural and functional characterization of tick anticoagulation peptide (TAP): a potent and selective inhibitor of blood coagulation factor Xa. Thromb Haemost 1993; 70:212–216.
84. Dunwiddie C, Thornburry NA, Bull HG, et al. Antistasin: a leech-derived inhibitor of factor Xa: kinetic analysis of enzyme inhibition and identification of the reactive site. J Biol Chem 1989; 264:16694-16699.
85. Bauer KA, Erissson BI, Lassen MR, Turpci AGG. Fondaparinux compared with enoxaparin for the prevention of venous thromboembolism after elective major knee surgery. N Engl J Med 2001; 345:1305–1310.
86. Eriksson BI, Bauer KA, Lassen MR, Turpic AGG, for the steering committee of the Pentasaccharide in Hip-Fracture Surgery Study. Fondaparinux compared with enoxaparin for the prevention of venous thromboembolism after hip-fracture surgery N Engl J Med 2001; 345:198–304.
87. Lassen MR, Bauer KA, Eriksson BI, Turpie AGG, for the European Pentasaccharide Hip Elective Surgery Study (EPHESUS) Steering Committee. Postoperative fondaparinux versus preoperative enoxaparin for prevention of venous thromboembolism in elective hip-replacement surgery: a randomised double-blind comparison. Lancet 2002; 359:1715–1720.
88. Turpie AGG, Eriksson BI, Lasen MR for the PENTATHLON 2000 Study Steering Committee. Postoperative fondaparinux versus postoperative enoxaparim for prevention of venous thromboembolism after elective hip-replacement surgery: a randomised double-blind trail. Lancet 2002; 359:1721–1726.
89. Buller HR, Davidson BL, Decousus H, Gallus A, Gent M, Piovella F, Prins MH, Raskob G, vanden Berg-Segers, AE, Cariou R, Leeuwenkamp O, Lensing AW, Matisse Investigators. Subcutaneous fondaparinux versus unfractionated heparin in the initial treatment of pulmonary embolism. N Engl J Med 2003; 349:1762–1764.
90. The PERSIST investigators. A novel long-acting synthetic factor Xa inhibitor (SanOrg34006) to replace warfarin for secondary prevention in deep vein thrombosis. A phase II evaluation. J Thromb Haemost 2004; Jan 2:47–53.
91. Baughman RA, Kapoor SC, Agarwal RK, et al. Oral delivery of anticoagulant doses of hepanin: a randomized, double-blind controlled study in humans. Circulation 1998; 98:1610–1615.

92. Gonze MD, Manord JD, Leone-Bay A, et al. Orally administered heparin for preventing deep venous thrombosis. Am J Surg 1998; 176:176–178.
93. Goldhaber SZ. Pulmonary embolism death rates. Am Heart J 1988; 115:342.
94. Sasahara AA, Sharma GVRK, McIntyre K, et al. A national cooperative trial of pulmonary embolism, phase I results of urokinase therapy. J Louisiana State Med Soc 1972; 124:130.
95. Tibbut DA, Dawes JA, Anderson JA, et al. Comparison controlled clinical trial of streptokinase and heparin in treatment of major pulmonary embolism. Br Med J 1974; 1:393.
96. Ly B, Arnesen J, Eie H, et al. A controlled trial of streptokinase and heparin in the treatment of major pulmonary embolism. Acta Med Scand 1978; 203:465.
97. Sharm GVRK, Folland ED, McIntyre KM, Sasahara AA. Long-term hemodynamic benefit of thrombolytic therapy in pulmonary embolic disease [abstract]. J Am Coll Cardiol 1990; 15:65A.
98. Goldhaber SZ, Vaughn ED, Markis JE, et al. Acute pulmonary embolism treated with tissue plasminogen activator. Lancet 1986; 2:886.
99. Goldhaber SZ, Meyerovitz MF, Markis JE, et al. Thrombolytic therapy of acute pulmonary embolism: current Status and future potential. J Am Coll Cardiol 1987; 10:96B.
100. Goldhaber SZ, Maris JE, Kessler CM, et al. Perspective in treatment of acute pulmonary embolism with tissue plasminogen activator. Semin Thromb Hemost 1987; 13:221.
101. Godhaber SZ, Kessler CM, Hert J, et al. A randomized controlled trial of recombinant tissue plasminogen activator versus urokinase in the treatment of acute pulmonary embolism. Lancet 1988; 2:293.
102. Goldhaber SZ, Recent advances in the diagnosis and lytic therapy of pulmonary embolism. Chest 1991; 99(suppl):179S.
103. Terren M, Goldhaber SZ, Thompson RO, TIPE investigators Selection of patients with acute pulmonary embolism for thrombolytic therapy. The Thrombolysis in Pulmonary Embolism (TIPE) survey. Chest 1989; 95(suppl):279S.
104. Hoaglund PM. Massive pulmonary embolism. In: Goldhaber SZ, ed. Pulmonary Embolism and Deep Venous Thrombosis. Philadelphia, PA: WB Saunders, 1985:179.
105. Mattox KL, Feldman RW, Beall AC, et al. Pulmonary embolectomy for acute massive pulmonary embolism. Ann Surg 1982; 195:726.
106. Sautter R, Myers WO, Ray JF, et al. Pulmonary embolectomy: review and current status. In: Sasahara AA, Sonncnblick EH, Lesch MI, eds. Pulmonary Emboli. New York: Grune and Stratton, 1974:143.
107. Masters RG, Koshal A, Higginson LAJ, et al. Ongoing role of pulmonary embolectomy. Can J Cardiol 1988; 4:347.
108. Cooper JD, Tearsdale S, Neems JM, et al. Cardiorespiratory failure secondary to peripheral pulmonary emboli. Survival following a combination of prolonged extracorporcal membrane oxygenation support and pulmonary embolectomy. J Thorac Cardiovasc Surg 1976; 761:876.
109. Krellenstein DJ, Bryan-Brown CW, Fayena AO, et al. Extracorporeal membrane oxygenation for massive pulmonary thromboembolism. Ann Thorac Surg 1977; 23:421.

30
Airway Management

Ian J. Gilmour
Anesthesia Associates of Martinsville, Inc., Martinsville, Virginia, USA

Airway management decisions should not be based solely on the patient's need for mechanical ventilatory support. Consideration also must be given to the maintenance of the patient's airway. Mental status, associated musculoskeletal disorders, and the amount of pulmonary toilet required all enter into the decision-making process. Approaches to airway support other than endotracheal tubes (ETTs) or tracheostomy tubes (TTs) include nasopharyngeal airways (Fig. 1), oropharyngeal airways (Fig. 2), and continuous positive airway pressure (CPAP) masks (Fig. 3). The intensivist must be familiar with these commonly used airway adjuncts. The laryngeal mask airway is another alternative (1).

INDICATIONS FOR ENDOTRACHEAL INTUBATION

Indications for endotracheal intubation (ETI) include (i) continuing threat to airway patency (trauma, edema, hemorrhage); (ii) risk for aspiration of gastric contents or other substances (blood, foreign objects); (iii) removal of substances (sputum, blood); (iv) diagnostic procedures (bronchoscopy); (v) general anesthesia requiring muscle relaxation; and (vi) mechanical ventilation.

ROUTE OF INTUBATION AND SELECTION OF TUBE

Translaryngeal intubation may be attempted through either the nares [nasotracheal intubation (NTI)] or the mouth [orotracheal intubation (OTI)]. The advantages and disadvantages of each route are listed in Table 1.

Several observations deserve emphasis. In an emergency, OTI is faster than NTI. If the use of the ETT will be required for longer than 48–72 h, the potential for sinus and middle ear infections is increased with NTI, and, therefore, OTI may be preferable. Establishment of the airway must take precedence over patient comfort; therefore, judicious use of sedatives and muscle relaxants is necessary, especially for the hypovolemic patient. NTI is not suitable for the patient at risk for regurgitation and aspiration of gastric contents or the patient with facial trauma, bleeding diathesis, sinusitis, or retropharyngeal abscess.

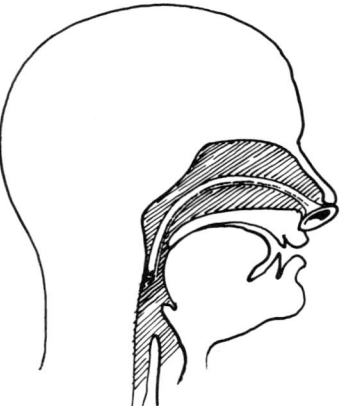

Figure 1 Nasopharyngeal airway in place. Airway passes through the nose and ends at a point just above the epiglottis. Redrawn from Dorsch JA, Dorsch SE. Understanding Anesthetic Equipment, 2d ed. Baltimore: Williams & Wilkins, 1984:326–337.

Because any manipulation of the airway can markedly increase intracranial pressure in patients with reduced intracranial compliance, intubation in these patients should follow adequate resuscitation and aggressive measures to obtund reflex responses. After three or four failed attempts, laryngoscopy may cause sufficient soft tissue trauma and edema that the physician may be unable to ventilate the patient. An alternative route should be considered if three or four efforts with laryngoscopy have been unsuccessful. Additional complications of intubations are listed in Boxes 1 and 2.

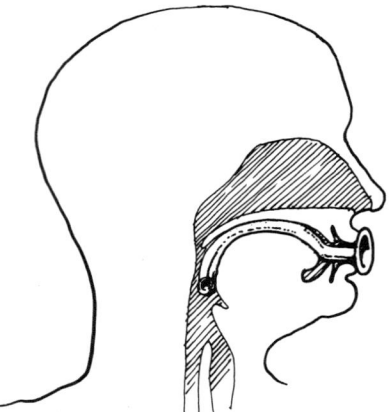

Figure 2 Oropharyngeal airway in place. Airway follows curvature of the tongue, pulling it and the epiglottis away from the posterior pharyngeal wall and providing a channel for air passage. Redrawn from Dorsch JA, Dorsch SE. Understanding Anesthetic Equipment, 2d ed. Baltimore: Williams & Wilkins, 1984:326–337.

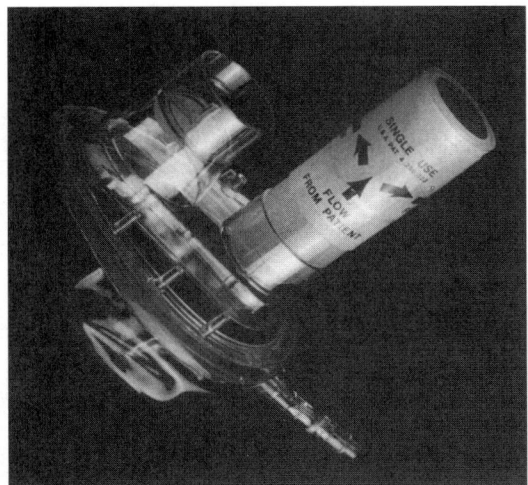

Figure 3 CPAP mask. Courtesy of Vital Signs, Inc., Tocowa, NJ.

STANDARD APPROACHES TO INTUBATION

Standard approaches to intubating patients include blind nasal or oral intubation, direct laryngoscopy, and fiberoptic bronchoscopy. With blind nasal or oral intubation, instrumentation of the oropharynx is not done, and patient comfort is improved. The procedure is useful in patients who have reduced movement of the mandible or the neck. However, it requires considerable practice. These methods should not be used in children or in patients with pathologic conditions of the upper airway or neck.

Table 1 Comparison of NTI and OTI

	Nasotracheal	Orotracheal
Specifications	Smaller diameter	Larger diameter
	Longer length	Shorter length
	Increased resistance	Decreased resistance
Instrumentation	May be done blind	Requires instrumentation
Usefulness	More useful in difficult airway	More easily used with adjuncts (i.e., bronchoscope)
Endobroncheal intubation	Decreased possibility	Increased possibility
Stability	More stable	Less stable
Possibility of sinus infection	Risk of sinusitus	Low risk
Risk of hemorrhage	Increased risk	Lesser risk
Cuff damage	Increased potential[a]	Less potential[a]
Trauma	To retropharynx, conchae, larynx	To tongue, teeth, larynx
Patient comfort	More comfortable	Less comfortable

[a]Inversely related to tube diameter.

Box 1 Complications of ETI

During intubation
  Laryngospasm
  Laceration, bruising of lips, tongue, and pharynx
  Fracture, chipping, dislodgment of teeth or dental appliances
  Perforation of trachea or esophagus
  Retropharyngeal dissection
  Fracture or dislocation of cervical spine
  Trauma to eyes
  Hemorrhage
  Aspiration of gastric contents or foreign bodies
  Endobronchial or esophageal intubation
  Dislocation of arytenoid cartilages or mandible
  Hypoxemia and hypercarbia
  Bradycardia and tachycardia
  Hypertension
  Increased intracranial or intraocular pressure
With tube in situ
  Accidental extubation
  Endobronchial intubation
  Obstruction or kinking
  Bronchospasm
  Ignition of tube by laser device
  Aspiration
  Excoriation of nose or mouth
Evident after extubation
  Laryngospasm
  Aspiration of secretions, gastric contents, blood, or foreign bodies
  Glottic, subglottic, or uvular edema
  Dysphonia, aphonia
  Paralysis of vocal cords or hypoglossal, lingual nerves
  Sore throat
  Noncardiogenic pulmonary edema
  Laryngeal incompetence
  Sore and dislocated jaw
  Tracheal collapse
  Sinusitis
  Glottic, subglottic, or tracheal stenosis
  Vocal cord granulomata or synechiae

Source: From Stehling LC. Management of the airway. In Barash PG, Cullen FB, Stoelting RK, eds. Clinical Anesthesia. Philadelphia: JB Lippincott, 1989; 989:543–561.

Direct laryngoscopy is the most familiar approach. Although easier to learn and less influenced by blood and secretions than other methods, this procedure is affected by the patient's anatomy. The instrumentation necessary produces a high level of patient discomfort.

Fiberoptic bronchoscopy/laryngoscopy is being used more frequently. This approach is useful when direct laryngoscopy is difficult or dangerous, and it permits visual confirmation of ETT tip location. The procedure produces less patient discomfort than does direct laryngoscopy. Fiberoptic approaches are more difficult to learn, are

Airway Management

Box 2 Complications of Nasotracheal Intubation

Epistaxis
Turbinectomy
Sinusitis
Nasal infection
Ulceration of ala nasi or septum
Otisis media
Nasal pain
Nasal adhesion
Bacteremia
Submucosal dissection
Pharyngeal perforation
Eustachian tube damage

Source: Modified from Ref. 3, p. 95.

difficult to perform in the unconscious or sedated patient, and may be more difficult to perform in the presence of large volumes of blood or mucus.

DIFFICULT AIRWAY

The goal of laryngoscopy is to position the head and neck so that the axes of mouth, pharynx, and larynx are aligned (Fig. 4). Syndromes and clinical conditions that may make ETI difficult are listed in Box 3 and Tables 2 and 3. Occasionally, even in the absence of predisposing factors, laryngoscopy will be difficult. However, by looking into the patient's open mouth, one can often predict the ease of laryngoscopy by which pharyngeal structures are visible (Figs. 5 and 6). If a Class III or IV anatomic configuration is seen (see Fig. 5), referral of the patient's intubation to an expert should be considered.

The most appropriate method of intubation depends on the circumstances. A variety of laryngoscope blades have been designed to be used in difficult airways. Intubating stylets, some with lights, allow easier manipulation of ETTs. Blind ETT should not be used in a patient with marked airway distortion (i.e., epiglottitis, soft tissue tumors). In skilled hands, fiberoptic laryngscopy may have a significant advantage when difficult airway access is expected. Intubation over a wire passed retrograde through the cricothyroid membrane and out through the mouth is also an option. For alternative approaches in the patient with an unstable cervical spine, see Table 4.

When the skill and experience necessary for the above methods are lacking, esophageal obturator airways are a practical alternative. For the difficult airway, the consultation of an anesthesiologist or otorhinolaryngologist may be lifesaving. Because the inability either to intubate or to ventilate is life-threatening, everyone in the SICU should be familiar with the necessary additional steps in airway management. The keys to successful emergency airway management in the SICU include,

1. Having immediately available: oxygen, functioning bag/valve/mask, a selection of oral/nasal pharyngeal airways, a selection of ETTs, a functioning laryngoscope, preferably with several different blades and suctions
2. Adequate evaluation of the patient and the patient's airway

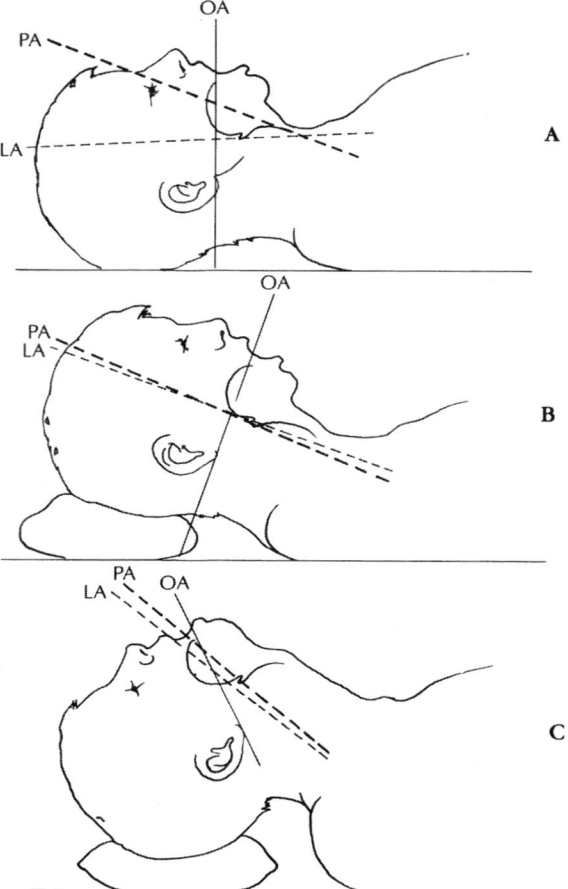

Figure 4 Demonstration of head position for ETI. A, Successful direct laryngoscopy for exposure of glottic opening requires alignment of oral (OA), pharyngeal (PA), and laryngeal (LA) axes. B, Elevation to head ~10 cm with pads underneath to occiput and shoulders remaining on table aligns laryngeal and pharyngeal axes. C, Subsequent head extension at atlanto-occipital joint serves to create shortest distance and straightest line possible from incisor teeth to glottic opening. Redrawn from Stone DJ, Gal TJ. Airway management. In Miller RD. Anesthesia, 3d ed. New York: Churchill Livingstone, 1990:1265–1292.

3. Knowledgeable assistance
4. Immediate, accurate confirmation of tube placement
5. Appropriate alternatives being immediately available
6. Recognition of limitations of the physician

CONFIRMATION OF SUCCESSFUL INTUBATION

Confirmation of correct placement must be undertaken immediately after intubation. Standard methods of confirming tube placement are shown in Table 5. Any of these methods depends on the skill and experience of the operator (fiberoptic bronchoscopy/laryngoscopy,

Box 3 Conditions in Which Intubation Is Potentially Dangerous

Conditions associated with atlantoaxial subluxation	*Syndromes associated with odontoid hypoplasia*
Congential	Morquio's syndrome
Down's syndrome	Klippel–Feil syndrome
Odontoid anomalies	Down's syndrome
Mucopolysaccharidoses	Spondyloepiphyseal dysplasia
Acquired	Dysproportionate dwarfism
Rheumatoid arthritis	Congenital scoliosis
Still's disease	Osteogenesis imperfecta
Ankylosing spondylitis	Neurofibromatosis
Psoriatic arthritis	
Enteropathic arthritis	
Crohn's disease	
Ulcerative colitis	
Reiter's syndrome	
Trauma	
Odontoid fracture	
Ligamentous disruption	

Source: From Crosby ET, Lui A. The adult spine: implications for airway management. Can J Anaesth 1990; 37:77–93.

auscultation), and the operator's knowledge of the inherent limitations of the technique (cuff palpation, capnometry, pulse oximetry). Capnometry is the best technique available, but it is not wholly reliable (2).

Incorrect placement of an ETT means that either the tube is in the esophagus or has been advanced too far or not far enough in the airway (Table 6). Neck flexion and extension can cause significant movement of the ETT. Furthermore, fixation of the external portion of the tube does not guarantee that, as the ETT becomes softer and more malleable with time and body heat, it will not migrate with coughing and tongue movements.

Table 2 Selected Congenital Syndromes Associated With Difficult Endotracheal Intubation

Syndrome	Difficulty
Down's	Large tongue, small mouth make laryngoscopy difficult; small subglottic diameter possible
	Laryngospasm frequent
Goldenhar's (oculoauriculovertebral anomalies)	Mandibular hypoplasia and cervical spine abnormality make laryngoscopy difficult
Klippel–Feil	Neck rigidity because of cervical vertebral fusion
Pierre Robin	Small mouth, large tongue, mandibular anomaly; awake intubation essential in neonate
Treacher Collins (mandibulofacial dysostosis)	Laryngoscopy difficult
Turner's	High likelihood of difficult intubation

Source: From Stone DJ, Gal TJ. Airway management. In Miller RD. Anesthesia, 3d ed. New York: Churchill Livingstone, 1990:1265–1292.

Table 3 Selected Pathologic States That Influence Airway Management

Infectious	
Epiglottis	Laryngoscopy may worsen obstruction
Abscess (submandibular, retropharyngeal, Ludwig's angina)	Distortion of airway renders mask ventilation or intubation extremely difficult
Croup, bronchitis, pneumonia (current or recent)	Airway irritability with tendency for cough, laryngospasm, bronchospasm
Papillomatosis	Airway obstruction
Tetanus	Trismus renders oral intubation impossible
Traumatic	
Foreign body	Airway obstruction
Cervical spine injury	Neck manipulation may traumatize spinal cord
Basilar skull fracture	Nasal intubation attempts may result in intracranial tube placement
Maxillary/mandibular injury	Airway obstruction, difficult mask ventilation, and intubation; cricothyroidotomy may be necessary with combined injuries
Laryngeal fracture	Airway obstruction may worsen during instrumentation; ETT may be misplaced outside larynx and worsen injury
Laryngeal edema (post intubation)	Irritable airway, narrowed laryngeal inlet
Soft tissue, neck injury (edema, bleeding, emphysema)	Anatomic distortion of airway, airway obstruction
Neoplastic	
Upper airway tumors (pharynx, larynx)	Inspiratory obstruction with spontaneous ventilation
Lower airway tumors (trachea, bronchi, mediastinum)	Airway obstruction may not be relived by tracheal intubation; lower airway distorted
Radiation therapy	Fibrosis may distort airway or make manipulations difficult
Inflammatory	
Rheumatoid arthritis	Mandibular hypoplasia, temporomandibular joint arthritis, immobile cervical spine, laryngeal rotation, cricoarytenoid arthritis all make intubation difficult and hazardous
Ankylosing spondylitis	Fusion of cervical spine may render direct laryngoscopy impossible
Temporomandibular joint syndrome True ankylosis "False" ankylosis (burn, trauma, radiation, temporal craniotomy)	Severe impairment of mouth opening
Scleroderma	Tight skin and temporomandibular joint involvement make mouth opening difficult
Sarcoidosis	Airway obstruction (lymphoid tissue)
Angioedema	Obstructive swelling renders ventilation and intubation difficult

(Continued)

Table 3 (*Continued*)

Endocrine/metabolic	
Acromegaly	Large tongue, body overgrowths
Diabetes mellitus	May have reduced mobility of atlano-occipital joint
Hypothyroidism	Large tongue, abnormal soft tissues (myxedema) make ventilation and intubation difficult
Thyromegaly	Goiter may produce extrinsic airway compression or deviation
Obesity	Upper airway obstruction with loss of consciousness; tissue mass makes successful mask ventilation difficult

Source: From Stone DJ, Gal TJ. Airway management. In Miller RD. Anesthesia, 3d ed. New York: Churchill Livingstone 1990:1265–1292.

Accordingly, position of the ETT can be monitored by daily X-ray examination. Approximate distances for ETT insertion can be found in Table 7.

CHANGING OF OROTRACHEAL TUBE

If, for some reason, the exchange of one orotracheal tube for another becomes necessary, consideration should be given to the use of an intubating stylet. Limitations of the intubating stylet procedure include laryngeal edema, which makes passage of the tube difficult; laryngospasm/coughing; and lack of patient co-operation (biting). The technique is not useful for NTT because of the narrowness of the airway and the large number of twists and turns encountered with NTI.

EXTUBATION

Extubation should not be equated with weaning. The indications for and the methods of weaning are described in Chapter 32. Extubation should be considered only when

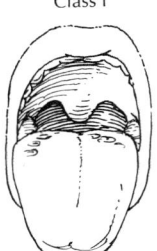 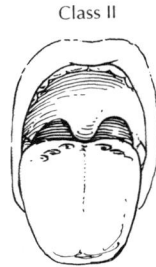 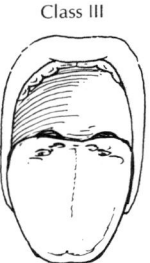 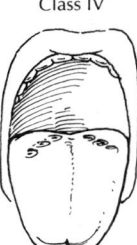

Figure 5 Classification of pharyngeal structures as seen during conduction of tests. Class III, soft palate visible; Class IV, soft palate not visible. Redrawn from Samsoon GLT, Young JRB. Difficult tracheal intubation: a retrospective study. Anesthesia 1987; 42:487–490.

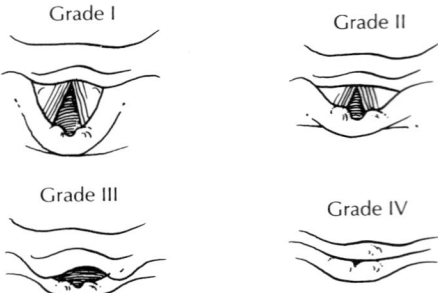

Figure 6 Classification of laryngoscopic views obtained by modifying drawings used by Cormack and Leane in their original classification. Redrawn from Samsoon GLT, Young JRB. Difficult tracheal intubation: a retrospective study. Anesthesia 1987; 42:487–490.

Table 4 Methods of Intubation for Unstable Cervical Spine

Patient state	Technique
Awake	Blind nasotracheal
	Fiberoptic orotracheal/nasotracheal
	Retrograde catheter
	Cricothyrotomy
Anesthetized; no relaxants	Blind nasotracheal
	Fiberoptic orotracheal/nasotracheal
Anesthetized; rapid sequence, muscle relaxants	Orotracheal laryngoscopic

Source: Modified from Crosby ET, Lui A. The adult spine: implications for airway management. Can J Anaesth 1990; 37:77–93.

Table 5 Methods of Confirmation of ETT Placement

Method	Esophageal	Endobronchial	How high
Auscultation	Not reliable	Decreased reliability in children	Good
Chest X-ray examination	Not reliable, very delayed	Very delayed	Very delayed
Observation of chest movement	Not reliable	Not reliable	Poor
Condensation in tube	Not reliable	N/A	N/A
Palpation of cuff	N/A for uncuffed tubes, not reliable for cuffed	Good	Good
Persistent expired CO_2 (capnometry)	Good	Not reliable	Not reliable
Pulse oximetry	Delayed	Very delayed	Not reliable
Direct visual confirmation			
Rigid	Good in experienced hands	N/A	Good in experienced hands
Fiberoptic	Good, delayed	Good, delayed	Good, delayed

Table 6 Consequences of Misplaced ETTs

Placement	Consequence
Esophageal intubation	No alveolar ventilation
	Rapid development of hypoxia, hypercapnea
Endobronchial intubation	May be continuous or intermittent
	May cause hypoxia, barotrauma
High ETT	May be continuous or intermittent
	May cause inadequate alveolar ventilation
	May allow loss of positive end-expiratory pressure, causing hypoxia
	Promotes accidental extubation
	May increase potential for aspiration

weaning goals have been reached *and* the patient is expected to have an unobstructed airway that they will be capable of protecting after extubation. Uncertainty regarding either of these conditions should lead to postponement of extubation and consideration of tracheostomy.

TRACHEOSTOMY

A tracheostomy is indicated in the following situations:

1. Prolonged necessity for mechanical ventilation/artificial airway
2. Airway obstruction/lack of access to airway at or above the larynx
3. Inadequate pulmonary toilet, particularly if reintubation is necessary
4. Inability to wean the patient from mechanical ventilation support

Table 7 ETT Size and Position Based on Patient Age

Age	Internal diameter (mm)	External diameter (mm)[a]	French unit	Distance inserted from lips (cm)[b]
Premature	2.5	3.3	10	10
Full-term newborn	3.0	4.0–4.2	12	11
1–6 months	3.5	4.7–4.8	14	11
6–12 months	4.0	5.3–5.6	16	12
2 years	4.5	6.0–6.3	18	13
4 years	5.0	6.7–7.0	20	14
6 years	5.5	7.3–7.6	22	15–16
8 years	6.0	8.0–8.2	24	16–17
10 years	6.5	8.7–9.3	26	17–18
12 years	7.0	9.3–10	28–30	18–20
≥14 years	7.0 (women)	9.3–10	28–30	20–24
	8.0 (men)	10.7–11.3	32–34	

[a]Approximate, varying among manufacturers.
[b]For tip placement in midtrachea. Add 2–3 cm for nasal tubes.
Source: From Stehling LC. Management of the airway. In Barash PG, Cullen FB, Stoelting RK, eds. Clinical Anesthesia. Philadelphia: JB Lippincott, 1989:543–561.

For many years, routine tracheostomy was undertaken whenever ETI was required for >24–48 h because the high-pressure, low-volume cuffs on older ETTs caused tracheal stenosis at the cuff site. With the advent of low-pressure, high-volume cuffs, long-term translaryngeal intubation has become common (3). Additional benefits, such as lower incidence of aspiration past the cuff with the ETT vs. the tracheostomy tube (TT), have supported the trend of delaying tracheostomy until the third or fourth week of intubation (4). Associated with this trend has been an increase in damage to the vocal cords and the larynx (3). However, that subsequent tracheostomy decreases laryngeal complications caused by prolonged translaryngeal intubation is not certain (5,6). For this reason, most authors recommend an anticipatory approach. Some suggest regular fiberoptic examination of the upper airway, with creation of a tracheostomy only when significant laryngeal injury becomes apparent. Other complications of tracheostomy are listed in Box 4.

Inadequate pulmonary toilet or inability to wean are judgments often made in debilitated patients with severe chronic obstructive pulmonary disease, in whom repeated attempts at extubation are foiled by the patient's failure to clear secretions or to wean past a low level of ventilator support. Such patients may benefit from tracheostomy because of the improved toilet or small decrease in airway resistance and dead space.

Tube Selection

Cuffed vs. Noncuffed

In adults, noncufffed tubes can be considered for patients who are capable of spontaneous ventilation and airway protection.

Box 4 Complications of Tracheostomy

First 48–72 h
    Bleeding (usually vein or thyroid vessel)
    Pneumothorax
    Pneumomediastinum
    Accidental decannulation
After 72 h
    Infection at stomal site
    Mucous plug obstruction
    Innominate artery fistula
    Sinusitis
    Otitis media
    Tracheobronchitis
    Pneumonia (nosocomial)
Late
    Dilation of trachea at cuff site
    Granulation tissue at stoma
    Tracheoesophageal fistula
Delayed
    Difficulty decannulating
    Persistent tracheocutaneous fistula
    Tracheal stenosis at stoma or cuff site

Source: From Ref. 7, p. 117.

Inner Cannula

For long-term tracheostomy, particularly when the patient is no longer in the hospital, an inner cannula that can be removed and cleaned can be very helpful. However, an inner cannula decreases the internal diameter and, consequently, increases airway resistance. In addition, a TT with a rigid inner cannula often has a larger outer diameter for a given inner diameter, a property that may increase the risk of stenosis at the stomal site following decannulation.

Shape and Construction of Tube

The length of the extratracheal portion of the TT is important when the distance between the incision and the tracheal stoma is longer than normal (due to obesity, edema, induration, or subcutaneous emphysema). A tracheostomy appliance that is too short greatly increases the risk of accidental decannulation. By adapting to the shape of the patient's airway, malleable TTs have fewer pressure points and thus reduce tracheal damage.

Special Considerations With Recent Tracheostomy

Accidental decannulation of a recent tracheostomy may be life-threatening. Just as for failed intubation, each SICU should have a procedure for avoiding accidental decannulation. Taking preventive measures is clearly superior to managing such a difficult problem. Attention to several features of tracheostomy placement is helpful.

1. All tracheostomies should have "stay" sutures inserted into the third or fourth tracheal rings (7). These sutures should extrude from the stoma to facilitate emergency recannulation.
2. The selected TT should be of appropriate size, length, and shape (Fig. 7).
3. Tracheal ties should be snug and secure so that the wings of the tube rest against the skin. As swelling dissipates, the ties may need to be tightened.

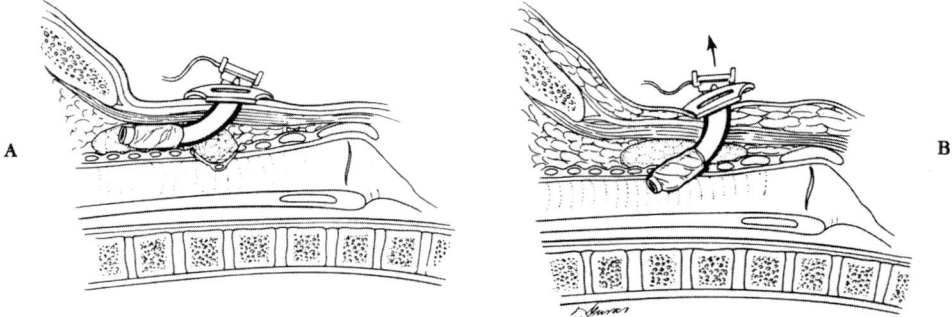

Figure 7 Accidental decannulation is one of the most common complications of tracheostomy. Proper size and length of tracheostomy tube and incision are important in preventing this complication. A, Fenstra can be lost during changing of a TT. B, A tube that is too short can decannulate. From Adams GL. Complications of tracheostomy. Perspect Crit Care 1990; 3(1):117.

4. Manipulation of the airway should be avoided for at least 72 h. Ventilator hoses/oxygen tubing should be disconnected when the patient is being moved. When the mouth is wired shut, wire cutters must be kept at the bedside.
5. Emergency airway materials, including a tracheostomy/cricothyrotomy tray with tracheostomy hooks, larygngoscope, and ETTs, and a bag/valve/mask setup, must be immediately available.

If the patient should be decannulated, the following steps must be taken:

1. Call for experienced airway assistance and emergency airway materials.
2. While help and equipment are arriving:
   a. If the patient is moving air, increase FIO_2 at the nose and the mouth or the tracheostomy site (if the stoma in the trachea is visible) and request indirect monitors (pulse oximetry, capnometry).
   b. If the patient is making respiratory efforts but not moving air, look for easily remediable problems, such as a blood clot in the tracheal stoma.
   c. If the patient is not making respiratory efforts and the upper airway is potentially available, attempt bag/valve/mask ventilation with oxygen. Blind passes with a suction catheter may cannulate the distal trachea. The catheter then can be used as a stylet to reintroduce the TT or an ETT.
3. Once equipment and personnel arrive, proceed as follows:
   a. If the patient is ventilating/being ventilated and if stay sutures were placed, use gentle traction on the sutures and suction to attempt recannulation. Adequate light is mandatory to visualize the tracheal stoma.
   b. If the patient is not being ventilated and the upper airway is potentially open (i.e., the patient has not had a laryngectomy), proceed with OTI.
   c. If (a) and (b) are not successful, use the emergency tracheostomy equipment.
   d. Although its use is difficult when blood and secretions are present, a fiberoptic laryngoscope occasionally may be used to replace the TT.
4. Do not attempt to ventilate the patient through the newly reestablished airway unless (i) correct position has been determined by fiberoptic laryngoscopy, (ii) a suction catheter can be passed freely through the tube, or (iii) the patient is ventilating spontaneously through the cannula. Capnometry will confirm appropriate placement. Subcutaneous/mediastinal/submucosal emphysema from positive pressure ventilation (PPV) through a misplaced tube can make subsequent intubation/ventilation impossible.

Changing of TT

Indications for Tube Change in Recent Tracheostomies (<72 h After Tracheostomy)

1. Obstructed tube
2. Inappropriate tube size or shape
3. Mechanical problems—leaky cuff, leaky inner cannula
4. Change in patient status—necessity for PPV, cuffed vs uncuffed tube

Procedure

1. Ensure that all ancillary equipment is available (intubation, tracheostomy, bag/valve/mask, replacement TT).

Airway Management

2. Procure a stylet about 12 in. long, malleable but not floppy.
3. Preoxygenate the patient; consider sedation/analgesia.
4. Loosen the tracheostomy ties and lubricate the replacement tube.
5. Consider application of a local anesthetic. Injection may cause bleeding.
6. Pass the stylet through the TT, deflate the cuff, and remove the old tube. Thread the replacement tube over the stylet into the trachea.
7. Establish correct placement as earlier.
8. Tie or suture the tube into place.

Fiberoptic laryngoscopes may be used for this procedure (Fig. 8), but their use necessitates losing the airway momentarily after the old TT has been removed.

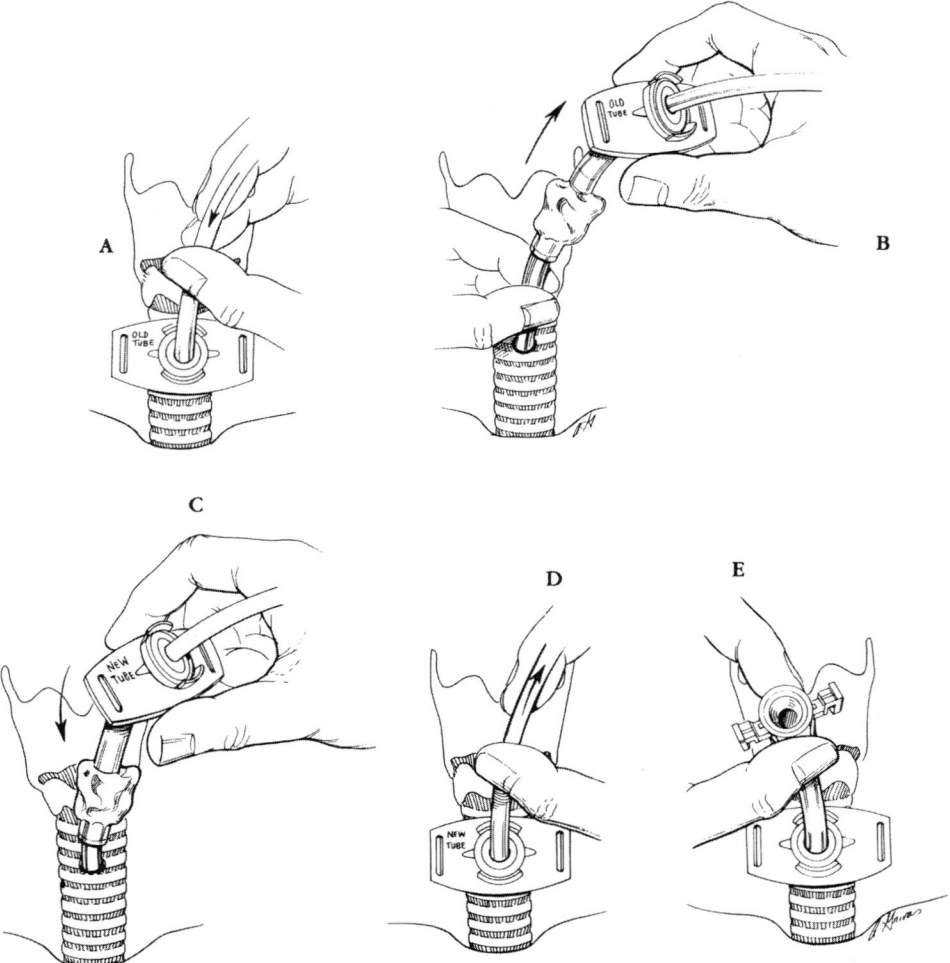

Figure 8 Safe method of changing a TT over a suction catheter. A, Catheter is inserted. B, Old TT is removed over catheter. C, New TT is placed over catheter. D, Catheter is removed. E, Inner cannula is inserted into new tube. From Adams GL. Complications of tracheostomy. Perspect Crit Care 1990; 3(1):117.

Tracheostomy instruments also may be used, but their use requires some knowledge and experience.

PULMONARY HEMORRHAGE/MASSIVE HEMOPTYSIS

Minor hemoptysis occurs frequently in the SICU. Typically, it is associated with a mucosal ulcer in the trachea and a concomitant mild bleeding diathesis (i.e., platelet dysfunction, renal failure). Although such bleeding occasionally warrants intervention, most commonly, correction of the bleeding disorder is sufficient. Bleeding in excess of 200 cc per 24 h is defined as massive hemoptysis. By this definition, massive hemoptysis is rare and occurs in only 1.5% of cases.

The most common causes of massive hemoptysis are tuberculosis, bronchiectasis (including cystic fibrosis), and lung cancer (see Box 5). The mortality rate may be as high as 78%; patients usually die of suffocation from airway obstruction (8). Underlying pulmonary dysfunction may make even minor hemoptysis life-threatening.

Approaches to the treatment of hemoptysis include ongoing life support and resuscitation, brochoscopy, ballon tamponade, angiography embolization, radio nuclear scanning, and surgery.

All Cases

All patients in need of airway management require ongoing life support and resuscitation, including oxygen, mechanical ventilation (if required), correction of coagulopathies, and consideration of the use of double-lumen ETTs or bronchi blockers if the bleeding site is known or suspected.

Box 5 Common Causes of Massive Hemoptysis

Infectious	Immunologic
Tuberculosis	Goodpasture's syndrome
Lung abscess	Collagen-vascular diseases
Bronchopneumonia	Congenital
Fungus ball	Cystic fibrosis
Parastic infestations	Bronchiectasis associate with Kartagener's
Neoplastic	syndrome
Bronchogenic carcinoma	Others
Bronchial adenoma	Bronchiectasis
Lymphoma	Retained foreign body
Metastatic disease	Broncholithiasis
Carcinoma of contiguous structures	Idiopathic pulmonary hemosiderosis
Cardiovascular	Iatrogenic
Mitral stenosis	Trauma
Arteriovenous malformation	Idiopathic
Thoracic aortic aneurysm	
Vasculitis	
Pulmonary hypertension	

Source: From Rudzinski JT, del Castillo J. Massive hemoptysis. Ann Emerg Med 1987; 16:561–564.

Bronchoscopy

Rigid bronchoscopy is the treatment of choice because it allows concomitant ventilation, suctioning, and application of local treatments (vasoactive agents, iced-saline lavage). This approach is particularly useful in massive bleeding. The disadvantages are the need for general anesthesia and transport to the operating room. When the source of bleeding is not in the large airways, rigid bronchoscopy allows localization of the bleeding.

Fiberoptic bronchoscopy is available in most SICUs. It allows for visualization of the smaller branches of the tracheobronchial tree, and some forms of localized treatment (Fogarty catheters, epinephrine, gel foam) can be applied. Fiberoptic bronchoscopy is less useful in the presence of massive or diffuse bleeding. The efficacy of either type of bronchoscopy is reduced when the patient is not actively bleeding.

Balloon Tamponade

Ballon tamponade is usually used in conjunction with bronchoscopy. Along with tamponade, balloon catheters allow distal irrigation with vasoactive substances or iced saline. Balloon tamponade is most useful when the site of bleeding has been localized. Although inflating the balloon blindly in a larger bronchus can be effective, it frequently leaves the patient with insufficient residual pulmonary function. When the bleeding source is thought to be a pulmonary artery rupture associated with the use of a Swan–Ganz catheter, leaving the catheter in position and inflating the balloon may be lifesaving (9).

Angiography/Embolization

Massive hemoptysis usually results from systemic (bronchial) artery bleeding. Unfortunately, the anatomy of the bronchial arteries is highly variable. Because the anterior spinal artery may arise close to the bronchial arteries, potential for embolic material to cause neurologic dysfunction exists. Although useful only in the presence of active bleeding, angiography with embolization can be highly effective and is associated with only a small recurrence rate. This approach has the added advantage of being minimally invasive, but it does require the patient to be moved to the radiology suite.

Radionuclear Scanning

Radionuclear scanning is noninvasive and relatively benign but can be used only with heavy, active bleeding (>60 mL/h) (10). This approach is diagnostic rather than therapeutic.

Surgery

Surgery is the treatment of last resort for massive hemoptysis, primarily because many patients with this disease have insufficient pulmonary reserve to allow resection of adequate amounts of lung tissue. For surgery to be effective, the site of the bleeding must be known, and the patient must be adequately resuscitated. Furthermore, surgery requires transport to the operating room, general anesthesia, and additional blood loss. In selected patients, however, surgery can be highly effective, with some studies showing a $>50\%$ decrease in mortality.

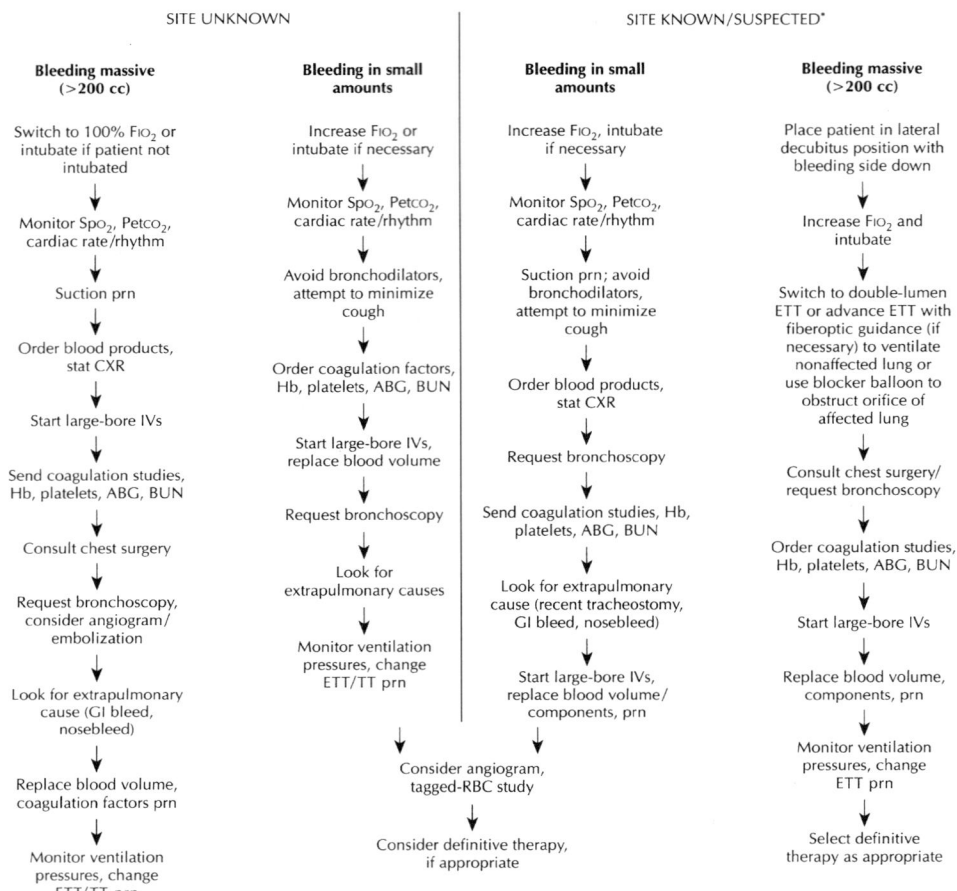

*Swan-Ganz catheter balloon rupture.

Figure 9 Treatment approach to pulmonary hemorrhage/massive hemoptysis.

For a presentation of the treatment of pulmonary hemorrhage/massive hemoptysis, see Fig. 9.

SUMMARY

- Use ETT for (i) trauma, edema, or hemorrhage that threatens airway patency, (ii) significant risk of aspiration; (iii) suctioning of airway repeatedly and frequently; (iv) diagnostic procedures; (v) general anesthesia requiring muscle relaxation; and (vi) mechanical ventilation.
- Standard intubating approaches include blind nasal or oral intubation, direct laryngoscopy, and fiberoptic bronchoscopy/laryngoscopy.

- Emergency airway management requires extensive preparation, evaluation of patient, skilled assistance, immediate and accurate determination of tube location, and necessary equipment for managing difficult airway.
- Indications for tracheostomy include prolonged mechanical ventilation, airway obstruction at or above larynx, and chronic suctioning for pulmonary toilet.
- Accidental decannulation of recent tracheostomy:
  - Minimize chance of decannulation by using tracheostomy appliance of appropriate size, length, and shape; securing tracheal ties; adjusting tracheal ties as edema resolves; and avoiding airway manipulation for at least 12 h.
  - Take precautions to avoid accidental decannulation. Have immediately available tracheostomy tray with tracheostomy hooks, laryngoscope, ETTs, bag/valve/mask, and wire cutter (if patient's mouth is wired shut).
  - If accidental decannulation occurs:
    1. Call for help. Increase FIO_2 at nose, mouth, or stoma (if visible). Look for blood clot in stoma. If upper airway is patent, attempt bag/valve/mask ventilation.
    2. If unable to ventilate patient, attempt oral intubation.
    3. Confirm correct position of newly established airway.
- Massive hemoptysis:
  - Establish a secure, patent airway.
  - Resuscitate with volume, oxygen and mechanical ventilation.
  - Correct coagulopathies (if present).
  - Rigid bronchoscopy is preferred with massive bleeding.
  - Balloon tamponade may be used to stop bleeding when bleeding site is known.
  - Angiography with embolization may be effective.

REFERENCES

1. Maltby JR, Loken RG, Watson NC. The laryngeal mask airway: clinical appraisal in 250 patients. Can J Anaesth 1990; 37:509–513.
2. Dunn SM, Mushlin PS, Lind CJ, Raemer D. Tracheal intubation is not invariably confirmed by capnography. Anesthesiology 1990; 73:1285–1287.
3. Berlauk JF. Intubation in the ICU: a review from a different perspective. Perspect Crit Care 1990; 3(2):89–107.
4. Stauffer JL, Olson DE, Petty TL. Complications and consequences of endotracheal intubation and tracheostomy: a prospective study of 150 critically ill patients. Am J Med 1981; 70:65–76.
5. Bishop MJ. Mechanisms of laryngotracheal injury following prolonged tracheal intubation. Chest 1989; 96:185–186.
6. Sasaki CT, Horiuchi M, Koss N. Tracheostomy related subglottic stenosis: bacteriologic pathogenesis. Laryngoscope 1979; 139:857–877.
7. Adams GL. Complications of tracheostomy. Perspect Crit Care 1990; 3(2):105–123.
8. Jones DK, Davies RJ. Massive hemoptysis. Br Med J 1990; 300:889–890.
9. Thomas R, Siproudhis L, Laurent JF, et al. Massive hemoptysis from iatrogenic balloon catheter rupture of pulmonary artery: successful early management by balloon tamponade. Crit Care Med 1987; 15:772–773.
10. Haponik EF, Rothfeld B, Britt ES, Bleecker ER. Radionuclide localization of massive pulmonary hemorrhage. Chest 1984; 86:208–212.

SUGGESTED READING

Airway Management

Stone DJ, Gal TJ. Airway management. In: Miller RD, ed. Anesthesia, 3d ed. New York: Churchill Livingstone, 1990, 1265–1292.

Wilson RS. Upper airway problems. Resp Care 1992; 37:533–550.

Difficult Intubation

Crosby ET, Lui A. The adult spine: implications for airway management. Can J Anaesth 1990; 37:77–93.

Davies JM, Weeks S, Crone LA, Pavlin EG. Difficult intubation in the parturient. Can J Anaesth 1989; 36:668–674.

King TA, Adams AP. Failed tracheal intubation. Br J Anaesth 1990; 65:400–414.

Mallampati SR, Gatt SP, Gugino LD, et al. A clinical sign to predict difficult tracheal intubation: a prospective study. Can Anaesth Soc J 1985; 32:429–434.

Samsoon GLT, Young JRB. Difficult tracheal intubation: a retrospective study. Anaesthesiology 1987; 42:487–490.

Tracheostomy

Adams GL. Complications of tracheostomy. Perspect Crit Care 1990; 3(2):105–123.

Berlauk JF. Intubation in the ICU: a review from a different perspective. Perspect Crit Care 1990; 3(2):89–107.

Hemoptysis

Metzdorff MT, Vogelzang RL, LoCicero J, et al. Transcatheter broncheal artery embolization in the multimodality management of massive hemoptysis. Chest 1990; 97:1494–1496.

Wedzicka JA, Pearson MC. Management of massive hemoptysis. Resp Med 1990; 84:9–12.

31
Mechanical Ventilator Support

Karl L. Yang
Herman Hospital, Louisville, Kentucky, USA

Guillermo Guiterrez
University of Texas Medical School, Houston, Texas, USA

The primary goal of mechanical ventilatory support in critically ill patients is to help the lungs eliminate carbon dioxide produced by cellular metabolic processes while waiting for the underlying disease to resolve. Furthermore, endotracheal intubation permits positive-pressure ventilation, which may improve oxygenation. Therefore, mechanical ventilation serves two functions: ventilation, or removal of carbon dioxide, and oxygenation, the enrichment of blood with oxygen (Table 1).

Management of respiratory failure begins with the identification of the patient with respiratory distress. Evaluation should begin with clinical findings. One of the most easily evaluated clinical variables is the respiratory rate. Nearly all patients with respiratory distress demonstrate tachypnea. A respiratory rate of 25 breaths/min or greater is a sensitive indicator of respiratory dysfunction. Tachypnea should be given careful consideration in all patients. Another important clinical sign of respiratory distress is the use of accessory muscles of breathing. These muscles include the strap muscles, the abdominal muscles, and the intercostal muscles. Further clinical signs of worsening respiratory failure include those of increased sympathetic tone. Tachycardia, hypertension, and diaphoresis, along with an increased respiratory rate, indicate impending respiratory collapse. When these signs are present, the patient will almost certainly require ventilatory support, and careful consideration should be given to instituting positive-pressure ventilation via endotracheal intubation. More commonly, the critical care physician must determine the need for intubation and mechanical ventilation when patients demonstrate some degree of decompensation, but not overt respiratory failure. If the patient is sufficiently stable to allow more information to be gathered, a decision concerning intubation and mechanical ventilation can be aided by obtaining information about gas exchange and the mechanics of ventilation.

GAS EXCHANGE

Adequate gas exchange requires saturation of the hemoglobin molecules with oxygen and elimination of carbon dioxide to prevent acid–base imbalance. Practically, arterial blood

Table 1 Arterial Blood Variables Affected by Ventilation and Oxygenation

	Ventilation	Oxygenation
Variables controlled by clinician	Minute ventilation	FIO_2
Variables affected	PCO_2	PO_2
	pH	O_2 saturation

gas measurements are used to assess gas exchange of both oxygen and carbon dioxide simultaneously. A useful clinical target for adequate oxygenation is a PaO_2 that provides an arterial oxygen saturation of 90% or more. Another helpful measure is the PaO_2/FIO_2. A ratio of less than 250 suggests serious ventilation/perfusion mismatch. Hypoxemia alone should raise another question. Is loss of functional residual capacity from atelectasis, for example, the cause of hypoxemia? Is compliance decreased enough to make a patient's work of breathing excessive and produce further loss of lung volume? Such patients may require an intervention to improve compliance. Some of these patients may be candidates for continuous positive airway pressure (CPAP). If CPAP is successful, endotracheal intubation and mechanical ventilation may be avoided. $PaCO_2$ provides a clinical measure of CO_2 elimination and alveolar ventilation. Inability to excrete sufficient CO_2 to maintain a normal blood pH results in respiratory acidosis. Chronic obstructive lung disease may produce respiratory acidosis, indicated by CO_2 retention and elevated $PaCO_2$, that is partially compensated by renal mechanisms and results in minimal acidemia. If the $PaCO_2$ is elevated such that an acute respiratory acidosis is present, the patient may require endotracheal intubation and mechanical ventilatory support. A pulse oximeter provides no information about $PaCO_2$. Use of the pulse oximeter alone, without the additional information of arterial blood gas analysis, may provide insufficient information in the SICU.

RESPIRATORY MECHANICS

Patients may require ventilator support if the effort required to maintain normal arterial blood gases is excessive. Variables that reflect the work of breathing include respiratory rate, vital capacity, and expired minute ventilation. For example, a patient is unlikely to maintain the effort necessary to continue a respiratory rate of 30–35 breaths/min. Patients who have markedly diminished vital capacity, <10–12 ml/kg, are unlikely to maintain adequate ventilation. Finally, patients with large minute ventilations, the product of respiratory rate and tidal volume, also are unlikely to sustain the effort necessary to maintain gas exchange. Average minute ventilation for unstressed individuals of average size is ~7 L/min, but somewhat more minute ventilation can be sustained. If gas exchange is adequate, the patient does not have signs of respiratory collapse, and respiratory mechanics appear to be compromised, a trial of CPAP may be worthwhile. If CPAP improves lung compliance and reduces the work of breathing, the patient may be able to avoid intubation and mechanical ventilation. Figure 1 summarizes clinical guidelines for ventilator support. The flowchart is meant as a guide: the clinician may need to deviate from the flowchart for specific patients.

Once the decision has been made to intubate and mechanically ventilate the patient, several additional decisions must be made, including modes of ventilation, recommended settings of respiratory rate, inspired gas concentration, the use of positive end-expiratory pressure (PEEP), and appropriate tidal volumes. Chapter 62 contains a discussion of variables that are useful in monitoring pulmonary function.

Ventilator Support

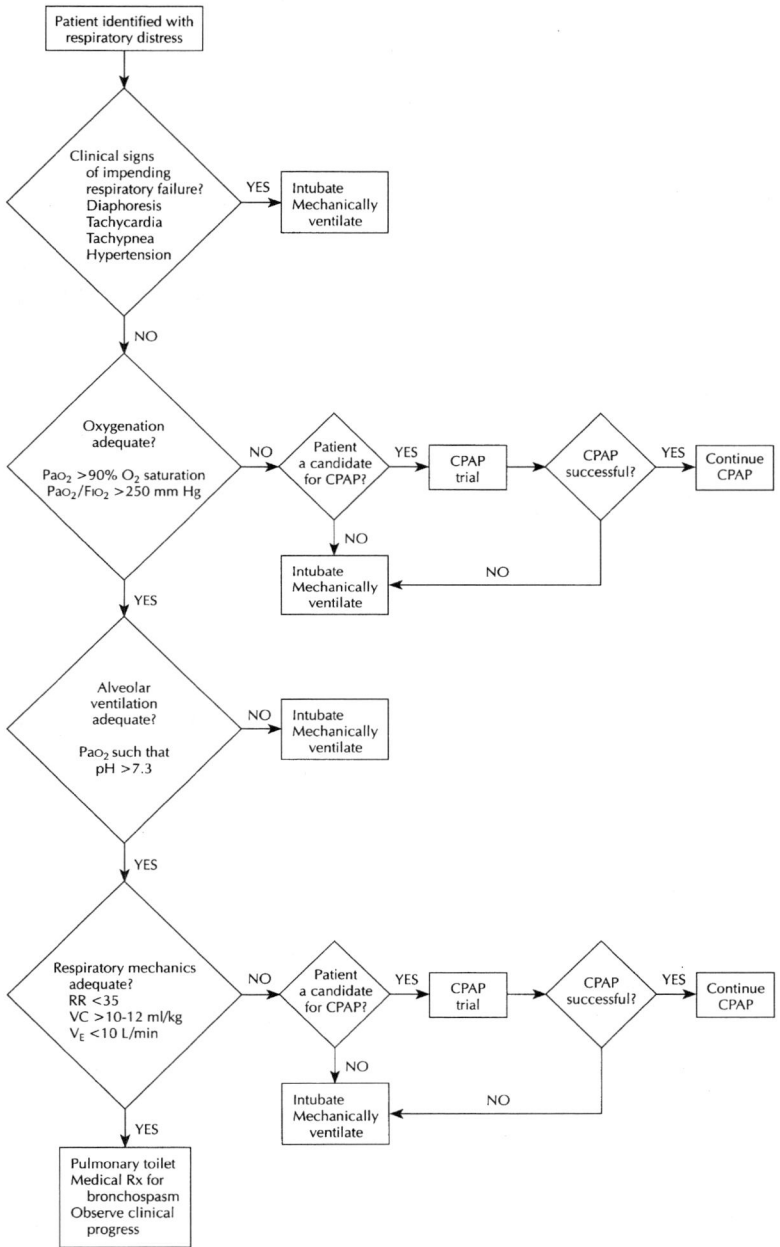

Figure 1 Criteria for instituting mechanical ventilator support.

MODES OF VENTILATION

The two major modes of mechanical ventilation are negative-pressure ventilation, akin to the normal physiologic function in which air moves into the lungs in response to negative pleural pressure, and positive-pressure ventilation, in which air is pushed onto the lungs by increases in airway pressure. Negative-pressure ventilation was widely used during the polio epidemic of the 1940s and 1950s (the "iron lungs"), and it remains a viable alternative in patients with neuromuscular disorders and compliant lungs. However, the vast majority of critically ill patients with respiratory failure have stiff lungs, and ventilating them with a negative-pressure device is impossible. Consequently, positive-pressure ventilation has been the standard ventilatory method for the last 25 years. This chapter reviews some modes of positive-pressure mechanical ventilation and the indications for their use.

Positive-pressure ventilators may be either volume cycled or pressure cycled. Although volume cycled ventilators have been used most frequently for ventilatory support in intensive care units, newer ventilators offer refined modes of pressure cycled ventilation. In volume cycled ventilation, a preset flow rate and volume are delivered by the ventilator. The pressure in the ventilator increases until the lungs and associated ventilator circuit reach the set volume. Inspiratory flow is a value set by the clinician in most volume cycled ventilators. With a preset volume and preset inspiratory flow rate, the inspiratory time is determined. Figure 2 shows typical pressure (PAW) vs. time and flow ($\dot{V}$) vs. time waveforms for volume cycled ventilation.

In contrast, pressure cycled ventilators deliver flow until a preset pressure is reached. The tidal volume that is delivered is determined by the patient's lung compliance. Inspiratory time varies and is determined by how rapidly the pressure limit is reached. Splinting or fighting the ventilator can terminate inspiration prematurely and produce an inadequate tidal volume. Because pressure cycled ventilation does not deliver a guaranteed tidal volume, volume cycled ventilators have been the mainstay in intensive care units. Figure 3 shows typical pressure (PAW) vs. time and flow ($\dot{V}$) vs. time waveforms for pressure cycled ventilation.

Three basic modes of positive-pressure mechanical ventilation are control-mode ventilation (CMV), assist-control ventilation (ACV), and intermittent mandatory ventilation (IMV).

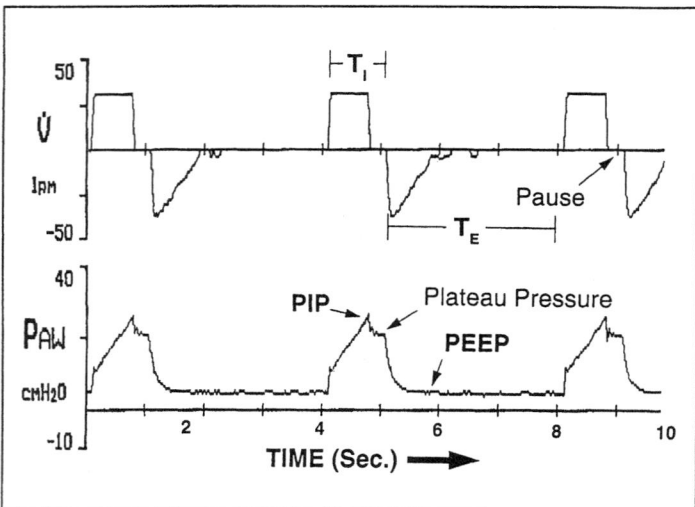

Figure 2 Volume limited ventilation.

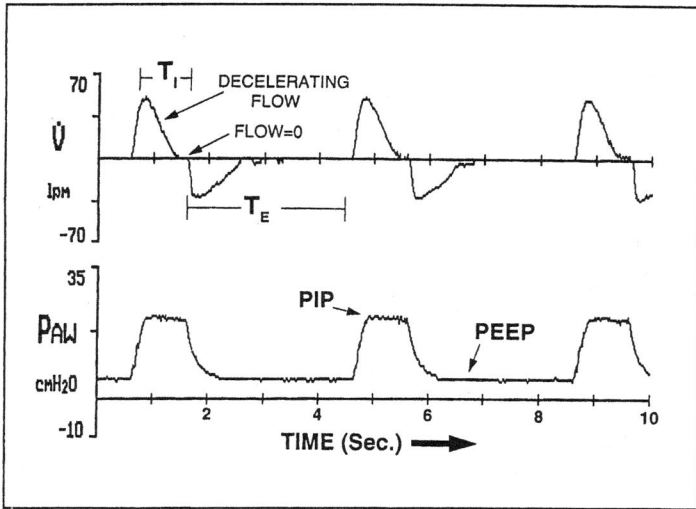

Figure 3 Pressure limited ventilation.

Control Mode Ventilation (CMV)

The oldest mode of ventilation is CMV, in which a preset tidal volume is delivered at specified time intervals and at a given flow rate. Total ventilation is regulated by the physician, who determines the respiratory rate and tidal volume delivered by the ventilator. With this mode of ventilation, spontaneous efforts by the patient do not trigger the ventilator to deliver a breath (1). CMV is rarely used today because the patient has no control of ventilator functions, and the support required may vary according to the metabolic activity of the tissues. As a result of this lack of cooperation between the patient and the ventilator, struggles against the ventilator can be extremely uncomfortable or dangerous unless the patient is sedated. This mode has little use in the intensive care unit. It should be used only if the patient is apneic, paralyzed, or deeply sedated and the respiratory drive is depressed. By assuming control of the patient's ventilation, the physician also becomes fully responsible for the maintenance of adequate gas exchange. Therefore, careful observation and frequent blood gas tests are mandatory.

Assist-Control Ventilation (ACV)

ACV was developed to overcome the major disadvantage of CMV, lack of patient–ventilator feedback interaction. This mode allows the patient to augment the preset minute ventilation by delivering additional tidal volume whenever the patient produces a negative inspiratory effort. A pressure transducer detects the reduced airway pressure and triggers the ventilator to deliver the preset tidal volume. In newer ventilators, a flow trigger may be used. If the patient fails to initiate a spontaneous effort, a predetermined number of breaths (backup rate) with a set tidal volume will be delivered to the patient to ensure adequate ventilation. In other words, the patient receives a guaranteed minimum minute ventilation. Because the ventilator assists on every spontaneous breath, minute ventilation can be increased with minimal increases in the work of breathing. ACV is frequently used for full ventilatory support of critically ill patients. Although the work of breathing is usually decreased with this mode of ventilation, a decrease in the work of breathing may not always be the case. Significant muscular effort may result from improper ventilator setup (2).

Intermittent Mandatory Ventilation (IMV)

IMV is a common mode of mechanical ventilation. With IMV, the ventilator delivers a fixed number of breaths at a predetermined tidal volume, but in between those breaths the patient is allowed to breathe spontaneously at the tidal volume developed by the patient's own efforts. To avoid air stacking of ventilator-initiated and spontaneous breaths, the ventilator-initiated breath is synchronized with the patient's own inspiratory effort. This mode is termed "synchronized intermittent mandatory ventilation" (SIMV). By initially setting a high ventilatory rate, most of the work of breathing is done by the ventilator. As the patient's respiratory function improves, the ventilator-initiated breaths may be gradually decreased. The patient then assumes a greater load of the work associated with breathing. The patient's minute ventilation during IMV is the sum of the ventilator-initiated breaths at the predetermined tidal volume and the patient's spontaneous breaths, with their associated tidal volumes. SIMV was originally developed as a method to wean difficult patients from mechanical ventilation. Such an approach avoids the stresses imposed on the patient and the demands imposed on the staff for close supervision by a T-tube weaning procedure, in which the patient is disconnected from the ventilator and observed for a short time. During these trials, breathing occurs through the endotracheal tube attached to a T piece (3). Clinical studies do not support the efficacy of IMV over other modes of ventilatory support for weaning, reducing detrimental hemodynamic side effects, preventing muscular atrophy, and reducing the incidence of respiratory alkalosis (4–13). The patient's underlying condition is more likely to be the major contributing factor to the development of respiratory alkalosis than the mode of ventilation chosen.

A major disadvantage of SIMV is the presence of a demand valve that is actuated by the patient's breathing effort. The purpose of this valve is to allow spontaneous breaths. It opens when the airway pressure becomes negative as the patient initiates a breath and allows the gas mixture to flow into the ventilator circuit and into the lungs. Because of the large negative pressure required to open this valve in some ventilators, and the delay of fresh gas inflow required to meet the demand of the patient, the work of breathing in a patient hungry for air may be extremely high. Note that improper selection of ventilator settings causes further distress to the already fatigued muscles of respiration by forcing them to work excessively. By carefully observing the patient and by appropriately adjusting the ventilator settings, the patient's discomfort during mechanical ventilation can be minimized, if not totally avoided.

Other Ventilator Variables

In addition to the mode of ventilation, a number of other settings should be specified when writing mechanical ventilation orders. These additional variables include the respiratory rate, FIO_2, PEEP, tidal volume, trigger sensitivity, ventilator flow pattern, and inspiratory time.

Respiratory Rate

One of the goals of mechanical ventilation is prevention of respiratory muscle from fatiguing. Selection of a respiratory rate that meets the patient's ventilatory requirement is important. Generally, the backup rate may be set 2–4 breaths/min fewer than the patient's spontaneous respiratory rate. This number of breaths should provide adequate ventilation and prevent serious hypoventilation if the patient becomes apneic.

Oxygen Concentration in Inspired Gas

An adequate FIO_2 is important to prevent arterial hypoxemia. How much oxygen should be given to a patient depends on the level of arterial oxygen saturation. As a guideline, use the lowest possible FIO_2 capable of maintaining an arterial oxygen saturation >90%. The rationale for using low levels of FIO_2 is the avoidance of oxygen toxicity, which may occur even at relatively low levels of FIO_2. An FIO_2 of 1 can produce toxicity in 24–48 h; whereas, the use of an FIO_2 of 0.50 or less for a long time (up to several weeks) is generally considered safe (14).

Positive End-Expiratory Pressure

If necessary, PEEP should be used to keep the FIO_2 at or below 0.50. The effects of PEEP on cardiac output and oxygen transport should be considered when using this therapeutic modality. The use of PEEP is indicated in patients with severe hypoxemia, such as those with adult respiratory distress syndrome, as it improves oxygenation and minimizes the risk of oxygen toxicity. PEEP improves oxygenation by recruiting previously closed alveoli for gas exchange (15). PEEP also may help redistribute the fluid in partially filled alveoli from the center to the periphery (16) to facilitate better gas exchange. The major complications of PEEP are hemodynamic compromise and barotrauma (17). PEEP levels of ≥ 10 cm H_2O can result in hemodynamic instability as venous return decreases, and the interventricular septum is either stiffened or displaced into the left ventricle. These changes impede diastolic filling and decrease stroke volume. A flow-directed pulmonary artery catheter can be of great value in monitoring the intrathoracic hemodynamics when using high levels of PEEP.

Patients with severe airway obstruction may exhibit a phenomenon termed "intrinsic PEEP." This term describes the presence of a positive intrathoracic pressure at the end of expiration when the expiratory time is not long enough to allow full exhalation of the tidal volume. In mechanically ventilated patients with obstructive airway disease, a significant level of intrinsic PEEP occurs 60% of the time (18). Hemodynamic compromise may also result from high levels of intrinsic PEEP. To decrease the effect of intrinsic PEEP, intensive bronchodilation, a longer expiratory time, or PEEP ventilation at a slightly lower level than the intrinsic PEEP may be tried (see Chapters 25 and 62).

Tidal Volume

Tidal volume may be set at 5–15 mL/kg body weight. The use of smaller tidal volumes is preferable, because an excessively large tidal volume can increase lung injury. High tidal volumes are also associated with increased intrathoracic pressure, which in some situations may cause hemodynamic instability. Proponents of using large tidal volumes argue that such a strategy prevents alveolar collapse, a phenomenon thought to be a consequence of the higher mean airway pressure (19,20). A recent but controversial study published by the Acute Respiratory Distress Syndrome (ARDS) Network demonstrated improved survival in patients with acute lung injury and ARDS who were treated with lower tidal volumes when compared with those managed with traditional tidal volumes (21).

Trigger Sensitivity

Trigger sensitivity is the level of negative pressure that a patient is required to generate before the ventilator senses the effort and delivers a breath in assist-control and pressure-support modes. Usually, the trigger sensitivity is set at -2 cm H_2O. The setting is important, because a large negative trigger sensitivity can increase the work of breathing by forcing the patient to generate large negative inspiratory pressures in order to trigger the ventilator. In such cases, the patient's work of breathing with a ventilator may exceed the work of spontaneous breathing (22,23). A more positive trigger sensitivity than -2 cm H_2O may be inappropriate and result in advertent triggering and hyperventilation. Trigger sensitivity should be carefully titrated by observing the patient's breathing pattern.

Ventilator Flow Patterns

Most ventilators have two flow patterns: the square wave flow, in which flow remains constant during much of inspiration, and decelerating flow pattern, in which an initial high inspiratory flow is gradually tapered. Conflicting information exists concerning the influence of flow pattern on the work of breathing and on gas exchange. One study showed no significant differences in gas exchange in patients ventilated with either flow pattern (24), although a decelerating pattern resulted in lower mean airway pressure. Another study showed that a decelerating flow pattern resulted in better oxygenation and increased respiratory system compliance (25). A high inspiratory flow rate also improves gas exchange and ventilation distribution (26) and reduces the work of breathing (23,27) in patients with chronic obstructive pulmonary disease. This improvement appears to be related to the prolongation of expiratory time. Excessively low flow rates may cause dyspnea, air-hunger, and tachypnea, despite adequate ventilation.

Safety Features

Every ventilator has a number of alarms designed to alert the health care team when certain ventilatory measurements of function are exceeded or not met. Given the importance of ventilation to the patient's survival, these alarms should be heeded immediately. If the caregiver is unsure of an alarm's origin, the patient should be disconnected from the ventilator and ventilated manually.

To prevent barotrauma, the peak airway pressure limit can be specified, and, when it exceeds the specified pressure, an expiratory valve opens to prevent further increase in airway pressure. However, adequate ventilation may not be delivered to the patient, if the high pressure limit is frequently exceeded and significant volume is lost through the expiratory valve. Peak airway pressure can be reduced by lowering the tidal volume, decreasing the inspiratory flow rate, and lowering airway resistance. Inspiratory flow rate is also important, because an inappropriate flow rate can increase the patient's work of breathing with the ventilator (2,23). For a normal lung, a respiratory flow rate of <60 L/min is adequate. For someone with increased respiratory drive, a higher flow rate (80 L/min) may be more appropriate (Table 2).

Table 2 Initial Settings for Mechanical Ventilation

Factor	Setting
Mode	ACV or SIMV
Respiratory frequency	Two breaths below spontaneous
Tidal volume	10 mL/kg body weight for height
FIO_2	1.0 initially, then titrate to keep $SaO_2 > 90\%$
Inspiratory flow rate	60–80 liters/min
Trigger sensitivity	-2 cm H_2O
PEEP	Use if required to maintain $SaO_2 > 90\%$ with $FIO_2 \leq 0.5$

Other Modes of Mechanical Ventilation

Pressure-Support Ventilation

Pressure-support ventilation (PSV) can be used to provide full ventilatory support and to wean patients from the ventilator. During PSV, each spontaneous breath is augmented by a predetermined pressure. PSV is triggered by the patient's effort to breathe, and inspiratory flow continues while the airway pressure rapidly approaches the predetermined level. The positive inspiratory pressure is terminated when the inspiratory flow rate has decreased to a specified rate (5 L/min in some ventilators and 25% of peak flow in others). PSV is not recommended in patients with high respiratory impedance (28). PSV in these patients leads to a severe respiratory acidosis when the patient is apneic. High-pressure support levels may be comparable to assist-control ventilation with respect to providing nearly all of the patient's work of breathing.

A major advantage of PSV over other modes of ventilation is that the patient can control the respiratory rate, duration of inspiration, and inspiratory flow rate; therefore, better synchronization between mechanical ventilation and spontaneous breathing can be achieved. This property may explain why PSV is better tolerated and more comfortable for the patient than other modes (29). A number of studies have demonstrated the usefulness of PSV in ventilatory support, especially during weaning. Furthermore, because of the increased airway resistance from the endotracheal tube, some physicians use a small amount of pressure support (usually 5–10 cm H_2O) to overcome this resistance. Extubation from this level of support is usually well tolerated.

Airway Pressure Release Ventilation

With airway pressure release ventilation (APRV), the patient receives CPAP that is transiently decreased during expiration. The duration of pressure release is ~ 1.5 s. The theory behind APRV is that airway pressure should be kept at a positive level for as much of the respiratory cycle as possible in order to stabilize those alveoli which tend to collapse. APRV theoretically should help improve oxygenation, although its major advantage is a lower peak airway pressure than conventional intermittent positive-pressure ventilation. Yet mean airway pressure may be higher. Its principal use is the support of patients with extremely poor lung compliance, for example, patients with severe ARDS.

High-Frequency Ventilation

High-frequency ventilation (HFV) is a concept totally different from that of intermittent positive pressure. With HFV, the respiratory frequency is substantially greater, and the tidal volumes are much less than those used in conventional ventilation. The three types of HFV are (1) high-frequency positive-pressure ventilation, (2) high-frequency jet ventilation, and (3) high-frequency oscillation.

HFV, with lower intrathoracic pressure swings as a result of the relatively small tidal volume delivered, results in lower peak airway pressure. On the other hand, the incidence of barotrauma with HFV has been reported to be similar to that of CMV in a number of studies (30). HFV has been reported to be more effective than conventional positive-pressure ventilation in patients with large bronchopleural fistulae (31). Clinical trials with HFV showed that patients with relatively normal lung compliance experienced better gas exchange than those with decreased lung compliance (32). Another theoretic advantage of HFV is less hemodynamic compromise than that found with CMV. As discussed in Chapter 25, the reduced magnitude of intrathoracic pressure swings may improve cardiac function. However, clinical studies have not supported these claims (33). Because HFV requires high flow rates, its operation can result in dangerous levels of air trapping and intrathoracic pressure increases. Patients with obstructive disease and those with increased lung compliance are especially at risk. In summary, HFV has no clear advantage over CMV, and its operation requires considerable expertise. Its application in clinical practice has been limited.

SUMMARY

- The major goals of mechanical ventilation are support of ventilation in a patient who cannot sustain the work of breathing and improved oxygenation through the use of positive pressure and increased FIO_2.
- Criteria for endotracheally intubating and mechanically supporting patients include clinical features, gas exchange, and respiratory mechanics (see Fig. 1).
- Positive-pressure ventilators are either volume cycled or pressure cycled. Volume cycled ventilators deliver a preset volume at a preset inspiratory flow. Pressure cycled ventilators deliver a tidal volume that is dependent on the compliance of the lungs with an inspiratory time determined by the rate at which the preset pressure is achieved.
- In general, when using volume cycled ventilation, use a backup respiratory rate of 2–4 breaths/min less than the patient's spontaneous respiratory rate.
- Use the lowest FIO_2 to produce an arterial oxygen saturation of >90%.
- PEEP is generally indicated in the management of severe hypoxemia.
- Lung protective strategies with lower tidal volumes and lower associated plateau pressures are likely to be beneficial.

REFERENCES

1. Bonner JT, Hall JR. Respiratory Intensive Care of the Adult Patient. St. Louis: CV Mosby, 1985:90.
2. Marini JJ, Capps JS, Culver BH. The inspiratory work of breathing during assisted mechanical ventilation. Chest 1985; 87:612.

3. Downs JB, Klein EF, Desautels et al. Intermittent mandatory ventilation: a new approach to weaning patients from mechanical ventilation. Chest 1973; 64:331.
4. Hastings PR, Bushnell LS, Skillman JJ, et al. Cardiorespiratory dynamics during weaning with IMV versus spontaneous ventilation in good-risk cardiac-surgery patients. Anesthesiology 1980; 58:429.
5. Schachter EN, Tucker D, Beck GJ. Does intermittent mandatory ventilation accelerate weaning? JAMA 1981; 246:1210.
6. Kirby RR, Downs JB, Civetta JM, et al. High level positive end-expiratory pressure (PEEP) in acute respiratory insufficiency. Chest 1975; 67:156.
7. Downs JB, Douglas ME, Sanfelippo PM, et al. Ventilatory pattern, intrapleural pressure, and cardiac output. Anesth Analg 1977; 56:88.
8. Hudson LD, Tooker J, Haisch C, et al. Comparison of assisted ventilation and PEEP with IMV and CPAP in ARDS patients [abstract]. Am Rev Respir Dis 1978; 177:129.
9. Downs JB, Block AJ, Venum KB. Intermittent mandatory ventilation in the treatment of patients with chronic obstructive pulmonary disease. Anesth Analg 1974; 55:437.
10. Petty TL. Intermittent mandatory ventilation reconsidered. Crit Care Med 1981; 9:620.
11. Christopher KL, Neff TA, Bowman JL, et al. Demand and continuous flow intermittent mandatory ventilation systems. Chest 1985; 87:625.
12. Op't Holt TB, Hall MW, Bass JB, et al. Comparison of changes in airway pressure during continuous positive airway pressure (CPAP) between demand valve and continuous flow devices. Respir Care 1982; 82:1200.
13. Culpepper JA, Rinaldo JE, Rogers RM. Effect of mechanical ventilator mode on tendency towards respiratory alkalosis. Am Rev Respir Dis 1979; 120:1039.
14. Bryan CL, Jenkinson SG. Oxygen toxicity. Clin Chest Med 1988; 9:141–152.
15. Katz JA, Ozanne GM, Zinn SE, et al. Time course and mechanisms of lung volume increase with PEEP in acute pulmonary failure. Anesthesiology 1981; 54:9.
16. Malo J, Ali J, Wood LDH. How does positive end-expiratory pressure reduce intrapulmonary shunt in canine pulmonary edema? J Appl Physiol 1984; 57:1002.
17. Quist J, Ponto PP, Idan H, Wilson RS, et al. Hemodynamic response to mechanical ventilation with PEEP. The effect of hypervolemia. Anesthesiology 1981; 55:53.
18. Rossi A, Gonfried SB, Zocchi L. Measurements of static lung compliance of the total respiratory system in patients with acute respiratory failure during mechanical ventilation: the effect of intrinsic positive end-expiratory pressure. Am Rev Respir Dis 1985; 131:672.
19. Burnham SC, Martin WE, Cheney FW. The effects of various tidal volumes on gas exchange in pulmonary edema. Anesthesiology 1972; 37:27.
20. Bendixen HH, Bulwinkle B, Hedley-White J, Laver MB. Atelectasis and shunting during spontaneous ventilation in anesthetized patients. Anesthesiology 1964; 25:297.
21. Ventilation with lower tidal volumes as compared with traditional tidal volumes for acute lung injury and the acute respiratory distress syndrome. New Engl J Med 2000; 342:1301–1308.
22. Ayres SM, Kozam RL, Lukas DS. The effects of intermittent positive pressure breathing on intrathoracic pressure, pulmonary mechanics, and the work of breathing. Am Rev Respir Dis 1976; 87:370.
23. Marini JJ, Rodriguez RM, Lamb V. The inspiratory workload of patient-initiated mechanical ventilation. Am Rev Respir Dis 1986; 134:902.
24. Johansson H. Effects of breathing mechanics and gas exchange of different inspiratory gas flow patterns in patients undergoing respiratory treatment. Acta Anaesth Scan 1975; 19:19.
25. Al-Saady N, Bennett ED. Decelerating inspiratory flow waveform improves lung mechanics and gas exchange in patients on intermittent positive pressure ventilation. Intens Care Med 1985; 11:68.
26. Connors AF, McCaffree DR, Gray BA. Effect of inspiratory flow rate on gas exchange during mechanical ventilation. Am Rev Respir Dis 1981; 124:537.

27. Sassoon CSH, Mahutte CK, Te T, et al. Work of breathing and airway occlusion pressure during assist-mode mechanical ventilation. Chest 1988; 93:571.
28. Marinin JJ. Mechanical ventilation. In: Simmons DH, ed. Current Pulmonology, Vol. 9. Chicago, Year Book, 1988:165.
29. MacIntyre NR. Respiratory function during pressure support ventilation. Chest 1986; 89:677.
30. High-frequency oscillatory ventilation compared with conventional mechanical ventilation in the treatment of respiratory failure in premature infants. N Engl J Med 1989; 320:88.
31. Carlon G, Ray C Jr, Klain M, et al. High frequency positive pressure ventilation in management of a patient with bronchopleural fistula. Anesthesiology 1980; 52:160.
32. Turnbull A, Carlton G, Howland W, et al. High frequency jet ventilation in major airway or pulmonary disruption. Ann Thorac Surg 1981; 32:468.
33. Traverse J, Korvenranta H, Adams E, et al. Cardiovascular effects of high frequency oscillatory and jet ventilation. Chest 1989; 96:1400.

32
Discontinuation of Mechanical Ventilation

Paul Druck
VA Medical Center, Minneapolis, Minnesota, USA

INTRODUCTION

Ideally, mechanical ventilatory support is discontinued as soon as it is no longer required. Unfortunately, identifying when this point is reached in the course of a patient's illness may be difficult. Failure to recognize that a patient is able to breathe spontaneously results in excess ventilator days, increased hospital and ICU lengths of stay and costs, added stress for the patient and family, and, of greatest importance, increased ventilator-associated complications, notably ventilator-associated pneumonia. On the other hand, premature discontinuation of support results in respiratory distress and the need for reintubation. Failed extubation is associated with significant morbidity and mortality (mortality as high as 40% in some series) (1–4). Although the marked morbidity and mortality among patients failing extubation undoubtedly reflect the morbidity of the underlying diseases causing the respiratory failure, reintubation itself is associated with complications such as airway trauma and aspiration (5,6). Additionally, the interval of respiratory distress preceding reintubation may cause respiratory fatigue, which can further delay ultimate weaning, as well as further deterioration in an already compromised patient. For all these reasons, the ability to accurately determine the earliest time when a patient is fully able to resume spontaneous ventilation is of great importance.

Several related issues must be considered. First, should the patient undergo a program of gradually reduced ventilatory support that leads to discontinuation, or should periodic tests of spontaneous breathing be tried? Second, if gradual reduction of support is chosen, which is the best support mode to use, and how should it be reduced? Third, if spontaneous breathing trials (SBTs) are used, what type of trial and of what duration is most appropriate?

Discussions of discontinuation of ventilator support demonstrate inconsistencies in terminology. The term "to wean" has been used in the literature to refer to both the gradual reduction of ventilatory support and the final discontinuation of it. The American College of Chest Physicians has defined weaning as "the gradual reduction of ventilatory support and its replacement with spontaneous ventilation (7)." For clarity and consistency, the term "to wean" will be used in this chapter to refer to a gradual reduction of ventilatory support; the term "to extubate" will refer to the final discontinuation of ventilatory support (whether delivered via endotracheal tube or tracheostomy tube).

Of note, the requirements for extubation exceed those for simple discontinuation of ventilatory support. A patient who is able to spontaneously ventilate may still require a secure airway if that patient is at especially high risk for aspiration, at risk for upper airway obstruction, or is unable to clear respiratory secretions.

APPROACHES TO DISCONTINUATION OF VENTILATORY SUPPORT

The Earliest Approach: Weaning Criteria and T-Piece Trials

The earliest forms of positive pressure ventilation (controlled and assisted-controlled ventilation) excluded significant patient effort and made determination of a patient's respiratory ability while still receiving support impossible. This feature of older modes of ventilator support required disconnecting the ventilator from the airway device (endotracheal or tracheostomy tube) and observing the patient during the complete absence of support. Because a patient who was still severely compromised might quickly develop respiratory distress, these so-called "T-piece trials" required constant patient supervision and were labor and resource intensive. These limitations made identifying clinical criteria, which would predict ventilatory (in)sufficiency and thus avoid repeated, unsuccessful T-piece trials, desirable. In pursuit of this goal, many "weaning criteria" were proposed. The criteria most frequently used were originally proposed by Sahn et al. in 1973 (8,9) (Table 1), and subsequently modified. These, and a multitude of later criteria, lacked sufficient predictive accuracy, in part because they were tests of *maximal* rather than *sustainable* effort. When these criteria are used, a final confirmatory SBT is still necessary.

The rapid shallow breathing index of Tobin and Yang is a quantification of an often-used qualitative assessment (10). It is often lumped with the other predictive criteria, although, unlike these other criteria, it is not used to predict the suitability of a patient for a T-piece trial. Rather, it is used to assess the progress of an ongoing weaning or spontaneous breathing trial. It is calculated as the respiratory rate divided by the tidal volume in liters and has good discriminative value at 105 breaths/min/L. Patients with higher values have a high likelihood of requiring continued ventilatory support, whereas patients with lower values have a high likelihood of successful spontaneous ventilation.

"Weaning Modes" of Ventilation: The Tapered Support Method

Since the 1970s, so-called "weaning modes" of ventilation such as synchronized intermittent mandatory ventilation (SIMV) and, later, pressure support ventilation (PSV)

Table 1 Traditional Weaning Criteria

1. Resting minute ventilation ≤ 10 L/min
2. Maximal voluntary ventilation greater than or equal to twice minute ventilation
3. Tidal volume ≥ 5 mL/kg
4. Vital capacity ≥ 10 mL/kg
5. Maximum inspiratory force more negative than -20 cm H_2O
6. Acceptable PaO_2 with $FiO_2 \leq 0.4$ and PEEP ≤ 5 cm H_2O

have been developed. These modes permit the gradual reduction of ventilatory support while the patient assumes increasing amounts of the work of breathing. When the patient has assumed all, or nearly all, of the work of breathing (stable with minimal ventilator support), the patient, logically, is ready for extubation. This tapering, empirical approach to discontinuation of support has become popular and widespread, and obviates the need for predictive criteria. However, the observation that >50% of patients who were "prematurely" extubated (either by self-extubation or inadvertent tube dislodgement during care) were able to breathe spontaneously and did not require reintubation has created concern that this approach may delay recognition that the patient is ready for extubation (11,12). In addition, a randomized, prospective trial has demonstrated that gradual reduction of support according to a rigid schedule may delay extubation when compared with repeated SBTs (see Protocol Weaning, below) (13).

If the tapered support method of weaning is to demonstrate in a *timely way* that the patient is ready for weaning, then ventilatory support must be reduced *each day* to the *lowest level* consistent with the patient's ability to adequately ventilate without distress or progressive fatigue. However, a commonplace approach is reduction of support according to some arbitrary schedule, such as decreasing IMV rate by 2 breaths per minute each day, or pressure support level by 2 cm H_2O daily, without attempting to determine if the patient would tolerate a more rapid reduction. These strategies may commit a patient who is rapidly improving to a longer course of ventilation than is required. Another problem with the gradual taper method is that in circumstances of frequently rotating physician responsibility, the taper "plan" may change repeatedly (with respect to either mode or rate of taper), with resulting confusion and delay in the weaning process. Arguably, reducing support each day to the minimal adequate level will result in timely recognition of readiness for extubation.

Protocol Weaning

During the last decade, numerous studies have been conducted in which assessment of a patient's ability to breathe spontaneously is performed by nurses or respiratory therapists according to a defined "protocol." These protocols (usually called "weaning protocols," although they do not involve gradual reduction of support but, rather, are tests of spontaneous breathing) are generally designed as follows. The responsible physician makes a determination that the patient is a suitable candidate for reduction of ventilator support. This determination may be based on individual judgment or explicitly defined criteria, including: resolution of the original indication for mechanical ventilation, hemodynamic stability, adequate oxygenation without requirement for high inspired oxygen or PEEP, and adequate arterial blood gas determination without dyspnea or tachypnea at current level of ventilatory support (Table 2). If the patient is deemed suitable, a SBT consisting of some form of monitored, minimal support [e.g., T-piece, pressure support = 5 cm H_2O, continuous positive airway pressure (CPAP) = 5 cm H_2O, or SIMV = 2 breaths/min, as described later] is conducted by bedside providers (generally ICU nurses and/or respiratory therapists). If the patient is able to breathe adequately (as assessed by respiratory rate, vital signs, comfort, and arterial blood gas determination) for the prescribed period of time (usually 30–120 min), extubation is performed. If not, ventilatory support is resumed, and the test is repeated daily or more frequently. This approach is designed to eliminate unnecessarily gradual weaning, continually changing weaning

Table 2 Typical Criteria for "Protocol Weaning"

Initial screening criteria for entry into protocol:
  Improvement or resolution of original indication for mechanical ventilation
  Respiratory rate <35/min or RR/V_T ≤ 105, no dyspnea or agitation, and adequate arterial blood gas on current ventilator settings
  PaO_2/FiO_2 ≥ 200 on PEEP ≤ 5 cm H_2O
  Hemodynamically stable without vasopressor agents
  Minute ventilation <15 L/min
  Patient is awake and oriented

Criteria for extubation after SBT:
  Respiratory rate <35/min or RR/V_T ≤ 105, no dyspnea or agitation, and adequate arterial blood gas
  No significant increase in heart rate or change in blood pressure (increase or decrease)
  No need for continued secure airway

approaches, and dependence on the presence of physicians at the ICU bedside when other duties may supervene. In four prospective, randomized, controlled trials (14–17), this approach, as well as the physician-directed approach of Esteban et al. (13), has reduced the duration of mechanical ventilation.

What Constitutes an Adequate Trial of Spontaneous Breathing

Regardless of the weaning approach used, a trial of spontaneous breathing will usually be the final determinant of readiness for extubation. Controversy exists over the most appropriate mode of SBT. T-piece, low PSV or CPAP, or low SIMV rates have all been used. Low SIMV rates are associated with increased work of breathing (18–20) and have not compared well with the other minimal support modes (13,21). Esteban et al. found that PSV = +7 cm H_2O resulted in more rapid extubation than T-piece trials with no additional support. In this study, the reintubation rates were similar (4).

Endotracheal or tracheostomy tubes, demand valve ventilator circuits, and ventilator humidifiers impose significant additional work of breathing. The magnitude of this additional work will depend on the diameter of the endotracheal tube, the inspiratory flow rate, and the ventilator used (22–25). Low levels of CPAP or PSV have been proposed to compensate for this additional imposed work of breathing. Inadequate compensation may lead to underestimation of the patient's readiness for extubation and cause delay. On the other hand, excessive support results in a false sense of respiratory adequacy and an increased rate of failed extubation. The precise amount of inspiratory support required to overcome imposed work of breathing will vary significantly from patient to patient, is difficult to predict, and will be influenced by the variables mentioned above. However, when the additional imposed work of breathing has been measured, compensatory levels of support have ranged from 5 to as high as 22 cm H_2O PSV (26–30).

The duration of the SBT can also affect its ability to predict successful unassisted breathing. Too short a trial may fail to demonstrate a lesser degree of ventilatory insufficiency and result in failed extubation and the need for reintubation. Too long a trial, particularly if the conditions are such that the imposed work of breathing is significant but not adequately compensated for, may result in fatigue and unnecessarily delayed extubation.

Most published weaning protocols utilize SBTs of 30–120 min and report similar reintubation rates. Esteban et al. (31) randomized patients undergoing SBTs to 30 *or* 120 min trials. The number extubated and the number requiring reintubation within 48 h were the same in both groups.

Current Recommendations

Current literature supports the use of intermittent SBTs (T-piece, or PSV = 5 cm H_2O, for 30–120 min) for patients satisfying typical screening criteria (Table 2), followed by extubation if the patient is ventilating adequately without dyspnea or tachypnea. Conducting these trials more frequently than once per day has not been shown to accelerate weaning (13) and may cause excess fatigue. As much as 24 h may be required for resolution of severe diaphragmatic fatigue (32). That a chronically ventilator-dependent patient who fails an SBT will, without correction of a significant adverse factor, be able to ventilate only a few hours later is unlikely.

Although widely accepted as appropriate to offset additional work of breathing imposed by endotracheal tubes and ventilator circuits, 5 cm H_2O PSV or 5 cm H_2O CPAP may be inadequate for patients with smaller endotracheal tubes or higher minute ventilation requirements (and thus higher inspiratory flow rates) (see What Constitutes an Adequate Trial of Spontaneous Breathing, above). Cavo et al. (22) found that the resistance of an artificial airway exceeded that of the native airway for tracheostomy tubes <8 mm in diameter at 30 L/min flow, a low to moderate flow rate. Note that the combination of higher flow rates and smaller tubes produces a more than additive increase in work of breathing (30). Consequently, use of higher levels of compensatory support to achieve an accurate SBT may be appropriate. As measurement of imposed work of breathing for every patient and subsequent provision of precise compensation is impractical, judgment is required. Fiastro et al. (30) measured the level of PSV needed to compensate for imposed work of breathing for a range of endotracheal tube sizes and flow rates, and these data may be used as a guide.

Alternatively, an argument can be made for reducing ventilatory support each day to the lowest level consistent with adequate ventilation and patient comfort, and extubating the patient when that level is "minimal." Although logic supports this strategy, no controlled trials have compared this manner of weaning with protocol weaning.

FAILURE TO WEAN

When a patient fails to wean or requires reintubation, adequate ventilatory support must be re-instituted. The responsibility of the managing physician does not end with re-intubation. Determining the cause of the patient's continued respiratory insufficiency is extremely important for two reasons. First, it is desirable that the patient no longer require mechanical ventilation so that the risk of ventilator-associated complications, ICU and hospital lengths of stay and costs, and distress to the patient and family may be minimized. Second, failure to wean is often a consequence of other inapparent or overlooked pathology, and thus may serve as an important diagnostic "red flag". Understanding failure to wean requires examining reasons for failure to oxygenate and failure to ventilate. There is a multitude of reasons for failure to wean, so an organized diagnostic approach will save time, effort, and resources.

Failure to Oxygenate

The most common causes of hypoxemia severe enough to require continued mechanical ventilation are listed in Table 3. Lung auscultation and chest radiograph will often suffice in making a diagnosis. Occasionally, a CT scan will help elucidate the nature of a localized but poorly defined pulmonary infiltrate.

Failure to Ventilate (CO₂ Retention)

Failure to adequately excrete CO_2, with resulting hypercarbia and acidemia, is the most common cause of chronic ventilator dependency in adults. The algorithm in Figure 1 depicts an approach to diagnosing the underlying disorder. The first discriminator is the minute ventilation required to maintain acceptable pH and $PaCO_2$. If this value is high (generally >10 L/min for an average size patient), one should consider increased CO_2 production or increased dead space ventilation. Increased CO_2 production [>250 mL/min for an average size adult (33)], which may be confirmed with a CO_2 detector, is usually a consequence of hypermetabolism, which in turn may result from sepsis, inflammation, injury, or agitation, and less commonly from overfeeding or metabolic acidemia. Increased dead space may be calculated by CO_2 detectors, or inferred from a minute ventilation requirement out of proportion to measured CO_2 production. It may result from exacerbation of underlying COPD, destructive lung processes such as necrotizing pneumonia, and, less commonly, from faulty ventilator circuit/tubing setup. Note that endotracheal and tracheostomy tubes actually *decrease* the dead space of the upper airway (34).

If the patient requires, but is unable to produce, normal minute volumes, then consider increased work of breathing or decreased inspiratory strength. Increased work of breathing is most commonly a result of decreased thoracopulmonary compliance or increased airway resistance. Pulmonary compliance may be reduced by atelectasis, pneumonia, pulmonary edema, large effusions, or acute or resolving ARDS. Thoracic compliance may be reduced by abdominal distention, marked obesity, neuromuscular disease, Trendelenburg positioning, splinting secondary to pain, and, rarely, improperly applied vest restraints. Airway resistance may be increased by endotracheal tube size that is too small relative to the inspiratory flow rate (which in turn depends on the minute ventilation), kinked, bitten, or partially obstructed endotracheal tubes, or

Table 3 Causes of Severe Hypoxemia

1. Atelectasis
2. Pneumonia
3. Hydrostatic pulmonary edema (CHF)
4. Adult respiratory distress syndrome (ARDS)
5. Pulmonary embolism
6. Bronchospasm
7. Exacerbation of chronic hypoxic pulmonary disease
8. Factors exacerbating hypoxemia:
    Hypoventilation/hypercarbia
    Low mixed venous PO_2

Discontinuation of Mechanical Ventilation 507

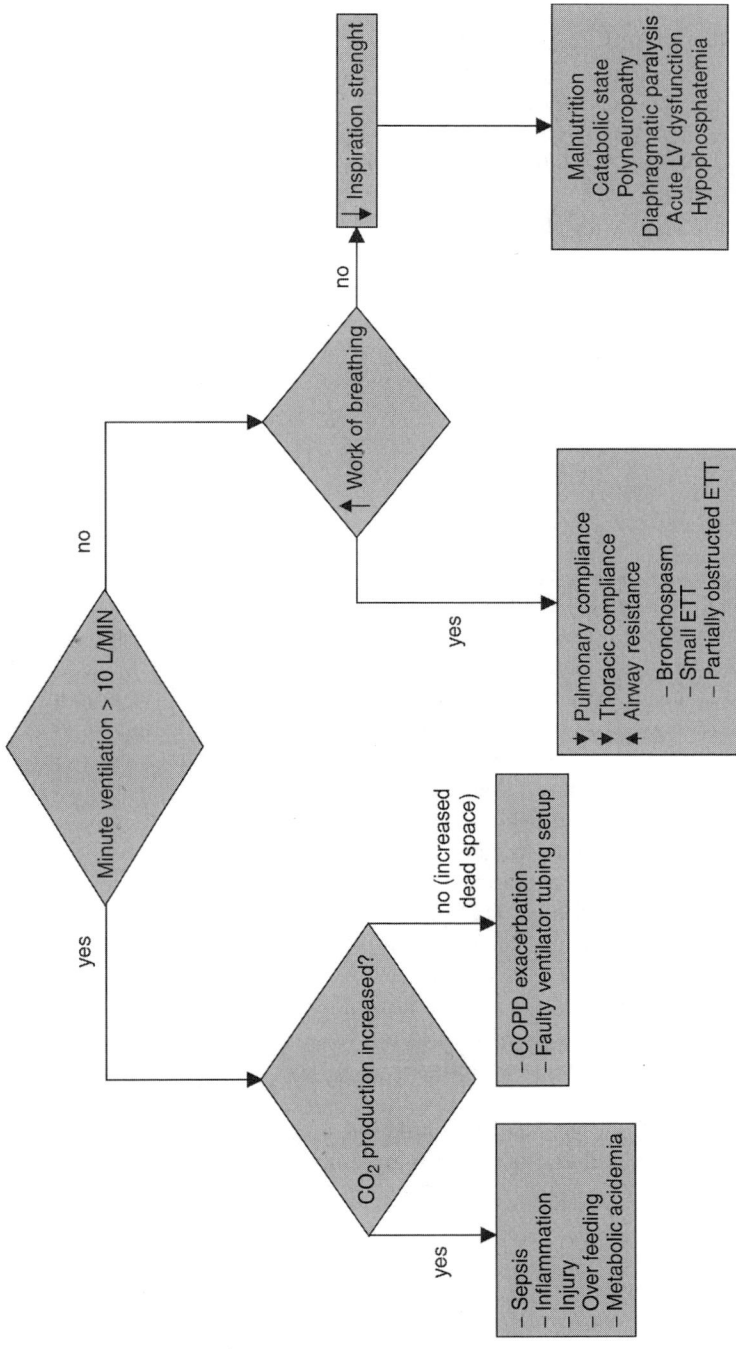

Figure 1 Algorithm for investigating ventilatory failure.

bronchospasm. High levels of intrinsic PEEP (PEEP$_i$) cause an inspiratory load and may cause increased work of breathing (35).

Decreased inspiratory muscle strength may be caused by deconditioning from long-standing mechanical ventilation, profound malnutrition, catabolism secondary to severe sepsis, critical illness polyneuropthy/myopathy, LV dysfunction, or diaphragmatic paralysis. Rarely, severe hypophosphatemia (<1 mmol/L) may impair inspiratory muscle contractility (36,37).

Finally, a patient with chronic, compensated CO_2 retention (usually secondary to COPD) who is mechanically ventilated to "normal" PCO_2 will gradually reduce his serum HCO_3^- to normal concentrations. When permitted to resume spontaneous ventilation, this patient will return to baseline PCO_2 and develop uncompensated respiratory acidemia. Baseline room air arterial blood gas measurements (e.g., in anticipation of planned surgery) can help prevent mistaking this situation for acute respiratory failure.

SUMMARY

- Mechanical ventilation should be discontinued as soon as the patient is able to assume the work of breathing. Premature extubation will lead to respiratory distress and necessitate reintubation, which is associated with complications and poorer outcome. Delayed extubation causes additional, unnecessary ventilator and ICU days with increased risk of ventilator-associated complications and increased costs.
- Readiness for extubation may be judged according to the patient's ability to ventilate and oxygenate during a trial of minimal or no support. This trial may consist of PSV or CPAP = +5 to +7 cm H_2O, or a T-piece trial lasting 30–120 min.
- SBTs or extubation should not be considered in patients (1) whose original indication for mechanical ventilation has not resolved, (2) who require high FiO_2, PEEP >5 cm H_2O, or high I:E ratios to maintain adequate oxygenation, (3) who are hemodynamically unstable, or (4) who have high minute ventilation requirements.
- Readiness for extubation may also be judged by reducing the level of "weanable" ventilatory support (PSV or SIMV) to the lowest level consistent with adequate ventilation and no dyspnea or fatigue, each day, until the patient is stable on minimal support.
- Failure to wean from mechanical ventilation should be investigated in an orderly manner. Keep in mind that the underlying problem is often extrapulmonary.

REFERENCES

1. Demling RH, Read T, Lind LJ, Flanagan HL. Incidence and morbidity of extubation failure in surgical intensive care patients. Crit Care Med 1988; 16:573–577.
2. Torres A, Gatell JM, Aznar E, El-Ebiary M, Puig de la Bellacasa J, Gonzalez J, Ferrer M, Rodriguez-Roisin R. Reintubation increases the risk of nosocomial pneumonia in patients needing mechanical ventilation. Am J Respir Crit Care Med 1995; 152:137–141.

3. Epstein SK, Ciubotaru RL, Wong JB. Effect of failed extubation on the outcome of mechanical ventilation. Chest 1997; 112:186–192.
4. Esteban A, Alia I, Gordo R, Fernandez R, Solsona JF, Vallverdu I, Macias S, Allegue JM, Blanco J, Carriedo D, et al. Extubation outcome after spontaneous breathing trials with T-tube or pressure support ventilation. Am J Respir Crit Care Med 1997; 156:459–465.
5. Rashkin MC, Davis T. Acute complications of tracheal intubation. Chest 1986; 89:165–167.
6. Beckman U, Gillies DM. Factors associated with reintubation in intensive care. Chest 2001; 120:538–542.
7. American College of Chest Physicians Consensus Conference: Mechanical Ventilation. Chest 1993; 104:1833–1859.
8. Sahn SA, Lakshminarayan S. Bedside criteria for discontinuation of mechanical ventilation. Chest 1973; 63:1002–1005.
9. Sahn SA, Lakshminarayan S, Petty TL. Weaning from mechanical ventilation. JAMA 1976; 235:2208–2212.
10. Yang KL, Tobin MJ. A prospective study of indexes predicting the outcome of trials of weaning from mechanical ventilation. NEJM 1991; 324:1445–1450.
11. Listello D, Sessler C. Unplanned extubation: clinical predictors for reintubation. Chest 1994; 105:1496–1503.
12. Tindol GA Jr, DiBenedetto RJ, Kosciuk L. Unplanned extubations. Chest 1994; 105:1804–1807.
13. Esteban A, Frutos F, Tobin MJ, Alia I, Solsona JF, Valverdu I, Fernandez R, de la Cal MA, Benuto S, Tomas R, et al. A comparison of four methods of weaning patients from mechanical ventilation. N Engl J Med 1995; 332:345–350.
14. Strickland JH, Hasson JH. A computer-controlled ventilator weaning system. A clinical trial. Chest 1993; 103:1220–1226.
15. Ely EW, Baker AM, Dunagan DP, Burke HL, Smoith AC, Kelly PT, Johnson MM, Browder RW, Bowton DL, Haponik EF. Effect on the duration of mechanical ventilation of identifying patients capable of breathing spontaneously. NEJM 1996; 332:1864–1869.
16. Kollef MH, Shapiro SD, Silver P, St. John RE, Prentice D, Sauer S, Ahrrens TS, Shannon W, Baker-Clinkscale D. A randomized, control trial of protocol-directed versus physician-directed weaning from mechanical ventilation. Crit Care Med 1997; 25:567–574.
17. Marelich GP, Murin S, Battistella, Inciardi J, Vierra T, Roby M. Protocol weaning of mechanical ventilation in medical and surgical patients by respiratory care practitioners and nurses. Chest 2000; 118:459–467.
18. Marini JJ, Smith TC, Lamb VJ. External work ouput and force generation during synchronized intermittent mandatory ventilation. Am Rev Respir Dis 1988; 138:1169–1179.
19. Gibney RTN, Wilson RS, Pontoppidan H. Comparison of work of breathing on high gas flow and demand valve continuous positive airway pressure systems. Chest 1982; 82:692–695.
20. Weisman IM, Rinaldo JE, Rogers RM, Sanders MH. Intermitent mandatory ventilation. Am Rev Respir Dis 1983; 127:641–647.
21. Brochard L, Rauss A, Benito S, Conti G, Mancebo J, Rekik N, Gasparetti A, Lemaire F. Comparison of three methods of gradual withdrawal from ventilatory support during weaning from mechanical ventilation. Am J Respir Crit Care Med 1994; 150:896–903.
22. Cavo J, Ogura JH, Sessions DG, Nelson JR. Flow resistance in traheostomy tubes. Ann Otol Rhinol Laryngol 1973; 82:827–830.
23. Shapiro M, Wilson RK, Casar G, Bloom K, Teague RB. Work of breathing through different sized endotracheal tubes. Crit Care Med 1986; 14:1028–1031.
24. Bolder PM, Healy TEJ, Bolder AR, Beatty PC, Kay B. The extra work of breathing through adult endotracheal tubes. Anesth Analg 1986: 65:853–859.
25. Wright PE, Marini JJ, Bernard GR. In vitro versus in vivo comparison of endotracheal tube airflow resistance. Am Rev Respir Dis 1989; 140:10–16.

26. Sassoon CSH, Light RW, Lodia R, Sieck GC, Mahutte CK. Pressure–time product during continuous positive airway pressure, pressure support ventilation, and T-piece during weaning from mechanical ventilation. Am Rev Respir Dis 1991; 143:469–475.
27. Banner MJ, Kirby RR, Blanch PB, Layon AJ. Decreasing imposed work of the breathing apparatus to zero using pressure-support ventilation. Crit Care Med 1993; 21:1333–1338.
28. Brochard L, Rua F, Lorino H, Lemaire F, Harf A. Inspiratory pressure support compensates for the additional work of breathing caused by the endotracheal tube. Anesthesiology 1991; 75:739–745.
29. Petrof BJ, Legaré M, Goldberg P, Milic-Emili J, Gottfried SB. Continuous positive airway pressure reduces work of breathing and dyspnea during weaning from mechanical ventilation in severe chronic obstructive pulmonary disease. Am Rev Respir Dis 1990; 141:281–289.
30. Fiastro JF, Habib MP, Quan SF. Pressure support compensation for inspiratory work due to endotracheal tubes and demand continuous positive airway pressure. Chest 1988; 93:499–505.
31. Esteban A, Alia I, Tobin MJ, Gil A, Gordo F, Vallverdu I, Blanch L, Bovet A, Vazquez A, de Pablo R, Torres A, de la Cal MA, Macius S. Effect of spontaneous breathing trial duration on outcome of attempts to discontinue mechanical ventilation. Am J Respir Crit Care Med 1999; 159:512–518.
32. Laghi F, D'Alfonso N, Tobin MJ. Pattern of recovery from diaphragmatic fatigue over 24 hours. J Appl Physiol 1995; 79:539–546.
33. Pierson DJ. Weaning from mechanical ventilation in acute respiratory failure: concepts, indications and techniques. Respir Care 1983; 28:646–662.
34. Habib MP. Physiologic implications of artificial airways. Chest 1989; 96:180–184.
35. Smith TC, Marini JJ. Impact of PEEP on lung mechanics and work of breathing in severe airflow obstruction. J Appl Physiol 1988; 65:1488–1499.
36. Agusti AG, Torres A, Estopa R, Agustividal A. Hypophosphatemia as a cause of failed weaning: the importance of metabolic factors. Crit Care Med 1984; 12:142–143.
37. Aubier M, Murciano D, Lecocguic Y, Viires N, Jacques Y, Squara V, Pariente R. Effect of hypophosphatemia on diaphragmatic contractility in patients with acute respiratory failure. NEJM 1985; 313:420–424.

F. Renal Function

33
Disturbances of Acid–Base Homeostasis

Jon F. Berlauk*

Jerome H. Abrams
VA Medical Center, Minneapolis, Minnesota, U.S.A.

Arterial blood gas (ABG) chemistries are among the laboratory tests most frequently ordered in the SICU, because ABG analysis provides a wealth of critical information about the SICU patient. Contained in the four variables measured [i.e., pH, partial pressure of carbon dioxide (PCO_2), partial pressure of oxygen (PO_2), and bicarbonate (HCO_3)] is an overall assessment of the patient's respiratory adequacy and cellular metabolic environment. Consequently, an accurate interpretation of ABGs, along with clinical and electrolyte data, can provide a circumscribed differential diagnosis of many significant medical problems. In addition, a patient's response to cardiovascular and respiratory support is monitored through the ABG values. This chapter provides a simplified approach to the interpretation of ABG values and the physiology of acid–base disturbances, along with diagnostic clues available to differentiate the disturbances of acid–base homeostasis. The emphasis is on diagnosis. Treatment of the specific acid–base disturbances is not discussed.

ABG INTERPRETATION

A brief review of acid–base physiology aids ABG interpretation. Under normal, *unstressed* metabolic conditions the human body produces excess acid. An adult produces 40–100 meq of organic acids and 13,000–15,000 mmol of CO_2 daily (Fig. 1).

To mediate the tissue pH changes that would accompany the continual organic acid production, intracellular and extracellular fluids in the body contain conjugate acid–base pairs.

These conjugate pairs act as buffers at normal physiologic pH of 7.40. The major extracellular buffer in blood and interstitial fluid is the HCO_3^- buffer system:

$$HCO_3^- + H^+ \longleftrightarrow H_2CO_3 \stackrel{CA}{\longleftrightarrow} CO_2 + H_2O \tag{1}$$

where CA is carbonic anhydrase and H_2CO_3 is carbonic acid.

---

*Deceased. Dr. Berlauk's contribution to the first edition was updated by Dr. Abrams.

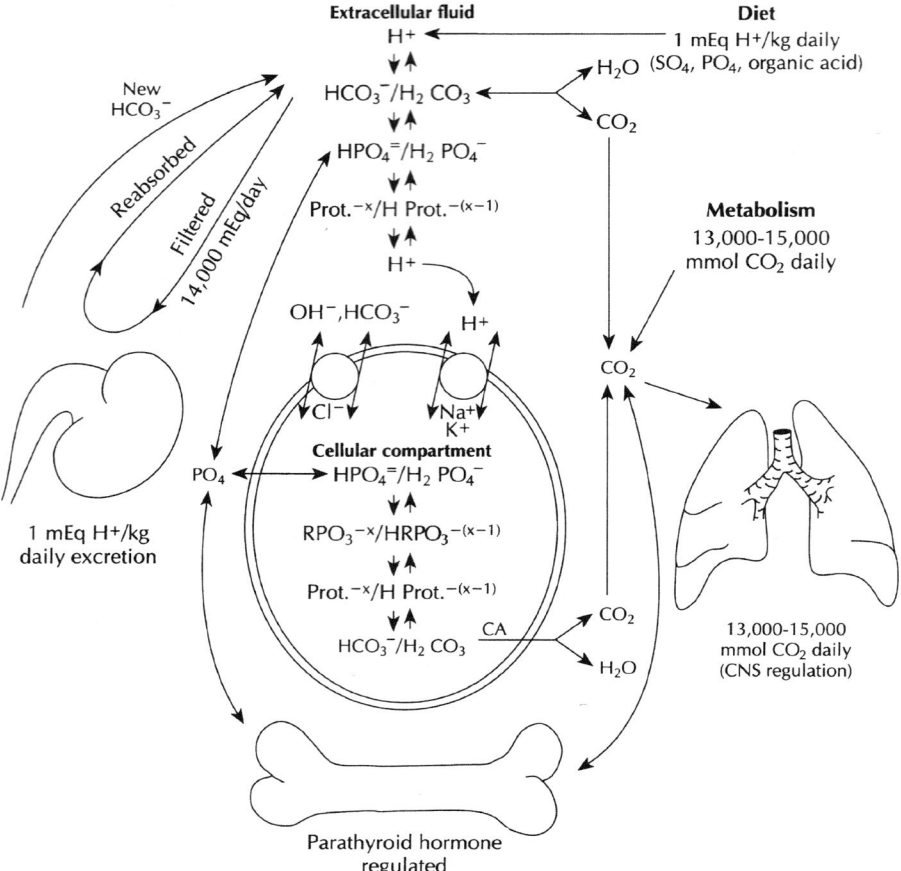

Figure 1 Interactions that occur between body fluid compartments with respect to buffering and major organ systems involved in maintenance of acid–base balance. Major buffers are shown in compartments in which they occur. Buffers within either intracellular or extracellular compartments are in equilibrium by isohydric principle; intracellular and extracellular compartments are linked by ion exchange systems indicated and by PCO_2. Carbonic anhydrase (CA) occurs only intracellularly. Not illustrated are renal and gut handling of phosphate and hormonal control of these processes. When normal balance is being maintained, daily production of "new" bicarbonate (HCO_3) by the kidney equals amount of HCO_3 consumed during acute buffering of acid loads ingested. *Source*: From Laski ME. Normal regulation of acid–base balance. Renal and pulmonary response and pulmonary response and other extrarenal buffering mechanisms. Med Clin North Am 1983; 67:771.

Once the organic acids are buffered (HCO_3^- is consumed), they are excreted by the kidney. New bicarbonate is regenerated through this hydrogen ion (H^+) excretion process (Fig. 2). This mechanism is the body's only source of endogenous bicarbonate. Abnormalities in HCO_3^-, as measured by the ABG analysis, will reflect *metabolic* acid–base disorders or metabolic compensation for a respiratory disorder.

The continuous cellular CO_2 production would cause drastic pH changes were it not for the intracellular hemoglobin buffer system. Reduced hemoglobin will absorb

Acid–Base Homeostasis

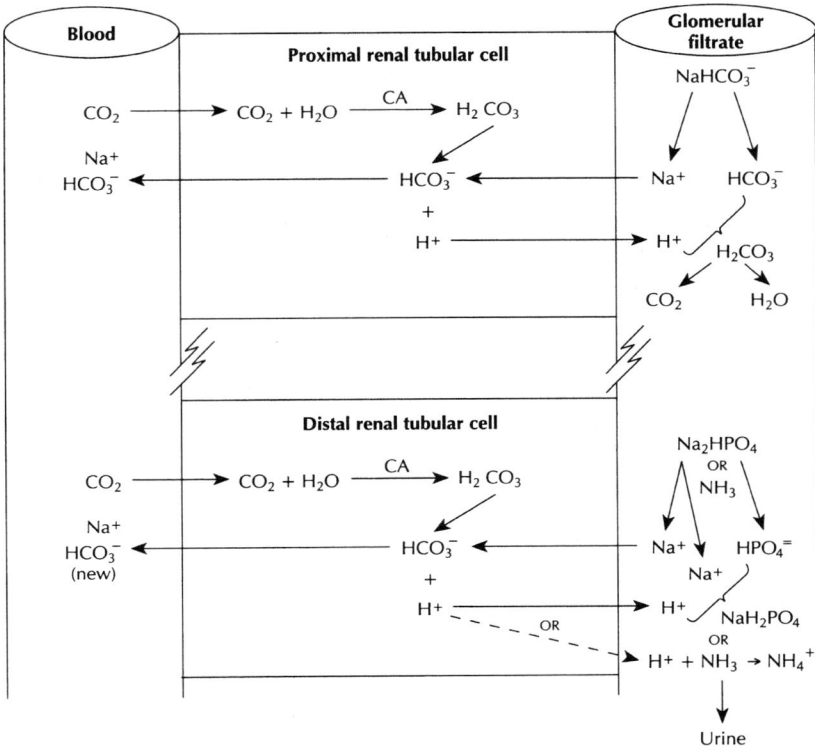

Figure 2 Proximal renal tubular cell: simplified mechanism for sodium (Na$^+$) and bicarbonate (HCO$_3$) reabsorption. Distal renal tubule cell: simplified mechanism for acidification of urine and new HCO$_3$ regeneration. CA, carbonic anhydrase.

~0.7 mmol H$^+$ for each millimole of oxygen released to the tissues without a subsequent change in serum pH. Although this H$^+$ buffering is mediated through the action of carbonic anhydrase, HCO$_3^-$ is not consumed in the process. The CO$_2$ ultimately is eliminated through pulmonary gas exchange. Therefore, abnormalities in PCO$_2$, as measured by the ABG analysis, will reflect *respiratory* acid–base disorders or respiratory compensation for a metabolic disorder.

This interplay of renal–pulmonary regulation of acid excretion is ultimately determined through the Henderson–Hasselbalch equation for the bicarbonate buffer system:

$$\text{pH} = 6.1 + \log \frac{[\text{HCO}_3^-]}{[\text{H}_2\text{CO}_3] + [\text{CO}_2]} \qquad (2)$$

CO$_2$ dissolved in the blood greatly exceeds the concentration of H$_2$CO$_3$ at equilibrium (809×); therefore, the equation can be simplified to:

$$\text{pH} = 6.1 + \log \frac{[\text{HCO}_3^-]}{[\text{CO}_2]} \qquad (3)$$

As HCO_3^- and H_2CO_3 are not clinically measured, but total CO_2 and PCO_2 are, this equation becomes:

$$pH = 6.1 + \log\frac{\text{Total } CO_2 - 0.03 PCO_2}{0.03 PCO_2} \qquad (4)$$

Changes in PCO_2 significantly affect pH and HCO_3^-. As indicated by the Henderson–Hasselbalch relationship, a change in any one variable results in simultaneous changes in the others. As CO_2 causes a predictable, nonlinear, change in pH through a wide physiologic range of pH, the key to interpreting ABG values is the PCO_2.

Finally, the Henderson–Hasselbalch equation has been rewritten as:

$$pH = \text{Constant} + \frac{\text{Kidneys}}{\text{Lungs}} \text{ or } \frac{\text{Metabolic}}{\text{Respiratory}} \qquad (5)$$

Equation (5) states that a change in either component of this equilibrium must be "compensated" by a similar change (increase or decrease) in the reciprocal component, if the pH is to remain near normal.

With these concepts in mind, those caring for ICU patients can rely on fairly simple and practical guidelines to interpret ABG data. Four steps are involved:

1. Check the pH.
2. Assume all perturbations in pH are due to an *acute* change in PCO_2.
3. Confirm or refute this assumption (diagnose the primary acid–base disorder).
4. Check for normal physiologic compensation (diagnose the secondary acid–base disorder, if present).

Step 1

Note the measured pH. (Analysis of PO_2 in conjunction with acid–base changes is discussed in Chapter 62.) By convention, a pH of 7.40 is considered neutral or "normal" (normal pH is actually within a range of values from 7.38 to 7.42). Likewise, a PCO_2 of 40 torr (mm Hg) is normal. *Acidosis* refers to any serum pH below 7.40 and *alkalosis* refers to pH values above 7.40. [As a memory aid: *alkalosis* (nine letters) is greater than *acidosis* (eight letters).] Yet, quite often, a patient with a normal serum pH is mistakenly believed to have an acidosis simply because the HCO_3^- reported on the ABG analysis is low.

ABG analysis should begin with pH, because there are only four primary acid–base disorders: metabolic acidosis, metabolic alkalosis, respiratory acidosis, and respiratory alkalosis. Of these four, only one, chronic respiratory alkalosis, ultimately compensates enough to result in a normal serum pH. The primary disorder will never "overcompensate;" therefore, the pH confirms the presence or absence of acidosis (metabolic vs. respiratory). With this information, half of the analysis is done.

Step 2

After the measured pH has been checked, the PCO_2 should be addressed. It should be assumed that the pH measured from the ABG was the result of an acute change in the PCO_2. Acute changes in the PCO_2 result in predictable changes in the serum pH (the converse is not true). For an acute 10 torr increase in PCO_2 above 40 torr, the pH will decrease by ~0.05 units. However, for an identical acute 10 torr decrease in PCO_2, the pH will

Acid–Base Homeostasis

increase ~0.1 units (Box 1). An equivalent change in PCO_2 results in different changes in pH. By using these two rules, a pH predicted by the assumption of an acute change in PCO_2 can be calculated from the measured PCO_2, resulting in both measured pH and predicted pH.

Step 3

By comparing the predicted pH with the measured pH, a primary acid–base diagnosis can be made.

- If the predicted pH and measured pH correlate very well, an acute respiratory disorder is present.
- If the predicted pH and measured pH lie in opposite directions of a pH of 7.40, a primary metabolic disorder exists. A secondary respiratory disorder is also possible (see Step 4).
- If the predicted pH and measured pH lie on the same side of a pH of 7.40, but otherwise do not correlate, several possibilities exist:
    - A primary (chronic) respiratory disorder exists, and renal compensation has occurred. The combination of a low PCO_2 and normal pH (7.38–7.42) almost always indicates chronic respiratory alkalosis.
    - A combined disorder exists (i.e., metabolic and respiratory acidosis). A combined disorder is easy to diagnose, because the measured pH is more acidotic or alkalotic than the predicted pH.
    - A mixed disorder exists.

Step 4

The first three steps determine whether an acid–base disorder exists and, if so, whether the primary disorder is respiratory or metabolic. If the primary disorder is respiratory (ΔPCO_2), physiologic compensation would be expected to occur through renal (ΔHCO_3^-) mechanisms. If the primary disorder is metabolic, respiratory compensation would be expected. This physiologic compensation has been well-defined, and does have limits (rules 3–8 in Box 1). Two principles apply: (1) only chronic respiratory alkalosis will completely compensate to a normal pH, and (2) without iatrogenic intervention, no primary disorder will overcompensate. *Establishing whether the physiologic compensation for a primary acid–base disorder falls within expected limits or not can determine if a second acid–base disorder exists.*

The metabolic (ΔHCO_3^-) compensation for a primary respiratory disorder (ΔPCO_2) occurs in two steps. First, there is a rapid re-equilibration of HCO_3^- as described by the Henderson–Hasselbalch equation. This acute compensation occurs within minutes. The subsequent loss or regeneration of HCO_3^- is much slower and occurs through renal mechanisms over 12–36 h. Rules 3–6 in Box 1 describe this compensation and the expected limits of normal compensation. If the compensation for a primary respiratory disorder is more or less than expected, a secondary acid–base disorder should be diagnosed. Again, compensation for alkalosis is greater than for acidosis.

The respiratory (ΔPCO_2) compensation for a primary metabolic (ΔHCO_3^-) disorder can occur rapidly. However, the rules defining this compensation (Box 1, rules 7 and 8) are unique and cannot be extrapolated from the previous rules. If the compensation for a primary metabolic disorder is more than or less than expected, a secondary acid–base disorder is present.

Box 1 Rules for ABG Analysis

1. Each acute 10 torr increase in PCO_2 above 40 torr will decrease blood pH $\sim$0.05 units.
2. Each acute 10 torr decrease in PCO_2 below 40 torr will increase blood pH $\sim$0.1 units.
3. An acute 10 torr increase in PCO_2 will be buffered by an increase in HCO_3 of $\sim$1 meq/L (upper limit, HCO_3 of 30 meq/L).
4. A chronic 10 torr increase in PCO_2 will be compensated by an increase in HCO_3 of $\sim$3.5 meq/L (upper limit, HCO_3 of 45 meq/L).
5. An acute 10 torr decrease in PCO_2 will be buffered by a decrease in HCO_3 of $\sim$2.5 meq/L (lower limit, HCO_3 of 18 meq/L).
6. A chronic 10 torr decrease in PCO_2 will be compensated by a decrease in HCO_3 of $\sim$5 meq/L (lower limit, HCO_3 of 12 meq/L).
7. For metabolic acidosis only:
   Expected $PCO_2 = 1.5[HCO_3] + 8 \pm 2$ (lower limit, PCO_2 of 10 torr) (modified Winter's formula).
   Expected PCO_2 approximates last two digits of the pH.
   Expected PCO_2 is $\sim 15 + [HCO_3]$.
8. For metabolic alkalosis only:
   Each 10 meq/L increase in HCO_3 will be compensated by an increase in PCO_2 of $\sim$6 torr (upper limit, PCO_2 of 55 torr).
9. Between 6 to 7 meq of HCO_3^- per liter of HCO_3^- distribution space will change the pH $\sim$0.1 units.

Once an ABG has been analyzed, it should be recalled that acid–base changes are dynamic. Especially in an SICU setting, the interplay of patient pathophysiology and physician intervention can create interesting ABG results. Previous ABG values, if they are available, often provide the additional information necessary to define a specific diagnosis.

METABOLIC ACID–BASE DISORDERS

Metabolic Acidosis

Metabolic acidosis is arguably the most interesting of the four primary acid–base disorders. By combining clinical information with ABG and serum electrolyte data, a precise diagnosis is very often possible.

Physiology

An unstressed adult produces 40–100 meq of acid daily as a by-product of intermediary metabolism. This acid is in the form of sulfuric, phosphoric, additional hydrogen phosphate, and other minor organic acids. Extracellular buffers are required to prevent dangerous pH changes that would result from continual acid production. These buffers are predominately HCO_3^-, proteins, and the skeletal system (Fig. 1). Eventually, the kidneys must excrete the acid load and, additionally, resynthesize HCO_3^- lost in the buffering process. Overproduction of acids, loss of buffer stores, or underexcretion of acid can disrupt this delicately balanced system and induce metabolic acidosis. Regardless of the mechanism of systemic acidosis, eventually the pH in the CSF also declines.

Medullary chemoreceptors respond to the elevated H$^+$ by stimulating respiration. Hyperventilation will cause hypocapnia, which will return the systemic pH toward normal, but compensation is never complete (1,2).

Winter's formula (3) relates the expected PCO_2 compensation for any degree of acidosis (as reflected in HCO_3^-). A simplified version of Winter's formula is given in Box 1. The lower limit of normal compensation is PCO_2 of ∼10 torr (4). If the actual PCO_2 deviates significantly from the expected PCO_2, a secondary disorder is possible.

When the acid load reaches the kidney, excretion depends on the ability of the renal tubule to excrete H$^+$ and ammonia (NH$_3$) normally. H$^+$ secretion occurs in both proximal and distal renal tubular cells. The amount secreted depends on intracellular production of H$^+$, cellular carbonic anhydrase concentration, and PCO_2. In the proximal tubule, H$^+$ secretion is most dependent on PCO_2. In the distal tubule, H$^+$ secretion is independent of PCO_2 and is primarily dependent on carbonic anhydrase concentration. In the renal tubular cell, carbon dioxide combines with water under the influence of carbonic anhydrase. H$^+$ is secreted into the tubular fluid (urine) in exchange for sodium. The HCO_3^- is reabsorbed into the blood (Fig. 2). To prevent secreted H$^+$ from recombining with tubular HCO_3^- to reverse the previous reactions, H$^+$ must be chemically "trapped" and excreted, a process accomplished through phosphate and ammonia secretion into the *distal* tubular lumen. For each H$^+$ that is trapped and excreted, one HCO_3^- is regenerated. This process is the only mechanism available for new HCO_3^- generation. Potassium-for-sodium exchange also occurs in the distal tubule, but will not generate new HCO_3^-.

Differential Diagnosis

Box 2 lists a broad classification of metabolic acidoses. These conditions are divided by their effect on the serum electrolytes, calculated by the anion gap (5,6). Acidoses are categorized as producing a normal anion gap or an elevated anion gap. The term "anion gap" is misleading, as it implies a disequilibrium (gap) between the concentration of serum anions and serum cations. One formula commonly used to calculate the anion gap (AG) is:

$$AG = [Na^+] - [Cl] + [HCO_3^-]$$

The normal anion gap, in this formulation, is ∼12 meq/L with the concentration of potassium omitted. The gap, in reality, arises from using only frequently measured serum anions and cations. The true anion gap, however, reflects the unmeasured anions (UA) and unmeasured cations (UC) in blood:

$$AG = UA = UC$$

Box 3 lists most of the common unmeasured anions and cations. On the basis of these observations, if chloride is ultimately the anion that accumulates during an acidosis, the resulting anion gap will be normal (or ∼12 meq/L). The result will be hyperchloremic metabolic acidosis. Although potassium does not play an important role in determining the anion gap, it provides valuable information to further differentiate the hyperchloremic metabolic acidoses. In contrast, elevated anion gap acidoses are characterized by the accumulation of an anion other than chloride (Box 3). Historically, these disorders are most frequently associated with metabolic acidosis.

Box 2 Metabolic Acidosis

Normal anion gap acidosis (10–12 meq/L)		Elevated anion gap acidosis (>12 meq/L)
Hypokalemia	*Normal to hyperkalemia*	*Hyperkalemia*
Renal tubular acidosis	Early renal failure	Chronic renal failure
Proximal	Hydronephrosis	Lactic acidosis
Distal	Hypoaldosteronism	Ketoacidoses
Buffer deficiency (phosphate or ammonia)	Acidifying agents	Diabetes mellitus
	Hydrochloric acid	Alcohol induced
Diarrhea	Ammonium chloride	Starvation
Posthypocapnic acidosis	Arginine chloride	Toxins
Carbonic anhydrase inhibitors	Lysine chloride	Methanol
Acetazolamide (Diamox)	Sulfur toxicity	Ethylene glycol
Mefenamide (Sulfamylon)		Paraldehyde
Ureteral diversions		Salicylates
Ureterosigmoidostomy		
Ileal bladder		
Ileal ureter		

Metabolic Alkalosis

Metabolic alkalosis is the most common acid–base disorder in the general hospital patient population (7). It is characterized by a sustained hyperbicarbonatemia. This condition can result from loss of acid, loss of volume (extracellular fluid), exogenously administered alkali, or imbalances in the renal–adrenal axis.

Physiology

Alkalinization of the serum by any of the above mechanisms eventually will lead to alkalinization of the CSF. Medullary chemoreceptors will respond by depressing

Box 3 Anion Gap

Increased anion gap (>12 meq/L)	**Decreased anion gap (<10 meq/L)**
Increased unmeasured anions	Decreased unmeasured anion
Organic anions (lactate, ketoacids)	Hypoalbuminemia
Exogenous anions (salicylate, formate, penicillin)	Laboratory error
	Falsely low sodium secondary to viscous serum (hyperglycemia, hyperlipidemia)
Inorganic anions (phosphate, sulfate)	Bromide intoxication
Hyperalbuminemia (transient)	Low sodium measured
Incompletely identified anion (paraldehyde poisoning)	High chloride or bicarbonate measured
Laboratory error	Increased unmeasured cation
High sodium measured	Normal cation (hyperkalemia, hypercalcemia, hypermagnesemia)
Low chloride or bicarbonate measured	Abnormal cation (IgG, lithium, TRIS buffer)
Decreased unmeasured cation	
Hypokalemia, hypocalcemia, hypomagnesemia	

respiration. Hypoventilation will cause hypercapnia, which will return the elevated serum pH toward normal, but pH compensation will never be complete. The PCO_2 will rise ~6 torr for each 10 meq/L rise in HCO_3^- (8). The maximum CO_2 compensation occurs at ~55 torr (9–12). If the measured PCO_2 falls outside these limits, a secondary disorder should be suspected. In patients with metabolic acidosis, renal tubular cell function is essential to eliminate the acid load. In contrast, the renal mechanism to eliminate excess bicarbonate depends on changes in glomerular filtration rate (GFR). Under normal conditions, bicarbonate reabsorption, like sodium reabsorption, changes directly with the GFR, and very little filtered bicarbonate is excreted. This bicarbonate reabsorption is probably mediated through a combination of H^+ secretion by tubular cells and alteration in tubular size. The most common mechanism for the development of metabolic alkalosis involves loss of chloride-rich fluid (13). When the kidney detects volume depletion, it attempts to protect renal blood flow through sodium (hence volume) reabsorption. The accompanying anion reabsorbed is the relatively more abundant HCO_3^-. Eventually, mild hyperbicarbonatemia occurs. If the volume deficit is not restored, this protective mechanism would initiate a vicious cycle, leading to increasingly severe alkalosis, were it not for the renal tubular maximum for HCO_3^- concentration. The normal renal tubular maximum for $[HCO_3^-]$ is 27–29 meq/L. If a higher concentration of HCO_3^- is filtered, it is promptly excreted. Although the elevated PCO_2 (respiratory compensation) will enhance H^+ secretion and HCO_3^- reabsorption in the proximal tubule (Fig. 2), this addition to serum HCO_3^- is minor. Therefore, if the GFR remains constant, large amounts of HCO_3 are excreted after the tubular maximum for HCO_3^- is reached. Severe systemic alkalosis is prevented, but once alkalosis is initiated, the kidney will perpetuate it (14). Mineralocorticoid hormones, serum calcium, and serum chloride also influence HCO_3^- homeostasis through poorly understood mechanisms. Under pathologic conditions, they are factors that elevate the renal tubular for maximum HCO_3^-. The result is sustained hyperbicarbonatemia and serious alkalosis.

Differential Diagnosis

The differential diagnosis for metabolic alkalosis involves extracellular fluid volume and mineralocorticoid hormones. The anion gap is not helpful as it is slightly elevated (5–9 meq/L) in all metabolic alkaloses (15). Rather, classification of metabolic alkaloses includes a saline-responsive group and a saline-resistant group (Box 4). These groups are separated by urinary chloride excretion. The majority of alkaloses in the SICU are saline responsive and are mediated through a chloride deficiency (Fig. 3). Avid chloride retention (with sodium) by the kidney results in little chloride excretion, with consequent low urinary chloride concentration. The majority of the saline-resistant alkaloses are mediated by imbalances in the renal–adrenal axis. Volume state and hypertension provide additional clues to these disorders.

RESPIRATORY ACID–BASE DISORDERS

Respiratory acid–base disorders result from alteration in normal CO_2 excretion. Therefore, the physiology of CO_2 transport and elimination is common to both respiratory acidosis and alkalosis. As stated previously, hemoglobin is the primary buffer against the pH

Box 4 Classification of Metabolic Alkaloses

Saline responsive (urinary chloride <15 meq/L)	Saline unresponsive (urinary chloride >15 meq/L)
Normotensive	*Normotensive*
Renal	Renal
Diuretic induced	Bartter's syndrome
Poorly reabsorbable anion therapy	Magnesium deficiency
(carbenicillin, sulfate, phosphate)	Severe potassium depletion
Posthypercapnic alkalosis	Refeeding alkalosis
Gastrointestinal	Hypercalcemia
Vomiting	Hyperparathyroidism
Nasogastric drainage	*Hypertensive*
Villous adenoma	Renal or adrenal
Congenital chloride diarrhea	Primary aldosteronism (Conn's syndrome)
Exogenous alkali	Hyperreninism
Baking soda (NaHCO$_3$)	Cushing's syndrome
Antacids	Liddle's syndrome
Salts of strong acids (citrate, lactate, acetate)	Adrenal 11-beta or 17-alpha hydroxylase deficiency
Blood product transfusion	Glycyrrhizinic acid (licorice, chewing tobacco)
"Overshoot" alkalosis	Carbenoxolone
Contraction alkalosis	

changes that would result from continual CO_2 production (16). HCO_3^- is not the best buffer in blood because the pK of the HCO_3^- buffer system (see Henderson–Hasselbalch equation) is remote from the physiologic pH of 7.40. The hemoglobin molecule serves as an important buffer because it is rich in the amino acid histidine. The imidazole group of histidine has a pK of 7, which is in the physiologic pH range of blood. On reduced hemoglobin, the imidazole group absorbs as much as 50% of the H^+ generated

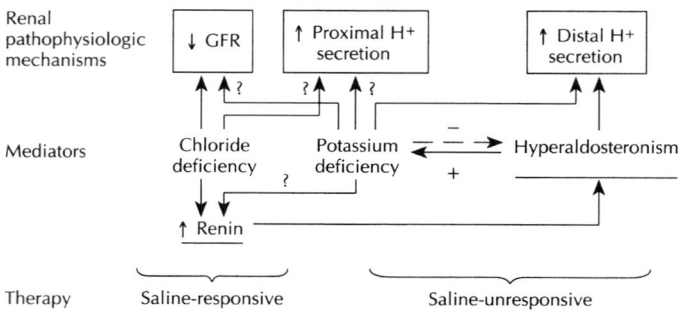

Figure 3 Factors contributing to the maintenance of metabolic alkalosis. Renal retention of bicarbonate can be affected by a decrease in GFR and/or an increase in proximal or distal bicarbonate reabsorption. These mechanisms in turn can be activated by combinations of chloride deficiency, potassium deficiency, and hyperaldosteronism. Saline therapy corrects only those pathophysiologic factors attributable to chloride deficiency. *Source*: From Cogan MG, Liu F, Berger BE, et al. Metabolic alkalosis. Med Clin North Am 1983; 67:903.

Acid–Base Homeostasis

by cellular CO_2 production. The total CO_2 produced is finally carried in one of four forms: (1) HCO_3^- (70%), (2) carbamino compounds (20%), (3) dissolved CO_2 (10%), and (4) H_2CO_3 (a small fraction) (Fig. 4). Once the venous blood reaches the lungs, the concentration gradients for oxygen and CO_2 are reversed from those present at the tissue level. Reactions that occurred at the tissue level are also reversed (Fig. 5). In contrast to reactions occurring in tissue, these reactions in the lung proceed against an unfavorable thermodynamic gradient. In the lung, the primary driving force is continual depletion of CO_2.

The healthy lung has an enormous capacity to excrete CO_2. Saturation of this excretion mechanism through overproduction of CO_2 is unknown. In addition, medullary chemoreceptors that control ventilation are exquisitely sensitive to changes in PCO_2. The result is a finely balanced feedback system to maintain stable PCO_2 by modulating CO_2 excretion in response to CO_2 production. Imbalances in the regulation of ventilation or the excretion of CO_2 result in respiratory acid–base disorders.

Respiratory Acidosis

If central respiratory centers are depressed or CO_2 is underexcreted relative to production, the PCO_2 becomes elevated. As renal compensation (increased HCO_3^-) for an acute rise in PCO_2 requires 36 h or more, buffering the acidemia produced by an abrupt and sustained elevation in PCO_2 is dependent on plasma and intracellular buffers described in previous sections. An acute 10 torr rise in PCO_2 is accompanied by $\sim$1 meq/L rise in HCO_3^-, described by the Henderson–Hasselbalch relationship (8). The maximal compensation through this mechanism occurs at a HCO_3^- level of $\sim$30 meq/L. Over the subsequent

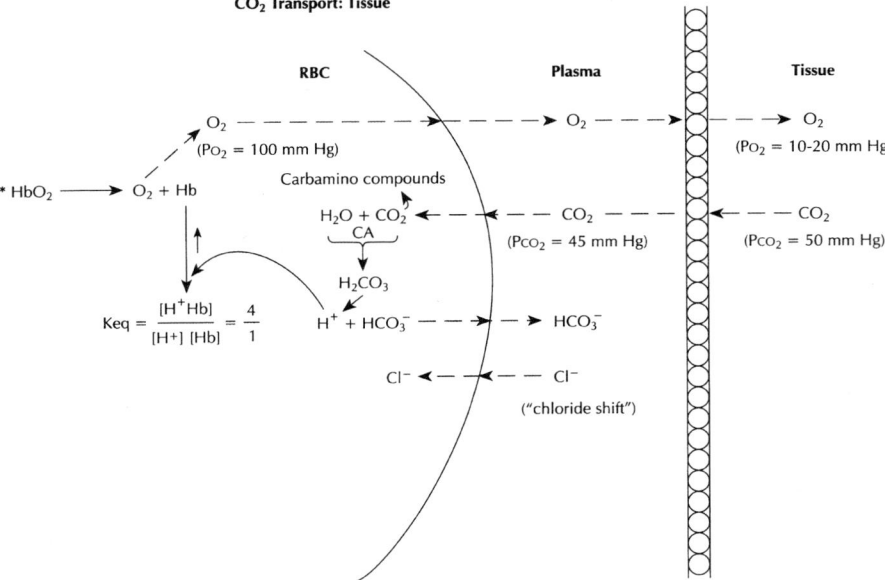

Figure 4 Reaction (*) favors dissociation to oxygen and reduced hemoglobin. However, main driving force is continual depletion of both end products. CA, carbonic anhydrase.

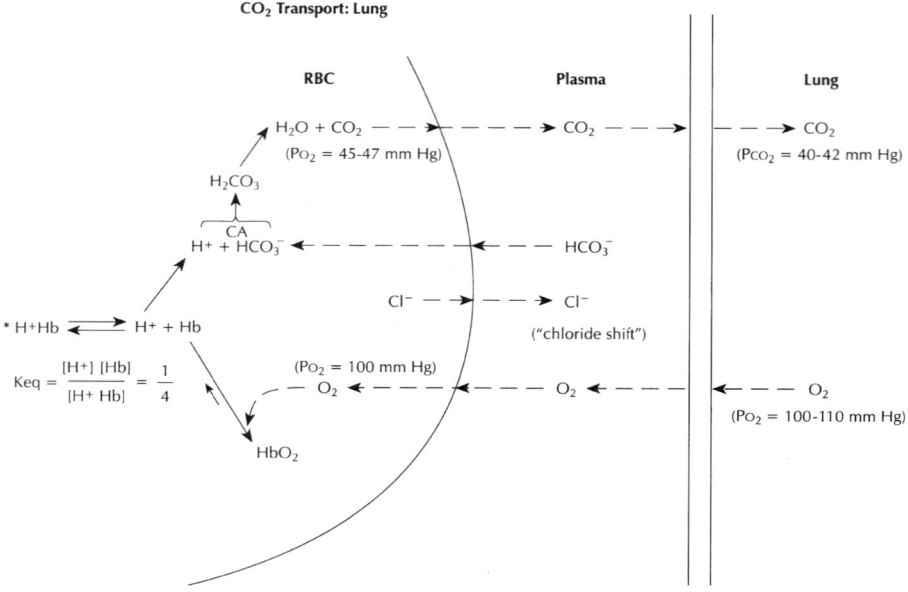

Figure 5 Reaction (*) does not favor dissociation to H^+ and reduced hemoglobin. Main driving force is continual depletion of both end products to form stable compounds.

hours to days, the kidney compensates for a sustained PCO_2 elevation by reabsorbing all filtered HCO_3^- and secreting H^+ into the distal tubule (17,18). The secreted H^+ is "trapped" by ammonia and excreted; one new HCO_3^- is generated and absorbed into the blood (Fig. 2). This sustained HCO_3^- reabsorption is accompanied by a chronic loss of chloride. This mechanism provides adequate, but never complete, pH compensation for chronic CO_2 retention. In addition, severe CO_2 elevation ($PCO_2 > 60$ torr) begins to impair renal tubular ammonia production, which reduces HCO_3^- regeneration and results in severe systemic acidosis. Overall, chronic renal compensation can be expected to raise the HCO_3^- $\sim$3.5 meq/L for each sustained 10 torr rise in PCO_2 (8,19,20). The limit of compensation is HCO_3^- level of $\sim$45 meq/L (17,21). If the actual HCO_3^- deviates from these expectations, a secondary disorder may exist.

Differential Diagnosis

The causes of acute and chronic respiratory acidosis are given in Box 5.

Respiratory Alkalosis

Simple respiratory alkalosis is characterized by a low PCO_2 induced by sustained hyperventilation. As in respiratory acidosis, compensation occurs in two phases. Intracellular and extracellular buffering are complete within 5–15 min, and renal compensation follows. An acute 10 torr fall in PCO_2 will be buffered by a decrease in HCO_3^- of $\sim$2.5 meq/L (8,22). The limit for acute compensation is $\sim$18 meq/L (23). Over the next 12–36 h, up to 5 meq/L of HCO_3^- are lost for a sustained 10 torr drop in PCO_2 (23).

Acid–Base Homeostasis

Box 5 Causes of Respiratory Acidosis

Acute
Secondary to respiratory control failure
  Central nervous system
    Cerebrovascular accident
    Drug overdose (sedatives, narcotics)
    Anesthesia
    Central sleep apnea
    Trauma
Secondary to carbon dioxide excretory failure
  Spinal cord
    Cervical cord trauma
    Guillan-Barré syndrome
  Neuromuscular
    Neurotoxins (botulism, tetanus, organophosphates)
    Neuromuscular blocking drugs (e.g., succinylcholine, curare, pancuronium)
    Neuromuscular blocking antibiotics (e.g., streptomycin, kanamycin, polymyxin)
    Myasthenic crisis
    Hypokalemic paralysis
    Hypophosphatemia
    Hypermagnesemia
  Thoracic
    Flail chest
    Pneumothorax
    Hemothorax
  Upper airway
    Obstructive sleep apnea
    Epiglottitis, laryngotracheitis
    Vocal cord paralysis
    Postintubation laryngeal edema
    Laryngospasm
    Foreign body aspiration
  Cardiovascular
    Massive pulmonary embolism
    Fat embolism
    Snake bite
    Cardiac arrest
  Lower airway or alveolar
    Gastric aspiration (particulate)
    Severe pulmonary edema
    Adult respiratory distress syndrome
    Severe pneumonia
    Severe bronchospasm (asthma)

Chronic
Secondary to respiratory control failure
  Central nervous system
    Obesity and hypoventilation (Pickwickian syndrome)
    Brainstem infarcts
    Tumor
    Chronic sedative or tranquilizer overdose
    Myxedema
    Metabolic alkalosis
    Bulbar poliomyelitis
Secondary to carbon dioxide excretory failure
  Spinal cord
    Poliomyelitis
    Amyotrophic lateral sclerosis
    Cervical cord trauma
  Neuromuscular
    Myasthenia gravis
    Multiple sclerosis
    Myxedema
  Thoracic
    Muscular dystrophy
    Kyphoscoliosis
    Spondylitis
  Lower airway or alveolar
    Chronic obstructive lung disease
    Severe interstitial lung disease
    Bronchiectasis

The renal mechanism involves the decreased serum H^+ and CO_2 concentrations presented to the renal tubular cells as a result of hypocapnia. The alteration in H^+ and CO_2 concentrations tends to decrease proximal tubular absorption of the filtered HCO_3^- and inhibit distal tubular regeneration of HCO_3^- (urinary acid excretion stops). Potassium (and sodium) is lost with HCO_3^-; whereas, chloride is retained. The resultant electrolyte pattern of hyperchloremia and hypokalemia can mimic some patterns seen with normal anion gap metabolic acidoses (24). Significant amounts of HCO_3^- are lost to a maximum quantity of HCO_3^- of $\sim$12–15 meq/L (23). This acid–base disorder can compensate to a normal pH through this mechanism. Respiratory alkalosis is the most frequently seen ABG abnormality in the SICU patient population (25).

Box 6 Causes of Respiratory Alkalosis

Central mechanisms	Pulmonary mechanisms
Central nervous system disorders	Pneumonia
Cerebrovascular accident	Asthma
Trauma	Pulmonary embolus
Infection	Congestive heart failure
Tumor	Interstitial lung disease
Hypoxemia	*Complex mechanisms*
Altitude	Cirrhosis
Ventilation–perfusion abnormalities	Gram-negative sepsis
Pulmonary shunts	Hyponatremia
Pulmonary diffusion abnormalities	Heat exposure
Hypotension, low cardiac output	Mechanical ventilation
Drugs or hormones	
Salicylates	
Nicotine	
Progesterone (pregnancy)	
Xanthines	
Thyroid hormone	
Anxiety, hysteria	
Fever	
Pain	

Differential Diagnosis

Hypocapnia does not result from abnormal CO_2 excretion; therefore, all causes of respiratory alkalosis involve disturbances in respiratory control. The causes of respiratory alkalosis involve central mechanisms, pulmonary mechanisms, and complex mechanisms (Box 6).

SUMMARY

- Abnormalities in PCO_2 reflect a respiratory acid–base disorder or respiratory compensation for a metabolic disorder.
- The key to interpreting ABG values is the PCO_2.
- Guidelines for interpreting ABG values include checking the pH (assuming all perturbations in pH are due to acute changes in PCO_2), confirming or refuting the assumption of acute changes, and checking for normal physiologic compensation.
- Primary acid–base disorders are metabolic acidosis, metabolic alkalosis, respiratory acidosis, and respiratory alkalosis.
- Only chronic respiratory alkalosis can compensate enough to produce a normal pH. No primary disorder will overcompensate without iatrogenic interventions.
- By determining whether physiologic compensation for a primary acid–base disturbance falls within expected limits, the clinician can identify the presence or absence of a second acid–base disorder.

REFERENCES

1. Pierce NF, Fedson DS, Brigham KL, Mitra RC, Sack RB, Mordal A. The ventilatory response to acute base deficit in humans: time course during development and correction of metabolic acidosis. Ann Intern Med 1970; 72:633–640.
2. Lennon EJ, Lemann J. Defense of hydrogen ion concentration in chronic metabolic acidosis: a new evaluation of an old approach. Ann Intern Med 1966; 65:265–274.
3. Albert MS, Dell RB, Winters RW. Quantitative displacement of acid–base equilibrium in metabolic acidosis. Ann Intern Med 1967; 66:312–322.
4. Relman AS. Metabolic acidosis. Med Times 1968; 96:1094–1105.
5. Emmett M, Narins RG. Clinical use of the anion gap. Medicine (Baltimore) 1997; 56:38, 197.
6. Oh MS, Carroll HJ. The anion gap. N Engl J Med 1977; 297:814–817.
7. Hodgkin JE, Soeprono FF, Chan DM. Incidence of metabolic alkalemia in hospitalized patients. Crit Care Med 1980; 8:725–728.
8. Narins RG, Emmett M. Simple and mixed acid–base disorders: a practical approach. Medicine (Baltimore) 1980; 59:161–187.
9. Goldring RM, Cannon PJ, Heinemann HO, Fishman AP. Respiratory adjustment to chronic metabolic alkalosis in man. J Clin Invest 1968; 47:188–202.
10. Bone JM, Cowie J, Lambie A, Robson JS. The relationship between arterial PCO_2 and hydrogen ion concentration in chronic metabolic acidosis and alkalosis. Clin Sci Mol Med 1974; 46:113–123.
11. Elkinton JR. Clinical disorders of acid–base regulation. A survey of seventeen years' diagnostic experience. Med Clin North Am 1966; 50:1325–1350.
12. Fulop M. Hypercapnia in metabolic alkalosis. NY State J Med 1976; 76:19–22.
13. Garella S, Chang BS, Kahn SI. Dilution acidosis and contraction alkalosis. Review of a concept. Kidney Int 1975; 8:279–283.
14. Seldin DW, Rector FC Jr. Symposium on acid–base homeostasis: the generation and maintenance of metabolic alkalosis. Kidney Int 1972; 1:306–321.
15. Madias NE, Ayus JC, Androgué HJ. Increased anion gap in metabolic alkalosis: the role of plasma protein equivalency. N Engl J med 1979; 300:1421–1423.
16. Giebisch G, Berger L, Pitts RF. The extrarenal response to acute acid–base disturbances of respiratory origin. J Clin Invest 1955; 34:231–245.
17. Schwartz WB, Brackett NC Jr, Cohen JJ. The response of extracellular hydrogen ion concentration to graded degrees of chronic hypercapnia. The physiologic limits of the defense of pH. J Clin Invest 1965; 44:291–301.
18. Van Ypersele de Strihou C, Brasseur CL, DeConinck J. The "carbon dioxide response curve" for chronic hypercapnia in man. N Engl J Med 1966; 275:117–122.
19. Brackett NC Jr, Cohen JJ, Schwartz WB. Carbon dioxide titration curve of normal man: effect of increasing degrees of acute hypercapnia on acid–base balance. N Engl J Med 1965; 272:6–12.
20. Schwartz WB, Cohen JJ. The nature of the renal response to chronic disorders of acid–base equilibrium. Am J Med 1978; 64:417–428.
21. Robin ED. Abnormalities of acid–base regulation in chronic pulmonary diseases with special reference to hypercapnia and extracellular alkalosis. N Engl J Med 1963; 268:917–922.
22. Arbus GS, Hebert LA, Levesque PR, Etsten BE, Schwarts WB. Characterization and clinical application of the "significance band" for acute respiratory alkalosis. N Engl J Med 1969; 280:117–123.
23. Gennari FJ, Goldstein MB, Schwartz WB. The nature of the renal adaption to chronic hypocapnia. J Clin Invest 1972; 51:1722–1730.
24. Brown EB, Campbell GS, Elam JO, Gollan F, Hemingway A, Visscher MB. Electrolyte changes with chronic passive hyperventilation in man. J Appl Physiol 1949; 1:848–855.
25. Mazzara JT, Ayres SM, Grace WJ. Extreme hyopcapnia in the critically ill patient. Am J Med 1974; 56:450–456.

34
Acute Renal Failure

Mark E. Rosenberg
University of Minnesota, Minneapolis, Minnesota, USA

INTRODUCTION

Acute renal failure (ARF) is a clinical syndrome characterized by rapid deterioration of renal function that results in the accumulation of nitrogenous wastes. This syndrome complicates the hospital course of 5% of hospitalized patients and 30% of patients admitted to the ICU. As an isolated organ system failure, ARF carries a low mortality of ~8%. However, ARF that accompanies multi-organ system failure, as is usually the case in the critically ill surgical patient, carries a much poorer prognosis. For example, ARF as part of two-organ system failure has a mortality of 75%. The mortality increases to 90–100% with involvement of more than two organs. The outcome of ARF is most often linked to the resolution of the patient's underlying problems. However, prompt recognition and management of renal failure is critical to improving patient survival. The terminology regarding ARF is confusing and selected terms are defined in Table 1.

DIFFERENTIAL DIAGNOSIS

ARF is first recognized by a decrease in urine output, a rising BUN and Creatinine (Cr), or both. The differential diagnosis of ARF is best approached by dividing the possible etiologies into prerenal, intrinsic renal, and postrenal causes (Fig. 1). This approach not only obviates the need to memorize long lists of possible etiologies but also provides a useful starting point for the diagnostic evaluation and management of the patient with failing kidneys. The common causes of ARF are listed in Table 2, and the clinical approach to the diagnosis of ARF is summarized in Table 3.

Prerenal ARF

Causes
A prerenal etiology for ARF is the most common cause of renal failure in the hospitalized patient. Recognition of prerenal causes is critical because they are potentially reversible, yet can lead to acute tubular necrosis (ATN) if left untreated. In addition, a prerenal factor often contributes to other forms of ARF. The fundamental abnormality is a decrease

Table 1 Definitions of Selected ARF Terms

Acute renal failure	A syndrome characterized by rapid deterioration of kidney function that results in the accumulation of nitrogenous wastes.
Acute tubular necrosis	The most common form of ARF caused by ischemic or nephrotoxic injury to the kidney with subsequent necrosis of tubules
Acute cortical necrosis	A rare form of ARF that is due to necrosis of all elements of the renal cortex and produces irreversible renal failure
Oliguric renal failure	ARF from any cause associated with a urine output <400 mL/day
Nonoliguric renal failure	ARF from any cause associated with a urine output >400 mL/day

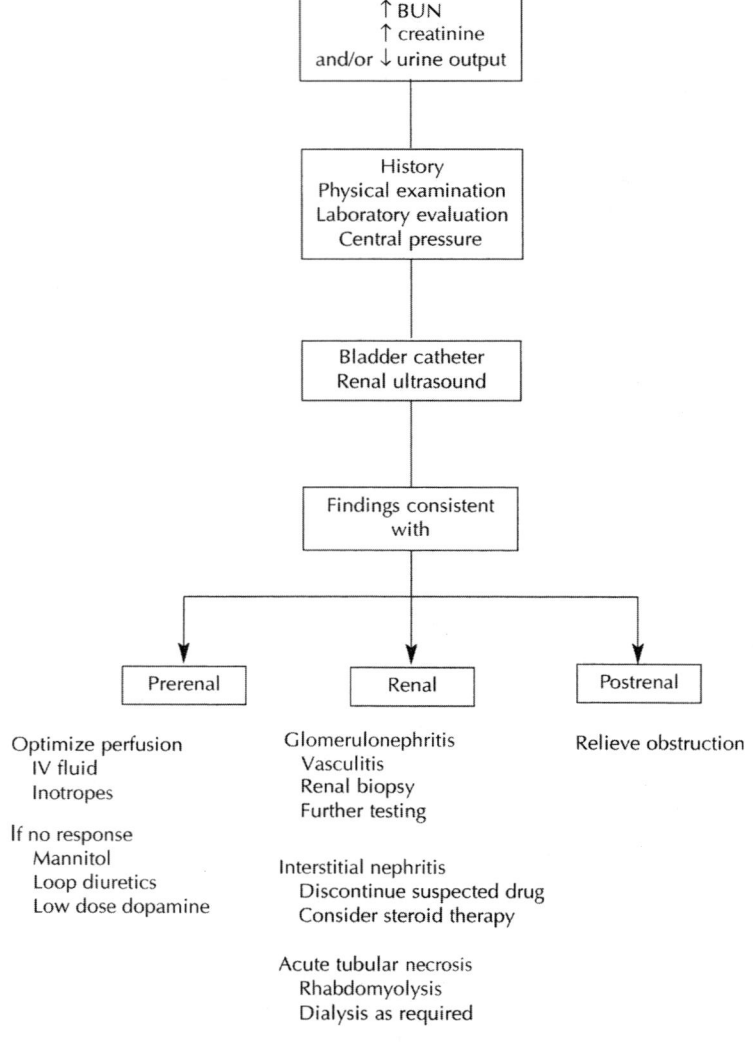

Figure 1 Differential diagnosis of acute renal failure.

Table 2 Differential Diagnosis of ARF

Prerenal ARF
    Decreased cardiac output
    Decreased circulating blood volume
        Decreased input
        External fluid losses (bleeding, gastrointestinal, renal, and skin)
        Redistribution (peritonitis, pancreatitis, and hypoalbuminemia)
        Peripheral vasodilation (sepsis, liver disease, and antihypertensives)
    Renal artery occlusion

Renal ARF
    Glomerular
        Glomerulonephritis
    Vascular
        Vasculitis
        Hemolytic uremic syndrome
        Malignant hypertension
        Cholesterol emboli
    Interstitial
        Allergic (methicillin, sulfonamide, and allopurinol)
        Infiltration (leukemia and lymphoma)
        Infections (staphylococcus, Gram negatives, and tuberculosis)
    Tubular (ATN)
        Ischemic (shock and cardiac failure)
        Nephrotoxic (drugs and pigment)

Postrenal ARF
    Obstructed urinary catheter
    Urethra (stricture)
    Bladder (prostatic disease, carcinoma, neurogenic, stones, and clot)
    Ureter and pelvis
        Intrinsic (stones, blood clot, papillary necrosis, and fungus)
        Extrinsic (retroperitoneal fibrosis, tumor, abscess, and ligation)

in renal perfusion, which results in a fall in the glomerular filtration rate (GFR). Some of the causes of prerenal ARF are listed in Table 2. Renal hypoperfusion can be caused by a decrease in cardiac output, effective circulating blood volume depletion, or renal artery occlusion. Although in some cases volume loss is obvious, such as with diarrhea, blood loss, or overdiuresis, in other cases the loss of fluid can be internal, for example, as with third spacing in the patient with peritonitis. "Effective circulating blood volume" is a term that takes into account the amount of circulating blood, how well the blood is being pumped throughout the body, and, most important, how well the tissues are being perfused. For instance, in the patient with sepsis, effective circulating blood volume depletion may occur as a result of peripheral vasodilation and shunting of blood despite a high cardiac output and no loss of extracellular fluid.

Diagnosis

The patient history should focus on the possible sources and quantity of fluid loss, symptoms of volume depletion (including orthostatic dizziness or weight loss), and the

Table 3 Evaluation of the Patient with ARF

History
   Predisposing medical conditions
   Pre-existing renal function
   Input, output, and weights
   Hypotensive episodes
   Anesthesia report
   Medications
   Toxin exposure
   Crush injury
Physical
   Postural BP and pulse
   Temperature
   Weight
   Fundi (exudates, hemorrhages, and Roth's spots)
   Skin (rash and jaundice)
   Jugular venous pressure (volume status, atrial fibrillation, and tamponade)
   Lungs (rales and pneumonia)
   Heart (gallop, rub, and new murmur)
   Abdomen (mass, ascites, and enlarged kidneys)
   Edema
Central pressure monitoring
   Central venous catheter
   Swan–Ganz catheter
Laboratory
   Serial BUN/Cr
   Urinalysis
   CBC and smear
   Electrolytes (anion gap)
   Arterial blood gas
   Urinary sodium or fractional excretion of sodium
X-ray
   Renal ultrasound (exclude obstruction)

existence of underlying cardiac or liver disease. In the hospitalized patient, the chart should be reviewed; particular attention should be given to input, output, and daily weight (the weight of the patient with third space losses may actually increase despite the presence of volume depletion). On physical examination, the volume status of the patient can be estimated by careful attention to postural blood pressure and pulse, height of the neck veins, and presence or absence of signs of congestive heart failure (pulmonary rales, S3, and edema). Often the volume status is difficult to define, particularly in the patient with sepsis, who may have vascular leak with peripheral edema, or in the patient with cardiac decompensation. When doubt exists, central pressures, preferably the pulmonary capillary wedge pressure, should be measured in an attempt to optimize circulating volume.

Laboratory evaluation of prerenal ARF is based on the ability of the functioning kidney to avidly conserve sodium and water when it senses a decrease in renal perfusion. Thus, measurement of blood and urinary variables not only provides an index of volume

Table 4 Prerenal ARF Versus ATN

	Prerenal	ATN
BUN/Cr	>20	10–20
Urine specific gravity	>1.020	<1.010
Urine osmolality (mOsm/kg)	>500	<350
Urinary sodium (mEq/L)	<20	>40
FENa (%)	<1	>1
Renal failure index	<1	>1

Note: $FENa = (U_{Na} \times P_{Cr}/U_{Cr} \times P_{Na}) \times 100$; renal failure index = $(U_{Na} \times P_{Cr}/U_{Cr})$.

status, but also helps differentiate prerenal ARF from ATN, where the kidney loses its ability to reabsorb sodium. Table 4 lists some useful variables to measure and the expected results in differentiating prerenal ARF from ATN. These measurements need to be performed prior to volume replacement or the administration of mannitol or diuretics.

Treatment

The treatment of prerenal ARF focuses on restoring the circulating blood volume to normal. If true volume depletion is present, normal saline or colloid should be infused, with the physical examination, central venous pressures, urine output, and improvement in BUN and creatinine used as clinical markers. Most important, therapy should be directed at the underlying disease, for example, vasodilator therapy for heart failure or antibiotics for sepsis.

Intrinsic ARF

Causes

The major structures in the kidney are the glomeruli, tubules, vasculature, and interstitium. Disease of any of these structures can lead to ARF. Although glomerular disease is rare in the surgical patient, it can occur. For instance, postinfectious glomerulonephritis can complicate chronic infections or bacterial endocarditis. Occlusion of the renal microvasculature can occur as part of vasculitis, in hemolytic uremic syndrome, in malignant hypertension, or following cholesterol embolization from an atheroma. Acute interstitial nephritis is characterized by an inflammatory infiltrate and edema in the interstitium accompanied by varying degrees of tubular injury.

The most common cause of ARF is ATN, a diagnosis made after prerenal and postrenal causes have been excluded and glomerulonephritis, interstitial nephritis, and intrarenal vascular disease have been ruled out. ATN is caused by ischemic or nephrotoxic injury to the kidney. Prolonged renal hypoperfusion from any prerenal cause can lead to ATN (Table 2). The most common nephrotoxins that cause ATN are drugs—particularly aminoglycosides, amphotericin B, *cis*-platinum, nonsteroidal anti-inflammatory drugs, and radiocontrast agents. Nephrotoxicity occurs in 10–25% of patients treated with aminoglycosides and is classically nonoliguric. Predisposing factors include older age, chronic kidney disease, the presence of liver disease, and concomitant use of cephalosporins. ARF is more common in patients treated with aminoglycosides for longer than 7 days, and in those patients with peak serum concentrations of gentamicin or tobramycin greater than 10 μg/mL or trough levels greater than 2 μg/mL. However, ARF has been observed in patients with drug serum concentrations in the range of 2–10 μg/mL and after discontinuation of aminoglycosides therapy. Once-daily high-dose therapy is associated with less nephrotoxicity.

Risk factors for radiocontrast-induced ARF include serum creatinine concentrations greater than 1.5 mg/dL, diabetic nephropathy, NSAID therapy, heart failure, multiple myeloma, volume depletion, high dose contrast (>40 mL), and two doses within 48 h. Amphotericin B causes ARF by direct tubular toxicity as well as renal vasoconstriction. A decrease in GFR can occur with the first dose, and the GFR is decreased in 40–50% of patients treated with amphotericin B.

Diagnosis

Prerenal ARF must be differentiated from ATN (see discussion of diagnosis of prerenal ARF). Volume infusion is crucial in the prerenal patient, but it is potentially hazardous in the oliguric patient with ATN. Comparison of the onset of renal failure with the start of a new medication may provide some clues to the cause of the renal disease. The analysis of a fresh urine specimen can be quite helpful in differentiating the causes of intrinsic ARF. The presence of proteinuria, hematuria, and red blood cell (RBC) casts is characteristic of glomerulonephritis and renal vasculitis. In allergic interstitial nephritis, urinary abnormalities may be minimal, or they can include the presence of small amounts of protein, white blood cells (WBC) and casts, eosinophils (in only 30–50% of cases), and renal tubular epithelial (RTE) cells and casts. In ATN the urine is classically a muddy brown color and contains RBCs, WBCs, RTE cells, and pigmented granular and RTE casts. In some circumstances, particularly if the diagnosis of ARF is unclear, a renal biopsy should be considered.

Treatment

If glomerulonephritis or vasculitis is suspected, a renal biopsy should be performed to help guide therapy. In drug-induced acute interstitial nephritis the offending agent (or any suspected drug) should be discontinued. The use of steroids to treat interstitial nephritis is controversial. Approaches to the management of ATN are discussed in the following sections.

Postrenal ARF

Causes

Obstruction of the urinary tract is an uncommon cause of ARF but one that is easily treatable and therefore crucial to recognize. The common causes of obstruction are listed in Table 2.

Diagnosis

Complete anuria suggests urinary tract obstruction. On abdominal examination careful palpation for abdominal masses, enlarged kidneys, and an enlarged bladder (requires >500 mL to be palpable) should be performed. The first diagnostic test is bladder catheterization, which yields a large volume of relatively normal urine (by urinalysis) in patients with urethral or bladder neck obstruction. Renal ultrasound is a safe, noninvasive, and sensitive method for diagnosing obstruction. The diagnosis is based on demonstration of dilation of the collecting system. Therefore, false negatives may occur when obstruction is present but dilation is not, such as with early obstruction (first 24–36 h) or encasement of the collecting system by tumor, which prevents dilation from occurring. Dilation of the collecting system in the absence of obstruction (false positive) is found in 15–20% of cases and may be due to vesicoureteral reflux, previous high urine flow states, pregnancy, adynamic ureter, pelvic cysts, or previously treated obstruction. Radiocontrast studies, particularly intravenous pyelography, should be avoided in patients in whom obstruction is suspected. Once obstruction has been diagnosed, the site of the obstruction needs to be localized, which may involve antegrade or retrograde pyelograms.

Treatment

Therapy must be directed at relieving the obstruction. This therapy may be as simple as inserting a urinary catheter, or it may involve more complex procedures such as percutaneous nephrostomy or internal ureteral stenting. Return of renal function can occur after 1–2 weeks of obstruction. Return of function after much longer time periods has been reported. The thinner the renal cortex is on ultrasound, the lesser the chance for recovery of function. In general, attempts should be made to salvage as much renal function as possible, which may involve decompression of both kidneys in patients with bilateral obstruction.

After relief of the obstruction, diuresis may occur as a result of sodium, urea, and water retention during the period of obstruction. Such diuresis is therefore appropriate and does not require fluid replacement above maintenance requirements. Matching of the urine output will maintain volume expansion, and the diuresis will continue.

PREVENTION

Prompt correction of prerenal factors is the most critical preventive measure for ARF. In the case of volume depletion, fluid should be administered. Time should be taken to optimize volume status prior to surgery. Sepsis should be promptly treated with volume expanders and antibiotics. In cardiac failure, therapy with inotropic agents, vasodilators, or an intra-aortic balloon pump should be instituted as necessary. Aminoglycoside drug serum concentrations should be closely monitored and drug dosages adjusted accordingly. Prophylaxis against radiocontrast-induced ARF is discussed in Chapter 11 and should include saline hydration and acetylcysteine (Mucomyst). With intravascular hemolysis or rhabdomyolysis, hydration and urinary alkalinization comprise the treatment of choice.

Mannitol and Loop Diuretics

These agents have been used for: (1) prophylaxis in clinical settings that have a high incidence of ARF (e.g., administration of radiocontrast agents, major cardiovascular surgery, and massive trauma); (2) in the oliguric patient whose urine volume remains low despite correction of prerenal factors such as volume depletion ("incipient ATN"); and (3) to hasten recovery of renal function in patients with established ATN. The efficacy of these agents is still unproven. Mannitol and loop diuretics are capable of increasing urine flow in some patients, but increased urine volume does not necessarily translate into improved GFR or reduced mortality. Furthermore, a response to these agents may simply indicate those patients with less severe renal dysfunction. Nonetheless, a trial of high dose diuretics is reasonable after prerenal factors are corrected. If no beneficial effect is seen in the urine output, these therapies should be discontinued. Loop diuretics can be given alone as bolus or continuous infusions, or used in combination with diuretics that act on other sites of the tubule such as metolazone (distal tubule).

Dopamine

Low dose dopamine (1–3 µg/kg per min) has no proven beneficial effect in the prevention or treatment of ARF. The dopamine A-1 receptor agonist fenoldopam is approved for the treatment of hypertension. This agent has been demonstrated to increase renal blood flow in normal and hypertensive subjects. Trials are underway to examine the effects of fenoldopam in the prevention and treatment of ARF.

MANAGEMENT

Complications of ARF can appear in almost any organ system and are often the major determinants of prognosis. The most common complications of ARF are listed in Table 5. General principles of management include careful monitoring of input and output, changes in the physical examination, serum electrolytes, drug dosages, and serum concentrations. Because of the high incidence of infection associated with invasive catheters, their use should be kept to a minimum. For example, a chronic indwelling urinary catheter is often not needed in the patient with ARF.

Fluid Balance

In the absence of fluid overload, the volume of maintenance fluids should equal measured fluid losses (urine, gastrointestinal fluids, surgical drains) and insensible losses, which can be estimated at 600 mL/day. Higher insensible losses occur with fever. Often a higher fluid intake is needed to deliver medications or hyperalimentation. In such cases, dialysis therapy is often necessary to manage volume. Whenever possible, excess fluid intake should be kept to a minimum. The electrolyte composition of infused fluids is dictated by the type of loss (which can be measured) and the serum electrolytes.

Table 5 Complications of ARF

Metabolic	Retention of nitrogenous wastes, hyperkalemia, hyponatremia, metabolic acidosis, hyperphosphatemia, hypocalcemia, hyperuricemia, and muscle catabolism
Cardiovascular	Fluid overload, pericarditis, arrythmias, hypertension, and myocardial infarction
Infectious	Urine, bacteremia, catheter, pneumonia, and surgical site infections
Neurologic	Disorientation, confusion, coma, and seizures
Hematologic	Anemia, coagulopathy, and platelet dysfunction
Gastrointestinal	Hemorrhage, nausea, vomiting, and gastritis
Pulmonary	Pulmonary edema, pneumonia, emboli, and ARDS

Hyperkalemia

Potassium should almost never be administered, particularly in the oliguric patient. Because of the potential for serious arrythmias, hyperkalemia should be treated promptly. Emergency therapy of hyperkalemia is outlined in Table 6.

Hyponatremia

Hyponatremia implies a disorder of osmolarity and not an abnormality of sodium metabolism. The patient with oliguric ARF has impaired free water excretion and is therefore susceptible to hyponatremia, particularly if large amounts of dilute solutions are administered. The therapy is free water restriction, which means limiting not only oral intake but also IV fluids (including hyperalimentation). Hypertonic sodium infusion can lead to pulmonary edema in the oliguric patient. Dialysis is often needed to correct hyponatremia.

Hypocalcemia and Hyperphosphatemia

Failure of urinary excretion of phosphate leads to hyperphosphatemia with a reciprocal decrease in serum calcium. Higher levels of phosphate are found in patients in a catabolic state or those with rhabdomyolysis. Phosphate intake should be minimized, and phosphate binders, such as aluminum-containing antacids, calcium carbonate or acetate, or sevelamer, should be administered. Magnesium-containing antacids should be avoided, because renal excretion of magnesium is impaired in ARF. The calcium-phosphate product should be kept <55. If symptoms of hypocalcemia, such as carpopedal spasm (Trousseau's sign), a positive Chvostek's sign, or dysrythmias are present, calcium needs to be administered.

Acidosis

Sodium bicarbonate should be administered if severe metabolic acidosis (serum bicarbonate concentration <15 mg/dL) is present.

Table 6 Therapy of Hyperkalemia

Treatment	Dosage	Time of onset	Mechanism
Calcium gluconate (10%)	5–10 mL IV over 2 min; a second dose may be repeated in 5 min	Immediate	Antagonize cardiac and neuromuscular effects of K
Glucose (50%) and insulin	50 mL of glucose and 5–10 units of regular insulin IV over 5 min	30–60 min	Shifts K into cells
Sodium bicarbonate (7.5%)	50 mL IV over 5 min	30–60 min	Shifts K into cells; particularly effective in acidotic patients
Cation-exchange resin	15–30 g of resin in 50–100 mL of 20% sorbitol PO (or by rectal catheter); may repeat q4 h	Hours	Removes 1 mEq K/g of resin by exchange for 1.5 mEq of Na
Dialysis	As Needed	Hours	Diffusive loss

Note: Cardiac monitoring at all times.

Nutrition

Although early studies demonstrated nutritional therapy improved survival and hastened recovery of renal function in patients with ARF, these studies have not been confirmed. Still, one of the goals of therapy in the patient with ARF is to maintain good general health, as the course of ARF is likely to last several weeks. The nutritional requirements of patients with ARF vary greatly and are largely dependent on the nature of the underlying disease and the integrity of other organ systems.

Dialysis

Dialytic therapy of ARF is discussed in detail in Chapter 35. The timing of dialysis is important, because early dialysis improves survival. Indications for initiation of dialysis are listed in Table 7. The absolute serum concentrations of BUN and Cr are not as important a factor in the decision to initiate dialysis as the patient's overall condition. Dialysis should probably be instituted when the BUN is >150 mg/dL, particularly if other metabolic abnormalities are present (e.g., acidosis or hyperkalemia). Many of the complications of uremia, such as the neurologic manifestations, nausea and vomiting, and bleeding disorders, are improved with dialysis.

Bleeding

A clotting defect from abnormal platelet function is present in ARF, and this defect may contribute to a bleeding tendency. Also, in the hemodialyzed patient, heparin is used to prevent dialyzer clotting. The treatment of the uremic platelet defect is discussed in Chapter 11. No-heparin dialysis can be performed, if necessary.

Drug Dosing

Dosage adjustments need to be made for many drugs according to the level of renal function and the degree of removal of drugs by dialysis. See Suggested Reading and Chapters 11 and 49 for more information.

COURSE AND PROGNOSIS OF ARF

The prognosis for the hospitalized patient with ARF is highly dependent on the resolution of the underlying disease, because no patient, if properly managed, should die of uremia or its associated metabolic disturbances. In the surgical patient with ARF, the prognosis is

Table 7 Indications for Dialysis

Volume overload
Uremia
Pericarditis
Hyperkalemia
Hyponatremia
Acid–base disturbance
Coma or seizures
Uremic bleeding

Table 8 Predictors of a Poor Prognosis in the Course of ARF

Dialysis requirement
Increment in serum Cr >3 mg/dL
Oliguria
Advanced age
Second episode of ARF
Number of complications
Multi-organ system failure
Respiratory failure
Cardiac failure
Sepsis
Jaundice
Coma

often poor, with a mortality rate of 30–60%. Predictors of poor prognosis are listed in Table 8. As shown in the table, the number and type of complications are often the most important determinant of a poor prognosis. The mortality in ARF is often underestimated by APACHE III scores, a finding that suggests renal failure itself is an independent prognostic factor.

In the oliguric patient with ARF whose underlying disease resolves, renal function begins to return after an average of 10–21 days. However, the course may be much shorter or prolonged for as much as several months. Recovery is heralded by an increase in urine volume followed by a delayed fall in BUN and Cr. In the nonoliguric patient recovery often occurs earlier. In 10% of patients no recovery of renal function occurs; in ∼30% only incomplete recovery is found, with a small percentage (5%) developing late deterioration of renal function.

SUMMARY

- ARF is a common problem in the hospitalized patient and is an independent risk factor for mortality.
- Determine whether ARF is prerenal, renal, or postrenal.
- Prerenal causes of ARF need to be promptly recognized and treated to prevent the development of ATN.
- Prerenal causes are suggested by postural blood pressure changes, acute weight loss, low central venous pressure, BUN/Cr >20, and FENa <1%.
- ATN is the most common cause of intrinsic ARF and is diagnosed by ruling out prerenal, other renal, and postrenal causes.
- In ATN, loss of tubular function is reflected in a FENa >1%.
- Examination of fresh urine for proteinuria, blood, WBCs, eosinophils, and RTE casts is important for the diagnosis of intrinsic renal failure.
- Complete anuria suggests obstruction. Perform bladder catheterization as the first diagnostic test followed by renal ultrasound.
- Loop diuretics can be administered in ARF once prerenal causes have been corrected. If there is no increase in urine output, they should be stopped.

- Saline hydration and acetylcysteine should be used to prevent radiocontrast-induced ARF.
- Low dose dopamine is ineffective in preventing or treating ARF.
- In the euvolemic patient with ARF, maintenance IV fluids should equal measured fluid losses and estimated insensible losses.
- Do not administer potassium to the oliguric patient with ARF.
- Hyponatremia implies free water excess and is often an indication for dialysis in the oliguric patient with ARF.
- Minimize phosphate intake and administer a phosphate binder if serum concentrations are elevated.
- Initiate dialysis early if indications are present (see Table 7).

SUGGESTED READING

Allgren RL, Marbury TC, Rahman SN, Weisberg LS, Fenves AZ, Lafayette RA, Sweet RM, Genter FC, Kurnik BRC, Conger JD, Sayegh MH. Anaritide in acute tubular necrosis. N Engl J Med 1997; 336:828–834.

Baldwin L, Henderson A, Hickman P. Effect of postoperative low-dose dopamine on renal function after elective major vascular surgery. Ann Intern Med 1994; 120:744–747.

Bellomo R, Chapman M, Finfer S, et al. Low-dose dopamine in patients with early renal dysfunction: a placebo-controlled randomised trial. Lancet 2000; 356:2139–2143.

Conger JD. Interventions in clinical acute renal failure: what are the data? Am J Kidney Dis 1995; 26:565–576.

DuBose TD, Warnock DG, Mehta RL, Bonventre JV, Hammerman MR, Molitoris BA, Palle MS, Siegel NJ, Scherbenske J, Striker GE. Acute renal failure in the 21st century: recommendations for management and outcomes assessment. Am J Kidney Dis 1997; 29:793–799.

Klahr S, Miller SB. Acute oliguria. N Engl J Med 1998; 338:671–675.

Lawman SHA, Cohen SL, Batson SD. Acute renal failure after cardiothoracic surgery: a review of three years experience. Blood Purif 2002; 20:293–295.

Liano F, Pascual J, and the Madrid Acute Renal Failure Study Group. Epidemiology of acute renal failure: a prospective, multicenter, community-based study. Kidney Int 1996; 50:811

Mueller C, Buerkle G, Buettner HJ, Petersen J, Perruchoud AP, Erikkson U, Marsch S, Roskamm H. Prevention of contrast media-associated nephropathy. Arch Intern Med 2002; 162:329–336.

Nolan CR, Anderson RJ. Hospital-acquired acute renal failure. J Am Soc Nephrol 1998; 9:710.

Pascual J, Liaño F, Ortuño J. The elderly patient with acute renal failure. J Am Soc Nephrol 1995; 6:144–153.

Racusen LC. Pathology of acute renal failure: structure/function correlations. Adv Ren Replace Ther 1997; 4(suppl 1):3–16.

Solomon R, Werner C, Mann D, D'Elia J, Silva P. Effects of saline and furosemide on acute decreases in renal function induced by radiocontrast agents. N Engl J Med 1994; 331:1416–1420.

Spurney RF, Fulkerson WJ, Schwab SJ. Acute renal failure in critically ill patients: prognosis for recovery of kidney function after prolonged dialysis support. Crit Care Med 1991; 19:8–11.

Star RA. Treatment of acute renal failure. Kidney Int 1998; 54:1817–1831.

Tepel M, van der Giet M, Schwarzfeld C, Laufer U, Liermann D, Zidek W. Prevention of radiographic-contrast-agent-induced reductions in renal function by acetylcysteine. N Engl J Med 2000; 343:180–184.

Webb JA. Regular review: ultrasonography in the diagnosis of urinary tract obstruction. Br Med J 1990; 301:944–946.

35
Support of Renal Function

Connie L. Manske
University of Minnesota, Minneapolis, Minnesota, USA

HEMODIALYSIS

In healthy individuals, the kidney serves the dual function of eliminating waste products and controlling fluid balance. Critically ill patients frequently sustain a loss of one or both of these renal functions and require support with dialysis. Dialysis therapy is initiated when the level of waste products in the blood is toxic, or when fluid balance cannot be maintained with the aggressive use of diuretics. The major indications for emergency dialysis include fluid overload that compromises oxygenation, hyperkalemia that cannot be managed with ion-exchange resins or diuretics, uncontrollable bleeding not attributable to a cause other than uremia, or anuria. Additional indications are summarized in Chapter 34.

The dialysis process alters the solute composition of blood by exposing it to a dialysis solution through a semipermeable membrane (Fig. 1). Water molecules and small-molecular-weight solutes in the blood can pass through the membrane pores into the dialysate, but large solutes, such as proteins, cannot pass through the membrane and remain in the plasma. The factors listed in Table 1 affect solute and water transport across the dialysis membrane.

The ability of dialysis to remove many solutes depends on the area of the dialysis membrane and the rate of blood flow through the dialyzer. However, large or highly protein-bound solutes cannot be removed well with dialysis. The ability of dialysis to remove fluid depends on the area of the dialysis membrane and the amount of pressure applied across the membrane. For both solute and water removal, increasing the amount of time a patient receives dialysis can increase efficiency. Because solute removal depends on the initial solute concentration, dialysis becomes progressively less efficient as the solute concentration is lowered. For this reason, dialysis is performed intermittently, when toxic levels of waste products have accumulated in the bloodstream. Successful dialysis depends on access to the bloodstream. Temporary access can be established using a double-lumen dialysis catheter in which the catheter contains both the venous and arterial ports. Access characteristics are summarized in Table 2.

The dialysis procedure is performed by a trained hemodialysis nurse or technician as specified by written orders from a nephrologist. Before dialysis, the nephrologist assesses the patient and determines an appropriate "dry" weight. Table 3 lists the variables that must be specified for dialysis. During the dialysis run, the nurse records the blood pressure every 15–30 min and sends laboratory tests as ordered.

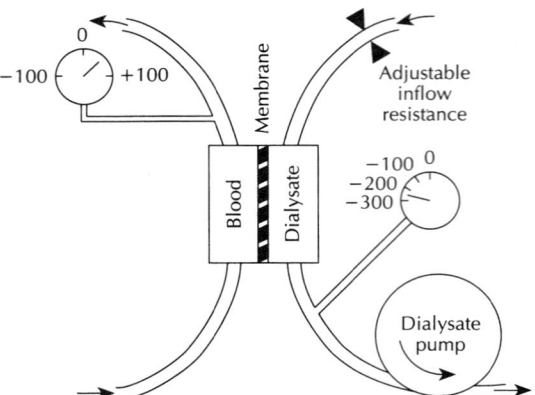

Figure 1 Dialyzer with blood flowing in one direction and dialysis solution flowing in opposite direction. Hydrostatic pressure across membrane (and ultrafiltration) is adjusted by varying resistance to inflow of dialysis solution. Position of gauges monitoring pressure at blood and dialysate outflow ports also is shown, along with typical operating pressures. In this case transmembrane pressure is 300 mg Hg [+50 at the blood outlet −(−250) at dialysate outlet]. (Redrawn from Daugirdas JT, Ing TS, eds. Handbook of Dialysis. Boston: Little, Brown, 1988:14.)

The expected fluid removal with dialysis is determined by the transmembrane pressure and is calculated as shown in Table 3. Newer dialysis machines can measure the actual quantity of fluid removed. A single dialysis procedure can remove up to 5 L of fluid, but many critically ill patients cannot tolerate this amount of fluid removal.

Removal of toxic waste products is less straightforward than removal of fluid. Although lower molecular weight substances such as potassium and magnesium can be easily removed, higher molecular weight compounds may be dialyzed less easily. The blood urea nitrogen (BUN) and creatinine concentrations are often used as indictors of dialysis adequacy. However, these values are often unreliable in critically ill patients (Table 4).

Regular dialysis, the current standard, done thrice weekly for 4 h at a time and at a blood flow rate of at least 200 mL/min, gives the patient the equivalent of an average weekly glomerular filtration rate (GFR) of 10–15 mL/min. However, a recent study suggests that daily dialysis of critically ill patients with acute renal failure reduces mortality and leads to more rapid resolution of renal failure than conventional thrice weekly dialysis.

A number of complications can occur while the patient is undergoing dialysis. The most common one is hypotension (Table 5). Less common complications include

Table 1 The Dialysis Process

Dialysis function	Factors affecting dialysis
Solute removal	Molecular size of solute
	Concentration gradient between blood and dialysate for solute
Fluid removal	Ultrafiltration capacity of dialysis membrane (K_{uf})
	Transmembrane pressure

Table 2 Access for Hemodialysis

Access mode	Advantages	Disadvantages	Relative contraindications
Tunneled internal jugular catheter	Usable for many weeks	Potentially life threatening complications: pneumothorax, air embolism, arterial puncture, superior cava puncture, tamponade	Patient cannot lie flat; coagulopathy; severe pulmonary compromise; lack of skilled operator to insert; bacteremic patient (risk of catheter seeding)
Femoral catheter	Low rate of catheter-associated bacteremia: easy to insert	Temporary (<72 h)	Agitated patient, previous lower extremity bypass procedure with prosthetic or vein graft

cramps, nausea, vomiting, headache, dialysis disequilibrium, anaphylactic reaction to the dialyzer, and air embolus. Dialysis also can be associated with hypoxemia. The PO_2 may fall 5–30 mm Hg, a decrease that may be dangerous in a critically ill patient who is not receiving mechanical ventilation. This hypoxemia is nearly always a result of hypoventilation induced by metabolic alkalosis caused by bicarbonate transfer from the dialyzer or by loss of carbon dioxide into the dialysate. Complement activation by the dialysis membrane may also disturb ventilation/perfusion matching when Cuprophane membranes are used.

Medication and hyperalimentation require special attention in dialysis patients. Because the major waste products removed by dialysis are derived from protein catabolism and because many critically ill patients are catabolic, excessively high protein loads should be avoided. (See Chapter 4 for metabolic support guidelines.) Drug metabolism is altered in patients with renal failure, and many unmeasured metabolites accumulate in the bloodstream. In addition, highly protein-bound drugs, such as warfarin and phenytoin, are displaced from albumin by organic acids. High concentrations of free drug then result.

Table 3 Dialysis Orders

Variables	Options available	Usual choice
Dialyzer K_{uf} (mL/h per mm Hg)	1.4–22	4–6
Dialyzer surface area (m^2)	0.5–1.9	1.4–1.8
Blood flow rate (mL/min)	200–450	Maximum obtainable
Transmembrane pressure (TMP) (mm Hg)	0–500	Calculate from desired fluid loss (F): TMP = $F/(K_{uf} \times$ h of d.)
Dialysate composition		
Potassium (mEq/L)	0–4	2 (varies with patient)
Base	Acetate or bicarbonate (35 mEq/L)	Bicarbonate
Dextrose (g/dL)	0–200	200
Anticoagulation	Administer heparin systemically or to dialyzer only	Administer heparin systemically
Length of dialysis (h)	2.5–5	4

Table 4 Factors Other Than Renal Function That Affect Creatinine and BUN Values

	Increase	Decrease
Creatinine	Muscle catabolism Diabetic ketoacidosis	Decreased muscle mass (immobilization, amputation, advanced age)
BUN	Gastrointestinal bleeding Catabolic state Steroid therapy Volume depletion Excessive protein intake Diuretics Acidosis	Hepatic failure

The number of medications should be minimized in dialysis patients. Specific guidelines for common drugs are summarized in Chapter 49. Clinical pharmacologists and nephrologists can help determine appropriate medication regimens. *The Physicians' Desk Reference* also includes information on drug use in renal failure.

Fluid removal with dialysis is limited by the patient's hemodynamic status and the time spent receiving dialysis. Because removal of more than 5 L of fluid at a time is generally not possible, the patient's total fluid intake, including blood products, should

Table 5 Causes of Hypotension During Dialysis

Common Causes
  Excessive decrease in blood volume because of high ultrafiltration rate, low target dry weight
  Lack of vasoconstriction from antihypertensives, acetate in dialysate, autonomic neuropathy
  Poor cardiac function (systolic dysfunction, diastolic dysfunction, right heart failure)
Uncommon causes
  Tamponade
  Myocardial infarction
  Hemorrhage
  Septicemia
  Dysrhythmias
  Anaphylaxis
  Air embolism
Possible solutions
  Evaluate patient for blood loss
  Increase target dry weight
  Reduce transmembrane pressure or decrease dialyzer size
  Increase pressor medications
  Stop antihypertensives
  Reduce temperature of dialysate
  Institute sodium modeling
  Transfuse any required blood products during dialysis
  Increase time on dialysis
  Give midodrine before run
  Obtain echocardiogram to evaluate cardiac function
  Consider uncommon causes listed above

be limited to no more than 2 L plus replacement of urine and nasogastric drainage. Urine output can frequently be increased by diuretic use. An effective strategy is to combine a loop diuretic, such as furosemide or bumetanide, with a thiazide diuretic, such as metolazone or hydrochlorothiazide. The use of large bolus doses of loop diuretics should be avoided because of the high risk of ototoxicity. Intravenous furosemide in doses >100 mg should be given as a controlled infusion of 4 mg/min. Alternatively, continuous low dose intravenous infusion of bumetanide may be effective in patients with chronic renal failure. The need for fluid removal with dialysis should be minimized by concentrating all medications and alimentation solutions in the smallest possible volume of fluid.

CONTINUOUS VENOVENOUS HEMOFILTRATION

Continuous venovenous hemofiltration (CVVH) is a method of continuous fluid removal. The ultrafiltrate passes through the membrane into the ultrafiltration space and drains into a collection bag. Gravity drainage creates subatmospheric pressure in the filter, which increases the ultrafiltration rate. In addition, a pump can be added to the circuit to control the ultrafiltration rate. The blood cells and proteins remaining in the blood chamber are then returned to the patient. The process is continued 24 h/day. Large volumes of fluid (up to 900 mL/h) can be removed with this therapy, and replacement fluid must be infused into the patient. Because of this fluid exchange, a limited clearance of waste products also occurs.

CVVH can be modified to slow continuous ultrafiltration (SCUF) if solute clearance is not necessary. Ultrafiltration rate is limited to <5 mL/min and replacement fluid is not given. With either procedure, volume status and medication dosages must be carefully monitored.

CONTINUOUS VENOVENOUS HEMOFILTRATION WITH DIALYSIS

Patients with severe renal failure cannot achieve adequate solute clearance with CVVH. In this situation, intermittent hemodialysis can be instituted or CVVH can be modified to include dialysis (CVVHD). Dialysate is infused into the dialyzer, countercurrent to blood flow. Solute removal is effected as in hemodialysis (see earlier discussion). However, the rate of solute removal is proportional to the dialysate flow rate (generally 1–2 L/h) rather than the blood flow rate. The ultrafiltration rate can be varied. If it is <5 mL/min, the need for replacement fluid is diminished. Alternatively, it may be increased as needed if the patient is volume expanded.

CHOOSING A METHOD OF RENAL REPLACEMENT THERAPY

Advantages and disadvantages of CVVHD compared with hemodialysis are summarized in Table 6. Unfortunately, randomized prospective studies are not available comparing the morbidity and mortality of these dialysis methods. Hemodialysis has the advantage of being widely available. CVVH and CVVHD require skilled nursing staff, specifically trained in their use, as well as clinical pharmacologists, to aid in the modification of medication doses. CVVHD may be useful in patients who do not tolerate hemodialysis or who

Table 6 CVVHD Compared to Hemodialysis

Advantages
  Well tolerated in hypotension
  Allows greater volume of fluid removal
  Does not require continuous presence of
    dialysis nurse
Disadvantages
  Requires anticoagulation
  Requires continuous bedrest
  Requires high volume of fluid replacement
  Has low efficiency in removing urea and other
    metabolic end products
  Not useful for acute hyperkalemia
  Medication dosage adjustment can be
    problematic
  Expensive

require large amounts of alimentation solutions or blood products. In addition, intriguing evidence exists that CVVHD may remove endotoxin-triggered mediators, such as thromboxane A2 and leukotrienes, and may possibly increase survival rates in patients with multiorgan system failure.

SUMMARY

- Monitor variables of fluid balance, including daily weights, blood pressure in lying and standing positions, pulse, and hemodynamic measurements, if available.
- Monitor variables of uremia, including creatinine and BUN values, pericardial rub, and anorexia and nausea.
- Be alert for serious complications of dialysis, including hypoxemia, hypotension, and anaphylactic reaction to dialyzer membrane.
- Monitor patient for evidence of bleeding.
- Limit intravenous fluid administration. The clinical target is no more than 2 L/day plus urine and insensible losses.
- Limit hyperalimentation to <1.5 g/kg per day of protein, if appropriate for level of metabolic stress.
- Check all medication dosages for necessary adjustments, including the need for a supplemental dose after hemodialysis.
- Consider use of CVVHD in patients with refractory volume overload or hypotension.

REFERENCES

1. Hamel M, et al. Outcomes and cost-effectivenes of initiating dialysis and continuing aggressive care in seriously ill hospitalized adults. Ann Intern Med 1997; 127:195–202.

2. Manns M, Sigler M, Teehan B. Intradialytic renal haemodynamics-potential consequences for the management of the patient with acute renal failure. Nephrol Dial Transplant 1997; 12:870.
3. Golper T, Marx M. Drug dosing adjustments during continuous renal replacement therapies. Kidney Int 1998; 53:S-165–S-168.
4. Manns M, Sigler M, Teehan B. Continuous renal replacement therapies: an update. Am J Kidney Dis 1998; 32:185–207.
5. Pastan S, Bailey J. Dialysis therapy. N Engl J Med 1998; 1428.
6. Dheenan S, Henrich W. Preventing dialysis hypotension: a comparison of usual protective maneuvers. Kidney Int 2001; 59:1175–1181.
7. Galland R, et al. Short daily hemodialysis rapidly improves nutritional status in hemodialysis patients. Kidney Int 2001; 60:1555–1560.
8. Butterly D, Schwab S. The case against chronic venous hemodialysis access. J Am Soc Nephrol 2002; 13:2195–2197.
9. Schiffel H, Lang S, Fischer R. Daily hemodialysis and the outcome of acute renal failure. N Engl J Med 2002; 346:305.

G. Gastrointestinal and Hepatic Function

36

Gut Function: Practical Considerations for the Intensivist

David C. Evans
McGill University Health Care, Montreal, Quebec, Canada

The mucosa of the human intestine covers an estimated 300 m^2 and provides a critical barrier against a reservoir of over 400 bacterial strains. In addition to digestion and nutrient absorption, the gut mucosa also presents an active immunologic interface, which plays a key role in host health. Reliable clinical variables to monitor the health of the gut mucosal barrier (GMB) currently do not exist. Consequently, current therapy aims at supporting the GMB's three major constituents: mucosal integrity, immunocompetence, and the balance of commensal microflora. Of practical concern to the intensivist are preservation of GMB, maintenance of normal gut ecology, awareness of the risk of antibiotic-associated (*Clostridium difficile*) colitis, optimization of nutritional support, and minimization of the risk of stress ulceration and bleeding.

THE GUT MUCOSAL BARRIER

GMB is a multi-tiered defense against potentially lethal systemic invasion by intestinally contained micro-organisms, which are potentially lethal to the host. While the stomach and upper GI tract are normally sparsely inhabited by *Lactobacillus* and gram-positive species, the colon harbors hundreds of bacterial strains, including *Enterobacteriaceae*, *Proteus*, *Enterococcus*, *Pseudomonas*, *Lactobacillius*, and a greater than 1000-fold predominance of anaerobic species. The consequences of failure to contain these strains and the toxins they elaborate are important in the care of the critically ill patient (1,2). Understanding all components of the GMB is essential for appropriate therapy.

Physical Barrier Function

Mechanical Barrier
The enterocyte's lipid membrane, bound to adjacent cells by tight junctions, is a physical barrier to bacterial invasion. The orderly turnover of healthy cells is crucial to the maintenance of this barrier. Malnutrition, hypoxia, and the reduced trophic stimulation of gut hormones, characteristic of the catabolic state, impair cell migration and regeneration and compromise this barrier. Coordinated intestinal motility, also commonly disrupted in

the ICU patient, is not only an essential stimulus to cellular turnover, but also maintains the flow of bacterial toxins through the digestive tract.

Chemical and Enzymatic Barriers

A gastric pH < 4.5 is antibacterial. Activation of pepsinogen to pepsin below this pH counters the action of microbes and their toxins. Intestinally produced mucus and secreted humoral factors protect the host from bacterial invasion. Like bile salts, mucin secreted throughout the GI tract nonspecifically binds bacteria and endotoxins within the bowel lumen. Substances such as lactoferrin, salivary lysozyme, and peroxidase also serve to inhibit the growth of sensitive organisms. Mucin protects the gastric enterocyte from acidity by maintaining an alkaline gradient of bicarbonate against the cell surface. The small, but real, risk of clinically important stress-related GI bleeding in at-risk ICU patients makes use of antacid regimens routine. Although alkalinization effectively reduces acid-induced mucosal ulceration, it promotes gastric overgrowth by enteric and extrinsic nosocomial flora (3). This bacterial overgrowth does not harm the stomach, but may predispose the patient to ICU-acquired pneumonia.

Immunologic Barrier

Local Barrier

The intestinal mucosa and submucosa are richly inhabited by macrophages, lymphocytes, neutrophils, eosinophils, and mast cells. Peyer's patches are strategically located in the distal ileum to sample the antigenic load of the gut contents. Along with the lymphoid tissue of the lamina propria, they give rise to activated B lymphocytes, which mature in mesenteric lymph nodes and reach the systemic circulation by way of the thoracic duct. These B cells, stimulated by IL-4 and IL-10, differentiate predominantly into secretory IgA-producing plasmocytes, which selectively relocate along mucosal surfaces to secrete antibodies into saliva, bile, and succus. Secretory IgA binds bowel bacteria, induces bacteriolysis, and prevents bacterial adherence to the mucosal surface. A population of T lymphocytes also resides alongside the enterocytes of the gut mucosa to provide a cytotoxic line of defense through cytokine production.

Systemic Barrier

Bacteria and toxins migrate across the GMB, enter the portal circulation, and filter through the Kupffer cell macrophage bed of the liver. After sampling portal antigens, these cells are involved in the mediation of systemic immune responses (4). Gram-negative bacteria, which either colonize the small bowel or are introduced into the portal circulation, depress the delayed-type hypersensitivity response to subcutaneously injected antigens (5). Kupffer cells appear to produce immunologic mediators in response to antigenic stimulation by the gut. These cells also prompt increased interleukin-1 and prostaglandin E_2 production when exposed to endotoxin. Unregulated antigenic stimulation possibly prompts an exaggerated immune response that culminates in the syndrome of multiple system organ failure (MSOF) (6).

The common mucosal immune hypothesis has been advanced to account for the observed immunity conferred by the extra-intestinal migration of lymphoid cells to, for example, lung mucosa, which is stimulated by antigen processing in gut-associated lymphoid tissue (GALT) (7). Experimentally, the gut in enterally fed animals supports secretory IgA-based immunity against pulmonary infections from *Haemophilus influenzae* and *Pseudomonas aeruginosa*. Parenteral nutrition is associated with GALT atrophy, reduced cytokine production (notably B cell stimulating IL-4 and IL-10), reduced intestinal IgA production, and a marked loss of existing IgA-based immunocompetence. A clinical trial randomizing trauma patients to parenteral vs. enteral feeds demonstrated a pneumonia rate of 31% and 11%, respectively. Mucosal immunity and intestinal priming of neutrophils are key elements of host defense mounted by GMB.

Bacteriologic Barrier

The maintenance of normal gut microbial ecology is critical in the prevention of enteric autoinfection. The intestinal microflora not only preserves barrier integrity and enhances mechanical function by stimulating and nourishing the mucosal cells but also acts to prevent overgrowth and colonization by potentially harmful organisms. The capacity of a balanced population of gut microflora to prohibit an abnormal proliferation of potentially harmful bacteria in the gut is termed *colonization resistance*. The stability of gut ecology, however, is greatly influenced by host antibiotic exposures. Enteric bacteria translocate across gut mucosa when antibiotic use has altered normal microbial populations (8). Furthermore, common SICU-acquired infections are linked to overgrowth of certain gut commensals, including *Enterococcus*, *Staphylococcus epidermidis*, *Pseudomonas*, and *Candida*. Alterations of gut microflora also impair local host immunity and increase the potential for GMB failure. Translocation of *Candida* across gut mucosa in debilitated surgical patients has been demonstrated (9,10).

Perturbations in the balance of gut flora are potentially harmful in many ways. Enteric bacteria have been shown to translocate across gut mucosa when antibiotic use has altered normal microbial populations (8). General patterns of antimicrobial use in an ICU, particularly the liberal use of broad-spectrum antibiotics, exert "antibiotic pressure" on gut flora and allow widespread colonization of ICU patients by multi-resistant organisms. The depopulation of the predominant anaerobic flora of the gut through anti-anaerobic antibiotic use, and particularly the widespread use of third-generation cephalosporins, is postulated to play a major role in the increasing prevalence of resistant strains (11). A rigorous program of fecal screening and subsequent isolation of identified carriers is essential to limit the colonization of other patients by these organisms.

Clostridium Difficile Colitis

One consequence of altered gut microflora is *C. difficile* colitis. *C. difficile* is a gram-positive spore-forming bacillus now recognized as the major cause of nosocomial diarrhea in North America. It colonizes up to 20% of hospitalized patients receiving antibiotic therapy and infects up to 3%. The clinical manifestations vary from an asymptomatic carrier state to mild inflammation to life-threatening toxic pseudomembranous colitis. Exotoxins A and B produced by the bacillus damage the enterocyte cytoskeleton, cause tight junction disruption, and increase mucosal permeability and fluid secretion to produce sometimes severe diarrhea. In severe cases, mucosal ulceration occurs and a proteinaceous inflammatory exudate mixed with overlying necrotic debris forms the characteristic pseudomembranes recognized during colonoscopy. Although all antibiotics are a risk, those agents most commonly associated with *C. difficile* infection are clindamycin, cephalosporins, ampicillin, and amoxicillin.

The standard diagnostic test for *C. difficile* is the tissue culture cytotoxin assay, in which a monolayer of cultured fibroblasts is inoculated with stool specimen filtrate. This test has 70–100% sensitivity and 85–100% specificity, but is costly and requires up to 48 h to complete. More commonly used are commercially available enzyme-linked immunoassays to detect exotoxin (usually type A). Only slightly less accurate, this test is cheaper and faster (2–6 h).

The treatment of *C. difficile* colitis is 98% effective with metronidazole 250 mg PO QID, 500 mg PO TID, or 500 mg IV TID for 7–10 days. Vancomycin 125 mg PO QID is recommended for patients not improving with metronidazole therapy. For severe pseudomembranous colitis, combination therapy with IV metronidazole, PO vancomycin, and vancomycin retention enemas (500 mg in 100 mL NS q6H) is recommended. Other treatment options include teicoplanin, bacitracin, elimination of antiperistaltic agents, cholestyramine anion exchange resin to absorb and clear toxins, immunoglobulin therapy, and biotherapy using yeast or fecal enemas to repopulate the gut with nonpathogenic flora. None of these adjuncts have been proven effective. Discontinuing antibiotics resolves 20% of cases without a need for further therapy. Discontinuing all non-essential antibiotics should always be attempted.

THE GUT AND MSOF

Enteric microflora enhance gut function by facilitating digestion, nutritionally supporting the mucosal epithelium, and maintaining a crucial balance of commensal organisms. They also represent a threat to the host should the gut fail to contain them adequately. The lipopolysaccharide component of the gram-negative bacterial cell wall known as endotoxin is a well-recognized trigger of the septic clinical state marked by fever, confusion, tachycardia, hyperdynamic circulation, water retention, hyperbilirubinemia, compromised renal function, and impaired respiratory function. Because endotoxin is a product of both viable and nonviable bacteria, the gut comprises the body's largest reservoir of potentially harmful bacterial products. "Autointoxication" by these microbial substances is regarded by many as the first step in a cascade of systemic events culminating in the often fatal syndrome of MSOF (12). One potential mechanism of this autointoxication is translocation, the migration of bacteria and toxins under conditions of compromised barrier function. Translocation has been convincingly demonstrated under experimental conditions that mimic those present in the critically ill (9,13). Gut bacteria have been isolated in homogenates of liver, spleen, and mesenteric lymph nodes in amounts proportional to the degree of imposed hypovolemic shock in laboratory animals (14). Bacteremia of enteric origin is also described as a fatal complication of chemotherapy in neutropenic patients. Other factors thought to enhance translocation are peritonitis, bowel obstruction, inflammatory bowel disease, thermal injury, bacterial overgrowth, immunosuppression, splanchnic low-flow states, and endotoxemia. Bacteremic organisms in patients with these conditions are often the predominant aerobic fecal strains.

Although untreated infection has been thought responsible for the progression of MSOF, the frequent failure to identify an infectious focus by routine cultures, postmortem studies, and blind laparotomy has resulted in the concept of nonbacterial clinical sepsis (2). The septic state can arise in the absence of infection by systemic exposure to endotoxin, a likely source of which is the compromised gut. A controlled prospective clinical trial using HA-IA human IgM antibody against the lipid A domain of endotoxin showed that monoclonal immunotherapy could reduce mortality in certain patients with gram-negative bacteremia (15). In other trials, this protection was not observed. Tumor necrosis factor, interleukin-1, interleukin-2, and prostaglandins are host-derived mediators in this process, which are capable of invoking the "septic response" independent of endotoxin. Therapy targeting these and other mediators of the septic response offers a logical approach to this complex physiologic problem, as illustrated by the recent demonstration of improved survival with activated protein C in septic ICU patients (16). Chapter 1 discusses some recent progress in understanding the pathophysiology and therapy of the organ failure syndrome.

The unhealthy gut must thus be recognized as a potential instigator of MSOF (9,17). As long as the treatment of MSOF remains primarily supportive, attempted prevention through intestinal support is paramount in the ICU setting. Although numerous prophylactic regimens have become well established, current thinking challenges common protocols, particularly the value of "bowel rest" and a pH–neutral stomach.

SUPPORTING GUT BARRIER FUNCTION

Assessment of intestinal function is based on clinical evaluation of the presence of ileus, diarrhea, gastritis, and stress ulceration. Maintenance of GMB per se has now become an important clinical goal. Although providing support for intestinal physiology as described below is important, the key for preserving mucosal function is control of the process initiating or contributing to its compromise. Rapid resolution of the inciting process, infection, ischemia, or graft rejection is pivotal to the effective management of sepsis. Sepsis, and ultimately MSOF, is a late-stage manifestation of the biologic response to some initial physiologic derangement, and effective therapy must integrate the concept that *infection is a process and sepsis is a response.*

To control the response, first the process must be controlled. This concept addresses the need for diligence in the clinical approach to the prevention and treatment of MSOF in which GMB dysfunction is but one of many components that may comprise either the primary inciting event or some secondary sequelae. Support of the GMB may be a factor that prevents MSOF and includes consideration of optimizing oxygen transport, enhancing gut motility, nutritional support, stress ulcer prophylaxis (SUP), and antibiotic prophylaxis.

Oxygen Transport

Breakdown of the GMB and bacterial translocation occurs in splanchnic low-flow states, such as hypovolemic shock or cardiac arrest. Hypoxia, enterocyte-protease activation, and superoxide-free-radical generation are postulated mechanisms. Experimental evidence supports a role for therapy with antiprostaglandins and free radical scavengers. In practice, therapy is limited to maintaining adequately oxygenated circulation to the splanchnic bed. Intravenous volume replacement, red blood cell transfusion to maintain oxygen carrying capacity, and maintaining an oxygen saturation >90% are essential. Hemodynamic monitoring and assisted ventilation should be used as required. Some investigators advocate pharmacologic dilation of the splanchnic vascular bed with low-dose dopamine. In the experimental setting beta-adrenergic agonists (2), cholinergic agents, and peptide hormones have all shown promise, but are rarely used clinically for this indication. Restoration of oxygen transport receives further discussion in Chapter 2.

Enhancing Gut Motility

Reduced sepsis, better wound healing, and lower costs make enteral feeding of the critically ill patient preferable to total parenteral nutrition (TPN). Efficacy of enteral feeding may be compromised by multiple factors that impair gut motility. These factors include narcotic analgesia, catecholamine administration, sepsis, hyperglycemia, recumbent position, and abdominal surgery. Three prokinetic agents are used to enhance gut motility: metoclopramide (10–20 mg IV), erythromycin (40 mg PO, 200 mg IV), and cisapride (20 mg). Erythromycin is a macrolide antibiotic that enhances phase III of the gut migrating myoelectric complex through activation of motilin receptors. Metoclopramide antagonizes dopamine inhibition of gut motility. Although effective, cisapride has the potential for causing lethal cardiac dysrhythmias and currently is not used.

A systematic review of evidence from 18 studies (18) concluded that enteral feeding can be improved by the use of promotility agents in critically ill patients intolerant to feeds and recommended metoclopramide over erythromycin. A one-time dose of erythromycin (200 mg) does appear useful to aid placement of jejunal feeding tubes.

Nutritional Support

The provision of adequate nutrition, either enterally or parenterally, is essential to maintaining immune competence and ameliorate the catabolic state of critical illness. For reasons of efficacy, simplicity, and cost, enteral nutrition is always preferred. Even when parenteral nutrition is indicated, concurrent administration of as many calories through the gut as safely possible is desirable. Chapter 4 discusses nutritional support in further detail.

Stress Ulcer Prophylaxis

Although the catastrophic bleeding episodes seen in the 1970s now rarely occur, ostensibly as a result of improved methods of resuscitation and supportive care, superficial gastric erosion causing serious hemorrhage remains a complication in ICU patients. A landmark epidemiological study determined that the greatest risk factors for stress-related GI hemorrhage are intubation >48 h and nonpharmacologic coagulopathy (19). Statistically significant associated relative *risk ratios* were 15.6 and 4.3, respectively. Other important factors appeared to be hypotension and sepsis. While the incidence of important bleeding in the presence of risk factors was 3.7%, it was <0.1% in the absence of risk factors. Clinically important bleeding was defined as overt bleeding with hemodynamic changes, a 2 gm/dL decrease in hemoglobin concentration, a 2-unit packed red blood cell transfusion, or a requirement for surgery. Because patients with clinically important bleeding have been found to have an increased mortality compared with patients without bleeding (48.5% vs. 9.1%, respectively), stress ulcer prophylaxis (SUP) is recommended for at-risk patients. To date, H2-blockers, antacids, sucralfate, and pirenzepine are the only agents to have been evaluated in randomized controlled trials, and they appear to be effective in stress ulcer prophylaxis.

A metanalysis of controlled trials evaluating SUP strategies suggested that both H2-blockers and sucralfate significantly reduced important bleeding (20). This report was followed by a prospective, multi-center, randomized controlled trial comparing ranitidine (50 mg IV q8H) with sucralfate (1 gm/NG q6H) (21). Ranitidine was found to reduce bleeding by more than 50%. The incidence of bleeding in the ranitidine group was 1.7%, whereas a 3.8% bleeding incidence was associated with sucralfate therapy. Proton pump inhibitors, such as omeprazole, have not yet been rigorously evaluated for the purpose of SUP, but are widely used in the belief that they offer the most effective acid inhibition.

A significant consequence of gastric alkalinization is colonizaztion of the stomach with enteric bacteria, which can gain access to the upper airways and cause pneumonia through the mechanisms of oropharyngeal reflux and micro-aspiration (22). Some investigators argue that the mortality increase attributable to nosocomial pneumonia may exceed the benefit of reduced GI bleeding in at-risk patients who have been given stress ulcer prophylaxis. One study showed that acidification of enteral feeds is effective in reducing gastric colonization, but the study was not adequately powered to reveal significant differences in pneumonia or mortality, despite the observation that the pneumonia rate was 9% higher without gastric acidification (23). Although classic work by Driks et al. (3) suggested that cytoprotective agents, such as sucralfate, preserve gastric acidity and relative gastric sterility in intubated patients compared with antacid therapy, the rate of nosocomial pneumonia in the previously cited trial comparing ranitidine with sucralfate demonstrated no statistically significant difference in the incidence of pneumonia (19.1% vs. 16.2%, respectively; $p = 0.19$). No study has rigorously investigated the relationship between stress ulcer prophylaxis and nosocomial pneumonia in order to adequately resolve this important issue.

A recently reported concern related to stress ulcer prophylaxis is the observation of an increased incidence of *Clostridium difficile* associated diarrhea (CDAD) linked to the use of proton pump inhibitors. This is worrisome given an increasing prevalence of CDAD in recent years, and an increase in its attributable mortality (24). Ingested clostridial spores are largely neutralized by normal gastric acidity, and alkalinization breaches this important defense. Good prospective data is presently required to confirm this potentially fatal threat to patients.

Antibiotic Prophylaxis

Selective Decontamination of the Digestive Tract

Selective decontamination of the digestive tract (SDD) was introduced by Stoutenbeck et al. (25) in 1984 as a means to control enteric sepsis by: (1) eliminating aerobic gram-negative gut bacteria, (2) preventing fungal overgrowth, and (3) preserving commensal anaerobic microflora of the oropharynx and gastrointestinal tract. The usual SDD regimen involves a combination of polymyxin E, tobramycin and amphotericin B, given both intragastrically and topically as an oral paste, plus a broad-spectrum systemic antibiotic, such as cefotaxime, given intravenously for four days. The use of a systemic cephalosporin to prevent infection before the triple-antibiotic regimen can attain a sterilizing effect may promote colonization with resistant organisms (26). Studies show that aminoglycoside-resistant strains can emerge in the SDD-treated patients, and early colonization with staphylococcus may be enhanced.

Microbiologic monitoring in the form of three times weekly cultures from the nasopharynx, tracheobronchial aspirate, gastric aspirate, urine, blood, and rectum is required to assess the efficacy of sterilization and the emergence of resistant bacterial strains. As concluded by numerous investigators, this intervention appears to sterilize the nasopharynx successfully and to reduce bacterial counts variably in the stomach and rectum (7,25,27). It is also useful in the elimination of resistant nosocomial strains of gut colonizing bacteria in the ICU patient (28). When compared with control results, SDD prophylaxis is associated with a low overall incidence of nosocomial infection in SICU patients (27). Pneumonia, the most common infectious complication in ICU patients, can be significantly reduced, and patients appear to suffer fewer septic episodes associated with gram-negative bacteremia. Presumably, the decreased rate of nosocomial infection in SDD patients is primarily due to sterilization of the upper oropharynx and digestive tract. In this way the results of SDD compare with similar findings in patients receiving cytoprotective sucralfate therapy, which preserves bacteriostatic gastric acidity (3).

Theoretically, SDD should diminish the risk of exposure to circulating endotoxin and attendant MSOF. Despite a meta-analysis of controlled prospective trials of SDD demonstrating a 30% mortality reduction in critically ill surgical patients (OR 0.7, 95% CI 0.52–0.93) (29), the study of Ledingham et al. (30) demonstrated that the mortality rate is reduced only in certain subgroups, namely, those patients with trauma, prolonged hospitalization, and midrange APACHE II scores. The precise role of SDD and the elucidation of effective regimens need further clarification.

GUT FAILURE: WHAT DO WE MEAN?

The common description of gut failure in the critically ill patient as the presence of ileus is inadequate. When compromised by microcirculatory failure, which is thought to be at the root of MSOF, the gut not only loses the mechanical function of peristalsis, but also demonstrates impaired nutrient absorption, mucosal breakdown with consequent hemorrhage, bacterial translocation, and diminished gut immune function. By unleashing a flood of bacteria and their byproducts into the systemic circulation, the gut may well be the "engine" of MSOF, but recognizing, defining, and measuring gut dysfunction have proven difficult. Not surprisingly, the widely cited *multiple organ dysfunction* score of Marshall et al. (31), used to measure multiple organ failure, excludes intestinal function in its six-system composite score. The mortality rate of nearly 50% associated with GI bleeding in critically ill patients, an extreme manifestation of gut failure that alone is a powerful marker for poor outcome, indicates the need for better definition and quantification of gut failure in outcome analysis.

Like the so-called "vital organs," the intestine must be regarded by the ICU physician as a target organ requiring aggressive support to ensure patient survival. Currently, therapeutic measures aimed at maintaining gut homeostasis still fall into the realm of generalized supportive care. That early adequate nutrition, preferably by the enteral route, is required to preserve both intestinal cell mass and function is not disputed. Judicious antibiotic use will increase the likelihood that the balanced ecology of valuable gut flora is not harmfully upset or that antibiotic-associated colitis does not develop. Also, a high index of suspicion must exist to ensure that irreversibly compromised bowel is not present in the deteriorating ICU patient. No clinical markers to identify this situation in a timely manner currently exist, and laparotomy remains the diagnostic and therapeutic standard when the gut is suspected to be significantly compromised by ischemia, bleeding, or superinfection. Advanced radiologic imaging is rarely definitive. Bedside mini-laparotomy and laparoscopy are emerging as diagnostic alternatives in these often enigmatic ICU patients.

SUMMARY

- The major components of GMB are mucosal integrity, immunocompetence, and balance of commensal flora.
- The enterocyte's lipid membrane, with its binding to adjacent cells by tight junctions, is a physical barrier to bacterial invasion.
- Intestinally secreted mucus and humoral factors are protective. Mucin binds bacteria and toxins, lysozyme and peroxidase inhibit bacterial growth, and acid production in the stomach is antibacterial.

- Immunologic components of the intestinal mucosa and submucosa include macrophages, lymphocytes, neutrophils, eosinophils, and mast cells. Peyer's patches and lymphoid tissue activate B lymphocytes.
- B lymphocytes differentiate into secretory IgA-producing cells. Secretory IgA binds bowel bacteria, induces bacteriolysis, and prevents bacterial adherence to the mucosa.
- T lymphocytes secrete cytokines to provide a cytotoxic defense.
- The common mucosal immune hypothesis accounts for the immunity seen in, for example, the lung that is conferred by the extra-intestinal migration of lymphoid cells stimulated by antigen processing in gut-associated lymphoid tissue.
- Translocation is the migration of bacteria and toxins across the GMB. It is increased under conditions of compromised intestinal mucosal barrier function.
- Normal intestinal microflora preserves barrier integrity, enhances mechanical function by stimulating and nourishing mucosal cells, and prevents overgrowth by potentially harmful organisms.

REFERENCES

1. Saadia R, Schein M, MacFarlane C, Boffard KD. Gut barrier function and the surgeon. Br J Surg 1990; 77:487–492.
2. Steinmetz OK, Meakins JL. Care of the gut in the surgical intensive care unit: Fact or function? Can J Surg 1991; 34:207–215.
3. Driks MR, Craven DE, Celli BR, Manning M, Burke RA, Garvin GM, Kunches LM, Farber HW, Wedel SA, McCabe WR. Nosocomial pneumonia in intubated patients given sucralfate as compared with antacids or histamine type-2 blockers. The role of gastric colonization. N Engl J Med 1987; 317(22):1376–1382.
4. Marshall J, Lee C, Meakins JL. Kupffer cell modulation of the systemic immune response. Arch Surg 1987; 122:191–196.
5. Marshall J, Christou NH, Meakins JL. Immunomodulation by altered gastrointestinal tract flora. Arch Surg 1988; 123:1465–1469.
6. Billiar TR, Maddaus MA, West MA, Curran RD, Wells CA, Simmons RL. Intestinal gram-negative overgrowth in vivo augments the in vitro response of Kupffer cells to endotoxin. Ann Surg 1988; 208(4):532–540.
7. Montejo JC. The Nutritional and Metabolic Working Group of the Spanish Society of Intensive Care Medicine and Coronary Units. Enteral nutrition-related gastrointestinal complications in critically ill patients: a multicenter study. Crit Care Med 1999; 27:1447–1453.
8. Berg RD. Promotion of the translocation of enteric bacilli from the gastrointestinal tracts of mice by oral treatment with penicillin, clindamycin or metronidazole. Infect Immun 1981; 33:854–861.
9. Deitch EA. The role of intestinal barrier failure and bacterial translocation in the development of systemic infection and multiple organ failure. Arch Surg 1990; 125:403–404.
10. Stone HH, Kolb LD, Currie, CA, Geheber CE, Cuzzell JZ. *Candida sepsis*: pathogenesis and principles of treatment. Ann Surg 1974; 179(5):697–711.
11. Bonten MJ, Willems R, Weinstein RA. Vancomycin-resistant enterococci: why are they here, and where do they come from? Lancet Infect Dis 2001; 1(5):314–25.
12. Fry DE. Multiple system organ failure. Surg Clin North Am 1988; 68:107–122.
13. Schweinburg FR, Seligman AM, Fine J. Transmural migration of intestinal bacteria—a study based on the use of radioactive *Escherichia coli*. N Engl J Med 1950; 242:747–752.
14. Baker JW, Deitch EA, Berg RD, Special RD. Hemodynamic shock induced bacterial translocation from the gut. J. Trauma 1988; 28:896–906.

15. Ziegler EJ, Fisher CJ Jr, Sprung CL, Straube RC, Sadoff JC, Foulke GE, Wortel CH, Fink MP, Dellinger RP, Teng NN, et al. Treatment of gram-negative bacteremia and septic shock with HA-IA human monoclonal antibody against endotoxin. A randomized, double-blind, placebo-controlled trial. The HA-1A Sepsis Study Group. N Engl J Med 1991; 324(7):429–436.
16. Bernard GR, Vincent JL, Laterre PF, LaRosa SP, Dhainaut JF, Lopez-Rodriguez A, Steingrub JS, Garber GE, Helterbrand JD, Ely EW, Fisher CJ Jr. Recombinant human Protein C worldwide Evaluation in Severe Sepsis (PROWESS) study group. Efficacy and safety of recombinant human activated protein C for severe sepsis. N Engl J Med 2001; 344(10):699–709.
17. Carrico CJ, Meakins JL, Marshall JC, Fry D. Maier RV. Multiple-organ-failure syndrome. Arch Surg 1986; 121(2):196–208.
18. Iverdy JC, Chi HS, Sheldon GF. The effect of parenteral nutrition on gastrointestinal immunity: the importance of enteral stimulation. Ann Surg 1985; 202:681–684.
19. Cook DJ, Fuller HD, Guyatt GH, Marshall JC, Leasa D, Hall R, Winton TL, Rutledge F, Todd TJ, Roy P, et al. Risk factors for gastrointestinal bleeding in critically ill patients. Canadian Critical Care Trials Group. N Engl J Med 1994; 330(6):337–381.
20. Cook DJ, Reeve BK, Guyatt GH, Heyland DK, Griffith LE, Buckingham L, Tryba M. Stress ulcer prophylaxis in critically ill patients. Resolving discordant meta-analyses. JAMA 1996; 275(4):308–314.
21. Cook D, Guyatt G, Marshall J, Leasa D, Fuller H, Hall R, Peters S, Rutledge F, Griffith L, McLellan A, Wood G. Kirby A. A comparison of sucralfate and ranitidine for the prevention of upper gastrointestinal bleeding in patients requiring mechanical ventilation. Canadian Critical Care Trials Group. N Engl J Med; 1998; 338(12):791–797.
22. du Moulin GC, Patterson DG, Hedley-Whyte J, Lisbon A. Aspiration of gastric bacteria in antacid-treated patients: a frequent cause of postoperative colonisation of the airway. Lancet 1982; 1(8266):242–245.
23. Heyland DK. The effect of acidified enteral feeds on gastric colonization in critically ill patients: results of a multicenter randomized trial. Canadian Critical Care Trials Group. Crit Care Med 1999; 27(11):2399–406.
24. Dial S, Alrasadi K, Manoukian C, Huang A, Menzies D. Risk of *Clostridium difficile* diarrhea among hospital inpatients prescribed proton pump inhibitors: cohort and case-control studies. Can Med Assoc J 2004; 171(1):33–38.
25. Stoutenbeck CP, Van Saene HKF, Miranda DR, Zandstra DF. The effect of selective decontamination of the digestive tract on colonization and infection rate of multiple trauma patients. Intensive Care Med 1984; 10:185–192.
26. Sanderson PJ. Selective decontamination of the digestive tract. Br Med J 1989; 299:1413–1414.
27. Blair P, Rowlands BJ, Lowry K, Webb H, Armstrong P, Smilie J. Selective decontamination of the digestive tract: a stratified, randomized prospective study in a mixed intensive care unit. Surgery 1991; 110(2):303–309 (discussion 309–310).
28. Brun-Buisson C, Legrand P, Rauss A. Intestinal decontamination for control of nosocomial multiresistant gram-negative bacilli—study of an outbreak in the intensive care unit. Ann Intern Med 1989; 110:873–881.
29. Nathens AB. Selective decontamination of the digestive tract in surgical patients: a systematic review of the evidence. Arch Surg 1999; 134(2):170–616.
30. Ledingham IM, Alcock SR, Eastway AT, McDonald JL, McKay IC, Ramsay G. Triple regimen of the selective decontamination of the digestive tract, systemic cefotaxime, and microbiological surveillance for prevention of acquired infection in intensive care. Lancet 1988; 2:785–790.
31. Marshall JC, Cook DJ, Christou N, Bernard GR, Sprung CL, Sibbald WJ. Multiple organ dysfunction score: a reliable descriptor of a complex clinical outcome. Crit Care Med 1995; 23(10):1638.

37
Acute Gastrointestinal Hemorrhage

Jerome H. Abrams
VA Medical Center, Minneapolis, Minnesota, USA

Acute gastrointestinal (GI) hemorrhage is a frequent cause for admission to the surgical intensive care unit. Upper gastrointestinal (UGI) causes are more common (85%) than lower gastrointestinal (LGI) causes (15%). The likelihood that emergency surgery will be necessary is estimated at 40% for UGI sources and at 30% for LGI sources (1). Clinically, the distinction between UGI and LGI sources is important. Practically, LGI bleeding is hemorrhage that occurs beyond the range of the UGI endoscope. Fortunately, bleeding ceases in ~85% of patients without intervention. The remaining 15% of patients require early, accurate diagnosis and therapy (2).

UGI HEMORRHAGE (Fig. 1)

In the United States, the estimated rate of hospitalization for UGI bleeding is ~100/100,000 patients per year. Typically, patients are >70 years of age and have one or more major chronic organ system diseases (3). Patients hospitalized for another reason before significant bleeding begins have a mortality of 70% (4). In the hospitalized patient, tachycardia, hypotension, or anemia should suggest the possibility of GI hemorrhage.

The most common causes of UGI hemorrhage are esophageal varices, gastric ulcer, and duodenal ulcers. In two large series, these entities accounted for >20% of UGI bleeding sources (4,5). Other causes included esophageal ulcers, malignant ulcers, hiatal herniae, and diverticula. Each of these entities was associated with a <5% chance of producing clinically significant hemorrhage. In the series of Chalmers et al. (5), esophageal varices were demonstrated in 33 of 44 patients with cirrhosis. In 16 of these 33 patients, no point of rupture of varices was found. Yet, in only one of these patients was another possible source of bleeding seen, a chronic duodenal ulcer. When faced with the unusual situation of a patient with apparent GI bleeding, known varices, no evidence of bleeding from the varices, and no other identifiable source, the clinician should continue to suspect variceal bleeding until another source can be found.

UGI endoscopy can locate a bleeding lesion, assess the risk of rebleeding, and, with increasing frequency, control bleeding. With respect to locating the lesion, diagnostic accuracy of 90–95% is typical (6,7). With respect to the risk of rebleeding, several observations have special importance. Active arterial bleeding with streaming of blood, clot adherence to a lesion, an exposed vessel that protrudes from the lesion, and staining of

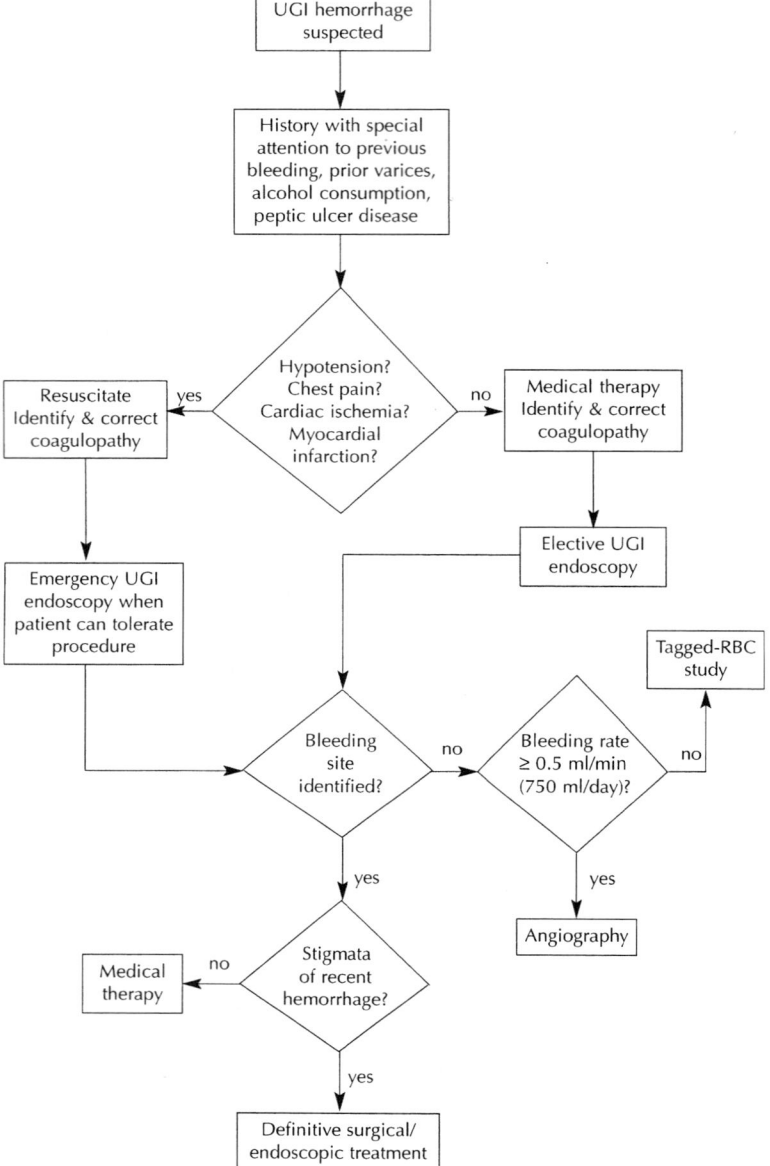

Figure 1 Approach to UGI hemorrhage.

the ulcer base within a lesion are collectively known as stigmata of recent hemorrhage (SRH) (8).

Presence of SRH is associated with increased rebleeding risk and increased mortality. For ulcers actively bleeding at the time of endoscopy, the rebleeding rate has been reported to range from 53% to 100%. For collected series, the mean rate is 66% (9). For patients with visible vessels in ulcers, the rebleeding rate is ~50%, and the emergency surgery rate has been reported at 52% (9,10). Other SRH have a lower incidence of rebleeding, ~10% (10). In one large series, mortality for patients with SRH was 12%; whereas, for patients without SRH, the mortality was 0% (11).

Early endoscopy in acutely bleeding patients presumably would have several advantages. First, surgery, when indicated, would be performed earlier. With more rapid definitive surgery, the patient is likely to receive fewer transfusions. Second, the surgical procedure could be directed at the specific lesion and site. Accurate preoperative diagnosis would reduce operating time and eliminate inappropriate surgical procedures. Accurate diagnosis also should eliminate the need for blind gastrectomy. Third, accurate preoperative diagnosis would eliminate surgical exploration to detect the bleeding source. Fourth, surgical risk could be predicted better, especially for treatments with an expected high morbidity, such as total gastrectomy for hemorrhagic gastritis. The lavage, which precedes endoscopy, may slow or stop bleeding. In addition, endoscopy can suggest long-term threapy, such as abstention from aspirin or alcohol (12). For patients with continued active bleeding, early and specific diagnosis with UGI endoscopy remains vital for selecting appropriate therapy (13).

COMMON CAUSES

Mallory-Weiss Lesion

The Mallory-Weiss lesion is a linear mucosal tear, usually found on the lesser curvature of the stomach, either at or below the gastroesophageal junction. The lesion is diagnosed by UGI endoscopy in ~95% of patients. Seventy percent of cases of Mallory-Weiss tears can be effectively treated with blood transfusion, control of gastric pH, and saline irrigation. If surgery is necessary, a gastrotomy is made high on the stomach to allow oversewing of the bleeding point. Endoscopic coagulation also has been used successfully (14). Although some authors advocate the use of a Sengstaken–Blakemore tube or other ballon tamponade device, the risk of converting a partial thickness lesion into a full thickness perforation is present and should relegate balloon tamponade to a treatment of last resort.

Esophageal Varices

The risk of bleeding from esophageal varices is increased with larger size, location at the gastroesophageal junction, presence of red stigmata at endoscopy, advanced liver failure, and advanced ascites. Patients with Child–Pugh class A cirrhosis have a lower incidence of variceal bleeding, 5–7%, than those with Child–Pugh class C cirrhosis, who have a 70% risk (15). Although 85–90% of patients with nonvariceal UGI bleeding will cease bleeding spontaneously, those patients with variceal bleeding have a 50% chance of spontaneous cessation of bleeding. Early rebleeding is common, and 50% of rebleeding events occur within 10 days of the index bleeding episode.

Treatment of esophageal varices is varied. Balloon tamponade is a decades old therapy and can provide temporary control of bleeding. For combined series, a 78% rate of bleeding control has been achieved, with a rebleeding rate of 42%. The combination of the high rebleeding rate after deflation of the balloon with the potential for serious complications, including esophageal necrosis and aspiration, relegates the use of balloon tamponade to cases not controlled by drug or endoscopic therapy (16). Should balloon tamponade be selected, the clinician should follow a careful protocol to achieve control of bleeding with minimum complications (Table 1).

Table 1 Protocol for Use of Sengstaken–Blakemore Tube

Before insertion
1. Consider nasotracheal intubation
2. Use new tube and check balloon for leaks
3. Attach No. 18 Salem sump tube above esophageal balloon
4. Evacuate blood from stomach with a large tube
5. Insert tube through nose using ring forceps, if necessary

After insertion
1. Apply low, intermittent suction to stomach tube
2. Apply constant suction to Salem sump
3. Inflate gastric balloon with 25-mL increments of air to 100 mL, observing patient for pain
4. Snug gastric balloon to gastroesophageal junction and affix to nose, under slight tension, with soft rubber pad
5. Add 150 mL of air to gastric balloon
6. Place two clamps (one taped close) on tube to gastric balloon
7. Inflate esophageal balloon to 24–45 mm Hg, clamp, and check every hour
8. Perform heavily penetrated upper abdomen–lower chest roentgenography (portable) to confirm balloon positions
9. Determine serial hematocrit levels every 4–6 h (gastric tube may occlude and fail to detect recurrent hemorrhage)
10. Tape scissors to head of bed so tube can be transected and rapidly removed if respiratory distress develops
11. Deflate esophageal and gastric balloons after 24 h
12. Remove tube in an additional 24 h if there is no recurrent hemorrhage

Source: From Rikkers LF, ed. Non-operative emergency treatment of variceal hemorrhage. Surg Clin North Am 1990; 70:297.

Vasoconstrictor therapy has been useful in controlling acute variceal bleeding. The American College of Gastroenterology recommends the empiric use of vasoactive therapy in the patient with a high likelihood of variceal bleeding before a definitive bleeding site is identified. Commonly used agents are octreotide and the combination of vasopressin and nitroglycerin. Octreotide, a longer acting analog of somatostatin, does not adversely affect cardiac function or blood pressure and can be used with safety in the patient with coexisting cardiac disease. Patients do not require special monitoring. The combination of safety and relative ease of use has made octreotide the initial choice for suspected or confirmed variceal bleeding. The infusion is generally continued for five days. Vasopressin reduces portal tributary inflow and, consequently, decreases portal pressure. In addition, vasopressin infusion may induce cardiac or splanchnic ischemia or cardiac bradydysrhythmias. Concomitant use of nitroglycerin can mitigate some of these side effects and allow higher doses of vasopressin to be used (16,17).

Endoscopic therapy includes endoscopic sclerotherapy and endoscopic variceal ligation (EVL). These two procedures are now commonly available and allow the possibility of definitive therapy at the time of endoscopic diagnosis. Because of the complications associated with sclerotherapy, including esophageal perforation, esophageal stenosis, and ulcer bleeding, EVL has been used with a lower complication rate. Both sclerotherapy and EVL control acute bleeding in ~80% of patients. Recent data favor EVL over sclerotherapy in the long-term prevention of rebleeding (18).

Sclerotherapy has been compared with surgical shunts in several studies. In controlled trials with follow-up of two to five years, sclerotherapy resulted in a decreased rebleeding rate or decreased transfusion requirements when compared with medical therapy. Despite improved control of bleeding, studies do not demonstrate a clear increase in survival (19–23). When compared with portacaval shunt, sclerotherapy has a significantly higher rebleeding rate. Despite better control of bleeding, portacaval shunt does not improve either encephalopathy or mortality (24). Three controlled trials have compared sclerotherapy with distal splenorenal shunt (DSRS). In all three trials, DSRS significantly decreased the rebleeding rate but did not change survival (25–27). Transhepatic internal jugular portosystemic shunts (TIPS), placed in the radiology suite, are now available. In four studies that compared TIPS with endoscopic treatment, rebleeding was reduced, encephalopathy was higher, and survival was comparable (28).

With acute bleeding, rapid control of hemorrhage is critical. As neither TIPS nor surgery can be performed as rapidly as endoscopic and pharmacologic therapies, these modalities are not recommended as first line therapy. TIPS has been successfully used as salvage therapy for patients who have failed endoscopic control of bleeding (29). A comprehensive review can be found in Ref. 30.

Gastritis

Association of ulceration of the gastric mucosa with subsequent stress bleeding and critical illness has a long history. Cushing reported acute duodenal ulceration in patients with major burn injury in 1842. Cushing's ulcer refers to the association of peptic ulcers with traumatic brain injury. With advances in resuscitation, metabolic support, and prophylaxis, the incidence of stress bleeding and surgical intervention for massive stress gastritis hemorrhage has decreased. The mortality for patients who require intervention for stress-related bleeding remains high, up to 50% (31,32).

Prophylaxis against stress bleeding is effective. Antacids, H2-receptor antagonists, and sucralfate all have demonstrated efficacy. Several studies demonstrate that antacids decrease stress bleeding when compared with placebo or control groups. For collected series, a bleeding rate of 18.9% in the placebo or control groups was reduced to 7.1% in the antacid group. H_2-receptor antagonists can provide a similar degree of bleeding prophylaxis. Again, from collected series, bleeding in control groups was 17.1%. In patients treated with H_2-blockers, the bleeding rates in collected series were 6% to 7%. Several studies confirm the efficacy of sucralfate for prophylaxis. From pooled data, the bleeding incidence in the sucralfate group was 3.8%; in the antacid/H_2-blocker groups, it was 8% (32).

These findings suggest that all patients in the ICU would receive benefit from stress ulcer prophylaxis. One shortcoming of the foregoing studies is that microscopic bleeding was not distinguished from clinically significant bleeding. The incidence of clinically significant bleeding was observed to be 1.5% in a multicenter trial of more than 2000 patients. Two independent risk factors for clinically significant bleeding were determined: respiratory failure and coagulopathy. The investigators concluded that stress ulcer prophylaxis could be safely withheld from patients in the ICU unless they have a coagulopathy or respiratory failure requiring mechanical ventilation (33). This conclusion arises from an estimation of the numbers needed to treat to prevent a complication. For those patients without coagulopathy and not requiring mechanical ventilation, more than 900 patients would need to receive prophylaxis to prevent a single bleeding episode. In contrast, in mechanically ventilated patients with coagulopathy, only 30 patients would need prophylaxis to prevent a bleeding complication. In a subsequent investigation, Cook et al. (34) compared the efficacy of ranitidine and sucralfate. The incidence of clinically important bleeding was 1.7% in the ranitidine group and 3.8% in the sucralfate group. The authors observed no significant differences in the incidence of ventilator associated pneumonia, ICU length of stay, or mortality. In both of these studies, the number of patients with head injury was small. Patients with CNS injuries, especially those involving the diencephalon and the brain stem, may have disinhibition of the medullary vagal system. Stress induced stimulation of brain neuropeptide production may directly affect the gut. The combination of these two effects may result in a higher incidence of stress ulceration and hemorrhage. For patients with head injury, especially those requiring mechanical ventilation, our practice is the use of stress ulcer prophylaxis. Lack of efficacy of H_2-receptor antagonists in controlling pH in patients with severe CNS injury has been shown. Sucralfate or antacids may be preferable to H_2-receptor antagonists in this population of patients (35).

Although effective prophylaxis can be achieved by alkalinizing stomach secretions to achieve a gastric pH $\geq$ 4, an increased incidence of nosocomial pneumonia with increasing pH has been demonstrated. The risk of gastric colonization and consequent nosocomial pneumonia may be comparable to the risk of stress bleeding. Selective decontamination of the digestive tract is effective in reducing nosocomial pneumonia and other infections (36). For critically ill patients who are expected to remain in ICU for at least 5 days, gut decontamination is effective in reducing nosocomial infection. The use of gut decontamination regimen should be considered for patients receiving gastric stress bleeding prophylaxis, especially if these patients are receiving broad-spectrum antibiotic therapy.

Peptic Ulcer Disease

The mainstay of peptic ulcer disease treatment is medical. Proton pump inhibitors, therapy aimed at *Helicobacter pylori*, and H_2-receptor antagonists are effective. With a rebleeding rate that is $\geq 65\%$, further therapy, including emergency surgery, is frequently necessary for ulcers that are acutely bleeding at the time of endoscopy. Other SRH are associated with an increased risk of rebleeding. In a meta-analysis of endoscopic therapy for acute nonvariceal UGI hemorrhage, Cook et al. found that endoscopic therapy results in a reduction in morbidity and mortality rates. In the series reviewed, the fraction of patients with peptic ulcer disease approached 1.0. Monopolar and bipolar electrocoagulation, injection therapy, and laser coagulation all significantly reduced rebleeding rates. With respect to mortality, all modalities reduced mortality, but only laser coagulation achieved statistical significance (37). A study of 100 patients with bleeding peptic ulcer diatheses in whom control of bleeding by endoscopic means was achieved demonstrated significantly decreased rebleeding when they received a proton pump inhibitor rather than an H_2-receptor antagonist (38). These findings were corroborated by Lau et al. Rebleeding after control of ulcer bleeding was decreased when the patient received intravenous proton pump inhibitor following control of the bleeding and oral proton pump inhibitor for 2 months (39).

Surgical treatment is indicated for severe or unrelenting bleeding. A definitive ulcer procedure can be performed; the choice of procedure depends on the condition of the patient and the severity of the bleeding. In a series of more than 1000 patients with bleeding duodenal ulcers, 250 patients had emergency surgery. Truncal vagotomy and antrectomy were performed in all. In the emergency surgery group, the mortality was 5.5% (29). A discussion of specific surgical considerations is beyond the scope of this chapter but may be found in Ref. 40.

LGI HEMORRHAGE (Fig. 2)

The most likely causes of LGI hemorrhage are related to age. In children, Meckel's diverticulum is common; whereas, in adults over 60 years of age, vascular ectasias are frequently associated with severe LGI hemorrhage (41). In one large series, the most common causes of LGI bleeding were diverticular disease, colon cancer, inflammatory bowel disease, and colonic polyps (31) (Table 2). Vascular ectasias, ischemic colitis, rectal cancer, and hemorrhoids all had an incidence of $\leq 10\%$. Although vascular ectasias had a 6% incidence, they accounted for one-third of patients requiring emergency surgery and 50% of patients requiring >4 units of blood in the first 24 h. Vascular ectasias are usually multiple and most commonly found in the cecum or proximal ascending colon. Two-thirds of affected patients are over 70 years old. The lesions are thought to be acquired (41).

Approximately 20% of patients with LGI bleeding have a transfusion requirement of ≥ 3 units. A transfusion requirement of 3–4 units or more of blood in the first 24 h is associated with an increased need for emergency surgery. In one large series, all patients who required emergency surgery needed ≥ 4 units of blood in the first 24 h (42).

Patient Evaluation

Evaluation of patients with suspected LGI hemorrhage should begin with a thorough physical examination, including a careful rectal examination. Coagulation studies and platelet counts should be obtained. A BUN/creatinine >25 distinguishes UGI bleeding from LGI bleeding in 90% of patients (32). In 10–15% of patients, the source of presumed LGI bleeding is actually a UGI source. UGI endoscopy or nasogastric tube aspiration is indicated. Absence of blood and presence of bile in the aspirate virtually exclude a bleeding source proximal to the ligament of Treitz (41).

In recent years, colonoscopy has become the diagnostic procedure of choice in the stable patient, in whom bleeding has stopped or significantly decreased. Some authors advocate colonoscopy in the patient with severe hematochezia and report 74–82% diagnostic accuracy (43,44). If colonoscopy cannot be performed or is unsuccessful, angiography should be performed in the patient with persistent, severe bleeding. If the patient's condition is stable or cessation of bleeding is not certain, colonoscopy should be followed by tagged-RBC study, if no diagnosis is made endoscopically. Although not as definitive as angiography in identifying the site of bleeding, the tagged-RBC study may be more sensitive in detecting bleeding. Increased sensitivity of the nuclear medicine study arises from the potential to accumulate radionuclide at the bleeding site over several hours. It does not depend on active bleeding during the brief period of colonoscopic examination or of injection of radiocontrast agent. Furthermore, several examinations can be obtained for up to 36 h after injection of the radionuclide (45). If the radionuclide study suggests a site of bleeding and the patient's condition is stable, colonoscopy is next performed. The examination should be abandoned if technical problems are encountered. If the patient continues to bleed actively, angiography is the next study. Bleeding rates of 0.5 mL/min can be detected. Angiography is successful in locating the source of bleeding

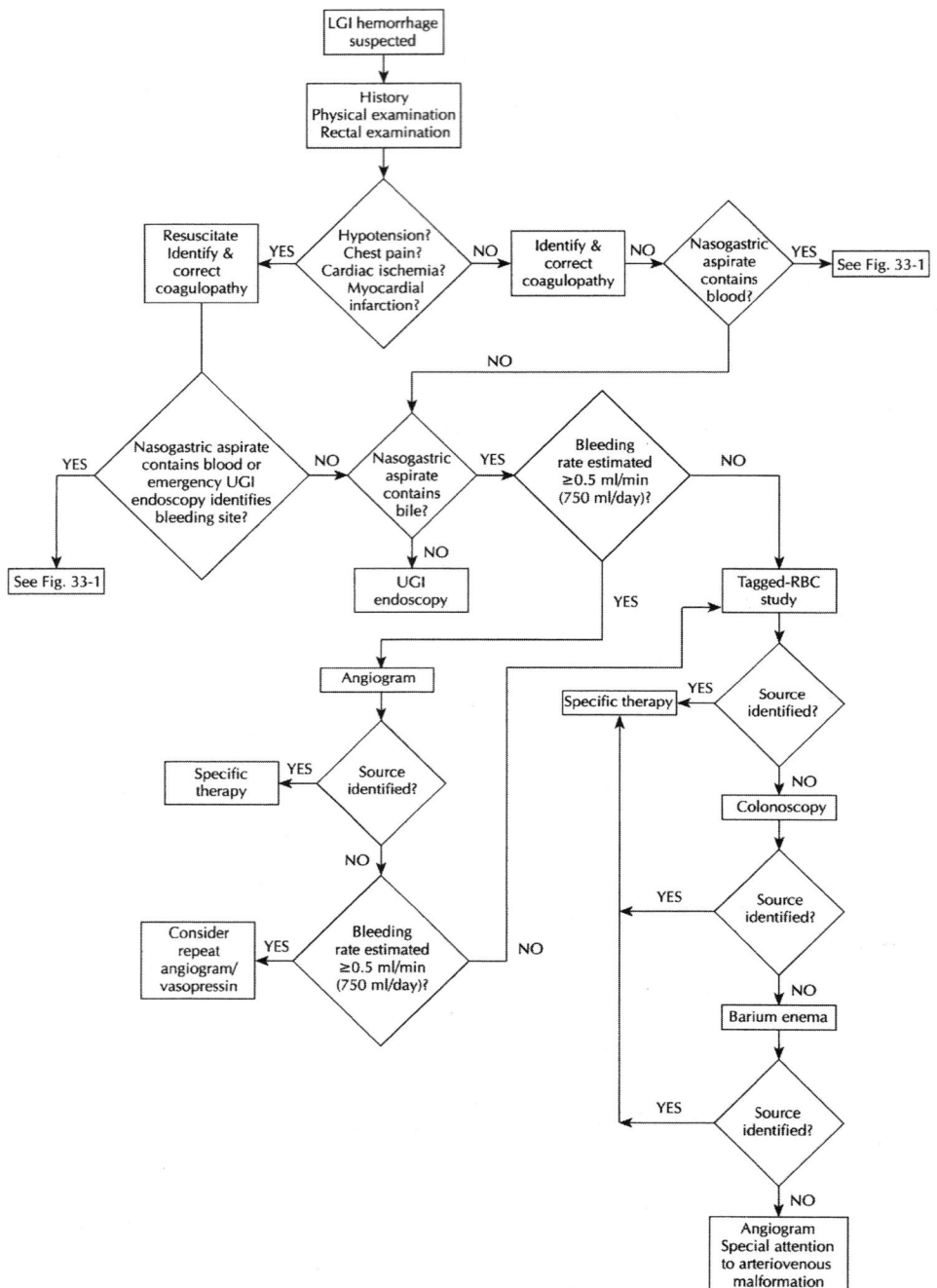

Figure 2 Approach to LGI hemorrhage.

Table 2 Causes of Acute LGI Hemorrhage in a Series of Patients During a 4-Year Period.

Diagnosis	No. of patients
Diverticular disease	30
Carcinoma of colon	28
Inflammatory bowel disease	17
Colonic polyps	10
Vascular ectasia	6
Ischemic colitis	3
Rectal ulcer	3
Hemorrhoids	2
Anticogulant treatment	1
Thrombocytopenia	1
Aortosigmoid fistula	1
Malignant histiocytosis	1
Anastomotic bleeding	1
Undetermined	1
Total	105

Source: From Ref. (42). Farrands PA, Taylor I. Management of acute lower gastrointestinal haemorrhage in a surgical unit over a 4-year period. J Royal Soc Med 1987; 80:79–82.

in one-half to two-thirds of patients. Angiographic diagnostic success is increased if angiography is performed within 24 h of the onset of bleeding (41,46).

In most patients, bleeding will spontaneously stop. If a source of bleeding has not been identified, repeat colonoscopy should be performed. Studies to evaluate the small bowel, including UGI with small bowel follow-through or enteroclysis, should be considered. In the small group of patients who continue to lack diagnosis, repeat angiography, including the celiac axis, should be performed. In an occasional patient, hemobilia may be the source of bleeding.

Conservative management of LGI hemorrhage is indicated initially. Approximately 90% of bleeding will stop before transfusion requirements exceed 2 units. If >4 units are required in 24 h, the chance that surgery will be necessary approaches 50%. An aggressive search for the source should be undertaken. If a bleeding source is clearly identified, segmental resection is recommended. If a bleeding source is not clearly identified, subtotal colectomy with or without ileorectal anastamosis should be done (42).

SUMMARY

- Acute GI hemorrhage can complicate critical illness. When GI bleeding occurs in hospitalized patients, mortality is high.
- Variceal bleeding is less likely to spontaneously cease than nonvariceal UGI bleeding. Vasoactive therapy, preferably with octreotide, should be instituted in the patient with suspected variceal bleeding before a definitive diagnosis is made. First line definitive therapy is EVL or sclerotherapy.

- Prophylaxis of acute GI bleeding is effective in those patients requiring mechanical ventilation or with coagulopathy.
- Nosocomial infection increases with rising gastric pH. Selective gut decontamination has been shown to decrease the nosocomial infection rate and should be considered in critically ill patients receiving pH prophylaxis, especially if the patients are concurrently receiving broad spectrum antibiotic therapy.
- SRH, especially bleeding at the time of endoscopy and a visible vessel, have a high rebleeding rate. These patients should receive definitive therapy and a proton pump inhibitor after bleeding is controlled.
- LGI bleeding requiring transfusion of ≥ 3 units of blood in 24 h has an $\sim 50\%$ likelihood of requiring emergency surgery. Rapid, accurate diagnosis is essential for therapy. Angiography in patients with a large transfusion requirement can establish the bleeding site in up to two-thirds of patients, especially when performed early in the hospital course. Angiographic embolization may be definitive therapy.

REFERENCES

1. Longstreth GF. Epidemiology of hospitalization for acute gastrointestinal hemorrhage: A population based study. Am J Gastroenterol 1995; 90:206–210.
2. Gostout CS. Acute gastrointestinal bleeding—A common problem revisited. Mayo Clin Proc 1988; 63:596–604.
3. Cutler JA, Mendeloff AI. Upper gastrointestinal bleeding: Nature and magnitude of the problem in the US Dig Dis Sci 1981; 26(suppl 7):90S–96S.
4. Chojkier M, Laine L, Conn HO, Lerner E. Predictors of outcome in massive upper gastrointestinal hemorrhage. J Clin Gastroenterol (1986); 8:16–22.
5. Chalmers TC, Zamcheck N, Curtins GW. Fatal gastrointestinal hemorrhage: Clincopathologic correlations in 101 patients. Am J Clin Pathol 1952; 22:633–645.
6. Dagradi AE, Arguello JF, Weingarten ZG. Failure of endoscopy to establish a source for upper gastrointestinal bleeding. Am J Gastroenterol 1979; 72:395–402.
7. Lieberman D. Gastrointestinal bleeding: Initial management. Gastroenterol Clin North Am 1993; 22:723–736.
8. Foster DN, Miloszewski KJA, Losowsky MS. Stigmata of recent haemorrhage in diagnosis and prognosis of upper gastrointestinal bleeding. Br Med J 1978; 1:1173–1177.
9. Pescovitz MD, Satterberg TL, Shearen JG. Endoscopic control of bleeding ulcers: The Minnesota experience with several methods. In: Najarian JS, Delaney JP, eds. Progress in Gastrointestinal Surgery. Chicago, IL: Year Book, 1989:247–254.
10. Swain CP, Storey DW, Bown SG, Heath J, Mills TN, Salmon PR, Northfield TC, Kirkham JS, O'Sullivan JP. Nature of the bleeding vessel in recurrently bleeding gastric ulcers. Gastroenterology 1986; 90:595–608.
11. Brearley S, Morris DL, Hawker PC, Dykes PW, Keighley MR. Prediction of mortality at endoscopy in bleeding peptic ulcer disease. Endoscopy 1985; 17:173–174.
12. Dagradi AE, Ruiz RA, Weingarten ZG. Influence of emergency endoscopy on the management and outcome of patients with upper gastrointestinal hemorrhage. Am J Gastroenterol 1979; 72:403–415.
13. Domschke W, Lederer P, Lux G. The value of emergency endoscopy in upper gastrointestinal bleeding: Review and analysis of 2014 cases. Endoscopy 1983; 15:126–131.
14. Todd GJ, Zikira BA. Mallory—Weiss Syndrome. Ann Surg 1977; 186:146–148.

15. Prediction of the first variceal hemorrhage in patients with cirrhosis of the liver and esophageal varices. A prospective multicenter trial. The North Italian Endoscopic Club for the study and Treatment of Esophageal Varices. N Engl J Med 1988; 319:983–989.
16. Carey WD, Grace ND, Reddy KR, Shiffman ML. Managing variceal hemorrhage in the cirrhotic: A primer. Am Coll Gastroenterol 1998; 1–12.
17. Burnett DA, Rikkers LF. Nonoperative emergency treatment of variceal hemorrhage. Surg Clin North Am 1990; 70:291–306.
18. Laine L, Cook D. Endoscopic ligation compared with sclerotherapy for treatment of esophageal variceal bleeding. A meta-analysis. Ann Intern Med 1995; 15:280–287.
19. Terblanche J, Bornman PC, Kahn D, Jonker MA, Campbell JA, Wright J, Kirsch R. Failure of repeated injection sclerotherapy to improve long-term survival after oesophageal variceal bleeding. A five-year prospective controlled trial. Lancet 1983; 2:1328–1332.
20. Copenhagen Esophageal Varices and Sclerotherapy Project. Sclerotherapy after first variceal hemorrhage in cirrhosis: A randomized multicenter trial. N Engl J Med 1984; 311:1594–1600.
21. Westaby D, MacDargall BRD, Williams R. Improved survival following injection sclerotherapy for esophageal varices: Final analysis of a controlled trial. Hepatology 1985; 5:827–830.
22. Korula J, Balart LA, Radvan G, Zweiban BE, Larson AW, Kao HW, Yamada S. A prospective, randomized controlled trial of chronic esophageal variceal sclerotherapy. Hepatology 1985; 5:584–589.
23. Soderlund C, Ihre T. Endoscopic sclerotherapy v. conservative management of bleeding oesophageal varices. A 5-year prospective controlled trial of emergency and long-term treatment. Acta Chir Scand 1985; 151:449–456.
24. Cello JP, Grendell JH, Crass RA, Weber TE, Trunkey DD. Endoscopic sclerotherapy versus portacaval shunt in patients with severe cirrhosis and acute variceal hemorrhage: Long-term follow-up. N Engl J Med 1987; 316:11–15.
25. Warren WD, Henderson JM, Millikan WJ, Galambos JT, Brooks WS, Riepe SP, Salam AA, Kutner MH. Distal splenorenal shunt versus endoscopic sclerotherapy for long-term management of variceal bleeding. Preliminary report of a prospective, randomized trial. Ann Surg 1986; 203:454–462.
26. Rikkers LF, Burnett DA, Volentine GD, Buchi KN, Cormier RA. Shunt surgery versus endoscopic sclerotherapy for long-term treatment of variceal bleeding. Early results of a randomized trial. Ann Surg 1987; 206:261–271.
27. Teres J, Bordas JM, Bravo D, Visa J, Grande L, Garcia-Valdecasas JC, Pera C, Rodes J. Sclerotherapy vs. distal splenorenal shunt in the elective treatment of variceal hemorrhage: A randomized controlled trial. Hepatology 1987; 7:430–436.
28. Luketic BA, Sanyal AJ. Esophageal varices II. TIPS (Transjugular Intrahepatic Portosystemic Shunt) and surgical therapy. Gastorenterol. Clin North Am. 2000; 29:387–421.
29. Sanyal AJ, Freedman AM, Luketic VA, Purdum PP, Shiffman ML, Tisando J, Cole PE. Transjugular portosystemic shunts for patients with active variceal hemorrhage unresponsive to sclerotherapy. Gastorenterol. 1996; 111:138–146.
30. Cappell MS. High risk gastrointestinal bleeding, part II. Gastroenterol. Clin North Am. 2000; 29:275–557.
31. Greenburg AG, Saik RP, Bell RH, Collins GM. Changing patterns of gastrointestinal bleeding. Arch Surg 1985; 120:341–344.
32. Gourdin TG, Smith BF, Craven DE. Prevention of stress bleeding in critical care patients: Current concepts on risk and benefit. Perspect Crit Care 1989; 2:44–73.
33. Cook DJ, Fuller HD, Guyatt GH, Marshall JC, Leasa D, Hall R, Winton TL, Rutledge F, Todd TJ, Roy P. Risk factors for gastrointestinal bleeding in critically ill patients. Canadian Critical Care Trials Group. N Engl J Med 1994; 330:337–381.

34. Cook D, Guyatt G, Marshall J, Leasa D, Fuller H, Hall R, Peters S, Rutledge R, Griffith L, McLellan A, Wood G, Kirby A. A comparison of sucralfate and ranitidine for the prevention of upper gastrointestinal bleeding in patients requiring mechanical ventilation. Canadian Critical Care Trials Group. N Engl J Med 1998; 338:791–797.
35. Lu WY, Rhoney DH, Boling WB, Johnson JD, Smith TC. A review of stress ulcer prophylaxis in the neurosurgical intensive care unit. Neurosurgery 1997; 41:416–426.
36. Ramsey G, van Saene RHKF. Selective gut decontamination in intensive care and surgical practice: Where are we? World J Surg 1998; 22:164–170.
37. Cook DJ, Guyatt GH, Salena BJ, Laine LA. Endoscopic therapy for acute nonvariceal upper gastrointestinal hemorrhage: A meta-analysis. Gastroenterology 1992; 102:139–148.
38. Lin HJ, Lo WC, Lee FY, Perng CL, Tseng GY. A prospective randomized comparative trial showing that omeprazole prevents rebleeding in patients with bleeding peptic ulcer after successful endoscopic therapy. Arch Intern Med 1998; 158:54–58.
39. Lau JY, Sung JJ, Lee KK, Yung MY, Wong SK, Wu JC, Chan FK, Ng EK, You JH, Lee CW, Chan AC, Chung SC. Effect of intravenous omeprazole on recurrent bleeding after endoscopic treatment of bleeding peptic ulcers. N Engl J Med 2000; 343:310–316.
40. Herrington JL, Davidson J III. Bleeding gastroduodenal ulcers: Choice of operations. World J Surg 1987; 11:304–314.
41. Dickstein G, Boley SJ. Severe lower intestinal bleeding in the elderly. In: Najarian JS, Delaney JP, eds. Progress in Gastrointestinal Surgery. Chicago: Year Book, 1989:525–542.
42. Farrands PA, Taylor I. Management of acute lower gastrointestinal haemorrhage in a surgical unit over a 4-year period. J Royal Soc Med 1987; 80:79–82.
43. Vernava AM III, Moore BA, Longo WE, Johnson FE. Lower gastrointestinal bleeding. Dis Colon Rectum 1997; 40:846–858.
44. Jensen DM, Machicado GA, Jutabha R, Kovacs TOG. Urgent colonoscopy for the diagnosis and treatment of severe diverticular hemorrhage. N Engl J Med 2000; 342:78–82.
45. Winzelberg GG, Froelich JW, McKusick KA, Strauss HW. Scintigraphic detection of gastrointestinal bleeding: A review of current methods. Am J Gastroenterol 1983; 78:324–327.
46. Nusbaum M, Baum S. Radiographic demonstration of unknown sites of gastrointestinal bleeding. Surg Forum 1963; 14:374–375.

38

Acute Pancreatitis in the Surgical Intensive Care Unit

Jeffrey G. Chipman
VA Medical Center, Minneapolis, Minnesota, USA

INTRODUCTION

Pancreatitis can tax all the resources of the surgical intensive care unit. Though some triggers of the disease are understood, the mechanism of progression remains uncertain. Most occurrences are mild and self-limited, but occasionally they progress to a more severe, fulminant form that causes tremendous metabolic and physiologic stress. The purpose of Ranson's classic criteria is identification of the patient at risk for the most severe disease and stratification of therapy to control disease progression and support the systemic effects of the resultant inflammation (1). Every physician, regardless of specialty, has frantically scrambled at some point in training to remember these criteria in preparation for a discussion of acute pancreatitis. What they identify are signs reflecting the severity of the inflammatory response to tissue injury. Similar responses are found in other inflammatory states, such as sepsis, severe trauma, and massive hemorrhage.

This chapter addresses acute pancreatitis in the surgical intensive care unit. As the discussion focuses on critical care, it will center primarily on the most severe forms of the disease. The pathophysiology of the disease and methods for its diagnosis will be reviewed. Treatment, with a focus on surgical intensive care, will review obtaining source control, restoring oxygen transport, and providing metabolic support. Finally, evidence for improved outcomes as a result of the intensive intervention will be presented.

PATHOPHYSIOLOGY

Etiology

The two most common causes of acute pancreatitis are alcohol and gallstones. The predominant etiology depends on the cohort studied. Among the other less common causes are various drugs, shock states, coronary bypass surgery, cardiopulmonary bypass, hyperparathyroidism, hypertriglyceridemia, and endoscopic retrograde cholangiopancreatography (ERCP) (2).

Pancreatitis caused by gallstones is estimated to occur in 3–8% of patients with symptomatic cholelithiasis. It is usually self-limited, although occasionally it escalates to more severe forms. Passage of stones through the ampulla of Vater is thought to be the mechanism. The means by which stone passage triggers pancreatitis is debated. One explanation is that a gallstone impacts and obstructs the ampulla. This obstruction blocks the pancreatic ducts and results in the build-up of pancreatic secretions, increased intraductal pressure, activation of pancreatic enzymes in tissues not normally exposed to enzymatic activity, and subsequent cellular injury. Another plausible explanation is that bile may reflux into the pancreatic duct if the gallstone obstruction is distal enough in the common distal pancreatic and common bile duct channel. The presence of bile in the pancreatic duct may prematurely activate pancreatic enzymes (2). Independent of the mechanism, the explanation for mild disease in one patient and severe disease in another remains a mystery.

The mechanism for alcohol-induced pancreatitis is less certain. It rarely occurs in isolated binge drinking. Instead, alcohol-induced pancreatitis usually appears after significant alcohol consumption in chronic drinkers. Causal theories include high pancreatic duct pressure, direct cellular toxicity, and alterations in vascular supply (2).

Whatever the cause of pancreatitis, activated pancreatic enzymes, usually found only in the intestinal lumen for the digestion of dietary lipid and protein, are present in tissues where they normally do not exist and in tissues that lack protection against their activity. In the normal pancreas, inactive enzyme precursors known as proenzymes are packaged in zymogen granules in the cytoplasm of acinar cells. When stimulated, the zymogens fuse with the acinar cell membrane and the proenzymes are released by exocytosis to collect in the pancreatic ductal system. They follow the alkalotic, bicarbinate-rich pancreatic fluid through the ducts into the duodenum. In the duodenum, the inactive proenzymes are then activated by the hydrolytic action of trypsin. Trypsin itself is activated from its inactive precursor trysinogen by the acidic environment of the duodenum, and by enterokinases that exist on intestinal mucosal cells (3). In pancreatitis, the enzymes are activated either in the acinar cell, the pancreatic interstitium, or the peripancreatic tissue of the retroperitoneum resulting in the autodigestion of the tissue they contact (2).

Pathology

As with many diseases, pancreatitis is a spectrum of disease ranging from mild to severe. In the mildest forms the pancreatic interstitium is edematous with few leukocytes. The acinar cells and capillary blood supply remain intact. In this form of pancreatitis, the inflammatory process is low grade and localized to the pancreas itself.

In about 10% of patients the process is more severe. In these individuals the interstitial edema extends to the retroperitoneum and even to adjacent organs. The edema can become so marked that fluid collections occur. The inflammatory process can result in obliteration of capillaries with subsequent necrosis of neighboring pancreatic cells. Necrosis of adjacent fatty tissue occurs with the spillage and activation of pancreatic enzymes. This process can extend into the lesser sac, into adjacent organs, including the stomach, colon, and spleen, and along other anatomic planes, for example, lateral to the left colon. With such an extensive and uncontrolled inflammatory process, the occurrence of systemic manifestations is not surprising (2).

Several methods to quantify severity of disease have been suggested. Ranson published 11 criteria to identify those patients with the most severe disease (Table 1). The first five are determined on admission, and the subsequent six are measured during the first 48 hours of therapy. In his original paper published in 1974, 62% of patients with more

Table 1 Prognostic Indicators of Severe Pancreatitis

On admission
  Age >55 years
  WBC >16,000/mm^3
  Glucose >200 mg/dL
  LDH >350 IU/L
  SGOT >120 IU/L
During first 48 h
  Hematocrit decrease >10%
  BUN increase >5 mg/dL
  Serum calcium >8 mg/dL
  Arterial PO_2 <60 mm Hg
  Base defecit >4 mEq/L
  Fluid sequestration >6 L

Source: From Ref. (1).

than three signs died (1). Subsequent methods to stratify disease, including the acute pathophysiology and chronic health evaluation (APACHE) scores, have been developed and validated (4).

The availability of newer evaluation methods like dynamic, helical computed tomography (CT) scanning, has refined stratification of patients. A 1992 conference in Atlanta, Georgia, attempted to create a uniform definition for the severity of disease. Acute pancreatitis was defined as "an acute inflammatory process of the pancreas, with variable involvement of other regional tissues or remote organ systems." Severe acute pancreatitis was defined as acute pancreatitis with "associated organ failure and/or local complications, such as necrosis, abscess, or pseudocyst." Additional features include three or more Ranson criteria or eight or more APACHE II points. The conference also concluded that description of pancreatitis should be specifically defined. For example, the term phlegmon is commonly used to describe the anatomic findings resulting from the disease; however, it does not provide the specific information needed for appropriate treatment, such as the presence of necrosis, peripancreatic fluid collections, infected tissues, or abscesses (5).

DIAGNOSIS

Signs and symptoms are rarely specific indicators of pancreatitis. The history and physical examination combined with radiologic and laboratory data can point toward the diagnosis of acute pancreatitis. Clinical details determine its severity. An important question requiring resolution is the presence or absence of pancreatic necrosis and/or infection. In the words of one author, "Diagnosis of infected necrosis remains a bit like recognizing that you have just stepped over the edge of a cliff in the dark: would that you could have seen ahead to change direction before getting to the precipice" (6).

History and Physical Information

Patients suffering from pancreatitis complain of pain in the epigastrium. The pain may have a component that radiates to the back. For some it has a slow onset, but for others it may have acute onset and may be associated with a meal or alcoholic binge. Pain is the most consistent complaint in patients with pancreatitis. Accompanying nausea and/or vomiting occurs in about half of the patients (2).

Pancreatitis can mimic many other diseases (Fig. 1). The differential diagnosis initially includes biliary disease, peptic ulcer disease, alcoholic gastritis, and, problematically, nearly every other abdominal pathology. If the chief complaint and initial history place pancreatitis in the differential diagnosis, then the clinician's questions can focus on

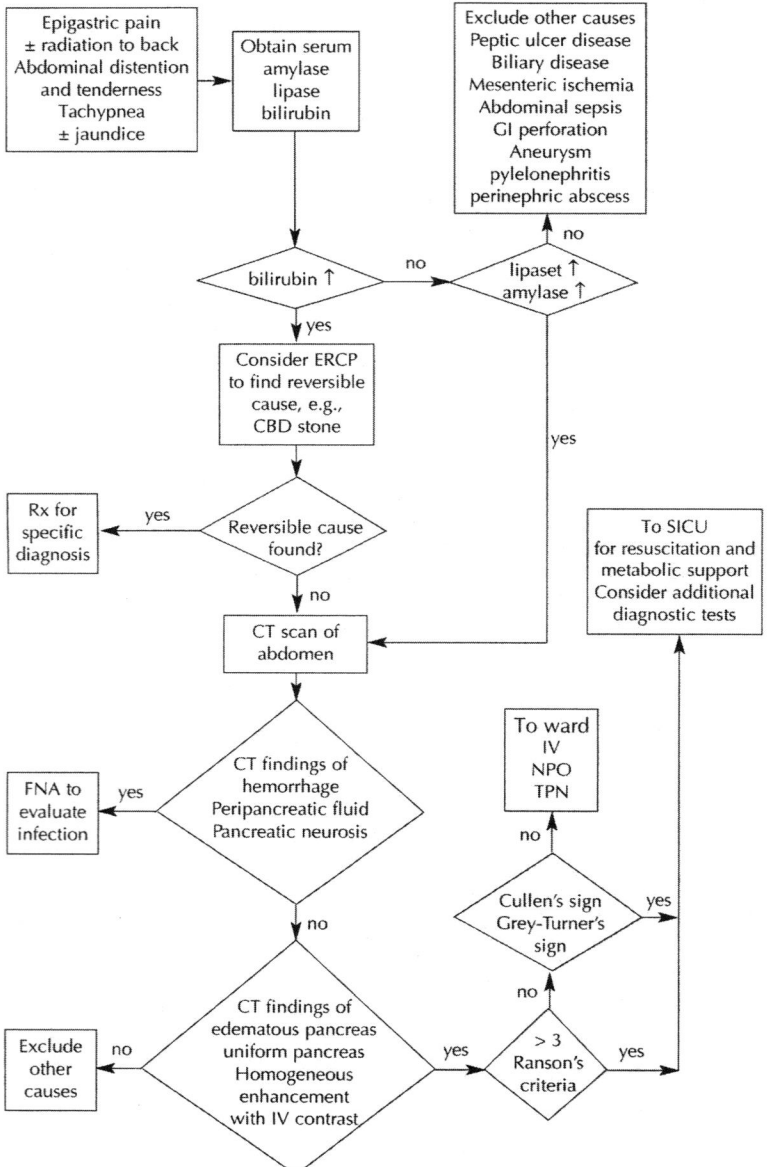

Figure 1 Diagnosis of acute pancreatitis and its complications.

the common causes of pancreatitis, most often alcohol and gallstones. Directed questions may probe the frequency and use of alcohol, previous episode of similar pain, a history of jaundice, acholic stools, or pain typical of biliary colic. For patients in the hospital, recent pharmacotherapy, shock, surgery or cardiopulmonary bypass support the diagnosis.

The physical examination can be helpful in focusing the differential diagnosis, as well as indicating the severity of disease. Inspection of the abdomen may indicate a fullness in the epigastrium, auscultation may reveal a paucity of bowel sounds, and palpation often reveals tenderness, especially in the epigastrium. Abdominal distention, or even a palpable mass, may indicate the extent of the inflammatory process. Other abdominal examination findings that may suggest severe disease are flank ecchymosis, known as Grey-Turner's sign, and periumbilical ecchymosis, known as Cullen's sign. They are cutaneous manifestations of hemorrhagic pancreatitis extending along planes in the retroperitoneum.

Additional aspects of the physical examination that indicate disease severity include vital signs. Ominous are vital signs consistent with a shock state. Tachycardia is present when extreme fluid sequestration by the inflammatory process depletes the vascular volume and produces hypovolemia. Inflammatory mediators can also cause increased heart rate. Hypotension may be seen with marked hypovolemia, a severe systemic inflammatory response, and/or sepsis. Tachypnea is present with each of these conditions as well. Other physical signs of shock include fever, mental status changes, and warm or cool extremities.

Laboratory Data

Laboratory data can help limit the differential diagnosis and determine the severity of disease as defined by Ranson's criteria. Leukocytosis is common, typically $10-25 \times 10^9$ per liter, although higher counts are also seen. As it can be elevated in any inflammatory state, the leukocyte count is not specific. Moreover, a leukocytosis does not distinguish infected pancreatitis from noninfected states, although a trend in the leukocyte count over time may be a helpful determinant of improvement or deterioration (2).

Amylase is an enzyme made by pancreatic acinar cells to break down sugars. It is not normally found in significant quantities in the serum, but is elevated early in pancreatitis. Amylase typically returns to normal serum concentration about 1 week after the onset of pancreatitis. The serum amylase concentration is not specific and can be elevated in other settings. It is made in salivary glands; fallopian tubes; lungs; prostate, breast, tear glands, and sweat glands. Amylase is largely cleared by the kidney; consequently, serum concentration may remain elevated in renal failure.

An additional pitfall with relying on hypermylasemia to define pancreatitis is its lack of sensitivity. Some patients with pancreatitis, on the basis of other criteria for pancreatitis, have a normal serum amylase concentration. This can occur late in the disease course, with increased renal clearance, or with extensive pancreatic destruction (2).

Lipase may be a more sensitive and specific marker of pancreatitis, especially in acute alcoholic pancreatitis. It has a longer half-life and may remain elevated later in the course of the disease, while the serum amylase concentration has returned to normal.

Elevations in hepatic transaminases are very nonspecific. Elevations may indicate the degree of hepatocellular injury from the inflammation. Elevations in the bilirubin concentration may also suggest hepatic dysfunction from sepsis. In this setting, both direct and indirect hyperbilirubinemia are observed. An increase in conjugated bilirubin is consistent with choledocholithiasis as the trigger of pancreatitis or obstruction of the common bile duct from edema in the inflamed gland. Recent studies have attempted to stratify severity of pancreatitis with serum cytokine concentrations. Further study is necessary before cytokine levels prove practical.

Radiologic Data

Plain radiographs are not specific and do not quantify the severity of disease. As the pancreas is usually not visualized, findings on plain film depend on changes in other organs as a result of the pancreatic inflammation. The bowel gas pattern may appear normal or may suggest a picture of an adynamic ileus. A distended loop of small bowel in the left upper quadrant (sentinel loop) may be found. A calcified pancreas may be visualized on plain radiographs and can be indicative of chronic pancreatitis.

Ultrasound may be useful in detecting fluid collections around the pancreas or elsewhere in the abdomen. It cannot, however, determine if the fluid is contaminated, or the cause of its accumulation.

CT is the most useful radiologic test in limiting the differential diagnosis to pancreatitis. It can also aid in determining severity of disease. Beside noting changes consistent with inflammation around the pancreas, the CT scan may also reveal periglandular fluid collections. This fluid may represent peripancreatic edema or fluid sequestration, a pancreatic pseudocyst, or an abscess. The CT scan cannot determine if the fluid is infected.

CT may be of additional benefit in suggesting necrotic pancreatic tissue if an appropriate protocol is used. Areas of the pancreas that fail to enhance with intravenous contrast are likely to have little to no blood flow and may represent necrosis. Though not an absolute determinant of necrosis, if the dynamic contrast enhanced CT shows well defined zones of nonenhancing pancreatic parenchyma that are >3 cm or make up >30% of the gland, necrosis is likely present. As mentioned, necrotic pancreatic or peripancreatic tissue is often present when the inflammation is caused by infection (7).

Though not in widespread use, magnetic resonance (MR) imaging has been utilized to help identify pancreatitis and local complications. Some authors consider MR to be equivalent to CT scanning. It may also be used as an alternative to ERCP to evaluate the biliary system for obstruction.

Fine Needle Aspiration

Fine needle aspiration (FNA) can diagnose infection in the setting of pancreatic necrosis and provide critical information for therapeutic decisions. Sensitivity is as high as 96% (8,9). As not all pancreatic necrosis is infected, a difficult question arises. When should FNA be performed? The answer to this question must consider the inherent risks of the procedure, including the possibility that previously sterile necrosis can be contaminated by the procedure (10). Clinical evidence suggesting infection, such as tachycardia, fever, tachypnea, and hypotension, are also present in noninfected inflammatory states and, therefore, are not useful indicators for FNA. Following the patient's clinical course may provide the indication to perform FNA. For example, FNA could be performed for the patient with evidence of pancreatic necrosis who deteriorates or ceases to improve.

TREATMENT

Treatment varies with the severity of disease. With simple inflammation, supportive care is sufficient. When disease is more severe and necrosis is present, therapy may also include antibiotics and methods to diagnose the presence of infection. Infection is an indication for surgical necrosectomy or debridement. As the presence of shock is the highest predictor of mortality in patients with pancreatitis, the goal of treatment at any stage is prevention of shock and rapid effective resuscitation when it does occur (6,11). When a patient with severe acute pancreatitis or one who is at risk for it is identified, treatment to limit shock has three aims: control of the disease source, restoration of oxygen transport to tissues, and metabolic support for healing.

Source Control

Surgeons should always be interested in whether control of the source disease has been achieved. For example, was the tumor completely resected with appropriate margins? Was the source of the infection removed and repaired in a way to limit future infection? Were all of the abscesses drained adequately? The same question is at the root of treating pancreatitis. In mild forms of the disease, the only question may be whether the cause has been eliminated. Source control in gallstone pancreatitis may be limited to removing the stone-laden gallbladder and performing cholangiography to verify a stone-free bile duct. If common duct stones are found, it may require an intervention to clear the common bile duct of remaining stones (ERCP with sphincterotomy or open common duct exploration).

For severe disease the questions about source control are more difficult. The morbidity of surgical necrosectomy and debridement is high. But, untreated infected pancreatic or peripancreatic tissue also has a high probability of multisystem organ failure and death (6,9,12). Determining if the necrosis is infected or sterile is a major challenge. FNA may be of great use in answering this question. Also challenging is balancing the potential benefits of prophylactic, broad-spectrum antibiotics to prevent infection with the consequences of prolonged use, such as emergence of resistant organisms and fungus.

Debridement and Drainage

Physicians and surgeons continue to debate the value of various treatments aimed at controlling the source or progression of the pancreatic inflammation. Options include percutaneous or open debridement and drainage. Treatment is successful when infected and necrotic tissue is sufficiently removed to allow healing of the remaining pancreas. The critical care provider's role is meticulous support of the patient until healing occurs.

Surgical debridement of infected pancreatic necrosis has long been the main treatment for infected pancreatitis. Methods to manage infected pancreatitis are as numerous as the surgeons who describe them. Some suggest wide debridement or necrosectomy with the placement of drains (12,13). Others propose frequent and repetitive debridement with or without intra-abdominal packing (12,14), still others argue for the placement of large drains with continual large volume lavage (15). Most agree that more than one operation is usually required. A less invasive method for drainage using percutaneous techniques has been suggested. It has not been extensively studied and is not widely practiced. Its effectiveness remains unproven (16,17).

Patients explored repeatedly for further debridement may return with intra-abdominal packing, an open abdomen, and potentially exposed bowel. Occasionally, if resources exist, the abdominal packs can be changed in the intensive care unit. These patients are at risk for other complications, including pancreatic fistulae, small and large bowel fistulae, and bleeding. Intestinal fistulas occur in 4–35% of patients and bleeding can occur in 20–26% (13).

Mortality after surgery for infected pancreatitis varies widely, but is historically in the range of 15–56%. Recently, some authors have suggested that rate can be lowered to around 6% (13). Of note, surgery in patients with sterile necrosis has a similar mortality rate of 10–14%. For this reason, surgery would ideally be limited to those with infected pancreatitis. Evidence for infected pancreatic necrosis may include a positive FNA (9), gas in the pancreatic bed on CT scan, or a worsening clinical picture (18). To this end surgeons have developed, studied, and advanced strategies for the treatment of severe acute pancreatitis aimed at avoiding surgery by preventing infection and avoiding organ dysfunction.

Antibiotics

Seven to twelve percent of cases of acute pancreatitis will become infected. The probability of infection increases to 30–70% if necrosis is present. Owing to the increased mortality associated with infected pancreatitis, prophylactic prevention with antibiotics has been advocated. In the 1970s prophylactic antibiotic use failed to demonstrate benefits and was abandoned. Most of these studies treated patients with ampicillin. Lack of benefit may be explained by the choice of ampicillin, which has poor penetrance into the pancreas and a limited spectrum of activity for organisms typically found in infected pancreatitis.

Over the last decade, antibiotics have again emerged as an option to prevent sterile necrosis from becoming infected. Evidence exists from several small prospective, randomized trials that fewer patients with pancreatitis who are treated with antibiotics progress to infected pancreatitis when compared with those who are not treated. The carbapenems (impienem) and fluouroquinolones (ofloxacin and norfloxacin) have the best penetrance into pancreatic tissue when compared with other antibiotics, such as aminoglycosides, and are capable of treating organisms typically producing pancreatic infection (19). The studies, which investigated small numbers of patients, did not show that antibiotics reduce the need for surgery or improve mortality. Other arguments against antibiotic treatment to reduce the risk of infected pancreatitis include: penetration into necrotic tissue, which lacks blood supply, is uncertain; antibiotic treatment may delay necessary surgery until such time as mortality is unavoidable; and indiscriminate antibiotic use increases the emergence of resistant bacterial and fungal infections (20).

Antifungal therapy has a role in the treatment of acute pancreatitis. Many patients with severe pancreatitis will be at risk for disseminated fungal infections. Further, mortality in pancreatitis complicated by fungal infection may be four-fold higher (21). Known risk factors for disseminated fungal infection, often present in patients with severe acute pancreatitis, include acute renal failure, long-term or broad-spectrum antibiotics, total parenteral nutrition, central lines, high APACHE II scores, and ventilator dependence (22,23). A decision for prophylactic, empiric, or therapeutic use of antifungals should consider these risk features, as well as cultures indicating disseminated fungal infection.

Although the benefit of prophylactic antibiotics may be controversial, a treatment principle that is not controversial is that infected pancreatic necrosis requires surgical intervention.

Restoration of Oxygen Transport

Cardiovascular Support

The mortality associated with severe acute pancreatitis increases with organ failure. Advanced organ dysfunction and failure may occur because of inadequate early resuscitation and support. Rapid identification of shock and early resuscitation may limit the degree of dysfunction.

Pancreatitis, depending on its severity, can evoke a significant inflammatory response both locally, in the adjacent tissue, and systemically. Patients can sequester a significant fraction of intravascular volume in the extravascular tissues. Ranson recognized early that the fluid volume needed to resuscitate a patient predicted severity of illness. Recall that one of his original criteria was a fluid requirement of >6 L in the first 48 h (1). With the obligate loss of intravascular fluid, preload may be decreased. Subsequent decrease in cardiac output can lead to potentially inadequate oxygen delivery. Therefore, initial treatment is restoration of intravascular volume with balanced salt solutions. The clinician must recognize that the required volume may be large. The choice of replacement fluid should consider red blood cell transfusions for symptomatic anemia. The need for colloid is controversial.

Adequacy of intravascular volume replacement should be measured and monitored. Urine output, as an indicator of organ perfusion, may be sufficient in the previously healthy patient with mild disease. Invasive monitoring with a pulmonary artery catheter to guide appropriate fluid replacement may be required in the patient who requires large replacement volumes, who has concurrent cardiovascular disease, or who demonstrates systemic inflammatory response syndrome (SIRS), or sepsis. Such invasive monitoring can also provide information about cardiac function, oxygen delivery, oxygen consumption, and shunt. Despite current opinions opposed to their use, many providers could never imagine caring for a patient with severe systemic inflammation and sepsis without the information provided by the pulmonary artery catheter.

Support of the cardiovascular system may require more than replacement of preload. Circulating inhibitors produced in sepsis and SIRS may directly impair cardiac contractility. Associated hypoxemia decreases myocardial compliance and causes diastolic dysfunction. These conditions may require inotropic and oxygen support in addition to effective volume replacement.

Pulmonary Support

Severe pancreatitis can cause acute lung injury. The patient with pancreatitis is also at risk for developing acute respiratory distress syndrome (ARDS), thought to be a result of circulating inflammatory cytokines.

Approximately 50% of patients with acute pancreatitis will have pulmonary insufficiency. It may be even higher in severe acute pancreatitis (24,25). The causes of respiratory failure include the inability to generate the required minute ventilation to eliminate

CO_2 created by the metabolically active inflammatory process. The inflammatory mediators released from the injured pancreas can directly injure lung tissue. The injured lung has increased extravascular lung water and decreased compliance. The patient may not be capable of increasing the work of breathing to maintain needed ventilation in the poorly compliant lung. In addition, the injury may impair diffusion and cause hypoxemia. Clinical observation of the patient's respiratory efforts combined with arterial blood gas monitoring can alert the physician to the need for ventilator support.

Renal Support

With inadequate or delayed resuscitation, the likelihood that the patient with pancreatitis may develop acute renal failure increases. Timely intravascular fluid replacement and optimization of cardiac pump function may be effective in reducing this risk. In one series, 21% of patients with severe acute pancreatitis needed dialysis for renal failure (25).

Metabolic Support

Nutritional

Nutrition for the patient with pancreatitis appears paradoxical. On the one hand, nutritional support in the critically ill patient is necessary for maintaining immunologic integrity and organ function. On the other hand, pancreatic function is stimulated by food, and enteral feeding may exacerbate the disease. One solution is parenteral nutrition. With parenteral nutrition, one assumes that intravenously delivered calories would not stimulate an injured pancreas. Few prospective studies of parenteral nutrition in pancreatitis have been performed. The available data suggest that positive nitrogen balance can be achieved with parenteral nutrition in pancreatitis at the cost of an increase in catheter-related infections (26,27).

The use of enteral feedings in pancreatitis has been pursued. Pancreatic stimulation is minimal if nutrients are delivered to the jejunum. Several prospective and randomized trials comparing TPN and enterally delivered nutrition have been performed. They suggest that enteral feeding is safe, and some suggest that enterally fed patients have fewer septic complications, fewer episodes of hyperglycemia, and a lower mortality. In pancreatitis, as with other severe disease, enteral nutrition is safe and perhaps superior to parenteral nutrition (28,29).

Antisecretory

Since pancreatitis is caused by the leakage and activation of pancreatic enzymes outside of the gland, which results in the destruction of peripancreatic tissue, a logical treatment is reducing the enzyme production and secretion by the pancreas. Somatostatin is a naturally occuring peptide that inhibits gastrointestinal endocrine and exocrine activities. Octreotide, a synthetic somatostatin analog, has been used to treat a variety of hyersecretory gastrointestinal diseases, such as Zollinger–Ellison syndrome, by minimizing secretions. Its potential benefit in treating pancreatitis by limiting pancreatic secretions was initially supported by animal models. Its benefit in humans remains questionable (30). In a prospective, randomized study of patients with severe, acute pancreatitis, Paran et al. showed reduced rates of sepsis and ARDS in patients treated with octreotide compared to patients treated with supportive therapy alone (31). The benefit of octreotide may be realized in severe pancreatitis only.

In addition to somatostatin analogs, other medications have been used to treat pancreatitis by limiting secretory stimulation. They include H_2 blockers, glucagon, calcitonin, and anticholinergic drugs. None has shown any benefit (2).

OUTCOMES

In the past, mortality rates for what was called necrotizing pancreatitis were as high as 80%. With today's advanced critical care and surgical therapy, survival has improved significantly. Contemporary evidence places mortality in severe acute pancreatitis at 25–30%.

The physical toll of a prolonged stay in the intensive care unit can be extreme. Patients with severe acute pancreatitis have prolonged ICU and hospital stays that can result in significant physical and emotional impairment. A recent study evaluated 21 of 39 hospital survivors of severe acute pancreatitis. Subjective and objective data showed quality of life was generally good. Health, compared to the previous year, was at least as good or better in 95%, and physical or mental health measures were comparable to age matched controls. The authors concluded that despite significant resource utilization and physical strain to patients, aggressive treatment of severe acute pancreatitis was justified by the result (25).

FUTURE CONSIDERATIONS

New methods to detect, diagnose, and treat pancreatitis are being evaluated. Novel markers of pancreatic injury and inflammatory activation have been studied to see if they might characterize the severity of disease and the need to diagnose, biopsy, and debride necrotic peripancreatic tissue. Some of the markers studied include: tumor necrosis factor-α, interleukin (IL)-1β, IL-6, IL-8, and IL-18. None has shown any clinical applicability (32).

Refinements in imaging technology continue to occur. Interventional radiology techniques are being applied not only to diagnose infection but also to drain peripancreatic fluid collections. The effectiveness of these techniques compared with surgery has yet to be evaluated. Endoscopy and laparoscopy are also being used to diagnose, biopsy, and debride necrotic peripancreatic tissue, but their role remains undefined.

SUMMARY

- Pancreatitis is a disease with several etiologies; the most common are alcohol and gallstones.
- A patient with abdominal pain and an elevated serum amylase concentration is concluded as having pancreatitis until proven otherwise. Note that GI perforation can produce hypermylasemia.
- Pancreatitis usually is a self-limited process but can progress to the organ dysfunction with or without local complications. Progression to severe organ dysfunction is termed severe acute pancreatitis and often requires the resources of the intensive care unit.

- CT scan is currently the best method used for imaging the pancreas.
- Source control may require debridment of devitalized pancreatic and peripancreatic tissue. The decision to operate is complex and is based on evidence that suggests infection. Resuscitation aims to limit progress of the inflammation, to prevent infection, and to avoid multisystem organ dysfunction. Determining the end points of the resuscitation may require invasive monitoring.
- Metabolic support assures adequate nutrition to optimize healing and immune function.
- Critical care provided to patients with these aims improves survival and results in outcomes acceptable to patients.

REFERENCES

1. Ranson JHC, Rifkind KM, Roses DF, Fink SD, Eng K, Spencer FC. Prognostic signs and the role of operative management in acute pancreatitis. Surg Gynecol Obstet 1974; 139:69–80.
2. Howard JM, Idezuki Y, Ihse I, Prinz RA. Surgical Diseases of the Pancreas. 3d ed. Baltimore: Williams and Wilkins, 1998.
3. Lee KKW, Durham SJ. Physiology of the exocrine pancreas. In: Simmons RL, Steed DL, eds. Basic Science Review for Surgeons. Philadelphia: WB Saunders, 1992:257–269.
4. Williams M, Simms HH. Prognostic usefulness of scoring systems in critically ill patients with severe acute pancreatitis. Crit Care Med 1999; 27:901–907.
5. Bradley EL III. A clinically based classification system for acute pancreatitis. Arch Surg 1993; 128:586–590.
6. Warshaw AL. Pancreatic necrosis: to debride or not to debride—that is the question. Ann Surg 2000; 232:627–629.
7. Piironen A. Severe acute pancreatitis: contrast-enhanced CT and MRI features. Abdom Imaging 2001; 26:225–233.
8. Beger HG, Bittner R, Block S, Buchler M. Bacterial contamination of pancreatic necrosis: a prospective clinical study. Gastroenterology 1986; 91:433–438.
9. Buchler M, Gloor B, Muller CA, Friess H, Seiler CA, Uhl W. Acute necrotizing pancreatitis: treatment strategy according to the status of infection. Ann Surg 2000; 232:619–626.
10. Paye F, Rotman N, Radier C, Nouira R, Fagniez P-L. Percutaneous aspiration for bacteriological studies in patients with necrotizing pancreatitis. Br J Surg 1998; 85:755–759.
11. Le Mee J, Paye F, Sauvanet A, O'Toole D, Hammel P, Marty J, Ruszniewski P, Belghiti J. Incidence and reversibility of organ failure in the course of sterile or infected pancreatitis. Arch Surg 2001; 136:1386–1390.
12. Savino JA, LaPunzina C, Agarwal N, Cerabona TD, Policastro AJ. Open versus closed treatement of necrotizing pancreatitis. Shock 1996; 6:S65–S70.
13. Castillo CF, Rattner DW, Makary MA, Mostafavi A, McGrath D, Warshaw AL. Debridment and closed packing for the treatment of necrotizing pancreatitis. Ann Surg 1998; 228:676–684.
14. Bosscha K, Hulstaert PF, Hennipman A, Visser MR, Gooszen HG, van Vroonhoven TJMV, vdWerken C. Fulminant acute pancreatitis and infected necrosis: results of open management of the abdomen and "planned" reoperations. J Am Coll Surg 1998; 187:255–262.
15. Beger HG, Buchler M, Bittner R, Oettinger W, Block S, Nevalainen T. Necroseetomy and postoperative local lavage in patient with necrotizing pancreatitis: results of a prospective clinical trial. World J Surg 1988; 12:255–262.
16. Freeny PC, Hauptmann E, Althaus SJ, Traverso LW, Sinanan M. Percutaneous CT-guided catheter drainage of infected acute necrotizing pancreatitis: techniques and results. Am J Roentgenol 1998; 170:969–975.

17. Baril NB, Ralls PW, Wren SM, Selby RR, Radin R, Parekh D, Jabbour N, Stain SC. Does an infected peripancreatic fluid collection or abcess mandate operation? Ann Surg 2000; 231:361–367.
18. Oleynikov D, Cook C, Sellers B, Mone MC, Barton R. Decreased mortality from necrotizing pancreatitis. Am J Surg 1998; 176:648–653.
19. Runzi M, Layer P. Nonsurgical management of acute pancreatitis: use of antibiotics. Surg Clin North Am 1999; 79:759–765.
20. Barie PS. A critical review of antibiotic prophylaxis in severe acute pancreatitis. Am J Surg 1996; 172:38S–43S.
21. Hoerauf A, Hammer S, Muller-Myhsok B, Rupprecht H. Intra-abdominal Candida infection during acute necrotizing pancreatitis has a high prevalence and is associated with increased mortality. Crit Care Med 1998; 26:2010–2015.
22. Burchard KW, Minor LB, Slotman GJ, Gann DS. Fungal sepsis in surgical patients. Arch Surg 1983; 118:217–221.
23. Savino JA, Agarwal N, Wry P, Policastro A, Cerabona T, Austria L. Routine prophylactic antifungal agents (clotrimazole, ketoconazole, and nystatin) in nontransplant/nonburned critically ill surgical and trauma patients. J Trauma 1994; 36:20–25.
24. Imrie CW, Ferguson JC, Murthy D, Blumgart LH. Arterial hypoxia in acute pancreatitis: Br J Surg 1977; 64:185–188.
25. Soran A, Chelluri L, Lee KKW, Tisherman SA. Outcome and quality of life of patients with acute pancreatitis requiring intensive care. J Surg Res 2000; 91:89–94.
26. Sitzmann JV, Steinborn PA, Zinner MJ, Cameron JL. Total parenteral nutrition and alternate energy substrates in treatment of severe acute pancreatitis. Surg Gynecol Obstet 1989; 168:311–317.
27. Sax HC, Warner BW, Talamini MA, Hamilton FN, Bell RH Jr, Fisher JE, Bower RH. Early total parenteral nutrition in acute pancreatitis: lack of beneficial effect. Am J Surg 1987; 153:117–124.
28. Windsor ACJ, Kanwar S, Li AGK, Barnes E, Guthrie JA, Spark JI, Welsh F, Guillou PJ, Reynolds JV. Compared with parenteral nutrition, enteral feeding attenuates the acute phase response and improves disease severity in acute pancreatitis. Gut 1998; 42:431–435.
29. Kalfarentzos F, Kehagias J, Mead N, Kokkinis K, Gogos CA. Enteral nutrition is superior to parenteral nutrition in severe acute pancreatitis: results of a randomized prospective trial. Br J Surg 1997; 84:1665–1669.
30. Wyncoll DL. The management of severe acute necrotizing pancreatitis: an evidence-based review of the literature. Intensive Care Med 1999; 25:146–156.
31. Paran H, Mayo A, Paran D, Neufeld D, Shwartz I, Zissin R, Singer P, Kaplan O, Skornik Y, Freund U. Octreotide treatment in patients with severe acute pancreatitis. Dig Dis Sci 2000; 45:2247–2251.
32. Lipsett PA. Serum cytokines, proteins, and receptors in acute pancreatitis: mediators, markers, or more of the same? Crit Care Med 2001; 29:1642–1643.

39

Biliary Complications During Critical Illness

Paul Druck
VA Medical Center, Minneapolis, Minnesota, USA

Critical illness may be complicated by a variety of intra- and extrahepatic biliary disorders unrelated to the original illness. These complications include acute cholecystitis, obstructive jaundice with or without cholangitis, and hepatic dysfunction manifested as nonobstructive hyperbilirubinemia [intensive care unit (ICU) jaundice] (Fig. 1).

ACUTE CHOLECYSTITIS

Epidemiology of Acute Cholecystitis in the Critically Ill

Acute cholecystitis may complicate the course of unrelated medical or surgical illness in 1–2% of critically ill postoperative patients. The high mortality rate of cholecystitis in the critically ill (>50% in some series) reflects the compromised condition of these patients as well as possible delays in diagnosis (1,2). Diagnostic uncertainty is a consequence of the absence or lack of specificity of the classic signs of cholecystitis, particularly in injured or postoperative patients in whom abdominal pain and tenderness, fever, leukocytosis, and hypermetabolism are common. Cholecystitis should be considered in any critically ill patient with unexplained abdominal pain or signs of sepsis.

Pathogenesis of Acute Cholecystitis in the Critically Ill

Acute cholecystitis may be classic *calculous* (obstructive) cholecystitis, or may occur in the absence of obstruction of the cystic duct, so-called *acalculous cholecystitis*. Postoperatively, cholecystitis is *acalculous* in ~50% of cases; in trauma or burn patients this figure exceeds 90% (3).

Acute calculous cholecystitis may occur as an unfortunate coincidence during a critical illness, possibly precipitated by prolonged fasting. The so-called total parenteral nutrition *(TPN)-associated cholecystitis* is not a consequence of TPN administration, per se, but of the underlying nil per os (NPO) status that necessitated the use of TPN. NPO status has been shown to lead to the rapid development or progression of gallbladder sludge and stones, which may result in calculous (obstructive) cholecystitis (4). Bile stasis secondary to NPO status may result in a nonobstructive, irritative cholecystitis unrelated to gallstones (5,6). Independent of gallbladder pathology, TPN is also associated with hepatocellular dysfunction and hyperbilirubinemia (see the following section on Hepatocellular Dysfunction).

Acalculous cholecystitis is distinguished pathologically from calculous cholecystitis by arterial occlusions and lack of venous filling rather than vascular engorgement (7). These findings, along with the strong association with hypotension (particularly after ruptured aortic aneurysm or cardiopulmonary bypass), the use of vasoconstrictor agents, gram-negative sepsis, and positive pressure ventilation (which can reduce splanchnic perfusion), support gallbladder ischemia as the precipitating cause (3,8,9). If stones or sludge are present in the gallbladder of a critically ill patient with cholecystitis, but conditions known to predispose to acalculous cholecystitis are present as well, the etiology of the cholecystitis may be unclear. If, at the time of operation, extensive gallbladder necrosis is encountered, the distinction between acalculous and gangrenous calculous cholecystitis may not be possible.

Diagnosis of Acute Cholecystitis in the Critically Ill

The clinical features of acute cholecystitis in outpatients—right-upper-quadrant pain and tenderness, fever, leukocytosis, and variable abnormalities in bilirubin, alkaline phosphatase, and occasionally transaminases and amylase—are often obscured by critically ill patients' underlying conditions. If acute cholecytitis is being considered, ultrasound with ~90% sensitivity and specificity is the preferred initial study. Positive findings include gallbladder wall thickening or edema, pericholecystic fluid, and intramural gas. False-positive scans may be caused by ascites, biliary sludge, or chronic gallbladder disease, which can contribute to exaggerated estimates of gallbladder wall thickness. The presence or absence of gallstones is of little diagnostic significance as not all gallstones cause cholecystitis and, conversely, *acalculous* cholecystitis can occur in the absence of gallstones. The computed tomography (CT) scan has comparable sensitivity and specificity to ultrasound, but requires transportation of the patient to the radiology department, the use of intravenous iodinated contrast, and is more expensive. The primary advantage of CT scanning lies in excluding nonbiliary intra-abdominal pathology when ultrasound is nondiagnostic (10,11).

Radionuclide cholescintigraphy can demonstrate cystic duct occlusion, present in almost all cases of acute *calculous* cholecystitis. Sensitivity and specificity have been reported to be as high as 97% and 95%, respectively (12). However, false positives (nonvisualized gallbladder in the absence of cholecystitis) are more frequent with prolonged NPO status (common in critically ill or postoperative patients), a condition that reduces specificity to 38% (10). Chronic alcoholism, severe chronic gallstone disease, and unsuspected prior cholecystectomy also may lead to false positives (13). False negatives (visualized gallbladder in the presence of acute cholecystitis) may occur in acalculous (nonobstructive) cholecystitis; therefore, a negative scan does not exclude cholecystitis in a critically ill patient. Thus, cholescintigraphy plays little role in the diagnosis of cholecystitis in postoperative or critically ill patients.

Percutaneous bile aspiration and culture is highly specific, but lacks sensitivity, especially in acalculous cholecystitis, where the bile may be sterile initially (10). Bedside diagnostic laparoscopy under intravenous sedation has been successfully used to diagnose acute cholecystitis. In some cases, cholecystostomy has been performed during the procedure as well (14).

Biliary Complications

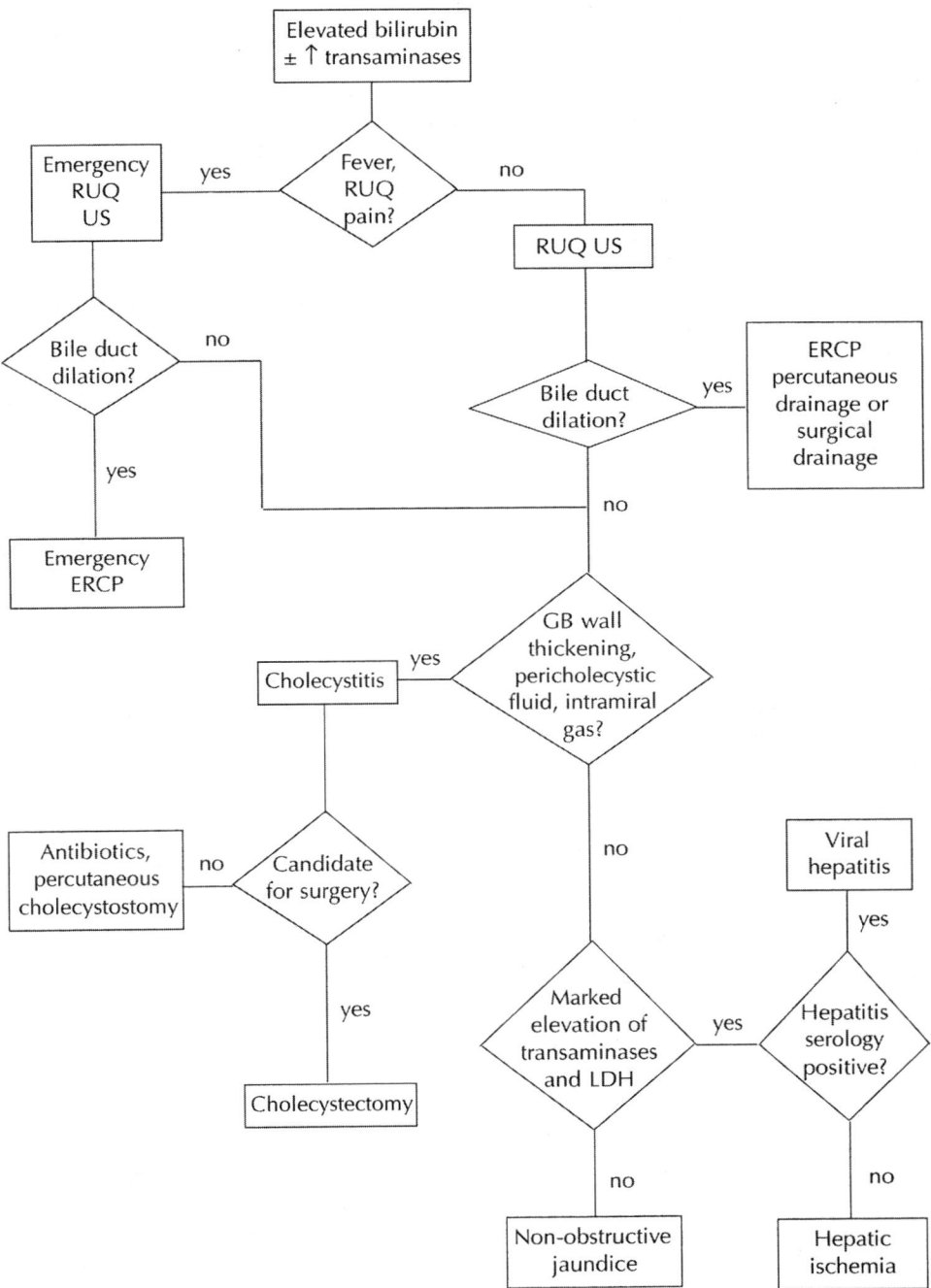

Figure 1 Treatment approach for biliary complications. *Abbreviations*: RUQ US, ultrasound of right upper quadrant; ERCP, endoscopic retrograde cholangio-pancreatography.

Treatment of Acute Cholecystitis in the Critically Ill

Cholecystectomy is the definitive treatment of cholecystitis. In a patient with acute cholecystitis, who is at high risk for general anesthesia and surgery and whose signs and symptoms of cholecystitis resolve completely with antibiotics, cholecystectomy may be deferred, but relapses are common. Intravenous antibiotics with activity against the organisms typically implicated (i.e., gram-negative rods, anaerobes, and *Enterococcus*) should be used. Prior colonization with resistant organisms is a common occurrence in ICU patients and should be considered. If the response to antibiotics is incomplete, or if relapse occurs, ultrasound-guided percutaneous cholecystostomy produces clinical improvement in 58–94% of patients, with a ~10% incidence of serious complications (bleeding, leakage of purulent bile with peritonitis, and catheter dislodgement) (15–19). If this procedure is not available, an alternative is open cholecystostomy through a minimal incision under local anesthesia. Patients with acalculous cholecystitis and gallbladder necrosis may continue to manifest hypermetabolism and signs of intra-abdominal sepsis after cholecystostomy, because necrotic gallbladder remains. After recovery from the critical illness, cholecystectomy can be performed with more acceptable risk.

OBSTRUCTIVE AND NONOBSTRUCTIVE JAUNDICE AND CHOLANGITIS

Hyperbilirubinemia is common in critically ill patients. It may be apparent as jaundice (icterus) when the serum bilirubin level exceeds 2–3 mg/dL. It is visible earliest in the sclerae and lingual frenulum, but artificial light may mask it (20). Etiologies are either obstructive (mechanical obstruction of the biliary tract) or nonobstructive (hepatocellular dysfunction or hemolysis) (see the section on Nonobstructive Jaundice). The term *cholestasis* refers to an arrest of the flow of bile, which may be a result of biliary obstruction or hepatocellular dysfunction. It is used inconsistently and will be avoided here in favor of more specific descriptors.

Initial Evaluation of the Jaundiced Patient

Mild degrees of hyperbilirubinemia that are not progressive are not consistent with acute biliary obstruction. On the other hand, a markedly elevated or steadily increasing bilirubin mandates further workup. Excluding biliary obstruction is imperative as this is a life-threatening but correctable condition. Obstructive jaundice is associated with >50% conjugated ("direct") bilirubin, variable increases in alkaline phosphatase and transaminase levels, acholic stools, bilirubinuria, and absence of urobilinogen from the urine. Bilirubin fractionation (conjugated vs. nonconjugated) and liver enzyme profiles may be suggestive of an etiology, particularly in advanced hyperbilirubinemia. Cholangiography is the gold standard for diagnosing or excluding extrahepatic biliary obstruction. This procedure may not be suitable for unstable patients, and can be technically impossible after some types of upper GI surgical reconstructions. Bedside abdominal ultrasound is the initial test of choice. It is rapid, noninvasive, universally applicable, and does not require patient transport. It has a reported sensitivity of 95% (12). Biliary dilation is the critical finding; failure to identify common bile duct stones on ultrasound does not rule out the diagnosis of choledocholithiasis. Biliary dilation may be seen on CT scan, and biliary obstruction inferred from radionuclide hepatobiliary scans, but these are not the preferred diagnostic modalities.

Obstructive Jaundice and Cholangitis

Obstructive jaundice in critically ill patients is most commonly caused by gallstones. Benign or malignant strictures of the extrahepatic bile ducts much less commonly complicate an unrelated critical illness. An exception would be a patient who is in the ICU immediately following biliary tract surgery. Hemobilia caused by liver trauma or hepatic aneurysms is occasionally identified as a cause of obstruction.

Relief of the obstruction is urgently required to prevent infection (cholangitis) and eventual hepatic dysfunction. Endoscopic transpapillary sphincterotomy is the method of choice in patients in general, and especially for critically ill patients. It is associated with a high success rate and significantly lower morbidity and mortality than surgical decompression (21). If ERCP is not technically feasible, percutaneous transhepatic cholangiography and drainage would be the next choice (22).

If infection develops in an obstructed bile duct (cholangitis) it is generally manifested by Charcot's triad (fever, right-upper-quadrant pain, and hyperbilirubinemia) and is usually accompanied by leukocytosis. The course may be indolent but is often fulminant; septic shock may develop within hours. The differential diagnosis includes but is not limited to: acute viral hepatitis (distinguished by marked elevations in transaminases—see the section on Hepatocellular Dysfunction); acute cholecystitis (rarely associated with bilirubin >3, and usually associated with marked right-upper-quadrant tenderness and suggestive findings on ultrasound or CT—see the section on Diagnosis of Acute Cholecystitis in the Critically Ill); appendicitis with coincidental nonobstructive hyperbilirubinemia (distinction can be made on the basis of CT or ultrasound findings of appendicitis with the lack of biliary dilation on ultrasound); and perforated peptic ulcer with coincidental nonobstructive hyperbilirubinemia (distinguished by free air on abdominal imaging studies). Definitive diagnosis is made via endoscopic retrograde cholangiography. If biliary obstruction and cholangitis are discovered, sphincterotomy and removal of obstructing stones or sludge should be performed. If ERCP is not technically feasible, percutaneous transhepatic cholangiography and drainage is an alternative. Surgical common bile duct exploration and clearance is associated with a higher morbidity and mortality and may be inadvisable in critically ill patients (21,22).

Patients with suspected cholangitis who demonstrate low to moderate fever and are hemodynamically stable should receive antibiotic coverage for enteric gram-negative organisms, *Enterococcus*, and anaerobes, and undergo biliary decompression (usually ERCP) as soon as feasible. Patients with signs of septic shock, such as hypotension and mental status changes, should undergo emergency decompression as soon as they are sufficiently stable hemodynamically to undergo the procedure. They should also receive antibiotic coverage as above.

Nonobstructive Jaundice

Nonobstructive hyperbilirubinemia may result from acute hepatocellular dysfunction or accelerated hemolysis. Nonobstructive jaundice is not associated with cholangitis.

Hepatocellular Dysfunction

Hepatocellular dysfunction is usually first recognized in a critically ill patient when hyperbilirubinemia, accompanied by variable abnormalities in transaminases and alkaline phosphatase, is noted. Hepatic dysfunction is often seen during severe sepsis or acute inflammatory conditions such as ARDS, and it may be one component of the syndrome of multiple organ dysfunction (23–25). Other etiologies include hepatic ischemia, drug toxicity, TPN, acute viral hepatitis, and inherited disorders of bilirubin metabolism.

The pathogenesis of hepatic dysfunction in sepsis has not been completely elucidated. Evidence supports contributions of hepatic hypoperfusion and direct hepatocyte or cholangiole injury mediated by Kupfer cell-attracted neutrophils (26,27). Postmortem examinations of patients succumbing to sepsis have revealed focal hepatocyte necrosis, intrahepatic cholestasis, inflammatory changes and neutrophil infiltration of the portal tracts and cholangioles, venous congestion, and Kupfer cell hyperplasia (28). Correlation of the degree of hyperbilirubinemia with prognosis is poor. The prognosis is that of the underlying condition; resolution of that condition is followed by gradual clearance of the hyperbilirubinemia, usually without lasting hepatic compromise.

Hepatitic ischemia is characterized by sudden, marked increases in transaminases [especially aspartate aminotransferase (AST)] and L-lactate dehydrogenase (LDH) levels. Etiologies include profound shock, prolonged supra-celiac aortic cross-clamping, and severe left or right ventricular failure. If extensive hepatic necrosis has not occurred and the ischemia is promptly corrected, hepatic function usually returns to baseline in 7–10 days (29,30).

A number of therapeutic agents have been associated with cholestasis, including antibiotics (e.g., amoxicillin/clavulanic acid, the sulfonamides, erythromycin, tetracycline, and trimethoprim/sulfamethoxazole), acetaminophen, anabolic and contraceptive steroids, and some antineoplastic agents (31).

TPN has been associated with elevations in transaminases, bilirubin, and alkaline phosphatase that often resolve without discontinuation of the TPN. Histologically, bile stasis, bile ductule proliferation, and portal inflammation and fibrosis may be seen. The precise mechanism is not clear; some evidence implicates either the free amino acids used or the large carbohydrate load (32).

Viral hepatitis is a common cause of jaundice but an uncommon complication of otherwise unrelated critical illness. Jaundice usually appears at the time of peak transaminase levels (which may reach several thousand International Units in severe cases). The hyperbilirubinemia is a mixture of conjugated and nonconjugated forms and is usually in the range of 5–10 mg/dL, although it may exceed 20 mg/dL on occasion. The diagnosis can be confirmed by a panel of hepatitis serologies (31).

Several inherited disorders of bilirubin metabolism may prompt a search for the cause of hyperbilirubinemia. *Gilbert's syndrome*, which may be inherited or sporadic, is a defect in hepatic bilirubin uptake, which results in chronic mild unconjugated hyperbilirubinemia that rarely exceeds 5 mg/dL. The hyperbilirubinemia is exacerbated by fasting, surgery, infection, fever, and ethanol. *Crigler–Najjar syndrome* is glucuronyl transferase deficiency, causing conjugated hyperbilirubinemia of 6–20 mg/dL [partial, or type II; complete deficiency (type I) is usually fatal in infancy]. *Dubin–Johnson syndrome* is a defect in the excretion of conjugated bilirubin, leading to predominantly conjugated bilirubin concentrations of 3–15 mg/dL. *Rotor syndrome* is a rare defect in hepatic storage capacity, causing variable degrees of conjugated hyperbilirubinemia (33).

Hemolysis

Markedly accelerated hemolysis in critically ill patients is most commonly due to hemolytic transfusion reactions, reabsorption of large hematomas from surgery, trauma, leaking aneurysms, accelerated hemolysis following massive blood transfusion, or inherited disorders, such as sickle cell anemia or hereditary spherocytosis. Hemolysis generally does not cause hyperbilirubinemia in excess of 5 mg/dL without simultaneous hepatic dysfunction or severe sickle cell crisis. Severe, necrotizing *Clostridia* infections may also cause accelerated hemolysis (32).

SUMMARY

- Biliary tract diseases that may complicate the course of a critical illness include acute cholecystitis, obstructive jaundice with or without cholangitis, and hepatocellular dysfunction leading to nonobstructive jaundice.
- Cholecystitis should be considered in a critically ill patient with new onset right upper quadrant pain or tenderness or otherwise unexplained signs of sepsis.
- Cholecystitis may be calculous or acalculous. Acalculous cholecystitis is ischemic in etiology and may occur in the absence or presence of gallstones. Right upper quadrant ultrasound is the initial diagonstic modality, but false negatives and positives are possible. Cholecystectomy is a definitive treatment; percutaneous cholecystostomy is useful in patients too ill or unstable to undergo general anesthesia and surgery.
- Bile duct obstruction should be excluded if jaundice develops in a critically ill patient. If right upper quadrant ultrasound is not diagnostic, ERCP is definitive. If obstruction is present, endoscopic drainage is the treatment of choice. If ERCP drainage is technically impossible, percutaneous transhepatic drainage is an alternative.
- Nonobstructive jaundice in a critically ill patient may represent hepatic dysfunction associated with sepsis, drug toxicity, hepatic steatosis from TPN, viral hepatitis, congenital hyperbilirubinemia, or markedly accelerated hemolysis. Management is treatment of the underlying infectious, inflammatory, or traumatic etiology and general supportive care, including nutritional support.

REFERENCES

1. Long TN, Heimbach TM, Carrico CJ. Acalculous cholecystitis in critically ill patients. Am J Surg 1978; 136:31–36.
2. Orlando R, Gleason E, Drezner AD. Acute acalculous cholecystitis in the critically ill patient. Am J Surg 1983; 145:472–476.
3. Barie PS, Fischer E. Acute acalculous cholecystitis. J Am Coll Surg 1995; 180:232–244.
4. Messing B, Bories C, Kunstlinger F, Bernier JJ. Does total parenteral nutrition induce gallbladder sludge formation and lithiasis? Gastroenterology 1983; 84:1012–1019.
5. Kouromalis E, Hopwood D, Ross PE, Milne G, Bouchier IA. Gallbladder epithelial hydrolases in human cholecystitis. J Pathol 1983; 139:179–191.
6. Niderheiser DH. Acute acalculous cholecystitis induced by lysophosphatidyl choline. Am J Pathol 1986; 124:559–563.
7. Warren BL. Small vessel occlusion in acute acalculous cholecystitis. Surgery 1992; 111:163–168.
8. Glenn F, Becker CG. Acute acalculous cholecystitis. Ann Surg 1982; 195:131–136.
9. Fabian TC, Hickerson WL, Mangiante EC. Posttraumatic and postoperative acute cholecystitis. Am Surgeon 1986; 52:188–192.
10. Mirvis SE, Vainright JR, Nelson AW, Johnston GS, Schorr R, Rodriguez A, Whitney NO. The diagnosis of acute acalculous cholecystitis: a comparison of sonography, scintigraphy, and CT. Am J Roentgenol 1986; 147:1171–1175.

11. Shuman WP, Rogers JV, Rudd TG, Mack LA, Plumley T, Larson EB. Low sensitivity of sonography and cholescintigraphy in acalculous cholecystitis. Am J Roentgenol 1984; 142:531–534.
12. Shea JA, Berlin JA, Escarce JJ, Clarke JR, Kinosian BP, Cabana MD, Tsai WW, Horangic N, Malet PF, Schwartz JS. Revised estimates of diagnostic test sensitivity and specificity in suspected biliary tract disease. Arch Int Med 1994; 154:2573–2582.
13. Shuman WP, Gibbs P, Rudd TG, Mack LA. PIPIDA scintigraphy for cholecystitis: false positives in alcoholism and total parental nutrition. Am J Roentgenol 1982; 138:1–5.
14. Almeida J, Sleeman D, Sosa JL, Puente I, McKenney M, Martin L. Acalculous cholecystitis: the use of diagnostic laparoscopy. J Laparosc Surg 1995; 5(4):227–231.
15. McGahan JP, Lindfors KL. Percutaneous cholecystostomy: an alternative to surgical cholecystostomy for acute cholecystitis? Radiology 1989; 173:481–485.
16. Werbel GB, Nahrwold DL, Joehl RJ, Vogelzang RL, Rege RV. Percutaneous cholecystostomy in the diagnosis and treatment of acute cholecystitis in the high risk patient. Arch Surg 1989; 124:782–786.
17. Lee MJ, Saini S, Brink JA, Hahn PF, Simeone JF, Morrison MC, Rattner D, Mueller PR. Treatment of critically ill patients with sepsis of unknown cause: value of percutaneous cholecystostomy. Am J Roentgenol 1991; 156:1163–1166.
18. van Sonnenberg E, D'Agostino HB, Goodacre BW, Sanchez RB, Casola G. Percutaneous gallbladder puncture and cholecystostomy: results, complications, and caveats for safety. Radiology 1992; 183:167–170.
19. Melin MM, Sarr MG, Bender CE, van Heerden JA. Percutaneous cholecystostomy: a valuable technique in high-risk patients with presumed acute cholecystitis. Brit J Surg 1995; 82:1274–1277.
20. DeGowin EL, DeGowin RL. Bedside Diagnostic Examination, 3rd ed. NewYork: Macmillan, 1976: 468–469.
21. Lai ECS, Mok FPT, Tan ES, Lo CM, Fan ST, You KT, Wong J. Endoscopic biliary drainage for severe acute cholangitis. N Engl J Med 1992; 326:1582–1586.
22. Pessa ME, Hawkins IF, Vogel SB. The treatment of acute cholangitis. Ann Surg 1987; 205:389–392.
23. Bone RC, Balk R, Slotman G, Maunder R, Silverman H, Hyers TM, Kerstein MD. Adult respiratory distress syndrome. Sequence and importance of development of multiple organ failure. Chest 1992; 101:320–326.
24. Maynard ND, Bihari DJ, Dalton RN, Beale R, Smithies MN, Mason RC. Liver function and splanchnic ischemia in critically ill patients. Chest 1997; 111:180–187.
25. Beal AL, Cerra FB. Multiple organ failure in the 1990's: systemic inflammatory response and organ dysfunction. JAMA 1994; 271:226–233.
26. Doi F, Goya T, Torisu M. Potential role of hepatic macrophages in neutrophil-mediated liver injury in rats with sepsis. Hepatology 1993; 17:1086–1094.
27. Dahn MS, Wilson RF, Lange P, Stone A, Jacobs LA. Hepatic parenchymal oxygen tension following injury and sepsis. Arch Surg 1990; 125:441–443.
28. Banks JG, Foulis AK, Ledingham IM, Macsween RM. Liver function in septic shock. J Clin Pathol 1982; 35:1249–1252.
29. Gitlin N, Serio KM. Ischemic hepatitis: widening horizons. Am J Gastroenterol 1992; 87:831–836.
30. Levy DK, Schwartz JM, Frishman WH, Schwartz ML, LeJemtel TH. Ischemic hepatitis in a patient with congestive cardiomyopathy: an innovative approach to therapy using intravenous dobutamine. J Clin Pharmacol 1994; 34:270–272.
31. Pratt DS, Kaplan MM. Jaundice. In: Braunwald E, Fauci AS, Kasper DL, Hauser SL, Longo DL, Jameson JL eds. Principles of Internal Medicine, 15th ed. New York: McGraw-Hill, 2001:255–259.
32. Quigley EM, Marsh MN, Schaffer JL, Markins RS. Hepatobiliary complications of total parenteral nutrition. Gastroenterol 1993; 104:286–301.
33. Berk PD, Wolkoff AW. Bilirubin metabolism and the hyperbilirubinemias. In: Braunwald E, Fauci AS, Kasper DL, Hauser SL, Longo DL, Jameson JL eds. Principles of Internal Medicine, 15th ed. New York: Mc Graw-Hill, 2001:1715–1720.

40
Acute Abdomen

Michael D. Pasquale
Lehigh Valley Hospital, Allentown, Pennsylvania, USA

Roderick A. Barke
VA Medical Center, Minneapolis, Minnesota, USA

Diagnosis and management of the acute abdomen are fundamental in general surgery. Few other conditions provide an equal challenge to the clinician's knowledge and judgment. This challenge becomes even more formidable when the patient is critically ill. The diagnosis of acute abdomen in the critically ill is made under two circumstances. The first is the patient for whom acute abdomen is the original medical indication for admission to the SICU; the second is in the setting of the postoperative surgical patient whose recovery is interrupted by an acute abdominal event. Although the diagnostic regimen for each is similar, the information available at the time of presentation to the surgical intensivist may be considerably different.

In a study done by the Department of Veterans Affairs, a typical presentation of potentially treatable abdominal pathologic conditions was revealed as a common cause of class I error (major unexpected findings at autopsy that would have led to a change in therapy and an improved survival rate had they been diagnosed before death) in veterans who received mechanical ventilation. The diagnoses were missed in two-thirds of patients because the clinicians failed to consider and pursue the diagnoses, not because they were misled by inconclusive or incorrect information from diagnostic procedures. This observation further reinforces the idea that identification of patients with an acute abdomen is of great importance for the surgical intensivist. A recommended approach to the patient with acute abdominal pain is shown in Fig. 1.

HISTORY AND PHYSICAL EXAMINATION

Despite the technologic advances in medicine, a detailed history and physical examination remain the most important tools in the initial evaluation of the patient. The history, obtained either from the patient or individuals close to the patient, directs further investigation. A complete medical history with attention to major illnesses, previous surgical procedures, and current medications is essential. In the subset of patients seen in the recovery room after a surgical procedure, historical details include the history of present illness

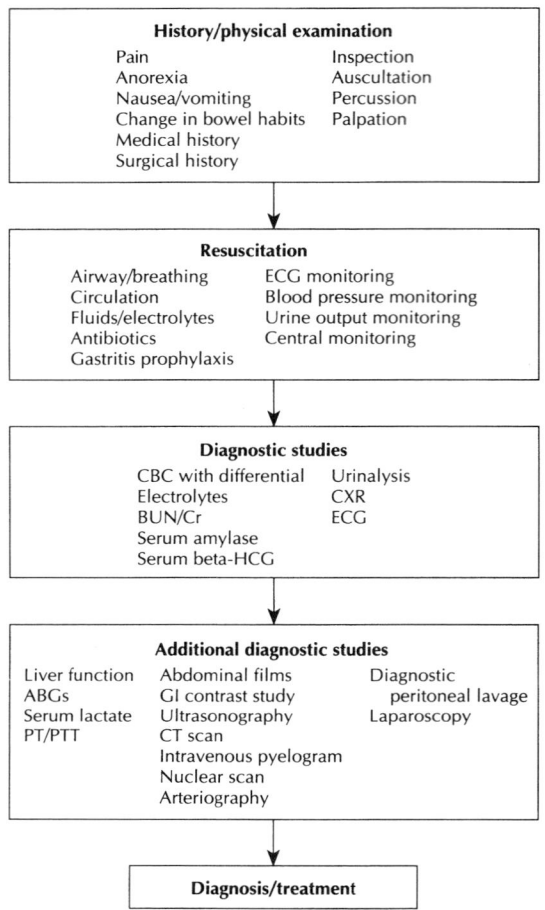

Figure 1 Approach to the patient with acute abdominal pain.

leading to the surgical procedure, operative notes, and anesthesia record. In addition, the classic historical details, such as the time course of the illness and associated constitutional symptoms (e.g., nausea, vomiting, diarrhea, chills, character of pain), provide the clues necessary for rapid definitive diagnosis and treatment.

Pain is often the presenting complaint of patients with acute abdomens, and knowing its location at onset and at the time of examination, its duration, quality, and aggravating factors is of substantial importance in the diagnostic process. Abdominal pain is mediated through both the autonomic and somatic sensory nervous systems.

Visceral pain is elicited from abdominal organs that are innervated by the autonomic system. This type of pain is usually crampy, poorly localized, and often associated with nausea and vomiting. Stimuli that produce visceral pain are increased hollow viscus wall tension, solid viscus capsule stretching, ischemia, and certain chemicals. Visceral pain usually is transmitted according to developmental patterns—foregut (stomach duodenum, liver, biliary tract, pancreas, spleen) radiating to the epigastrium, midgut (small bowel, appendix, right side of the colon) radiating to the periumbilical region, and hindgut (left side of the colon, rectum) radiating to the hypogastrium. This pattern is seen because the autonomic nerves follow the distribution of the blood supply from the major splanchnic arteries (celiac, superior mesenteric, and inferior mesenteric). Severe visceral pain also results in autonomic reflexes such as sweating, tachycardia or bradycardia, hypotension, cutaneous hyperalgesia, hyperesthesia, and involuntary spastic contractions of the abdominal musculature.

Somatic pain arises from irritation of parietal peritoneum, mesentery, or respiratory diaphragm. It is transmitted through somatic sensory nerves and is sharper, more distinct, and well localized to the site of stimulation. This pain is often associated with the classic "peritoneal" signs of rigidity: spasm of overlying muscles and rebound tenderness from inflammation of the parietal peritoneum. Referred pain arises at a distance from the pathologic site and follows neural pathways, often dermatome distributions. It is important to document when pain began, where it originated, what was its character, what precipitated it, what was associated with it, and whether it has varied.

Anorexia, nausea, and vomiting often occur in the setting of intra-abdominal pathology. Paralytic ileus accompanies most intraperitoneal inflammatory processes. Anorexia may be caused by a variety of organic and psychologic disturbances that are poorly understood. Nausea and vomiting may occur separately, but usually are closely related. Nausea generally precedes vomiting. The act of vomiting is controlled by the vomiting center and the chemoreceptor trigger zone (CTZ) in the medulla. The CTZ receives afferent stimulation from the gastrointestinal (GI) tract and sends impulses to the vomiting center. In some cases, afferent impulses from the GI tract bypass the CTZ. Emesis without antecedent nausea suggests a CNS lesion with increased intracranial pressure. Emesis that relieves epigastric pain usually is associated with intragastric lesions or pyloric spasm associated with pyloric channel ulcer. Immediate postprandial vomiting may represent a toxic or psychogenic cause, hyperemesis gravidarum, gastritis, high intestinal obstruction, or a gastric neoplasm. Vomiting larger amounts of undigested food at 12–24 h intervals suggests chronic pyloric obstruction. Vomiting ≥ 1 h after meals is consistent with gastric outlet obstruction, diabetic gastropathy, and postvagotomy disorders. Feculent emesis often indicates either a gastrocolic fistula or a complete low intestinal obstruction.

Change in bowel habits, typically constipation or obstipation, occurs in a patient with obstruction or ileus. Diarrhea also may occur in a patient with intra-abdominal inflammation, although diarrhea is more common with enterocolitis syndromes.

In females, the menstrual history is important. Amenorrhea, hypogastric pain, or uterine bleeding suggests ectopic pregnancy.

When the patient is unable to communicate (sedation, paralysis, intubation, or previous cerebrovascular accident), the history may prove inconclusive. Physical examination in this situation achieves greater importance in directing further diagnostic procedures. The initial physical examination of the critically ill patient must be complete to provide the basis for further comparisons. Ideally, the patient should be reassured and a good rapport established before the examination is begun. A sense of trust in the examiner serves to relax the patient and allow the evaluation to proceed without undue discomfort. Routine vital signs should be taken and evaluated. Both fever and hypothermia are significant signs of intra-abdominal sepsis. The rate and quality of the pulse should be noted, as should the character of respirations. Tachycardia and tachypnea with shallow inspirations suggest the possibility of impending instability or abdominal catastrophe. Blood pressure should be documented and compared with the patient's preillness value. The abdominal examination should be conducted in a systematic manner with attention to the fundamentals of inspection, auscultation, percussion, and palpation.

The first step in a thorough examination is careful inspection of the anterior and posterior abdominal wall, perineum, and flank areas. Defects (e.g., hernias, scars), ecchymoses (e.g., retroperitoneal bleeding), abnormal pulsations (e.g., abdominal aneurysm), engorged subcutaneous veins (e.g., from portal hypertension), jaundice (e.g., from hepatobiliary disease), and umbilical deformities [e.g., Sister Joseph's nodule (metastatic intra-abdominal carcinoma), eversion, ascites, fistula (either urachal or enterocutaneous)] should be sought. Surgical wounds should be inspected to evaluate them for bleeding, purulent drainage, crepitus, and/or dehiscence.

Auscultation should be performed next. The character of the bowel sounds and presence of bruits should be noted. Hypoactive or absent bowel sounds may indicate an ileus associated with an intra-abdominal infection, whereas hyperactive sounds with rushes are characteristic of intestinal obstruction. Bruits may signify the presence of aneurysms or significant hemangiomas, especially hepatic hemangiomas.

Percussion, which is performed next, is useful as a means to assess organ size, determine the presence of ascites (shifting dullness), and evaluate bladder fullness. Tympany over the midabdomen suggests obstruction, whereas tympany over the lateral liver is a clue to bowel perforation. Percussion is also useful in demonstrating peritoneal irritation.

Palpation of the abdomen is last and should be performed in a systematic fashion. If possible, the area of most discomfort should be evaluated last. Attempts to localize pain and to detect the presence of rigidity and rebound tenderness should be made. The presence of any masses should also be noted. A rectal and genital examination, and a pelvic examination in females, should be considered a part of the abdominal examination. The presence of blood, mass, or tenderness in these areas provides invaluable clues about the cause of acute abdominal pain.

After completion of a thorough history and physical examination, the intensive care physician should be able to formulate a working differential diagnosis for the patient. At this point several questions must be addressed. (1) Is the patient adequately resuscitated? (2) Does the patient require invasive monitoring? (3) What further diagnostic studies are required? (4) Should the patient be taken to the operating room, and if so, when?

RESUSCITATION AND MONITORING

Resuscitation first involves attention to airway, breathing, and circulation. The patient with an acute abdomen may have altered pulmonary function with atelectasis, hypoxia, and increased work of breathing. Patients with pre-existing pulmonary disease may not tolerate this pulmonary compromise, and early respiratory support may be needed. In general, most patients with an acute abdomen have had limited oral intake and associated GI losses via diarrhea, emesis, bleeding, or "third space" fluid shifts. They usually are dehydrated and demonstrate alterations in electrolyte balance. Early IV fluid and electrolyte replacement is mandatory. When the possibility of intra-abdominal sepsis exists, empiric antibiotic administration becomes an important early treatment. Before administering antibiotics, a definitive plan should be made. Antibiotics may mask the signs and symptoms of the intra-abdominal disease and delay other appropriate therapies.

All patients in the SICU with an acute abdomen should have ECG, blood pressure, and urinary output monitoring. Invasive monitoring generally is not required to resuscitate the patient with an acute abdomen. Selected patients (i.e., those with underlying cardiac,

Acute Abdomen

pulmonary, or renal disease) may require more sophisticated monitoring both to ensure adequate restoration of oxygen transport and to determine when the patient's condition is optimal for surgery. The guidelines for invasive monitoring set forth in Chapters 8, 60, and 61 of this text also apply to the patient with an acute abdomen.

DIAGNOSTIC EVALUATION

The availability of a laboratory or radiologic test does not mandate its use. Cope's classic treatise on the diagnosis of the acute abdomen states that "overreliance on laboratory tests and radiologic evaluations will very often mislead the clinician, especially if the history and physical examination are less than complete." This observation applies equally well to the critically ill patient.

Laboratory Tests

A complete blood count with differential should be done on all patients to detect anemia, chronic blood loss, and hemoconcentration. Elevation or depression of the WBC count with a shift to more immature forms suggests an inflammatory process. This leukocyte response can be masked by dehydration. Platelet counts frequently are elevated by chronic infection and usually are depressed with overwhelming sepsis or disseminated intravascular coagulopathy (DIC).

Electrolyte values are useful in evaluating all patients with a possible acute abdomen. Electrolyte concentrations may be abnormal with GI losses and dehydration. A low serum bicarbonate value suggests metabolic acidosis. Hypokalemia and hypochloremia, with metabolic alkalosis, suggest upper intestinal obstruction. Hyperglycemia can be the first sign of uncontrolled sepsis. Blood urea nitrogen and serum creatinine levels often are determined along with serum electrolyte values and are helpful in determining whether a patient has prerenal azotemia or renal failure.

Urinalysis is useful in differentiating genitourinary causes of abdominal pain. The urinalysis may reveal the presence or absence of WBC, RBC, bacteria, bilirubin, and ketone bodies. Pyuria also may be associated with intra-abdominal inflammatory conditions.

Serum amylase evaluation usually is obtained because elevations are common with acute pancreatitis. Hyperamylasemia, however, also may occur with cholecystitis, intestinal obstruction with strangulation, perforated viscus, ectopic pregnancy, and renal failure.

Serum beta-human chorionic gonadotropin (beta-HCG) levels should be obtained in all women of childbearing age. The complications of pregnancy associated with the acute abdomen include ectopic gestation and concurrent intra-abdominal pathology (e.g., appendicitis, cholecystitis).

Liver function studies (bilirubin, alanine and aspartate transaminases, lactate dehydrogenase, alkaline phosphatase) can be deranged by any hepatobiliary disorder. Marked elevations of the transaminases usually are associated with hepatitis, whereas increases in alkaline phosphatase and bilirubin are more commonly associated with biliary tract obstruction. Milder elevations of these test results are seen with cholecystitis and other nonobstructive causes.

Arterial blood gas values are useful when an acid–base abnormality is suspected. Metabolic acidosis, particularly lactic acidosis, often occurs in the patient with intra-abdominal sepsis. A serum lactate concentration also is helpful in this setting. It not only provides a clue to diagnosis but also helps to evaluate resuscitation efforts. Ongoing lactic acidosis, despite resuscitative efforts, is associated with a poorer prognosis. Diabetic ketoacidosis may also be seen. Glucose metabolism is dysregulated in the setting of sepsis. Unexplained metabolic acidosis is characteristic of intestinal ischemia.

Assessment of coagulation by determination of the prothrombin time (PT or INR) and partial tissue thromboplastin time (PTT) is useful in patients with advanced liver disease or DIC. Correction of coagulopathy should be done before any invasive therapy.

Stool studies for WBCs and *Clostridium difficile* toxin should be obtained in all critically ill patients with unexplained diarrhea. The use of broad-spectrum antibiotics has led to a dramatic increase in pseudomembranous colitis, which, if untreated, can progress to toxic megacolon and colonic perforation.

Radiologic Tests

The single, most valuable film for the evaluation of an abdominal process is an upright chest film. This film allows inspection of abnormalities above the diaphragm (e.g., pneumonia, atelectasis, effusion) and below the diaphragm (e.g., free intraperitoneal air). Abdominal films (supine and upright) are useful in evaluating bowel gas patterns and in assessing ascites, blurring of psoas shadows, stones, vascular calcification, or foreign bodies. Despite the potential for providing significant clinical information, the use of plain abdominal radiographs in assessing the acute abdomen influences management in only 4% of cases; thus, abdominal films should be used selectively.

GI constrast studies are useful when evaluating patients with suspected obstruction or perforation. In the critically ill patient, water-soluble contrast agents should be used when perforation of the GI tract is suspected. These contrast studies have been of great value in ruling out perforated gastric or duodenal ulcers and in differentiating mechanical large bowel obstruction from the so-called pseudo-obstruction. Enteroclysis, on the other hand, better delineates pathologic conditions of the jejunum and ileum.

Intravenous pyelograms are used to rule out ureteral obstruction as the cause of abdominal pain and to define genitourinary involvement in intra-abdominal infections. Genitourinary disease is an important diagnostic possibility in the differential diagnosis of the acute abdomen. In the critically ill patient, genitourinary disease presenting as an acute abdomen is usually associated with pyonephrosis or hydronephrosis from obstruction of the renal pelvis or ureter. Abdominal pain also may be associated with severe cystitis or bladder outlet obstruction.

Ultrasonography has been used increasingly to investigate both acute and chronic abdominal conditions. It can identify gallstones, biliary dilation, pancreatic pseudocysts, hydronephrosis, aortic aneurysms, intraperitoneal fluid collections, and pelvic pathology. It is also useful for directing percutaneous drainage of fluid collections.

CT scans may be of value in patients with acute abdominal pain but generally only when routine radiographic studies are not diagnostic and the patient's condition allows the time to complete the study. An important use of the CT scan in critically ill patients is to search for intra-abdominal abscesses. Additional information about the urinary and GI tracts is obtained when IV and intra-luminal contrast agents are used. Percutaneous drainage of fluid collections can be guided by CT imaging.

Nuclear medicine studies (technetium-99 radionuclide scan) have been used to aid in the diagnosis of acute cholecystitis and postoperative biliary leaks (HIDA scan), to evaluate pulmonary embolism as a cause of abdominal pain (V/Q scan), and to diagnose possible Meckel's diverticulum (Meckel scan). Aside from these specific conditions, nuclear studies are of limited use in the diagnosis of the acute abdomen.

Angiography, although not routinely used in the evaluation of the acute abdomen, is invaluable for assessing the cause of mesenteric ischemia (e.g., embolism, thrombosis, nonthrombotic occlusion).

Miscellaneous Tests

An ECG, although not routinely required when evaluating abdominal pain, is probably warranted in all critically ill patients. Associated diseases in this group of patients, along with the possibility of underlying heart disease, place increased stress on the myocardium. A patient with myocardial infarction may initially present with epigastric pain; thus, it should be ruled out.

Fine-needle aspiration or diagnostic peritoneal lavage (DPL) in patients with a suspected acute abdomen is useful. Alverdy et al. (1) demonstrated a sensitivity of 100% and specificity of 88% in a study of 68 patients who underwent DPL in the evaluation of critically ill patients with a possible acute abdomen. Criteria for a positive tap were >50,000 RBC/mL, >500 WBC/mL, the presence of bile in lavage fluid, and the presence of bacteria by Gram stain. This group concluded that a negative DPL made intra-abdominal disease requiring surgical treatment highly unlikely; however, a positive DPL result may require further diagnostic evaluation. Similar results have been reported with fine-needle aspiration.

The use of preoperative laparoscopy for acute abdominal pain is not new. Use of laparoscopy in diagnostic decision making in the patient with an acute abdomen has been strongly suggested by a number of studies. Most of these studies found laparoscopy particularly useful in differentiating the cause of acute right iliac fossa or pelvic pain. Evidence exists that a selective policy of using laparoscopy in patients with acute abdominal pain, for whom the decision to operate is in doubt, significantly decreases management errors. Laparoscopy and DPL are invasive diagnostic techniques and are not suited to all patients.

DIAGNOSIS AND TREATMENT

The management of the critically ill patient with a suspected acute abdomen depends on the diagnosis that has been formulated at the conclusion of the diagnostic evaluation. The question that must be answered at this point is whether a surgically treatable cause of the abdominal pain is present (Fig. 2). In general, patients fall into one of the following four categories (Fig. 3):

1. Diagnosis known—immediate operation. Patients with peritonitis and patients with an abdominal catastrophe (i.e., ruptured or dissecting aneurysms, mesenteric infarction, strangulated intestinal obstruction, volvulus, GI perforation, testicular or adnexal torsion, ectopic pregnancy, splenic rupture) fall into this

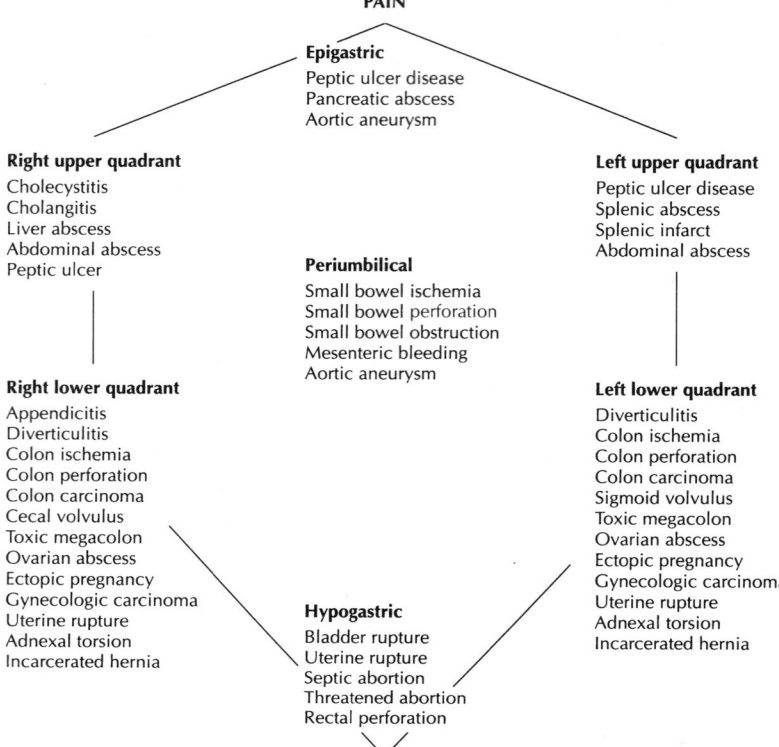

Figure 2 Surgically treatable causes of abdominal pain.

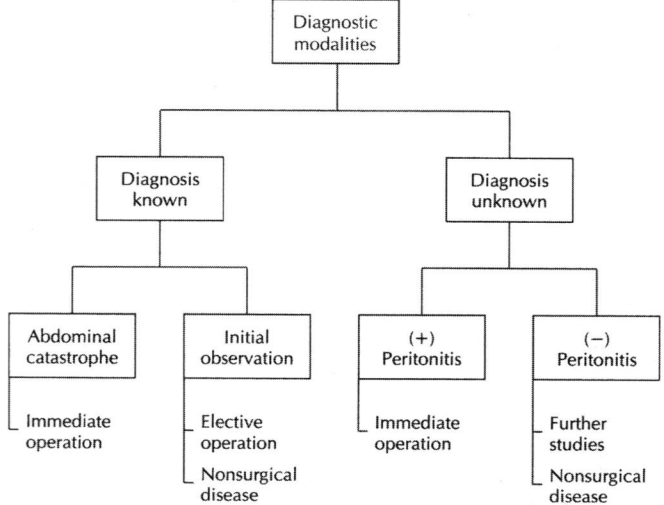

Figure 3 Determination of whether surgery is necessary.

class. After the initial stabilization of the patient, urgent operative intervention is required to prevent excessive morbidity and mortality.
2. Diagnosis known—initial management nonsurgical. Patients with cholecystitis, diverticulitis, small bowel obstruction, and continuous abdominal peritoneal dialysis catheter-related peritonitis fall into this category. These patients undergo initial resuscitation and are followed closely to either resolution of their problem or deterioration requiring urgent intervention. The majority of these patients will require an elective operation at some time after the acute condition resolves.
3. Diagnosis unknown—presence of peritonitis. In this group of patients, a definitive diagnosis has not been made; however, presence of peritonitis mandates an urgent operation. A classic example is the patient who is taken to the operating room to rule out acute appendicitis. In the critically ill patient, once a diagnosis of peritonitis is made, the patient should be prepared for operation, and time should not be wasted on further diagnostic studies.
4. Diagnosis unknown—absence of peritonitis. In this group of patients, the physician is able to observe or perform further diagnostic studies. If peritonitis develops or a diagnosis mandating surgery is made, the patient should be treated expeditiously. A nonsurgical cause of the abdominal pain (Box 1), once identified, should dictate appropriate therapy.

DIAGNOSTIC DIFFICULTIES IN THE CRITICALLY ILL PATIENT

Despite the advances that have been made in medical technology and the improved diagnostic tools currently available to the surgical intensivist, several entities pose particular diagnostic problems.

Acalculous Cholecystitis

Acalculous cholecystitis is an acute inflammation of the gallbladder not caused by gallstones. Its incidence as a cause of cholecystitis is estimated at 4–8%; however, recent evidence suggests that its incidence is rising. It occurs in patients with burns or major trauma and after major operative procedures. Although not a constant association, a low-flow state is often an antecedent event. Other causative factors include biliary stasis and sepsis. The incidence of gangrene and perforation is higher than with acute *calculous* cholecystitis. The diagnosis is difficult to make, and a high degree of suspicion based on clinical history is necessary for successful treatment. Nuclear scans have a higher incidence of false positive studies. The reduced diagnostic value of nuclear scans is due to the inadequate oral intake of these patients. Their bile usually is viscid and stagnant, because the gallbladder does not contract. Ultrasonographic evidence for acalculous disease includes thickening of the gallbladder wall and the presence of pericholecystic fluid. Again, these imaging tests may be helpful, but the diagnosis rests largely on clinical suspicion. Acalculous cholecystitis mandates urgent intervention; accurate and early diagnosis is important (see Chapter 39).

Acute Mesenteric Ischemia

The *bête noire* of acute abdominal conditions is acute mesenteric ischemia. Diagnosing this entity is difficult, not only because laboratory and noninvasive tests tend to be

Box 1 Nonsurgical Causes of Abdominal Pain

Pulmonary	Musculoskeletal
Pneumonia or pleurisy	Rectus sheath hematoma
Pulmonary embolus	Osteomyelitis
Pneumothorax	Arthritis
Cardiac	Neurologic
Angina or myocardial infarct	Multiple sclerosis
Congestive heart failure (on right side)	Tabes dorsalis
Pericarditis or myocarditis	Herpes zoster
Gastrointestinal	Abdominal epilepsy
Mesenteric adenitis	Miscellaneous
Gastritis or enteritis	Porphyria
Inflammatory bowel disease	Familial Mediterranean fever
Hepatitis	Hemochromatosis
Pancreatitis	Diabetic ketoacidosis
Ileus	Addison's disease
Pseudo-obstruction	Thyroid disease
Genitourinary	Hyperparathyroidism
Pyelonephritis	Sickle cell anemia
Renal infarct	Leukemia
Urolithiasis	Pernicious anemia
Cystitis	Measles or mumps
Prostatitis	Malaria
Epididymitis or orchitis	Rocky Mountain spotted fever
Obstetric	Rheumatic fever
Mittelschmerz	Connective tissue disorders
Ovarian cyst	Poisons
Salpingitis	Lead
Endometritis or endometriosis	Mercury
Dysmenorrhea	Arsenic
Threatened abortion	Mushroom
	Spider bite
	Narcotic withdrawal
	Psychosis

inconclusive, but also because the patient's history usually is vague, and a paucity of physical findings is present. Three causes of acute mesenteric ischemia are common: embolism, thrombosis, and nonocclusive mesenteric insufficiency. Emboli to the superior mesenteric artery arise from the heart (90%) or atherosclerotic plaques. The emboli generally lodge in the proximal superior mesenteric artery, a few centimeters from its origin, thus sparing the middle colic artery and the proximal jejunal branches of the superior mesenteric artery. Thrombosis of the superior mesenteric artery usually is associated with generalized atherosclerotic disease and occurs at the origin of the vessel. Thus the gut is ischemic from duodenum to midtransverse colon. Nonocclusive mesenteric insufficiency occurs in a patient with cardiac failure or dysrhythmia, digitalis intoxication, hemoconcentration, and other conditions that lead to a decrease in cardiac output and mesenteric flow.

Because of its insidious onset and the lack of obvious findings, early diagnosis of acute mesenteric ischemia is difficult. The classic findings of pain out of proportion to the examination and a "doughy" abdomen are difficult to identify in the SICU patient. Several observations that lead to early diagnosis are a markedly increased WBC count, unexplained metabolic acidosis, and an elevated serum phosphate level. On the basis of these findings and clinical suspicion, the surgeon should decide whether a visceral angiogram is indicated. Treatment is based on the angiographic findings.

Pancreatitis

Although patients may come to the SICU with a diagnosis of severe pancreatitis, occult acute pancreatitis may complicate any major surgical procedure. A high degree of suspicion is necessary to suggest the diagnosis, as classic historical details and physical signs may be absent in the critically ill patient. Clinical clues include unexplained tachycardia, abdominal tenderness, and pleural effusion on the left side. Laboratory evidence of hyperamylasemia and elevated lipase may be helpful but are nonspecific. In patients with pancreatitis who do not appear to improve with conservative management, the possibility of evolution to necrotizing pancreatitis with abscess formation must be considered. This possibility can be confirmed with dynamic CT and needle aspiration under CT guidance. Unexplained decreases in the hemoglobin concentration in a patient with severe pancreatitis suggest the development of hemorrhagic pancreatitis. Classic diagnostic clues such as Grey Turner's sign (flank ecchymosis in retroperitoneal hemorrhage) are rare.

Immunosuppression

Acute abdominal catastrophes can complicate immunosuppression associated with cancer chemotherapy, transplantation, and AIDS. In every instance the diagnostic possibilities must be placed in the context of the overall disease. For example, certain historical details are important, such as the temporal relationship of the nadir of blood counts with the onset of neutropenic colitis. Although the physical examination is always important, physical signs usually associated with acute abdominal catastrophes are often confusing or absent. Similarly, typical defense responses (e.g., increased WBC count) may also be absent. Disease in critically ill patients who are immunosuppressed may be complicated by a number of unusual entities. Reported infectious complications include acalculous cholecystitis secondary to *Cryptosporidium* or *Candida*, toxic colitis with perforation caused by cytomegalovirus, or GI metastases from Kaposi's sarcoma. Although unusual infectious complications may occur, immunosuppressed patients should be treated bearing in mind the thought that common causes of acute abdominal pain are more frequent.

SUMMARY

- Accurate and timely diagnosis of the acute abdomen can be very difficult in critically ill patients, especially those receiving mechanical ventilation.
- History and physical examination remain of greatest importance. Details of the onset of pain, character of pain, associated nausea and vomiting, location of pain, and radiation of pain are valuable diagnostic clues.

- Nausea that precedes emesis suggests abdominal pathology, whereas emesis without preceding nausea should raise the possibility of increased intracranial pressure.
- The availability of a laboratory or radiologic test does not mandate its use. Findings of the history and physical examination should guide further testing.
- Serum beta-HCG should be measured in women of childbearing age.
- In critically ill patients, CT scans may be useful in identifying and percutaneously draining intra-abdominal abscesses when an abscess is suspected.
- Acalculous cholecystitis, acute mesenteric ischemia, and pancreatitis may complicate the clinical course of SICU patients. These entities are difficult to diagnose and should be part of the differential diagnosis of abdominal pain in the critically ill patient.
- Acute abdominal crises can complicate immunosuppression. Unusual problems in the immunosuppressed patient include acalculous cholecystitis from *Cryptosporidium* or *Candida*, cytomegalovirus colitis with perforation, or GI metastases from Kaposi's sarcoma.

REFERENCE

1. Alverdy JC, Saunders J, Chamberlin WH, et al. Diagnostic peritoneal lavage in intra-abdominal sepsis. Am Surg 1998; 54:456.

SUGGESTED READING

Davies AH, Mastorakou I, Cobb R, et al. Ultrasonography in the acute abdomen. Br J Surg 1991; 78:1178.

Diethelm AG. The acute abdomen. In: Sabiston's Textbook of Surgery, 13th ed. Philadelphia, PA: WB Saunders, 1986.

Gregor P, Prodger JD. Symposium on mesenteric ischemia—abdominal crisis in the intensive care unit. Can J Surg 1988; 31:331.

Hiatt JR. Management of the acute abdomen—a test of judgement. Postgrad Med 1990; 87:38.

Hiatt JR, Calabria RP, Passaro E Jr, et al. The amylase profile—a discriminant in biliary and pancreatic disease. Am J Surg 1987; 154:490.

Hickey MS, Kiernan GJ, Weaver KE. Evaluation of abdominal pain. Emerg Med Clin N Am 1989; 7:437.

Hoffman J, Lanng C, Shokouh-Amiri H. Peritoneal lavage in the diagnosis of acute peritonitis. Am J Surg 1988; 155:359.

Jamieson WG. Symposium on mesenteric ischemia—acute intestinal ischemia. Can J Surg 1988; 31:200.

Papadakis MA, Mangione CM, Lee KK, et al. Treatable abdominal pathologic conditions and unsuspected malignant neoplasmas at autopsy in veterans who received mechanical ventilation. J Am Med Assoc 1991; 265:885.

Paterson-Brown S, Vipond MN. Modern aids to clinical decision-making in the acute abdomen. Br J Surg 1990; 77:13.

Rosemurgy AS, McAllister E, Karl RL. The acute surgical abdomen after cardiac surgery involving extracorporeal circulation. Ann Surg 1988; 207:323.

Schroeder T, Christoffersen JK, Andersen J, et al. Ischemic colitis complicating reconstruction of the abdominal aorta. Surg Gynecol Obstet 1985; 160:299.

Silen W. Cope's Early Diagnosis of the Acute Abdomen, 18th ed. New York, NY: Oxford University Press, 1991.

Stower MJ, Amar SS, Mikulin T, et al. Evaluation of the plain abdominal X-ray in the acute abdomen. J R Soc Med 1985; 78:630.

Vipond MN, Paterson-Brown S, Tyrrell MR, et al. Evaluation of the catheter aspiration cytology of the peritoneum as an adjunct to decision making in the acute abdomen. Br J Surg 1990; 77:86.

Vogt DP. The acute abdomen in the geriatric patient. Cleve Clin J Med 1990; 57:125.

Wilson SE, Robinson G, Williams RA, et al. Acquired immune deficiency syndrome (AIDS): indications for abdominal surgery, pathology, and outcome. Ann Surg 1989; 210:428.

Young GP. Abdominal catastrophes. Emerg Med Clin N Am 1989; 7:699.

41

A Pathophysiologic Approach to Fulminant Hepatic Failure in the Intensive Care Unit

Kambiz Kosari and Timothy D. Sielaff
University of Minnesota, Minneapolis, Minnesota, USA

INTRODUCTION

Decompensation of liver function is potentially life threatening: its presentation in the intensive care unit is an urgent management problem. Acute liver failure occurs in two general settings. First, and more commonly, a patient with preexisting chronic liver disease or cirrhosis develops an acute decompensation called acute-on-chronic liver failure (ACLF). Most such patients have alcoholic or viral hepatitis cirrhosis; one of several comorbid factors change the patient from the compensated to the decompensated state.

Second, a smaller number of patients with no prior history of liver problems develop fulminant hepatic failure (FHF). The incidence of FHF is about 2000 cases per year in the US (1). This relatively rare group of patients presents the clinician with unique challenges. These patients demonstrate high mortality and morbidity, complex pathophysiologic features of their disease process, and potential for tremendous improvement in outcome with such interventions as orthotopic liver transplants, supportive intensive care, and, in the near future, bioartificial liver treatment. Identification of the cause and type of liver failure, prompt and proper treatment, adequate support of failed vital processes, and realistic evaluation of the potential role of liver transplant is critical to patient survival.

This chapter reviews the diagnosis and management principles of ACLF and FHF, with attention to recent advances in liver transplantation and artificial liver support.

DEFINITIONS

Acute-on-Chronic Liver Failure (ACLF)

As the name implies, ACLF is the development of encephalopathy from the sudden decompensation of liver function in the setting of chronic liver disease. In the US, ACLF most commonly occurs in patients with chronic alcoholic or viral cirrhosis. They can develop ACLF within days to weeks. Chronic liver disease may make the exact time of the onset of ACLF difficult to determine. These patients typically develop ACLF after an inciting event, such as infection or gastrointestinal bleeding. The stress of illness exceeds the chronically diseased liver's ability to compensate. Since these patients may not be identified as having cirrhosis, all patients with encephalopathy must be evaluated for occult cirrhosis. If present, it can have a significant impact on the appropriateness of a liver transplant.

Fulminant Hepatic Failure (FHF)

FHF is defined as progression to hepatic encephalopathy and severe hepatic dysfunction, without prior history of liver disease, within 8 weeks after the onset of jaundice (2). Development of the same pattern of illness more than 8 weeks after the onset of hepatic insufficiency is referred to as subfulminant hepatic failure. Usually, FHF patients demonstrate hepatic encephalopathy. They often have severe coagulopathy, elevated serum bilirubin concentrations, and other metabolic abnormalities. Several time-dependent patterns of acute liver failure have been described (Table 1). O'Grady et al. (5), for example, divided acute liver failure into *hyperacute* (hepatic encephalopathy within 7 days), *acute* (between 8–28 days), or *subacute* (between 29 days and 12 weeks). Patients with hyperacute liver failure (seen more with hepatitis A and B than with non-A/non-B hepatitis) have the best prognosis (5). Consensus has not been reached regarding classification schemes (4–6).

Even though a standard definition of acute liver failure has not been adopted, accurate staging of liver failure is important. Most experts agree that the keys to optimizing treatment are quick identification of patients in FHF, and then prompt transfer to a center that has both an intensive care unit and access to liver transplant services. In general, FHF patients have a worse prognosis than chronic liver failure patients. However, FHF patients, unlike most chronic liver failure patients, do have potentially reversible conditions; if they survive, they can usually recover completely. Thus, rapid identification and prompt transfer of these patients to appropriate facilities can significantly affect outcome. Accurate staging of acute liver failure will help investigators to standardize and interpret data among centers, thereby facilitating rigorous studies.

Hepatic Encephalopathy

One of the common, usually devastating, complications of acute liver failure is hepatic encephalopathy. Sherlock and Dooley (2) described a hepatic encephalopathy as "a reversible neuropsychiatric state that complicates liver disease." This definition emphasizes the *psychiatric* and the *neurologic* components of hepatic encephalopathy. Psychiatric abnormalities include disturbed consciousness, personality changes, intellectual deterioration, and speech irregularities. Neurologic manifestations include asterixis, exaggerated deep tendon reflexes, increased muscle tone, sustained ankle clonus, pre-coma rigidity, flaccidity and

Table 1 Time-Dependent Definitions of Acute Liver Failure

Bernuau (3)	Fulminant or subfulminant (jaundice to encephalopathy; cutoff time, 2 weeks)
Gimson (4)	Fulminant or late onset (cutoff time, 8 weeks)
O'Grady (5)	Hyperacute (0–7 days), acute (8–28 days), subacute (29 days to 12 weeks)

Table 2 Grades of Hepatic Encephalopathy

I	Slowness of thought, asterixis, and altered mood or behavior
II	Drowsiness, inappropriate behavior, and confusion
III	Somnolence to semistupor, some response to stimuli, obedience of simple commands, and marked confusion
IV	Coma and no or minimal response to painful stimuli

Source: From Ref. (5).

areflexia (during coma), and visual disturbances such as reversible cortical blindness (7). Hepatic encephalopathy is subdivided into four grades (Table 2), starting with confusion and progressing to drowsiness, stupor, and finally coma (8). Once coma occurs, both FHF and subfulminant hepatic failure are associated with a >80% mortality rate (9).

CAUSES

Acute-on-Chronic Liver Failure

ACLF patients usually have an inciting event that changes the patient from the compensated to the decompensated state. Major causes include infection (e.g., spontaneous bacterial peritonitis, urinary tract infection, pneumonia), gastrointestinal bleeding, toxin exposure (e.g., EtOH), dietary indiscretion, electrolyte abnormalities, hypovolemia, portal vein thrombosis, and malignancy. The reduced hepatocyte functional volume and abnormal hepatic hemodynamics render the diseased liver unable to compensate for even minor insults.

Fulminant Hepatic Failure

Except for the UK where acetaminophen toxicity ranks number one, the most common cause of FHF worldwide (including in the US) is viral hepatitis (2,10,11). Table 3 lists possible causes. In a recent study by Shakil et al. (11) of 177 patients treated for acute liver failure during a 13-year period at the University of Pittsburgh, 31% had viral hepatitis. The next two most common causes were acetaminophen toxicity (19%) and idiosyncratic drug reactions (12%). Of interest, almost 30% of the patients had an indeterminate cause. A similar study in the UK (226 FHF patients, 1973–1985) found acetaminophen to be the causative agent more than 60% of the time. Viral hepatitis ranked second (26%), compared to drug-induced (other than acetaminophen) causes (7%) (10) (Table 4).

Of the diagnosed viral causes of FHF, hepatitis A and B rank the highest. Of the nearly 30% of patients in FHF with an undetermined cause, many have an illness whose course mimics that of viral hepatitis even though they never test positive for a specific hepatitis virus (8). Regarding these so-called non-A and non-B FHF patients, controversy exists as to the role of hepatitis C virus (HCV). Some series from Japan and Taiwan report higher HCV rates (43–52%) when compared with the US or the UK (0–25%) (2,12). Sergi et al. (12) amplified HCV and hepatitis G virus (HGV) RNA from the explanted livers of 26 consecutive patients undergoing orthotopic liver transplants for FHF. Their data showed a 25% correlation between HCV and FHF with an unknown cause ($n = 12$), but no specific correlation between HGV and the cause of FHF was observed. Similarly, an Australian group concluded that HGV infection is unlikely to be the primary cause of FHF (13).

Table 3 Possible Causes of Fulminant Hepatic Failure

Infective	Hepatitis virus A, B, C, D, E, ?G
	Herpes simplex
	Epstein–Barr virus
	Cytomegalovirus
	Adenovirus
	Varicella
	Parvovirus B19
Drug reactions and toxins	Acetaminophen (paracetamol) overdose
	Halothane
	Isoniazid
	Rifampin
	Antidepressants
	Nonsteroidal anti-inflammatory drugs
	Valproic acid
	Mushroom poisoning
	Herbal remedies
	Trimethoprim/sulfamethoxazole
	Chemotherapy agents
	Designer drugs (e.g., Ecstasy)
	Dilantin
	Hydroxycholoroquine
	Ketoconazole
	Lepiota helveola poisoning
	Nicotinic acid
	Octreotide
	Sulfasalazine
	Tetracycline
	Tricyclics
	Vicodin
	Ampicillin/clavulanate
	Antabuse
	Ciprofloxacin
	Dipyridium
	Erythromycin
	Fialuridine
	Flutamide
	Gold
	Lovastatin
	Nitrofurantoin
	Phenytoin
Ischemic	Ischemic hepatitis
	Surgical "shock"
	Acute Budd–Chiari syndrome
Metabolic	Wilson's disease
	Fatty liver of pregnancy
	Reye's syndrome
Miscellaneous (rare)	Massive malignant infiltration (leukemia and lymphoma)
	Severe bacterial infection
	Heat stroke
	Sea anemone stings

Table 4 Comparison of Causes of Fulminant Hepatic Failure

US	UK
Viral hepatitis (31%)	Acetaminophen (63%)
Acetaminophen toxicity (19%)	Non-A and non-B hepatitis (20%)
Idiosyncratic drug reactions (12%)	Hepatitis A (3%)
Miscellaneous causes (11%)	Hepatitis B (3%)
Indeterminate (28%)	Drug-induced (other than acetaminophen) (7%)
	Miscellaneous (5%)

PATHOPHYSIOLOGIC FEATURES

Although ACLF and FHF differ from one another according to the presence or absence of chronic liver injury, the pathophysiologic features behind most of the clinical manifestations of either disease are similar. Both diseases arise from necrosis of parenchymal and nonparenchymal liver cells.

Tissue Hypoxia

Although not completely understood, loss of liver function and then multiorgan failure are consequences of hepatic necrosis. A "vicious cycle of events" (14) follows massive destruction of hepatocytes. Failure of clearance of toxins, along with increased risk of infection, can lead to endotoxemia and to activation of macrophages. The result is release of cytokines, such as tumor necrosis factor (TNF) and interleukins (IL-1 and IL-6), into the systemic circulation. The ensuing clinical changes resemble septic shock. Patients typically exhibit elevated cardiac output, decreased peripheral vascular resistance, and arterial hypotension. The culmination of these events is tissue hypoxia at a cellular level in extrahepatic organ systems, and in the liver itself. The damaged hepatocytes and their accompanying nonparenchymal cells, including Kupfer cells and Pit cells (highly mobile natural killer lymphocytes attached to the sinusoidal surface of the endothelium), play a central role.

Kupffer cells, derived from blood monocytes, are highly mobile macrophages that live inside the luminal side of the sinusoid. They are the body's largest group of macrophages in direct contact with the blood and serve as a filter for gut-derived bacteria and endotoxins, as well as for tumor cells, yeast, viruses, parasites, old cells, and other foreign particles (15). Once activated by infection, trauma, or injury, Kupfer cells secrete a series of factors such as TNF, IL-1, and IL-6. The result is circulatory changes similar to those seen in septic shock. Secretion of these cytokines reduces the systemic vascular resistance causing tissue hypoxia at a cellular level.

Mechanical Obstruction

One cause of tissue hypoxia can be explained on a *mechanical* basis. Serum concentration of cytokines and free radicals are elevated in FHF patients (16,17). This elevation is thought to originate both from activated macrophages in response to massive hepatic damage and from decreased clearance of the cytokines and free radicals by the dysfunctional Kupfer cells. Activation of endothelial cells via TNF, IL-1, and IL-6 can contribute to activation and aggregation of platelets and to enhanced leukocyte adhesion. In turn, microthrombi can be produced and propagated within small vessels. The resulting shunt diverts blood away from respiring tissue and into normally present, but functionally inactive and nutritionally poor, arteriovenous shunts. Release of cytokines, unmetabolized toxins, or other agents (see later) also mediates dysregulation of the vasogenic tone and cause systemic hypotension. Furthermore, most patients with FHF suffer loss of appetite, nausea, and vomiting before they seek medical care. The resulting dehydration further exacerbates systemic hypotension.

Role of Nitric Oxide

Nitric oxide (NO) is likely a second cause of tissue hypoxia. The effects of NO are potent but short lived and local. Synthesized in the endothelial cells from L-arginine via NO synthase, NO activates guanylate cyclase and causes vasodilatation. Cytokines, bacterial endotoxins, or both can induce NO synthase. Serum concentrations of the end products (such as citrulline, nitrite, and nitrate) of NO metabolism are elevated in FHF patients (18). This apparent elevation in NO production may contribute to the systemic vasodilation seen in FHF patients. The L-arginine analog NG-monomethyl-L-arginine (L-NMMA) inhibits NO synthase-mediated conversion of L-arginine to NO. In rats with portal hypertension, this analog has reduced peripheral vasodilatation and systemic capillary hypotension (19). Yet, when such analogs are administered to human FHF patients, oxygen consumption decreases, a finding that suggests detrimental changes at a microcirculatory level (20).

A plausible explanation for the findings in humans hypothesizes that, despite its increased production in FHF patients, NO may fail to be excreted in sufficient amounts or may fail to exert its effects locally. The presence of microthrombi and damaged endothelial cells in the microcirculation is thought to inhibit excretion and activity of NO. Supporting evidence for this hypothesis comes from a clinical trial in which improved kidney function and reduced hepatic encephalopathy followed the administration of intravenous N-acetylcysteine (NAC) in acetaminophen-induced hepatic failure patients (21). The effects of NAC were evident after acetaminophen metabolites ceased to circulate. Thus, NAC is thought to function as more than just an antidote. In another clinical study, NAC increased serum concentrations of cyclic *guanosine* 3,5-monophosphate, (cGMP), the second messenger in vascular smooth-muscle relaxation, in FHF patients (20). As NO also functions through stimulation of soluble guanylate cyclase to form cGMP (22), the effects of NAC may lead to improved production or activation of NO within the local microvasculature, leading to enhanced blood flow.

Pathologic Supply Dependency

Aside from mechanical obstruction and possible derangements in NO function, FHF patients also demonstrate what has been termed "pathologic supply dependency" for oxygen. Bihari et al. (6) in 1986 observed that infusion of epoprostenol, a microcirculatory vasodilator with no inotropic properties, reduced peripheral vascular resistance, increased oxygen delivery, and significantly increased oxygen consumption. Oxygen delivery in non-FHF patients is around 525–675 mL/min per m^2 (14). Once this delivery drops below the critical level of 330 mL/min per m^2, tissue oxygen consumption will drop, and tissue hypoxia, anaerobic metabolism, and lactate accumulation will ensue (Fig. 1). With delivery between 330 and 525 mL/min per m^2, tissue hypoxia does not usually occur, because the amount of oxygen extraction is increased. FHF patients have

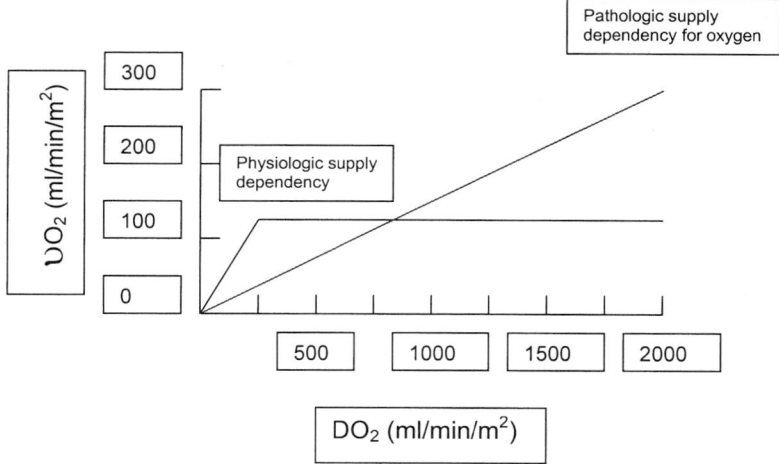

Figure 1 Pathologic supply dependency for oxygen.

abnormal capacity for oxygen extraction and thus become "pathologically dependent on the supply" of oxygen. As oxygen delivery is increased, oxygen consumption is increased. In Bihari's observation, the patients who did not survive had lower baseline oxygen consumption as well as increased oxygen consumption in response to epoprostenol infusion. This apparent "oxygen debt" can worsen with inappropriate use of inotropes. This idea suggests instropes should be used in conjunction with vasodilator agents. The oxygen consumption and arterovenous oxygen content difference must be frequently monitored.

Hepatic Encephalopathy

Hepatic encephalopathy in the presence of liver failure is thought to result from swelling of astrocytes and from impaired expression of glutamate transporter GLT-1. These events increase extracellular glutamate concentration (23). Swelling of astrocytes and of astrocytic end-feet was shown in clinical electron microscopic studies of brain tissue in FHF patients. This swelling is consistent with cytotoxic (as opposed to vasogenic) causes of edema. Ammonia and manganese have been implicated in the development of hepatic encephalopathy. Evidence suggests that the blood–brain barrier becomes increasingly permeable to ammonia in liver failure. Ammonia alters postsynaptic inhibition in the cerebral cortex by blocking chloride extrusion from postsynaptic neurons. It can also decrease excitatory synaptic transmission via a direct, as yet unknown, postsynaptic action. Ammonia, or one of its metabolites, causes swelling of cerebral cortical astrocytes in primates, possibly through the ensuing increase in glutamine synthesis, which is used to remove ammonia from astrocytes.

Ammonia has also been implicated in the impairment of cerebral energy consumption. Note that impaired brain energy metabolism is a late phenomenon. It is thought to be due mainly to decreased neuronal activity and not to primary energy failure.

The serum concentration of manganese also is elevated in FHF patients. Increased manganese had been implicated in the development of Alzheimer's type II astrocytosis, which is considered as a neuropathologic hallmark of hepatic encephalopathy.

However, similar changes are also seen in cirrhotic patients who do not have hepatic encephalopathy. Thus, the role of manganese needs further delineation.

In addition to astrocyte swelling and to the detrimental effects of increased ammonia and manganese, impairments of multiple neurotransmitter systems have been linked to hepatic encephalopathy. The amount of glutamate, a major excitatory neurotransmitter in the central nervous system, is elevated in patients with hepatic encephalopathy, probably as a consequence of decreased uptake by astrocytes and the loss of postsynaptic receptor sites. Recent experimental studies have demonstrated the loss of gene expression of GLT-1 protein in the cerebral cortex of animals in acute hepatic failure (23). Another experimental study demonstrated decreased densities of postsynaptic glutamate receptors, including *N*-methyl-D-aspartate (NMDA) receptors [formerly known as the amino-3-hydroxy-5-methyl-4-isoxazole propionic acid (or AMPA)/kinase subtype], and of the metabo-tropic glutamate receptors. The decreased densities were demonstrated in the brains of rabbits with galactosamine-induced FHF (24).

Concentrations of both serotonin (5HT), a neurotransmitter implicated in many neuropsychiatric symptoms of early portosystemic encephalopathy, and of its metabolite, 5-hydroxyindoleacetic acid (5HIAA), were elevated in the cerebrospinal fluid (CSF) and brain tissue of experimental animals and of human patients with chronic liver disease who manifest with hepatic encephalopathy. Concentrations of the 5HT-metabolizing enzyme monoamine oxidase (MAO-A) were also elevated, a finding that suggests increased oxidation, rather than increased turnover, as a possible cause of the increased 5HIAA concentrations in hepatic encephalopathy. Abnormal serotonin receptor binding has been implicated in the development of hepatic encephalopathy; however, further studies are needed to delineate the exact role of 5HT.

Catecholamines, such as dopamine and norepinephrine, have been studied as possible agents in hepatic encephalopathy. Because of some similarities between the symptoms and signs of Parkinson's disease (e.g., rigidity and tremor) and porto-systemic encephalopathy, derangements in dopamine neurotransmission have been suggested as possible contributors to the symptoms of hepatic encephalopathy. Concentrations of dopamine metabolites, such as homovanillic acid (HVA), were elevated in the autopsied brain tissue of cirrhotic patients who died in hepatic coma (25). In the brain tissue of similar patients, postsynaptic dopamine D_2 binding sites were decreased in the globus pallidus (26). Similar derangements in norepinephrine concentrations have been described in rats with FHF.

Recently, administration of the benzodiazepine receptor antagonist flumazenil has demonstrated neurologic improvement in a subset of patients with grade IV hepatic encephalopathy (27). Endogenous benzodiazepines may potentiate the effect of GABA; flumazenil is thought to block this effect (23). However, investigation of the inhibitory neurotransmission system involving GABA has revealed no abnormalities in the brain tissue of humans with portosystemic encephalopathy. Futhermore, the effects of flumazenil are short lived and incomplete.

Another benzodiazepine-related system, the peripheral-type benzodiazepine receptor (PTBR), was once thought to be strictly a peripheral nervous system receptor. It has recently been identified on the outer mitochondrial membrane of astrocytes. Increased concentrations of PTBR in the brains of both experimental animals and human patients who died of hepatic encephalopathy have been partially linked to exposure to ammonia or manganese. Increased PTBR densities on the outer membrane of the mitochondria of astrocytes may contribute to hepatic encephalopathy through oxidative metabolism and possibly through production of neurosteroids. Depending on their type, neurosteroids may have inhibitory (pregnenolone sulfate and dehydroepiandrosterone sulfate) or stimulatory (3α-hydroxy-5α-pregnane-20-one and 3α-21-dihydroxy-5α-pregnane-20-one) effects on the GABA-ergic system (23). Some evidence suggests that neurosteroids may modulate the ammonia-induced swelling seen in astrocytes (28).

MANAGEMENT

Because of the differences in treatment strategies between the two disease processes, the first important decision is distinguishing patients with FHF from those with ACLF. ACLF patients need to have the cause of their acute failure identified and then treated; they also need support and treatment for their chronic liver dysfunction. Most ACLF patients can be cared for locally unless they are transplant candidates. FHF patients require quick identification and transfer to specialized liver centers with advanced intensive care unit and liver transplant facilities.

Before Transfer to a Liver Center

FHF or subfulminant hepatic failure patients can exhibit a variety of nonspecific symptoms and signs, including abdominal pain, nausea, vomiting, and dehydration. Some may have jaundice. Hepatic encephalopathy may or may not be present; consequently, a careful neurologic assessment is required. Of prognostic importance is the interval between the onset of the symptoms of jaundice and hepatic encephalopathy (see later). ACLF patients can have similar symptoms and signs, but they tend to have the additional stigmata of chronic liver disease such as ascites, weight loss, jaundice, easy bruisability, muscle wasting, and weakness.

A complete history and physical examination, with an emphasis on findings related to the liver and with a high index of suspicion for hepatic encephalopathy, can significantly accelerate recognition and transfer of acute liver failure patients to appropriate facilities. The history should focus on prior episodes of liver problems, albeit often absent in FHF patients, on travel to areas where viral hepatitis is endemic, and on the presence of any high-risk behaviors, such as alcohol or drug use or abuse, and unsafe sexual practices. ACLF patients generally have a known history of liver disease. For some ACLF patients, acute failure is the first sign of their chronic disease. These patients need a thorough evaluation to identify the nature of their liver dysfunction. The following causes should be considered in ACLF patients who do not already have a diagnosis for the cause of their cirrhosis: alcoholic or viral hepatitis; biliary disease (e.g., chronic gallstone disease or pancreatitis leading to large bile duct obstruction, primary biliary cirrhosis); venous obstruction (e.g., portal vein thrombosis); idiopathic hemochromatosis; hereditary diseases (e.g., Wilson's disease, α_1-antitrypsin deficiency, cystic fibrosis); and other toxins or drugs.

Physical examination can further distinguish FHF from ACLF patients. As opposed to FHF patients who are mostly otherwise healthy, ACLF patients can have signs of chronic liver disease (e.g., testicular atrophy, gynecomastia, palmar erythema, asterixis), needle track marks in their extremities, pigmented skin, and clubbing of fingernails. Hepatosplenomegaly, periumbilical venous engorgement (caput medusa), hemorrhoids, and ascites indicate the presence of portal hypertension, which is rare in FHF patients, except for those suffering from acute Budd–Chiari syndrome. Protein synthesis problems may produce leg edema or anasarca (i.e., total body edema) and bruising. Both FHF and ACLF patients have focal or generalized neurologic deficits.

Adjunctive studies should include a complete blood count and chemistry panel to look for blood dyscrasias, electrolyte abnormalities, hypoglycemia, and renal insufficiency. Liver function should be assessed by measuring the international normalized ratio (INR), albumin concentrations, bilirubin concentrations, liver injury markers (e.g., alanine transferase levels), and canalicular markers (e.g., alkaline phosphatase levels). Serologic markers for viral hepatitis and toxicologic studies to screen for such drugs as acetaminophen can be of value. Reduced serum α_1-antitrypsin concentrations support the diagnosis of α_1-antitrypsin deficiency. Patients with Wilson's disease may have decreased serum ceruloplasmin and increased urinary copper concentration. Elevated serum iron saturation and serum ferritin concentration support the diagnosis of hemochromatosis. Appropriate tumor markers such as α-fetoprotein or carcinoembryonic antigen should be obtained. FHF patients usually exhibit elevated liver injury markers and electrolyte abnormalities. In contrast, ACLF patients usually have a host of other hepatic and hematologic derangements. Initially, FHF patients tend to have normal serum albumin levels. When clinically indicated, arterial blood gas analysis and blood lactate concentration can reveal metabolic acidosis. Microbiologic studies should be obtained because the incidence of infection is high with FHF (29). Imaging modalities, such as helical computed tomography and right upper quadrant abdominal Doppler ultrasound, may be of benefit in the pretransplant evaluation of patients. These studies help to assess the anatomy as well as the flow pattern within the portal triad. Liver biopsies should be avoided unless the suspected cause is Wilson's disease (in which case copper deposition should be checked), α_1-antitrypsin deficiency (a PAS stain will yield definitive results), lymphoproliferative disease (such as lymphoma), or autoimmune hepatitis. If bleeding is a concern, the biopsy should be done through a transjugular route.

Treatment of ACLF Patients

As an inciting event converts liver function in ACLF patients from the compensated cirrhotic state to the decompensated state, diligent efforts should be made to find and eliminate the source. Infection must be ruled out. Appropriate use of antimicrobials with broad coverage is essential for treating spontaneous bacterial peritonitis and pneumonia. Hepatic and abdominal abscesses should be drained. Variceal bleeding should be treated with endoscopic ablation. Electrolyte abnormalities require careful correction. Ascites should be treated with large-volume paracentesis, the use of trasjugular intrahepatic shunts (TIPS), or surgical shunts.

Full coverage of the therapeutic interventions needed in the face of chronic liver disease is beyond the scope of this chapter. Because many of the acute-care aspects of treating ACLF patients are similar to the care of FHF patients, the rest of this chapter will focus on FHF patients.

Issues Regarding Patient Transfer

As FHF has a high mortality rate (>80%), most investigators agree that once the signs and symptoms of acute liver failure are recognized, the patient must be transferred to a liver center. Liver transplantation, with survival rates of 60–80%, is the only treatment that significantly alters mortality (Table 5) (2). Shakil et al. (11) reported that, of

Table 5 Survival Rates After Liver Transplants

Transplant city	Main author(s)	Date	Number of patients	Survival (%)
Birmingham, UK	Vickers et al.	1988	16	56
Chicago	Edmond et al.	1989	19	58
London/Cambridge	Williams and O'Grady	1990	56	58
Paris	Devictor et al.	1992	19	68
San Francisco	Ascher et al.	1993	35	92
Madrid	Moreno Gonzalez et al.	1994	35	47
Pittsburgh	Dodson et al.	1994	115	60
Paris	Bismuth et al.	1995	116	68
US (12 liver transplant centers)	Schiodt et al.	1999	121	76
Pittsburgh	Shakil et al.	2000	87	55

Source: From Ref. (2).

177 patients treated at the University of Pittsburgh for FHF, 96% were referred from outside hospitals. The median interval between the onset of jaundice and patients' arrival at a liver intensive care unit was 4 days. The median waiting time for a liver transplant was 3 days. Of the patients who did not undergo a liver transplant, 72% died within 48 h after admission. Of those who died, 80% had been designated to receive a liver transplant but never did. Thus, many more lives could be saved if FHF patients could be more quickly diagnosed and transferred to appropriate centers.

Deciding who needs to be transferred to a liver center can be difficult. Different criteria have been proposed. The most widely quoted criteria are those of the King's College Hospital (KCH) in London (30) where investigators analyzed various prognostic factors in 588 medically treated patients (1973–1985) (Table 6). Patients who had a poor outcome were divided into two major groups categorized by the cause of their acute liver failure. For patients with acetaminophen-induced acute liver failure, poor outcome was associated with a blood pH <7.30, independent of degree of encephalopathy and with a prothrombin time (PT) >100 s (corresponding to an INR >6.5), a serum creatinine (Cr) >300 μmol/L (>3.4 μg/dL), and grade III or IV hepatic encephalopathy. For all other causes of FHF, poor outcome was associated with the following: PT >100 s (INR >6.5), independent of the degree of encephalopathy, or any three of (i) age <10 or >40 years, (ii) jaundice >7 days before the onset of encephalopathy, (iii) PT >50 s (INR >3.5), and (iv) serum billirubin >300 μmol/L (>17.5 mg/dL) (11,30).

Liver Center Care

The general approach to patients with altered mental status after onset of jaundice and elevated PT is outlined in Fig. 2 (31). The complex pathophysiologic causes of FHF demand frequent monitoring to detect rapid changes in encephalopathy, sepsis, and multiorgan failure. Furthermore, such patients often require respiratory, hemodynamic, and kidney support. FHF patients should be monitored in an ICU, especially when their hepatic encephalopathy is rapidly worsening or when grade II status is progressing. The ICU allows these severely sick patients to receive appropriate *cause-specific treatment* and proper care for the *complications* that frequently accompany acute liver failure.

Table 6 Criteria for Selection of Patients Most Likely to Benefit from Liver Transplants

King's College Hospital of London
1. Acetaminophen toxicity
   a. pH <7.3 regardless of grade of encephalopathy or
   b. PT[a] >100 s (INR[b] > 6.5) and creatinine >300 μmol/L (>3.4 mg/dL) in patients with grade III or IV encephalopathy
2. Viral hepatitis, drug reaction (non-acetaminophen causes)
   a. PT >100 s (INR > 6.5), regardless of the grade of encephalopathy
      or
   b. Any three of the following, regardless of the grade of encephalopathy:
      1. Age <10 or >40 years
      2. Duration of jaundice before the onset of encephalopathy >7 days
      3. Etiology is non-A/non-B hepatitis, halothane hepatitis, or idiosyncratic drug reaction
      4. PT >50 s (INR >3.5)
      5. Serum bilirubin >300 μmol/L (>17.5 mg/dL)

Beaujon Hospital in France
1. Low factor V
   a. <20% if age <30 years
   b. <30% if age >30 years

Source: Adapted from Ref. (11).
[a]PT, Prothrombin time.
[b]INR, International normalized ratio.

Cause-Specific Treatment

Although many of the agents that cause acute liver failure have no specific treatment, some toxins may have dose-dependent effects reduced by immediate intervention (32). For this reason, a working knowledge of the following "antidotes" is required. The beneficial effects of NAC in the setting of acetaminophen-induced hepatic failure have been described earlier (21). In addition, NAC administration might improve hepatic failure resulting from ingestion of hydrocarbons, such as trichloroethylene and carbon tetrachloride (33,34). In the case of mushroom poisoning (*Amanita phalloides*), early intravenous administration of penicillin and silibilin might be helpful (35). Steroid use in the setting of FHF from autoimmune hepatitis is advocated by some investigators but remains controversial (36). Immediate delivery of the baby after a pregnant woman is diagnosed with an acute fatty liver is beneficial (37). Thrombolytic therapy for acute Budd–Chiari syndrome may be useful (38). Better outcomes are achieved with early diagnosis and early treatment.

Management of Complications

Systemic Circulation: Principles of resuscitation are discussed in Chapter 2 where strategies to avoid tissue hypoxia receive further examination. Hypotension should be avoided. Low mean arterial pressure (MAP) adversely affects cerebral perfusion pressure (CPP). Inadequate CPP may worsen hepatic encephalopathy. A clinical target is a MAP ≥60 mm Hg. Use of vasoconstrictive agents may reduce splanchnic blood flow. Restoration of preload before administering vasoconstrictive agents may increase blood pressure while maintaining liver perfusion.

Despite their theoretical advantages, supported by some anecdotal data, prostaglandins (e.g., prostaglandin E) have not been found to have significant beneficial effects in acute hepatic failure patients (39). Further trials are needed to substantiate the observed

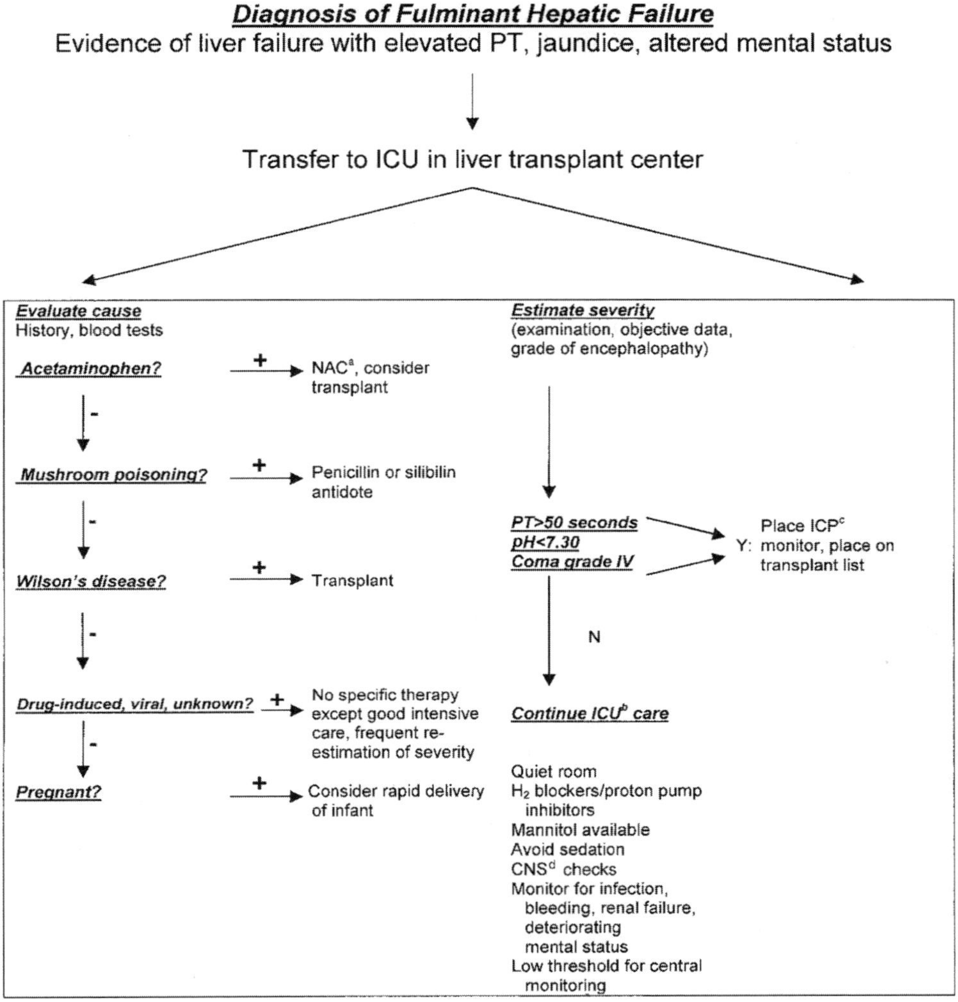

Diagnosis of Fulminant Hepatic Failure
Evidence of liver failure with elevated PT, jaundice, altered mental status

↓

Transfer to ICU in liver transplant center

Evaluate cause
History, blood tests

Acetaminophen? — + → NAC[a], consider transplant
| −
↓
Mushroom poisoning? — + → Penicillin or silibilin antidote
| −
↓
Wilson's disease? — + → Transplant
| −
↓
Drug-induced, viral, unknown? — + → No specific therapy except good intensive care, frequent re-estimation of severity
| −
↓
Pregnant? — + → Consider rapid delivery of infant

Estimate severity
(examination, objective data, grade of encephalopathy)

↓

PT>50 seconds
pH<7.30
Coma grade IV
→ Place ICP[c]
Y: monitor, place on transplant list

↓ N

Continue ICU[b] care

Quiet room
H₂ blockers/proton pump inhibitors
Mannitol available
Avoid sedation
CNS[d] checks
Monitor for infection, bleeding, renal failure, deteriorating mental status
Low threshold for central monitoring

Figure 2 Algorithm for the initial approach to patients in acute liver failure (31). [a]N-acetylcysteine, [b]intensive care unit, [c]intracranial pressure, [d]central nervous system.

hemodynamic improvement that is anecdotally seen in patients with NAC-treated, non-acetaminophen-induced liver failure. Agents, such as dopexamine (not available in the US), have shown some promise in improving support of acute liver failure patients by increasing splanchnic and kidney blood flow and exerting anti-inflammatory effects (40). The use of dopexamine is associated with protection of the kidney.

Kidney Failure: More than half of the patients with acute liver failure have concomitant kidney dysfunction. Altered kidney function ranges from prerenal azotemia and acute tubular necrosis secondary to drug toxicity, to the ominous hepatorenal syndrome seen mostly in association with chronic hepatic failure. A useful classification divides patients into those with oliguria and those with anuria and signs of metabolic imbalance.

For the oliguric patients, the most important intervention is to maintain adequate preload by proper, timely administration of intravenous fluid. Use of such agents as "low-dose" dopamine, loop diuretics, and terlipresin (not available in the US) continues to be controversial (41–43). Oliguric patients who do not respond to adequate maintenance of preload usually develop anuria or metabolic derangements and fluid overload. They frequently require dialysis. Some authors recommend continuous venovenous hemofiltration or high-volume exchange plasmapheresis (instead of conventional hemodialysis). These procedures have the advantages of relatively smaller volume shifts, less electrolyte alteration, and possibly less aggravation of cerebral edema (44).

Respiratory Failure: For the patient with acute liver failure, respiratory failure is often coupled with worsening encephalopathy. Patients with grade I or II encephalopathy generally do not require mechanical ventilatory support. Most FHF patients with grade III or IV hepatic encephalopathy will need endotracheal intubation and mechanical ventilation. To add to the complexity of the problem, up to 30% of such patients will eventually develop adult respiratory distress syndrome (ARDS). The concern about worsening intracranial pressure with the use of positive end-expiratory pressure is controversial (45,46).

Hepatic Encephalopathy: Dividing patients according to the presence or absence of cerebral edema has practical clinical implications. FHF patients with altered mental status but without signs and symptoms of cerebral edema often suffer from other non-central nervous system (CNS) problems, such as electrolyte disturbances, infection, or gastrointestinal bleeding. Identification and treatment of these disorders is a priority.

Patients with papillary abnormalities, decerebrate posturing, epileptiform activity, and hemodynamic derangements (such as bradycardia, systemic hypertension, and brainstem respiratory patterns) suffer from cerbral edema and will need specific interventions (47). Patients with grade III or IV hepatic encephalopathy often require one-on-one nursing, with hourly charting of mental status. By eliminating enteral protein intake and by using phosphate enemas, ammonia production can be decreased. The goal of inducing two soft bowel movements should be attempted by judiciously giving lactulose through the nasogastric tube.

Some authors advocate the use of nonabsorbable antibiotics (such as neomycin) to decrease the amount of ammonia-producing gut flora. As opposed to the long-acting agents advocated for treating encephalopathy in alcoholic cirrhotic patients, the use of short-acting benzodiazepines (e.g., midazolam) is indicated only when necessary. As mentioned above, the benzodiazepine-inhibitor flumazenil may have a limited role in a subset of patients with hepatic encephalopathy (27). All attempts should be made to minimize interventions or situations that could exacerbate intracranial pressure elevation (e.g., traumatic endotracheal intubation, hypoxia, hypercapnia). Endotracheal tube suctioning should be accompanied by the use of lidocaine gel and light sedation and should be limited to a few seconds at a time. A quiet room may be beneficial. Avoidance of infection, hypoglycemia, and hemodynamic instability will also help treat the encephalopathy.

Intracranial pressure (ICP) monitoring is a potentially useful procedure in caring for hepatic encephalopathy patients. The clinical goal is an ICP below 25–30 mm Hg, while keeping central perfusion pressure (CPP) above 60 mm Hg. Such measures as elevation of the head of the bed between 20° and 30°, hyperventilation, and mannitol (and/or hemofiltration for patients with concomitant kidney failure) all may be useful. Complications related to placement of an ICP monitor, such as sepsis and intracranial bleeding, occur in about 4% of patients. Fatal hemorrhage occurs in 1% of patients (3).

Of all the interventions to reduce ICP, mannitol has been the most studied. By causing an osmotic diuresis, it subsequently decreases cerebrospinal fluid volume. Its use is limited once serum osmolarity reaches 320 mOsm/L. In patients with kidney failure, care must be taken to maintain the serum osmolarity below 320 mOsm/L through the kidney support measures discussed previously. Otherwise, a rise in ICP can ensue. For patients with elevated ICP despite administration of mannitol, the use of barbiturates such as thiopental is advocated by some authors. Barbiturates are thought to reduce ICP through cerebral vasoconstriction and consequent reduction in the amount of hyperemia. In addition, their anticonvulsant and antioxidant effects are thought to be of benefit. Hyperventilation, which is often employed in trauma patients, can reduce ICP by decreasing carbon dioxide (CO_2) tension; however, it has also been shown to concomitantly increase cerebral lactate formation. Moreover, the overuse of hyperventilation can decrease CPP potentiating vasospasm. Therefore, its use is controversial in FHF patients. Mild (35°C) hypothermia has been reported to help reduce ICP in rats (47), whereas moderate hypothermia (32–33°C) is of benefit in acute liver failure patients (48). Further studies are needed to validate and define the value of hypothermia. As a last-resort for the most resistant intracranial hypertension, total hepatectomy with portocaval anatomosis with expeditious liver transplantation has been described (49).

Corticosteroids have no known benefits in patients with hepatic encephalopathy, and their use may even be harmful (50). An electroencephalogram can be used to document epileptiform activity. If present, appropriate treatment with diazepam, phenytoin, or both can be initiated to reduce the resulting cerebral oxygen consumption.

Infection: In FHF patients, Kupfer cells, the largest group of macrophages in direct contact with blood, are functionally impaired. Patients have an increased susceptibility to Gram-positive bacterial, Gram-negative bacterial, fungal, and viral infections. Some authors advocate obtaining daily cultures of blood, urine, and sputum to detect infection as soon as possible. In a prospective controlled trial, Rolando et al. (29) examined the controversial issue of selective administration of parenteral and enteral antibiotics. In that trial, 108 patients with FHF or severe acetaminophen toxicity were randomized to receive parenteral ceftazidime and flucloxacillin plus either: (i) concomitant oral and enteral colistin, tobramycin, and amphotericin B, or (ii) enteral amphotericin B alone. No significant difference in the incidence of infection was noted for the two groups (21% vs. 20%). Prophylactic parenteral antibiotic treatment reduced the rate of infection typically seen in this group of patients. Enteral antibiotics did not contribute to this reduction. Furthermore, prophylactic administration of enteral antifungal treatment did decrease the incidence of fungal infections. Of interest, this trial corroborated the recently recognized phenomenon of an increased incidence of infection in patients with hepatic encephalopathy. These findings lend support to the hypothesis that CNS dysfunction modulates the immune system and makes the host susceptible to infectious agents.

Coagulopathy: Most authors agree that routine correction of coagulopathy is not indicated and may even have negative effects. Achieving a normal INR in acute liver failure patients is difficult, unless large volumes of blood products are used. Furthermore, INR has prognostic value in the care of such patients (such as transfer criteria or transplant status). Therefore, fresh-frozen plasma, cryoprecipitate, and platelets should be used for specific indications (e.g., bleeding, hemodynamic instability) or for invasive procedures (e.g., placement of ICP monitors, liver biopsy). In addition, FHF patients should be given vitamin K supplementation and prophylaxis against gastrointestinal hemorrhage with acid-blocking agents.

Patients who may have a gastrointestinal source of bleeding should undergo endoscopic examination (upper and lower) in search of the source. Even though bleeding from esophageal varices is rare in FHF patients, this possibility should be considered in the presence of acute Budd–Chiari syndrome.

Metabolic Complications: Hypoglycemia is frequent and occurs in 40–50% of FHF patients. It must be avoided. Frequent serum glucose monitoring can detect hypoglycemia and infusion of appropriate dextrose solutions (10–20% dextrose) will correct it. These patients need nutritional support, and enteral nutrition is the preferred route of delivery. When enteral feeding is not feasible, total parenteral nutrition should be employed.

Given the frequent association of kidney failure with acute liver failure, electrolyte abnormalities are also common. In one study, maintenance of normal serum sodium concentration was shown to improve cerebral edema and hepatic encephalopathy. Hypomagnesemia, hypophosphatemia, and hyperkalemia are common and need to be corrected. Replacement of potassium in FHF patients with hypokalemia should be reserved for low concentration (e.g., <3 mmol/L) or for the presence of cardiac arrhythmias. The reason is important: if such patients were to undergo a liver transplant, they could experience sudden onset of hyperkalemia once the revascularization phase of the liver transplant is reached (1). Finally, acid–base abnormalities are very common in FHF patients and need to be vigilantly monitored and treated. Metabolic acidosis, which is observed in late phases of liver failure, carries a poor prognosis.

Liver Transplantation

Liver transplantation has been the only mode of treatment to significantly decrease the 80% mortality observed in FHF. Successful liver transplantation has been reported to have survival rates of 60–80% (Table 5) (2). In comparison, only 14% of FHF patients in study of Shakil et al. (11) spontaneously recovered. The potentially rapid progress of FHF mandates early liver transplantation, but the severe organ shortage prevents all who need liver transplantation from receiving this therapy. A well-defined set of criteria to identify patients with FHF who are candidates for liver transplantation could result in earlier placement on the transplant list and perhaps a decrease in mortality.

The most widely studied criteria for liver transplantation are the KCH criteria (Table 6) (2). Demographic differences between acute liver failure patients in the UK and the US (Table 4) may limit the suitability of the KCH criteria for patients in the US. A retrospective review of the 13-year Pittsburgh experience (11) examined the applicability of the KCH criteria in the US. In Pittsburgh's acetaminophen group, the sensitivity for predicting death in patients with pH <7.30 was 90% and the specificity was 50%. The positive predictive value (PPV) was 69%, whereas the negative predictive value (NPV), was 80%. Including the KCH criteria, INR >6.5, serum Cr to >3.4 mg/dL, and grade III to IV encephalopathy improved specificity and PPV to 100%. The NPV remained 80%. In Pittsburgh's nonacetaminophen group, an INR >6.5 had the highest PPV (98%), but the NPV remained ~50%. Shakil et al. (11) concluded that the KCH criteria had high specificity and high PPV but low NPV, for a poor outcome. In other words, if patients fulfill the KCH criteria, their likelihood of dying is high. Not matching the KCH criteria does not predict survival. Thus, patients who fulfill the KCH criteria should undergo immediate liver transplantation, but other factors should be taken into consideration for those patients who do not fulfill the criteria. For example, using serum factor V level as a prognostic tool has been advocated by Bernuau et al. (51) (Table 6) in France. It has not gained widespread popularity in the US because the assay for factor V is unavailable in most American hospitals.

Contraindications to liver transplantation for acute liver failure patients include irreversible neurologic damage accompanied by increased ICP, refractory hypotension, severe cardiac or pulmonary disease, sepsis without source control, advanced malignancy, and other serious pathophysiologic processes such as active acquired immunodeficiency syndrome (AIDS). Relative contraindications may include advanced age, portal-venous thrombosis, pulmonary hypertension, active substance abuse (e.g., alcohol), hepatic or biliary malignancies (e.g., cholangiocarcinoma), and chronic conditions [e.g., human immunodeficiency virus (HIV)].

The most common type of liver transplant performed for acute liver failure patients has been an orthotopic liver transplant (OLT) from a cadaver donor. Other types have been described. For example, an auxiliary partial OLT involves transplantation of a small donated liver in place of a partially resected native liver, with the hope that the auxiliary transplanted liver will give the remaining native liver enough time to regenerate. Partial liver transplantation can also be done in a heterotopic fashion, which would then eliminate the need for partial resection of the native liver. The advantage of such procedures is that immunosuppression of the recipient is only temporary. The disadvantages are the donor shortage and the uncertainty surrounding the capacity of the native liver to regenerate. Other types of liver transplantation under investigation are living donor and split-cadaver OLTs. Finally, liver assist devices are being studied intently for the purpose of serving as "bridges" to liver transplantation in patients waiting on the liver transplant list.

Liver Assist Devices

Liver assist devices have been developed to provide FHF patients with a "bridge" to either liver transplantion or spontaneous regeneration of their native livers. These devices provide substitute liver function. Several different designs have been tested, the earliest of which were mechanical liver support devices, used alone or in combination. These devices included: hemodialysis, hemofiltration, hemodiabsorption, plasma exchange, resin perfusion, albumin dialysis, charcoal hemoperfusion, and plasma perfusion. Although some transient benefit has been reported in small cohorts of FHF patients with mechanical devices, physical detoxification fails to provide sufficient liver support. In the clinical setting of the complex metabolic derangements of FHF, additional factors may be necessary to support these patients. Extracorporeal liver, perfusion, first tested by Otto et al. (52) in 1958 and further investigated by Eiseman et al. (53), involves circulating the blood of an FHF patient through an *ex vivo* organ. Various attempts used livers from different species, including pig, baboon, human cadaver, calf, and Macaca monkey (54) (Table 7). Despite improvements in neurologic and biochemical variables, no definitive survival benefit was demonstrated in any of these studies (55,56). The advent of OLTs in the mid-1980s and the shortage of donor organs have severely limited further extracorporeal liver studies using human livers. In addition, the development of the cell-based bioartificial devices has shifted attention away from this mode of liver support.

Table 7 Published Clinical Trials for Bioartificial Livers for Fulminant Hepatic Failure (54)

Main author	Year	Artificial support	Hepatocyte source	Survival rates Treatment	Survival rates Control
Matsumura	1987	Plate dialyzer, cell suspension	Rabbit	100% (1/1)	—
Margulis	1989	AV shunt, cell suspension	Porcine	63% (37/59)	41% (27/67)
Li	1993	Glass bead packed	Porcine	67% (2/3)	—
Li	1998	Bed reactor	Hepatocytes		
Sussman	1994	Hollow fiber	Cultured	45% (5/11)	—
Ellis	1996	Bioreactor	Human hepatoma line	78% (7/9)[a] 33% (1/3)[b]	75% (6/8)[a] 25% (1/4)[b]
Gerlach	1997	Multiple compartment hollow fiber bioreactor	Cultured porcine hepatocytes	100% (6/6)	—
Demetriou	1995	Hollow fiber	Porcine	89% (8/9)	—
Watanabe	1997	Bioreactor	Hepatocytes	94% (17/18)[c] 100% (3/3)[d]	

[a]Patients not expected to require a liver transplant.
[b]Patients expected to require a liver transplant.
[c]Patients with fulminant hepatic failure.
[d]Patients with primary nonfunction of their transplanted liver.

Hybrid Bioartificial Livers

Reports on the efficacy of whole-organ perfusion indicated that the replacement of functional hepatocyte mass is the critical factor in the support of FHF patients. The logistical limitations to the widespread use of whole-organ perfusion encouraged an alternative approach based on recent advances in tissue engineering. Current procedures use isolated and cultured hepatocytes to create hybrid bioartificial livers (BALs) (57–61). With hybrid BALs, a synthetic substrate (a bioreactor) is combined with a biologic component (hepatocytes) to support liver function. Hepatocytes can be harvested from various sources (e.g., rat, rabbit, pig) and then infused into the BAL fresh, cryopreserved, or cold-stored (not frozen) for later use. Cold storage of hepatocytes is a current focus of intense research, because it potentially could simplify logistical problems of mass production and delivery to remote sites. When hepatocytes are cultured, the individual cells aggregate and form *spheroids*. Spheroids have increased differentiated function (e.g., increased albumin secretion, ammonia removal, urea synthesis) when compared to cultures of single or plated hepatocytes (62). Immortalized human cell lines have been developed that potentially can present unlimited sources of genetically engineered, nonimmunogenic, functional surrogates for native hepatocytes.

The bioreactor is composed of a plastic shell that usually houses a semipermeable membrane. The membrane serves as the interface between the patient's blood or plasma and the cultured hepatocytes. The hollow-fiber bioreactor, similar to the type

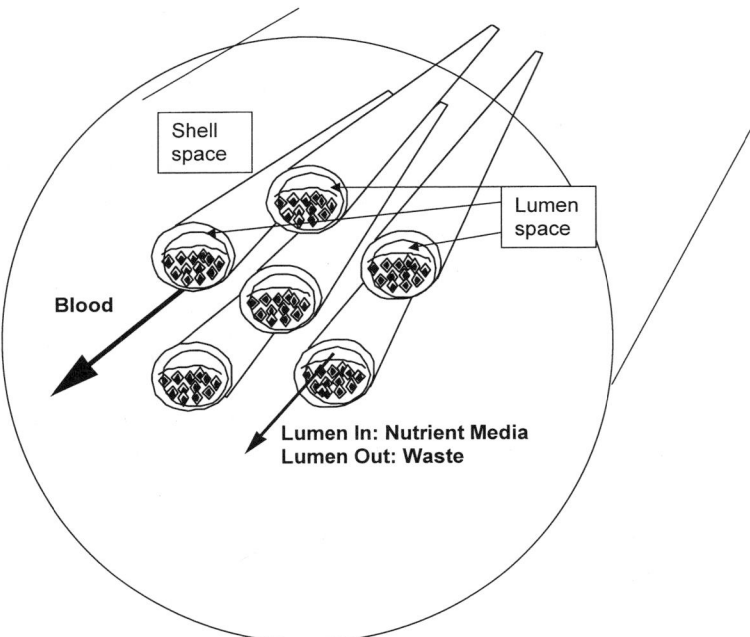

Figure 3 Three-compartment gel entrapment BAL: collagen-entrapped porcine hepatocytes are loaded into the lumen space. Gel contraction recreates a lumen channel, allowing delivery of nutrient media.

employed in conventional hemodialysis, has been studied most intensively. In the hollow fiber bioreactor, the patient's whole blood or just the centrifuge-separated plasma portion circulates through either the lumen space or the shell space (Fig. 3). The most extensively studied clinical BAL was developed by Demitriou et al. (57). In that series, 31 patients were treated with the BAL. They were separated into three groups. Group I ($n = 18$) consisted of FHF patients who were candidates for liver transplantation. Group II ($n = 3$) had primary nonfunction of a transplanted liver. Group III ($n = 10$) had acute exacerbations of chronic liver disease. Of the 18 patients in Group I, 16 were successfully bridged to liver transplantion. One patient recovered fully without a transplant and one died of pancreatitis. All three patients in Group II were supported to a second transplant. As predicted by the pathophysiology of the process, the efficacy of BAL support in ACLF patients (Group III) was less. Only 2 of 10 patients survived to receive a liver transplant. Measurement of ICP pre- and post-BAL application demonstrated a significant reduction, from 17 to 10 mm Hg. A significant improvement in the comprehensive level of consciousness score also was seen. The authors concluded that the provision of hepatocyte support by the BAL, in addition to aggressive medical support, can prevent intracranial hypertension and the adverse effects of cerebral edema. Results of an ongoing Phase II study are pending. Several other designs of the bioreactor being tested (63–66) have been limited to experimental settings. In the near future, liver assist devices will likely become an important tool in the care of FHF patients.

CONCLUSIONS

Acute liver failure is a highly fatal disorder if only treated medically. Rapid diagnosis is crucial, with special attention to the time interval between the onset of jaundice and the first signs of altered mental status. A careful history and physical examination, along with appropriate adjunctive studies, can differentiate FHF and ACLF patients. ACLF patients need medical attention to their inciting factors as well as to their chronic liver disease process. FHF patients should receive care at centers that have specialized ICU teams and access to liver transplant services. Using such criteria as the KCH criteria, appropriately selected patients should be placed on the transplant list to minimize the time interval between ICU admission and liver transplant. Clearly, of all available treatment modalities, only liver transplants have significantly reduced the high mortality associated with FHF.

Meticulous attention to detail in caring for these patients is of utmost importance. The high incidence of sepsis, hypoglycemia, and hemodynamic compromise makes the care of these patients challenging. New advances in the field of artificial support, such as the cell-based BAL, represent exciting new frontiers in the field of surgery, medicine, and science. BALs currently under investigation have higher expectations than previously developed support systems. Current tissue-engineering techniques allow the culture of large masses of viable hepatocytes on biocompatible blood interfaces, which promote efficient mass transfer. However, as with other support systems developed in the past, carefully designed clinical studies are necessary to assess efficacy.

SUMMARY

- Patients with ACLF have pre-existing liver disease that decompensates in response to physiologic and metabolic stress. It is defined as development of encephalopathy from sudden decompensation of chronic liver disease.
- Patients with FHF have no pre-existing liver disease. It is defined as progression to hepatic encephalopathy and severe dysfunction within 8 weeks of the onset of jaundice in a patient with no pre-existing liver disease.
- FHF patients have potentially reversible disease. Rapid identification and transfer to centers with appropriate resources can produce good outcomes.
- Psychiatric abnormalities of encephalopathy include disturbed consciousness, personality changes, intellectual deterioration, and speech irregularities.
- Neurologic manifestations of encephalopathy include asterixis, exaggerated deep tendon reflexes, increased muscle tone, sustained ankle clonus, pre-coma rigidity, and visual disturbances.
- Causes of ACLF include: spontaneous bacterial peritonitis, urinary tract infection, gastrointestinal hemorrhage, portal vein thrombosis, and malignancy.
- The most common cause of FHF is viral hepatitis.
- Acute liver failure can mimic septic shock. Pathologic delivery-dependent oxygen consumption has been identified in patients with acute liver failure.
- Astrocyte swelling, glutamate, ammonia, manganese, serotonin, dopamine, norepinephrine, GABA, and endogenous benzodiazepines have been implicated in hepatic encephalopathy.

Fulminant Hepatic Failure

- History and physical examination should be thorough and should focus on the presence or absence of signs of chronic liver disease to help distinguish patients with ACLF from those with FHF.
- In addition to routine blood chemistry analysis, obtain INR, albumin, bilirubin, AST, ALT, alkaline phosphatase, and serologic markers for viral hepatitis. Obtain toxicology screening including acetaminophen. If Wilson's disease is suspected, obtain serum ceruloplasmin and urinary copper concentrations. If hemochromatosis is suspected, obtain iron saturation and serum ferritin concentrations.
- Mortality with FHF is >80%. Transfer to a center that can provide support and liver transplantation may represent the best option for the patient.
- For acetaminophen induced FHF, poor outcomes were associated with blood pH <7.30 or with PT >100 s, serum creatinine >3.4 mg/dL, and grade III or grade IV hepatic encephalopathy.
- For other causes of FHF, poor outcomes were associated with PT >100 s or any three of the following:
    Age <10 years or >40 years
    Onset of jaundice greater than 7 days before the onset of encephalopathy
    PT >50 s
    Serum bilirubin >17.5 mg/dL
- *N*-acetyl cysteine may be beneficial in acetaminophen-induced FHF.
- Penicillin and silibilin may be beneficial in *Amanita phallodies* (mushroom) poisoning.
- Steroid treatment for autoimmune hepatitis producing FHF is controversial.
- Thrombolytic therapy may be useful in Budd–Chiari syndrome.
- Principles of resuscitation as described in Chapter 2 should be followed.
- Patients with liver failure often require renal support with dialysis, CVVH, or plasmapheresis. Respiratory support is frequently necessary.
- Patients with evidence of cerebral edema may benefit from ICP monitoring.
- Fresh frozen plasma, cryoprecipitate, and platelets should be used for bleeding and invasive procedures. See also Chapters 52 and 53.
- Enteral metabolic support is the preferred route. Hypoglycemia should be avoided.
- Successful liver transplantation is associated with survival rates of 60–80%. King's College Hospital of London criteria are useful in identifying patients who may benefit from liver transplantation.
- Liver assist devices will be valuable as a bridge to liver transplantation. Bioartificial livers have been used with success.

REFERENCES

1. Wood RP, Ozaki CF, Clark J. Acute fulminant hepatic failure. In: Cameron JL, ed. Current Surgical Therapy. St. Louis: Mosby, 1998:362–367.
2. Sherlock S, Dooley, J. Fulminant hepatic failure. In: Sherlock S DJ, ed. Diseases of the Liver and Biliary System. Oxford: Blackwell Science Ltd, 1997:103–117.
3. Bernuau J, Rueff B, Benhamou JP. Fulminant and subfulminant liver failure: definitions and causes. Semin Liver Dis 1986; 6:97–106.
4. Gimson AE, O'Grady J, Ede RJ, Portmann B, Williams R. Late onset hepatic failure: clinical, serological and histological features. Hepatology 1986; 6:288–294.

5. O'Grady JG, Schalm SW, Williams R. Acute liver failure: redefining the syndromes. Lancet 1993; 342:273–275.
6. Bihari DJ, Gimson AE, Williams R. Cardiovascular, pulmonary and renal complications of fulminant hepatic failure. Semin Liver Dis 1986; 6:119–128.
7. Miyata Y, Motomura S, Tsuji Y, Koga S. Hepatic encephalopathy and reversible cortical blindness. Am J Gastroenterol 1988; 83:780–782.
8. Reynolds TB, Telfer BR. Acute hepatic failure. In: Grenvik A, Ayres S, Holbrook PR, ed. Textbook of Critical Care. Philadelphia: W.S. Saunders Company, 2000:1616–1621.
9. Sielaff TD, Cerra F, Cattral M. Extracorporeal support of the failing liver. Current Opinion in Critical Care 1998; 4:125.
10. Anand AC, Nightingale P, Neuberger JM. Early indicators of prognosis in fulminant hepatic failure: an assessment of the King's criteria. J Hepatol 1997; 26:62–68.
11. Shakil AO, Kramer D, Mazariegos GV, Fung JJ, Rakela J. Acute liver failure: clinical features, outcome analysis, and applicability of prognostic criteria. Liver Transpl 2000; 6:163–169.
12. Sergi C, Jundt K, Seipp S, Goeser T, Theilmann L, Otto G, Otto HF, Hofmann WJ. The distribution of HBV, HCV and HGV among livers with fulminant hepatic failure of different aetiology, J Hepatol 1998; 29:861–871.
13. Moaven LD, Locarnini SA, Bowden DS, Kim JP, Breschkin A, McCaw R, Yun A, Wages J Jr, Jones B, Angus P. Hepatitis G virus and fulminant hepatic failure: evidence for transfusion-related infection. J Hepatol 1997; 27:613–619.
14. Williams R. Acute hepatic failure. In: Webb AR, Shapiro M, Singer M, et al., ed. Oxford Textbook of Critical Care. Oxford: Oxford University Press, 1999; 362–378.
15. Sherlock S, Dooley J. Anatomy and function. In: Sherlock S DJ, ed. Diseases of the Liver and Biliary System. Oxford: Blackwell Science Ltd, 1997:1–16.
16. Muto Y, Nouri-Aria KT, Meager A, Alexander GJ, Eddleston AL, Williams R. Enhanced tumour necrosis factor and interleukin-1 in fulminant hepatic failure. Lancet 1988; 2:72–74.
17. Sheron N, Goka J, Whendon J, et al. Highly elevated levels of plasma cytokines in fulminant hepatic failure: correlations with multi-organ failure and death. Hepatology 1990; 12:939.
18. Chase RA, Davies M, Trewby PN, Silk DB, Williams R. Plasma amino acid profiles in patients with fulminant hepatic failure treated by repeated polyacrylonitrile membrane hemodialysis. Gastroenterology 1978; 75:1033–1040.
19. Lee FY, Colombato LA, Albillos A, Groszmann RJ. N omega-nitro-Larginine administration corrects peripheral vasodilation and systemic capillary hypotension and ameliorates plasma volume expansion and sodium retention in portal hypertensive rats. Hepatology 1993; 17:84–90.
20. Ellis A, Wendon J. Circulatory, respiratory, cerebral, and renal derangements in acute liver failure: pathophysiology and management. Semin Liver Dis 1996; 16:379–388.
21. Keays R, Harrison PM, Wendon JA, Forbes A, Gove C, Alexander GJ, Williams R. Intravenous acetylcysteine in paracetamol induced fulminant hepatic failure: a prospective controlled trial. Bmj 1991; 303:1026–1029.
22. Harrison P, Wendon J, Williams R. Evidence of increased guanylate cyclase activation by acetylcysteine in fulminant hepatic failure. Hepatology 1996; 23:1067–1072.
23. Hazell AS, Butterworth RF. Hepatic encephalopathy: an update of pathophysiologic mechanisms. Proc Soc Exp Biol Med 1999; 222:99–112.
24. Michalak A, Butterworth RF. Selective loss of binding sites for the glutamate receptor ligands [3H]kainate and (S)-[3H]5-fluorowillardiine in the brains of rats with acute liver failure. Hepatology 1997; 25:631–635.
25. Bergeron M, Reader TA, Layrargues GP, Butterworth RF. Monoamines and metabolites in autopsied brain tissue from cirrhotic patients with hepatic encephalopathy. Neurochem Res 1989; 14:853–859.
26. Mousseau DD, Perney P, Layrargues GP, Butterworth RF. Selective loss of pallidal dopamine D2 receptor density in hepatic encephalopathy. Neurosci Lett 1993; 162:192–196.

27. Layrargues GP, Butterworth R. Efficacy of Ro-15–1788 in cirrhotic patients with hepatic coma: results of a randomized, double blind placebo-controlled crossover tria. Hepatology 1992; 16:311.
28. Bender AS, Norenberg MD. Effect of benzodiazepines and neurosteroids on ammonia-induced swelling in cultured astrocytes. J Neurosci Res 1998; 54:673–680.
29. Rolando N, Wade JJ, Stangou A, Gimson AE, Wendon J, Philpott-Howard J, Casewell MW, Williams R. Prospective study comparing the efficacy of prophylactic parenteral antimicrobials, with or without enteral decontamination, in patients with acute liver failure. Liver Transpl Surg 1996; 2:8–13.
30. O'Grady JG, Alexander GJ, Hayllar KM, Williams R. Early indicators of prognosis in fulminant hepatic failure. Gastroenterology 1989; 97:439–445.
31. Lee WM. Management of acute liver failure. Semin Liver Dis 1996; 16:369–378.
32. Rahman T, Hodgson H. Clinical management of acute hepatic failure. Intensive Care Med 2001; 27:467–476.
33. Valles EG, de Castro CR, Castro JA. N-acetyl cysteine is an early but also a late preventive agent against carbon tetrachloride-induced liver necrosis. Toxicol Lett 1994; 71:87–95.
34. Commandeur JN, Vermeulen NP. Identification of N-acetyl(2,2-dichlorovinyl)- and N-acetyl(1,2-dichlorovinyl)-L-cysteine as two regioisomeric mercapturic acids of trichloroethylene in the rat. Chem Res Toxicol 1990; 3:212–218.
35. Montanini S, Sinardi D, Pratico C, Sinardi AU, Trimarchi G. Use of acetylcysteine as the life-saving antidote in Amanita phalloides (death cap) poisoning. Case report on 11 patients. Arzneimittelforschung 1999; 49:1044–1047.
36. Al-Khalidi JA, Czaja AJ. Current concepts in the diagnosis, pathogenesis, and treatment of autoimmune hepatitis. Mayo Clin Proc 2001; 76:1237–1252.
37. Ockner SA, Brunt EM, Cohn SM, Krul ES, Hanto DW, Peters MG. Fulminant hepatic failure caused by acute fatty liver of pregnancy treated by orthotopic liver transplantation. Hepatology 1990; 11:59–64.
38. Slakey DP, Klein AS, Venbrux AC, Cameron JL. Budd–Chiari syndrome: current management options. Ann Surg 2001; 233:522–527.
39. Sterling RK, Luketic VA, Sanyal AJ, Shiffman ML. Treatment of fulminant hepatic failure with intravenous prostaglandin E1. Liver Transpl Surg 1998; 4:424–431.
40. Baguneid MS, Welch M, Bukhari M, Fulford PE, Howe M, Bigley G, Eddleston JM, McMahon RF, Walker MG. A randomized study to evaluate the effect of a perioperative infusion of dopexamine on colonic mucosal ischemia after aortic surgery. J Vasc Surg 2001; 33:758–763.
41. Power DA, Duggan J, Brady HR. Renal-dose (low-dose) dopamine for the treatment of sepsis-related and other forms of acute renal failure: ineffective and probably dangerous. Clin Exp Pharmacol Physiol Suppl 1999; 26:S23–S28.
42. Shilliday IR, Quinn KJ, Allison ME. Loop diuretics in the management of acute renal failure: a prospective, double-blind, placebo-controlled, randomized study. Nephrol Dial Transplant 1997; 12:2592–2596.
43. Hadengue A, Gadano A, Moreau R, Giostra E, Durand F, Valla D, Erlinger S, Lebrec D. Beneficial effects of the 2-day administration of terlipressin in patients with cirrhosis and hepatorenal syndrome. J Hepatol 1998; 29:565–570.
44. Davenport A, Finn R, Goldsmith HJ. Management of patients with renal failure complicated by cerebral oedema. Blood Purif 1989; 7:203–709.
45. McGuire G, Crossley D, Richards J, Wong D. Effects of varying levels of positive end-expiratory pressure on intracranial pressure and cerebral perfusion pressure. Crit Care Med 1997; 25:1059–1062.
46. Georgiadis D, Schwarz S, Baumgartner RW, Veltkamp R, Schwab S. Influence of positive end-expiratory pressure on intracranial pressure and cerebral perfusion pressure in patients with acute stroke. Stroke 2001; 32:2088–2092.

47. Larsen FS, Knudsen GM, Hansen BA. Pathophysiological changes in cerebral circulation, oxidative metabolism and blood-brain barrier in patients with acute liver failure. Tailored cerebral oxygen utilization. J Hepatol 1997; 27:231–238.
48. Jalan R, Damink SW, Deutz NE, Lee A, Hayes PC. Moderate hypothermia for uncontrolled intracranial hypertension in acute liver failure. Lancet 1999; 354:1164–1168.
49. Hammer GB, So SK, Al-Uzri A, Conley SB, Concepcion W, Cox KL, Berquist WE, Esquivel CO. Continuous venovenous hemofiltration with dialysis in combination with total hepatectomy and portocaval shunting. Bridge to liver transplantation. Transplantation 1996; 62:130–132.
50. Rakela J, Mosley JW, Edwards VM, Govindarajan S, Alpert E. A double-blinded, randomized trial of hydrocortisone in acute hepatic failure. The acute hepatic failure study group. Dig Dis Sci 1991; 36:1223–1228.
51. Bernuau J, Samuel D, Durand F. Criteria for emergency liver transplantation in patients with acute viral hepatitis and factor V below 50% of normal: a prospective study. Hepatology 1991; 14:49A.
52. Otto J, Pender J, Cleary J, Sensenig D, Welch C. The use of a donor liver in experimental animals with elevated blood ammonia. Surgery 1958; 43:301.
53. Eiseman B, Liem DS, Raffucci F. Heterologous liver perfusion in treatment of hepatic failure. Ann Surg 1965; 162:329–345.
54. McLaughlin BE, Tosone CM, Custer LM, Mullon C. Overview of extracorporeal liver support systems and clinical results. Ann N Y Acad Sci 1999; 875:310–325.
55. Chari RS, Collins BH, Magee JC, DiMaio JM, Kirk AD, Harland RC, McCann RL, Platt JL, Meyers WC. Brief report: treatment of hepatic failure with ex vivo pig-liver perfusion followed by liver transplantation. N Engl J Med 1994; 331:234–237.
56. Chari RS, Meyers WC. Extracorporeal xenogenetic liver support. In: Bussutil R, Klintmalm G, eds. Transplantation of the Liver. Philadelphia: W.B. Saunders, 1996:806–812.
57. Watanabe FD, Mullon CJ, Hewitt WR, Arkadopoulos N, Kahaku E, Eguchi S, Khalili T, Arnaout W, Shackleton CR, Rozga J, Solomon B, Demetriou AA. Clinical experience with a bioartificial liver in the treatment of severe liver failure. A phase I clinical trial. Ann Surg 1997; 225:484–491 (discussion 491–494).
58. Rozga J, Holzman MD, Ro MS, Griffin DW, Neuzil DF, Giorgio T, Moscioni AD, Demetriou AA. Development of a hybrid bioartificial liver. Ann Surg 1993; 217:502–509 (discussion 509–511).
59. Rozga J, Podesta L, LePage E, Morsiani E, Moscioni AD, Hoffman A, Sher L, Villamil F, Woolf G, McGrath M, et al. A bioartificial liver to treat severe acute liver failure. Ann Surg 1994; 219:538–544 (discussion 544–546).
60. Rozga J, Williams F, Ro MS, Neuzil DF, Giorgio TD, Backfisch G, Moscioni AD, Hakim R, Demetriou AA. Development of a bioartificial liver: properties and function of a hollow-fiber module inoculated with liver cells. Hepatology 1993; 17:258–265.
61. Demetriou AA, Watanabe FD, Rozga J. Artificial hepatic support systems. Prog Liver Dis 1995; 13:331.
62. Kamihira M, Yamada K, Hammamoto R. Spheroid formation of hepatocytes using synthetic polymer. Annals of New York academy of science 1999; 875:389.
63. Sielaff TD, Hu MY, Amiot B, Rollins MD, Rao S, McGuire B, Bloomer JR, Hu WS, Cerra FB. Gel-entrapment bioartificial liver therapy in galactosamine hepatitis. J Surg Res 1995; 59:179–184.
64. Sussman NL, Finegold MJ, Barish JP, Kelly JH. A case of syncytial giantcell hepatitis treated with an extracorporeal liver assist device. Am J Gastroenterol 1994; 89:1077–1082.
65. Gerlach JC. Development of a hybrid liver support system: a review. Int J Artif Organs 1996; 19:645–654.
66. Ellis AJ, Hughes RD, Wendon JA, Dunne J, Langley PG, Kelly JH, Gislason GT, Sussman NL, Williams R. Pilot-controlled trial of the extracorporeal liver assist device in acute liver failure. Hepatology 1996; 24:1446–1451.

H. Endocrine System

42
Endocrine Emergencies

Paul Druck
VA Medical Center, Minneapolis, Minnesota, USA

ADRENAL INSUFFICIENCY

Adrenocortical hormones, which include the glucocorticoid cortisol (hydrocortisone) and the mineralocorticoid (aldosterone), have a wide range of life-sustaining effects that include the regulation of carbohydrate, protein, lipid, and nucleic acid metabolism, modulation of immune responses, and control of body water, sodium, and potassium distribution and excretion. During physiologic stress, glucocorticoids help maintain hemodynamic stability by enhancing the response of cardiac and vascular smooth muscle to catecholamines and angiotensin II (1–5). Glucocorticoid deficiency can thus aggravate or precipitate critical illness. Some degree of adrenal insufficiency (AI) is present in as many as 30% of critically ill patients (6).

Etiology of AI

AI occurs when the physiologic glucocorticoid requirement exceeds the functional reserve of the hypothalamic–pituitary–adrenal (HPA) axis. Severe loss (>90%) of adrenal responsiveness is required before symptoms develop in a stable, unstressed patient; lesser degrees of dysfunction may become symptomatic during a physiologic stress such as sepsis, inflammation, injury, or the postoperative state, when adrenocortical hormone requirement is greater (relative AI). AI may be primary (intrinsic adrenal disorder) or secondary (impaired hypothalamic or pituitary regulation of adrenal function). It may be a mild, slowly progressive disorder (Addison's disease), or an acute, life-threatening hypoadrenalism (adrenal crisis).

Slowly progressive AI, which may remain subclinical until a sudden physiologic stress occurs, may be caused by metastatic replacement of the adrenal glands (particularly with malignancies of the breast, lung, or prostate), autoimmune atrophy (adrenalitis), infection (mycobacteria, fungi), sarcoid, amyloidosis, or hypopituitarism secondary to neoplastic replacement or granulomatous disease of the pituitary (1). Chronic ethanol ingestion is associated with decreased ACTH production and consequently decreased adrenal responsiveness (7). Varying degrees of AI also have been observed in patients with AIDS. In this group, the etiology is not clear but may involve adrenal cytomegalovirus infection (8,9). Ketoconazole, often used to treat fungal infections in AIDS patients, can interfere with cortisol synthesis (10,11). Other drugs interfere with cortisol synthesis (etomidate) or increase the metabolism of glucocorticoids (phenytoin, phenobarbital, and rifampin) (12). The administration of exogenous steroids will cause suppression of the HPA axis, but symptoms of AI will not become apparent unless the exogenous steroids are suddenly withheld, or a stress occurs that demands an amount of glucocorticoid in excess of that provided by the exogenous steroids.

Sudden hypoadrenalism is caused by spontaneous adrenal hemorrhage, which may occur during anticoagulation, pregnancy, or overwhelming sepsis (Waterhouse–Friderichsen syndrome), surgical removal of or trauma to the adrenal glands, or acute hypopituitarism (surgery, trauma, radiation, postpartum necrosis).

Clinical Features and Diagnosis of AI

Clinical Features

The diagnosis should be considered in any patient with profound hypotension that is unexplained or not improved with administration of fluids and vasopressor agents. Hyponatremia, hyperkalemia, and less commonly hypoglycemia, may be present. Associated clinical findings are lethargy or somnolence, nausea, vomiting, diarrhea, and abdominal pain, which may be severe enough to suggest an acute abdomen. Unexplained eosinophilia has also been observed. Subclinical AI of sufficient duration, unmasked by a sudden physiologic stress, may produce hyperpigmentation of the skin or mucosae, loss of axillary and pubic hair in females, and a history of weakness, anorexia, weight loss, and personality changes (13). A history of any of the etiologic factors mentioned in the section on Etiology of AI, particularly recent steroid use, supports the diagnosis. The lack of specificity of the clinical features makes empiric therapy essential.

When to Suspect AI as a Consequence of Prior Steroid Therapy

The severity and persistence of HPA suppression secondary to exogenous steroids depends, with considerable individual variation, on the dose and duration of therapy. Suggested thresholds for suspicion of steroid-induced adrenal suppression have included: use of glucocorticoid equivalent to 20 mg prednisone (Table 1) daily for more than 1 week (14), 12.5 mg of prednisone daily for 6 months, 10 mg of prednisone daily for over 2 years, or 5 mg of prednisone daily for >5 years (15). Streck and Lockwood (16) demonstrated blunted HPA responses after only 5 days of 25 mg/day prednisone. However, in a study of 279 patients undergoing provocative testing of adrenal function during steroid therapy, 63% of patients receiving <5 *mg per day* of prednisone or equivalent had blunted or absent adrenal responsiveness, whereas 24% of patients receiving >25 mg

Table 1 Relative Glucocorticoid Potencies[a]

Hydrocortisone	1
Prednisone	4
Methylprednisolone	5
Dexamethasone	30–40

[a]Significant mineralocorticoid activity not associated with long-acting steroids such as dexamethasone.

of prednisone or equivalent per day had normal responsiveness. Cumulative dose had some discriminative value, but in this study, duration of therapy did not (17).

The rate of recovery of HPA function after discontinuation of steroids is similarly unpredictable. Livanou et al. demonstrated progressive recovery of responsiveness beginning 48 h after steroid discontinuation, but a significant number of patients still exhibited subnormal basal serum concentrations of cortisol after 1 month and blunted adrenal response to hypoglycemic challenge (a measure of maximal adrenal output) after 1 year (18). A marked difference among patients receiving >10 mg of prednisone or <7.5 mg was noted. Graber confirmed that suppression may last as long as 9 months (19).

In summary, a patient receiving any amount of glucocorticoid for more than a few days may experience some degree of HPA axis suppression, ranging from only blunting of maximal response to inadequate basal secretion. After steroids have been discontinued, the time to recovery of function will be unpredictable and can last as long as 12 months. Adequate basal function will return before the reserve necessary for maximal response to stress is again present.

Biochemical Tests of Adrenal Function

The most common screening test for AI has been the rapid high-dose ACTH stimulation test. This test is not affected by circadian rhythm and may be performed at any time of day by administering 250 µg of a synthetic ACTH analog (cosyntropin) IV or IM, and determining plasma cortisol serum concentrations before and 30–60 min after administration. The normal response, as defined in *unstressed subjects*, is considered to be a rise in plasma cortisol of at least 9 µg/dL over baseline or an absolute concentration of 18–20 µg/dL (13,20–22).

Unfortunately, these criteria lack both specificity and sensitivity. Highly stressed patients with maximally stimulated HPA axes may have such high circulating cortisol levels that they are unable to augment serum concentration by an additional 9 µg/dL, yet may not be experiencing glucocorticoid deficiency (false positive). On the other hand, a stressed patient with only partial loss of adrenal reserve may achieve a stimulated plasma cortisol of 20 µg/dL but, if this response is inadeaquate relative to very high physiologic requirements, may experience relative AI (false negative). Mean cortisol serum concentration of 45–60 µg/dL have been observed in sepsis, septic shock, severe trauma, and hypotension secondary to gastrointestinal bleeding (5,23–25). Finally, the test dose of 250 µg of corticotropin is markedly supraphysiologic and may overcome subnormal adrenal responsiveness to physiologically achievable ACTH levels. A 1 µg ("low dose") cosyntropin test may be more sensitive and more indicative of physiologic response (26–28).

Treatment of Adrenal Crisis

Acute AI is life threatening; therefore, empiric therapy with glucocorticoids should be initiated *as soon as the diagnosis is considered* (Table 2). Dexamethasone 4 mg IV should be administered immediately; hydrocortisone will interfere with interpretation of subsequent tests of adrenal function. Intravascular fluid and sodium depletion should be corrected by rapid infusion of saline. Hypoglycemia, if present, should be treated with glucose infusion. Following initial stabilization, an ACTH stimulation test may be performed (see the section on Biochemical Tests of Adrenal Function). Within hours of the administration of glucocorticoids, resistant hemodynamic instability may improve spontaneously or become more responsive to the administration of fluids, inotropes, or vasoactive agents.

If the ACTH stimulation test suggests AI, or if the patient has a positive response to glucocorticoids but test results are still pending, continued steroid therapy is warranted. As

Table 2 Treatment of Acute AI

Administer dexamethasone 4 mg IV once diagnosis is considered
Treat hypotension, if no evidence of fluid overload, with isotonic fluid and pressors as needed
Perform ACTH stimulation test when patient is stable
Continue glucocorticoid supplementation with 100 mg hydrocortisone IV every 6–8 h for 24 h, then reduce by half every 24–48 h, as tolerated
If patient remains glucocorticoid-dependent after resolution of illness, continue maintenance steroids at 5–15 mg/m^2 hydrocortisone or equivalent in two divided doses per day. Consider fludrocortisone 0.1–0.2 mg daily

discussed in the section on Biochemical Tests of Adrenal Function, an ACTH-stimulated cortisol level of 20 μg/dL may not exclude AI in a highly stressed patient. Even a random cortisol determination *in excess of 25 μg/dL* may not always exclude relative AI. For example, among hypotensive patients, a random serum cortisol <25 μg/dL identifies a group most likely to improve hemodynamically with steroids (29). A salutary response to steroids may be considered a practical, empirical, and diagnostic criterion of AI.

Hydrocortisone, 100 mg every 6–8 h, is administered during the first 24 h. If the patient's condition permits, this dose is reduced by 50% on each of the subsequent 2–3 days and then discontinued. If the patient had been receiving therapeutic steroids previously, that dose should be continued. If signs of hypoadrenalism persist after the acute stress has resolved, continued maintenance therapy is required and, traditionally, has consisted of hydrocortisone 12–15 mg/m^2 (~25 mg), with two-thirds of the total dose given in the morning and one-third in the late afternoon. Recent studies suggest that 5–6 mg/m^2 (10 mg) may be more physiologic (30). A number of drugs, such as phenytoin, barbiturates, and rifampin accelerate cortisol metabolism and may necessitate higher maintenance doses (11,31). Mineralocorticoid supplementation with fludrocortisone, 0.1–0.2 mg daily, should be considered for the treatment of long-term AI. In addition, additional testing may be required to distinguish between primary and secondary AI (13).

During critical illness, a longer course of "stress dose" steroids may be required than during simple postoperative recovery (13). The time course of resolution of physiologic stress in critically ill patients can only be estimated and may require cautious tapering of dosage and observation of response. Severely injured patients also have been noted to have prolonged cortisol elevations of ≥7 days (25). Postoperative complications such as infection, need for mechanical ventilation, and complications requiring return to the operating room, may require continuing perioperative steroid supplementation. Outside of the context of AI, no benefit has been demonstrated for the routine use of steroids therapeutically during sepsis (32–34).

Prevention of Perioperative AI

Acute AI may occur intra- or postoperatively if: (i) ongoing steroid therapy is interrupted for surgery, (ii) steroids are continued, but the stress of surgery requires higher glucocorticoid serum concentrations than are provided by the current dose, or (iii) the patient is not taking steroids at the time of surgery but is still experiencing HPA-axis suppression as the result of previously administered steroids, and the stress of surgery exceeds current adrenal reserve. The incidence of acute AI in unselected perioperative patients has ranged from 0.01% to 0.1% in large retrospective reviews (35,36). Small studies of patients at high risk on the basis of ongoing steroid therapy or documented HPA-axis suppression have failed to document any cases of proven symptomatic AI, a finding that demonstrates the low incidence even in high-risk groups (37–40). A recent review has summarized 57 case reports over the last 50 years (41).

To prevent perioperative AI, one must provide sufficient glucocorticoid to compensate for the discrepancy between the glucocorticoid requirement imposed by the stress of surgery and the actual adrenal reserve. Requirements only can be estimated on the basis of probable physiologic stress. Adrenal reserve can be estimated only if HPA axis function has been tested preoperatively. Thus, the appropriate prophylactic regimen will be an *estimate* based on the observations to follow. Little evidence exists that a *very* brief course of steroids will adversely affect outcome. One should, therefore, err on the side of caution (assume greater steroid requirement where uncertainty is present), as the consequences of acute glucocorticoid deficiency outweigh the probable adverse effects of 24–48 h of *slightly* excessive steroid administration.

The perioperative increase in serum cortisol is related to the magnitude of surgical stress. Chernow et al. (42) divided patients into three groups, stratified by the magnitude of their cortisol (and other hormone) responses to anesthesia and surgery. Group 1 patients underwent brief, uncomplicated procedures such as inguinal herniorrhaphy, often under local anesthesia, and exhibited no significant increases in serum cortisol concentrations. Group 2 patients underwent more involved intra-abdominal procedures, such as cholecystectomy, hysterectomy, or appendectomy, and exhibited mean cortisol serum concentrations of 30 μg/dL postoperatively, which returned to baseline within 24 h. Group 3 patients underwent extensive procedures such as gastrectomy, colectomy, or aorto-bifemoral bypass. These patients had the greatest increases in cortisol (mean > 45 μg/dL), which persisted beyond 24 h but returned to baseline by the fifth postoperative day (POD). Similar data have been recorded by others (15,43,44).

Patients should receive perioperative glucocorticoid supplementation if they currently have documented HPA axis suppression. If they are at risk (i.e., have completed a several day course of steroids during the last year), presumptive coverage can be given or an ACTH stimulation test may be performed and coverage reserved for suppressed patients. The current recommendations for glucocorticoid supplementation (Table 3) (12,31,41) are:

1. For minor surgery (local or regional anesthesia, ≤1 h, not involving entry into the thoracic or abdominal cavities), continue the patient's current therapeutic steroid dose (if any) on the day of surgery. No additional steroids are required.
2. For moderately stressful procedures (lesser intra-abdominal procedures such as cholecystectomy, colectomy, laparoscopy, hysterectomy, or major extremity or head and neck procedures etc.), continue the current therapeutic steroid dose (if any) up to the time of surgery and add 50–75 mg hydrocortisone pre- or intraoperatively. On POD 1, 20–25 mg of hydrocortisone should be given every 8 h. On POD 2, supplementation should be discontinued and the usual preoperative steroid dose (if any) resumed.
3. For severely stressful procedures (esophagectomy, gastrectomy, pancreaticoduodenectomy, hepatectomy, total proctocolectomy, cardiac procedures involving cardiopulmonary bypass, etc.) continue the current steroid dose (if any) up to the time of surgery and add 50–75 mg hydrocortisone intraoperatively and every 8 h thereafter for 48–72 h. Reduce this dose by half for an additional 24 h, then discontinue supplementation and return to the usual preoperative steroid dose (if any).

Table 3 Perioperative Glucocorticoid Supplementation

Low-stress procedures (minor surgery, local or regional anesthesia, short duration)
    Continue ongoing therapeutic steroid dose up to time of surgery
    No additional steroids are indicated
    Resume preoperative therapeutic steroids, if any, postoperatively
Moderate-stress procedures (abdominal/thoracic surgery, major extremity/head/neck surgery, general anesthesia)
    Continue ongoing therapeutic steroid dose up to time of surgery
    Give additional 50–75 mg hydrocortisone IV pre- or intraoperatively
    POD 1: Give 20–25 mg hydrocortisone IV every 8 h
    POD 2: Discontinue supplementation, resume preoperative therapeutic steroids, if any
High-stress procedures (esophagectomy, gastrectomy, pancreatectomy, hepatectomy, aortic surgery, cardiopulmonary bypass)
    Continue ongoing therapeutic steroid dose up to time of surgery
    Give additional 50–75 mg hydrocortisone IV pre- or intraoperatively
    POD 1–3: Give 50–75 mg hydrocortisone IV every 8 h
    POD 4: Give 25–35 mg hydrocortisone IV every 8 h
    POD 5: Discontinue supplementation (as tolerated), resume preoperative therapeutic steroids, if any

Complications such as infections, respiratory failure, postoperative pancreatitis, hemorrhage, reoperation, etc., may necessitate higher doses or more prolonged supplementation. Suspicion of acute AI, regardless of whether perioperative supplementation has been given, should prompt empiric treatment, as described in the section on Treatment of Adrenal Crisis.

THYROID DYSFUNCTION

Thyroid Storm

Thyroid storm, hyperthyroidism or thyrotoxicosis in its most severe form, is a life-threatening disorder that occurs when a physiologic stress causes decompensation in a patient with established hyperthyroidism. Typical precipitating events include infection, surgery, trauma, childbirth, stroke, myocardial infarction, or withdrawal of antithyroid medication. Thyroid storm also has been precipitated by exposure to iodine from iodinated radiocontrast material or amiodarone (which can deliver 100 times the daily iodine requirement at therapeutic dosages) (45) or, rarely, during lithium therapy (46). Mortality has been as high as 100% without prompt treatment; even with early diagnosis and treatment, mortality is as high as 20–50% (47).

Clinical Features and Diagnosis

The cardinal features of thyroid storm are refractory tachyarrhythmias (usually atrial fibrillation with rapid ventricular response), mental status changes (usually agitation, but may be as severe as delirium or psychosis and may progress to coma), hyperpyrexia (may be as high as 106°F), and occasionally, ventricular dysfunction and congestive heart failure. Nausea, vomiting, diarrhea, and jaundice may be seen (48). This hyperadrenergic state may be due to an upregulation of beta-adrenergic receptors mediated by thyroid hormone excess, as well as by postreceptor response modification (49). Unfortunately, the prominent clinical features are common to many critical illnesses. Furthermore, the signs and symptoms are often blunted in elderly patients (see below), and in patients who have received symptomatic treatment with beta blockers and sedatives prior to considering the diagnosis. The suspicion of thyroid storm should arise when these signs and symptoms are observed in a patient with a known history of hyperthyroidism or thyroid surgery, thyromegaly, signs and symptoms of chronic hyperthyroidism (proptosis, eyelid lag, hyperreflexia, proximal muscle weakness, recent onset of nervousness, tremors, heat intolerance, palpitations, or unexplained weight loss), if these new symptoms cannot be otherwise explained or if the patient fails to respond to appropriate treatment. An uncommon variant, seen primarily in elderly patients, is so-called "apathetic hyperthyroidism," in which most of the common features are absent or mild, with the exception of new onset tachyarrhythmias, weight loss, and muscle weakness (50). Thyroid storm is at the extreme end of the spectrum of worsening hyperthyroidism; considerable variation in criteria exists among published reviews. Burch and Wartofsky (48) have suggested a point-score system that integrates severity of pyrexia and cardiovascular, CNS, and gastrointestinal manifestations to stratify patients according to probability of true thyroid storm.

Thyroid function tests can only support, not confirm, the diagnosis because considerable overlap is found between thyroid hormone serum concentrations in uncomplicated hyperthyroidism and in thyroid storm. Elevation of free thyroid hormone serum concentration may correlate better with symptoms than total hormone serum concentrations (free and bound) (51). Treatment should be initiated on the basis of suspicion; treatment should not be delayed for return of laboratory results.

Management

Management consists of urgent supportive therapy, administration of antithyroid medication, and identification and correction of the precipitating event (Table 4). Hyperthermia

Table 4 Management of Acute Thyroid Dysfunction

Thyroid storm
Correct hyperthermia: external cooling and acetaminophen
Treat tachyarrhythmias with IV beta blockers:
    Esmolol: start at 50–100 μg/min IV, titrate to control ventricular rate, or
    Propranolol: 2–5 mg/h IV, titrate to control ventricular rate, or
    Diltiazem: 5 mg/h IV if intolerant of beta blockers, or 120 mg PO every 8 h
Restore intravascular volume with isotonic fluids
Block hormone synthesis and release:
    PTU 600–1000 mg PO × 1, then 200–250 mg every 4–8 h, or methimazole 20 mg PO every 4–6 h
    One hour after antithyroid drugs: Lugol's iodine 8 drops PO every 6 h, or SSKI* 5 drops PO every 6 h, or 1000 mg iodinated soluble radiocontrast material PO per day. If iodine allergic, lithium carbonate 300 mg PO every 6 h.
Adjunctive measures: sedation, dexamethasone 2 mg every 6 h

Myxedema coma
Treat hypothermia: passive external warming
Treat hypovolemia: isotonic fluids, monitor serum sodium concentration, avoid overload
Treat respiratory failure with mechanical ventilation if indicated
Hormone replacement: thyroxine up to 300 mg/m^2 IV initially, then 50–100 μg/day, maintenance as guided by TSH and clinical findings. Avoid cardiotoxicity
Adjunctive measures: dexamethasone 2–4 mg IV, continue every 6 h if favorable response

*SSKI = saturated solution of potassium iodide.

must be rapidly corrected with external cooling and acetaminophen. Salicylates may increase free thyroid hormone serum concentrations by reducing hormone binding and should be avoided (48). Shivering during external cooling should be suppressed with meperidine, 25 mg intravenously. Marked hypovolemia, the result of gastrointestinal losses and diaphoresis, is often present and should be corrected with isotonic fluids. Initial hyperglycemia may become hypoglycemia as hepatic stores are exhausted. To prevent hypoglycemia, glucose should be added to IV fluids. Thiamine should be administered to correct possible deficiency.

Tachyarrhythmias are treated with beta-adrenergic blockade in the form of a continuous infusion of propranolol at 2–5 mg/h or esmolol at 50–100 μg/min, titrated to achieve reduction of the rapid ventricular rate. Electrical cardioversion is usually ineffective until the patient has been rendered euthyroid (52). Patients intolerant of beta blockade, for example, those individuals with bronchospastic disease, may be treated with calcium channel blockers such as diltiazem 120 mg PO every 8 h (53). A continuous infusion of diltiazem, beginning at 5 mg/h, is an option.

Congestive heart failure, particularly in patients with underlying heart disease, may occur as a result of rate-related impairment of ventricular filling or rate-related ischemia. Although most hyperthyroid patients have increased cardiac contractility, long-standing hyperthyroidism also may produce hypertrophic cardiomyopathy, which predisposes the patient to ventricular dysfunction during an episode of thyroid storm (54). Such patients often respond favorably to beta blockade, but invasive hemodynamic monitoring may be necessary to guide therapy. In the event that ventricular failure fails to respond favorably to beta blockade and intravascular fluid management guided by invasive monitoring, digitalis and diuresis are indicated (55). Rarely, refractory hypotension with marked peripheral vascular dilation may require treatment with alpha-adrenergic agents.

Prompt blockade of thyroid hormone synthesis is accomplished with a loading dose of 600–1000 mg propylthiouracil (PTU) followed by maintenance doses of 200–250 mg every 4–8 h. Alternatively, methimazole may be given at a rate of 20 mg every 4–6 h, but PTU has the added advantage of blocking peripheral conversion of T_4 to T_3. Neither drug is available in parenteral form and must be given orally to alert patients or via nasogastric tube to obtunded patients. An aqueous solution of methimazole may be given rectally. A history of agranulocytosis secondary to either of these drugs contraindicates their use. Release of preformed hormone may be inhibited by the administration of iodine [Lugol's solution 8 drops every 6 h or saturated solution of potassium iodide (SSKI) 5 drops every 6 h], *provided further hormone synthesis has already been blocked.* This intervention usually requires a delay of at least 1 h following administration of PTU or methimazole. Iodinated radiocontrast material (sodium ipodate or sodium iopanoate), 1 g daily or 500 mg twice daily, is an effective alternative, which is associated with a rapid drop in circulating T_3 (56). If a patient has a history of iodine-induced anaphylaxis, lithium carbonate, which impairs thyroid hormone release, may be given at the rate of 300 mg every 6 h. Lithium serum concentration should be monitored, and the dose should be adjusted to maintain serum lithium serum concentrations of 1 meq/L (48).

Agitation may be reduced by sedatives. The marked hypermetabolism of thyroid storm increases demand for circulating glucocorticoids; administration of glucocorticoid is associated with reduced mortality. Steroids also reduce peripheral conversion of T_4 to T_3. Dexamethasone 2 mg every 6 h or hydrocortisone 100 mg every 6 h is recommended (48,57). Finally a search for and correction of the precipitating stress should be undertaken.

Myxedema Coma

Myxedema coma, or acutely decompensated hypothyroidism, is an uncommon condition that may occur when a physiologic stress is superimposed on subclinical or well-compensated hypothyroidism. The cardinal features of myxedema coma are altered mental status (not necessarily true coma, despite the name), hypothermia without shivering, and cardiovascular instability. Clinical suspicion should be raised by a known diagnosis of hypothyroidism, the presence of a goiter, or a thyroidectomy ("necklace") incision. Typical precipitating events include infection, surgery, trauma, hemorrhage, stroke, overmedication with sedatives, tranquilizers, or diuretics, lithium therapy, hypoglycemia, or hypothermia (58,59). This condition is highly morbid. Even with prompt treatment mortality is reported as 15–20% (60).

Clinical Features and Diagnosis

Hypothermia is the result of decreased metabolic rate, which in turn leads to decreased heat generation. Peripheral vasoconstriction permits some body heat conservation and produces the typical findings of cool, pale, dry extremity skin. Beta-adrenergic receptor down-regulation, increased phosphodiesterase activity, and altered second messenger function lead to decreased responsiveness to beta-adrenergic stimulation with bradycardia and depressed myocardial contractility (49,58). The resulting unbalanced alpha-adrenergic tone leads to further peripheral vasoconstriction and intravascular volume contraction, which, in turn, lead to regional hypoperfusion manifested by falling mixed venous oxygen saturation despite diastolic hypertension. Additional, sudden loss of blood volume, vasodilation from sepsis or unwise administration of vasodilators, or development of myocardial ischemia with further reduction of cardiac function may cause cardiovascular collapse. Normal or low blood pressure in a patient with signs of intense peripheral vasoconstriction heralds hemodynamic decompensation. Restoration of intravascular volume may unmask or exacerbate the anemia and hyponatremia of chronic hypothyroidism.

Respiratory failure with hypercarbia and hypoxia, the result of reduced central respiratory drive and respiratory muscle weakness, may require intubation and mechanical ventilation. Myxedema may be manifested by failure to wean from mechanical ventilation after general anesthesia or after resolution of a pulmonary problem that precipitated the myxedema coma.

Altered mental status is a *sine qua non* of myxedema coma (58). The underlying pathogenesis is unclear. The mechanism may be primary neurological dysfunction aggravated by superimposed symptomatic hyponatremia. Hypoadrenalism may accompany hypothyroidism, either as a consequence of a generalized autoimmune disorder (autoimmune hypothyroidism and autoimmune adrenalitis), or as another manifestation of hypopituitarism (61).

Management

Management consists of urgent supportive therapy, hormone replacement, and identification and correction of the precipitating event. Prompt supportive therapy includes hemodynamic stabilization, intubation and mechanical ventilation if indicated by clinical respiratory findings or arterial blood gas determination, and treatment of hypothermia. Presumptive hormone replacement should not be delayed until definitive biochemical testing is completed.

Hypothermia is best treated with passive measures, such as keeping the patient covered and in a warm environment to prevent further heat loss. Use of active external warming may cause peripheral vasodilation with hypotension, and a drop in core temperature, and should be avoided. Core temperatures lower than 30°C are unusual without concomitant exposure; active rewarming with warmed intravenous fluids and inspired gases should be reserved for such patients.

Volume contraction should be treated with isotonic fluid resuscitation. Care should be taken to avoid water intoxication and hyponatremia, as well as fluid overload in patients with poor ventricular function. Invasive hemodynamic monitoring may be necessary for patients with known congestive heart failure or for those who have not responded adequately to judicious fluid replacement. Treat hypoglycemia, if present, with glucose-containing IV fluids. If adrenal insufficiency is present, glucocorticoids may help sustain cardiovascular responsiveness, and should precede the administration of thyroid hormone, which will increase metabolic rate. Dexamethasone 2–4 mg IV should be given initially. If hemodynamic instability appears to respond favorably to dexamethasone, an ACTH stimulation test should be performed and maintenance glucocorticoids (see earlier) continued pending test results.

Initial thyroid hormone replacement should begin with intravenous L-thyroxine, 300 mg/m^2 (~500 mg for an average size adult). Over-zealous thyroid hormone replacement may precipitate tachyarrhythmias in patients with a propensity to such arrhythmias or ischemia in patients with significant coronary artery disease. More gradual replacement may be undertaken for patients with such risk factors, especially if the patient responds promptly to supportive measures. Once the patient is stabilized, serum TSH should be measured; an elevated TSH is diagnostic but does not distinguish between primary hypothyroidism and less common hypopituitarism. Maintenance thyroid replacement should then begin with L-thyroxine 50–100 μg/day as dictated by TSH determinations and clinical findings. Oral administration may replace intravenous therapy as soon as the patient is tolerating oral intake (58). A search should begin for precipitating factors such as occult infection (see precipitating factors mentioned earlier).

Sick-Euthyroid Syndrome

Seriously ill patients may be found to have low (but detectable) TSH serum concentrations, normal to low T_4, low T_3, and elevated reverse T_3, (rT_3) yet appear euthyroid clinically. Collectively these findings are termed the "sick-euthyroid syndrome." This syndrome is not a true endocrine emergency but is seen with sufficient frequency in the critically ill to warrant a brief description.

The underlying abnormality appears to be central hypothyroidism, with low TSH despite low T_4 and T_3 serum concentrations (62). This hypothesis is supported by the observation that exogenous TRH restores normal TSH secretion in sick-euthyroid patients (63). The characteristic hormone changes have been reproduced by infusion of recombinant tumor necrosis factor in normal volunteers, an observation suggesting that cytokines act on the hypothalamus to reduce TRH secretion and are ultimately the cause of this syndrome (64). Other abnormalities associated with this syndrome are reduced plasma binding of T_4, which results in normal serum concentrations of free T_4 (hence the clinical euthyroidism), reduced peripheral deiodination of T_4 to T_3, and reduced serum clearance of rT_3 (62). Treatment with thyroid hormone replacement has resulted in unchanged or worsened outcomes and cannot be recommended at this time (65,66).

DISORDERS OF GLUCOSE HOMEOSTASIS

Maintenance of Normoglycemia in Critically Ill Patients

Subclinical glucose intolerance is often unmasked and overt diabetes mellitus is frequently exacerbated by illness, particularly infection or circulatory shock. Traditionally, the aim of glucose control in hospitalized and especially in critically ill patients has been to maintain reasonable, but not stringent, control because clinicians feared hypoglycemic episodes in patients with unstable metabolic conditions and unpredictable absorption of and sensitivity to insulin. Even mild to moderate hyperglycemia, however, is associated with numerous physiologic derangements, such as impaired phagocytosis and oxidative burst by neutrophils and alveolar macrophages (67,68), enhanced adhesion of pathogenic micro-organisms such as *Candida* spp. (69), interference with immunoglobulin function (70), and impaired wound healing as a result of glycosylation of collagen and increased collagenase activity (71).

Numerous studies have demonstrated an association between stricter glycemic control during hospitalization and reduced morbidity and mortality (71–75). A large, randomized, prospective trial has demonstrated that maintaining blood glucose between 80 and 110 mg/dL in surgical ICU patients is associated with reduced mortality, ICU length of stay, duration of mechanical ventilation, episodes of bacteremia, and incidence of renal failure and critical-illness polyneuropathy. Only 5% of patients experienced hypoglycemia, and those patients suffered no significant complications (76).

Glucose control is best maintained in critically ill patients with continuous intravenous insulin titrated to achieve the desired blood glucose level (see the following). For a patient with type II diabetes, oral hypoglycemics should be withheld in favor of insulin until the patient is stable and ready to resume oral nutrition. Blood glucose must be monitored frequently, and IV fluids should contain glucose once the hyperglycemia is under control. Continuous intravenous insulin is preferred in critically ill patients because the absorption of subcutaneous insulin is unpredictable, especially if peripheral hypoperfusion is present, intermittent bolus insulin produces wide fluctuations in blood glucose, and, finally, most regimens do not call for insulin injection for normal or near-normal blood glucose, which results in rebound hyperglycemia. An excellent way to manage hyperglycemia in patients receiving TPN is to add the daily insulin requirement to the TPN solution (as regular insulin). Patients receiving continuous enteral feedings also should receive continuous, rather than intermittent, bolus insulin. Once the patient is stable, a long-acting insulin preparation such as NPH or lente, with intermittent supplementation with regular insulin, may be substituted for the insulin infusion (77).

Diabetic Ketoacidosis and Hyperglycemic Hyperosmolar Nonketotic Syndrome (Hyperosmolar Coma)

Diabetic ketoacidosis (DKA) and hyperglycemic hyperosmolar nonketotic syndrome (HHNS) (hyperosmolar coma) are related syndromes of uncontrolled diabetes. The cardinal features of dehydration, hyperglycemia, and hyperosmolality are common to both. Diabetic ketoacidosis tends to occur in younger, type I diabetic patients with absent or minimal insulin secretion and is characterized by mild-to-moderate hyperglycemia, ketonemia and ketonuria, nonanion gap acidemia, severe dehydration, sodium and potassium depletion, and mild-to-moderate degrees of serum hyperosmolality (generally <320 mOsm/L). Clinical features include signs of profound dehydration,

Kussmaul breathing if acidemia is present, vomiting, and abdominal pain in 30% of patients (78,79). Depressed mental status suggests more severe hyperosmolality (see the following) or another problem.

The HHNS tends to occur in older, type II diabetic patients with preserved but inadequate insulin secretion and peripheral insulin resistance. It is characterized by extreme hyperglycemia (usually >600 mg/dL but may approach 1000 mg/dL), severe dehydration, sodium and potassium depletion, plasma hyperosmolality (≥ 320 mOsm/L), and obtundation (hence the term "hyperosmolar coma"). True coma occurs at osmolalities >340 mOsm/L (79). Acidemia and ketonemia are usually absent.

Precipitating events are most commonly infection, noncompliance with treatment, or dehydration, although 25% of cases of DKA occur as the first clinical manifestation of diabetes, and as many as half of the cases of HHNS occur in undiagnosed diabetic individuals in whom the signs and symptoms of worsening hyperglycemia and osmotic diuresis were not recognized (78). Steroid therapy, myocardial infarction, stroke, pancreatitis, alcohol or cocaine intoxication, burns, and renal failure have also been implicated (77,79,80). Mortality, usually from sepsis, thromboembolic disorders, or cardiovascular complications, occurs in 2–4% of DKA patients and increases to 20% for patients above age 65 (78,81). Mortality has been higher in HHNS than in ketoacidosis, an observation that probably reflects the older age and greater prevalence of comorbid conditions in patients with HHNS.

Treatment consists of restoration of intravascular volume with attention to electrolyte abnormalities, insulin administration, and prophylaxis against thromboembolism (Table 5). Fluid deficits can exceed 10% of body weight and must be urgently replaced. Controversy exists over whether the rate of fluid administration is related to the development of cerebral edema and possibly death (82,83). Cerebral edema can be minimized by correcting the fluid deficit over 12–24 h. A practical regimen in adults is administration of 1000 mL of 0.9% saline during the first hour, followed by 250–500 mL/h until the deficit is corrected. If the initial serum sodium concentration is >150 meq/L, 0.45% saline should be used. Once intravascular volume is restored, hypotonic fluid should be used to avoid sodium overload or subsequent hyperchloremic acidemia (77). Potassium deficits

Table 5 Management of Diabetic Ketoacidosis and Hyperglycemic Hyperosmolar Nonketotic Syndrome (Hyperosmolar Coma)

Restore intravascular volume: 0.9% Saline 1 L in first hour, then 250–500 mL/h to correct fluid deficit in 12–24 h. Change to 0.45% saline thereafter.

Correct electrolyte abnormalities: Add potassium 20–30 mEq/L to IV fluids if $K^+ < 5.0$ mEq/L and urine output is adequate; if $K^+ \leq 5.0$ mEq/L or patient oliguric, do not administer potassium initially.

Monitor serum K^+ closely: Replace magnesium and phosphorus if serum concentration is severely depressed.

Give regular insulin loading dose of 0.1–0.2 units/kg: Begin regular insulin infusion at 5–10 units/hr and titrate to keep blood glucose $\sim$250 mg/dL until ketoacidosis is resolved. IM route acceptable if IV access not initially available. Monitor blood glucose closely. Add 5% glucose to IV fluids once hyperglycemia controlled.

Bicarbonate therapy: Although traditionally used for acidemia, no demonstrable benefit and possible adverse effects.

Severe headache and mental status changes: May indicate rare cerebral edema; treat urgently with mannitol 0.5–2.0 g/kg IV.

of 200–300 mEq may be obscured initially by hypovolemia and acidemia; fluid resuscitation may rapidly precipitate dangerous hypokalemia. If serum potassium is <5 mEq/L and urine output is adequate at the start of fluid administration, 20–30 mEq potassium should be added to each liter of IV fluid. If hyperkalemia is initially present, or if urine output is minimal, potassium should be withheld until the serum concentration of potassium begins to decline. Magnesium and phosphorus should be replaced only if serum concentrations are markedly low. Acidemia is usually improved by fluid and insulin administration; bicarbonate therapy is rarely (if ever) indicated, and may actually be detrimental, even during severe acidemia (77,84,85).

Insulin should not be administered until fluid resuscitation has begun and is best administered as an initial loading dose of 0.1–0.2 units/kg followed by continuous infusion of 5–10 units/h, with adjustments as indicated by hourly monitoring to achieve a blood glucose of ~250 mg/dL (77–79). Lower glucose serum concentrations during the first 24 h have been associated with cerebral edema, although this is controversial (82,83). If intravenous access is not available initially, an intramuscular loading dose of 10–20 units, followed by hourly injections of 1–5 units as needed may be substituted (78). Subcutaneous administration of insulin should be avoided. If signs of cerebral edema (headache, deterioration in mental status) develop, mannitol 0.5–2.0 g/kg body weight IV should be given immediately and repeated as necessary. Once glucose serum concentration has declined to 250 mg/dL, 5% glucose should be added to the IV fluids and continued along with the IV insulin until ketonemia and acidemia have resolved. At that point, stricter glucose control may be instituted.

SUMMARY

Adrenal Insufficiency

- AI should be considered in any patient with refractory hypotension of unclear etiology. Hyponatremia, hyperkalemia, and hypoglycemia may be associated. Nausea, vomiting, and severe abdominal pain may occur. Precipitating factors include withdrawal of chronic steroids, sudden loss of adrenal function (adrenal hemorrhage, trauma), or physiologic stress in a patient with partial adrenal suppression.
- Suspected AI must be treated promptly with glucocorticoids; dexamethasone 4 mg IV is preferred, as it will not interfere with subsequent adrenal axis testing. If the patient responds favorably, or if testing confirms adrenal suppression, supplementation should continue with hydrocortisone 100 mg every 6–8 h for at least 24 h, and then be progressively reduced as the patient's condition permits.
- Patients who have received steroids within the last 6–12 months have unpredictable adrenal function and may develop symptomatic AI during or after a surgical procedure. The degree of adrenal suppression and the time to return of full adrenal function depends, in a complex and unpredictable way, on dosage and duration of therapy and is most accurately determined by a preoperative ACTH simulation test.
- Patients at risk for AI who undergo minor procedures under local anesthesia do not require supplementation. Patients who undergo more significant surgical stress (general anesthesia, intra-abdominal or intrathoracic procedures, etc.) should receive perioperative supplementation scaled to the anticipated magnitude of stress.

Thyroid Disorders

- Myxedema (decompensated hypothyroidism) is characterized by impaired mental status, hypothermia, respiratory insufficiency and hemodynamic instability. Hyponatremia, anemia, hypoglycemia, and adrenal insufficiency may be seen as well.
- Supportive treatment consists of respiratory support, cautious fluid resuscitation, slow correction of hyponatremia, and passive control of external body heat loss. Specific therapy is thyroid hormone administration with monitoring of clinical signs and thyroid function tests, and presumptive glucocorticoid treatment pending results of adrenal function testing.
- Thyroid storm (decompensated hyperthyroidism) is characterized by mental status changes, hyperpyrexia, and signs of adrenergic overstimulation, with severe and often refractory tachyarrhythmias, and occasional ventricular dysfunction and congestive heart failure.
- Supportive therapy consists of external cooling and antipyretics, restoration of intravascular volume, sedation, and adjunctive glucocorticoids. Tachyarrhythmias are initially treated with beta-adrenergic blockade. Congestive heart failure usually improves with control of heart rate and reduction of excess circulating thyroid hormone. Thyroid hormone excess is reduced with PTU or methimazole followed by iodine administration.

Disorders of Glucose Homeostasis

- Strict control of hyperglycemia during critical illness and in the postoperative period has been demonstrated to reduce morbidity and mortality. Insulin infusions should be used to maintain blood glucose between 80 and 110 mg/dL.
- Diabetic ketoacidosis and HHNS (hyperosmolar coma) are consequences of severe, uncontrolled diabetes mellitus, and may be precipitated by infection, dehydration, noncompliance with treatment, or as the first presentation of unsuspected diabetes. Clinical features are dehydration, sodium and potassium depletion, hyperglycemia (worse in HHNS), and hyperosmolality (worse in HHNS and often associated with obtundation). Acidemia and ketonemia are generally seen only in ketoacidosis.
- Treatment of DKA and HHNS consists of urgent restoration of intravascular volume, monitoring for and correction of electrolyte abnormalities, gradual correction of hyperglycemia with intravenous insulin, and prophylaxis against thromboembolism.

REFERENCES

1. Williams GH, Dluhy RG. Disorders of the adrenal cortex. In: Braunwald E, Fauci AS, et al., eds. Principles of Internal Medicine, 15th ed. New York: McGraw-Hill, 2001:2084–2105.
2. Ramey ER, Goldstein MS, et al. Action of norepinephrine and adrenal cortical steroids on blood pressure and work performance of adrenalectomized dogs. Am J Physiol 1951; 165:450–455.
3. Fritz I, Levine R. Action of adrenal cortical steroids and nor-epinephrine on vascular responses of stress in adrenalectomized rats. Am J Physiol 1951; 165:456–465.
4. Besse JC, Bass AD. Potentiation by hydrocortisone of responses to catecholamines in vascular smooth muscle. J Pharmacol Exp Ther 1966; 154:224–238.

5. Marik PE, Zaloga GP. Adrenal insufficiency in the critically ill. Chest 2002; 122:1784–1796.
6. Zaloga GP, Marik PE. Hypothalamic–pituitary–adrenal insufficiency. Crit Care Clin 2001; 17:25–42.
7. Bernan JD, Cook DM, et al. Diminished adrenocorticotropin response to insulin-induced hypoglycemia in nondepressed, actively drinking male alcoholics. J Clin Endocrinol Metab 1990; 71:712–717.
8. Greene LW, Cole W, et al. Adrenal insufficiency as a complication of the acquired immunodefficiency syndrome. Ann Int Med 1984; 101:497–498.
9. Glascow BJ, Steinsapir KD, et al. Adrenal pathology in the acquired immune deficiency syndrome. Am J Clin Pathol 1985; 84:1975–1988.
10. Pont A, Williams PL, et al. Ketoconazole blocks adrenal steroid synthesis. Ann Int Med 1982; 97:379–382.
11. Farwell AP, Devlin JT, et al. Total suppression of cortisol excretion by ketoconazole in the therapy of ectopic adrenocorticotropic hormone syndrome. Am J Med 1988; 84:1063–1066.
12. Lamberts SWJ, Bruining HA, et al. Corticosteroid therapy in severe illness. N Engl J Med 1997; 337:1285–1292.
13. Werbel SS, Ober KP. Acute Adrenal insufficiency. Endocrinol Metab Clin North Am 1993; 22:303–328.
14. Axelrod L. Glucocorticoid therapy. Medicine 1976; 55:39–63.
15. Kehlet H, Binder CHR. Adrenocortical function and clinical course during and after surgery in unsupplemented glucocorticoid-treated patients. Br J Anaesth 1973; 45:1043–1048.
16. Streck WF, Lockwood DH. Pituitary adrenal recovery following short term suppression with corticosteroids. Am J Med 1979; 66:910–914.
17. Schlaghecke R, Kornely E, et al. The effect of long-term glucocorticoid therapy on Pituitary–adrenal responses to exogenous corticotropin-releasing hormone. N Engl J Med 1992; 326:226–230.
18. Livanou T, Ferriman D, et al. Recovery of hypothalamo–pituitary–adrenal function after corticosteroid therapy. Lancet 1967; 2:856–859.
19. Graber AL, Ney RL, et al. Natural history of pituitary–adrenal recovery following long term suppression with corticosteroids. J Clin Endocrinol 1965; 25:11–16.
20. May ME, Carey RM. Rapid adrenocorticotropic hormone test in practice—retrospective review. Am J Med 1985; 79:679–684.
21. Clark PM, Neylon I, et al. Defining the normal cortisol response to the short synacthen test: implications for the investigation of hypothalamic–pituitary disorders. Clin Endocrinol 1998; 49:287–292.
22. Streeten DHP. What test for hypothalamic–pituitary adrenocortical insufficiency? Lancet 1999; 354:179–180.
23. Melby JC, Spink WW. Comparative studies on adrenal cortial function and cortisol metabolism in healthy adults and inpatients with shock due to infection. J Clin Invest 1958; 37:1791–1798.
24. Schein RMH, Sprung CL, et al. Plasma cortisol levels in patients with septic shock. Crit Care Med 1990; 18:259–263.
25. Vermes I, Beishuizen A, et al. Dissociation of plasma adrenocorticotropin and cortisol levels in critically ill patients: possible role of endothelin and atrial natriuetic hormone. J Clin Endocrinol Metab 1995; 80:1238–1242.
26. Dickstein G, Shechner C, et al. Adrenocorticotropin stimulation test: effect of basal cortisol level, time of day, and suggested new sensitive low dose test. J Clin Endocrinol Metab 1991; 72:773–778.
27. Richards ML, Caplan RH, et al. The rapid low dose (1 microgram) cosyntropin test in the immediate postoperative period: results in elderly subjects after major abdominal surgery. Surgery 1999; 125:431–440.

28. Abdu TA, Elhadd TA, et al. Comparison of the low dose short synacthen test (1 microg), the conventional dose short synacthen test 250 microg), and the insulin tolerance test for assessment of the hypothalamo–pituitary–adrenal axis in patients with pituitary disease. J Clin Endocrinol Metab 1999; 84:838–843.
29. Rivers EP, Gaspari M, et al. Adrenal insufficiency in high-risk surgical ICU patients. Chest 2001; 119:889–896.
30. Esteban NV, Loughlin T, et al. Daily cortisol production rate in man determined by stable isotope dilution/mass spectrometry. J Clin Endocrinol Metab 1991; 72:39–45.
31. Coursin DB, Wood KE. Corticosteroid supplementation for adrenal insufficiency. JAMA 2002; 287:236–240.
32. The Veterans Administration Systemic Sepsis Cooperative Study Group. Effect of high-dose glucocorticoid therapy on mortality in patients with clinical signs of systemic sepsis. N Engl J Med 1987; 317:659–665.
33. Lefering R, Neugebauer EAM. Steroid controversy in sepsis and septic shock: a meta-analysis. Crit Care Med 1995; 23:1294–1303.
34. Cronin L, Cook DJ, et al. Corticosteroid treatment for sepsis: a critical appraisal and meta-analysis of the literature. Crit Care Med 1995; 23:1430–1439.
35. Mohler JL, Flueck JA, et al. Adrenal insufficiency following unilateral adrenalectomy: a case report. J Urol 1986; 135:554–556.
36. Alford WC, Meador CK, et al. Acute adrenal insufficiency following cardiac surgical procedures. J Thorac Cardiovasc Surg 1979; 78:489–493.
37. Plumpton FS, Besser GM, et al. Corticosteroid treatment and surgery. An investigation of the indications for steroid cover. Anaesthesia 1969; 24:3–11.
38. Bromberg JS, Alfrey EJ, et al. Adrenal suppression and steroid supplementation in renal transplant recipients. Transplantation 1991; 51:385–390.
39. Friedman RJ, Sciff CF, et al. Use of supplemental steroids in patients having orthopedic operations. J Bone Joint Surg 1995; 77:1801–1805.
40. Glownaik JV, Loriaux DL. A double-blind study of perioperative steroid requirements in secondary adrenal insufficiency. Surgery 1997; 121:123–129.
41. Salem M, Tainsh RE, et al. Perioperative glucocorticoid coverage. Reassessment 42 years after emergence of a problem. Ann Surg 1994; 219:416–425.
42. Chernow B, Alexander R, et al. Hormonal response to surgical stress. Arch Int Med 1987; 147:1273–1278.
43. McIntosh TK, Lothrop DA, et al. Circadian rhythm of cortisol is altered in postsurgical patients. J Clin Endocrinol Metab 1981; 53: 117–122.
44. Mohler JL, Michael KA, et al. The serum and urinary cortisol response to operative trauma. Surg Gynecol Obstet 1985; 161:445–449.
45. Meurisse M, Gollogly L, et al. Iatrogenic thyrotoxicosis: causal circumstances, pathophysiolgy, and principal of treatment—review of the literature. World J Surgery 2000; 24:1377–1385.
46. Yassa R, Sanders A, et al. Lithium-induced thyroid disorders: a prevalence study. J Clin Psychiatry 1988; 49;14–16.
47. Mazzaferri EL, Skillman TJ. Thyroid storm. A review of 22 episodes with special emphasis on the use of guanethidine. Arch Int Med 1969; 124:684–690.
48. Burch HB, Wartofsky L. Life-threatening thyrotoxicosis. Endocrinol Metabol Clin North Am 1993; 22:263–277.
49. Bilezikian JP, Loeb JN. The influence of hyperthyroidism and hypothyroidism on alpha-and beta-adrenergic receptor systems and adrenergic responsiveness. Endocr Rev 1983; 4:378–388.
50. Dabon-Almirante L,Surks MI. Clinical and laboratory diagnosis of thyrotoxicosis.Endocrinol Metabol Clin North Am 1998; 27:25–35.
51. Brooks MH, Waldstein MS. Free thyroxine concentrations in thyroid storm. Ann Int Med 1980; 93:694–697.

52. Klein I, Ojamma K. Mechanisms of disease: thyroid hormone and the cardiovascular system. N Engl J Med 2001; 344:501–509.
53. Roti E, Montermini M, et al. The effect of diltiazem, a calcium channel-blocking drug, on cardiac rate and rhythm in hyperthyroid patients. Arch Int Med 1998; 148:1919–1921.
54. Forfar JC, Muir Al, et al. Abnormal left ventricular function in hyperthyroidism: evidence for possible reversible cardiomyopathy. N Engl J Med 1982; 307: 1165–1167.
55. Klein I, Ojamma K. Thyrotoxicosis and the heart. Endocrinol Metab Clin North Am 1998; 27:51–62.
56. Sharp B, Reed AW, et al. Treatment of hyperthyroidism with sodium ipodate (Orografin) in addition to propylthiouracil and propranolol. J Clin Endocrinol Metab 1981; 53:622–625.
57. Cooper DS. Antithyroid drugs for the treatment of hyperthyroidism caused by Graves' disease. Endocrinol Metab Clin North Am 1998; 27:225–247.
58. Nicoloff JT, LoPresti JS. Myxedema coma: a form of decompensated hypothyroidism. Endocrinol Metab Clin North Am 1993; 22:279–290.
59. Waldman S, Park D. Myxendema coma associated with lithium therapy. Am J Med 1989; 87:355–356.
60. Jordan R. Myxedema coma. Pathophysiology, therapy, and factors affecting prognosis. Med Clin North Am 1995; 79:185–194.
61. Ross DS. Serum thyroid-stimulating hormone measurement for assessment of thyroid function and disease. Endocrinol Metab Clin North Am 2001; 30:245–264.
62. DeGroot LJ. Dangerous dogmas in medicine: the non-thyroidal illness syndrome. J Clin Endocrinol Metab 1999; 84:151–164.
63. Romijn JA, Wiersinga WM. Decreased nocturnal surge of thyrotropin in non-thyroidal illness. J Clin Endocrinol Metab 1990; 70:35–42.
64. Van der Poll T, Romijn JA, et al. Tumor necrosis factor: a putative mediator of the sick-euthyroid syndrome in man. J Clin Endocrinol Metab 1990; 71:1567–1572.
65. Brent GA, Hershman JM. Thyroxine therapy in patients with severe non-thyroidal illnesses and low serum thyroxine concentration. J Clin Endocrinol Metab 1986; 63:1–8.
66. Acker CG, Singh AR, et al. A trial of thyroxine in acute renal failure. Kidney Int 2000; 57:293–298.
67. Nielson CP, Hindson DA. Inhibition of polymorphonuclear leukocyte respiratory burst by elevated glucose concentrations in vivo. Diabetes 1989; 38:1031–1035.
68. Kwoun MO, Ling PR, et al. Immunologic effects of acute hyperglycemia in nondiabetic rats. J Parenter Enteral Nutr 1997; 21:91–95.
69. Hostetter MK, Lorenz JS, et al. The iC3b receptor on *Candida albicans:* subcellular localization and modulation of receptor expression by glucose. J Infect Dis 1990; 161:761–768.
70. Black CT, Hennessey PJ, et al. Short-term hyperglycemia depresses immunity through nonenzymatic glycosylation of circulating immunoglobulin. J Trauma 1990; 30:830–832.
71. Funary AP, Zerr KJ, et al. Continuous intravenous insulin infusion reduces the incidence of deep sternal wound infection in diabetic patients after cardiac surgical procedures. Ann Thorac Surg 1999; 67:352–360.
72. Capes SE, Hunt D, et al. Stress hyperglycemia and increased risk of death after myocardial infarction in patients with and without diabetes: a sytematic overview. Lancet 2000; 355:773–778.
73. Capes SE, Hunt D, et al. Stress hyperglycemia and prognosis of stroke in nondiabetic and diabetic patients. Stroke 2001; 32:2426–2432.
74. Malmberg K, Norhammar A, et al. Glycometabolic state at admission: important risk marker of mortality in conventionally treated patients with diabetes mellitus and acute myocardial infarction. Circulation 1999; 99:2626–2632.
75. Finney SJ, Zekveld C, et al. Glucose control and mortality in critically ill patients. JAMA 2003; 290:2041–2047.
76. Van den Berghe G, Wouters P, et al. Intensive insulin therapy in critically ill patients. N Engl J Med 2001; 345:1359–1367.

77. Boord JB, Graber AL, et al. Practical management of diabetes in critically ill patients. Am J Resp Crit Care Med 2001; 164:1763–1767.
78. Lebovitz HE. Diabetic ketoacidosis. Lancet 1995; 345:767–772.
79. Siperstein MD. Diabetic keoacidosis and hyperosmolar coma. Endocrinol Metab Clin North Am 1992; 21:415–432.
80. Fujikawa LS, Meisler DM, et al. Hyperosmolar hyperglycemic nonketotic coma. A complication of short-term systemic corticosteroid use. Ophthalmol 1983; 90:1239–1242.
81. Delaney MF, Zisman A, et al. Diabetic ketoacidosis and hyperglycemic hyperosmolar nonketotic syndrome. Endocrinol Metab Clin North Am 2000; 29:683–705.
82. Harris GD, Fiordalisi I, et al. Minimizing the risk of brain herniation during treatment of diabetic ketoacidemia: a retrospective and prospective study. J Pediatric 1990; 117:22–31.
83. Rosenbloom AL. Intracerebral crises during treatment of ketoacidosis Diabetes Care 1990; 13:22–33.
84. Lever E, Jaspan JB. Sodium bicarbonate therapy in severe diabetic ketoacidosis. Am J Med 1983; 75:263–268.
85. Morris LR, Murphy MB, et al. Bicarbonate therapy in severe diabetic ketoacidosis. Ann Int Med 1986; 105:836–840.

43
Divalent Ions

Jeffrey A. Bailey
St. Louis University School of Medicine, St. Louis, Missouri, USA

John E. Mazuski
Washington University School of Medicine, St. Louis, Missouri, USA

Disorders of calcium, magnesium, and phosphorus metabolism are frequently observed in SICU patients. Although divalent ion abnormalities are usually asymptomatic, they have the potential to impair cardiovascular and neuromuscular function. A high index of suspicion for these disorders should be maintained, and routine monitoring of serum calcium, magnesium, and phosphorus levels is warranted in most critically ill patients.

CALCIUM

Calcium is the most abundant electrolyte in the body, with a total content of ~1300 g in the average-sized person. Over 99% of the body's calcium is deposited in the skeleton and, with the exception of a small pool of calcium that can be readily mobilized, skeletal calcium does not enter into routine homeostasis (1).

The normal total serum calcium concentration is 8.5–10.5 mg/dL. However, only 0.03% of the body's calcium is present in the plasma. Approximately 50% of plasma calcium is present as free ionized form; ~40% is bound to proteins, primarily albumin, and ~10% is complexed with other ions, including bicarbonate, citrate, phosphate, carbonate, and lactate. Only the free ionized form actively participates in the physiologic reactions involving calcium (2).

A number of factors can affect the relationship between the ionized calcium concentration and the total serum calcium concentration. A reduction in the serum albumin concentration usually decreases the total serum calcium without affecting the ionized calcium concentration. Changes in plasma pH alter the binding of calcium to protein. Acidosis decreases the binding of calcium to albumin, whereas alkalosis promotes increased binding of calcium to the protein. The ionized calcium concentration also may be depressed by increased concentrations of chelating ions, such as phosphate or citrate. This latter ion is especially important in patients who have received massive blood transfusions (2).

A number of algorithms have been developed to estimate the serum ionized calcium concentration from the total serum concentration and the total protein or albumin concentration. These algorithms do not appear to adequately estimate the ionized calcium concentration in critically ill patients (3,4). Therefore, in most cases, the serum ionized calcium concentration should be directly measured rather than relying on one of these estimates (2).

Calcium homeostasis is normally regulated tightly by the actions of parathyroid hormone (PTH) and calcitriol (1,25-dihydroxy vitamin D). Gastrointestinal absorption of calcium is promoted by calcitriol, and both PTH and calcitriol interact with the skeleton to maintain normal extracellular calcium concentrations. PTH acts on the kidney both to increase calcium reabsorption and to stimulate hydroxylation of 25-hydroxy vitamin D, an action that produces the hormonally active compound, calcitriol (1,2,5,6). Thus, disorders of both the parathyroid glands and of vitamin D metabolism may profoundly affect serum calcium concentrations.

The mechanisms underlying calcium homeostasis have become better understood with the cloning of the calcium sensing receptor (CaSR). The CaSR is most abundantly expressed by renal and parathyroid cells and is expressed at lower levels in thyroid "C" cells, intestine, lung, and brain (7). By binding to this receptor, calcium inhibits PTH secretion and stimulates calcitonin secretion (8). By these actions calcium acts as a bidirectional first messenger for its own regulation. The importance of the CaSR in calcium homeostasis has been documented by finding mutations in the CaSR gene in certain inherited disorders of calcium metabolism. These conditions include familial hypocalciuric hypercalcemia (FHH) and neonatal severe hyperparathyroidism. Both of these disorders demonstrate persistent hypocalciuric hypercalcemia despite parathyroidectomy, a finding supporting an intrinsic abnormality of renal calcium homeostasis associated with mutations in the CaSR (9).

Hypocalcemia

In the SICU, hypocalcemia is most often seen in patients with acute illnesses, such as trauma, pancreatitis, sepsis, and burns. Decreases in total and ionized calcium occur frequently after massive blood transfusion (10,11), especially in patients who have had a significant period of hypovolemic shock. These changes may be partially due to the complexing of calcium with unmetabolized citrate, and partially as a result of the shock process itself, which promotes the uptake of ionized calcium into the intracellular compartment. In most of these patients, ionized calcium concentrations return to normal within 48 h, although persistent hypoalbuminemia may reduce total serum calcium concentrations.

The association of hypocalcemia with pancreatitis is well known. Defects in the hormonal regulation of calcium concentrations and intracellular uptake of calcium probably account for the hypocalcemia. In the past, hypocalcemia was erroneously attributed only to the depositions of calcium in areas of fat necrosis. Similar mechanisms also contribute to the decreases in total and ionized calcium concentrations observed with sepsis and burns (2,5).

Hypocalcemia occurs in the presence of metabolic disorders, such as hypomagnesemia and hyperphosphatemia. In addition, hypermagnesemia, through its impact on PTH secretion, may also produce hypocalcemia. Hypocalcemia is relatively common in patients with chronic renal failure and is related to decreased hydroxylation of 25-hydroxy vitamin D and to concomitant hyperphosphatemia and hypermagnesemia. Hypoparathyroidism as a cause of hypocalcemia is rare in the SICU, except for the reactive hypocalcemia seen after surgery for hyperparathyroidism. Chronic diseases associated with vitamin D deficiency, such as alcoholism and malnutrition, also may produce hypocalcemia (2,5).

Symptoms and signs of acute hypocalcemia are most often observed in the neuromuscular and cardiovascular systems. Neuromuscular manifestations include tetany, muscle spasms, weakness, and paresthesias, as well as nonspecific mental status changes. Chvostek's sign and Trousseau's sign may be elicited, but these responses are not necessarily reliable, particularly in the SICU. Cardiovascular manifestations include ECG changes, such as prolongation of the QT and ST intervals, nonspecific T-wave changes, bradycardia, and ventricular dysrhythmias. Severe hypocalcemia may lead to hypotension, cardiac insufficiency unresponsive to catecholamines and digoxin, and eventually circulatory collapse (2,5,6).

If clinical findings of hypocalcemia are present, or if the clinical setting is appropriate, total and ionized serum calcium concentrations should be obtained (Fig. 1). If hypocalcemia is diagnosed, serum phosphorus and magnesium concentrations also should be checked, since concomitant disorders of these ions are common. If no obvious cause for the hypocalcemia can be found, an endocrinologic evaluation should be initiated and may include determinations of PTH and vitamin D concentrations.

Patients with symptomatic or severe hypocalcemia should be treated urgently. In the critical care setting, intravenous calcium is the preferred treatment, with the administration of 100–200 mg of elemental calcium given as 10–20 mL of 10% calcium gluconate or 4–8 mL of 10% calcium chloride. Maintenance therapy, given as an intravenous infusion of 1–2 mg/kg per h of elemental calcium (2,6), will be needed for patients with severe

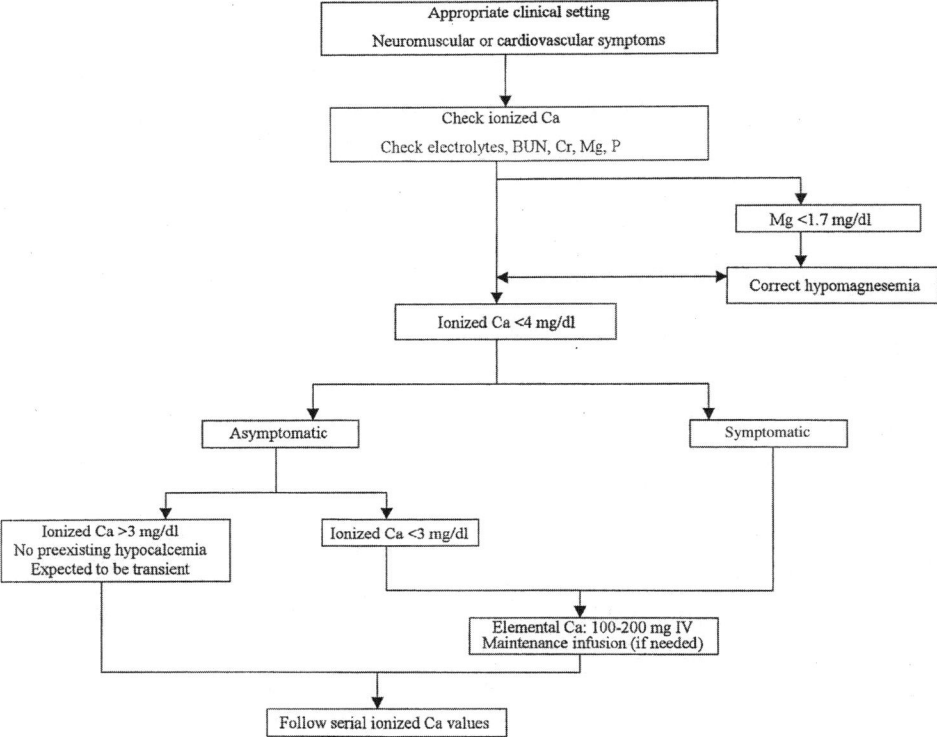

Figure 1 Treatment approach to hypocalcemia.

hypocalcemia. Patients receiving total parenteral nutrition (TPN) should receive maintenance dosages of calcium, generally 250–450 mg (6–11 mmol) of elemental calcium per day (12).

Hypercalcemia

Although not as common as hypocalcemia, hypercalcemia is occasionally seen in the SICU. Most often it is associated with malignancy or immobilization, or it is produced inatrogenically by the administration of calcium salts or drugs such as thiazides, that promote hypercalcemia. Hypovolemia also contributes to hypercalcemia. Hyperparathyroidism rarely warrants placing the patient in SICU unless it is associated with severe symptomatic hypercalcemia. Other causes of hypercalcemia include familial hypercalcemia, granulomatous diseases such as sarcoidosis, and endocrine disorders such as hyperthyroidism, pheochromocytoma, and acromegaly. Patients with renal failure occasionally develop hypercalcemia, although hypocalcemia is more typical (2,5).

The clinical manifestations of hypercalcemia are protean. Acute hypercalcemia is more likely to be symptomatic than is chronic hypercalcemia. With acute hypercalcemia, cardiovascular and neuromuscular symptoms predominate. The QT interval is shortened, but this finding may not be a reliable sign of hypercalcemia. Dysrhythmias and increased sensitivity to digitalis preparations may be seen. In addition, calcium exerts an inotropic effect on the heart and may lead to vascular smooth muscle contraction. The result is increased systemic vascular resistance and hypertension. Neuromuscular symptoms include weakness and hyporeflexia. CNS problems, such as personality changes, depression, and disorientation, progressing to obtundation and frank coma, are frequently observed. Chronic hypercalcemia may produce only vague complaints, such as anorexia, constipation, nausea and vomiting, or skeletal pain. In patients with long-standing hypercalcemia, nephrolithiasis and nephrocalcinosis may occur along with renal osteodystrophy (2,5).

Diagnosis of hypercalcemia is determined by the serum calcium concentration (Fig. 2). Generally, an elevated total serum calcium concentration indicates an elevated ionized calcium concentration. In patients with depressed serum protein concentrations, an ionized calcium concentration should be obtained, since this component may be elevated despite a normal total serum calcium concentration. Magnesium and phosphorus concentrations also should be checked, since the incidence of concomitant disorders in relatively high. If the cause of hypercalcemia is not immediately clear, a diagnostic evaluation, including a PTH determination, should be initiated.

Acute symptomatic hypercalcemia should be treated as a medical emergency. General measures include correction of any volume deficits present, discontinuation of calcium or medications contributing to hypercalcemia, and treatment of the underlying disorder, if at all possible. The mainstay of therapy for acute symptomatic hypercalcemia is forced diuresis with 1–2 L of saline administrated over a few hours, and furosemide supplementation as needed to promote diuresis. Serum potassium and magnesium concentrations must be monitored along with calcium concentrations during this intervention. In patients with significant renal dysfunction, dialysis may be the only method with which to acutely lower serum calcium concentrations (2,5).

A number of other agents that treat hypercalcemia by inhibiting bone reabsorption are available for use. These agents include mithramycin, salmon calcitonin, glucocorticoids, and bisphosphonates. Because of their inhibitory effect on osteoclastic bone resorption, bisphosphonates have become the preferred therapy for the treatment of

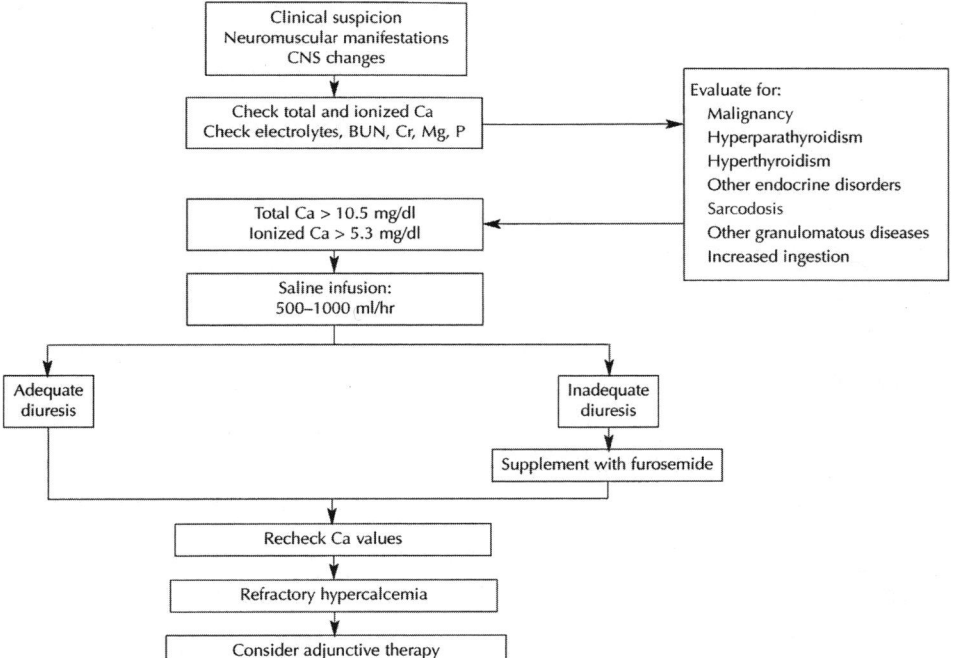

Figure 2 Treatment approach to hypercalcemia.

hypercalcemia associated with metastatic bone disease and postmenopausal osteoporosis (13). Generally, these agents require several hours to days to have an effect, but their use may be initiated, if needed, in conjunction with forced diuresis. Infrequently, calcium chelators such as EDTA and phosphates have been used for acute hypercalcemia, but they are not generally recommended. Calcium channel blockers such as verapamil may be of value for the treatment of life-threatening cardiovascular manifestations of hypercalcemia (2,5).

MAGNESIUM

Magnesium is distributed throughout the body, but approximately two-thirds of the body's magnesium is present in the skeleton. One-third of this magnesium is potentially available for exchange with the extracellular fluid. Most of the remaining magnesium is found intracellularly, where it represents the second most common intracellular cation after potassium. Again, only a portion of this intracellular magnesium is actually available for exchange with extracellular fluid, since much of the intracellular magnesium is complexed with proteins or phosphates. Approximately 1.3% of the body's magnesium is found in the extracellular fluid (2,14).

Although not readily available for clinical applications, methods using ion-specific electrodes, atomic absorption spectroscopy, and ultrafiltration allow measurement of both ionized and complexed plasma magnesium. Free magnesium makes up ∼67% of the total magnesium concentration, with 19% being complexed with proteins and 14% with smaller organic and inorganic ions (15). The normal total serum magnesium concentration is 1.7–2.4 mg/dL. However, serum concentrations of magnesium may not reflect total body magnesium stores, since much of the ion is present intracellularly. A normal serum magnesium concentration may mask a significant deficiency or excess of magnesium.

Plasma magnesium concentrations are regulated by some of the same factors, including PTH and vitamin D, that regulate calcium concentrations. In general, plasma magnesium concentrations are not as tightly regulated as are calcium concentrations. In adults, the average magnesium intake is 6–10 mg/kg per day (15). Magnesium is absorbed from the intestine by both vitamin D-dependent and vitamin D-independent transport systems (16). The amount of magnesium in the diet and the overall body stores of magnesium regulate the amount absorbed from the intestine (17). Plasma magnesium concentrations are primarily regulated by the kidney. Although both PTH and calcitriol promote tubular reabsorption of magnesium, the majority of magnesium reabsorption depends on intrinsic renal mechanisms, which are in turn regulated by the serum magnesium concentration. The glomerular filtration rate affects renal magnesium excretion and may account in part for the hypermagnesemia seen with renal failure (11). Evidence indicates that renal clearance of magnesium depends, at least in part, on the previously mentioned CaSR.

Patients with FHH who have mutation in the CaSR gene manifest reductions in renal clearance of magnesium in addition to PTH-independent hypocalciuric hypercalcemia (9).

Hypomagnesemia

Hypomagnesemia is a relatively common disorder that is found in 9–12% of hospitalized patients. The incidence of this disorder in the SICU may be substantially higher (2,18). Hypomagnesemia is usually due to inadequate uptake of magnesium from the gastrointestinal tract or due to increased losses of the ion from the kidneys or intestines. Malabsorption caused by bowel or pancreatic disease; gastrointestinal losses from fistulas, diarrhea, or prolonged nasogastric suction; and reduced intake from prolonged bowel rest without magnesium replacement may all lead to a magnesium deficiency. Increased renal losses are common with the use of diuretics and other drugs such as aminoglycosides and amphotericin B. Hypomagnesemia is also seen in alcoholics, in whom both gastrointestinal and renal causes may play a role in the development of deficiency. Nutritional repletion causes magnesium to shift intracellularly; thus an occult magnesium deficiency may become manifested in many patients when such repletion is undertaken (2,14,18,19).

The primary manifestations of magnesium deficiency are observed in the neuromuscular and cardiovascular systems. Hyperreflexia, tetany, and muscle spasms may be seen. Neurologic disturbances, such as disorientation, obtundation, and seizures also occur. Of greater importance are the cardiovascular manifestations. The ECG changes mimic those of hypokalemia and include QT prolongation, ST segment abnormalities, broadening of T-waves, and occasionally the development of U-waves. Myocardial irritability is increased, and frequent premature ventricular contractions are commonly seen. More severe dysrhythmias, such as ventricular tachycardia and ventricular fibrillation, may occur; these latter arrhythmias may be unresponsive to conventional antiarrhythmic therapy. Hypomagnesemia is also associated with other electrolyte abnormalities, such as hypocalcemia and hypokalemia, and with an anemia of unexplained origin (2,18).

Diagnosis is based on the serum magnesium concentration. However, magnesium deficiency is still possible even with a normal serum magnesium concentration, since the serum concentration may not accurately reflect intracellular stores. Serum calcium concentration, phosphorus concentration, standard electrolyte concentration, and renal function tests also should be checked once the diagnosis of hypomagnesemia has been entertained (Fig. 3).

Asymptomatic mild hypomagnesemia may be treated with parenteral administration of 2 g (8 mEq) of magnesium sulfate every 4–6 h or with oral supplements such as magnesium oxide, if the patient can tolerate them. Since magnesium equilibrates relatively slowly with the intracellular compartment, therapy may have to be continued for several days to adequately replace a significant deficiency (2). For maintenance purposes, patients receiving only parenteral fluids should receive 8–10 mEq of magnesium daily (12), and supplemental amounts should be given to patients with significant gastrointestinal or renal losses of the ion (2). Dysrhythmias and other manifestations of symptomatic magnesium deficiency may require more aggressive parenteral magnesium therapy. For severe hypomagnesemia, up to 6 g of magnesium sulfate or 5 g of magnesium chloride can be given intravenously over a 3 h period (2). For acute life-threatening dysrhythmias, 2–4 g of magnesium sulfate can be given over a 15 min period (18). In patients with normal serum magnesium concentrations, prophylactic treatment of dysrhythmias with 1 g of magnesium sulfate every 6 h has been used. This therapy has been recommended specifically for dysrhythmias associated with digitalis toxicity, those related to long QT intervals, and in patients with acute myocardial infarction (20,21).

Hypermagnesemia

Hypermagnesemia produces significant clinical problems much less commonly than does hypomagnesemia. Most often, hypermagnesemia is caused by renal failure. Occasionally,

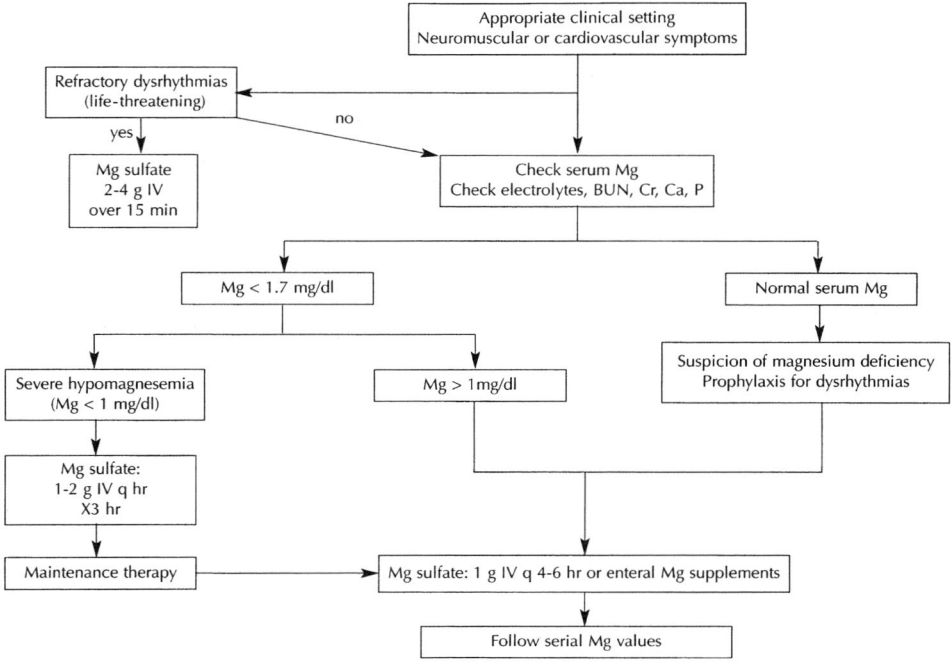

Figure 3 Treatment approach to hypomagnesemia.

hypermagnesemia is the result of iatrogenic administration. For instance, elevated serum magnesium concentrations are expected as part of the treatment of pre-eclampsia and eclampsia.

Symptoms of hypermagnesemia usually do not occur until serum magnesium concentrations approach 5 mg/dL. Above that point, muscle weakness becomes evident; with concentrations of 13 mg/dL, frank paralysis may be seen. CNS changes, including somnolence, are associated with magnesium concentrations of 9 mg/dL. ECG changes, such as prolonged PR, QRS, and ST intervals, may be seen at serum concentrations of 5–8 mg/dL. Bradycardia and hypotension become apparent as the serum magnesium concentration increases further. Heart block and cardiac arrest may occur when serum magnesium concentrations approach 20 mg/dL. Because of its effect on PTH release, hypermangnesemia may produce hypocalcemia. Nonspecific gastrointestinal symptoms (e.g., nausea, vomiting) also are associated with elevated serum magnesium concentrations.

For asymptomatic patients, treatment consists of restriction of magnesium-containing solutions and medications. For symptomatic patients, 100–200 mg of elemental calcium may be given to transiently block some of the effects of hypermagnesemia. Forced diuresis helps to remove excessive magnesium in patients with functioning kidneys. However, for patients with renal failure, hemodialysis may be the only method for treating acute hypermagnesemia.

PHOSPHORUS

Phosphorus is present in the body primarily as organic and inorganic phosphate. At physiologic pH, inorganic phosphate consists of a 4:1 mixture of monobasic (HPO_4^-) and dibasic ($H_2PO_4^{-2}$) forms of the ion. Approximately 80% of the body's phosphate is found in the skeleton, and most of the remaining phosphate is present intracellularly, where it represents the most common intracellular anion. A small fraction of the body's phosphate is present in the extracellular compartment. In the plasma, 85% of the inorganic phosphate is present as free ion, 5% is complexed with other cations, primarily magnesium and calcium, and 10% is bound to protein (22). The serum phosphorus concentration is used to measure the concentration of inorganic phosphate in the plasma (normal range, 2.7–4.5 mg/dL or 0.8–1.5 mmol/L) (2).

The serum phosphorus concentration is regulated by both the absorption of phosphate from the intestines and by the excretion of phosphate by the kidneys. Although intestinal absorption of phosphate is enhanced by vitamin D, adequate amounts of phosphate can usually be absorbed even in the presence of vitamin D deficiency. The kidneys play the primary role in the regulation of plasma phosphate. PTH sets the tubular maximum for phosphate reabsorption, but the intrinsic renal mechanisms also play a role in phosphate regulation. Serum phosphorus concentrations also are altered by intracellular shifting of the ion, which can be induced directly by insulin or produced indirectly by carbohydrate loading (2,22).

Hypophosphatemia

Although hypophosphatemia is another common disorder in the SICU, in many instances, it does not represent a true phosphorus deficiency. Hypophosphatemia may be observed in as many as 29% of postoperative patients (23). Hypophosphatemia occurs as part of the treatment or recovery from a number of conditions, including burns, sepsis, malnutrition, ketoacidosis, and hypothermia. Acute hypophosphatemia may be life-threatening in patients undergoing nutritional repletion following prolonged starvation ("refeeding syndrome"; see also Chapter 4). With these conditions, hypophosphatemia usually reflects a transcellular shift of phosphates rather than a true phosphate deficiency. Hypophosphatemia is also common among alcoholics and can occur with both acute alcohol intoxication (24) and chronic alcoholism (25). Other causes of hypophosphatemia include hyperparathyroidism, hypomagnesemia, and the administration of certain drugs that bind phosphates, such as antacids and sucralfate (2,26).

Hypophosphatemia rarely causes symptoms unless the serum phosphorus concentration is less than 2 mg/dL. Below this concentration, weakness, malaise, and anorexia may be observed. As the concentration approaches 1 mg/dL, muscle weakness becomes more pronounced, and clinical impairment in respiratory and cardiac function may be exhibited. With severe hypophosphatemia (<1 mg/dL), muscle cell injury and rhabdomyolysis may occur. Blood components also are affected by severe hypophosphatemia, which may produce platelet dysfunction, leukocyte dysfunction, and hemolysis. Because of the importance of phosphates in intermediary metabolism, hypophosphatemia also produces a host of metabolic abnormalities. The most common manifestations are insulin resistance and impaired glucose tolerance. Hypercalcemia and hypermagnesemia are both causes and consequences of hypophosphatemia (2,26).

Therapy of hypophosphatemia is based on the degree of the disorder (Fig. 4). With severe hypophosphatemia, intravenous phosphate preparations are the treatment of choice. Consensus on initial phosphate replacement has not yet been reached. Zaloga and Chernow (2) recommend an infusion of intravenous sodium or potassium phosphate at a rate of 0.6 mg (0.02 mmol)/kg per h for acute hypophosphatemia and an infusion of 0.9 mg (0.03 mmol)/kg per h in cases of chronic phosphorus depletion. Others have used infusions of as much as 0.25–0.5 mmol/kg of phosphate given over a 4 h period (27). In addition to phosphate replacement, agents contributing to hypophosphatemia, such as antacids and diuretics, should be stopped, and, if possible, glucose and insulin infusions should be curtailed. Serum phosphorus concentrations should be monitored frequently during phosphate replacement. Once a serum phosphorus concentration ≥2 mg/dL has been achieved, phosphorus supplementation should be continued by the enteral route, if possible. In cases of severe phosphorus deficiency, phosphate supplements should be continued for several days to adequately replete intracellular stores (2). In patients receiving TPN, ~30 mmol of phosphorus should be supplied per day for maintenance. Additional supplemental phosphorus may be needed for repletion of deficiencies or if acute refeeding syndrome develops (2,12).

Hyperphosphatemia

Renal failure is the most common cause of hyperphosphatemia, but it is occasionally observed with overvigorous administration of phosphate supplements, particularly in patients with borderline renal insufficiency. Hyperphosphatemia also is seen with disorders in which cell destruction occurs, such as rhabdomyolysis, hemolysis, malignant hyperthermia, and severe hypothermia, as well as with metabolic problems such as lactic acidosis. Rare causes of hyperphosphatemia include hypoparathyroidism, pseudohypoparathyroidism, and vitamin D excess (2,26).

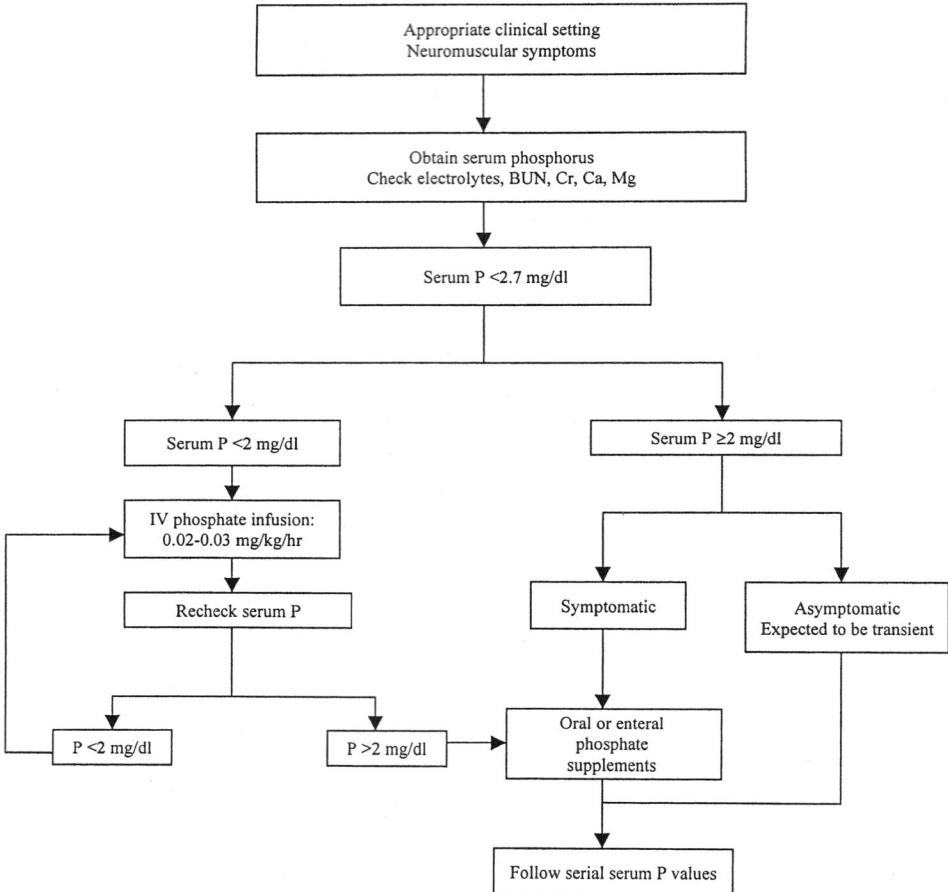

Figure 4 Treatment approach to hypophosphatemia.

Hyperphosphatemia usually produces relatively few symptoms. Symptoms usually are a result of metastatic calcifications, which may occur when the calcium–phosphorus product exceeds 75. Other acute symptoms are related to concomitant hypocalcemia. The latter symptoms represent the strongest indication for therapy (2,26).

Chronic treatment of hyperphosphatemia consists of controlling the absorption of phosphates from the gastrointestinal tract, usually by direct phosphate restriction and the use of oral phosphate binders. With acute hyperphosphatemia, treatment of the associated hypocalcemia is the first priority. However, the high phosphorus concentrations may make it difficult to provide adequate calcium supplementation. Under these circumstances, phosphate excretion can be promoted by saline diuresis and concomitant acetazolamide therapy in patients with normally functioning kidneys. In patients with renal failure, hemodialysis may be needed to assist phosphate removal. The effect of dialysis is usually transient: serum phosphorus concentrations typically rebound within a few hours as a consequence of phosphate release from intracellular stores (2,26).

SUMMARY

- Divalent ion abnormalities can cause cardiovascular and neuromuscular dysfunction.
- Routinely measure serum concentrations of calcium, magnesium, and phosphorus in most SICU patients.

Hypocalcemia

- Neuromuscular irritability, tetany, muscle spasms, paresthesis, Chvostek's sign, and Trouseau's sign suggest hypocalcemia.
- ECG changes include prolonged QT and ST intervals, T-wave changes, and ventricular dysrhythmias.
- Symptomatic hypocalcemia requires urgent treatment with intravenous calcium.
- Hypomagnesemia should be treated concomitantly.
- Asymptomatic, transient hypocalcemia may not require treatment.

Hypercalcemia

- Malignancy and immobilization are common causes of hypercalcemia.
- Weakness, hyporeflexia, and shortened QT interval suggest hypercalcemia.
- Acute symptomatic hypercalcemia is a medical emergency treated by forced diuresis.

Hypomagnesemia

- Hypomagnesemia is common in SICU patients. Many factors promote urinary and gastrointestinal losses of magnesium.
- Ventricular dysrhythmias are common and may include ventricular tachycardia and ventricular fibrillation.
- Magnesium deficiency may exist despite a normal serum magnesium concentration.
- Hypomagnesemia should be treated.
- Many cardiac dysrhythmias respond to magnesium treatment.

Hypermagnesemia

- Renal failure is the most common cause.
- Very high magnesium concentrations may produce muscle weakness and ECG changes.
- Magnesium restriction and dialysis are the mainstays of therapy.

Hypophosphatemia

- Phosphorus concentration ≥ 2 mg/dL rarely produce symptoms.
- Severe hypophosphatemia (<1 mg/dL) may result in rhabdomyolysis and respiratory or cardiac insufficiency.

- Acute, life-threatening hypophosphatemia may occur upon institution of nutritional repletion of the severely malnourished patient (refeeding syndrome).
- Use intravenous phosphorus replacement for severe hypophosphatemia; enteral phosphorus replacement may be used once serum phosphorus concentration is ≥2 mg/dL.

Hyperphosphatemia

- Renal failure is the most common cause.
- Restriction of phosphate intake and oral phosphate binders is the usual therapy.
- Associated hypocalcemia may require treatment.

REFERENCES

1. Bourdeau JE, Atttie MF. Calcium metabolism. In: Maxwell MH, Kleeman ER, Narin RG. eds. Clinical Disorders of Fluid and Electrolyte Metabolism 5th ed. New York: McGraw-Hill, 1994:243–306.
2. Zaloga GP, Chernow B. Divalent ions: calcium, magnesium, and phosphorus. In: Chernow B, Holaday JW, Zaloga GP, Zaritsky AL, eds. The Pharmacologic Approch to the Critically Ill Patient. Baltimore: Williams & Wilkins, 1988:603–636.
3. Ladenson JH, Lewis JW, Boyd JC. Failure of total calcium corrected per protein, albumin, and pH to correctly assess free calcium status. J Clin Endocrinol Metab 1978; 46:986–993.
4. Zaloga GP, Chernow B, Snyder R, Clapper M, O'Brian JC. Assessment of calcium homeostasis in the critically ill surgical patient. The diagnostic pitfalls of McLean–Hastings nomogram. Ann Surg 1985; 202:587–594.
5. Benabe JE, Martinez-Maldonado M. Disorders of calcium metabolism. In: Maxwell MH, Kleeman Er, Narins RG, eds. Clinical Disorders of Fluid and Electrolyte Metabolism 5th ed. New York: McGraw-Hill, 1994:1009–1044.
6. Zaloga GP, Chernow D. Hypocalcemia in critical illness. JAMA 1986; 256:1924–1929.
7. Brown EM, Vassilev PM, Hebert SC. Calcium ions as extracellular messengers. Cell 1955; 83:679–682.
8. Chattopadhyah N, Vassilev PM, Brown EM. Calcium-sensing receptor: roles in and beyond systemic calcium homeostasis. Biol Chem 1997; 378:759–768.
9. Hebert SC, Brown EM, Harris WM. Role of the Ca^{2+}-screening receptor in divalent mineral ion homeostasis. J Exp Biol 1997; 200:295–302.
10. Howland WS, Schweizer O, Carlon GC, Goldiner PL. The cardiovascular effect of low levels of ionized calcium during massive transfusion. Surg Gynecol Obstet 1977; 145:581–586.
11. Harrigan C, Lucas CE, Ledgerwood AM. Significance of hypocalcemia following hypovelmic shock. J Trauma 1983; 23:488–493.
12. Inadomi BW, Kopple JD. Fluid and electrolyte disorders in total parenteral nutrition. In: Maxwell MH, Kleeman ER, Narins RG, eds. Clinical Disorders of Fluid and Electrolyte Metabolism 5th ed. New York: McGraw-Hill, 1994:1437–1462.
13. Finely RS. Biophosphonates and the treatment of bone metastasis. Semin Oncol 2002; 29(suppl 4):132–138.
14. Quamme GA, Dirks JH. Magnesium metabolism. In: Maxwell MH, Kleeman ER, Narins RG, eds. Clinical Disorders of Fluid and Electrolyte Metabolism 5th ed. New York: McGraw-Hill, 1994:373–397.
15. Noronha JL, Matuschak GM. Magnesium in critical illness: metabolism, assessment, and treatment. Intensive Care Med, 2002; 28:667–679.

16. Lee C, Zaloga GP. Magnesium metabolism. Semin Respir Med 1985; 7:70–80.
17. Gums JG. Clinical significance of magnesium: a review. Drug Intell Clin Pharm 1987; 21:240–246.
18. Agus ZS, Massry SG. Hypomagnesemia and hypermagnesemia. In: Maxwell MH, Kleeman ER, Narins RG, eds. Clinical Disorders of Fluid and Electrolyte Metabolism 5th ed. New York: McGraw-Hill, 1994:1099–1119.
19. Rude RK, Singer FR. Magnesium deficiency and excess. Ann Rev Med 1981; 32:245–259.
20. Roden DM. Magnesium treatment of ventricular arrhythmias. Am J Cardiol 53:45G–46G.
21. Sheehan J. Importance of magnesium chloride repletion after myocardial infarction. Am J Cardiol 1989; 63:35G–38G.
22. Yonagawa N, Nakhoul F, Kurokawa K, Lee DBN. Physiology of phosphorus metablism. In: Maxwell MH, Kleeman ER, Narins RG, eds. Clinical Disorders of Fluid and Electrolyte metabolism 5th ed. New York: McGraw-Hill, 1994:307–371.
23. Swaminathan R, Bradley P, Morgan DB, Hill GL. Hypophosphatemia in surgical patients. Surg Gynecol Obstet 1979; 148:448–454.
24. Stein JH, Smith WO, Ginn HE. Hypophosphatemia in acute alcoholism. Am J Med Sci 1966; 252:78–83.
25. Territo MC, Tanaka KR. Hypophosphatemia in chronic alcoholism. Arch Intern Med 1974; 134:445–447.
26. Levine BS, Kleeman CR. Hypophosphatemia and hyperphosphatemia: clinical and pathophysiologic aspects. In: Maxwell MH, Kleeman ER, Narins RG, eds. Clinical Disorders of Fluid and Electrolyte Metabolism 5th ed. New York: McGraw-Hill, 1994:1045–1097.
27. Kingston M, Al-Siba'r MB. Treatment of severe hypophosphatemia. Crit Care Med 1985; 13:16–18.

44
Chemical Homeostasis

Roderick A. Barke
VA Medical Center, Minneapolis, Minnesota, USA

BODY COMPARTMENTS AND DISTRIBUTION OF WATER AND ELECTROLYTES

Insight into the normal distribution of water and electrolytes in the unstressed state is necessary for an understanding of disordered fluid and electrolyte balance in the critically ill patient. The distribution of the extracellular fluid (ECF) and intracellular fluid (ICF) spaces in the normal state is described by the Yannet–Darrow diagram, as is the normal electrolyte distribution of the plasma and ICF (Fig. 1). Normal fluid homeostasis

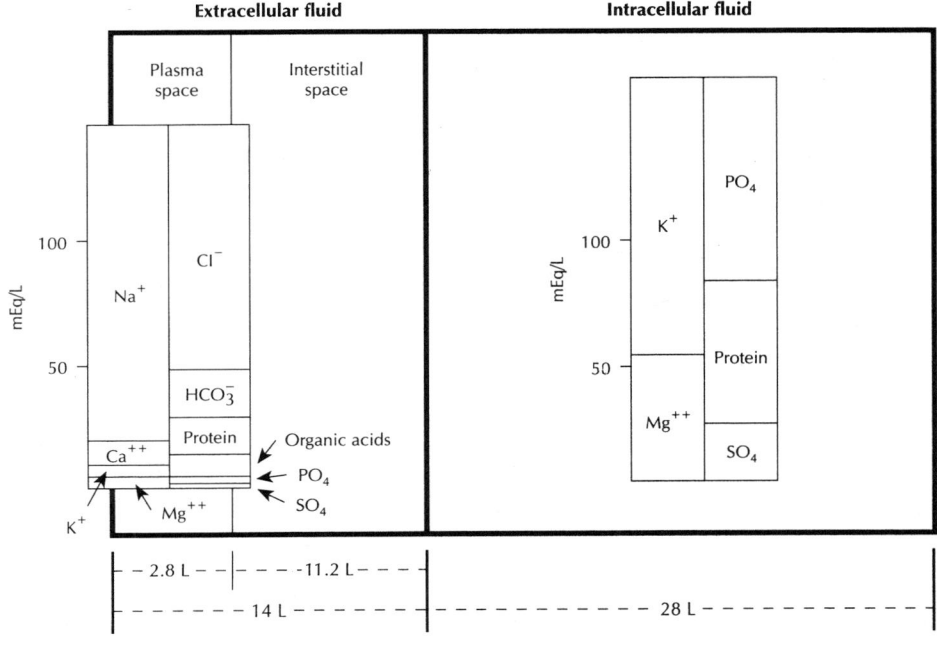

Figure 1 Yannet–Darrow diagram of distribution of ECF and ICF volumes in the normal state. Values are for a 70 kg person with 60% water content.

Table 1 Fluid Balance in the Normal State

Input	Amount (mL)	Output	Amount (mL)
Oral fluid	1300–2300	Urine	800–1600
Water of oxidation	300	Feces	100
		Insensible loss	
		Skin	300–400
		Respiratory	300–400
		Sweat	100
Total gain	1600–2600	Total loss	1600–2600

assumes both the ability to take fluid orally as desired and normal kidney function. Assuming normal activity, temperature, and humidity, fluid balance for a 70 kg adult in the normal state is outlined in Table 1. Critical illness alters the input–output equation, with resultant effects on volume, concentration, and composition of the body compartments. For example, insensible respiratory-free water loss effectively is minimized during mechanical ventilation. Common measurable losses in terms of GI secretions are outlined in Table 2. The mechanisms by which injury alters salt and water balance during critical illness, surgery, and trauma are important in managing critically ill patients.

EFFECT OF STRESS OF SURGERY OR TRAUMA ON FLUID HOMEOSTASIS

Although anesthesia alone is associated with decreased renal plasma flow, glomerular filtration rate (GFR), and urinary volume, the anesthesia-related renal effects return to normal rapidly after the termination of anesthesia. The addition of a surgical procedure to the effect of anesthesia markedly alters the homeostatic response. The depression in renal function that results in salt and water retention lengthens and persists 3–10 days. Compromise of renal function depends on the magnitude of the stress. The retention of sodium and water after surgery and trauma has been attributed to a change in the hormonal environment following stress. However, the relationship between the alterations in salt and water physiology and the associated change in the hormonal environment do not fully answer the question of whether surgical stress results in an obligate hormonal response with increased production of 17-hydroxycorticosteroids, aldosterone, and antidiuretic

Table 2 Composition of Common Gastrointestinal Secretions

Secretion	Sodium (mEq/L)	Potassium (mEq/L)	Chloride (mEq/L)	HCO_3^- (mEq/L)
Saliva	10	20	15	30
Stomach	30–90	4–12	50–150	0
Pancreatic	135–155	4–6	60–110	70–90
Bile	135–155	4–6	80–110	35–50
Jejunal	70–125	3.5–6.5	70–125	10–20
Ileostomy	90–140	4–10	60–125	15–50
Diarrhea	25–50	35–60	20–40	35–45

hormone (ADH). Rather, the major factor may relate to a redistribution of the ECF to the ICF and interstitial space. The next section reviews the evolution of present thinking on this relationship.

Evolution of Understanding of Hormonal Response

At the time of Coller and Hardy (1–3), surgeons thought that surgical stress or trauma evoked an adrenocortical response, the so-called classic stress response. This concept led to a recommendation that salt and water be restricted after surgical stress. Further study of the adrenal response to surgery and trauma led to remarkable contradictory data challenging this concept. Although some temporal correlation between the alteration in renal fluid and electrolyte handling and 17-hydroxycorticosteroid response exists, the correlation was out of phase with respect to the real-time retention of salt and water after injury. In fact, data from animals (4) or Addisonian patients (5) who had undergone an adrenalectomy suggested that an increased 17-hydroxycorticosteroid response was not necessary for poststress fluid and sodium retention. These and other data cast doubt on 17-hydroxycorticosteroid response as a principal mechanism of altered renal response after injury. The discovery of aldosterone and insight into the renin–angiotensin–aldosterone response provided another possible mechanism for altered renal function after stress. On careful analysis, although the adosterone level increases after surgery or trauma, the temporal relationship between plasma aldosterone concentration and renal salt and water retention correlated only initially during the postoperative course (6–8). As in the 17-hydroxycorticosteroid case, patients who had undergone an adrenalectomy had a degree of fluid and electrolyte retention similar to that of normal patients. These findings suggest that a factor other than aldosterone may be active. ADH was an attractive possibility. Although ADH activity was noted to increase after stress, data collected from surgical patients with diabetes insipidus suggested the renal fluid-handling after stress was not wholly consistent with increased ADH activity alone (9–11). These data suggested that the altered renal response to stress should not be interpreted solely as an adrenocortical response to injury, but that it may represent a homeostatic mechanism in response to a deficit in ECF volume.

The thesis that inadequate resuscitation in response to injury decreases plasma volume and renal plasma flow by internal redistribution of fluid to the interstitial space and ICF space was tested using numerous dilution techniques. The measurement of the functional ECF volume (FECV), as determined by the sulfate dilution equilibrium volume after hemorrhagic shock and resuscitation (12), demonstrated that simple isovolemic replacement on the basis of shed blood led to a marked deficit in FECV. These and other studies suggested the adrenal response to surgical stress and trauma may be secondary to decreased circulating plasma volume and could not be assumed to be strictly an adrenal phenomenon. Currently, fluid therapy after injury should be directed at repletion of the fluid internally redistributed plus insensible and sensible losses.

This discussion may be expanded from surgery or trauma to critical illness in general. Critical illness such as sepsis, unrelated to operative or traumatic injury, can result in a loss of ECF to the ICF and interstitial spaces by altering endothelial and cell membrane permeabilities. This mechanism results in a similar condition of low renal plasma flow from both decreased circulating plasma volume and depleted FECV. The approach to fluid and electrolyte therapy in critical illness, in general, should also correct possible losses, insensible losses, and internally redistributed fluid.

Table 3 Crystalloid Solutions

Solutions	Glucose (g/L)	Sodium (mEq/L)	Chloride (mEq/L)	Potassium (mEq/L)	Calcium (mEq/L)	Lactate (mEq/L)
D5%/W	50					
D10%/W	100					
D5%/0.2% NaCl	50	34	34			
D5%/0.33% NaCl	50	56	56			
D5%/0.45% NaCl	50	77	77			
D5%/0.9% NaCl	50	154	154			
0.9% NaCl		154	154			
Lactated Ringer's		130	109	4	3	28
3% NaCl		513	513			

Table 4 Colloid Solutions

Solutions	Glucose (g/L)	Sodium (mEq/L)	Chloride (mEq/L)
5% Albumin	5	130–160	130–160
25% Albumin	25	130–160	130–160
5% Hetastarch	5	154	154

GOAL OF FLUID AND ELECTROLYTE THERAPY

From the foregoing discussion, a proper treatment plan after injury or critical illness should restore renal plasma flow by replacement of the FECV deficit. Intravenous replacement solutions, the tools available to accomplish this goal, may be divided into crystalloid or colloid groups. Table 3 lists commonly used crystalloid solutions. Colloid solutions are used for special purposes as indicated in the management of fluid and electrolytes. Table 4 lists commonly used colloid solutions. Fluid and electrolyte therapy may be analyzed further according to disorders common to the critical care setting.

HYPEROSMOLALITY, HYPERTONICITY, AND HYPERNATREMIA

Although both osmolality and tonicity describe plasma solute concentration, they represent fundamentally different concepts that are important to the understanding of altered fluid and electrolyte homeostasis. Osmolality is defined as the number of osmoles per kilogram of water and includes substances, such as urea, that equilibrate across cell membranes. Tonicity excludes these substances. Osmotic concentration can be measured directly by freezing point depression or vapor pressure measurement or indirectly by using the serum sodium concentration. The relationship of serum sodium concentration to water balance makes several important assumptions:

- The total amount of crystalloids is constant. Important exceptions include hyperglycemia and azotemia.

Chemical Homeostasis

- No significant water-insoluble substances exist in the plasma. Clinical exceptions include hyperproteinemia (e.g., with multiple myeloma) or hyperlipidemia.
- The relationship of sodium ions to total cations is normal (normal ratio, 142 mEq of sodium ions to 155 mEq total cations).

With these assumptions, the plasma osmolarity can be estimated from measurement of plasma sodium, glucose, and BUN concentration by using the following equation:

$$\text{Serum osmolarity (mOsm/L)} = 2Na^+ (mEq/L)_{plasma} + \frac{\text{Glucose (mg\%)}}{18} + \frac{\text{BUN (mg\%)}}{2.8}$$

Assuming no other osmotically active solutes, the measured osmolarity will be <10 mOsm/L greater than the calculated osmolarity. Although plasma osmolarity can be calculated in hyperproteinemic and hyperlipidemic states, plasma osmometry should be performed if the diagnosis of a hypertonic or hypotonic (the most common cause) state will be seriously considered.

Sodium and glucose are distributed in the ECF, whereas urea is distributed in total body water. Solute can be classified as "effective" or "ineffective." Effective solute is distributed only in the ECF, whereas ineffective solute is distributed in total body water. Effective solutes include sodium, glucose, mannitol, and glycerol. Ineffective solutes include urea, ethanol, methanol, and ethylene glycol. Tonicity is calculated by modifying the previous equation as follows:

$$\text{Serum tonicity (mOsm/L)} = 2Na^+ (mEq/L)_{plasma} + \frac{\text{Glucose (mg\%)}}{18}$$

The distinction between osmolality and tonicity is important to differentiate a hyperosmolar, hypertonic state from a hyperosmolar, nonhypertonic state. In the hyperosmolar, hypertonic state, ICF water is redistributed to the ECF. Consequently, the ICF compartment decreases in size. The signs and symptoms of a decreased ICF compartment are a consequence of cellular dehydration and are expressed primarily as neurologic signs and symptoms (e.g., weakness progressing to lethargy, disorientation or delusional states, obtundation, coma) (13). Acute rapid changes in ICF can result in mechanical disruption of the cerebral blood vessels (i.e., subarachnoid and subcortical hemorrhage).

To compensate for changes in osmolality, the brain generates "idiogenic osmols," which are isolated to the brain. These idiogenic osmols represents a partial compensation for the changes in brain parenchymal volume and occur within hours (hyperglycemia) to days (hypernatremia) of the onset of the abnormal tonicity. In the hyperosmolar, nonhypertonic state, the change in ICF volume is minimized. As the solute is distributed in total body water, CNS alteration is produced by the solute toxicity itself (i.e., ethanol) and not by the change in the ICF volume.

Hyperosmolar, hypertonic states can result from pure water loss, hypotonic water loss, or an increase in effective solute. Pure water loss results in a decrease in both the ICF and the ECF, according to the distribution of solute. Pure water loss can result from exaggerated insensible losses through the skin and lungs as a result of environmental conditions or extensive burns, hyperpyrexia, or mechanical hyperventilation. As critically ill patients generally cannot correct losses through thirst mechanisms, careful monitoring is necessary in patients with these conditions to prevent and correct fluid loss.

Another cause of almost pure water loss is diabetes insipidus—either central or nephrogenic (Fig. 2). Central diabetes insipidus can occur as a result of blunt head trauma, anoxic encephalopathy, vascular disorders (e.g., intraventricular hemorrhage, cerebral aneurysms), hypophysectomy, brain tumors (especially metastatic breast cancer), infectious causes (e.g., encephalitis, meningitis), or drug use (e.g., ethanol, opiate antagonist, clonidine). The presentation of central diabetes insipidus may be partial or complete. With access to water as desired, patients who are affected with complete central diabetes insipidus generally have urinary osmolality <100 mOsm/L and massive polyuria (14).

Nephrogenic diabetes insipidus results from insufficient water conservation by the kidney despite a normal ADH signal (15). Nephrogenic diabetes insipidus can result

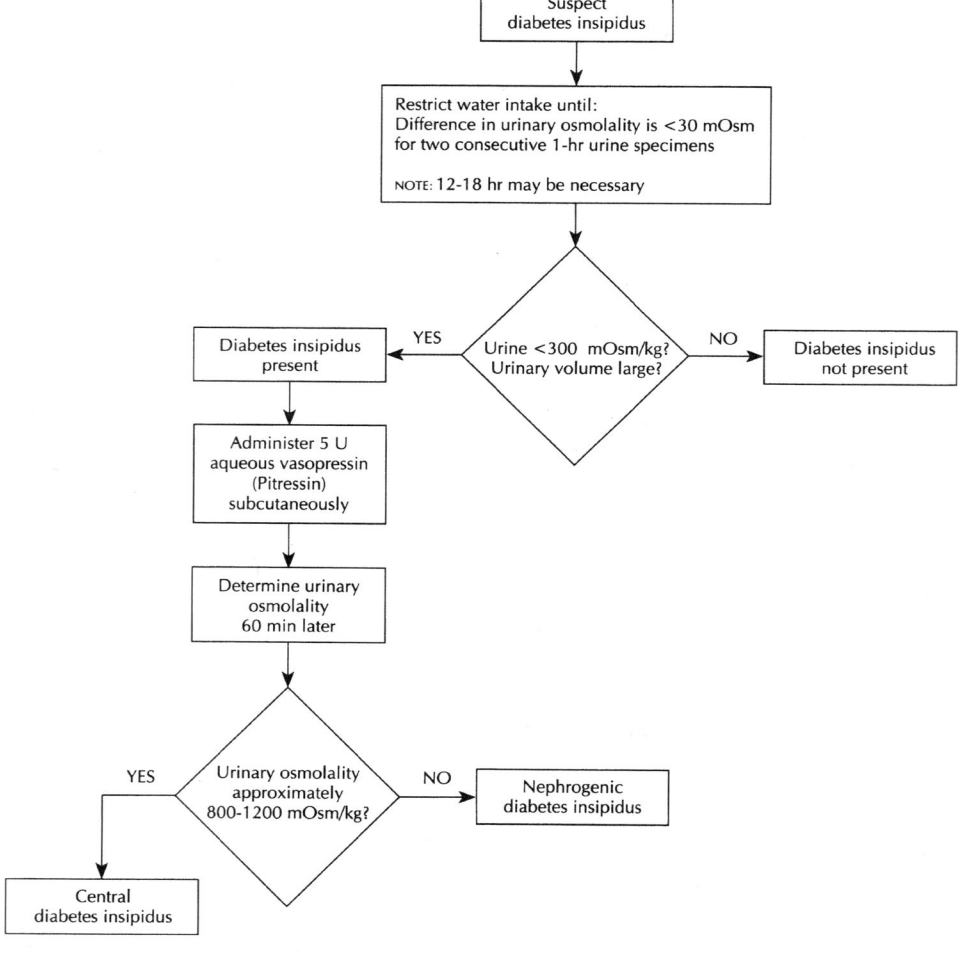

Figure 2 Diagnosis of diabetes insipidus.

from interruption of the normal corticomedullary gradient or from acquired insensitivity of the distal tubule and collecting duct to ADH. Interruption of the normal corticomedullary gradient occurs with protein or caloric malnutrition, diuretic use, and renal failure. Acquired insensitivity to ADH can result from nephrotoxic drugs (e.g., aminoglycosides), hypercalcemia, and hypokalemia. The diagnosis of either nephrogenic or central diabetes insipidus is made clinically under the conditions of controlled dehydration. Demonstration of inappropriate urinary volume and hypo-osmolality (<200 mOsm/kg) in the presence of increasing plasma hyperosmolality (>300 mOsm/kg) over the period of 12–18 h confirms the presence of diabetes insipidus.

Differentiation of nephrogenic diabetes insipidus from central diabetes insipidus is made by administration of aqueous vasopressin (Pitressin) (5 U SC). In patients with central diabetes insipidus, urinary osmolality will concentrate to 800–1200 mOsm/kg after vasopressin administration, whereas in patients with nephrogenic diabetes insipidus, little or no increase in urinary osmolality occurs. Compromised renal function may make the diagnosis of diabetes insipidus difficult, as the usual endpoints cannot be reached.

The time needed for rehydration of the patient with pure water loss should approximate the time it took to develop the dehydrated state. Too rapid and potentially hazardous volume loading must be avoided. The volume loss is approximated as follows (16):

$$\text{Water deficit (L)} = 0.6 \text{ Body weight (kg)} \times \left(\frac{\text{Plasma Na}^+(\text{mEq/L})}{140 \text{ mEq/L}} - 1 \right)$$

The first half of the calculated deficit is administered over one-third of the interval thought to produce the dehydration. Electrolyte values are measured at the end of this period, and the water deficit again is calculated at this time.

Hypotonic fluid losses result in marked decreases in the ECF and in plasma volume. As opposed to pure water loss, hypotonic fluid loss is associated with hypovolemia, hypotension, tachycardia, azotemia, and oliguria. Renal mechanisms are the most common causes of the clinical findings that occur with hypotonic losses. Hyperglycemia (e.g., hyperosmolar hyperglycemic nonketotic coma), polyuric acute tubular necrosis, postobstructive uropathy, loop diuretic administration, or mannitol administration is commonly implicated. Urinary losses are diagnosed by measuring the urinary sodium concentration. Generally, for hypotonic fluid loss of renal origin, the sodium concentration is >40 mEq/L, and for that of nonrenal origin it is <20 mEq/L. Hypovolemia and hypotension are corrected by replacement of volume deficits; hypertonicity is corrected once the volume deficit is corrected.

The most common cause of hypertonicity (effective solute gain) is hypernatremia (Table 5) resulting from the administration of sodium bicarbonate during cardiac arrest. The osmolal gap (osmolality minus tonicity) is <10 mOsm/kg in this state. Another cause for hypertonic solute gain is the treatment of cerebral edema with administration of mannitol or glycerol. In this state, the osmolal gap is >10 mOsm/kg, as mannitol or glycerol is usually an unaccounted effective solute. The administration of osmotic diuretics results in further hypotonic fluid loss and increased hypertonicity.

Finally, hyperosmolality without hypertonicity is by default associated with the presence of an ineffective solute such as azotemia that complicates acute renal failure. In the proper clinical context in patients with increased plasma osmolality, normal tonicity, an osmolal gap >10 mOsm/kg, and the presence of a BUN concentration <40 mg%,

Table 5 Causes and Treatment of Hypernatremia

Water loss	Hypotonic fluid loss	Effective solute increases
Mechanism		
Renal losses	Renal loses	Hypertonic sodium and sodium bicarbonate
Diabetes insipidus	Acute tubular necrosis with polyuria	Primary hyperaldosteronism
Central	Postobstructive uropathy	Cushing's syndrome
Nephrogenic	Loop diuretics	
	Mannitol	
Increased insensible losses		
Burns		
Respiratory infection or injury		
Fever		
Treatment		
Judicious water replacement	Hypotonic saline solution replacement	Diuretics and judicious water replacement

ingestion of ethanol, methanol, or ethylene glycol is suspected because these solutes distribute in total body water.

Hypo-Osmolality and Hyponatremia

Water excess is produced when either excess water is administered or renal water clearance is insufficient [e.g., in a patient with syndrome of inappropriate antidiuretic hormone (SIADH)]. The symptoms of water intoxication are related to the shifting of water from the ECF space into the ICF space. In a closed space such as the skull, the edema produced can be life-threatening. The symptoms of hypotonicity are, consequently, mainly neurologic and ophthalmologic:

> *Neurologic*: headache, nausea and vomiting, muscle fasciculation, hyperactive reflexes (early), loss of reflexes (late), obtundation, convulsions, and hypertension or bradycardia
> *Ophthalmologic*: blurred vision, blindness, and papilledema

The severity of symptoms is related more to the rate at which the hypotonicity is produced than to the serum sodium concentration. The more gradual the process, the more mild are the signs and symptoms. In addition, the hypotonic state is almost never one of pure water excess at a constant solute concentration. Mixed states are the rule rather than the exception. The differential diagnosis of hypotonic states common to the SICU includes the following:

- The administration of excess hypotonic fluid during states with excess ADH (e.g., in the postoperative period with inadequate resuscitation)
- SIADH (e.g., with carcinoma of the lung, Hodgkin's disease, leukemia, CNS disorders)
- Hypertonic fluid loss with hypotonic fluid replacement
- The clinical use of oxytocin
- Patients admitted to the SICU with cardiovascular or hypertensive diagnoses who are receiving diuretic therapy

Table 6 Causes and Treatment of Hyponatremia

Mechanism	ECF changes	Causes	Urinary sodium	Treatment
Excess total body water	ECF increase, no edema	SIADH Glucocorticoid insufficiency Thyroid insufficiency	>20 mg/L	Water restriction

Total body water deficit and larger total body sodium deficit	ECF volume depletion	Renal
		  Diuretics
		  Mineralocorticoid insufficiency
		  Salt-wasting nephropathy
		  Renal tubular acidosis
		  Osmotic diuresis
		Nonrenal
		  Vomiting
		  Diarrhea
		  Third-space losses
			Renal, >20 mg/L,
			Nonrenal, <10 mg/L
				Isotonic saline solution

Total body sodium excess and larger total body water excess	ECF increase, edema	CHF Cirrhosis Nephrotic syndrome Chronic renal failure	<10 mg/L If chronic renal failure, >20 mg/L	Water restriction

Source: Modified from Berl T, Anderson RJ, McDonald KM, et al. Clinical disorders of water metabolism. Kidney Int 1976; 10:117–132.

In some conditions, such as pregnancy, mild to moderate hypotonicity is a normal response and requires no action by the physician. The diagnosis is established by evidence of hypotonicity (decreased osmolality) and hyponatremia (Table 6). Other laboratory findings are of little value unless one of the previously mentioned conditions is present. Treatment depends on the severity of the symptoms and the acid–base disorder present in association with the dilutional disorder. In many cases simple water restriction is all that is required. In moderate to severe situations, hypertonic salt solution may be given. Generally, the hypotonic state should be corrected over a length of time similar to that which produced the hypotonic state. Rapid correction of a hypotonic state can be lethal and must be avoided. The serum concentration should not be increased more than 2 mEq/L per h unless severe symptoms exist (convulsions). In the presence of normal acid–base balance, a mixture of 3% normal saline solution and sodium lactate solution, in equal volumes, may be given. In the presence of alkalosis, a 3% normal saline solution should be administered. With acidosis, 0.5 or 1 M sodium lactate may be given in an equal volume mixture with 3% normal saline solution. Critically ill patients may not tolerate the fluid shifts that result from hypertonic fluid loading, and another strategy should be used. One such strategy uses a loop diuretic (e.g., furosemide) and replaces the urinary loss with hypertonic saline solution, while cardiovascular status is carefully monitored.

Potassium

Hyperkalemia and hypokalemia are common electrolyte disturbances in the critically ill. Hypokalemia is common in the SICU and can result from many causes, including the following:

- Nasogastric suction, which removes gastric secretion containing ~20 mEq/L potassium
- Insulin-mediated glucose transport and glycogen synthesis, which involve an obligate intracellular potassium store (i.e., the treatment of diabetic hyperglycemia and ketoacidosis)
- Alkalosis, which results in a shift of potassium from the ECF to the ICF. Gastrointestinal losses (e.g., from diarrhea, ileostomy), pancreatic juice losses (pancreatic fistula), and biliary losses (biliary fistula, T-tube drainage), which can contain 5–15 mEq/L of potassium

Renal losses of potassium are prominent: (1) because obligate urinary potassium losses occur even in the presence of hypokalemia, and (2) because of the frequent use of thiazide and loop diuretics. Hypokalemia can be secondary to other electrolyte disorders such as hypomagnesemia. Beta-adrenergic agonists decrease serum potassium through beta-2-mediated stimulation of cellular potassium uptake. Epinephrine therapy in patients with acute myocardial infarction or terbutaline–albuterol therapy in obstetric patients with premature labor has been associated with hypokalemia.

Hyperkalemia can occur from: (1) a shift of potassium from the ICF to the ECF, as in acidosis; (2) massive cell lysis (chemotherapy with extensive rapid cell death); (3) rhabdomyolysis (crush injury and extreme exercise); (4) rapid hemolysis; and (5) iatrogenic mechanisms. Finally, the most common cause of hyperkalemia in the critically ill is renal failure.

The signs and symptoms of hypokalemia may be subtle and depend on whether the deficit is acute or chronic. The clinical signs and symptoms of hypokalemia are as follows:

Cardiovascular: depression of the ST segment; lengthening of the PR interval; flattening or inversion of the T-wave; presence of a U-wave; widening of the QRS complex; ventricular fibrillation; cardiac arrest with the heart in diastole
Gastrointestinal: paralytic ileus
Renal: impaired ability to concentrate urine; increased hepatic encephalopathy (increased renal ammoniagenesis)
Skeletal muscle: weakness; decreased reflexes
Metabolic: glucose intolerance
Central nervous system: confusion

In patients with chronic hypokalemia the ECG signs are often absent, and skeletal muscle weakness is the most prominent finding. Knowledge of the nature of the signs and symptoms and the magnitude of the potassium deficit are needed to treat hypokalemia. Treatment of serious cardiac or neurologic signs constitutes an emergency. However, the calculation of the actual potassium deficit is at best a crude estimation, as total potassium stores and serum potassium concentration can vary independently. As mentioned previously, severe hypokalemia often is accompanied by metabolic alkalosis from renal tubular conservation of potassium and obligate retention of bicarbonate.

Thus, the more profound the metabolic alkalosis, the greater is the potassium deficit. It is better to know that hypokalemia with metabolic alkalosis is often associated with a deficit as large as 450–600 mEq of potassium than to use one of the many mathematic approaches to the calculation of the potassium deficit based on serum potassium and serum pH levels. In patients with severe hypokalemia, treatment should be parenteral through a centrally placed catheter with cardiac monitoring. In the critically ill adult patient, 20 mEq of potassium chloride in 100 mL of 0.9% normal saline solution may be administered safely over 1 h. Infusions >20 mEq potassium chloride over 1 h periods must be administered only with great care and monitoring in patients with severe symptomatic hypokalemia. Obtaining serial measurements of serum potassium concentration is imperative.

Certain special situation should be noted in the treatment of hypokalemia. Hypokalemia in the presence of metabolic acidosis should be treated before treatment of the acid–base disorder, as bicarbonate therapy will exacerbate the potassium deficit. Digoxin inhibits the transport of potassium into the cell. Patients receiving cardiac glycoside therapy are more likely to have transient hyperkalemia during potassium administration. Potassium administration in the patient with impaired renal function must be done with extreme caution.

The clinical signs and symptoms of hyperkalemia are as follows:

Cardiovascular (in order of appearance): peaking of the T-wave; prolonged PR interval, widening of the QRS complex, loss of the P-wave; "sine-wave" configuration; ventricular fibrillation or cardiac arrest with asystole

Renal: decreased renal ammoniagenesis and mild metabolic hyperchloremic acidosis

Skeletal muscle: weakness progressing to flaccid paralysis; decreased reflexes

As with hypokalemia, the treatment of hyperkalemia should be matched to the severity of the signs and symptoms. Emergency treatment is necessary if ECG signs of hyperkalemia are present (independent of the serum potassium concentration) or if the serum potassium concentration is >6 mEq/L. Treatment of hyperkalemia is divided into several categories: membrane antagonism, temporary potassium redistribution, and potassium removal. The mainstay of membrane antagonism is calcium treatment (gluconate or chloride, 10–20 mL IV of 10% solution). The effect is immediate, and calcium adminstration should be the initial treatment unless special circumstances such as cardiac glycoside therapy or associated hypercalcemia exist. Temporary redistribution of potassium from the ECF to the ICF is accomplished with either sodium bicarbonate (50–150 mEq IV over 5 min) or insulin–glucose therapy (10 U regular insulin in 50 mL $D_{50}W$ over 30–60 min). Temporary redistribution by these methods results in an onset of action of 5–30 min, with a duration of action of $\sim$1–2 h in the case of bicarbonate therapy or 4–6 h with insulin–glucose therapy. Profound alkalosis, hyperglycemia, or hypoglycemia would limit such therapy. The foregoing treatments provide only a temporary reprieve from severe hyperkalemia. These treatments must be followed by potassium removal. Potassium elimination is accomplished by diuretic therapy [furosemide, 40–80 mg IV, or bumetanide (Bumex), 1–2 mg IV], use of cationic exchange resins [sodium polystyrene sulfonate (Kayexalate), 50 g in 500–1000 cc 70% sorbitol solution orally or as a retention enema], and dialysis (hemodialysis or peritoneal dialysis) (see Box 1).

Box 1 Treatment of Hyperkalemia

Membrance antagonism
Calcium gluconate or calcium chloride, 10–20 mL 10% solution IV
Temporary redistribution of potassium from ECF to ICF
Sodium bicarbonate, 50–150 mEq IV over 5 min
Insulin and glucose, 10 U regular insulin in 50 mL $D_{50}W$ IV over 30–60 min
Potassium removal
Dialysis
Cationic exchange resins (sodium sulfonate, 50 g in 500–1000 mL 70% sorbitol solution orally or as retention enema)
Diuretic therapy

SUMMARY

- Anesthesia and surgery result in salt and water retention. Corticosteroid, aldosterone, and ADH increases exist after surgery, but they do not fully explain salt and water retention.
- A major goal of fluid therapy is replacement of the FECV deficit to restore renal and other organ perfusion.
- Hyperosmolar, hypertonic states result from pure water loss, hypotonic water loss, or effective solute increase (see Table 5).
- Pure water loss can result from diabetes insipidus (see Fig. 2).
- Excess water administration or deficient renal water clearance causes hyponatremic, hypotonic states. Hyponatremia should be corrected gradually (increase sodium not more than 2 mEq/L/h unless severe symptoms exist).
- Treat hypokalemia before metabolic acidosis when both conditions exist. Use caution when administering potassium to patients with renal failure.
- Treatment of hyperkalemia includes memberane antagonism, potassium redistribution, or potassium removal (see Box 1).

REFERENCES

1. Coller FA, Campbell KN, Vaughan HH, et al. Postoperative salt intolerance. Ann Surg 1944; 119:533.
2. Hardy J. The role of the adrenal cortex in the postoperative retention of salt and water. Ann Surg 1950; 132:189.
3. Hardy J, Ravdin I. Some physiological aspects of surgical trauma. Ann Surg 1952; 136:345.
4. Ingle DJ, Meeks RC, Thomas KE. The effect of fractures upon urinary electrolytes in non-adrenalectomized and in adrenalectomized rats treated with adrenal cortex extract. Endocrinology 1951; 49:703.
5. Rosenbaum JD, Paper S, Ashley MM. Variation in renal excretion of sodium independent of change in adrenocortical hormone dosage in patients with Addison's disease. J Clin Endocrinol Metabol 1955; 15:1459.
6. Moran WH Jr, Rosenberg JC, Schloff L, et al. The relationship of adrenal steroids to postoperative electrolyte metabolism. Surgery 1959; 46:109.

7. Jepson RP, Jordon A, Levell MJ, et al. Metabolic response to adrenalectomy. Ann Surg 1957; 145:1.
8. Mason AS. Metabolic response to total adrenalectomy and hypophysectomy. Lancet 1955; 2:632.
9. Ariel IM. Effects of a water load administered to patients during the immediate postoperative period. Arch Surg 1951; 62:303.
10. Kennedy JH, Sabga GA, Hopkins RW, et al. Urine volume and osmolality. Arch Surg 1964; 88:155.
11. Hayes MA, Coller RA. The neuroendocrine control of water and electrolyte excretion during surgical anesthesia. Surg Gynecol Obstet 1952; 95:142.
12. Shires GT, Carrico CT, Cohn D. The role of extracellular fluid in shock. Int Anesthesiol Clin 1964; 2:435.
13. Feig PU, McCurdy DK. The hypertonic state. N Engl J Med 1977; 297:1444–1454.
14. Miller M, Dalakos T, Moses Am, et al. Recognition of partial defects in antidiuretic hormone secretion. Ann Intern Med 1970; 73:731–729.
15. Cox M, Geheb M, Singer I. Disorders of thirst and renal water excretion. In: Arieff AL, DeFronzo RA, eds. Fluid, Electrolyte, and Acid–Base Disorders. New York: Churchill Livingstone, 1985, 119–183.
16. Geheb MA. Clinical approach to the hyperosmolar patient. Crit Care Clin 1987; 3:805.

SUGGESTED READING

Bernards WC. Fluid therapy in surgery, shock, and trauma: an historical survey. Crit Care Updates 1991; 2:1–9.
Vanatta JC, Fogelman MJ. Moyer's Fluid Balance, A Clinical Manual, 4th ed. Chicago, IL: Year Book Medical Publishers, 1988.

I. Infectious Diseases

45

Antibiotic Resistance in the Intensive Care Unit

Jan E. Patterson
University of Texas at San Antonio, San Antonio, Texas, USA

Daniel L. Dent
University of Texas Health Science Center at San Antonio, San Antonio, Texas, USA

INTRODUCTION

The problem of antimicrobial resistance has increased significantly in the past decade and is now a major issue in most hospitals. A number of factors magnify this problem in the intensive care unit (ICU). These factors include the multiple invasive devices and procedures predisposing the ICU patient to infection, the widespread use of broad-spectrum antibiotics, lapse of infection control technique in the care of critically ill patients, and economic pressures that lead to understaffing. Antimicrobial resistance is a greater urgency for those multidrug-resistant organisms for which only a few antibiotic alternatives remain, such as vancomycin-resistant *Enterococci* and carbapenem-resistant *Acinetobacter baumannii*. Multiple drug resistance also increases health care costs, adds isolation precautions to the care of an already complicated patient, and results in inadequate empiric therapy that increases mortality. Understanding the current problems of antibiotic resistance will enhance the care and management of individual patients with these organisms in the ICU and lead to better prevention and control measures to decrease the prevalence of this problem.

EPIDEMIOLOGY OF ANTIMICROBIAL RESISTANCE IN THE ICU

To address antimicrobial resistance in the ICU, the factors contributing to the problem in this setting should be understood. ICU patients typically have multiple invasive devices, including central lines, arterial lines, urinary catheters, and endotracheal tubes, that bypass the usual host defenses and predipose the patient to infection. In fact, the rate of hospital-acquired infection in the ICU patient can be correlated with the use of invasive devices (1). Colonization of the skin and respiratory tract with resistant organisms occurs relatively quickly in the hospital, and this process can be enhanced by the selection pressure of broad-spectrum antimicrobials. An evaluation of ventilator-associated pneumonia showed that 57% of episodes were caused by antibiotic-resistant bacteria. The most significant risk factors for the antibiotic-resistant infections were previous antibiotic use and previous use of broad-spectrum antibiotics (third-generation cephalosporin, fluoroquinolone, carbapenem, or a combination of these drugs) (2).

Antibiotic Utilization in the ICU

Antibiotic Use and Resistance

The use of antibiotics has long been linked to emergence of resistance (3,4). In the ICU where broad-spectrum antibiotics are ubiquitous and duration of therapy may be long, resistant organisms are a particular problem. Studies have also documented the correlation of increased use of certain classes of broad-spectrum agents with higher rates of resistance in ICU compared with non-ICU areas (Table 1) (5,6). Among the top eight pathogens causing hospital-acquired infection (coagulase-negative staphylococci, *Staphylococcus aureus*, *Pseudomonas aeruginosa*, *Enterococcus*, *Enterobacter*, *Escherichia coli*, *Candida*, and *Klebsiella pneumoniae*), the rates of resistance for each of these pathogens is higher in ICU patients than in non-ICU patients. Not surprisingly, these findings were reported by the Centers for Disease Control and Prevention (CDC) National Nosocomial Infection Surveillance (NNIS) Program, which tracks national trends in antibiotic resistance using a database of more than 300 hospitals (Table 2) (5). Recent NNIS data show that, among ICU patients with nosocomial infections, the largest increase in resistance in the past decade have been in fluoroquinolone-resistant *P. aeruginosa* (53% increase), vancomycin-resistant *Enterococci* (31% increase), methicillin-resistant *S. aureus* (MRSA) (29% increase), third-generation cephalosporin-resistant *P. aeruginosa* (24% increase), imipenem-resistant *P. aeruginosa* (23% increase), and third-generation cephalosporin-resistant *E. coli* (15% increase) (6).

Table 1 Rates of Antibiotic-Resistant Pathogens and Association with Use of Types of Antibiotics in ICU Compared with Non-ICU Areas

Higher resistance in ICUs	Higher use in ICUs
Escherichia coli, *Pseudomonas aeruginosa* Third-generation cephalosporins	Third-generation cephalosporins (ceftazidime, cefotaxime, ceftriaxone)
Pseudomonas aeruginosa Piperacillin	Antipseudomonal penicillins (piperacillin, piperacillin/tazobactam, ticarcillin/clavulanate)
Fluoroquinolones	Fluoroquinolones
Imipenem	Carbapenems
Enterococci Vancomycin	Vancomycin
Similar or less resistance in ICUs	Similar or less use in ICUs
Streptococcus pneumoniae Penicillin	Ampicillin
E. coli Fluoroquinolones	Fluoroquinolones

Source: Adapted from Refs. 5,6.

Table 2 Prevalence of Infecting Pathogen Resistant to Antibiotics: ICU Compared with Non-ICU Isolates

Pathogen, antibiotic	% Resistance[a] ICU	Non-ICU
Staphylococcus aureus, methicillin	37	33
Coagulase-negative *Staphylococcus*, methicillin	85	75
Enterococci, vancomycin	23	15
Klebsiella pneumoniae, third-generation cephalosporins	12	8
Enterobacter spp., third-generation cephalosporins	36	27
Pseudomonas aeruginosa, imipenem	15	8
P. aeruginosa, ofloxacin or ciprofloxacin	16	12

[a]Approximate, based on trends.
Source: Data from Ref. 5.

Monitoring Antibiotic Resistance

Although nationwide rates identify trends, institution-specific data on antibiotic susceptibilities by organism and drug, are crucial. Trends can vary widely from institution to institution since local flora and antibiotic practices vary as well. Hospital-wide susceptibility data are useful, and unit-specific data are very valuable, especially in the ICU, because antibiotic susceptibilities can vary between ICU and non-ICU isolates (5,7). Such data are helpful in making empiric antibiotic choices. Most inadequate antibiotic treatment of hospital-acquired infections is due to antibiotic-resistant organisms, and inadequate empiric antibiotic treatment can affect mortality (8).

Antibiotic Utilization and Guidelines for Infection Treatment

Recent studies indicate that improvements in antibiotic utilization can decrease the emergence of antibiotic resistance. Practice guidelines or protocols for the use of antibiotics may be helpful in decreasing unnecessary antibiotic use and in improving the use of necessary ones (9,10). Locally developed guidelines are best accepted by practicing clinicians and have the best chance for implementation (11,12). Automated, computerized guidelines have improved empiric antibiotic use and can reduce overall antibiotic utilization (9,10,13). Unnecessary antibiotic use can also be minimized by the use of standardized criteria for infection treatment. An example is ventilator-associated pneumonia. The definitive diagnosis of this infection is difficult: patients requiring mechanical ventilator support for several days have colonization of the sputum with nosocomial flora and multiple reasons for abnormal chest radiographs obtained in the ICU setting. Recent studies have demonstrated the utility of quantitative bronchoalveolar lavage cultures and risk assessments for ventilator-associated pneumonia risk in reducing prolonged unnecessary antibiotic exposure (14–17). Another example is asymptomatic bacteriuria or candiduria. In patients with urinary catheters, the presence of organisms in a urine culture may simply reflect colonization of the catheter rather than infection of the urinary tract. An assessment of the patient's overall status, including determination of fever, pyuria, or other signs or symptoms of urinary tract infection, should be done prior to starting antibiotics for a positive urine culture.

Duration of antibiotic use has also been implicated in the development of resistance (18,19). A study of the duration of antibiotic therapy for penetrating abdominal trauma showed that prolonged use of antibiotics (5 days vs. 1 day) did not reduce subsequent infection rates and, in fact, resulted in more infections with resistant organisms (19). Major abdominal infections occurred in 8% of those with 1 day therapy and 14% of those with 5 day therapy. In addition, a study of short (<48 h) vs. prolonged (>48 h) antibiotic prophylaxis following cardiovascular surgery showed that prolonged antibiotic prophylaxis did not decrease the risk of surgical site infection and was correlated with an increased risk of acquired antibiotic resistance (20). In a study of the effects of short-course empiric treatment on antibiotic resistance in an SICU, a 72 h course of empiric broad-spectrum antibiotics was followed by culture-directed therapy or discontinuation of antibiotics if cultures were negative (21). This approach was not associated with the emergence of antibiotic-resistant bacteria. Thus, although early empiric antibiotic therapy may be life-saving in the ICU patient, re-examination of the need for antibiotics, when culture results are available, is of great importance.

Hospital Antibiotic Restriction

Hospital antibiotic restriction, scheduled antibiotic changes, and antibiotic cycling have been considered as options for controlling antibiotic resistance. An increasing amount of evidence indicates that these strategies may be useful for certain types of resistance. As an intervention for an outbreak of multidrug resistant (extended-spectrum beta-lactamase-producing) *Klebsiella pneumoniae* in New York City, ceftazidime was restricted and imipenem was instituted (22). This change in treatments resulted in a decrease in resistant *K. pneumoniae*. Unfortunately, an outbreak of imipenem-resistant *Acinetobacter baumannii* occurred, which was difficult to control. Multidrug resistant *K. pneumoniae* recurred in this same hospital, and a class restriction of all cephalosporins, with certain exceptions such as cefazolin for surgical prophylaxis and ceftriaxone in the emergency room, was imposed. Cephalosporin use decreased by 80%, and imipenem use increased by 140%. This strategy led to a 44% decrease in multidrug resistant *K. pneumoniae* and imipenem-resistant *P. aeruginosa* (23). Observing a problem with *Clostridium difficile* and vancomycin-resistant *Enterococci* (VRE), Quale et al. (24) restricted vancomycin and cefotaxime (both classes of agents associated with emergence of VRE). The beta-lactamase inhibitors, ampicillin/sulbactam and piperacillin/tazobactam, were added to the formulary, and their use was encouraged in place of both third-generation cephalosporins and clindamycin (associated with the emergence of VRE and *C. difficile*). Cephalosporin, clindamycin, and vancomycin use decreased, and clinical cultures, as well as surveillance cultures for VRE, decreased significantly. Cases of *C. difficile* colitis also declined.

Scheduled Changes of Antibiotic Class

Kollef et al. (25) reported the effect of scheduled change of antibiotic class during 1995–1996 as a strategy to decrease the incidence of ventilator-associated pneumonia in a cardiothoracic ICU (25). During the 6-month "before" period, their usual practice of prescribing ceftazidime for a suspected Gram-negative bacterial infection was continued. During the 6-month "after" period, a fluoroquinoline (ciprofloxacin) was used instead of the cephalosporin. The occurrence of ventilator-associated pneumonia decreased significantly from 11.6% to 6.7%, and the decrease was primarily due to a significant reduction in infections from antibiotic-resistant Gram-negative bacteria. While useful in the mid-1990s, a scheduled change to fluoroquinolones may be of limited utility in many institutions today, because fluoroquinolone resistance in Gram-negatives has increased. Two studies document the utility of an antibiotic "switch" to decrease the prevalence of multidrug resistant (extended-spectrum beta-lactamase-producing) *K. pneumoniae*. Rice et al. (26) report an increase in multidrug resistant *K. pneumoniae* from 5% to 30% over a 2-year period. Interventions to decrease the rate of resistance included physician education about the association of ceftazidime with this type of resistance and avoidance of ceftazidime as an antibiotic for empiric Gram-negative coverage. Piperacillin/tazobactam was added to the formulary, and use of this agent for empiric Gram-negative coverage was encouraged. As ceftazidime use decreased and piperacillin/tazobactam use increased, resistance in *K. pneumoniae* to both of these agents decreased. Patterson et al. (27) reported a similar experience with substitution of piperacillin/tazobactam for ceftazidime as an empiric Gram-negative antibiotic. They observed a decline in *K. pneumoniae* resistance as well (27). In both of these institutions, rather than instituting antibiotic restriction the changes in antibiotic prescribing were accomplished by education with the assistance of infectious disease specialists and clinical pharmacists.

Antibiotic Cycling

One of the early experiences in antibiotic cycling was reported by Gerding et al. in the 1980s, who described cycling gentamicin and amikacin using time cycles of 12–51 months over a 10-year period. This strategy resulted in a decrease in gentamicin resistance among Gram-negative bacteria (28). Dominguez et al. (29) studied the cycling of regimens for patients with febrile neutropenia every 4–6 months in a hematology–oncology unit. Cycled regimens included: (1) ceftazidime + vancomycin, (2) imipenem, (3) aztreonam + cefazolin, and (4) ciprofloxacin + clindamycin. No change was noted in resistance rates. Since none of these regimens had activity against VRE, an increase in enterococcal infections was noted, that was likely related to the existence of VRE in this unit. *Enterobacter cloacae* infections decreased. This finding was attributed to the two regimens with better activity for *Enterobacter* spp. (the imipenem and ciprofloxacin regimens) than the ceftazidime and aztreonam containing regimens. Bradley et al. (30) noted a decrease in VRE in their hematology–oncology unit when piperacillin/tazobactam was used as the febrile neutropenia regimen in place of ceftazidime (30).

Two recent studies have evaluated antibiotic cycling in the ICU. Gruson et al. (31) reported their experience in a medical ICU in France. Owing to an increase in Gram-negative resistance, ceftazidime and ciprofloxacin were restricted, and the following empiric regimens were selected for rotation: (1) cefipime + amikacin, (2) piperacillin/tazobactam + tobramycin, (3) imipenem + netilimicin, and (4) ticarcillin/clavulanate + isepamycin (an aminoglycoside used in Europe). Clinicians in the ICU received daily input and evaluation from infectious disease specialists regarding antibiotic issues, and weekly infection control evaluations were done. They noted an overall decrease in antibiotic use. In particular, the use of fluoroquinolones, third-generation cephalosporins, vancomycin, and imipenem was decreased. There was increased use of piperacillin/tazobactam and cefipime. The number of potentially resistant Gram-negative bacteria (*P. aeruginosa*, *Burkholderia cepacia*, *Stenotrophomonas maltophilia*, and *Acinetobacter baumannii*) decreased, and there was decreased resistance in the *P. aeruginosa* and *B. cepacia* isolates from specimens for culture obtained from the ICU patients. Decreased oxacillin resistance was noted in *S. aureus*. The incidence of ventilator-associated pneumonia also decreased significantly.

Raymond et al. (32) have studied antibiotic cycling in a surgical ICU in the United States. Antibiotic regimens for pneumonia and peritonitis or sepsis were scheduled to change every 3 months. Regimens for pneumonia were: (1) ciprofloxacin ± clindamycin, (2) piperacillin/tazobactam, (3) a carbapenem, and (4) cefipime ± clindamycin. Regimens for peritonitis or sepsis were: (1) a carbapenam, (2) cefipime + metronidazole, (3) ciprofloxacin + clindamycin, and (4) piperacillin/tazobactam. Results showed a decrease in oxacillin resistance among Gram-positive organisms and decreased resistance in Gram-negative organisms. Another positive outcome was decreased mortality after infection. Antibiotic rotation was noted to be an independent predictor of survival.

Infectious Disease Specialists

Input from infectious disease specialists was deemed "indispensable" in the Gruson ICU study (31). Previous studies have shown that infected patients are less likely to receive inadequate antibiotic therapy if evaluation of the patient by an infectious disease specialist is done (33,34). In addition, routine input from infectious disease specialists and a multidisciplinary approach have been associated with less use of broad-spectrum agents and a decrease in antibiotic-resistant infections (27,33,35).

Thus, the use of antibiotics has a major impact on antibiotic resistance in the ICU. A program of antibiotic resistance monitoring, antibiotic stewardship consistent with locally developed treatment guidelines, and antibiotic rotation in response to current resistance patterns can be important in preventing the emergence of resistant pathogens.

The Role of Infection Control

Hand Hygiene

In addition to antibiotic selection pressures, cross-transmission of resistant clones in the ICU is common and contributes to further emergence of resistance. Factors that contribute to lapses in good infection control technique in the ICU include the multiple invasive devices that become colonized with microbes and require manipulation, the acuity of care of these patients, the need for urgent or emergency procedures, and decreased staffing. Hand hygiene either by handwashing or antiseptic handrub has been recognized since the time of Semmelweiss as an important measure in preventing hospital infections (36,37). Several studies have shown reduced rates of nosocomial infections, including those from resistant pathogens, with improved hand hygiene (38). Despite its simplicity and importance, non-compliance with this measure has been documented repeatedly (39,40). Features associated with non-compliance with hand hygiene include physicians with a high workload. While the lack of physician compliance remains inexplicable, high workload is a serious problem, particularly in an ICU, where as many as 40 opportunities for hand hygiene may occur in 1 h period (41,42). Handwashing at the sink is effective but is more time-consuming when compared with antiseptic handrub. Frequent handwashing can also result in skin reactions (43). These factors have led to studies that have documented the efficacy of antiseptic handrubs as a method for hand hygiene. Pittet et al. (43) documented an improvement in hand hygiene compliance from 48% to 66% with use of the handrub. This study also documented a consistent decrease in nosocomial infection rates including decreased rates of MRSA (43) hospital-wide. For these reasons, the antiseptic handrub is becoming increasingly accepted, particularly in high-risk units such as the ICU. If hands are visibly soiled, handwashing at the sink is mandatory.

Contact Precautions

The CDC currently recommends contact precautions for preventing the spread of multidrug resistant organisms in hospitals (44). These precautions include the use of a gown and gloves for contact with the patient or their immediate environment, if the patient is colonized or infected with a multi-drug resistant pathogen. Hand hygiene should be used after removing gloves. The use of gowns has been shown to prevent the spread of multi-drug resistant pathogens (45). Gloves should be changed routinely between patients. Using the same gloves for multiple patients has been implicated in nosocomial transmission of resistant organisms (46).

SPECIFIC PATHOGENS

Methicillin-Resistant *S. aureus* (MRSA)

Epidemiology

MRSA is an important pathogen in the ICU, since it is one of the leading causes of ventilator-associated pneumonia and catheter-related infection (5). The prevalence of MRSA among *S. aureus* isolates in hospitals continues to be of serious concern; many of these MRSA isolates are obtained from patients on admission to the hospital (47,48). Estimated nationally, the prevalence of MRSA in ICUs ranges from 37% to 51%, and is usually higher than the prevalence of MRSA among non-ICU isolates (5,6). Recent reports identify MRSA with intermediate and high-level resistance to vancomycin. These organisms were obtained from patients with MRSA infections who received long courses of vancomycin (49,50).

Therapy

Vancomycin remains the drug of choice for most MRSA infections. Due to the prevalence of MRSA or coagulase-negative *Staphylococci* among catheter-related infections, this agent is usually started for empiric therapy of such infections while information about cultures and susceptibilities is sought. For the patient with ventilator-associated pneumonia with Gram-positive cocci on Gram stain, vancomycin may be used for empiric therapy, depending on local rates of MRSA, until cultures and susceptibilities are available. If the *Staphylococcus* is determined to be susceptible to oxacillin, this therapy is preferred for two reasons. First, oxacillin is more rapidly bactericidal for *Staphylococci* than vancomycin, and, second, decreased vancomycin use in the ICU may decrease selection pressure for vancomycin-resistant *Enterococci* or *Staphylococci*. While vancomycin is usually well-tolerated, occasional patients with MRSA infections are intolerant to it or do not respond. Newer options for therapy include linezolid, an oxazolidinone antibiotic, and quinupristin/dalfopristin, a streptogramin antibiotic (51). Currently, these agents are costly and not without toxicity. Notable adverse effects of linezolid include cytopenias, especially thrombocytopenia and anemia. Adverse effects of quinupristin/dalfopristin include arthralgias/myalgias and drug interactions with the cytochrome P450 system (51).

Control and Prevention

Contact precautions for patients colonized or infected with MRSA are usually maintained, particularly in the ICU, where there is high potential for spread from patient to patient by the hands of health care workers. *S. aureus*, including MRSA, is spread primarily by hand carriage; therefore, hand hygiene with appropriate glove use is the most important control measure. Although transient hand carriage is the most common mechanism for cross-transmission, occasionally chronic nasal MRSA carriage in a health care worker has been associated with an outbreak of MRSA. In this case, nasal eradication of MRSA in the health care worker may be indicated. Although the environment is thought to be a minor reservoir for MRSA, cross-transmission environmental contamination with MRSA has been associated with cross-transmission in the setting of extensive skin infections, such as burn units or dermatology wards (52,53).

Vancomycin-Resistant Enterococci (VRE)
Epidemiology
Rates of VRE among hospital enterococcal isolates increased markedly during the 1990s and were notably higher among ICU isolates (5). Notably, in the most recent data, the prevalence of VRE has decreased somewhat for reasons that are not entirely clear. Recent national rates in the non-ICU setting (12%) are nearly equal to that in the ICU (12.5%) (6). Nevertheless, VRE remains a significant problem. It is easily cross-transmitted and, when it is the cause of infection, therapeutic options are severely limited. Risk factors for acquisition of VRE in the ICU include proximity to a patient colonized or infected with VRE, the rate of VRE colonization in the unit, the prevalence of VRE in non-ICU patients in the same hospital, amount of previous antibiotic use, and type of previous antibiotic therapy. Vancomycin, broad-spectrum cephalosporins, and anti-anaerobic agents such as clindamycin and metronidazole have demonstrated increased risk (18,54–56).

Enterococcus faecium, the second most common species of *Enterococci* overall, is the most common species to have vancomycin resistance. This finding is significant, because 80% of *E. faecium* isolates are ampicillin resistant, whereas 80% of *E. faecalis* isolates are ampicillin susceptible. Vancomycin resistance has been identified in *E. faecalis* and other enterococcal species, but it is much less common.

There are two major types of VRE: vanA and vanB phenotypes. These types are distinguished by their susceptibility in the laboratory to teicoplanin, a glycopeptide antibiotic similar to vancomycin that is used for susceptibility testing. The vanA phenotype isolates are resistant to teicoplanin, and the vanB phenotype isolates are susceptible to teicoplanin. These phenotypes are usually reported by the microbiology laboratory for epidemiologic, rather than therapeutic, significance. Although used for treatment is some countries, teicoplanin is not used for patients in the United States. Of significance, the vanA phenotype is readily transferable to other enterococci. It is the most common type of VRE in the United States.

Therapy
Two newer agents have been released in recent years with an indication for vancomycin-resistant *E. faecium*: linezolid and quinupristin/dalfopristin. Linezolid is available in oral and injectable form and is less expensive than quinupristin/dalfopristin in most hospitals. It has activity against *Enterococci* (*E. faecalis* as well as *E. faecium*), methicillin-sensitive *Staphylococci*, MRSA, and *Pneumococci*. Its significant adverse effects include anemia, thrombocytopenia, and headache. Structurally, it is a weak monoamine oxidase (MAO) inhibitor. The label suggests avoiding foods and drugs that can interact with these agents, although clinically MAO inhibition is not a significant side effect (51). However, serotonin syndrome associated with linezolid when given with selective serotonin reuptake inhibitors (SSRI) has been reported (57). Quinupristin/dalfopristin has

activity against *E. faecium* but has poor activity against *E. faecalis*. It should not be used for empiric enterococcal coverage but can be used for vancomycin-resistant *E. faecium* infection. It also has activity against other Gram-positive organisms such as *Staphylococci* and *Pneumococci*. Its adverse effects include phlebitis (if administered via a peripheral line), arthalgias/myalgias, elevated liver function tests, and drug interactions related to the cytochrome P450 system. VRE isolates that are resistant to these agents have already been reported. Laboratory susceptibility should be confirmed before using these agents in serious infections (58).

Control and Prevention

Contact precautions are recommended for controlling cross-transmission of VRE in the ICU. Transient hand carriage is a common mode of spread, but in contrast to *S. aureus*, these organisms are very hardy in the environment. Consequently, environmental reservoirs have been associated with ICU outbreaks (59–61). For this reason, cleaning of the VRE patient's immediate environment on a daily basis with a hospital-approved germicide is recommended (44). Antiseptic hand hygiene (chlorhexidine hadwash or antiseptic handrub) is recommended instead of routine soap for control of VRE (44). In addition to hand hygiene, the use of gowns has been shown to be associated with control of VRE in recent studies (45). In some units with cross-transmission of VRE, surveillance cultures (perirectal or stool swab cultures) for the early identification of VRE colonization may assist in controlling this problem (62,63).

In addition to infection control measures, scheduled antibiotic changes, from broad-spectrum cephalosporins to extended-spectrum penicillins, have been associated with decreases in rates of VRE (24,30).

Pseudomonas aeruginosa

Epidemiology

P. aeruginosa is the third most common ICU isolate after coagulase-negative staphylococci and *S. aureus* (5). It is a leading cause of ventilator-associated pneumonia (16%) and urinary tract infection (11%) in the ICU (5). This organism's tenacity makes it an important pathogen with significant therapeutic implications. Fluoroquinolone resistance has increased in *P. aeruginosa* over the past decade, and national data suggest that rates of ciprofloxacin/ofloxacin- and levofloxacin-resistant *P. aeruginosa* are 36% and 37%, respectively (5). In the same study, imipenem resistance increased (19%); ceftazidime and piperacillin resistance were 13% and 17%, respectively. Many ICU clinicians have encountered *P. aeruginosa*, which has become resistant to all of the usual therapeutic alternatives.

Therapy

Among the anti-pseudomonal penicillins, piperacillin and piperacillin/tazobactam have better activity than ticarcillin or ticarcillin/clavulanate, although the latter agents may still have adequate susceptibilities at some institutions. Among the cephalosporins, the third-generation antipseudomonal cephalosporin ceftazidime and the fourth-generation cephalosporin cefipime are generally the best agents. The monobactam, aztreonam, has the same side chain structure as ceftazidime and typically has very similar susceptibilities.

Among the carbapenems, meropenem has slightly better anti-pseudomonal activity than imipenem. The recently released ertapenem lacks anti-pseudomonal activity. Owing to the emergence of fluoroquinolone resistance in *P. aeruginosa* during the 1990s, these agents may have limited utility, but ciprofloxacin has the best anti-pseudomonal activity. Of note, recent studies of higher dosing of levofloxacin (750 mg daily) suggest pharmacodynamics that approach those of ciprofloxacin for this pathogen (64,65). Among the aminoglycosides, tobramycin typically has the best anti-pseudomonal activity when compared with gentamicin and amikacin. Local susceptibility patterns will be important in determining empiric anti-pseudomonal therapy at an individual institution and in an individual ICU. The rate of emergence of antibiotic-resistant *P. aeruginosa* during the course of therapy is 10–25% and may vary by antibiotic used (66,67). Imipenem has been associated with higher overall risk of emergence of resistance than other anti-pseudomonal agents (66). Combination therapy is often discussed. More data support this approach in treating serious *P. aeruginosa* infections than infections from other pathogens (67,68). A study of therapy for *P. aeruginosa* bacteremia showed that monotherapy with an antipseudomonal antibiotic was associated with increased risk of emergence of resistance to the single agent (69). In general, combination therapy should be used for serious *P. aeruginosa* infections, such as pneumonia and bacteremia.

Control and Prevention

A *P. aeruginosa* isolate with typical susceptibilities does not require contact precautions. Standard precautions should be followed for patients with typical *P. aeruginosa*; hand hygiene and barriers (gloves, gowns as needed) for contact with blood or body fluids should be used. Multidrug resistance in *P. aeruginosa* may be defined locally by each institution but typically is defined as an isolate that is resistant to multiple drug classes (i.e., resistant to antipseudomonal penicillins, cephalosporins, and aminoglycosides). Patients colonized or infected with such strains of multidrug resistant *P. aeruginosa* should be placed in contact precautions.

Enterobacter spp.

Epidemiology

Enterobacter spp. is the fifth most common nosocomial pathogen in the ICU and is a leading cause of ventilator-associated pneumonia and catheter-related bloodstream infection. Resistance to third-generation cephalosporins became common during the late 1980s and continued at a rate of 30–35% during the 1990s. Cephalosporin use is a documented risk factor for colonization or infection with *Enterobacter* spp. (3,70). It is important to understand that the resistance characteristics of this organism have therapeutic implications for serious infections. *Enterobacter* spp. contains a Type I (Group I) beta-lactamase that is usually resistant to the beta-lactamase inhibitors, such as clavulanate, sulbactam, and tazobactam. This beta-lactamase enzyme is inducible and produced at low levels by cells unexposed to cephalosporins; thus, *Enterobacter* spp. may initially appear susceptible to cephalosporins. However, once exposure to cephalosporins occurs (*in vitro* and in the clinical situation), a subpopulation of organisms that produce the Type I beta-lactamase at high levels becomes predominant, and resistance to cephalosporins can occur during the course of therapy (71,72).

Therapy

Owing to the problem of emergence of resistance during therapy, third-generation cephalosporins are not recommended for therapy of serious *Enterobacter* spp. infections. The carbapenems (imipenem, meropenem, and ertapenem) have a beta-lactam ring that is very stable to the Type I beta-lactamase. Typically, these agents have excellent activity against *Enterobacter* spp. Cefipime, the fourth-generation cephalosporin, also has a beta-lactam ring that is usually stable to the Type I beta-lactamase. It may also be used for therapy of *Enterobacter* infections, although there is currently less experience with cefipime than with the carbapenems.

Control and Prevention

Enterobacter spp., with a typical susceptibility pattern, do not require contact precautions. If the organism becomes multidrug resistant (as defined by the institution or resistant to multiple classes of antibiotics), contact precautions are recommended.

Extended-Spectrum Beta-Lactamase (ESBL)-Producing *Klebsiella pneumoniae*

Epidemiology

Extended-spectrum beta-lactamases (ESBLs) produce resistance to the broad-spectrum cephalosporins such as ceftazidime, cefotaxime, ceftriaxone, and the monobactam aztreonam. They are most often found in *K. pneumoniae*, but the trait is transferable to other genera and can also be found in *E. coli* and other Gram-negative bacteria. The resistance to cephalosporins typically results in a cross-resistance to other beta-lactam agents, including extended-spectrum penicillins and beta-lactamase inhibitors. Trimethoprim-sulfamethoxazole and gentamicin resistance are often co-transferred with the ESBL trait to produce a problem of multidrug resistance (73).

Fluoroquinolone resistance is commonly associated as well (74). Rates of ESBL-producing *K. pneumoniae* can vary widely from institution to institution.

Therapy

Cephalosporin failures, when used to treat serious ESBL-producing *K. pneumoniae* infections, have been reported (22,75). Although some ESBL-producing organisms are susceptible to cephamycins (cefoxitin and cefotetan), resistance has emerged during therapy with these agents (76).

The carbapenems are considered drugs of choice for serious infections from ESBL-producing *K. pneumoniae* (75,77). The use of these agents should be reserved for culture-documented infections, since widespread empiric use of carbapenems can lead to resistance (23,78). Fluoroquinolones may be also be used, if susceptibility testing results support their efficacy.

Control and Prevention

As many isolates of ESBL-producing *K. pneumoniae* are multidrug resistant, contact precautions are advised. Outbreaks of these organisms have been controlled with infection-control precautions, antibiotic utilization measures, and a combination of both (22,26,27). Optimally, a combination of infection control and antibiotic utilization techniques are used (79). As discussed in the section of Antibiotic Utilization, control of ESBL-producing *K. pneumoniae* has been facilitated by decreased cephalosporin use and use of an alternative agent, such as an extended-spectrum penicillin/beta-lactamase inhibitor combination (piperacillin/tazobactam) or imipenem (22,26,27).

Acinetobacter baumannii

Epidemiology

Emergence of multidrug resistant *A. baumannii* is of great concern, since no ideal alternative agents for treatment of serious infections with these strains are available. Emergence of carbapenem-resistant *A. baumannii* has occurred in association with imipenem use and is difficult to control (23,78). Areas of New York City are experiencing an increase in these organisms, including strains that are completely resistant to all the usual antibiotic choices. Sporadic outbreaks have occurred throughout the United States (80,81). A survey of Brooklyn hospitals showed that 10% of Gram-negative rod isolates were *A. baumannii*. Of these, 50% were resistant to carbapenems and 10% were resistant to all commonly used antibiotics (78). Third-generation cephalosporin use was a common risk factor (78). Fluoroquinolone and cephalosporin resistance are common in these organisms (64,78,80).

Therapy

A. baumannii may be susceptible to ampicillin/sulbactam, as a consequence of the sulbactam component. This agent may be an alternative for therapy in more susceptible strains (82,83). For multidrug resistant isolates that are resistant to commonly used antibiotics including carbapenems, colistin or polymyxin B are used for patients with serious infections (84,85).

Control and Prevention

Contact precautions are advised for multidrug resistant strains. Emergence of such strains has been associated with widespread use of carbapenems, a finding that suggests antibiotic utilization patterns can be helpful in control of this pathogen. The lack of good alternative agents for therapy makes prevention and control measures particularly important for these organisms.

SUMMARY

- Antibiotic resistance is associated with multiple invasive devices, use of broad spectrum antibiotics, lapses of infection control procedures, and understaffing.
- Recent data demonstrate large increases in fluoroquinolone-resistant *P. aeruginosa*, vancomycin-resistant *Enterococci*, methicillin-resistant *S. aureus*, third generation cephalosporin-resistant *P. aeruginosa*, imipenem-resistant *P. aeruginosa*, and third generation-resistant *E. coli*.
- Resistance trends can vary widely from institution to institution.
- Practice guidelines or protocols for use of antibiotics may decrease unnecessary antibiotic use.
- Reducing duration of broad-spectrum antibiotic empirical coverage in favor of culture directed therapy may reduce antibiotic resistance.
- Hospital antibiotic restriction, scheduled changes of antibiotic class, and antibiotic cycling may be helpful measures in controlling certain types of antibiotic resistance.

- Important infection control measures include hand hygiene and contact precautions.
- MRSA isolates are increasing. Vancomycin is generally effective. Oxacillin should be used for susceptible organisms. Contact precautions should be instituted.
- VRE is easily transmitted. Therapeutic options are limited. *E. faecium* is the most common vancomycin-resistant species. The vanA phenotype, the most common type of VRE, is readily transferable to other *Enterococci*. Linezolid and quinupristin/dalfopristin may be effective. Contact precautions are recommended.
- *P. aeruginosa* is the leading cause of ventilator associated pneumonia. Widespread resistance to many classes of antibiotics makes local susceptibility patterns important in determining empiric therapy.
- Combination therapy should be reserved for serious *P. aeruginosa* infection. Standard precautions should be followed.
- *Enterobacter* has an inducible beta-lactamase enzyme. Although it may appear susceptible to cephalosporins initially, induction of beta-lactamase may change resistance patterns during the course of therapy. Carbapenems are generally used. Contact precautions are recommended for multidrug resistant organisms.
- Carbapenems are the antibiotics of choice for extended spectrum beta-lactamase producing *Klebsiella pneumonia*. Contact precautions are advised for multidrug resistant strains.
- Multidrug resistant *Acinetobacter baumanii* is increasing. Resistance to carbapenems is of great concern. Ampicillin/sulbactam, colistin, or polymyxin B may be useful agents. Contact precautions are recommended for multidrug resistant strains.

REFERENCES

1. Jarvis WR, Edwards JR, Culver DH, Hughes JM, Horan T, Emori TG, Banerjee S, Tolson J, Henderson T, Gaynes RP, Martone WJ. The National Nosocomial Infections Surveillance System. Nosocomial infection rates in adult and pediatric intensive care units in the United States. Am J Med 1991; 91:185S–191S.
2. Trouillet JL, Chastre J, Vuagnat A, Joly-Guillou ML, Combaux D, Dombret MC, Gibert C. Ventilator-associated pneumonia caused by potentially drug-resistant bacteria. Am J Respir Crit Care Med 1998; 157:531–539.
3. Ballow CH, Schentag JJ. Trends in antibiotic utilization and bacterial resistance. Report of the National Nosocomial Resistance Surveillance Group. Diag Microbiol Infect Dis 1992; 15:37S–42S.
4. McGowan JE Jr. Antimicrobial resistance in hospital organisms and its relation to antibiotic use. Rev Infect Dis 1983; 5:1033–1048.
5. Fridkin SK, Gaynes RP. Antimicrobial resistance in intensive care units. Clin Chest Med 1999; 20:303–316.
6. National Nosocomial Infections Surveillance (NNIS) System Report, Data Summary from January 1992 to June 2001, issued August 2001. Am J Infect Control 2001; 29:404–421.
7. White AC Jr, Atmar RL, Wilson J, Cate TR, Stager CE, Greenberg SB. Effects of requiring prior authorization for selected antimicrobials: expenditures, susceptibilities, and clinical outcomes. Clin Infect Dis 1997; 25:230–239.
8. Kollef MH, Sherman G, Ward S, Fraser VJ. Inadequate antimicrobial treatment of infections: a risk factor for hospital mortality among critically ill patients. Chest 1999; 115:462–474.

9. Pestotnik SL, Classen DC, Evans RS, Burke JP. Implementing antibiotic practice guidelines through computer-assisted decision support: clinical and financial outcomes. Ann Intern Med 1996; 124:884–890.
10. Leibovici L, Gitelman V, Yehezkelli Y, Poznanski O, Milo G, Paul M, Ein-Dor P. Improving empirical antibiotic treatment: prospective, nonintervention testing of a decision support system. J Intern Med 1997; 242:395–400.
11. Onion CW, Bartzokas CA. Changing attitudes to infection management in primary care: a controlled trial of active versus passive guideline implementation strategies. Fam Pract 1998; 15:99–104.
12. Clemmer TP, Spuhler VJ, Berwick DM, Nolan TW. Cooperation: the foundation of improvement. Ann Intern Med 1998; 128:1004–1009.
13. Bailey TC, Ritchie DJ, McMullin ST, Kahn M, Reichley RM, Casabar E, Shannon W, Dunagan WC. A randomized, prospective evaluation of an interventional program to discontinue intravenous antibiotics at two tertiary care teaching institutions. Pharmacotherapy 1997; 17:277–281.
14. Croce MA, Fabian TC, Schurr MJ, Boscarino R, Pritchard FE, Minard G, Patton JH Jr, Kudsk KA. Using bronchoalveolar lavage to distinguish nosocomial pneumonia from systemic inflammatory response syndrome: a prospective analysis. J Trauma 1995; 39:1134–1139 (discussion 1139–1140).
15. Fagon JY, Chastre J, Wolff M, Gervais C, Parer-Aubas S, Stephan F, Similowski T, Mercat A, Diehl JL, Sollet JP, Tenaillon A. Invasive and noninvasive strategies for management of suspected ventilator-associated pneumonia. A randomized trial. Ann Intern Med 2000; 132:621–630.
16. Singh N, Rogers P, Atwood CW, Wagener MM, Yu VL. Short-course empiric antibiotic therapy for patients with pulmonary infiltrates in the intensive care unit. A proposed solution for indiscriminate antibiotic prescription. Am J Respir Crit Care Med 2000; 162:505–511.
17. Namias N, Harvill S, Ball S, McKenney MG, Sleeman D, Ladha A, Civetta J. A reappraisal of the role of Gram's stains of tracheal aspirates in guiding antibiotic selection in the surgical intensive care unit. J Trauma 1998; 44:102–106.
18. Tokars JI, Satake S, Rimland D, Carson L, Miller ER, Killum E, Sinkowitz-Cochran RL, Arduino MJ, Tenover FC, Marston B, Jarvis WR. The prevalence of colonization with vancomycin-resistant enterococcus at a Veterans' Affairs institution. Infect Control Hosp Epidemiol 1999; 20:171–175.
19. Fabian TC, Croce MA, Payne LW, Minard G, Pritchard FE, Kudsk KA. Duration of antibiotic therapy for penetrating abdominal trauma: a prospective trial. Surgery 1992; 112:788–794 (discussion 794–795).
20. Harbarth S, Samore MH, Lichtenberg D, Carmeli Y. Prolonged antibiotic prophylaxis after cardiovascular surgery and its effect on surgical site infections and antimicrobial resistance. Circulation 2000; 101:2916–2921.
21. Namias N, Harvill S, Ball S, Mckenney MG, Salomone JP, Sleeman D, Civetta JM. Empiric therapy of sepsis in the surgical intensive care unit with broad-spectrum antibiotics for 72 hours does not lead to the emergence of resistant bacteria. J Trauma 1998; 45:887–891.
22. Meyer KS, Urban C, Eagan JA, Berger BJ, Rahal JJ. Nosocomial outbreak of Klebsiella infection resistant to late-generation cephalosporins. Ann Intern Med 1993; 119:353–358.
23. Rahal JJ, Urban C, Horn D, Freeman K, Segal-Maurer S, Maurer J, Mariano N, Marks S, Burns JM, Dominick D, Lim M. Class restriction of cephalosporin use to control total cephalosporin resistance in nosocominal *Klebsiella*. J Am Med Assoc 1998; 280:1233–1237.
24. Quale J, Landman D, Saurina G, Atwood E, DiTore V, Patel K. Manipulation of a hospital antimicrobial formulary to control an outbreak of vancomycin-resistant enterococci. Clin Infect Dis 1996; 23:1020–1025.
25. Kollef MH, Vlasnik J, Sharpless L, Pasque C, Murphy D, Fraser V. Scheduled change of antibiotic classes: a strategy to decrease the incidence of ventilator-associated pneumonia. Am J Respir Crit Care Med 1997; 156:1040–1048.

26. Rice LB, Eckstein EC, DeVente J, Shales DM. Ceftazidime-resistant Klebsiella pneumoniae isolates recovered at the Cleveland Department of Veterans Affaris Medical Center. Clin Infect Dis 1996; 23:118–124.
27. Patterson JE, Hardin TC, Kelly CA, Garcia RC, Jorgensen JH. Association of antibiotic utilization measures and control of multiple-drug resistance in *Klebsiella pneumoniae*. Infect Control Hosp Epidemiol 2000; 21:455–458.
28. Gerding DN, Larson TA, Hughes RA, Weiler M, Shanholtzer C, Peterson LR. Aminoglycoside resistance and aminoglycoside usage: ten years of experience in one hospital. Antimicrob Agents Chemother 1991; 35:1284–1290.
29. Dominguez EA, Smith TL, Reed E, Sanders CC, Sanders WE Jr. A pilot study of antibiotic cycling in a hematology-oncology unit. Infect Control Hosp Epidemiol 2000; 21:S4–S8.
30. Bradley SJ, Wilson AL, Allen MC, Sher HA, Goldstone AH, Scott GM. The control of hyperendemic glycopeptide-resistant *Enterococcus* spp. on a haematology unit by changing antibiotic usage. J Antimicrob Chemother 1999; 43:261–266.
31. Gruson D, Hilbert G, Vargas F, Valentino R, Bebear C, Allery A, Gbikpi-Benissan G, Cardinaud JP. Rotation and restricted use of antibiotics in a medical intensive care unit. Impact on the incidence of ventilator-associated pneumonia caused by antibiotic-resistant gram-negative bacteria. Am J Respir Crit Care Med 2000; 162:837–843.
32. Raymond DP, Pelletier SJ, Crabtree TD, Gleason TG, Hamm LL, Pruett TL, Sawyer RG. Impact of a rotating empiric antibiotic schedule on infectious mortality in an intensive care unit. Crit Care Med 2001; 29:1101–1108.
33. Byl B, Clevenbergh P, Jacobs F, Struelens MJ, Zech F, Kentos A, Thys JP. Impact of infectious diseases specialists and microbiological data on the appropriateness of antimicrobial therapy for bacteremia. Clin Infect Dis 1999; 29:60–66 (discussion 67–68).
34. Herchline T, Gros S. Implementation of consensus guidelines for the follow-up of positive blood cultures. Infect Control Hosp Epidemiol 1997; 18:38–41.
35. Montecalvo MA, Jarvis WR, Uman J, Shay DK, Petrullo C, Rodney K, Gedris C, Horowitz HW, Wormser GP. Infection-control measures reduce transmission of vancomycin-resistant enterococci in an endemic setting. Ann Intern Med 1999; 131:269–272.
36. Larson EL. APIC guideline for handwashing and hand antisepsis in health care settings. Am J Infect Control 1995; 23:251–269.
37. Jarvis WR. Handwashing—the Semmelweis lesson forgotten? Lancet 1994; 344:1311–1312.
38. Larson E. Skin hygiene and infection prevention: more of the same or different approaches? Clin Infect Dis 1999; 29:1287–1294.
39. Albert RK, Condie F. Hand-washing patterns in medical intensive-care units. N Engl J Med 1981; 304:1465–1466.
40. Pittet D, Mourouga P, Perneger TV. Compliance with handwashing in a teaching hospital. Infection Control Program. Ann Intern Med 1999; 130:126–130.
41. Vandenbroucke-Grauls CM. Clean hands closer to the bedside. Lancet 2000; 356:1290–1291.
42. Voss A, Widmer AF. No time for handwashing!? Handwashing versus alcoholic rub: can we afford 100% compliance? Infect Control Hosp Epidemiol 1997; 18:205–208.
43. Pittet D, Hugonnet S, Harbarth S, Mourouga P, Sauvan V, Touveneau S, Perneger TV. Effectiveness of a hospital-wide programe to improve compliance with hand hygiene. Infection Control Programme. Lancet 2000; 356:1307–1312.
44. Recommendations for preventing the spread of vancomycin resistance. Hospital Infection Control Practices Advisory Committee (HICPAC). Infect Control Hosp Epidemiol 1995; 16:105–113.
45. Srinivasan A, Song X, Ross T, Merz W, Brower R, Perl TM. A prospective study to determine whether cover gowns in addition to gloves decrease nosocomial transmission of vancomycin-resistant enterococci in an intensive care unit. Infect Control Hosp Epidemiol 2002; 23:424–428.

46. Patterson JE, Vecchio J, Pantelick EL, Farrel P, Mazon D, Zervos MJ, Hierholzer WJ Jr. Association of contaminated gloves with transmission of *Acinetobacter calcoaceticus* var. *anitratus* in an intensive care unit. Am J Med 1991; 91:479–483.
47. Naimi TS, LeDell KH, Boxrud DJ, Groom AV, Steward CD, Johnson SK, Besser JM, O'Boyle C, Danila RN, Cheek JE, Osterholm MT, Moore KA, Smith KE. Epidemiology and clonality of community-acquired methicillin-resistant *Staphylococcus aureus* in Minnesota, 1996–1998. Clin Infect Dis 2001; 33:990–996.
48. Moreno F, Crisp C, Jorgensen JH, Patterson JE. Methicillin-resistant *Staphylococcus aureus* as a community organism. Clin Infect Dis 1995; 21:1308–1312.
49. *Staphylococcus aureus* with reduced susceptibility to vancomycin—Illinois, 1999. MMWR Morb Mortal Wkly Rep 2000; 48:1165–1167.
50. Public health dispatch: Vancomycin resistant *Staphylococcus aureus*—Pennsylvania, 2002. MMWR Morb Mortal Wkly Rep 2002; 51:902.
51. Patterson JE. New Gram-positive agents in nosocomial infection. Curr Opin Infect Dis 2000; 13:593–598.
52. Sheridan RL, Weber J, Benjamin J, Pasternack MS, Tompkins RG. Control of methicillin-resistant *Staphylococcus aureus* in a pediatric burn unit. Am J Infect Conrol 1994; 22:340–345.
53. Layton MC, Perez M, Heald P, Patterson JE. An outbreak of mupirocin-resistant *Staphylococcus aureus* on a dermatology ward associated with an environmental reservoir. Infect Control Hosp Epidemiol 1993; 14:369–375.
54. Donskey CJ, Chowdhry TK, Hecker MT, Hoyen CK, Hanrahan JA, Hujer AM, Hutton-Thomas RA, Whalen CC, Bonomo RA, Rice LB. Effect of antibiotic therapy on the density of vancomycin-resistant enterococci in the stool of colonized patients. N Engl J Med 2000; 343:1925–1932.
55. Fridkin SK, Edwards JR, Courval JM, Hill H, Tenover FC, Lawton R, Gaynes RP, McGowan JE Jr. The effect of vancomycin and third-generation cephalosporins on prevalence of vancomycin-resistant enterococci in 126 U.S. adult intensive care units. Ann Intern Med 2001; 135:175–183.
56. Patterson JE. Antibiotic utilization: is there an effect on antimicrobial resistance? Chest 2001; 119:426S–430S.
57. Wigen CL, Goetz MB. Serotonin syndrome and linezolid. Clin Infect Dis 2002; 34:1651–1652.
58. Gonzales RD, Schreckenberger PC, Graham MB, Kelkar S, DenBesten K, Quinn JP. Infections due to vancomycin-resistant *Enterococcus faecium* resistant to linezolid. Lancet 2001; 357:1179.
59. Hanna H, Umphrey J, Tarrand J, Mendoza M, Raad I. Management of an outbreak of vancomycin-resistant enterococci in the medical intensive care unit of a cancer center. Infect Control Hosp Epidemiol 2001; 22:217–219.
60. Sample ML, Gravel D, Oxley C, Toye B, Garber G, Ramotar K. An outbreak of vancomycin-resistant enterococci in a hematology-oncology unit: control by patient cohorting and terminal cleaning of the environment. Infect Control Hosp Epidemiol 2002; 23:468–470.
61. Livornese LL Jr, Dias S, Samel C, Romanowski B, Taylor S, May P, Pitsakis P, Woods G, Kaye D, Levison ME, et al. Hospital-acquired infection with vancomycin-resistant *Enterococcus faecium* transmitted by electronic thermometers. Ann Intern Med 1992; 17:112–116.
62. Muto CA, Giannetta ET, Durbin LJ, Simonton BM, Farr BM. Cost-effectiveness of perirectal surveillance cultures for controlling vancomycin-resistant *Enterococcus*. Infect Control Hosp Epidemiol 2002; 23:429–435.
63. Mayall CG. Control of vancomycin-resistant enterococci: it is important, it is possible, and it is cost-effective. Infect Control Hosp Epidemiol 2002; 23:420–423.

64. Sahm DF, Critchley IA, Kelly LJ, Karlowsky JA, Mayfield DC, Thornsberry C, Mauriz YR, Kahn J. Evaluation of current activities of fluoroquinolones against gram-negative bacilli using centralized *in vitro* testing and electronic surveillance. Antimicrob Agents Chemother 2001; 45:267–274.
65. Drusano GL. Fluoroquinolone pharmacodynamics: prospective determination of relationships between exposure and outcome. J Chemother 2000; 12(suppl 4):21–26.
66. Carmeli Y, Troillet N, Eliopoulos GM, Samore MH. Emergence of antibiotic-resistant Pseudomonas aeruginosa: comparison of risks associated with different antipseudomonal agents. Antimicrob Agents Chemother 1999; 43:1379–1382.
67. Moellering RC Jr. Antibiotic resistance: lessons for the future. Clin Infect Dis 1998; 27(suppl 1):S135–S140 (discussion S141–S132).
68. Allan JD, Moellering RC Jr. Antimicrobial combinations in the therapy of infections due to gram-negative bacilli. Am J Med 1985; 78:65–76.
69. El Amari EB, Chamot E, Auckenthaler R, Pechere JC, Van Delden C. Influence of previous exposure to antibiotic therapy on the susceptibility pattern of Pseudomonas aeruginosa bacteremic isolates. Clin Infect Dis 2001; 33:1859–1864.
70. Chow JW, Fine MJ, Shales DM, Quinn JP, Hooper DC, Johnson MP, Ramphal R, Wagener MM, Miyashiro DK, Yu VL. *Enterobacter bacteremia*: clinical features and emergence of antibiotic resistance during therapy. Ann Inter Med 1991; 115:585–590.
71. Heusser MF, Patterson JE, Kuritza AP, Edberg SC, Baltimore RS. Emergence of resistance to multiple beta-lactams in *Enterobacter cloacae* during treatment for neonatal meningitis with cefotaxime. Pediatr Infect Dis J 1990; 9:509–512.
72. Sanders WE Jr, Sanders CC. Inducible beta-lactamases; clinical and epidemiologic implications for use of newer cephalosporins. Rev Infect Dis 1988; 10:830–838.
73. Jacoby GA. Extended-spectrum beta-lactamases and other enzymes providing resistance to oxyimino-beta-lactams. Infect Dis Clin North Am 1997; 11:875–887.
74. Sader HS, Pfaller MA, Jones RN. Prevalence of important pathogens and the antimicrobial activity of parenteral drugs at numerous medical centers in the United States. II. Study of the intra-and interlaboratory dissemination of extended-spectrum beta-lactamase-producing Enterobacteriaceae. Diagn Microbiol Infect Dis 1994; 20:203–208.
75. Paterson DL, Ko WC, Von Gottberg A, Casellas JM, Mulazimoglu L, Klugman KP, Bonomo RA, Rice LB, McCormack JG, Yu VL. Outcome of cephalosporin treatment for serious infections due to apparently susceptible organisms producing extended-spectrum beta-lactamases: implications for the clinical microbiology laboratory. J Clin Microbiol 2001; 39:2206–2212.
76. Martinez-Martinez L, Pascual A, Hernandez-Alles S, Alvarez-Diaz D, Suarez AI, Tran J, Benedi VJ, Jacoby GA. Roles of beta-lactamases and porins in activities of carbapenems and cephalosporins against *Klebsiella pneumoniae*. Antimicrob Agents Chemother 1999; 43:1669–1673.
77. Paterson DL. Recommendation for treatment of severe infections caused by Enterobacteriaceae producing extended-spectrum beta-lactamases (ESBLs). Clin Microbiol Infect 2000; 6:460–463.
78. Manikal VM, Landman D, Saurina G, Oydna E, Lal H, Quale J. Endemic carbapenem-resistant *Acinetobacter* species in Brooklyn, New York: citywide prevalence, interinstitutional spread, and relation to antibiotic usage. Clin Infect Dis 2000; 31:101–106.
79. Patterson JE. Extended-spectrum beta-lactamases. Semin Respir Infect 2000; 15:299–307.
80. Landman D, Quale JM, Mayorga D, Adedeji A, Vangala K, Ravishankar J, Flores C, Brooks S. Citywide clonal outbreak of multiresistant *Acinetobacter baumannii* and *Pseudomonas aeruginosa* in Brooklyn, NY: the preantibiotic era has returned. Arch Intern Med 2002; 162:1515–1520.
81. Mahgoub S, Ahmed J, Glatt Completely resistant *Acinetobacter baumannii* strains. Infect Control Hosp Epidemiol 2002; 23:477–479.

82. Levin AS. Multiresistant *Acinetobacter* infections: a role for sulbactam combinations in overcoming an emerging worldwide problem. Clin Microbiol Infect 2002; 8:144–153.
83. Wood GC, Hanes SD, Croce MA, Fabian TC, Boucher BA. Comparison of ampicillin-sulbactam and imipenem-cilastatin for the treatment of acinetobacter ventilator-associated pneumonia. Clin Infect Dis 2002; 34:1425–1430.
84. Jimenez-Mejias ME, Pichardo-Guerrero C, Marquez-Rivas FJ, Martin-Lozano D, Prados T, Pachon J. Cerebrospinal fluid penetration and pharmacokinetic/pharmacodynamic parameters of intravenously administered colistin in a case of multidrug-resistant *Acinetobacter baumannii* meningitis. Eur J Clin Microbiol Infect Dis 2002; 21:212–214.
85. Levin AS, Barone AA, Penco J, Santos MV, Marinho IS, Arruda EA, Manrique EI, Costa SF. Intravenous colistin as therapy for nosocomial infections caused by multidrug-resistant *Pseudomonas aeruginosa* and *Acinetobacter baumannii*. Clin Infect Dis 1999; 28:1008–1011.

46
Intra-abdominal Infection

Ori D. Rotstein
University of Toronto, Toronto, Ontario, Canada

Jerome H. Abrams
VA Medical Center, Minneapolis, Minnesota, USA

The principles of management of the patient initially seen with an intra-abdominal infection include providing: (1) resuscitation, (2) nutritional and metabolic support, (3) broad-spectrum antibiotic therapy directed against a polymicrobial bacterial flora, and (4) surgical or radiologic intervention to treat the underlying pathology. This chapter reviews the host response to infection in the peritoneal cavity and describes an approach to the management of both bacterial peritonitis and intra-abdominal abscesses.

ANATOMY AND PHYSIOLOGY OF ABDOMINAL CAVITY

The peritoneum is a smooth, translucent membrane lining the abdominal cavity. Its surface consists of a single layer of flat mesothelial cells that reside on a basement membrane, which in turn overlies a bed of connective tissue. The overall surface area of the peritoneum approximates that of the total cutaneous surface area ($\sim 1.7 \, m^2$). The peritoneal cavity is normally sterile and contains <50 mL of fluid. The fluid has a specific gravity <1.016 and a protein concentration <3 g/dL. It contains fewer than 3000 cells/mm^3, predominantly macrophages and lymphocytes. The peritoneal membrane permits bidirectional diffusion of water and most solutes. In addition, particulate matter can be cleared through stomata between specialized peritoneal mesothelial cells that overlie lymphatic channels on the diaphragmatic surface of the peritoneal cavity. These intercellular stomata correspond with fenestrations in the basement membrane, and together they serve as channels from the peritoneal cavity to underlying specialized diaphragmatic lymphatics called lacunae (1). In concert with the one-way valves in the thoracic lymphatics, this unit serves as an important clearance mechanism of bacteria from the peritoneal cavity. Bacteria pass easily through the large stomata and can be recovered from the thoracic lymph duct within 6 min and from the blood within 12 min of intraperitoneal inoculation (2). This mechanism is facilitated by an intraperitoneal flow of fluid and particles toward the diaphragm, an effect presumably produced by suction caused by the pull of gravity on the upper abdominal viscera away from the diaphragmatic surface.

DEFENSE AGAINST PERITONEAL INFECTION

Local Response

Three local defense mechanisms contribute to the ultimate clearance of bacteria from the peritoneal cavity (3). They are (i) mechanical clearance of bacteria through the diaphragmatic lymphatics; (ii) phagocytosis and destruction of suspended or adherent bacteria by phagocytic cells; and (iii) sequestration and walling off of bacteria, coupled with delayed clearance by phagocytic cells. The first mechanism involves the physical removal of bacteria. Microorganisms are carried cephalad by the intraperitoneal circulation, absorbed into the diaphragmatic lymphatics, and carried to the bloodstream. The interaction of bacteria and their products with macrophage populations distant from the peritoneal cavity is presumably responsible for the development of the systemic response to intraperitoneal infection.

The peritoneal response is otherwise typified by the development of local inflammation, including hyperemia of the vasculature underlying the peritoneum, exudation of fluid into the peritoneal cavity, and a marked influx of phagocytic cells.

Within the first 2–4 h, bacteria not cleared by the peritoneal lymphatics are mostly cell associated and are presumably attached to or ingested by resident peritoneal macrophages (4). After 4 h, neutrophils become the predominant phagocytic cell in the peritoneal cavity (5). The events surrounding the development of the peritoneal response can be surmised from a combination of *in vitro* and *in vivo* studies of inflammation. For example, inflammatory exudates derived from subcutaneously implanted sponges contain measurable levels of interleukin-1, interleukin-6, tumor necrosis factor, and macrophage colony-stimulating factor (6). The combined effects of these cytokines clearly contribute to the inflammatory response observed during peritonitis (Table 1).

Table 1 Role of Cytokines in Peritoneal Response to Infection

Cytokine	Action
Tumor necrosis factor	Causes vascular leak
	Increases influx of neutrophils into the peritoneal cavity by augmenting neutrophil–endothelial interactions and transendothelial migration of neutrophils
	Stimulates and primes neutrophil functions
	Stimulates release of other cytokines
	Slight stimulation of macrophage procoagulant activity
Interleukin-1	Increases influx of neutrophils to peritoneum by augmenting neutrophil–endothelial interactions and transendothelial migration of neutrophils
	Chemotactic for neutrophils
	Primes neutrophil function
	Stimulates macrophage procoagulant activity
	Stimulates release of other cytokines
Cellular procoagulants	Induce intraperitoneal fibrin deposition
Interleukin-8	Strong neutrophil chemotactic activity
Colony-stimulating factor 1	Primes neutrophil function

Source: Modified from Rotstein OD. Peritonitis and intraabdominal abscesses. In: Wilmore DW, Brennan MF, Harken AH, et al. eds. Care of the Surgical Patient. New York: Scientific American Publications, 1992 (all rights reserved).

Other inflammatory mediator molecules such as leukotriene B_4, platelet-activating factor, and components of a complement cascade augment these effects by virtue of their ability to attract, prime, and activate cells in the peritoneal cavity.

Finally, a procoagulant response, manifested by the deposition of fibrinous exudates, is observed during peritoneal infection. Fibrin deposition apparently is important in sequestering infection, not only by incorporating large numbers of bacteria within the fibrin matrix (7), but also by causing loops of intestine and omentum to create a physical barrier against dissemination. Fibrin deposition is promoted by the procoagulant actions of mesothelial cells and peritoneal macrophages (8) on the fibrinogen-rich peritoneal exudate and by the loss of the intrinsic fibrinolytic activity of the peritoneal surface (9). Although under some circumstances sequestration of bacteria within these fibrinous exudates predisposes to residual infection, appropriate antibiotic therapy and surgery in combination with local mechanisms more commonly are able to effect clearance of bacteria with complete resolution of the infection.

Systemic Response

Several factors contribute to the systemic response to intra-abdominal infection. Dehydration caused by third-space fluid loss may cause altered hemodynamics, if it is of sufficient magnitude. In addition, particularly in the resuscitated patient, the synthesis and release of various mediator molecules in response to systemic endotoxemia and bacteremia cause marked hemodynamic and metabolic alterations. They are discussed in Chapter 1 in greater detail.

DIAGNOSIS AND MANAGEMENT OF INTRA-ABDOMINAL INFECTION

Intra-abdominal infection is most commonly manifested by the development of secondary peritonitis. Secondary bacterial peritonitis is defined as peritoneal infection caused by perforation of a hollow viscus or transmural necrosis of the gastrointestinal (GI) tract. Under most circumstances, the combination of appropriate antibiotic therapy and timely surgical intervention results in complete resolution of the intraperitoneal infection. When infection persists or recurs, the ability of the host to localize the infection results in the formation of discrete abscesses within the peritoneal cavity. A small proportion of patients with secondary peritonitis are unable either to clear or to contain infection and develop persistent diffuse peritonitis, that is, *tertiary peritonitis*. The approach to diagnosis and management of each of these three entities is discussed below.

Secondary Peritonitis

Diagnosis

The most common causes of secondary bacterial peritonitis are perforated appendix; perforated duodenal ulcer; perforated sigmoid colon as a result of diverticulitis, volvulus, or cancer; strangulation obstruction of the small bowel; and postoperative peritonitis from anastomotic disruption. The diagnosis of peritonitis is almost always clinical. The symptom complex of anorexia, nausea, and abdominal pain associated with the physical findings of fever, tachycardia, and abdominal tenderness is diagnostic of peritonitis. The hemodynamic and metabolic responses to intra-abdominal infection vary depending on the severity of the infectious process and the magnitude of the patient's response to the infection.

Laboratory and radiologic tests may support the diagnosis of peritonitis. Specifically, the leukocyte count characteristically is elevated with a left shift. Plain abdominal X-ray films may show evidence of ileus with distended loops of large and small bowel, air–fluid levels, and free fluid in the peritoneal cavity. Upright films demonstrate free air under the diaphragm in 80% of patients with perforated duodenal ulcer, but free air is evident in a smaller percentage of patients after perforation of other intra-abdominal organs.

Management

The principles of therapy in patients with secondary peritonitis are (i) resuscitation, (ii) appropriate antimicrobial therapy, and (iii) surgical intervention. All patients with peritonitis have some degree of hypovolemia related to third-space fluid loss into the peritoneal cavity. Patients should be resuscitated with crystalloid solution before surgery. The microbiology of secondary peritonitis is invariably polymicrobial (10) and consists of a mixture of gram-negative enteric bacteria and anaerobes (Box 1). Both experimental and clinical studies suggest that antimicrobial therapy should be directed against both the aerobic and anaerobic components of these infections, typified by *Escherichia coli* and *Bacteroides fragilis* (11,12). Single agents or combination regimens that fulfill this requirement are effective for treating secondary peritonitis. Table 2 summarizes the guidelines proposed by the Surgical Infection Society for the use of anti-infective agents during intra-abdominal infection (13). The need to treat enterococci specifically remains controversial. Although experimental studies suggest that this microorganism can act as a significant copathogen with *E. coli* (14), clinical studies demonstrate that antibiotic coverage directed against coliforms and anaerobes is sufficient treatment for intra-abdominal infection and usually does not result in treatment failure or relapse from enterococci. In contrast, enterococcal bacteremia or the recovery of enterococci from residual or recurrent intra-abdominal infection represents an indication for the treatment with the appropriate antienterococcal therapy (15). Current recommendations from the Surgical Infection

Box 1 Bacteria Causing Secondary Peritonitis and Intra-abdominal Abscess

Facultative gram-negative bacilli	Facultative gram-positive cocci
E. coli	Enterococci
Klebsiella species	*Staphylococcus* species
Proteus species	*Streptococcus* species
Enterobacter species	Aerobic gram-negative bacilli
Morganella morganii	*Pseudomonas aeruginosa*
Other *Enterococci* gram-negative species	
Obligate anaerobes	
B. fragilis	
Bacteroides species	
Fusobacterium species	
Clostridium species	
Peptococcus species	
Peptostreptococcus species	
Lactobacillus species	

Source: From Bohnen JMA, Solomkin JS, Dellinger EP, Bjornson HS, Page CP. Guidelines for clinical care: anti-infective agents for intra-abdominal infection. Arch Surg 1992; 127:83–89.

Table 2 Antibiotic Therapy for Secondary Peritonitis and Intra-abdominal Abscesses (Recommended Antimicrobial Regimens for Patients with Intra-abdominal Infections)

Single agents
  Ampicillin/sulbactam
  Cefotetan
  Cefoxitin
  Ertapenem
  Imipenem/cilastatin
  Meropenem
  Piperacillin/tazobactam
  Ticarcillin/clavulonic acid
Combination regimens
  Aminoglycoside (amikacin, gentamicin, netilmicin, tobramycin) and antianaerobe
  Aztreonam and clindamycin
  Cefuroxime and metronidazole
  Ciprofloxacin and metronidazole
    Third/fourth generation cephalosporin (cefepime, cefotaxime, ceftazidime, ceftizoxime, ceftriaxone) and antianaerobe

Source: From Ref. 13.

Society include agents with enterococcal coverage for high-risk patients (13). Similarly, *Candida* species may be recovered as part of the polymicrobial flora from the peritoneal exudate of patients with secondary peritonitis. As for enterococci, no indication exists for specific therapy directed against *Candida* species in patients with otherwise uncomplicated secondary peritonitis. Empiric antifungal therapy may be indicated for patients at high risk for candidiasis (13).

    The duration of antibiotic therapy following operative management of secondary peritonitis should be based on the clinical status of the patient. If the patient is afebrile, has a normal leukocyte count, and a band count <3%, the chance of recurrent sepsis after discontinuation of antibiotic therapy is virtually zero (16,17). In contrast, if the patient demonstrates a fever or leukocytosis, the probability of recurrent or residual infection ranges from 33% to 50%. With this approach, antibiotics may be discontinued as early as postoperative day 4. However, if leukocytosis or fever persists after postoperative days 7–10, the clinician should investigate the patient for the presence of residual infection, rather than simply extending antimicrobial therapy. Several clinical circumstances exist in which the duration of antibiotic therapy may be as short as 1 day. They include simple acute and suppurative appendicitis, small bowel infarction without perforation, and traumatic enteric perforations operated on within 12 h of injury (13). The common feature of these diagnoses is the minimal degree of peritoneal soiling and inflammatory response present at the time of laparotomy. A preoperative dose of antibiotics followed by two doses within 24 h of surgery is appropriate therapy for these conditions.

    The goals of the surgical management of peritonitis are to eliminate the source of contamination, to reduce the bacterial inoculum, and to prevent recurrent or persistent infection. The technique used to control contamination depends on the location and the nature of the pathologic condition. In general, continued peritoneal soiling is controlled by closing, excluding, or resecting the perforated viscus. Colonic pathology is handled most effectively by resection of the diseased segment with exteriorization of the proximal end as an end colostomy, and by creating a mucous fistula or oversewing the distal end. A primary anastomosis in a patient with diffuse peritonitis is associated with an increased rate of dehiscence and should be avoided (18). Small intestinal pathology should be dealt with similarly by resection of the diseased segment. As the risk of anastomotic dehiscence is reduced, a primary anastomosis may be considered in this circumstance. However, if peritoneal soiling is particularly extensive or the viability of the intestine is uncertain, the creation of stomas is preferable. A perforated duodenal ulcer caused by peptic ulcer disease is either patched with a piece of omentum or included in the creation of pyloroplasty. In the latter situation, simultaneous vagotomy should be performed. A perforated gastric ulcer is either included in a distal gastric resection with subsequent gastroduodenal or gastrojejunal anastomosis or excised locally with primary closure. Appendicitis is treated by appendectomy.

In addition to treating the underlying pathology, gross purulent exudates are aspirated, and loculations in the pelvis, paracolic gutters, and subphrenic regions are gently opened and debrided. Adjuvant materials, including fecal matter, barium, necrotic tissue, and blood, should be removed as part of this procedure. Intraoperative peritoneal lavage with saline solution will augment the debridement process. The addition of antibiotics to the lavage solution has not been shown to be of clear benefit. Drains are not generally necessary unless a well-defined abscess cavity is discovered at the time of abdominal exploration. Using either running or interrupted monofilament sutures, abdominal closure is performed in a single fascial layer. In heavily contaminated cases, wound infection is avoided by leaving the skin and subcutaneous tissues open, and closing them in a delayed fashion.

Intra-abdominal Abscess

Diagnosis

Abscesses are well-defined collections of purulent material that are walled off from the rest of the peritoneal cavity by inflammatory adhesions, loops of intestines, mesentery, the greater omentum, or other abdominal viscera. Intra-abdominal abscesses occurring outside of the solid viscera arise in two situations: (i) after resolution of diffuse peritonitis in which a loculated area of infection persists and evolves into an abscess and (ii) after perforation of a viscus or an anastomotic breakdown that is successfully walled off by peritoneal defense mechanisms. In the latter situation, the abscess most frequently is located in apposition to the defect in the GI tract (19). Intermesenteric perforation of the colon or perforation of the retroperitoneal aspects of the GI tract may result in retroperitoneal abscesses.

The diagnosis of an intra-abdominal abscess is based on clinical suspicion with radiologic confirmation. Abdominal pain, localized tenderness, and a diffuse mass are characteristic of intra-abdominal abscess formation. However, the clinical findings may be somewhat more insidious and manifested only by anorexia and mild abdominal tenderness. As previously noted, a patient recovering from peritonitis who has a persistent fever or leukocytosis should be investigated for the presence of residual infection. Ultrasonography and computed tomography (CT) scanning are clearly the examinations of choice for the diagnosis of intra-abdominal abscess formation (20). Techniques such as gallium scans, white blood cell scans, and plain X-ray studies are of minimal value in this situation.

Management

The basic approach to management of intra-abdominal abscesses is very much the same as that for secondary peritonitis, with the exception that the abscess cavity frequently is drained by radiologically guided percutaneous catheters. The microbiology is similar, and antibiotic recommendations are the same (Box 1 and Table 2).

Drainage, either percutaneous or surgical, represents the mainstay of the management of intra-abdominal abscesses. The ability to accurately localize abscesses not only allows the use of percutaneous techniques, but also significantly facilitates the approach to abscess drainage when surgery is necessary. Percutaneous drainage is highly effective when the abscess is a single, well-defined cavity without enteric communication (21,22). In contrast, multiple abscesses, the presence of extremely viscous abscess contents such as those found in patients with fungal infections or pancreatic necrosis, and infected hematomas have a lesser chance of success by the percutaneous route. When approaching abscesses surgically, the accurate localization of the abscess by CT prevents the need for a general abdominal exploration and permits a direct (often extraserous) approach to the abscess. Drains, whether placed surgically or percutaneously, should be left in place until the patient is clinically improved, minimal drainage from the catheter is demonstrated, and radiologic evidence of resolution of the abscess by CT scan or sinogram is found. A sinogram also identifies a connection to the GI tract.

Percutaneous abscess drainage has become the initial procedure of choice for the treatment of most intra-abdominal abscesses. Typically, the abscess is detected by CT scanning or by ultrasonography. Needle aspiration may be performed for diagnosis. If purulent fluid is obtained, catheter drainage is instituted (21). The outcome is optimized if the approach to the abscess is individualized for each patient and appropriate abscess drainage occurs early.

Tertiary Peritonitis

The combination of appropriate antibiotic therapy and timely surgical intervention is sufficient to effect complete resolution of an infection in the majority of patients with secondary peritonitis. Even when infection persists or recurs, the ability of the host to localize the infection results in a discrete abscess that can be treated by percutaneous or surgical drainage. However, some patients demonstrate an inability to wall off and resolve intraperitoneal infection and go on to develop persistent diffuse peritonitis. The clinical picture is characterized by poorly localized intra-abdominal infection, altered microbial flora, the development of progressive organ dysfunction, and higher mortality (23). The microbiology of tertiary peritonitis differs significantly from that reported for secondary peritonitis (Table 3). Specifically, *Staphylococcus epidermidis*, *Enterococcus*, and *Candida* species are predominant microorganisms recovered from these patients (23). Accordingly, antimicrobial therapy should be focused rather than empiric and broad-spectrum, as described for secondary peritonitis.

Optimal therapy for patients with tertiary peritonitis is limited by the poorly defined pathogenesis of this disease. Although microorganisms are regularly recovered from the peritoneal cavity, their precise contribution to the ongoing disease process is not well understood. Confounding observations include the fact that focused antimicrobial therapy is frequently unable to eradicate the microorganism, and the practice of performing repeat laparotomies to control residual infection has little impact on outcome in these

Table 3 Microbiology of Tertiary Peritonitis

Organisms[a]	Number of positive cultures	Number of patients
Aerobes		
S. epidermidis	24	16
Enterococcus	14	8
α-Hemolytic Streptococcus	4	3
P. aeruginosa	16	12
Facultative gram-negative bacilli		
E. coli	11	6
Klebsiella pneumoniae and K. oxytoca	8	6
Enterobacter cloacae and E. aerogenes	16	8
Anaerobes		
B. fragilis	4	3
Clostridium perfringens, C. clostridiiforme, and unidentified clostridial species	5	3
Fungus		
Candida albicans	19	10
C. glabrata	10	5
C. tropicalis	2	2

[a]Isolates from the peritoneal cavity of 25 patients with persistent peritonitis.
Source: Modified from Ref. 24.

patients and frequently does not reveal evidence of infection (25). These discrepancies have led to the development of alternate hypotheses to explain the development of organ dysfunction associated with tertiary peritonitis. First, tertiary peritonitis may be a consequence of undrained foci of infection in patients with secondary peritonitis being colonized with organisms under selection pressure from initially selected antimicrobials that become relatively resistant to antibiotics. Second, tertiary peritonitis may result from the spread of intensive care unit (ICU)-acquired infection from other sites. The predominant organisms of tertiary peritonitis are the same as those commonly causing bacteremia in the ICU. Third, the role of the GI tract as a source for bacteria and/or endotoxin has been the subject of recent interest (26). The flora of tertiary peritonitis includes those organisms that overgrow and colonize the proximal GI tract in the critically ill patient (23). Translocation of bacteria and endotoxin from the GI tract in response to an inflammatory stimulus, such as diffuse peritonitis, has been postulated to lead to distant organ dysfunction. Altering this process by using techniques such as selective digestive decontamination (27) or enhancing the integrity of the mucosal barrier with specific nutrients (28) may become important components of the therapy for these patients.

Tertiary peritonitis may not be the failure of infection control, but instead may represent the inadequacy of host defenses despite therapeutic efforts (29). It may be similar to other ICU-acquired infections, such as nosocomial pneumonia, in which antimicrobial or surgical therapy may result in only modestly improved outcome (30). Patients may die with, rather than of, tertiary peritonitis (23). At present, the best outcomes in this patient population are achieved by providing aggressive hemodynamic monitoring and support, adequate nutrition, directed antibiotic therapy, and timely surgical intervention.

SUMMARY

> **Patient with Peritonitis**
>
> - Resuscitate.
> - Start therapy with broad-spectrum antibiotics that are active against gram-negative enteric bacteria and anaerobic bacteria; continue antibiotic therapy until patient is afebrile and leukocyte count is normal for 48 h (band count <3%).
> - During surgical intervention, resect, close, or patch site of intestinal pathology.
>
> **Patient with Intra-abdominal Abscesses**
>
> - Resuscitate with crystalloids/colloids.
> - Provide broad-spectrum antibiotic therapy as per peritonitis until culture results are available.
> - Drain the abscess either percutaneously or surgically, depending on the clinical situation.

REFERENCES

1. Allen L, Weatherford T. Role of fenestrated basement membrane in lymphatic absorption from the peritoneal cavity. Am J Physiol 1956; 197:551.
2. Steinberg B. Infections of the Peritoneum. New York: Hoeber, 1944.
3. Hau T, Ahrenholz, DH, Simmons RL. Secondary bacterial peritonitis: the biologic basis of treatment. Curr Probl Surg 1979; 16:1.
4. Dunn DL, Barke RA, Ewald DC, Simmons RL. Macrophages and translymphatic absorption represent the first line of host defense of the peritoneal cavity. Arch Surg 1987; 122:105.
5. Hau T, Hoffman R, Simmons RL. Mechanisms of the adjuvant effect of hemoglobin in experimental peritonitis. I. *In vivo* inhibition of peritoneal leukocytosis. Surgery 1978; 83:223.
6. Ford HR, Hoffman RA, Wing EJ, et al. Characterization of wound cytokines in the sponge matrix model. Arch Surg 1989; 124:1422.
7. Dunn DL, Simmons RL. Fibrin in peritonitis. III. The mechanism of bacterial trapping by polymerizing fibrin. Surgery 1982; 92:513.
8. Sinclair SB, Rotstein OD, Levy GA. Disparate mechanisms of induction of procoagulant activity by live and inactivated bacteria and viruses. Infect Immun 1990; 58:182.
9. Hau T, Payne WD, Simmons RL. Fibrinolytic activity of the peritoneum during experimental peritonitis. Surg Gynecol Obstet 1979; 148:415.
10. Lorber B, Swenson RM. The bacteriology of intraabdominal infections. Surg Clin North Am 1975; 55:1349.
11. Berne TV, Yellin AW, Appleman MD, Heseltine PNR. Antibiotic management of surgically treated gangrenous or perforated appendicitis. Comparison of gentamicin and clindamycin versus cefamandole versus cefoperazone. Am J Surg 1982; 144:8.
12. Bartlett JG, Louie TJ, Gorbach SL, Onderdonk AB. Therapeutic efficacy of 29 antimicrobial regimens in experimental intraabdominal sepsis. Rev Infect Dis 1981; 3:535.
13. Mazuski JE, Sawyer RG, Nathens AB, Dipiro JT, Schein M, Kudsk KA, Yowler C. The Surgical Infection Society guidelines on antimicrobial therapy for intra-abdominal infections: an executive summary. Surg Infect 2002; 3:161–173.

14. Fry DE, Berberich S, Garrison RN. Bacterial synergism between the *enterococcus* and *Escherichia coli.* J Surg Res 1985; 38:475.
15. Barie PS, Christou NV, Dellinger EP, et al. Pathogenicity of the *enterococcus* in surgical infections. Ann Surg 1990; 212:155.
16. Lennard ES, Dellinger EP, Wertz MJ, et al. Implications of leukocytosis and fever at conclusion of antibiotic therapy for intraabdominal sepsis. Ann Surg 1982; 195:19.
17. Stone HH, Bourneuf AA, Stinson LD. Reliability of criteria for predicting persistent or recurrent sepsis. Arch Surg 1985; 120:17.
18. Schrock TR, Deveney CW, Dunphy JE. Factors contributing to leakage of colonic anastomoses. Ann Surg 1973; 197:513.
19. Altemeier WA, Culbertson WR, Shook CD. Intraabdominal abscesses. Am J Surg 1973; 125:70.
20. Baker ME, Blinder RA, Rice RP. Diagnostic imaging of abdominal fluid collections and abscesses. Crit Rev Diagn Imaging 1986; 25:233.
21. vanSonnenberg E, Wittich GR, Goodacre BW, Casola G, D'Agostino HB. Percutaneous abscess drainage. World J Surg 2001; 25:362–372.
22. Olak J, Christou NV, Stein LA, et al. Operative vs. percutaneous drainage of intraabdominal abscesses. Arch Surg 1986; 121:141.
23. Nathens AB, Rotstein OD, Marshall JC. Tertiary peritonitis: clinical features of a complex nosocomial infection. World J Surg 1998; 22:158–163.
24. Rotstein OD, Pruett TL, Simmons RL. Microbiologic features and treatment of persistent peritonitis in the intensive care unit. Can J Surg 1986; 29:247.
25. Norwood SN, Civetta JM. Abdominal CT scanning in critically ill surgical patients. Ann Surg 1985; 202:166.
26. Carrico CJ, Meakins JL, Marshall JC. Multiple-organ-failure syndrome: the gastrointestinal tract—the motor of "MOF". Arch Surg 1986; 121:197.
27. Ramsay G, van Saene RHKF. Selective gut decontamination in intensive care and surgical practice: where are we? World J Surg 1998; 22:164–170.
28. Wilmore DW, Smith RJ, O'Dwyer ST. The gut: a central organ of after-surgical stress. Surgery 1988; 104:917.
29. Reemst PH, van Goor H, Goris RJ. SIRS, MODS, and tertiary peritonitis. Eur J Surg 1996; 576(suppl):47–48.
30. Rello J, Ausina V, Ricart M, Castella J, Prats G. Impact of previous antimicrobial therapy on the etiology and outcome of ventilator associated pneumonia. Chest 1993; 104:1230–1235.

SUGGESTED READING

Ahrenholz DH, Simmons RL. Peritonitis and other intra-abdominal infections. In: Simmons RL, Howard RJ, eds. Surgical Infectious Diseases. Norwalk, Conn.: Appleton & Lange, 1988 (Excellent comprehensive discussion of intra-abdominal infection.)

Rotstein OD. Peritonitis and intraabdominal abscesses. In: Wilmore DW, Brennan MF, Harken AH, Holcroft JW, Meakins JL, eds. Care of the Surgical Patient. New York: Scientific American Publications, 1992 (A comprehensive overview of the pathophysiology, diagnosis, and management of intra-abdominal infection, with many references.)

47
HIV/AIDS and the Surgeon

Omobosola Akinsete and Edward N. Janoff
VA Medical Center, Minneapolis, Minnesota, USA

INTRODUCTION

Many surgeons have extensive experience with immunocompromised patients. Prominent among these patients are those with cancer, those who receive radiation and chemotherapy, and those who develop profound malnutrition following surgery in association with infectious and other complications in the intensive care unit (ICU). In addition, the induction and management of immunodeficiency among patients following organ transplantation (particularly kidney, liver, heart, and other sites) has long been the purview of surgical specialists. However, over the last two decades, the emergence of the human immunodeficiency virus (HIV) and the acquired immunodeficiency syndrome (AIDS) as the leading causes of severe and prolonged immune insufficiency in the United States has provided new medical, social, and ethical challenges for the surgical community. Physicians who attended medical school and completed residencies before the mid-1980s later found themselves confronted with novel clinical problems for which no precedents and no clear guidelines existed. More recently, the clinical experience associated with HIV infection, including both presentations and outcomes of different syndromes, has been well documented and analyzed. Increasingly effective interventions have been implemented to diagnose HIV infection, to prevent and treat the secondary opportunistic infections that complicate HIV disease, and to treat HIV infection itself. The incidence of HIV infection in the United States has remained stable or decreased, but the prolonged survival associated with highly active antiretroviral therapy (HAART) (1,2) has also introduced new variables, such as an increased rate of cardiac disease and liver failure, and non-HIV-associated age-related conditions that may require surgical evaluation and intervention.

In this chapter, we discuss the epidemiology of HIV infection to understand the rates and risk of infection, the common clinical signs and symptoms, and the laboratory data that suggest the presence of the disease. We examine the known risk of HIV infection to the surgeon associated with surgical procedures, as well as the risk to the patient during surgery from an infected practitioner. Common presenting symptoms that may elicit surgical attention are considered, as is the outcome of patients, particularly those in the ICU. Finally, we list the complications of specific antiretroviral drug regimens that may have an impact on the diagnosis and management of these patients.

EPIDEMIOLOGY

Since the first reports in 1981, HIV/AIDS has become the most devastating disease in the history of humankind. Over 60 million people worldwide have been infected, of whom 20 million have died. As this new century begins, an estimated 5 million individuals in the world become infected each year, of whom 10% are children (approximately 1500 children per day, or about 1 per min) (3). The World Health Organization and Joint United Nations Program on AIDS (UNAIDS) estimate that HIV/AIDS is the fourth leading cause of death worldwide, and accounts for approximately 3 million deaths annually. AIDS is the leading cause of death in sub-Saharan Africa, where 5–35% of the population is infected in many areas. In 2001, this region was home to 70% of the current cases and 68% of the HIV-related deaths. In southern Africa, the disease is disrupting food production, commerce, infrastructure, social stability, and the lives of every family. India and the former Soviet republics are also fast-expanding targets for HIV/AIDS. Among the last two countries, unprotected sex, poorly controlled sexually transmitted diseases, and intravenous drug use are prominent risks for new HIV infections (3).

Despite the remarkable rates of infection in resource-poor nations, HIV/AIDS remains a prominent health problem in the United States. Once the leading cause of death among men 15–45 years of age (4), both the incidence of HIV and its associated mortality had begun to decline at the end of the 20th century, mainly as a result of extensive public health prevention efforts and new effective antiretroviral therapy (1,5). However, that rate of decline appears to be leveling off, and the rate of new infections may be on the rise in some populations (3,4). To date, almost 800,000 Americans have developed AIDS, among whom more than 450,000 have died (4). The majority of the estimated 1 million HIV-infected Americans living with HIV (~35% with AIDS) belong to identifiable ethnic and behavioral risk groups. Among these patients, 38% were white, 20% were Hispanic, and 41% were black (4). Comprising only 12% of the U.S. population, African-Americans accounted for 47% of HIV/AIDS cases in 2000 (3). Although the overall incidence rates have decreased, the distribution of cases among racial groups has shifted to increasing rates in young ethnic minorities—blacks, Hispanics, and persons infected through heterosexual contact (3,4,6).

Homosexual transmission accounted for 53% of new infections in the United States in 2000 and is still the main mode of transmission. A recent increase in high-risk sexual activity and the incidence of HIV among men who have sex with men (e.g., from 0.6% between 1995 and 1999 to 3.7% in 2000 in Vancouver, Canada) (3) has been associated with misconceptions about the efficacy of HIV therapy and its unrealized potential for cure (4). Unfortunately, advances in treatment and care have not matched with progress on the prevention front. In addition to homosexual men, almost one-third of new cases are women whose high-risk behaviors include intravenous drug use, trading or selling sex for drugs, and heterosexual contact with intravenous drug users. Indeed, 30% of new HIV cases in the United States are identified intravenous drug users (3).

Health care workers (HCWs) are susceptible to HIV transmission in the occupational setting (7). As of September 1997, 94 documented and 170 possible cases of HIV seroconversion associated with HIV percutaneous exposure had been identified worldwide among HCWs (8). As of 2000, the Centers for Disease Control and Prevention (CDC) had received 56 additional reports of HCWs in the United States with documented HIV seroconversion temporally associated with an occupational HIV exposure. An additional 138 episodes were considered possible occupational HIV transmissions (4). The great majority of these were nurses who had experienced a needle stick (9), but several were surgeons. The great majority of infections among surgeons occurred in areas with a very high prevalence of HIV, such as sub-Saharan Africa.

TRANSMISSION OF HIV

HIV is transmitted by three principal mechanisms: sexual; vertical (mother to child); and by blood exposure through transfusion, intravenous drug use, or accidental needle stick (e.g., to HCWs). Sexual transmission, either heterosexual or homosexual, accounted for 75–85% of the nearly 28 million HIV infections reported by 1997 (10). Overall, the risk of HIV transmission from contact ranges from ∼1 in 100 to 1 in 1000 per high-risk exposure (10). The risk of sexual transmission appears to be lower than other routes of transmission, and some data suggest a relatively low efficiency of transmission in penile–vaginal intercourse, especially from women to men (4). Factors that have been shown to enhance the sexual transmission of HIV include higher levels of viremia (especially greater than 10,000 copies of HIV per milliliter of blood) or more advanced disease in the source person, receptive anal intercourse and genital tract trauma, sexual contact during menstruation, the presence of a foreskin in men, and other sexually transmitted diseases—both ulcerative and non-ulcerative (11). Despite high rates of exposure, some commercial sex workers and homosexual men have remained uninfected with HIV (12–15). Such resistance has been proposed to relate, in part, to the development of local mucosal HIV-specific IgA, which may prevent initial infection, virus-specific CD8+ cytotoxic lymphocytes (CTL), which kill infected cells, as well as a mutation in a common co-receptor for HIV (CCR5Δ32) on target cells. People who are homozygous for this mutation appear to be routinely resistant to most HIV infections, and those who are heterozygous may experience slower progression of the disease.

Mother-to-child transmission (MTCT) of HIV (vertical transmission), which accounts for 90% of pediatric AIDS cases and almost all newly diagnosed HIV infections in children (16), can occur during pregnancy, during delivery, or post partum via breast feeding. In the United States, the perinatal rate of HIV infection, in the absence of antiretroviral treatment or intervention, was ∼25% (17). However, the risk for pre- and perinatal MTCT may be reduced by at least 65% with Cesarian section and antiretroviral therapy in industrialized nations and, to a lesser extent, in developing countries (18–20). As a result of these and other interventions, the rates of vertical transmission of HIV have declined from ∼25% to <2% in the United States. Thus, far fewer than 500 children in the United States are infected with HIV per year by vertical transmission (rate <2%). Nevertheless, up to 1500 children are infected per day worldwide (rate of ∼20–35%) (21). Moreover, postnatal transmission through breast feeding accounts for a third of vertical transmission, particularly in sub-Saharan Africa (infection rate 3–10% per year) (22,23). Children who remain uninfected in these countries often become orphans by five years of age. Thus, the loss of socially and economically productive adults seriously impedes efforts to control the HIV epidemic in many parts of the world.

Direct blood exposure in both industrialized and resource-poor nations (particularly Asia and the former Soviet block) via intravenous drug use constitutes a prominent risk for HIV infection and accounts for a quarter of cases in men and over a third of cases in women in the United States (24). Moreover, in developing countries, infected medical equipment such as scalpels, needles, and syringes that are reused for procedures are also a significant mode of transmission, as is infection by contaminated blood transfusions when the prevalence of infection is high (>5%) and serologic screening procedures are limited (3). In contrast, the risk of HIV infection by blood transfusion is less than one per million units transfused in the United States, particularly since detection of HIV-specific antibodies by enzyme immunoassay and immunoblot became available in 1985. Detection of HIV antigen [p24 by polymerase chain reaction (PCR)] in blood units further reduced the risk by identifying infected donors early in the course of their infection, before antiviral antibodies had developed (a "window" period, typically from 3 weeks to 4 months from initial infection). Infection rates are 100% following transfusion of contaminated blood.

Rates of transmission are much lower following needle stick/occupational exposure. In the United States and other developed countries, such exposures usually occur in the setting of a medical or related institution, and HCWs of various skills are at risk of occupational exposure. Percutaneous injuries are defined as exposure to blood-borne pathogens, including HIV. They are caused by a needle stick or cut with a sharp object. Other means of occupational exposure include contact of potentially infectious fluids with the mucous membrane or nonintact skin, for example, abraded or chapped skin. These fluids include blood and blood products, and tissue or other body fluids, such as cerebrospinal fluid, synovial fluid, pleural fluid, peritoneal fluid, pericardial fluid, and amniotic fluid. Seminal and vaginal secretions not containing blood have not been proven to be infectious in the occupational setting. Infectivity of other fluids such as sweat, saliva, sputum, and urine has not been determined in occupational transmission, unless they contain blood, and are considered to be of very low risk (25).

In prospective studies, the average risk of HIV transmission after a percutaneous exposure to HIV-infected blood has been estimated as $\sim$0.3% (25,26) and after a mucous membrane exposure as $\sim$0.09% (25). The average risk of transmission after nonintact skin exposure is estimated to be lower than that of mucous membrane exposure. The risk of transmission from other body fluids has not been determined but is probably much lower than that for blood exposures. This risk is increased with exposure to a large quantity of blood, such as when a device is visibly contaminated with the source patient's blood, or from a procedure that involved a needle being placed directly into a vessel, or with a deep injury (8,25). Hollow-bore needles carry a higher risk of transmission than do solid needles; however, a low volume exposure can involve blood with a very high titer of infectious HIV and transmission may occur (27).

Needle sticks and other percutaneous injuries in the health care setting are very common but are frequently not reported (7). In 1996, of 590 (164 percutaneous and 426 mucocutaneous) exposures to blood or risky biologic substances, up to 39% of incidents were not reported (7,28). Surgeons are at particular risk of being infected with HIV by their patients during procedures, since percutaneous injuries occur regularly during surgical procedures (29,30). Surveys of orthopedic surgeons found that 39.2% had had percutaneous blood injuries in the preceding month (29), and another survey of surgeons from the United States and the University of Toronto found that the respondents averaged 11 needle stick injuries over a 3-year period (31). A CDC review of nine different prospective observational studies reported that a surgical team member sustained at least one percutaneous injury during 1.3–15.4% of procedures (32). A rate of 6.9% during 1382 surgical procedures was observed in one study (29).

The risk of percutaneous injury varies according to surgical specialty and procedure, from 4–5% of procedures in orthopedics and trauma surgery to 8–10% in the general, gynecologic, and cardiac surgery services (29). Seventy-seven percent of exposures were caused by suture needles and affected the nondominant hand, especially the distal

Table 1 Risk Factors for the Transmission of HIV to Surgeons

The HIV prevalence in the patient population (the probability that the patient is infected)
The probability of a percutaneous injury from a sharp instrument used on an HIV-infected patient resulting in infection (0.3%)
The number of percutaneous injuries the surgeon experiences in his career
Whether postexposure prophylaxis (PEP) is administered to the exposed surgeon

Source: Ref. 32.

forefinger. The risk was highest during vaginal hysterectomies, probably as a result of poor visibility and the tendency of surgeons to guide or palpate suture needles with their fingers. The risk was lowest for orthopedic procedures. The use of fingers rather than an instrument to hold the tissue being sutured was associated with 35% of injuries. Resident surgeons with 4 or more years of training were at highest risk of injury (OR 1.6). The high risk in this group was probably due to the frequency of their involvement in surgical procedures.

In another observational study of 1307 patients (33), accidental exposure of surgical personnel to patients' blood occurred at a rate of 6.4%. The rate of parenteral exposure was 1.7%. The risk of exposure was highest when procedures lasted over 3 h, when blood loss exceeded 300 mL, and when major vascular and intra-abdominal gynecologic surgery was performed (34). The risk of percutaneous injuries was 13.6% per 1000 surgical hours in plastic surgeons and slightly lower in orthopedic, obstetric, and gynecological surgery. Most authorities conclude that surgeons are likely to have multiple blood exposures during their careers (33). The risk of infection of surgeons with blood-borne pathogens, including HIV, is estimated to be 0.0024–0.024 per 1000 patients (32). Only one seroconversion is documented of a surgeon who became infected when he cut his gloved finger while incising a perianal abscess in 1996 (35). However, another surgeon, who subsequently was reported to have infected one of his patients, may have also acquired his infection from a needle stick during orthopedic surgery in 1983 (36). In summary, the higher the prevalence of HIV in the population served and the higher the number of percutaneous injuries, the greater the risk of HIV transmission to the surgeon (Table 1). In the event of a potential HIV exposure, rapid tests are widely accessible for the presence of the virus [p24 antigen and HIV ribonucleic acid (RNA)] and HIV-specific antibody, results of which should be available within hours.

TRANSMISSION OF HIV FROM SURGEON TO PATIENT

In addition to the risk to the surgeon, a risk also exists for transmission of HIV, as well as hepatitis B, from the surgeon to the patient during invasive procedures. These exposures appear to be related to "recontact" injuries following penetration of the HCWs skin (29) or when instruments or gloves that are possibly contaminated with an HCWs blood enter an open wound (7). The probability of transmission of HIV from an infected surgeon to at least one patient during 3500 procedures (the CDC's estimate of the number of procedures performed during a surgeon's career) is 0.81–8.1% (7). Between 1990 and 1992, a dentist in Florida was documented to have infected six of his patients (37) after having been diagnosed with AIDS in 1986. Epidemiologic and deoxyribonucleic acid (DNA) sequencing of his virus showed that he was likely the source of each of their infections. In 1999, an orthopedic surgeon in Paris was reported to have infected one of his patients during a prolonged procedure involving the placement of a hip prosthesis with bone graft (36). The exact date and mechanism of the transmission was not established, but the patient was a 67-year-old woman with no significant risk factors, and genetic sequencing of the virus in both parties showed them to be closely linked (30,36,38). Since 1990, at least 22,759 patients who received medical care from 53 United States health providers with HIV infection (including 29 dental workers and 15 surgeons and obstetricians) have been evaluated in retrospective studies monitored by the CDC. No new nosocomial HIV infections from surgeons to their patients have been identified to date (30). Thus, the probability of transmission from an HIV-infected provider to a patient is below the threshold of detection by even very intensive surveillance methods, and transmission is exceedingly rare in the United States (30). As a result, routine testing of HCWs, including surgeons, for evidence of active viral hepatitis B (HBV) or C (HCV), or HIV, is not recommended. Nevertheless, that infected surgeons inform their patients of their HIV status before surgery conforms with the highest and most appropriate ethical standards (39).

PREVENTION OF OCCUPATIONAL HIV INFECTION

Nosocomial HIV infection can be prevented by integrating two strategies. The first is prevention of exposure to the virus. Routinely observing universal blood and body substance precautions is a major obstacle to HIV exposure during and after surgical procedures. Immunization against hepatitis B, which carries ~100-fold the transmission risk of HIV, serves as a reasonable adjunct to preventing infection with blood-borne pathogens. The use of double gloves and blunt needles appears to decrease the risk of percutaneous injuries during surgical procedures (40). The use of hand protection and safe manipulation techniques for suturing and closing wounds, including using instruments to hold suture needles as opposed to fingers, and the improved equipment design currently in use in most operating rooms in the United States may also limit risk (30). Intraoperative exposures should be reported immediately and managed via risk assessment, PEP with antiretroviral therapy as indicated (Table 2), and follow-up. Protocols for evaluating and managing percutaneous injuries should be in place in emergency rooms, employee health clinics in every medical institution, and many outpatient clinics. Prompt reporting can facilitate risk assessment and access to PEP in a timely fashion (30). When the patient is exposed to the surgeon's blood, such as in a recontact type injury, the patient may also be exposed to a risk of which they are unaware. In this setting, the provider should be tested for HIV, antibody to HCV, and if not immune, antibody to HBV. The patient should be informed and followed. Controversy surrounds the question of whether surgeons should test themselves for HIV periodically.

The second strategy for prevention is the use of PEP. Owing to the random nature of HIV exposures in the workplace and the low number of resultant infections, animal models have provided the most consistent experience in predicting and preventing these infections. Factors associated with successful infection include increased viral inoculum (both the volume and the concentration of HIV), the interval between exposure and PEP, and the duration and specific drug selection for treatment (25). These studies have shown that infection with HIV requires time for migration to and proliferation in initial target cells such as lymph nodes. A window of opportunity exists for administration of PEP to inhibit viral replication in its early stages. On the basis of the level of risk for transmission represented by the exposure (Tables 2 and 3) a combination of two or three

Table 2 Recommended HIV PEP

	Status of source		
Exposure	Low risk[a]	High risk[b]	Unknown
Percutaneous			
Not severe: solid needle, superficial	Basic two-drug PEP	Expanded three-drug PEP	Usually none; consider basic two-drug PEP[c]
Severe: large bore, deep injury, visible blood in device, needle in patient artery/vein	Expanded three-drug PEP	Expanded three-drug PEP	Usually none; consider basic two-drug PEP[c]
Mucous membrane, nonintact skin (dermatitis, abrasion, wound)			
Small volume (drops)	Consider basic two-drug PEP	Basic two-drug PEP	Usually none; consider basic two-drug PEP[c]
Large volume (major blood splash)	Basic two-drug PEP	Basic three-drug PEP	Usually none; consider basic two-drug PEP[c]

[a] Low risk, asymptomatic HIV or viral load >1500 c/mL.
[b] High risk, symptomatic HIV, AIDS, acute seroconversion, and high viral load.
[c] Consider two-drug PEP if source is high risk for HIV or exposure is from an unknown source with HIV likely.
Source: Ref. 41–43.

Table 3 Basic and Expanded Regimens of PEP Against HIV Infection

Regimen	Doses
Basic	
Zidovudine (Retrovir) plus lamivudine (Epivir)[a]	600 mg of zidovudine daily in two or three divided doses; 150 mg of lamivudine twice daily
Lamivudine plus stavudine (Zerit)	150 mg of lamivudine twice daily; 40 mg of stavudine (if body weight is <60 kg, 30 mg) twice daily
Didanosine, available as a chewable or dispersable buffered tablet (Videx) or as a delayed-release capsule (Videx EC), plus stavudine	400 mg of didanosine daily, taken on an empty stomach if a buffered tablet is used (if body weight is <60 kg, 125 mg twice daily if a buffered tablet is used), or 250 mg daily if a delayed-release capsule is used; 40 mg of stavudine twice daily
Expanded (basic regimen plus one of the following)	
Indinavir (Crixivan)	800 mg every 8 h, taken on an empty stomach
Nelfinavir (Viracept)	750 mg three times daily, with a meal or snack, or 1250 mg twice daily, with a meal or snack
Efavirenz (Sustiva)	600 mg daily, at bedtime
Abacavir (Ziagen)[b]	300 mg twice daily

[a] A combined formulation is also available (Combivir); the recommended dose is one tablet twice a day.
[b] Abacavir is available as a combined formulation with zidovudine and lamivudine (Trizivir).
Source: Adapted from the recommendations issued in 2001 by the Public Health Service in Refs. 42 and 43.

Table 4 HIV/AIDS-Related Resources

Resource	Contact information
Managing occupational exposure to blood	
National Clinicians' Post-Exposure Prophylaxis Hotline (PEPline), University of California, San Francisco, San Francisco General Hospital	Telephone: +1 888-448-4911 http://www.ucsf.edu/hivcntr
Needlestick! (online decision-making support for clinicians), Emergency Medicine Center, UCLA School of Medicine	http://www.needlestick.mednet.ucla.edu
CDC	
Hepatitis information line	Telephone: +1 888-443-7232 http://www.cdc.gov/hepatitis
To report occupational HIV infection and failure of prophylaxis	Telephone: +1 800-893-0485
Food and Drug Administration (FDA), to report severe or unusual toxic effects of antiretroviral drugs	Telephone: +1 800-332-1088 http://www.fda.gov/medwatch
HIV/AIDS general information	
Center for HIV Information	http://hivinsite.ucsf.edu
AIDS information	http://www.aidsinfo.nih.gov
Johns Hopkins AIDS Service	http://hopkins-aids.edu

antiretroviral medications is given. Uncontrolled but aggregated international data suggest that appropriate PEP, which should begin within 24–36 h of exposure (25), can prevent 81% (confidence intervals 43–94%) of such nosocomial infections. However, failure of PEP to prevent seroconversion has been documented in at least 21 cases (4). These failures may result from the presence of drug-resistant virus, lack of efficacy of the drugs, or poor compliance. Indeed, up to half of patients report side effects, and a third discontinue therapy before the 4 week regimen is completed. Exposed persons are monitored for the presence of HIV-specific antibody by enzyme-linked immunosorbent assay (ELISA) (later confirmed by Western blot) at six weeks, three months, and six months to ensure seroconversion has not occurred. Questions about protocols or initial evaluation and management can be directed to several readily accessible sites (Table 4).

RECOGNIZING HIV INFECTION

The majority of HIV-infected patients are unaware of their infection when they initially seek medical attention for a primary compliant. Thus, the ability to identify features of HIV infection facilitates the safe and effective management of such immunocompromised patients. These features comprise epidemiologic, clinical, and laboratory components. Epidemiologically, the great majority of HIV-infected patients will describe relevant risk factors, such as men who have sex with men, sex with prostitutes, intravenous drug use, sex for money or drugs, or high-risk behavior among populations or in countries with high endemic rates of HIV infection. Clinical features can vary depending on whether patients exhibit an acute retroviral syndrome or chronic infection. A recognizable symptomatic early primary infection occurs in half to three-quarters of patients. Symptoms included a mononucleosis-like syndrome with fever, myalgias/arthralgias, and malaise present in 50–90% of patients, and lethargy, sore throat, weight loss, and headache occurring in greater than or equal to half of patients (44–47). Night sweats, a maculopapular rash, and diarrhea are also common. Laboratory features include the presence of detectable, and often very high, levels of HIV RNA in plasma, but CD4+ T cell counts of <300 cells/μL are uncommon (normal value is ∼1000 cells/μL). Transient neutropenia and lymphopenia (<1500 lymphocytes/μL) with atypical lymphocytosis may be present. Rates of abnormalities of erythrocytes, platelets, and hepatic transaminases are variable. Whether therapy with at least three different drugs from at least two classes should be initiated at this time is controversial.

Patients with chronic HIV infection may have no overt manifestations. About 10 years on average can elapse from primary infection to the onset of AIDS, and no symptoms are present for the majority of this period. In the presence of the same epidemiologic risk features, several physical findings suggest the presence of underlying HIV infection. These signs include the presence of diffuse lymphadenopathy (especially early), white lesions on a red base with oral candidiasis, white plaques on the tongue with oral hairy leukoplakia, and purple papules on the skin or oral mucosa from Kaposi's sarcoma (48). Facial seborrheic dermatitis in the eyebrow and nasolabial fold and molluscum contagiosum may also serve as premonitory signs, as do the presence of diffuse perirectal herpes simplex infection and condylomata. Other skin manifestations include xerosis (dry skin), folliculitis, and onycholysis. Psychomotor retardation (delayed but appropriate responses) may be recognized if sought. Lymphopenia is typically present and may be accompanied by anemia, thrombocytopenia, elevated plasma concentration of serum IgG, and with advanced disease, elevated plasma concentration of serum IgA (49). Viral RNA should be present in plasma, and CD4+ T cell counts range from >500 cells/μL in early and asymptomatic infection to 200–500 cells/μL as disease begins to progress to <200 cells/μL in patients with advanced disease and AIDS. Acute or chronic respiratory infections that are due to, for example, *Streptococcus pneumoniae* or *Pneumocystis carinii*, respectively, sinusitis, and diarrheal disease are common complaints. However, the syndromes that may prompt surgical consultation differ from the most common HIV-related presentations (Table 5) (50). As can be discerned from Table 5, the options for causes of common syndromes can be quite different in patients with HIV disease,

Table 5 Clinical Presentations of HIV/AIDS to the Surgeon

Abdominal pain	Infectious organ disease, non-Hodgkin lymphoma, pancreatitis, and typhilitis
Acute abdomen	Appendicitis (fecalith or Kaposi's sarcoma), perforation [cytomegalovirus (CMV), also Kaposi's sarcoma and lymphoma)
Hepatobiliary	Acalculous cholecystitis, sclerosing cholangitis, and papillary disorders
Pancreatitis	Drugs (pentamidine and ddI, d4T), infections [CMV, herpes simplex virus (HSV), mycobacteria, and neoplasms (non-Hodgkin's lymphoma and Kaposi's sarcoma)]
GI bleeding	Upper tract: infections, esophagitis, Kaposi's sarcoma, and lymphoma
	Lower tract: infectious colitis, idiopathic colonic ulcers, non-Hodgkin's lymphoma, and Kaposi sarcoma
Neoplasms	Non-Hodgkin's lymphoma (especially GI) and Kaposi's sarcoma
Anorectal disease	Anus: condylomata, infection, fistula, fissure, and squamous cell carcinoma
	Rectum: nonspecific proctitis, infectious proctitis, and perirectal abscess

Source: Adapted from Ref. 47.

among whom hepatobiliary disease and pancreatitis may be more often due to cancer (lymphoma or Kaposi's sarcoma), infections (e.g., *Cryptosporidium*, cytomegalovirus, or mycobacteria), and, particularly, drug reactions than the more typical gall stones or ethanol ingestion. Thus, the ability to suspect and recognize HIV infection is an important feature of sophisticated and effective surgical care for the estimated three quarters of a million Americans with HIV disease.

ANTIRETROVIRAL THERAPY

Recent data have confirmed that cure or total eradication of HIV infection is not possible. The virus may remain in an inactive state in a cell's cytoplasm as proviral DNA or after integration into chromosomal DNA (51). Moreover, the virus is readily detected in lymphoid tissue, even when plasma viremia is undetectable on antiretroviral therapy (52). Therefore, the goals of antiretroviral therapy for HIV management are the maximal and durable suppression of HIV RNA replication, restoration and preservation of immunologic function, improvement of quality of life, and reduction of HIV-related morbidity and mortality (53). Many of these goals are approachable with current antiretroviral regimens.

The first antiretroviral drug for the treatment of HIV infection, zidovudine (AZT; ZDV), was approved by the FDA in 1987. In the 15 years that followed, almost a score of other drugs in five different classes with different mechanisms of action have been approved by the U.S. FDA (Table 6). Reiterating the experience of an earlier generation with therapy of tuberculosis, HIV was initially treated with monotherapy or dual therapy with only modest and very transient success. Recognition of the structure, life cycle and replication of the virus, and the mechanisms by which drug resistance has emerged has mandated the use of combination therapy with at least three different drugs of at least two different classes. This combination is now the standard of therapy known as HAART, the goal of which, as noted above, is maximal reduction of the virus to undetectable levels by the current assays (less than 50 HIV copies/mL of plasma). The first of these five classes of antiretroviral medications are the nucleoside reverse transcriptase inhibitors (NRTIs). NRTIs were the first class of antiretroviral drugs established for the treatment of HIV. They interfere with the function of the enzyme reverse transcriptase in the transcription phase of infection by incorporating into the growing DNA chain and preventing conversion of the viral RNA to double stranded DNA. These drugs require phosphorylation by nucleoside kinases within the host cells before they can be activated. Nonnucleoside reverse transcriptase inhibitors (NNRTIs) are nonnucleoside competitors of reverse transcriptase that bind to the enzyme at other sites distinct from those of NRTIs and do not require phosphorylation to become active. Nucleotide inhibitors are similar to NRTIs except that they require only the last two steps of phosphorylation within the host cells for activation, a feature that allows antiviral activity in a wider range of infected cells.

Working by a very different mechanism, protease inhibitors (PIs) block the cleavage of immature polyproteins in the last stages of the viral replicative cycle and cause the production of immature, defective, noninfectious viral particles. The introduction of PIs allowed the dramatic and sustained reduction in viral replication and burden in a substantial proportion of patients with HIV infection when used in combination with other medications. This viral control has resulted in a significantly enhanced quality of life for those who tolerate and respond to HAART, decreased rates of opportunistic infection, and

Table 6 Complications of Antiretroviral Therapy and Potential Interactions with Other Common Medications

Type of medication	Medication	Trade name	Primary GI toxicity[a]	GI-associated drug interactions
Nucleoside analog RTI (NRTI)	Zidovudine (AZT, ZDV)	Retrovir	Anorexia; nausea (4–26%); vomiting (3–8%) (rare hepatitis, steatosis, lactic acidosis)	Activity may be inhibited by ribavirin
	Didanosine (ddI)	Videx	Pancreatitis (4–8%); diarrhea (16%); ↑ ALT/AST (6–20%)	Potential increased rate of pancreatitis with pentamidine, azathioprine); buffers assoc. with ↓ absorption of itraconazole, ketoconazole, dapsone; tetracycline, ciprofloxacin; ddI levels ↑ with ranitidine, ganciclovir
	Zalcitabine (ddC)	HIVID	Stomatitis (self-limited) (2–17%); pancreatitis (0.5–9%)	Few; possible ↑ neuropathy with metronidazole, disulfuram
	Stavudine (d4T)	Zerit	Diarrhea (33%), nausea/vomiting (26%), abdominal pain (23%); ↑ ALT/AST (65%); significant GI symptoms and hepatic abnormalities in 4–10%	Few; possible ↑ neuropathy with ethanol; ribavirin may increase activity (in vitro data)
	Lamivudine (3TC)	Epivir	Limited; mild and transient diarrhea, nausea, abdominal pain	Few
	Abacavir (ABC)	Ziagen	Nausea (45%), diarrhea (25%), vomiting (15%), and abdominal pain (15%) may decrease over weeks of therapy; hypersensitivity reaction with fever ± rash, malaise, nausea, vomiting, ↑ ALT/AST in 2–5% within 1 month	None reported
	Emtricitabine (FTC)	Emtriva	Headache; diarrhea, nausea, rash (only 1% severe)	None identified

(Continued)

Table 6 Continued

Type of medication	Medication	Trade name	Primary GI toxicity[a]	GI-associated drug interactions
Nucleotide analog RTI (NtRTI)	Adefovir dipivoxil	Preveon	Usually mild nausea, diarrhea, occasional vomiting (1–8%); ↑ ALT/AST (4%); (renal toxicity 38%)	None reported
	Tenofovir (PMPA)	Viread	Nausea, vomiting, diarrhea (renal insufficiency)	
Nonnucleoside RTI (NNRTI)	Nevirapine (NVP)	Viramune	Nausea; ↑ ALT/AST (1%); isolated ↑ GGT common; (rash most common)	Level ↓ with rifampin, rifabutin (P-450 system) and antacids (↑ gastric pH); level ↑ with clarithromycin, rifabutin, cisapride
	Delavirdine (DLV)	Rescriptor	Nausea (7%); diarrhea (4%); ↑ ALT/AST (≤5%) (rash most common; usually transient)	
	Efaviernz (EFV)	Sustiva	Transient rash and CNS symptoms of headache, dizziness, impaired concentration	Avoid cisapride; should not be taken within 2 h of antacids; not recommended with clarithromycin (interacts with other PI)
Protease inhibitors (PI)[b]	Saquinivir (SQC); Saquinavir-SGC (soft gel capsule)	Invirase; Fortovase	Nausea, diarrhea, abdominal pain, dyspepsia (5–10%)	Cisapride contraindicated; SQC level ↑ with ketoconazole, clarithromycin; SQC level ↓ with rifampin, rifabutin; clarithromycin level ↑ with SQC; (interacts with other PI)
	Ritonavir (RTV)	Norvir	Nausea, diarrhea, vomiting, anorexia, abdominal pain (20–40%), esp. in first few weeks of therapy; taste perversion (10%); increased triglycerides (60%, but >1500 mg/dL in 2–8%); ↑ ALT/AST (10–15%), esp. with NRTI	Cisapride contraindicated; caution with dronabinol, ondansetron, cimetidine, promethazine, corticosteroids; RTV level ↑ with ketoconazole, itraconazole; RTV level ↓ with rifampin; Clarithromycin, erythromycin, rifampin, rifabutin levels increased with RTV (interacts with other PI)

	Indinavir (IDV)	Crixivan	Nausea, vomiting, diarrhea, abdominal pain (4–15%); increased indirect bilirubin (10%); nephrolithiasis (5–10%)	Cisapride contraindicated; IDV level ↓ with rifabutin; IDV level ↑ with ketoconazole; rifabutin level ↑ with IDV (interacts with other PI)
	Nelfinavir (NLF)	Viracept	Diarrhea (usually mild) (2–19%)	Cisapride and rifabutin contraindicated; NLF levels ↓ with rifampin; rifabutin levels ↑ with NLF (interacts with other PI)
	Amprenavir	Agenerase	Diarrhea, nausea, vomiting (7–33%); rash (18%)	Cisapride and rifampin contraindicated; amprenavir levels ↓ with rifabutin; rifabutin levels ↑ with amprenavir; (interacts with other PI)
	ABT 378 (Lopinavir-Ritonavir)	Kaletra	Diarrhea (10–20%); ↑ ALT/AST (8%)	Similar to other PI
	Atazanavir	Reyataz	Jaundice (10%); nausea, diarrhea; ± increased ALT/AST; no change in lipids	Interacts with drugs metabolized by cytochrome P450 3A4 isoenzyme, rifabutin, clarithromycin, lipid-lowering agents; ritonavir, tenofovir
Fusion inhibitor	Enfuvirtide (T20)	Fuzeon	Decreased appetite, injection site reactions; peripheral neuropathy	
Other	Interleukin-2	Proleukin	Diarrhea, abdominal pain, stomatitis (7%); nausea; vomiting; isolated ↑ bilirubin (8%); ↑ ALT/AST; acalculous cholecystitis; constitutional flu-like symptoms (fever, chills, muscle/joint pain) (45%)	
	Hydroxyurea	Hydrea	Nausea (12%); ↑ ALT/AST (2%); stomatitis (8%); diarrhea; occasional anorexia, vomiting, diarrhea, constipation (myelosuppression; rash)	

(Continued)

Table 6 Continued

Type of medication	Medication	Trade name	Primary GI toxicity[a]	GI-associated drug interactions
Alternative	Vitamin C, allicin (garlic extract), Malaleuca (tea tree extract), N-acetylcysteine (Mucomyst)			

[a]Rates may vary among studies.
[b]As with other inhibitors of cytochrome p450 system, specifically CYP 3A4, protease inhibitors should not be given with cisapride (Propulsid), astemizole (Hismanal), terfenadine (Seldane), midazolam (Versed), or triazolam (Halcion), or ergot derivatives.
Abbreviations: RTI, reverse transcriptase inhibitors; ↑ALT/AST, alanine/asparate transminase elevation >2.5–5-fold above normal values; GGT, g-glutamyl transpeptidase. Combination medications include Combivir (AZT + 3TC) and Trizivir (AZT + 3TC + Abacavir).
Source: Adapted from Ref. 50.

discontinuation of the medications previously required to suppress them, as well as prolonged survival. The newest class of drugs, known as fusion inhibitors, inhibits the ability of a component of the viral envelope, gp41, to fuse with the cell membrane of target cells, such as CD4+ T cells or macrophages.

Despite many benefits, HAART is not without risks. In most clinical settings, only 50–60% of patients achieve effective viral suppression. This limited efficacy is due in part to poor adherence to regimen, a treatment with complex dosing schedules and cumulative toxicities (Table 6), and in part to viral resistance to the drugs. Resistance is emerging in the community and emerges in the individual patient with less-than-optimal viral suppression. A variety of serious metabolic toxicities have also accompanied HAART therapy, such as the disfiguring lipodystrophy syndrome. On the basis of the serious risks, the dramatic potential benefits, as well as the substantial cost of medications, decisions about when in the course of infection to initiate antiretroviral therapy are difficult. Expert panels convene regularly and produce yearly guidelines for effective and appropriate care (53) (www.aidsinfo.nih.gov; Table 4). A list of drug toxicities is provided (Table 6). Note that some of these reactions, particularly abdominal complaints, may form the basis of surgical consultation. Complications such as lactic acidosis with the nucleoside analog stavudine have resulted in prolonged admissions in ICUs (54).

COMPLICATIONS AND OUTCOME OF SURGERY AMONG HIV-INFECTED PATIENTS

HIV is a chronic disease. With improved therapy, patients with HIV/AIDS are living longer in industrialized nations. As a result, HIV-infected patients frequently require surgery (55), including cardiac surgery, kidney transplantation, and liver transplantation (56). The need for liver transplantation is due in large part to high rates of co-infection of HIV with HCV. Early in the epidemic surgeons debated whether HIV-infected patients had higher perioperative complication rates, whether surgical wounds would heal poorly as a consequence of reduced immune status, and whether patients with HIV infection, particularly those with advanced disease and AIDS, would spend a prolonged period postoperatively in the ICU only to die of sepsis and multiple organ failure. Of particular relevance and concern was the question of whether the surgical mortality rate in these patients would be so high that HCWs would ultimately be exposed to the virus unnecessarily (33).

Indeed, several early reports suggested that HIV/AIDS patients had poor postoperative outcomes and significant problems with wound healing and morbidity. High complication rates and mortality rates of 55–70% were observed (33). The poor operative results from these studies were attributed to general features: advanced stages of the patients' disease, delay in decision to operate since AIDS was in its infancy, and the relatively poor ability to diagnose and treat specific AIDS-related infections (57).

The literature provides inconsistent answers about whether HIV infection is associated with worse outcomes than those in uninfected adults. A retrospective review of 101 patients who underwent anorectal surgery, the most common surgery in patients with HIV/AIDS, showed that wound healing was significantly decreased; only 40% of patients had healed their wounds by 3 months postoperatively (58). Such delays were most prominent among patients with fewer than 50 CD4+ T cells/μL. Burke et al. (59), however, did not find any statistically significanct difference between wound healing rates among asymptomatic patients and AIDS patients. Emparan et al. (60) retrospectively examined 24 HIV-infected patients who had undergone abdominal surgery and found an overall infection rate of 58.3%. Rates were highest among patients with fewer than 200 CD4+ T cells/μL. However, Carillo et al. (61) in their examination of 21 patients who underwent 24 emergency operations after sustaining penetrating trauma, did not find a significant problem with delayed wound healing. Finally, Bizer et al. (62), whose 1989 study reported the highest complication and mortality rates, have now published another surgical series with markedly improved outcomes and an "encouraged" attitude (33). In a careful and critical review, Rose et al. (54) lament that "the literature on postoperative complications is descriptive and inconsistent and does not support a firm conclusion on the association between mortality rates and HIV serostatus or disease stage" (57). Nonanalytic methods and a failure to control for confounding variables limited the validity of most results. He concludes that outcomes of surgery are multifactorial and not directly related to the presence of HIV infection alone.

Consistent with the conclusion that overall outcomes are similar in patients with HIV infection and controls, mortality was similar in 52 patients with HIV disease and 350 control subjects admitted to a surgical ICU (63). Similarly, 3- and 30-day mortality was comparable in matched patients (26 per group) undergoing surgery, independent of HIV status, although long-term survival was lower in the HIV-infected group (64). An evaluation of HIV-infected and seronegative patients matched for age, sex, lung injury, and the severity of their burns reported that outcomes were comparable (65). The overall message of almost a dozen studies in medical ICUs reiterates that, although long-term survival may be decreased among patients with advanced HIV disease, treatment in an ICU should not be considered futile (66–75). The patients with HIV do as well as others. Overall predictors of outcome are those that are heavily weighted from APACHE II scores, such as age and creatinine.

Thus, decisions to treat patients with HIV infection in the ICU, whether surgical or medical, should be determined by their overall clinical status and not on the presence of HIV infection. HIV disease in and of itself does not appear to serve as a significant independent risk factor for delayed wound healing and infection. Rather, this relationship exists with multiple other factors, such as concurrent infections or diseases, malnutrition, neutropenia, wasting, multiple organ dysfunction, sepsis (61), type of surgery, extent of surgery, CD4+ T cell count (76), and indication for surgery (57). Just as for other surgical patients, factors predictive of poor prognosis include the presence of an opportunistic infection, serum albumin <2.5 g/dL, and the presence of concurrent organ failure (33). The risk of surgery can be reduced with aggressive prophylactic treatment for AIDS-related diseases, early diagnosis and treatment of the surgical problem, and nutritional assessment and support (33,55).

HIV/AIDS: ETHICAL AND LEGAL ISSUES

The moral and legal issues surrounding the care of the HIV-infected patient have been debated upon since the onset of the epidemic. Surgery for these patients would appear to confer an increased risk of transmission to the surgeon, but only two cases have been documented to date (35,36). Does this risk justify the refusal of surgeons to perform surgery on HIV-infected individuals? The consensus is that the moral and ethical obligation of any physician is to offer lifesaving or emergency treatment to any patient, independent of HIV infection status, as highlighted in the American Medical Association (AMA) code of ethics (77). The issues are less clear regarding elective surgery. In 1989 the American Society of Plastic and Reconstructive Surgery ruled that it was ethically acceptable to refuse cosmetic surgery to HIV-infected patients, but the society now considers such refusal unacceptable, as does the American College of Surgeons (78–80). The opinions of individual plastic surgeons, though, as with physicians in other fields, are divergent (78,80,81). Under the American Disabilities Act (ADA) of 1990, several suits have been filed against physicians who refused to provide care to HIV-infected patients (80–82). Whereas most courts agree that HIV infection constitutes a disability, they have ruled that relief under the ADA may be available only if there is a threat that the discrimination against the patient will persist in the future by the same physician or facility.

In the case of HIV-infected surgeons, several lawsuits have been filed by patients who have been operated on by HIV-infected surgeons (83–88) and there does not appear to be a general consensus on policy and the law governing this practice, even though there is evidence that risk of transmission is minimal if universal precautions are taken.

In summary, the most recent code of medical ethics for physicians written by both the AMA and the American College of Physicians (77,89) generally states that a physician may not ethically refuse to treat a patient whose condition is within the physician's current realm of competence solely because the patient is HIV seropositive, and that persons who are HIV-seropositive should not be subjected to discrimination based on fear or prejudice.

SUMMARY

- HIV infection and AIDS are the leading causes of severe and prolonged immunodeficiency in the United States.
- AIDS is the fourth leading cause of death worldwide and the leading cause of death in sub-Saharan Africa.
- High-risk behaviors include intravenous drug use, trading or selling sex for drugs, heterosexual contact with intravenous drug users, and men having sex with men.
- HIV is transmitted principally by three mechanisms: sexual, vertical (mother to child), and blood exposure.
- Risk of percutaneous injury and subsequent exposure to HIV is highest in providers who use a finger to guide suture needles. Risk of exposure is highest for procedures longer than 3 h, for procedures with blood loss >300 mL, and with vascular and gynecologic surgery.
- Estimated risk of infection of a surgeon by a blood borne pathogen is estimated to be 0.0024–0.024/1000 patients.
- Universal blood and body precautions and postexposure prophylaxis (PEP) are effective in the prevention of occupational HIV infection. Infection with HIV requires time for migration and proliferation in target cells. PEP can inhibit viral replication in this interval.

- Epidemiologic features that are helpful in recognizing HIV infection include men who have sex with men, sex with prostitutes, intravenous drug use, sex for money or drugs, or high-risk behavior in populations with high endemic rates of HIV infection.
- Clinical features useful in identifying HIV infection include fever, myalgias/arthralgias, malaise, lethargy, sore throat, weight loss, headache, night sweats, maculopapular rash, and diarrhea.
- Laboratory features of HIV infection include high levels of HIV RNA in plasma, neutropenia, lymphopenia, and atypical lymphocytosis. CD4+ cell counts fewer than 3 cells/μL are uncommon.
- Patients with chronic HIV infection may have no overt manifestations. In the presence of the foregoing epidemiologic features, diffuse adenopathy, candidiasis, white plaques on the tongue with oral hairy leukoplakia, purple papules on skin and oral mucosa (Kaposi's sarcoma), and perianal herpes simplex or condylomata may indicate HIV infection. Acute and chronic respiratory infections, sinusitis, and diarrhea are common.
- CD4+ cell counts are usually:
  - greater than 500 cells/μL in early disease
  - 200–500 cells/μL in early progression
  - less than 200 cells/μL in advanced disease
- HIV infection cannot be totally eradicated; the virus may remain in an inactive state in the cell.
- Goals of antiretroviral therapy for HIV are maximal and durable suppression of HIV RNA replication, restoration and preservation of immunologic function, and improvement in quality of life.
- Current therapy employs at least three different drugs from at least two different classes (HAART).
- Nucleoside reverse transcriptase inhibitors block reverse transcriptase and conversion of viral RNA to double stranded DNA.
- Nonnucleoside reverse transcriptase inhibitors are competitors of reverse transcriptase and do not require phosphorylation to become active.
- Nucleotide inhibitors are similar to nucleoside reverse transcriptase inhibitors but work in a wider range of cells. They have reduced phosphorylation requirements to become active.
- Protease inhibitors block cleavage of immature polyproteins in the viral replication cycle.
- Fusion inhibitors block the fusion of the viral envelope with target cell membranes.
- The moral and ethical obligation of any physician is to offer lifesaving or emergency treatment to any patient without regard to HIV status.

REFERENCES

1. Palella FJ Jr, Delaney KM, Moorman AC, et al. Declining morbidity and mortality among patients with advanced human immunodeficiency virus infection. N Engl J Med 1998; 338:853–860.
2. Mocroft A, Katlama C, Johnson AM, et al. AIDS across Europe, 1994–98: the EuroSIDA Study. Lancet 2000; 356:291–296.

3. UNAIDS and WHO. Report on the Global HIV/AIDS Epidemic. Geneva: UNAIDS/AIDS, 2001.
4. Centers for Disease Control and Prevention. HIV/AIDS Surveillance Report. Morb Mortal Wkly Rep 1998; 9:2.
5. Jain MK, Skiest DJ, Cloud JW, Jain CL, Burns D, Berggren RE. Changes in mortality related to human immunodeficiency virus infection: comparative analysis of inpatient deaths in 1995 and in 1999–2000. Clin Infect Dis 2003; 36:1030–1038.
6. Del Rio C, Curran JW. Epidemiology and prevention on acquired immunodeficiency syndrome and human immunodeficiency virus infection. Mandell, Douglas and Bennett's Principles and Practice of Infectious Disease. 5th ed. Churchill Livingstone, 2000.
7. Moloughney BW. Transmission and postexposure management of bloodborne virus infections in the health care setting: where are we now? Can Med Assoc J 2001; 165:445–451.
8. Ippolito G, Puro V, Heptonstall J, Jagger J, De Carli G, Petrosilo N. Occupational human immunodeficiency virus infection in health care workers: worldwide cases through September 1997. Clin Infect Dis 1999; 28:365–383.
9. Goldberg D, Johnson J, Cameron S, et al. Risk of HIV transmission from patients to surgeons in the era post-exposure prophylaxis. J Hosp Infect 2000; 44:99–105.
10. Royce RA, Sena A, Cates W Jr, Cohen MS. Sexual transmission of HIV. N Engl J Med 1997; 336:1072–1078.
11. Piot P, Merson MH. Global perspectives on human immunodeficiency virus infection and acquired immunodeficiency syndrome. Mandell, Douglas and Bennett's Principles and Practice of Infectious Disease. 5th ed. Churchill Livingstone, 2000.
12. Dragic T, Litwin V, Allaway GP, et al. HIV-1 entry into CD4+ cells is mediated by the chemokine receptor CC-CKR-5. Nature 1996; 381:667–673.
13. Shearer GM, Clerici M. Protective immunity against HIV infection: has nature done the experiment for us? Immunol Today 1996; 17:21–24.
14. Willerford DM, Bwayo JJ, Hensel M, et al. Human immunodeficiency virus infection among high-risk seronegative prostitutes in Nairobi. J Infect Dis 1993; 167:1414–1417.
15. Dean M, Carrington M, Winkler C, et al. Genetic restriction of HIV-1 infection and progression to AIDS by a deletion allele of the CKR5 structural gene. Science 1996; 273:1856–1862.
16. Lindegreen ML, et al. HIV/AIDS in infants, children and adolescents. Pediatr Clin N Am 2000; 47:1–20.
17. Davis SF, Byers RH Jr, Lindegren ML, Caldwell MB, Karon JM, Gwinn M. Prevalence and incidence of vertically acquired HIV infection in the United States. J Am Med Assoc 1995; 274:952–955.
18. Connor EM, Sperling RS, Gelber RG, et al. Reduction of maternal-in-transmission of human immunodeficiency virus type 1 with zidovudine treatment. N Engl J Med 1994; 331:1174–1180.
19. De Cock KM, Fowler MG, Mercier E, et al. Prevention of mother-to-child HIV transmission in resource-poor countries. J Am Med Assoc 2000; 283:1175–1182.
20. The European Mode of Delivery Collaboration. Elective caesarean-section versus vaginal delivery in prevention of vertical HIV-1 transmission: a randomised clinical trial. Lancet 1999; 353:1035–1039.
21. Peckham C, Gibb D. Mother-to child transmission of the human immunodeficiency virus. N Engl J Med 1995; 333:298–302.
22. Dunn DT, Newell ML, Ades AE, Peckham CS. Risk of human immunodeficiency virus type 1 transmission through breastfeeding. Lancet 1992; 340:585–588.
23. Burgess T. Determinants of transmission of HIV from mother to child. Clin Obstetr Gynecol 2001; 44:198–209.
24. Centers for Disease Control and Prevention. HIV/AIDS Surveillance Report. Morb Mortal Wkly Rep 2001; 13:1–44.

25. Centers for Disease Control and Prevention. Public Health Service guidelines for the management of health care worker exposure to HIV and recommendations for post-exposure prophylaxis. Morb Mortal Wkly Rep 1998; 47:1–33.
26. Bell DM, Shapiro CN, Culver DH, Martone WJ, Curran JW, Hughes JM. Risk of hepatitis B and human immunodeficiency virus transmission to a patient from an infected surgeon due to percutaneous injury during an invasive procedure: estimates based on a model. Infect Agents Dis 1992; 1:263–269.
27. Mast ST, Woolwine JD, Gerberding JL. Efficacy of gloves in reducing blood volumes transferred during simulated needlestick injury. J Infect Dis 1993; 168:1589–1592.
28. University of Virginia International Health Care Worker Safety Center. Annual number of occupational percutaneous injuries and mucocutaneous exposures to blood or potentially infective biological substance, Charlottesville, VA. June 1998: Available at www.med.virginia.edu/med.
29. Tokars JI, Bell DM, Culver DH, et al. Percutaneous injuries during surgical procedures. J Am Med Assoc 1992; 267:2899–2904.
30. Gerberding J. Provider-to-patient HIV transmission: how to keep it exceedingly rare. Ann Intern Med 1999; 130:64–65.
31. Patterson JM, Novak CB, Mackinnon SE, Patterson GA. Surgeons' concern and practices of protection against bloodborne pathogens. Ann Surg 1998; 228:266–272.
32. Bell DM, Shapiro CN, Ciesielski CA, Chamberland ME. Preventing bloodborne pathogen transmission from health-care workers to patients. The CDC perspective. Surg Clin North Am 1995; 75:1189–1203.
33. Harris HW, Schecter WP. Surgical risk assessment and management in patients with HIV disease. Gastroenterol Clin North Am 1997; 26:377–391.
34. Maas CS, Sussman SA, Hewett JJ. The human immunodeficiency virus and facial plastic surgery. Ear Nose Throat J 1995; 74:364–368.
35. Ippolito G, The Studio Italiano Rischio Occupationale da HIV (SIROH). Scalpel injury and HIV infection in a surgeon. Lancet 1996; 347:1042.
36. Lot F, Seguier JC, Fegueux S, et al. Probable transmission of HIV from an orthopedic surgeon to a patient in France. Ann Intern Med 1999; 130:1–6.
37. Ciesielski C, Marianos D, Ou CY, et al. Transmission of human immunodeficiency virus in a dental practice. Ann Intern Med 1992; 116:798–805.
38. Robert LM, Chamberland ME, Cleveland JL, et al. Investigations of patients of health care workers infected with HIV. The Centers for Disease Control and Prevention database. Ann Intern Med 1995; 122:653–657.
39. Daniels N. HIV-infected professionals, patient rights, and the "switching dilemma". J Am Med Assoc 1992; 267:1368–1371.
40. Mingoli A, Sapienza P, Sgarzini G, et al. Influence of blunt needles on surgical glove perforation and safety for the surgeon. Am J Surg 1996; 172:512–516 (discussion 16–17).
41. Bartlett JG, Gallant JE. Medical Management of HIV Infection. Baltimore, MD: Port City Press, 2000.
42. Gerberding JL. Clinical practice. Occupational exposure to HIV in health care settings. N Engl J Med 2003; 348:826–833.
43. Centers for Disease Control and Prevention. Updated U.S. Public Health Service Guidelines for the Management of Occupational Exposures to HBV, HCV, and HIV and Recommendations for Postexposure Proplylaxis. Morb Mortal Wkly Rep 2001; 50:1–52.
44. Tindall B, Barker S, Donovan B, et al. Characterization of the acute clinical illness associated with human immunodeficiency virus infection. Arch Intern Med 1988; 148:945–949.
45. Schacker T, Collier AC, Hughes J, Shea T, Corey L. Clinical and epidemiologic features of primary HIV infection. Ann Intern Med 1996; 125:257–264.
46. Quinn TC. Acute primary HIV infection. J Am Med Assoc 1997; 278:58–62.

47. Russell ND. Primary HIV infection: clinical, immunologic, and virologic predictors of progression. AIDS Reader 1998; 8:164–172.
48. Paauw DS, Wenrich MD, Curtis JR, Carline JD, Ramsey PG. Ability of primary care physicians to recognize physical findings associated with HIV infection. J Am Med Assoc 1995; 274:1380–1382.
49. Polk BF, Fox R, Brookmeyer R, et al. Predicators of the acquired immunodeficiency syndrome developing in a cohort of seropositive homosexual men. N Engl J Med 1987; 316:61–66.
50. Smith PD, Janoff EN. Gastrointestinal complications of the acquired immunodeficiency disease syndrome. In: Yamada T, Alpers DH, Owyang C, Powell DW, Silverstien FE, eds. Textbook of Gastroenterology, Chapter 124. Philadelphia, PA: Lippincott-Raven, 2002; 2567–2589.
51. Chun TW, Engel D, Berrey MM, Shea T, Corey L, Fauci AS. Early establishment of a pool of latently infected, resting CD4(+) T cells during primary HIV-1 infection. Proc Natl Acad Sci USA 1998; 95:8869–8873.
52. Cavert W, Notermans DW, Staskus K, et al. Kinetics of response in lymphoid tissues to antiretroviral therapy of HIV-1 infection. Science 1997; 276:960–964.
53. Guidelines for the use of antiretroviral agents in HIV-infected adults and adolescents. Available at http://www.hivatis.org 2002.
54. Miller KD, Cameron M, Wood LV, Dalakas MC and Kovacs JA. Lactic acidosis and hepatic steatosis associated with use of stavudine: report of four cases. Ann Intern Med 2000; 133:192–196.
55. Burns J, Pieper B. HIV/AIDS: impact on healing. Ostomy Wound Manage 2000; 46:30–40, 42, 44.
56. Roland ME, Havlir DV. Responding to organ failure in HIV-infected patients. N Engl J Med 2003; 348:2279–2281.
57. Rose DN, Collins M, Kleban R. Complications of surgery in HIV-infected patients. Aids 1998; 12:2243–2251.
58. Lord RV. Anorectal surgery in patients infected with human immunodeficiency virus: factors associated with delayed wound healing. Ann Surg 1997; 226:92–99.
59. Burke EC, Orloff SL, Freise CE, Macho JR, Schecter WP. Wound healing after anorectal surgery in human immunodeficiency virus-infected patients. Arch Surg 1991; 126:1267–1270 (discussion 70–71).
60. Emparan C, Iturburu IM, Ortiz J, Mendez JJ. Infective complications after abdominal surgery in patients infected with human immunodeficiency virus: role of CD4+ lymphocytes in prognosis. World J Surg 1998; 22:778–782.
61. Carrillo EH, Carrillo LE, Byers PM, Ginzburg E, Martin L. Penetrating trauma and emergency surgery in patients with AIDS. Am J Surg 1995; 170:341–344.
62. Bizer LS, Pettorino R, Ashikari A. Emergency abdominal operations in the patient with acquired immunodeficiency syndrome. J Am Coll Surg 1995; 180:205–209.
63. Bhagwanjee S, Muckart DJ, Jeena PM and Moodley P. does HIV status influence the outcome of patients admitted to a surgical intensive care unit? A prospective double blind study. Br Med J 1997; 314:1077–1081 (discussion 81–84).
64. Ayers J, Howton MJ, Layon AJ. Postoperative complications in patients with human immunodeficiency virus disease. Clinical data and a literature review. Chest 1993; 103:1800–1807.
65. Edge JM, Van der Merwe AE, Pieper CH, Bouic P. Clinical outcome of HIV positive patients with moderate to severe burns. Burns 2001; 27:111–114.
66. Casalino E, Mendoza-Sassi G, Wolff M, et al. Predictors of short- and long-term survival in HIV-infected patients admitted to the ICU. Chest 1998; 113:421–429.
67. Rosen MJ, Clayton K, Schneider RF, et al. Intensive care of patients with HIV infection: utilization, critical illnesses, and outcomes. Pulmonary Complications of HIV Infection Study Group. Am J Respir Crit Care Med 1997; 155:67–71.

68. De Palo VA, Millstein BH, Mayo PH, Salzman SH, Rosen MJ. Outcome of intensive care in patients with HIV infection. Chest 1995; 107:506–510.
69. Nickas G, Wachter RM. Outcomes of intensive care for patients with human immunodeficiency virus infection. Arch Intern Med 2000; 160:541–547.
70. Afessa B, Green B. Clinical course, prognostic factors, and outcome prediction for HIV patients in the ICU. The PIP (pulmonary complications, ICU support, and prognostic factors in hospitalized patients with HIV) study. Chest 2000; 118:138–145.
71. Gill JK, Greene L, Miller R, et al. ICU admission in patients infected with the human immunodeficiency virus—a multicentre survery. Anaesthesia 1999; 54:727–732.
72. Leifeld L, Rockstroh J, Skaide S, et al. Indication, outcome and follow up of intensive care in patients with HIV-infection. Eur J Med Res 2000; 5:199–202.
73. Bonarek M, Morlat P, Chene G, et al. Prognostic score of short-term survival in HIV-infected patients admitted to medical intensive care units. Int J STD AIDS 2001; 12:239–244.
74. Morris A, Creasman J, Turner J, Luce JM, Wachter RM and Huang L. Intensive care of human immunodeficiency virus-infected patients during the era of highly active antiretroviral therapy. Am J Respir Crit Care Med 2002; 166:262–267.
75. Masur H. Acquired immunodeficiency syndrome in the intensive care unit: will human immunodeficiency virus-related admissions continue to decline? Am J Respir Crit Care Med 2002; 166:258–259.
76. Consten EC, Slors FJ, Noten HJ, Oosting H, Danner SA, van Lanschot JJ. Anorectal surgery in human immunodeficiency virus-infected patients. Clinical outcome in relation to immune status. Dis Colon Rectum 1995; 38:1169–1175.
77. Code of medical ethics. American Medical Association. Chicago. 2001. s E-8.11, E-10.05. Available: www.ama-assn.org/ama/pub/category/2503.html (accessed 2004 September).
78. Clarke SR, Gonsoulin TP. Elective surgery and the HIV-positive patient: medical legal, and ethical issues. J Louisiana State Med Soc 1999; 151:245–249.
79. American College of Surgeons. Statement on the surgeon and HIV infection. Bull Am Coll Surg 1991; 76:28–31.
80. Friedland B. The Americans with Disabilities Act: should it compel cosmetic treatment for HIV-positive individuals? Plastic & Reconstructive Surgery 1997; 100(4):1061–1069.
81. The Americans with Disabilities Act of 1990. Pub L No. 101-336, 104 Stat 327 Council on Ethical and Judicial Affairs. American Medical Association. Ethical issues involved in the growing AIDS crisis. JAMA 1988; 259:1360–1361.
82. Manuel C, Charrel J, Larher MP et al. AIDS: the rights and duties of health-care providers. AIDS Public Policy J 1991; 6:37–40.
83. Faya v Alamaraz, 620 A2d 327 (Md 1993).
84. Estate of Behringer v Medical Center at Princeton, 249 NJ Sup 597, 592 A2d 1251 (1991).
85. Scoles v Mercy Health Corporation of Southeastern Pennsylvania, 887 FSupp 765.
86. Mauro v Borgess Medical Center, Ct App (6th Cir), No. 95-1544 (February 25, 1998).
87. Doe v Washington University, 780 F Supp 628.
88. Bradley v U of Texas MD Anderson Cancer Center, 3 F3d 922.
89. American College of Physicians Ethics of Manual. Ann Intern Med. 1998; 128:576–594.

48

Infection in the Immunocompromised Patient

Gregory A. Filice
VA Medical Center, Minneapolis, Minnesota, USA

Most patients in critical care have host defense defects ranging from minor, trivial ones to substantial ones that profoundly increase the risk of infectious disease. Multiple defects, which may interact to further enhance the risk, are often found in the same patient. This chapter explains host defense defects likely to occur in critical care. The goals for the intensivist should be to minimize infection risk, recognize and diagnose infectious diseases that occur, and manage infections promptly and efficiently.

BASIC CONCEPTS

Humans are protected by a broad array of host defenses that fall into two major categories. Innate host defenses operate continuously without specific antigenic stimulation, and immune host defenses are primed by and respond to antigenic stimulation. Innate host defenses are concentrated at body surfaces, both skin and mucous membranes. Skin constitutes a physical barrier that is supplemented by antimicrobial properties of fatty acids, dryness and desiccating effects of skin on microorganisms, and continuous desquamation of dead squamous cells. Very few pathogens can penetrate intact, healthy skin. On the other hand, patients in critical care units frequently have breaches in the skin caused by traumatic injuries, surgical wounds, transcutaneous catheters, and burns.

Microorganisms penetrate mucous membranes more easily than skin, and mucous membranes are frequently impaired in critically ill patients. Tubes inserted through the mouth or nose into the respiratory or gastrointestinal tracts or into the urinary tract or rectum damage mucous membranes. Certain drugs, especially antiproliferative ones, and gastric acid in the esophagus can damage mucous membranes. A wide variety of molecules, including natural antibodies, lysozyme, fibronectin, and iron-binding proteins, add to host defenses at mucous membrane surfaces. Mucous membranes are protected by a mucus layer that can be up to 200 μm thick and physically prevents organisms from gaining access to the mucous membranes. Neutrophils and macrophages ingest particles on healthy mucous membranes in the absence of a specific immune response. Other innate host defenses include such diverse structures and mechanisms as the ability of the upper respiratory system to prevent aspiration, the ability of the gastroesophageal junction to prevent reflux, the ability of the urinary bladder to empty frequently and completely, and the capability of the urethra to keep potential pathogens external.

Adequate nutrition is important for complete, competent host defenses. Periods of malnutrition lasting just a few days have measurable effects on host defenses. The longer nutrition lags behind metabolic needs, the greater the impairment of host defenses and susceptibility to infectious disease.

Body cavities normally inhabited by microbial flora, and to a lesser extent the skin, are protected from infectious diseases by resistance to colonization exhibited by the normal bacterial flora. The large intestine is inhabited by 10^{11}–10^{12} bacteria per gram of colonic contents, consisting of 450 species belonging to over 30 genera. The indigenous microorganisms repel colonization by or disease from exogenous microorganisms, many of which are less well adapted to survival or growth in ordinary body niches. In critically ill patients, several interventions disrupt the usual flora and diminish colonization resistance. The most important of these interventions is antimicrobial therapy.

Immune host defense mechanisms develop in response to specific pathogens or other antigens. Key elements of this complex system include lymphocytes, antibodies, and facilitated phagocytosis. Immune mechanisms developed later in evolution than innate ones and collectively contribute a focused, powerful antimicrobial attack, but immune mechanisms take days to weeks to develop. Immune and innate host defense systems interact extensively with both positive and negative regulatory effects on inflammation and immunity.

Host defenses undergo substantial changes throughout human development, maturation, and senescence. For example, fetuses, neonates, and infants are at greater risk for congenital rubella syndrome, congenital toxoplasmosis, *Escherichia coli* meningitis, and group B streptococcal infections. The elderly are at greater risk for listeria meningitis and urinary-tract infections. The greatest impact of aging is on cell-mediated immunity (CMI) and some innate host defenses. Humoral immunity suffers less. The intensivist must take the critically ill patient's stage of development into account in the approach to prevention, evaluation, and treatment of infectious diseases.

Infectious diseases that occur from host defense defects in an individual patient are usually predictable. The reason is that each host defense mechanism protects against a specific set of potential pathogens. For example, antibody or complement deficiencies predispose patients to disease with encapsulated organisms but not fungi. Defects in CMI increase the likelihood of infections with mycobacteria or cytomegalovirus, but not *E. coli* or influenza virus. The intensivist with a patient suspected of having an infectious disease must review the patient's host defects. Treatment generally includes antimicrobial therapy against likely pathogens. In the evaluation and management of these patients, antimicrobial therapy should be targeted against likely diseases but not all conceivable pathogens so as to maximize effectiveness and minimize adverse effects.

Multiple host defenses can combine to broaden susceptibility. For example, multiple myeloma usually leads to immunoglobulin (Ig) deficiency, and cytotoxic chemotherapy for this disease typically adds neutropenia. Patients with multiple myeloma who have just received chemotherapy are at risk for pneumococcal infections as a consequence of the antibody deficiency, and staphylococcal or gram-negative enteric bacillary infection from neutropenia (1). Defects in one host defense mechanism might impair another mechanism or exacerbate another defect. For example, mucous membranes may be intact but would not function effectively in the patient without normal concentrations and functionality of IgA antibodies.

Infection in the Immunocompromised Patient

In some conditions with host defense defects, the prevalences of specific infectious diseases change substantially over the course of the disease or condition. For example, in solid-organ transplant recipients, early infections, within the first few weeks, are related to surgical procedures and hospitalization (2,3) (Fig. 1). Typical pathogens include streptococci, *Staphylococcus aureus*, enterobacteriaciae, and *Pseudomonas aeruginosa*. Immunosuppressive therapy to prevent rejection of the transplanted organ begins near the time of surgery, but it takes days to weeks for the defect in CMI to develop. More time elapses before patients become exposed to potential pathogens and then for these

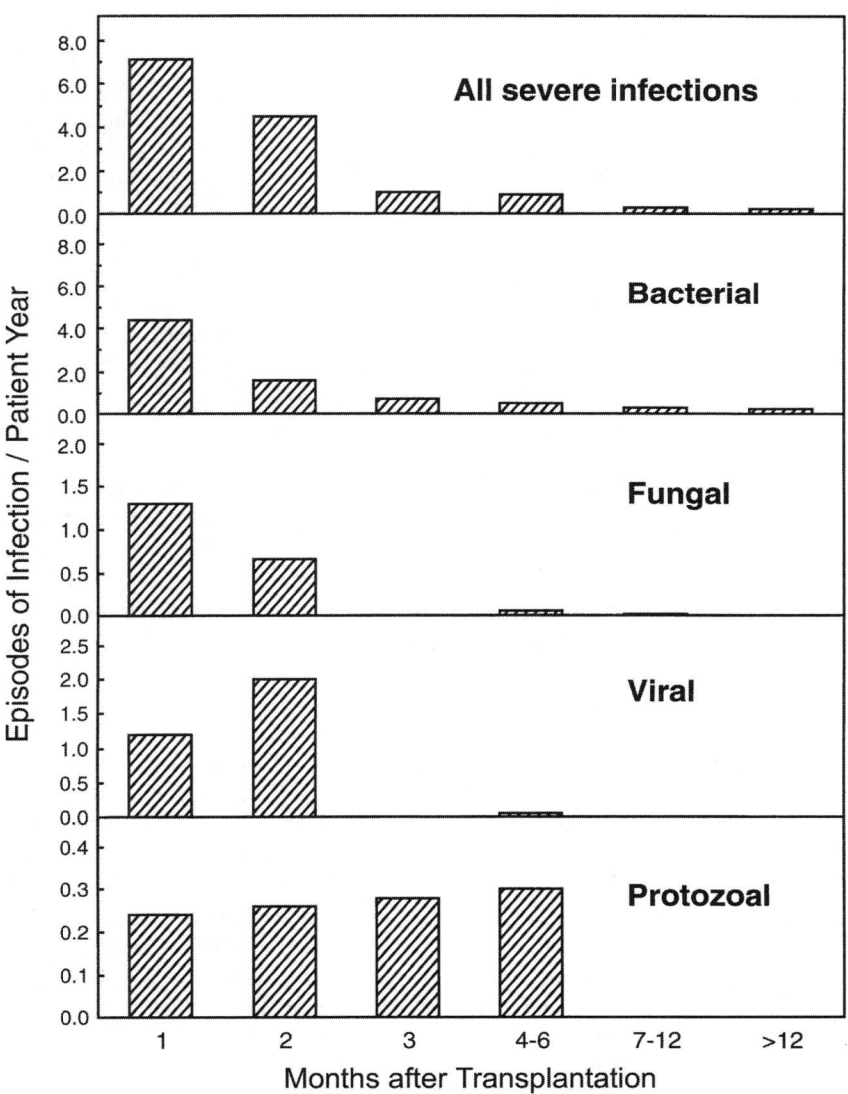

Figure 1 Severe infectious diseases after liver transplantation. Incidence for each time period is shown above each bar.

pathogens to infect the patient and for disease to develop. The peak time for infections related to cellular immunity defects is from six weeks to six months after transplantation. In most patients, immunosuppression diminishes beyond six months after transplantation. The risk of infection diminishes as well, but rarely approaches the risk in healthy persons.

INNATE DEFECTS

Neutropenia

Neutropenia is one of the more important defects leading to increased susceptibility to infection in critically ill patients. Approximately 10^{11} neutrophils are made per day in healthy persons. The marrow normally contains up to 10 times the normal daily neutrophil requirement in reserve. As a result, infectious diseases are not substantially more common until absolute neutrophil concentrations (mature neutrophils and band forms) are <1000 cells/μL blood. The risk of infectious diseases increases progressively as concentrations drop below 500 cells/μL and accelerates as concentrations drop below 100 cells/μL. The risk increases directly with the duration of neutropenia.

Neutrophil function may be impaired in patients who have received cytotoxic chemotherapy or irradiation. Numerous other drugs used widely in medical care occasionally impair neutrophil numbers or function in patients. Glucocorticoid therapy enhances granulopoiesis and demargination, but it also interferes with neutrophil function in subtle ways. Intrinsic defects in neutrophil function are much less common than acquired ones, and a discussion of the nature of these defects and their management is beyond the scope of this chapter. When patients with intrinsic defects require critical care, specialists familiar with the defects should be involved in management.

Pathogens likely to cause disease in patients with neutropenia or severe dysfunction include *S. aureus*, streptococci, aerobic or microaerophilic gram-negative bacilli including *E. coli*, klebsiella, proteus, and *P. aeruginosa*, *Candida*, *Aspergillus*, mucor fungi, and less commonly, other fungi. Coagulase-negative *Staphylococci*, including *Staphylococcus epidermidis*, become pathogens when they colonize plastic or metal surfaces inside the body but are not likely pathogens in patients without indwelling devices. The most common problem with coagulase-negative staphylococci in the critical care unit is intravascular catheter-associated septicemia.

When patients with neutropenia or neutrophil dysfunction develop febrile illnesses, they should be treated with an antimicrobial agent or combination active against the foregoing organisms. Many single drugs or drug combinations have been studied, and those that cover the majority of pathogens show similar effectiveness. No advantage has been realized when additional drugs are added so as to cover every conceivable pathogen. Such a regimen will increase the risk of toxicity and the pressure for selection of resistant flora. Leading drugs or combinations used in this setting are shown in Table 1.

Once antimicrobial therapy has been initiated for treatment of a febrile illness in a neutropenic patient, several decisions are usually necessary in the next few days or weeks. Antimicrobials are often adjusted to respond to new information, added for evidence suggesting or indicating continued infectious disease or superinfection, or discontinued. Decisions should be guided by the following general principles: (i) Monitor the patient carefully for the first three–five days of antimicrobial treatment and adjust therapy based on new information. Defervescence often takes from two to seven days (average five days) in severely neutropenic patients. (ii) Continue antimicrobials until signs or symptoms of infection

Table 1 Treatment of a Febrile Illness in a Patient with Neutropenia

Single drug[a]
  Ceftazidime, cefepime, imipenem, or meropenem
Combination[a] therapy
  Aminoglycoside + antipseudomonal penicillin, cefepime, ceftazidime, imipenem, or meropenem
Vancomycin[b] with one or two drugs
  Vancomycin + (cefepime or ceftazidime or imipenem or meropenem) ± aminoglycoside
  Vancomycin + antipseudomonal penicillin + aminoglycoside

[a]Selection should take into account patient characteristics and knowledge of the hospital flora, and the flora and susceptibilities of bacteria typically associated with infectious diseases in similar patients in the hospital. Many studies have shown that the clinical efficacies of single-drug and combination therapy used to treat febrile illnesses in neutropenic patients are empirically equivalent.
[b]Criterion for vancomycin use is (i) clinically suspected severe catheter-related infections (e.g., bacteremia, cellulitis); (ii) known colonization with penicillin- and cephalosporin-resistant pneumococci or methicillin-resistant *Staphylococcus aureus* (MRSA), positive results of blood culture for gram-positive bacteria before final identification and susceptibility testing; or (iii) hypotension or other cardiovascular impairment.
Source: Adapted from Ref. 4.

have been eradicated and usually until the absolute neutrophil count is ≥ 500 cells/μL. (iii) If fever persists for five days without a clear explanation, consider adding or modifying antibacterial therapy or adding antifungal therapy. These decisions are complicated and often difficult, and consultation with an infectious disease or hematology–oncology specialist is recommended.

Antiviral drugs usually are not necessary in febrile neutropenic patients without evidence of viral diseases. Herpes simplex or herpes zoster infections should be treated primarily to reduce the opportunities for bacteria to enter through lesions in skin or mucous membranes and cause severe bacterial infection. Cytomegalovirus infections are usually not clinically important except in bone-marrow-transplant recipients who typically have both neutropenia and CMI defects.

Colony-stimulating factors (CSFs) consistently shorten the duration of neutropenia but do not clearly affect outcomes of infectious diseases during neutropenia. CSFs in clinical use include granulocyte colony-stimulating factor (G-CSF, filgrastim) and granulocyte-macrophage colony-stimulating factor (GM-CSF, sargramostim). These factors should not be used except when neutropenia will be prolonged and documented infections do not respond to optimal antimicrobial therapy.

Antimicrobial prophylaxis against bacterial or fungal infections reduces the incidence of documented infection but does not reduce infection-related mortality. The benefits of reduced morbidity are countered by the strong likelihood that antimicrobial prophylaxis selects resistant flora to create a major problem in critical care units. Antimicrobial prophylaxis should not be used to prevent most bacterial or fungal infections. *Pneumocystis carinii* disease is an exception in patients with both neutropenia and defects in CMI, and trimethoprim–sulfamethoxazole (one double-strength tablet once or twice per day) should be given to such patients. *P. carinii* disease is uncommon in persons who have isolated defects in granulocyte number or function.

Granulocyte transfusions were used to prevent or treat infectious diseases in patients with granulocytopenia or granulocyte dysfunction in the 1960s and 1970s. These early clinical trials demonstrated no improvement in outcomes but significant associated costs and toxicities. Those studies were conducted with neutrophils collected by filtration, a process that activated many of the neutrophils and reduced their function. In some studies, the number of neutrophils infused were small compared with the ordinary output of a healthy bone marrow. Recently, centrifugation technologies have been developed that produce relatively large numbers of granulocytes that appear to retain their function after isolation and infusion into a recipient. The clinical efficacy, when these granulocytes are transfused into patients with infectious diseases, has not been adequately studied. For patients with inadequate neutrophil numbers or function, granulocyte transfusions might be considered to treat documented infectious diseases refractory to surgical drainage, antimicrobial therapy, or G-CSF therapy. This use should be considered experimental and may be accompanied by significant toxicity.

Complement Deficiency

Inherited complement deficiency occurs in ~3 in 10,000 persons. Substantial variations exist among different ethnic groups. Secondary complement deficiency is more common in patients with connective tissue diseases than in the general population. Complement deficiency leads to increased risk of disease with certain encapsulated organisms, including *Neisseria meningitidis*, *Neisseria gonorrhea*, *Streptococcus pneumoniae*, and *Haemophilus influenzae*. When patients with complement deficiency develop febrile illnesses, they should be treated with a drug active against the encapsulated organisms mentioned earlier, for example ceftriaxone.

Asplenia or Splenic Dysfunction

A functional spleen is important for defense against certain organisms, mainly encapsulated bacteria. The incidence of severe infectious disease in some subsets of splenectomized patients is as great as 600 times that among persons with normal splenic function. Most persons with inadequate splenic function have had their spleens removed as a consequence of trauma or surgery. Certain medical conditions are associated with inadequate splenic function, and rare individuals have congenital absence of the spleen. For those who lose a spleen, the risk of severe infection is greatest in the first year after splenectomy, diminishes over time, and approaches, but never reaches, the risk in the general population. The risk of severe infection is related to the reason for splenectomy. The risk is lowest in those who lost the spleen from traumatic injury; intermediate in those who had splenectomy for spherocytosis, idiopathic thrombocytopenic purpura, or portal hypertension; and greatest in those undergoing splenectomy for thalassemia or Hodgkin's disease.

Septicemia in persons with hyposplenism often produces subtle manifestations, including fever, chills, aches, and malaise. After a few hours or days of these symptoms, infection can accelerate rapidly and produce serious illness and death in hours or a few days. Antimicrobials active against the most likely pathogens should be given for any person with hyposplenism and a febrile illness. The most common bacterial pathogens include *S. pneumoniae*, *H. influenzae*, and *N. meningitidis*. Other less common bacteria pathogens include *Capnocytophaga canimorsus* and *Salmonella* spp. Babesiosis is more common in persons with splenectomy but does not initially produce overwhelming sepsis. When patients with splenic dysfunction develop febrile illnesses, they should be treated with a drug active against the encapsulated organisms mentioned earlier, for example ceftriaxone.

Malnutrition

Inadequate nutrition is common in many patients in critical care units. Profound malnutrition can lead to substantial host defense defects and calls for vigorous replacement. The impact of mild or moderate degrees of malnutrition on the risk of infections and other substantial outcomes are subtle and difficult to quantify. Decisions about when to intervene in regard to mild or moderate degrees of malnutrition are controversial. Ideally, correction is accomplished by feeding the patient by mouth. Tube feeding is the next best choice for a variety of reasons, but nutritional support through a tube has risks. Tubes that go from the mouth into the gastrointestinal tract interfere with the ability of the esophagus to prevent reflux. Tubes inserted through the abdominal wall directly into the upper gastrointestinal tract have less risk of reflux, but reflux can still occur if gastric and intestinal mobility are not sufficient to move food promptly into the small intestines. Despite these risks, tube feeding is clearly superior to parenteral nutrition if no contraindication to tube feeding exists. Parenteral nutrition requires a central venous catheter, and intravenous nutrition solutions support the growth of bacteria and fungi that frequently become pathogens in patients receiving intravenous metabolic support (see Chapter 4).

Malignancy

Tumors interfere with host defenses in many ways. For example, bronchogenic carcinomas obstruct airways and lead to atelectasis and pneumonia. Gastrointestinal tumors can induce overgrowth syndromes or disrupt mucous membrane integrity and allow colonic contents to enter the peritoneum or the bloodstream.

Diabetes Mellitus

Hyperglycemia increases the risk of infectious diseases throughout the course of diabetes mellitus. The mechanisms are incompletely understood. Young patients with diabetes are more prone to urinary-tract infections. In later stages of diabetes, end-organ dysfunction leads to substantially increased infectious disease risks. For example, impaired nerve and circulatory function leads to foot ulcers. Infection in the ulcers may result in cellulitis, abscesses, osteomyelitis, local deformities and dysfunction, or dissemination. Neuropathy of the urinary bladder predisposes to cystitis or ascending urinary-tract infections. Although complications of diabetes cannot be changed during critical illness, evidence indicates that optimal control of blood sugar improves infectious disease outcomes and prevention (see Chapter 42).

Neurological Dysfunction

In patients with neurological dysfunction, several aberrant behaviors increase the risk of infectious diseases. For example, obtunded or comatose patients are unable to keep weight off dependent tissues; pressure necrosis and decubitus ulcers develop as a result. Atelectasis is common in obtunded patients who cannot breathe deeply or cough. If these patients are intubated, the airway is compromised and the risk for infection is compounded.

Tobacco Use

Tobacco use increases the risk for several infectious diseases. The risk is greatest for cigarette smokers and is related to daily dose and duration of tobacco use. People who have smoked cigarettes for years are likely to have chronic lung disease and are at increased risk for pneumonia. They are also at risk for infectious disease with several microorganisms including *S. pneumoniae*, *L. pneumophila*, and *M. tuberculosis*.

Stress

Stress impairs host defenses and increases the risk of infectious diseases (5). Critically ill patients usually are profoundly stressed. The risk with stress is subtle, and the defects are nonspecific. The effects of stress probably act in concert with other host defense defects.

Hypochlorhydria

Diminished gastric acid secretion allows proliferation of bacteria in the stomach and a change in the flora to include several potentially pathogenic organisms. These changes probably increase the risk of nosocomial pneumonia. Efforts to preserve gastric acidity or selectively decontaminate the upper gastrointestinal tract have produced inconclusive results. Selective decontamination remains controversial and is not routinely recommended.

Altered Microbial Flora

The usual human flora becomes altered as soon as patients are admitted to hospitals. Changes occur more rapidly in patients admitted to intensive care units (ICUs). For example, gram-negative bacilli become the predominant organisms in the nasopharynx during the first few days in an ICU. Changes in the usual flora are magnified by antimicrobial use. The effects are greater with broad-spectrum antimicrobial therapy than with narrow-spectrum therapy and are dependent on the duration of antimicrobial use. With increasing duration of antimicrobial use, patients become colonized with gram-negative bacilli resistant to multiple antimicrobials, MRSA, vancomycin-resistant enterococci (VRE), and pneumococci resistant to penicillin and erythromycin.

Candida albicans and other *Candida* spp. are normal inhabitants of skin and mucous membranes. Antimicrobial use leads to overgrowth of candida species, especially in the gastrointestinal tract. Breaks in skin or mucous membranes, for example, with vascular catheters, lead to colonization and invasion. As a result, candidal infections have increased dramatically in the antibiotic era. Disease with *Aspergillus* spp. and other molds is also more common in persons who have received antimicrobials, but such persons nearly always have additional profound host defense defects, typically profound neutropenia or severe burns.

Diarrhea occurs in 3% to 30% of hospitalized patients who receive antimicrobials. Approximately one-quarter of these cases are attributable to *Clostridium difficile*. When colitis is present, one-half to three-fourths of cases are attributable to *C. difficile*, and if pseudomembranes are present, over 90% are attributable to *C. difficile*. Most patients with *C. difficile* disease have diarrhea, but a small fraction have ileus or megacolon. Nearly all cases occur in patients with recent antimicrobial use, but cases have occurred in patients taking antineoplastic drugs with antimicrobial properties. Colonization with

C. difficile precedes antimicrobial use, and disruption of the flora allows elaboration of toxin A and toxin B, both of which induce cytoskeletal derangements in intestinal epithelial cells, mucosal injury, and inflammation.

DEFECTS IN IMMUNITY

Antibody Deficiency

Antibodies are important for complement activation, phagocytosis, antibody-dependent cellular cytotoxicity, neutralization of toxins and viruses, prevention of adhesion, and agglutination. Severe disease with the encapsulated bacteria *S. pneumoniae*, *H. influenzae*, and *N. meningitidis* are more common in persons with profound antibody deficiencies.

Children may have a variety of inherited, genetically determined antibody deficiencies. A full discussion of these entities is beyond the scope of this chapter. Adults are more likely to acquire antibody deficiency from another disease, for example, chronic lymphocytic leukemia, multiple myeloma, Waldenström macroglobulinemia, protein wasting states, bone marrow transplantation, and human immunodeficiency virus (HIV)-related antibody deficiency.

IgG can be replaced in patients with severe deficiency. IgM and IgA cannot be replaced with current technology. The available preparations contain 95–99% IgG, and the half-life of IgG is 20 days. Much larger doses can be given intravenously than intramuscularly, and intravenous immune globulin (IVIg) is used for treatment of severe infection and to prevent infections in many patients.

When symptoms or signs suggest the presence of an infectious disease in a patient with clinically significant IgG deficiency, antimicrobials active against *S. pneumoniae*, *H. influenzae*, and *N. meningitidis* should be given immediately. When severe disease is diagnosed, IVIg should be administered in doses of 100–400 mg/kg every three–four weeks. For difficult cases, trough IgG levels should be measured during therapy and doses adjusted to maintain serum concentrations at 400–500 mg/dL during therapy.

CMI Defects

CMI refers to a complex set of cells and molecules that kill, suppress, or clear certain viruses, bacteria, fungi, protozoa, and helminthes. The major effector cells are T cells, NK cells, and macrophages. Some of these pathogens evade other host defenses by invading, multiplying, or persisting inside host cells. Hematological malignancies, congenital abnormalities, HIV infection, and cytotoxic drug therapy are important causes of reduced CMI.

Infections with organisms in Table 2 are more likely or more severe in persons with diminished CMI. Most infectious diseases that occur with greater frequency in patients with CMI defects are indolent or subacute. Signs and symptoms are often subtle. Note that signs or symptoms that might signify an infectious disease in a patient with deficient CMI should be promptly and thoroughly investigated, but the approach can be deliberate. In patients with defective CMI, empirical therapy is rarely necessary before a diagnosis has been made.

Infection-Induced Immune Dysfunction

HIV infection is the most common microbiological cause of immunosuppression. Nearly all people with late HIV infection have CMI defects. HIV infects T cells, which have

Table 2 Important Pathogens in Patients with Deficient CMI

Viruses
    Respiratory syncytial virus, adenovirus, parainfluenza, cytomegalovirus, herpes simplex virus, varicella-zoster virus, human herpes virus 6, human herpes virus 8
Bacteria
    Listeria monocytogenes, Legionella pneumophila, Mycobacterium tuberculosis, Mycobacterium avium complex, *Nocardia* species, *Rhodococcus equi, Salmonella* species, *Shigella* species
Fungi
    Histoplasma capsulatum, Penicillium marneffei, Coccidioidomyces immitis, Cryptococcus neoformans
Protozoa
    Cryptosporidium parvum, Leishmania species, *Microsporidia* species, *Toxoplasma gondii*
Helminth
    Strongyloides stercoralis

---

important immunoregulatory functions. As a result, HIV-infected patients typically have impaired antibody responsiveness to new antigens as well. Persons with late HIV infection often have other complications that impair host defenses, which include granulocytopenia, malnutrition, and skin and mucosal defects. Infectious diseases common in HIV infection are well known and are discussed in Chapter 47. Most of them are controlled by CMI. These diseases are typically subacute, and a deliberate approach to diagnosis and treatment is needed. *P. carinii* pneumonia is an exception and can progress rapidly. When patients with ≤ 250 CD4$^+$ cells/μL blood demonstrate typical manifestations of pneumocystis pneumonia, induced sputum should be sent for cytology. However, sputum specimens yield the diagnosis in $\leq 50\%$ of cases. Many physicians initiate empirical therapy against *P. carinii* disease in patients with typical manifestations and negative sputum tests and perform invasive tests to confirm diagnosis only when pneumonia does not respond to empirical therapy.

Other infectious diseases that cause generalized immunosuppression include cytomegalovirus infection, toxoplasmosis, and measles. Some infectious diseases cause local host defense defects. For example, acute influenza impairs lung host defenses and predisposes the patient to bacterial pneumonia. Most of these diseases are not prominent problems in patients in critical care units.

Transplantation

Persons with transplanted organs are at substantial risk of infectious diseases. The risk varies and is associated with diseases present before transplantation, latent infections with the potential to reactivate, colonization with nosocomial pathogens, lack of immunity to infections that occur after transplantation, immunosuppressive medications, type of organ implanted, type of surgery, immunosuppressive infections, and allograft reactions. Certain localized infections are more common as a result of the presence of the transplanted organ and alterations in local anatomy. Most transplant recipients develop a fever with opportunistic infections, but some do not. In this group of patients, fevers are often associated with noninfectious causes, including drug reactions, deep venous thrombosis, and rejection.

The approach to suspected infection in transplant recipients should be deliberate and systematic. Evaluation should start with a careful history and physical examination, chest roentgenogram, urinalysis, complete blood count, liver function tests, and blood cultures. Clues identified in this evaluation should be pursued. Empirical therapy without substantial evidence for the cause of fever is usually not necessary and is often counterproductive. In some centers, patients are given trimethoprim–sulfamethoxazole to prevent urinary-tract infections and other opportunistic infections in renal transplant and other transplant recipients (6). Trimethoprim–sulfamethoxazole clearly prevents *P. carinii* disease, toxoplasmosis, and probably nocardiosis and listeriosis. These diseases are less likely to occur in patients receiving trimethoprim–sulfamethoxazole who demonstrate signs or symptoms of infection.

FEVER AND INFECTIOUS DISEASES IN CRITICAL CARE

Altered host defenses add complexity and challenge to the evaluation and management of suspected or proved infection in patients in critical care. Optimal management includes an appropriate level of suspicion for infectious diseases, aggressive attempts at diagnosis, judicious use of antimicrobial agents for treatment of suspected or proved infectious diseases, and prevention of infections. Infectious diseases are common in critically ill patients, a circumstance that leads to widespread use of antimicrobial agents. Several studies have documented that antimicrobials are overused in critical care units, and that antimicrobial use results in antimicrobial resistance and worse outcomes for patients. For the sake of current and future patients, wise use of antimicrobials is critical.

Fever and other signs of inflammation are common in critically ill patients. Fever is due to infectious disease about half of the time (7–9). Other signs and symptoms of infection include chills, malaise, aches and pains, hypotension, or obtundation. Signs and symptoms of infectious diseases derive both from the pathogen and its effect on tissues and from the host response. In patients with host defense defects, signs or symptoms may be subtle or absent. Diminished signs or symptoms are particularly likely in persons with neutropenia, antibody or complement deficiency, splenectomy, and advanced age. Infectious diseases should be included in possible etiologies of most unexplained new clinical events that occur in patients in ICUs.

Leukocytosis also is common in critically ill patients who have inflammation. As with other manifestations of inflammation, leukocytosis is due to infection only about one-half of the time. In a recent study of patients with more than 25,000 leukocytes/μL and in which the majority of leukocytes were granulocytes, infection was present in only 48% (10). The other major causes were malignancy, bleeding, corticosteroid therapy, and shock syndromes.

Patients with chronic illness or who have had extensive exposure to clinics or hospitals are likely to be colonized with typical hospital flora resistant to commonly used antimicrobials. Gram-negative bacilli colonize the upper respiratory tract within a few days of hospitalization, especially for patients in ICUs. MRSA and VRE are likely to colonize patients in ICUs after a few days. Length of stay in the ICU is directly associated with the likelihood that a patient is colonized with gram-negative bacilli (11), resistant gram-positive cocci, and fungi (12). Colonization does not equate to disease. Gram-negative bacilli, *S. aureus*, and enterococci often colonize without causing disease.

Infections are more likely with increased ICU length of stay. Urinary-tract infections (13), ventilator-associated pneumonia (14), and *C. difficile* disease are all more common as length of stay increases. Asymptomatic bacteruria is also common in critically ill patients. Asymptomatic bacteruria is present in more than half of adults over the age of 65 years. It is almost always observed in patients with indwelling urinary catheters. No benefit from treating asymptomatic bacteruria has been demonstrated. The challenge for the intensivist is to differentiate between colonization and disease.

Although appropriate antimicrobial therapy is necessary for many patients in the ICU and substantially reduces morbidity and mortality, evidence exists that excessive antimicrobial use is harmful. In one medical/surgical critical care unit study (15), patients with infiltrates and clinical pneumonia infection scores ≤6 [evidence suggestive, but not conclusive, of the presence of bacterial pneumonia (16)] were randomized to one of two arms. In the first (short-term monotherapy group), patients received three days of therapy with a quinolone. If the clinical infection score remained ≤6 after three days, antimicrobial therapy was stopped. In the other arm, patients received usual care, which usually included multiple antimicrobials given for 10–21 days. When the study was terminated, the ICU stay was 9.4 days in the short-term monotherapy group compared with 14.7 days in the control arm in which patients received usual care ($p = 0.04$). Thirty-day mortality was 13% in patients in the short-term monotherapy group vs. 31% in the control group ($p = 0.06$). Resistance or superinfection developed in 14% of patients in the short-term monotherapy group vs. 38% in the control group ($p = 0.017$). Mean antimicrobial costs in short-term monotherapy cases were only 40% of mean costs in control cases.

The prevalence of resistance in the microbiological flora in the ICU is heavily influenced by the overall antimicrobial use. All decisions made throughout the course of a patient's stay in the unit are important. A tendency exists to focus more on antimicrobials used for initial, empirical therapy than on subsequent decisions. Initial antimicrobials are often continued when more narrowly tailored therapy would be just as effective and less likely to select resistant organisms. Antimicrobials given for suspected infection are often continued long after infection has been excluded, even when another cause for the signs and symptoms has been identified. In the interest of each patient in an ICU and for the overall flora, each day the clinical team should consider whether antimicrobials given to each patient continue to be necessary and whether they are tailored as much as possible to the patient's infectious problems. Occasional reviews of aggregate antimicrobial use in a unit often lead to important insights into how well principles of antimicrobial therapy are applied in individual patients.

Various approaches to antimicrobial prophylaxis have been studied in patients to prevent infectious diseases in critical care units. Generally, they have not been successful, and they have a negative impact on the resistance of the unit microbiological flora. Antimicrobial prophylaxis should not be used except in highly specific circumstances where the benefit has been clearly demonstrated.

Preventive antifungal therapy with fluconazole is often prescribed to prevent invasive disease in patients who are infected with *Candida* spp. at one or more skin or mucous membrane sites. However, many patients with multiple positive yeast cultures never develop deep infection, the prevalence of imidazole resistance is increasing among hospital candida isolates, and many patients receiving fluconazole develop toxicity. Until better tools are available to predict which patients will develop disease, patients with yeast isolates from skin and mucous membrane sites should be observed carefully for the development of disease. Blood cultures should be obtained at the first signs or symptoms of invasive disease. Antifungal therapy should be administered if deep candida infection is strongly suspected or proved.

MANAGEMENT

The first step for any patient with one or more signs or symptoms that might be associated with an infectious disease is to establish a diagnosis (7,9). The process should begin with a careful history, which should include events, possible exposures, and risk factors identified before hospitalization, and events that have occurred since admission. In patients who are not fully conscious or intubated, important historical information is often obtained from the record, nursing notes, and from conversations with family members, nurses, respiratory therapists, and other staff.

Every patient with suspected infectious disease should have a careful physical examination. Signs of infection should be sought at any site where local host defense defects might be compromised. Likely sites would include breaks in the skin, vascular insufficiency, and burns. For most patients, a complete blood count and urinalysis should be performed. Urine culture should be performed if there is pyuria or another reason to suspect urinary-tract infection, but asymptomatic bacteriuria is common and of little consequence. Blood cultures should be performed from at least two sites in most cases.

If symptoms refer to the chest, or if pneumonia is at all likely, a chest roentgenograph should be performed. If an infiltrate is present or there is other evidence of pneumonia, a sputum specimen should be obtained and submitted for Gram stain and bacterial culture. If the patient has a defect in CMI, or the pneumonia is subacute, and findings suggest mycobacterial or fungal disease, smears and cultures should be done to detect mycobacteria and fungi. In patients with pneumonia in which the pathogens are not quickly identified, or in which the patient does not respond to empirical antimicrobial therapy, bronchoscopy should be considered for further attempts at diagnosis. In some studies, quantitative cultures of bronchial secretions have been helpful for diagnosis of bacterial infection. These studies are difficult to interpret, because no good standard for comparison exists. This approach has not proved useful in all studies. Bronchoscopy is most clearly indicated in patients with deficient CMI and subacute pneumonia in whom sputum smears and cultures have not provided a diagnosis.

Once initial information has been gathered, the intensivist should construct a differential diagnosis involving infectious and noninfectious conditions that might be associated with the patient's signs or symptoms (7,9). The list should include infections with organisms likely to cause disease in the presence of any specific host defense defects. If clues to the presence of an infectious disease are uncovered during the initial evaluation, further tests should be done to document or exclude it. Extensive testing or imaging done in the absence of clues that the tests will be positive is usually not helpful and often turns up spurious or misleading findings.

If initial or subsequent studies provide evidence that an infectious disease is present and causing signs or symptoms, the clinician should usually initiate specific therapy. Bacterial and fungal infectious diseases are usually treated with antimicrobials, whereas many viral infectious diseases are not amenable to therapy. Colonization with potential pathogens in the oropharynx, tracheal secretions, skin, urine, or stool does not mean that disease is present and should not lead to antimicrobial treatment.

A number of factors should influence the antimicrobials that are chosen to treat infectious disease in a particular case. The intensivist should incorporate information about organisms likely to be involved in the type of infectious disease, microbiological findings for the patient being treated, and experience with similar cases in the ICU and hospital. The antimicrobial choice should be guided by susceptibility patterns of pathogens associated with similar cases in the ICU, hospital, and locality, in that order.

When signs or symptoms of infectious disease occur in a patient with a profound defect in antibody, complement, or splenic function, or in a patient with profound granulocytopenia or granulocyte dysfunction, empirical antimicrobials should be given immediately to treat infections likely to occur as a consequence of the specific defect. Without early empirical antimicrobial therapy, patients with these kinds of defects are at risk for rapid deterioration and death. If any patient appears to be critically ill from a new infectious disease, antimicrobials should be given immediately that are directed against likely pathogens.

Appropriate use of antimicrobials in the ICU depends as much on monitoring and decisions made after antimicrobial therapy is begun as on decisions involved in initial empirical therapy. Once an infectious disease has been diagnosed, the clinical response, new or updated microbiological results, evidence of antimicrobial toxicity, and other information that will help refine the diagnosis and approach to treatment should be reviewed daily. Where possible, the spectrum of antimicrobials used should be narrowed to focus treatment with the least possible impact on individual patient and hospital flora. If initial suspicions of infectious disease are not confirmed, or another cause for the signs or symptoms present in the patient becomes apparent, antimicrobials should be discontinued. When an infectious disease has been adequately treated, antimicrobials should be stopped.

Theoretically, reductions or elimination in immunosuppressive therapy would provide an advantage to an immunosuppressed patient who is being treated with antimicrobials for an infectious disease. In practice, the evidence to support this practice is mixed. For severe cytomegalovirus disease and invasive aspergillosis, stopping or reducing immunosuppressive therapy seems to be beneficial. In tuberculosis, nocardiosis, and *P. carinii* disease, no benefit from reducing immunosuppressive therapy has been shown. Indeed, outcomes of some diseases, like pneumocystis pneumonia and tuberculous meningitis, are enhanced by short-term, high-dose therapy with corticosteroids.

Optimal management of immunocompromised patients is especially complicated in an ICU. When patients with substantial immune compromising conditions are admitted to ICU, experts in the care of such patients should be involved from the time of admission. When infectious diseases are suspected or proved, both these experts and an infectious disease consultant should become involved in management.

PREVENTION

More than two million patients are diagnosed with nosocomial infections each year. The risk is greater in patients in ICU. In a recent study of patients in medical and surgical ICUs in a university hospital, 13% of patients developed nosocomial infections (17). Prevention of infection is much preferable to treatment, especially for patients with substantial defects in host defenses. Many of the pathogens involved in infections in ICUs are acquired within the units from flora of other patients, health care workers, and inanimate objects. Appropriate hand hygiene is critically important in the prevention of nosocomial infection and includes appropriate hand washing, disinfection, and use of gloves. Special isolation procedures should be established for organisms with unusual transmissibility or that pose significant threats to other patients or personnel. Each ICU should have well-publicized standards and protocols and should educate health care workers and monitor compliance (18).

Intravenous and intra-arterial catheters are a major source of infectious disease in critical care units, and these cases are often severe. Vascular catheters should be used when needed and removed promptly when no longer needed. Catheters should not be left in place for convenience or in anticipation of the possibility that they will be needed in the future. ICUs should have protocols and kits for device insertion, care, and removal. The Centers for Disease Control and Prevention recently published a set of guidelines and protocols for vascular catheter care (19).

Indwelling urinary catheters are another major source of infectious morbidity and mortality in critically ill patients. Urinary catheters are needed for patients who are unstable or for whom fluid status is unknown or needs careful monitoring. However, urinary catheters are often left in long after they are needed and long after physicians are paying close attention to input and output. Urinary catheters should be removed as soon as intensive monitoring is no longer needed. Because catheters are often left in place inadvertently, ICUs should have protocols that ask the physician in charge of each patient with an indwelling catheter whether the catheter is still needed. Urinary catheters should not be used for convenience of the patient or ICU staff. For patients who are incontinent and empty their bladders frequently, diapers are frequently an adequate solution. For patients whose bladders do not empty often enough, scheduled, frequent straight catheterization is preferred to indwelling urinary catheters.

Patients undergo many other procedures in ICUs. Clean or sterile techniques should be used during all procedures. The hospital infection control department and unit staff should decide which procedures should be done with each kind of technique. The unit should have protocols, prepackaged kits, and other systems in place to facilitate procedures likely to be done in the units. Units should also have protocols for skin and wound care and oral hygiene. Surveillance of nosocomial infections should be performed periodically and analyzed to detect problems and suggest solutions.

SUMMARY

- Innate host defenses operate without specific antigenic stimulation and are concentrated at body surfaces, including both skin and mucous membranes.
- Breaches of skin and mucous membranes are frequent in critically ill patients and increase susceptibility to infection.
- Immune host defenses develop in response to specific pathogens or other antigens. This defense system includes lymphocytes, antibodies, and facilitated phagocytosis. Immune defenses require days to weeks to develop.
- Adequate nutrition is crucial for complete, competent host defenses.
- Aging is associated with decreased CMI.
- Antibody or complement deficiencies increase the likelihood of disease from encapsulated organisms but not from fungi.
- Defects in CMI increase the likelihood of infections with mycobacteria or cytomegalovirus but not *E. coli* or influenza virus.
- Early infections in solid-organ transplant recipients are usually related to surgical procedures and hospitalization. Infections related to CMI occur six weeks to six months after transplantation.

- Risk of infectious disease in neutropenic patients is increased when neutrophil concentrations are <1000 cells/μL blood. Risk increases with severity and duration of neutropenia.
- See Table 1 for recommended antimicrobial therapy for febrile illnesses in neutropenic patients. Monitor these patients carefully, continue treatment until infection is eradicated and absolute neutrophil count is >500 cells/μL blood, and consider additional diagnostic procedures, antimicrobial therapy, or antifungal therapy if fever persists for ≥5 days without an identified cause.
- Antiviral drugs usually are not necessary in febrile neutropenic patients.
- Trimethoprim–sulfamethoxazole is given to some patients with neutropenia and CMI deficiency to prevent *P. carinii* disease.
- Complement deficiency increases the risk of infections with *N. meningitidis, N. gonorrhea, S. pneumoniae,* and *H. influenza*.
- Patients with splenic dysfunction who develop febrile illnesses should receive antimicrobials active against *S. pneumoniae, H. influenzae,* and *N. meningitidis*.
- Hyperglycemia is associated with increased risk of infectious disease. Control of blood sugar in the critically ill patient is associated with improved outcomes.
- Neurologic dysfunction may lead to increased risk of infection as a consequence of pressure ulcers and poor pulmonary toilet.
- Tobacco use, stress, and hypochlorhydria are associated with increased infectious risk.
- Antibiotic use is associated with transition to resistant nosocomial bacteria, candida overgrowth, and *C. difficile* colitis.
- Chronic lymphocytic leukemia, multiple myeloma, Waldenstrom macroglobulinemia, protein wasting states, bone marrow transplantation, and HIV infection are associated with antibody deficiency. IgG can be administered to IgG-deficient patients. Antimicrobials active against *S. pneumoniae, H. influenzae,* and *N. meningitidis* should be administered empirically for acute febrile illnesses.
- Important pathogens in patients with CMI deficiency are listed in Table 2.
- Late HIV infection is associated with CMI defects. When *P. carinii* infection is suspected, patients should receive empiric therapy.
- Risk of infection in solid-organ transplant recipients is associated with diseases present before transplantation, latent infections, colonization with nosocomial pathogens, immunosuppressive medications, type of organ transplant, type of surgery, and allograft reactions.
- Most transplant recipients develop fever with opportunistic infections. Empirical therapy without evidence for infection usually is not necessary.
- The likelihood of infection in a critically ill patient with fever alone is approximately one-half. Presence of obtundation, chills, malaise, or hypotension increases the likelihood of infection.
- Signs of infection may be subtle or absent in patients with neutropenia, antibody deficiency, complement deficiency, splenectomy, and advanced age.
- In the critically ill patient, the likelihood that leukocytosis arises from infection is approximately one-half.
- Length of ICU stay is directly correlated with colonization of patients with gram-negative bacilli, resistant gram-positive cocci, and fungi and with likelihood of infection.

- In addition to careful selection of antimicrobials when therapy is initiated, daily review of clinical course, additional microbiologic information, and continued need for antibiotics can maximize efficacy and minimize risks, including development of resistant microorganisms in the ICU.
- Antimicrobial prophylaxis should not be used except in selected circumstances where benefit is clear. An example is antibiotic prophylaxis for elective colon resection.
- Antifungal therapy should be administered only if deep candida infection is proved or is strongly suspected.
- When selecting antimicrobial therapy incorporate information about organisms likely to be involved in an infectious disease, microbiological findings, and experience with similar cases in a given ICU.
- In the patient with profound deficiency in antibody, complement, splenic function, or granulocytes, empirical therapy is urgent if signs or symptoms of infectious disease are present.
- For severe cytomegalovirus infection and for invasive aspergillosis, discontinuing or reducing immunosuppressive therapy is beneficial.
- Prevention of infection is superior to treatment of established infection. Hand hygiene is of critical importance. Hand washing, disinfection, and the use of gloves are measures demonstrated to decrease infection.
- Intravenous catheters should be removed when no longer needed. They should not be left in place for convenience or anticipation of an untoward event.
- Indwelling urinary catheters present an infectious risk and should be removed at the earliest possible time.
- Optimal management includes appropriate level of suspicion for infectious diseases, aggressive efforts at diagnosis, judicious use of antimicrobials, and prevention of infections.

REFERENCES

1. Perri RT, Hebbel RP, Oken MM. Influence of treatment and response status on infection risk in multiple myeloma. Am J Med 1981; 71:935–940.
2. Kusne S, Dummer JS, Singh N, et al. Infections after liver transplantation. An analysis of 101 consecutive cases. Medicine 1988; 67:132–143.
3. Peterson PK, Anderson RC. Infection in renal transplant recipients. Current approaches to diagnosis, therapy, and prevention. Am J Med 1986; 81:2–10.
4. Hughes WT, Armstrong D, Bodey GP, et al. 2002. Guidelines for the use of antimicrobial agents in neutropenic patients with cancer. Clin Infect Dis 2002; 34:730–751.
5. Peterson PK, Chao CC, Molitor T, Murtaugh M, Strgar F, Sharp BM. Stress and pathogenesis of infectious disease. Rev Infect Dis 1991; 13:710–720.
6. EBPG Expert Group on Renal Transplantation. European best practice guidelines for renal transplantation. Section IV: long-term management of the transplant recipient. IV.7.1 Late infections. *Pneumocystis carinii* pneumonia. Nephrol Dial Transpl 2002; 17(suppl 4):36–39.
7. Rizoli SB, Marshall JC. Saturday night fever: finding and controlling the source of sepsis in critical illness. Lancet Infect Dis 2002; 2:137–144.
8. Circiumaru B, Baldock G, Cohen J. A prospective study of fever in the intensive care unit. Intensive Care Med 1999; 25:668–673.

9. O'Grady NP, Barie PS, Bartlett JG, et al. Practice parameters for evaluating new fever in critically ill adult patients. Task force of the American College of Critical Care Medicine of the Society of Critical Care Medicine in collaboration with the Infectious Disease Society of America. Crit Care Med 1998; 26:392–408.
10. Reding MT, Hibbs JR, Morrison VA, Swaim WR, Filice GA. The clinical significance of extreme leukocytosis. Am J Med 1998; 104:12–16.
11. Blot S, Vandewoude K, Blot K, Colardyn F. Prevalence and risk factors for colonisation with Gram-negative bacteria in an intensive care unit. Acta Clin Belg 2000; 55:249–256.
12. McKinnon PS, Goff DA, Kern JW, et al. Temporal assessment of Candida risk factors in the surgical intensive care unit. Arch Surg 2001; 136:1401–1408; discussion 1409.
13. Laupland KB, Zygun DA, Davies HD, Church DL, Louie TJ, Doig CJ. Incidence and risk factors for acquiring nosocomial urinary tract infection in the critically ill. J Crit Care 2002; 17:50–57.
14. Sofianou DC, Constandinidis TC, Yannacou M, Anastasiou H, Sofianos E. Analysis of risk factors for ventilator-associated pneumonia in a multidisciplinary intensive care unit. Eur J Clin Microbiol Infect Dis 2000; 19:460–463.
15. Singh N, Rogers P, Atwood CW, Wagener MM, Yu VL. Short-course empiric antibiotic therapy for patients with pulmonary infiltrates in the intensive care unit. A proposed solution for indiscriminate antibiotic prescription. Am J Respir Crit Care Med 2000; 162:505–511.
16. Pugin J, Auckenthaler R, Mili N, Janssens JP, Lew PD, Suter PM. Diagnosis of ventilator-associated pneumonia by bacteriologic analysis of bronchoscopic and nonbronchoscopic "blind" bronchoalveolar lavage fluid. Am Rev Resp Dis 1991; 143:1121–1129.
17. McCusker ME, Perisse AR, Roghmann MC. Severity-of-illness markers as predictors of nosocomial infection in adult intensive care unit patients. Am J Infect Control 2002; 30:139–144.
18. Centers for Disease Control and Prevention. Guideline for hand hygiene in health-care settings: recommendations of the healthcare infection control practices advisory committee and the HICPAC/SHEA/APIC/IDSA hand hygiene task force. MMWR 2002; 51(No. RR-16):1–48.
19. Centers for Disease Control and Prevention. Guidelines for the prevention of intravascular catheter-related infections. MMWR 2002; 51(No. RR-10):1–36.

Part IV
Systemic Dysfunction

# J. Critical Care Pharmacology

49
Optimization of Drug Doses

Pamela K. Phelps and Bruce C. Lohr
University of Minnesota, Minneapolis, Minnesota, USA

The optimization of drug doses in acutely ill patients is a difficult and multifactorial process. The correct dose is one that exerts a desired therapeutic effect while producing minimal undesirable side effects. Critically ill patients may experience physiologic and pharmacokinetic changes that affect the disposition of medications (e.g., heart failure, renal failure, hepatic failure, trauma, sepsis, and burns). To optimize doses, the critical care practitioner first must evaluate these possible physiologic conditions for their effects on the absorption, distribution, metabolism, and excretion of drugs. Other crucial factors to consider include both the condition being treated and other disease states; drug interactions, tolerance, and penetration to the site of action; other drug therapies; the therapeutic index of the drug; toxic effects; and dose–response relationships. These factors are discussed in this chapter in a general way, and a more specific examination is provided for cardiotonic drugs and agents for treating hypertension, since use of these classes of drugs is prevalent in the SICU setting.

ABSORPTION

Absorption and bioavailability of a drug are dependent on the drug compound, its vehicle of delivery, its "first-pass" metabolism, and the site of absorption. Bioavailability is defined as the amount of drug that reaches the bloodstream when a drug is given by a chosen route, when compared with the amount of the drug reaching the bloodstream when the same drug is given intravenously. Site of absorption depends on route of delivery, which may be oral, rectal, topical, intramuscular (IM), subcutaneous (SC), transdermal, sublingual (SL), or intravenous (IV).

Physiologic changes in a critically ill patient can affect both the first-pass effects and the site of absorption. Drugs absorbed enterically first must be cycled through the portal vein and the liver before reaching the systemic circulation. If a drug is highly metabolized, this enterohepatic cycling results in first-pass metabolism and reduced bioavailability. If a critically ill patient has severe liver disease, first-pass metabolism may be reduced, resulting in *increased* bioavailability of the drug. One author advocates a 50% reduction in dosages of highly metabolized ("high-extraction") drugs such as lidocaine, meperidine, metoprolol, morphine, propranolol, and verapamil in patients with chronic liver disease or cirrhosis (1).

Vasoconstriction and reduced peripheral blood flow in patients with cardiac disease or multisystem organ failure may render the topical, transdermal, IM, or SC routes of administration erratic and ineffective. The presence of ileus or diarrhea may also limit the enteral absorption of drugs given by the oral or rectal route. The presence of enteral feedings can affect the absorption of certain drugs and reduce the bioavailability of phenytoin, for example, by 72% (2). To ensure adequate drug delivery in SICU patients, the IV route is preferred. Exceptions to this rule include drugs not available in an injectable dosage form (e.g., metolazone, spironolactone, captopril, diltiazem, nifedipine), drugs that exert a local effect (nonabsorbable antibiotics, vancomycin solution, nystatin suspension, antacids), drugs whose pharmacodynamic effects are easily measured (transdermal clonidine, antacids, H_2-receptor antagonists), and drugs whose pharmacokinetic changes can be monitored with serum concentrations.

DISTRIBUTION

The volume of distribution (Vd) of a drug is the theoretic volume of serum, tissues, and protein to which a drug is distributed. Vd is expressed in liters or liters per kilogram. For drugs that remain for the most part in the serum, or central compartment, Vd may be quite small. For drugs extensively bound to tissues or serum proteins, Vd may be quite large, reaching 100 times the blood volume in some cases. Vd is used to calculate the effect that an amount of drug administered will have on the serum concentrations according to the following equation:

$$\text{Change in concentration} = \frac{\text{Dose}}{\text{Vd}}$$

Changes in the volume of distribution can occur in critically ill patients as a result of altered tissue binding, increased or decreased protein binding, or changes in body composition that alter distribution compartments of a drug. For instance, altered body fluid composition has been suggested as a mechanism for increased aminoglycoside Vd in critically ill patients (3). Critically ill patients frequently need larger than usual doses of aminoglycosides to achieve desired therapeutic serum concentrations because of larger Vd. Likewise, patients with significant fluid shifts (e.g., burns, ascites) may also require larger doses of drugs that freely distribute into these fluid compartments. Protein-binding changes frequently occur in critically ill patients. Most acidic drug compounds bind to albumin, and protein binding can be reduced or altered as a result of hypoalbuminemia, malnutrition, or renal disease. Basic drugs such as lidocaine bind to alpha-1 acid glycoprotein, and protein binding can increase as a result of release of acute-phase reactants. The end result is an increase or decrease in the amount of free, or unbound, drug available to exert a therapeutic effect. The impact of an increase or decrease in free drug is probably significant only in drugs whose protein binding is 90% or greater, or those with a narrow therapeutic range. The classic examples include phenytoin and warfarin. Phenytoin free concentrations should be monitored if protein-binding changes are suspected. During renal failure, endogenous substances may compete with digoxin for tissue-binding sites, resulting in a 30–50% reduction in Vd.

METABOLISM

Altered metabolism of drugs can occur in critically ill patients as a result of hepatocellular damage or reduced hepatic blood flow. The impact of liver failure on absorption, first-pass metabolism, and protein binding has already been discussed. The point at which altered metabolism of drugs should cause concern is not clear. A reliable indicator of hepatic clearance of drugs is lacking in the clinical setting. High-extraction drugs are those for which the liver has a large metabolic capacity. The rate-limiting step of the metabolism of these drugs is the rate at which the drug is presented to the liver. The metabolism of these drugs, including lidocaine, meperidine, metoprolol, propranolol, and verapamil, is reduced when hepatic blood flow is reduced, or altered, as in a patient with cirrhosis (1). Low-extraction drugs are those for which metabolism is more sensitive to hepatic enzyme capacity and protein binding than to hepatic blood flow. Hepatocellular damage may reduce the metabolism of low-extraction drugs such as ampicillin, chloramphenicol, cimetidine, diazepam, furosemide, prednisone, theophylline, and warfarin. Metabolism of certain benzodiazepines through glucuronidation (e.g., lorazepam and oxazepam) is unaffected by chronic hepatic disease (1). Drugs for which serum concentration monitoring is not routinely available require monitoring for clinical response and signs of toxicity. Drugs of this nature commonly used in the SICU include nitroprusside, fentanyl, midazolam, morphine, calcium channel blockers, meperidine, and beta-blockers. Box 1 lists hepatically cleared drugs commonly used in the SICU that may require dosage reduction in hepatic failure.

EXCRETION

Altered excretion of drugs commonly occurs in critically ill patients. Renal failure can occur as a result of sepsis, shock, or the administration of nephrotoxic drugs such as amphotericin B, aminoglycosides, and contrast agents. The estimation of the glomerular filtration rate (GFR) and the effects of renal insufficiency on the elimination of drugs present a challenge to the clinical practitioner. Judging the degree of renal dysfunction based on a serum creatinine concentration alone could lead to significant dosing errors. In critically ill patients, the serum creatinine concentration is not a reliable indicator of changes in the elimination rate of renally excreted drugs. Fuhs et al. (4) found no correlation between changes in physiologic variables, such as serum creatinine and actual body weight or temperature, and the measured pharmacokinetic parameters of aminoglycosides. Drug dosages frequently are altered on the basis of creatinine clearance, either estimated or measured. The best approximation of creatinine clearance is a 24 h collection of urine for creatinine measurement. Even this method may overestimate actual GFR (5). Creatinine clearance is estimated by the methods of Cockcroft and Gault (6) or Jeliffe (7,8). These equations use body weight, age, and serum creatinine to estimate an individual creatinine clearance.

$$\text{CrCl (mL/min)} = \frac{(140 - \text{age})(\text{Weight in kilograms})}{(72 \times \text{Serum creatinine})}$$

For females, multiply the above equation by 0.85.

$$\text{CrCl (mL/min)} = \frac{114 - (\text{Age} \times 0.8)}{\text{Serum creatinine}}$$

For females, multiply the above equation by 0.9.

The assumption made when using these equations is that the elimination of creatinine is at steady-state. In a patient with rapidly declining renal function, the assumption is false, and the result is an overestimation of creatinine clearance.

Box 1 Drugs That May Require Dose Reduction in Patients with Hepatic Failure

Clindamycin	Procainamide
Chloramphenicol	Disopyramide
Erythromycin	Verapamil
Rifampin	Diazepam
Nafcillin	Midazolam
Lidocaine	Theophylline
Labetalol	Nitroprusside
Metropolol	Fentanyl
Pindolol	Morphine
Prazosin	Meperidine
Propranolol	Dilitazen
Quinidine	Nifedipine

Source: Modified from Williams RL. Drug administration in hepatic disease. N Engl J Med 1983; 309:1616. McEvoy GK, ed. American Hospital Formulary Service Drug Information. Bethesda, MD: American Society of Hospital Pharmacists, 1991.

Once an estimate of creatinine clearance has been obtained, Table 1 can be used for guidance in initiating drug therapy. The drug therapy must be re-evaluated on at least a daily basis for changes in renal function, serum concentration monitoring, evidence of drug efficacy, and signs of toxicity. Initial dosages can then be modified to meet the therapeutic needs of individual patients. Hepatically metabolized drugs can also be affected by renal failure. Meperidine's active metabolite, normeperidine, requires elimination by the kidney. Normeperidine has the ability to cause central nervous system (CNS) excitation. In the presence of compromised renal function or high doses of meperidine, the accumulation of the active metabolite normeperidine has caused seizure (9). Procainamide is metabolized to an active metabolite, *N*-acetylprocainamide (NAPA). Although NAPA shares some of the therapeutic benefits of the parent drug, it also shares the potential toxicities. Renal failure patients typically accumulate NAPA, even when procainamide serum concentrations alone are "therapeutic" (10). Both procainamide and NAPA serum concentrations must be measured to ensure that the total (procainamide plus NAPA) does not exceed 30–35 µg/mL.

USE OF SERUM CONCENTRATIONS

Serum drug concentrations can be useful in guiding drug therapy. They are often used for drugs with a narrow therapeutic index, that is, the drug dose or concentrations producing a desirable effect are very close to, or overlap, the dose or concentration producing an undesirable, or toxic, effect. Serum drug concentrations are also used for drugs for which a proven benefit is observed for a certain peak, trough, or average steady-state concentration. In general, it is desirable to wait until a drug reaches steady-state before obtaining serum drug concentrations. Steady-state indicates that the drug is in equilibrium with the blood and tissue compartments to which it distributes, and it is achieved after approximately five half-lives of a particular drug. Timing of serum drug concentrations is also

Table 1 Dosage Modification of SICU Drugs in Patients with Renal Impairment

Drug	Usual dose	CrCl 30–50 mL/min	CrCl 10–30 mL/min	<10 mL/min
Acyclovir IV	5–10 mg/kg IV q8 h	5–10 mg/kg q12 h	5–10 mg/kg q24 h	2.5–5 mg/kg q24 h
Amphotericin B	0.3–1.5 mg/kg IVQD	Unchanged	Unchanged	Unchanged
Amphotericin B (lipid products)	3–5 mg/kg IV QD	Unchanged	Unchanged	Unchanged
Ampicillin IV	1–2 gm IV q4–6 h	1–2 gm q6–8 h	1–2 gm q8–12 h	1–2 gm q12–24 h
Ampicillin plus sulbactam (Unasyn)	1.5–3 gm IV q6–8 h	Unchanged	1.5–3 gm q12 h	1.5–3 gm q24 h
Atenolol PO	50–100 mg PO QD	Unchanged	50 mg QD	50 mg QOD
Aztreonam	1–2 gm IV q6–8 h	Unchanged	500 mg–1 gm q6–8 h	250–500 mg q6–8 h
Captopril PO	25–50 mg PO bid or tid	Unchanged	Unchanged	12.5–25 mg bid or tid
Cefazolin	1 gm IV q8 h	1 gm q12 h	1 gm q12 h	500 mg–1 gm q24 h
Cefotaxime	1–2 gm IV q6–8 h	Unchanged	1–2 gm q8–12 h	1–2 gm q12–24 h
Cefotetan	1–2 gm IV q12 h	Unchanged	1–2 gm q24 h	1–2 gm q48 h
Cefoxitin	1–2 gm IV q6 h	1–2 gm q8–12 h	1–2 gm q12–24 h	500 mg–1 gm q12–24 h
Ceftazidime	1–2 gm IV q8 h	Unchanged	1–2 gm q12 h	1–2 gm q24 h
Ceftriaxone	1–2 gm IV q24 h	Unchanged	Unchanged	Unchanged
Cefuroxime	750 mg–1.5 gm IV q8 h	Unchanged	750 mg–1.5 gm q12 h	750 mg–1.5 gm q24 h
Cimetidine	300 mg IV/PO q6–8 h	Unchanged	300 mg q12 h	300 mg q12–24 h
Ciprofloxacin PO	500 mg–750 mg PO q12 h	250–500 mg PO q12 h	250–500 mg PO q24 h	250–500 mg q24 h
Ciprofloxacin IV	200–400 mg IV q8–12 h	Unchanged	200–400 mg q 18–24 h	200–400 mg q24 h
Clindamycin	600–900 mg IV q8 h	Unchanged	Unchanged	Unchanged
Clonidine	0.1–0.4 mg PO bid	Unchanged	Unchanged	0.05–0.2 mg PO bid
Corticosteroids	Variable	Unchanged	Unchanged	Unchanged
Digoxin	0.125–0.375 mg IV QD	0.125 mg alternating with 0.25 mg QD	0.125 mg QD	0.125 mg QOD

(Continued)

Table 1 Dosage Modification of SICU Drugs in Patients with Renal Impairment (*Continued*)

			CrCl	
Drug	Usual dose	30–50 mL/min	10–30 mL/min	<10 mL/min
Diltiazem	Variable	Unchanged	Unchanged	Unchanged
Dofetilide PO	500 µg bid	250 µg bid	125 µg bid	Contraindicated if <20 mL/min
Enalapril	2.5–20 mg PO QD or bid	Unchanged	Unchanged	1.25–10 mg QD or bid
Fluconazole	100–400 mg IV/PO QD	100–200 mg QD	50–100 mg QD	50–100 mg qod
Flucytosine PO	37.5 mg/kg PO q6 h	37.5 mg/kg q8–12 h	37.5 mg/kg q12–24 h	37.5 mg/kg q24–48 h
Gabapentin PO	400 mg tid	300 mg bid	300 mg QD	300 mg qod
Ganciclovir IV	5 mg/kg q12 h	2.5 mg/kg q12 h	2.5 mg/kg q24 h	1.25 mg/kg q24 h
Gatifloxacin	400 mg IV/PO QD	400 mg QD	400 mg × 1, then 200 mg QD	400 mg × 1, then 200 mg QD
Gentamicin	1.5–2 mg/kg IV q8 h	1.5–2 mg/kg q12–18 h	1.5 mg/kg q24–48 h	Follow serum concentrations
Haloperidol	1–4 mg IM q4–6 h	Unchanged	Unchanged	Unchanged
Hydralazine	10–100 mg PO qid	Unchanged	Unchanged	10–100 mg q8–24 h
Imipenem/Cilastatin (Primaxin)	500 mg–1 gm IV q6 h	500 mg q6–8 h	500 mg q8–12 h	250–500 mg q12 h
Itraconazole IV	200 mg q12 h × 4 doses, then 200 mg QD	Unchanged	Contraindicated	Contraindicated
Ketorolac IV	30 mg q6 h, if age >65, 15 mg q6 h	15 mg q6 h	Avoid	Avoid
Labetalol	100–200 mg PO q12 h	Unchanged	Unchanged	Unchanged
Levofloxacin	250–500 mg PO/IV q24 h	Give 50% of dose q24 h	Give 25% of dose q24 h	Give 25% of dose q24 h

Optimization of Drug Doses

Linezolid	600 mg PO/IV q12 h	Unchanged	Unchanged	Unchanged, give supplemental 200 mg after dialysis
Meperidine injection	Variable	Give 50% of dose	Avoid due to toxic metabolites/seizures	Avoid due to toxic metabolites/seizures
Meropenem (Merrem IV)	1 gm IV q8 h	1 gm q12 h	500 mg q12 h	500 mg q24 h
Metformin	500–1000 mg PO bid	Avoid due to lactic acidosis	Contraindicated	Contraindicated
Metoprolol PO	50–100 mg PO bid	Unchanged	Unchanged	Unchanged
Metoprolol IV	2.5–7.5 mg IV q6 h	Unchanged	Unchanged	Unchanged
Metronidazole	500 mg IV/PO q6 h	Unchanged	Unchanged	500 mg IV/PO q8 h
Nafcillin IV	1–2 gm IV q4–6 h	Unchanged	Unchanged	Unchanged
Nifedipine	30–60 mg SR QD or bid	Unchanged	Unchanged	Unchanged
Penicillin G IV	Variable q2–8 h	Q4–8 h	Q6–8 h	Q12 h
Pentamidine IV	3–4 mg/kg IV? q12 h	Unchanged	Unchanged	Q48 h
Piperacillin IV	2–4 gm IV q4–6 h	2–4 gm q8 h	2–4 gm q12 h	2–4 gm q12 h
Piperacillin/ Tazobactam (Zosyn)	3.375–4.5 gm IV q6 h	2.25 gm q6 h	2.25 gm q8 h	2.25 gm q8 h
Procainamide PO	250 mg–1 gm PO q4–6 h	750 mg–1 gm q6 h	375–500 mg q6 h	375 mg q8 h
Procainamide IV	2–3 mg/min infusion	2 mg/min infusion	1 mg/min infusion	0.5 mg/min infusion
Quinupristin/ Dalfopristin (Synercid)	7.5 mg/kg IV q8 h	Unchanged	Unchanged	Unchanged
Ranitidine IV	50 mg IV q6–8 h	Unchanged	50 mg q12 h	50 mg q12–24 h
Rifampin PO	600 mg PO QD	Unchanged	Unchanged	Unchanged
Sotalol PO	80 mg PO q12 h	80 mg PO q24 h	80 mg PO q48 h	Per response

(Continued)

Table 1 Dosage Modification of SICU Drugs in Patients with Renal Impairment (*Continued*)

Drug	Usual dose	CrCl 30–50 mL/min	CrCl 10–30 mL/min	CrCl <10 mL/min
Ticarcillin	3–4 gm IV q4–6 h	2 gm q4 h	2 gm q8 h	2 gm q12 h
Ticarcillin/ Clavulanate	3.1 gm IV q4–6 h	3.1 gm q6–8 h	2 gm q8 h	2 gm q12 h
Tobramycin IV	1.5–2 mg/kg IV q8 h	1.5–2 mg/kg q12–18 h	1.5–2 mg/kg q24–48 h	Follow serum concentrations
Trimethoprim/ Sulfamethoxazole	2–7.5 mg/kg (TMP) IV q6–12 h (Bactrim)	Unchanged	2–7.5 mg/kg q12 h	1–7.5 mg/kg q24 h
Valacyclovir PO	1 gm PO q8 h	1 gm q12 h	1 gm q24 h	0.5 gm q24 h
Vancomycin	15 mg/kg IV q12 h	15 mg/kg q24–48 h	15 mg/kg q2–7 days follow concentrations	15 mg/kg q7–10 days follow concentrations
Verapamil	80–120 mg PO tid or 120–240 mg SR PO QD or bid	Unchanged	Unchanged	Reduce dose 50–75%
Voriconazole	6 mg/kg IV q12 h for two doses, then 4 mg/kg q12 h. When PO, switch to 200 mg PO q12 h	Unchanged	Avoid due to accumulation of drug vehicle	Avoid due to accumulation of drug vehicle
Warfarin	1–10 mg PO QD	Unchanged	Unchanged	Unchanged

important. Drug concentrations are usually either at a peak (immediately after a dose) or at a trough (immediately before a dose). For drugs given by a continuous infusion, blood used to determine serum drug concentrations can be drawn at any time once steady-state is achieved. Exceptions to these rules include drugs, such as digoxin, that take a long time to distribute to tissues. Digoxin concentrations should be drawn at least 6 h after a dose is given to allow for distribution of the drug. Consideration must be given to the timing of a sample when evaluating serum drug concentrations. If a desired peak concentration is based on a trough measurement, gross dosing errors would occur.

A serum drug concentration is evaluated on the basis of a desirable therapeutic range. Patient response should be evaluated in conjunction with the serum drug concentration. The clinician should use the lowest dose and concentration that will produce the desirable patient response. Table 2 provides recommendations for serum concentration monitoring of drugs used frequently in SICU.

The clinical practitioner must constantly re-evaluate the risks and benefits of a drug therapy regimen, especially with drugs exhibiting a narrow therapeutic index. As stated previously, the first step is the evaluation of physiologic processes in a patient having pharmacokinetic disposition of a drug. Box 2 provides a useful summary of pharmacokinetic relations (Fig. 1). Although the drug-dosing tables provided give initial guidelines and considerations for acutely ill patients, the therapeutic and toxic effects, serum concentrations, and patient response must be monitored continually to guide further dosage modifications. Because of their frequent use by SICU patients, certain classes of drugs warrant special consideration. Helpful dosing guidelines for neuromuscular blocking agents and narcotic analgesic agents are listed in Tables 3 and 4.

Box 2 Pharmacokinetic Relations

Volume of distribution	*Half-life*
Vd = Amount of drug in body/C	$T_{1/2} = 0.693/\lambda_z$
where	where
Vd = Volume of distribution (vol/kg)	λ_z (Fig. 1)
C = Concentration of drug (mass/vol)	$T_{1/2} \sim 0.693 \, Vd/CL$
Clearance	*Loading dose*
CL = Rate of elimination,	Loading dose = $Vd \times C_p/S \times F$
where	where
CL = Clearance	C_p = Desired plasma concentration
Concentration	S = Fraction of drug that is active
C = Rate of elimination/CL	F = Bioavailability
$C = (Dose/Vd)e^{-kt}$	*Maintenance dose*
where	Maintenance dose = $CL \times C_p \times \tau/S \times F$
C = Concentration of drug	where
k = Rate constant for elimination	τ = Dosing interval
Rate constant for elimination	
$k = 0.693/T_{1/2}$	
where	
$T_{1/2}$ = Half-life of drug	

Source: Modified from Benet LZ, Massoud N. Pharmacokinetics. In: Benet LZ, Massoud N, Gambertoglio JG, eds. Pharmacokinetic Basis for Drug Treatment. New York: Raven Press, 1984:1–28.

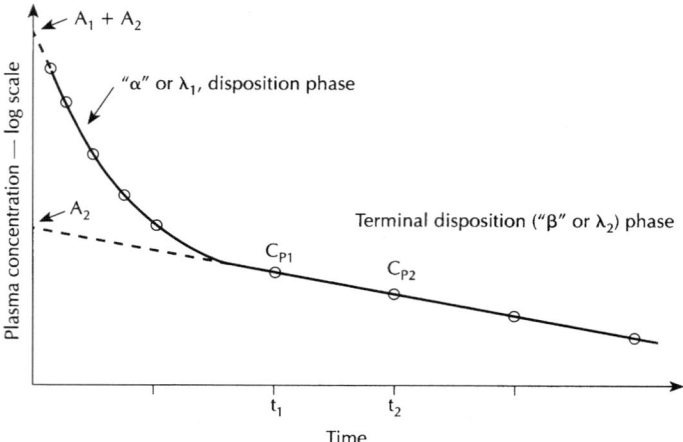

Figure 1 $\lambda_z = \ln(C_{P1}/C_{P2})/t_2 - t_1$. This equation allows one to calculate the elimination rate of a drug, given two serum concentrations drawn at two different times, or once the elimination rate is known, a future concentration can be calculated on the basis of a given concentration at time (t_1). *Source*: From Benet LZ, Massoud N. Pharmacokinetics. In: Benet LZ, Massoud N, Gambertoglio JG, eds. Pharmacokinetic Basis for Drug Treatment. New York: Raven Press, 1984:1–28.

Inotropic/Vasoactive Agents

Drugs with positive inotropic and/or vasoactive effects are frequently used in SICU for management of shock states. Positive inotropic agents increase the force of myocardial contraction and improve blood flow to vital areas such as the CNS, liver, heart, and kidneys. Vasoactive agents are used for their vasoconstrictive or vasodilatory effects on the blood vessels.

Inotropic Agents

A number of parenteral positive inotropes are available. Currently, no potent oral inotrope is available. Dobutamine, dopamine, and milrinone are considered first-line inotropes. Epinephrine is considered a second-line inotropic agent and is used primarily in pediatric patients. The older agents, norepinephrine and isoproterenol, should no longer be used as inotropes, because better agents are available. Table 5 summarizes the cardiac and vascular effects of these agents.

Dopamine: Dopamine is an endogenous catecholamine with activity on several different receptor types. Its hemodynamic effects are dose-dependent. It acts both directly as a beta-1 receptor agonist to increase cardiac contractility and heart rate and indirectly to release norepinephrine from storage sites in sympathetic nerve endings. A unique effect of dopamine is its activity on postsynaptic dopamine-1 and dopamine-2 receptors of the kidney. This property results in increases in GFR, renal blood flow, and sodium excretion. Dopamine also stimulates alpha-1 and alpha-2 receptors to produce vasoconstriction in arterial and venous vascular beds. Vasoconstriction generally affects blood vessels in skeletal muscle, mesentery, and kidneys. Dopamine has little or no action on beta-2 receptors. Dopamine produces markedly different pharmacologic effects as a result of the infusion rate, the receptor types activated, and the variability of patient response.

Table 2 Guidelines for Serum Concentration Monitoring

Drug	Primary route of elimination	Half-life (h)	Sampling time	Therapeutic range	Toxicity and comments
Amikacin	Renal	1.5–3	Peak Trough	15–30 µg/mL <10 µg/mL	Nephrotoxicity, ototoxicity
Carbamazepine	Hepatic	10–25	Trough	4–12 µg/mL	Induces own metabolism, dose escalation necessary
Chloramphenicol	Hepatic	2–4	PO: 2–3 h after dose IV: 1–2 h after dose	10–25 µg/mL	Peaks greater than 25 µg/mL associated with bone marrow depression, anemia
Cyclosporine	Hepatic	12–24	Trough	50–150 ng/mL	Hypertension, nephrotoxicity, many drug interactions
Digoxin	Renal	36–44	Trough (or at least 6 h after dose)	0.5–2 ng/mL	Dysrhythmias, CNS toxicity, hypokalemia predisposes to toxicity
Disopyramide	Hepatic, renal	5–8	Trough	2–4 µg/mL	Nausea, drowsiness, dizziness
Ethosuximide	Hepatic	60 (adult) 30 (children)	Trough	40–80 µg/mL	
Flucytosine	Renal	3–6	2 h after dose	50–100 µg/mL	Bone marrow depression at concentrations >100 µg/mL
Gentamicin	Renal	1.5–3	Peak Trough	4–10 µg/mL <2 µg/mL	Nephrotoxicity, ototoxicity
Lidocaine	Hepatic	1.2–2.2	Steady-state 5–10 h	2–5 µg/mL	Metabolite accumulation in renal disease; half-life prolonged after first 24 h of therapy (dose reduction necessary)

(Continued)

Table 2 Guidelines for Serum Concentration Monitoring (*Continued*)

Drug	Primary route of elimination	Half-life (h)	Sampling time	Therapeutic range	Toxicity and comments
N-Acetyl procainamide (NAPA)	Renal	6–8	Same as procainamide	15–25 μg/mL	Procainamide and NAPA concentrations should not exceed 35 μg/mL
Procainamide	Hepatic, renal	2.5–4.9	PO: Trough IV: at steady-state	4–10 μg/mL	Accumulation of NAPA in renal failure
Phenobarbital	Hepatic	48	Peak or trough	20–40 μg/mL	Ataxia, nystagmus, drowsiness
Phenytoin	Hepatic	24	Trough	Total: 10–20 μg/mL Free: 1–2 μg/mL	Measure free concentrations in patients with renal failure and hypoalbuminemia
Quinidine	Hepatic	5–7.2	Trough	2–5 μg/mL	Cinchonism at high concentrations
Sirolimus	Hepatic	60	Trough	10 ng/mL	CSA-like drug interactions
Tacrolimus	Hepatic	8–12 h	Trough	5–20 ng/mL	CSA-like drug interactions
Theophylline	Hepatic	3–12	PO: 1–2 h after dose IV: at steady-state	10–20 μg/mL	Dysrhythmias, convulsions at concentrations exceeding 35 μg/mL
Tobramycin	Renal	1.5–3 h	Peak Trough	4–10 μg/mL <2 μg/mL	Nephrotoxicity, ototoxicity
Valproic acid	Hepatic	8–17	2–4 h after dose	50–100 μg/mL	Tremor, irritability at concentrations >100 μg/mL

Table 3 Neuromuscular Blocking Agents

	Pancuronium	Vecuronium	Atracurium	Cisatracurium	Rocuronium
Type	Nondepolarizing	Nondepolarizing	Nondepolarizing	Nondepolarizing	Nondepolarizing
Loading dose	0.03–0.1 mg/kg	0.08–0.1 mg/kg	0.3–0.5 mg/kg	0.15–0.2 mg/kg	450–600 μg/kg
Continuous infusion	0.3–0.6 μg/kg per min	1.25 μg/kg per min	2–9 μg/kg per min	1–3 μg/kg per min	—
Half-life	4 h	1 h	20 min	22–31 min	1–3 h
Duration of action	30–40 min (12–24 h with continuous infusion)	20–25 min	20–25 min	30–45 min	30 min
Elimination	Renal	Hepatic (25% renal)	Enzymatic	Enzymatic	Biliary excretion
Cardiovascular effects	Tachycardia, increased blood pressure, increased pulmonary vascular resistance	None	Slight	None	No hemodynamic effects, <1% arrhythmias, tachycardia
Special considerations	Prolonged effect in renal insufficiency	Prolonged effect in hepatic failure	May be used in renal or hepatic failure. Metabolite laudanosine may accumulate in hepatic insufficiency and cause seizures	Half-life prolonged in chronic renal failure. Metabolite laudanosine may accumulate in hepatic insufficiency and cause seizures	No routine dose adjustment in renal or hepatic failure. Monitor response in hepatic failure
	Reversal with atropine, neostigmine, edrophonium, pyridostigmine	Reversal with atropine, neostigmine, edrophonium, pyridostigmine	Reversal with atropine, neostigmine, edrophonium, pyridostigmine	Reversal with atropine, neostigmine, edrophonium, pyridostigmine	Reversal with atropine, neostigmine, edrophonium, pyridostigmine

(Continued)

Table 3 Neuromuscular Blocking Agents (*Continued*)

Pancuronium	Vecuronium	Atracurium	Cisatracurium	Rocuronium
Potentiated by local anesthetics, quinidine, propranolol, aminoglycosides, tetracyclines, steroids, calcium blockers, procainamide, vancomycin, lithium, magnesium	Potentiated by local anesthetics, quinidine, propranolol, aminoglycosides, tetracyclines, steroids, calcium blockers, procainamide, vancomycin, lithium, magnesium	Potentiated by local anesthetics, quinidine, propranolol, aminoglycosides, tetracyclines, steroids, calcium blockers, procainamide, vancomycin, lithium, magnesium	Potentiated by local anesthetics, quinidine, propranolol, aminoglycosides, tetracyclines, steroids, calcium blockers, procainamide, vancomycin, lithium, magnesium	Potentiated by local anesthetics, quinidine, propranolol, aminoglycosides, tetracyclines, steroids, calcium blockers, procainamide, vancomycin, lithium, magnesium

Table 4 Narcotic Analgesic Agents

	Morphine	Hydromorphone	Fentanyl	Buprenorphine	Nalbuphine	Meperidine
Class	Opiate agonist	Opiate agonist	Opiate agonist	Partial antagonist and agonist	Partial antagonist and agonist	Opiate agonist
Dosage	2–5 mg IV q2–4 h Infusion: Load 0.1 mg/kg followed by 0.05–0.3 mg/kg per h	0.3–0.5 mg IV slowly; may repeat q20 min to a max dose of 1.5 mg in 60 min	25–50 μg IV over 2–3 min; may repeat q5–10 min to a max dose of 200 μg in 60 min	0.3–0.6 mg IV or IM q4–6 h	10–20 mg IM or IV q3–6 h	10–30 mg IV slowly (may repeat q10 min to a max of 100 mg in 60 min)
Duration of effect	2–6 h	4–5 h	30–60 min	6–8 h	3–6 h	2–4 h
Half-life	2–4 h	1.8–3.5 h	1–6 h	3 h	5 h	3–6 h
Elimination	Hepatic	Hepatic	Hepatic	Hepatic	Hepatic	Hepatic
Equivalent dosages	10 mg IV	1.5 mg IV	100 μg IV	0.3 mg IV	10 mg IV	75 mg IV

(*Continued*)

Table 4 Narcotic Analgestic Agents (Continued)

	Morphine	Hydromorphone	Fentanyl	Buprenorphine	Nalbuphine	Meperidine
Side effects	Respiratory depression, bradycardia, hypotension, sedation, cough suppression, decreases gut motility, potentiation of CV respiratory effects of other sedatives and analgesics, increased tone of anal and biliary sphincters, urinary retention, nausea, vomiting	Same as morphine, less nausea, constipation, and euphoria	Same as morphine, less nausea and vomiting	Sedation, dizziness, headache, nausea, vomiting, hypotension, respiratory depression, hypoventilation, miosis, diaphoresis	Sedation, dizziness, vertigo, miosis, headache, nausea, vomiting, dry mouth, CV effects, respiratory depression	Same as morphine. Use with caution in SVT, acute MI. Anticholinergic effects
Considerations	Metabolite can accumulate in renal failure, causing prolonged sedation		Highly lipophilic, accumulates with prolonged use; skeletal and thoracic muscle rigidity and hypotension can be caused by rapid infusions; available as transdermal delivery system	Can produce withdrawal in opioid-dependent patients; large doses of naloxone required for reversal	Can produce withdrawal in opioid-dependent patients	Accumulation of normeperidine metabolite may lead to CNS excitation (tremors, myoclonus, seizures)

Table 5 Relative Cardiac and Vascular Effects of Positive Intrope/Vasoactive Drugs

Drug and usual IV dose	Relative receptor activity effects					Hemodynamic effects					Remarks
	Beta-1 (inotropic)	Beta-1 (chronotropic)	Alpha-1 (vasoconstriction)	Beta-2 (vasodilation)	Dopaminergic (vasodilation)	CO	SVR	MAP	PCWP	HR	
Dopamine (Intropin) low dose: 0.5–2 µg/kg per min	0/+	0/+	0	0/+	+++	0	−	−	0	0	May induce or exacerbate supra ventricular dysrhythmias; extravasation may produce tissue necrosis similar to that of norepinephrine
Dopamine medium dose: 3–9 µg/kg per min	+++	+	+	0/+	+	+	−	+	+	+	
Dopamine high dose: >9 µg/kg per min	+++	++	+++	0	0	+	+	+	+	+	
Dobutamine (Dobutrex): 2–25 µg/kg per min	+++	+	+	+	0	+	−	0/+	−	0/+	Ventricular dysrhythmias and increased HR may occur but less likely than with other catecholamines

(Continued)

Table 5 Relative Cardiac and Vascular Effects of Positive Intrope/Vasoactive Drugs (*Continued*)

Drug and usual IV dose	Relative receptor activity effects					Hemodynamic effects					Remarks
	Beta-1 (inotropic)	Beta-1 (chronotropic)	Alpha-1 (vasoconstriction)	Beta-2 (vasodilation)	Dopaminergic (vasodilation)	CO	SVR	MAP	PCWP	HR	
Milrinone (Primacor) 50 µg/kg load over 10 min, then 0.25–0.75 µg/kg per min	0	0	0	0	0	+	−	0/+	−	0/+	May give load over longer period (20 min) to avoid hypotension
Epinephrine (Adrenaline) low dose: 0.01–0.06 µg/kg per min	+++	++	+	++	0	+	−	−/+	0/−	+	May induce or exacerbate ventricular ectopy, especially in patients receiving digoxin
Epinephrine high dose: >0.06 µg/kg per min	+++	+++	+++	0/+	0	+	+	+	+	+	
Norepinephrine (Levophed) 0.03–0.2 µg/kg per min	++	++	+++	0	0	−/+	+	+	+	−/+	Administer into a central vein; avoid extravasation; if it occurs, infiltrate area with 5–10 mg of phentolamine diluted in 10 mL normal saline

Optimization of Drug Doses

Drug							
Vasopressin 1–10 units/h	0	0	0	0/−	+	0	Works on vasopressin-1 receptor. Has no inotropic effects
Phenylephrine (Neosynephrine) 0.5–3 µg/kg per min	0	0	+++	0/−	+	0/−	Pure alpha agonist
Isoproterenol (Isuprel) 0.01–0.1 µg/kg per min	+++	+++	0	+++	0	+	−	0/−	−	+	Should not be used as an inotrope. Avoid use in patients with ischemic heart disease; may exacerbate tachyarrhythmias from digoxin toxicity or hypokalemia

Receptor effects: +++, pronounced effect; ++, moderate effect; +, slight effect; 0, no effect. Hemodynamic effects: +, increase; −, decrease; 0, no change.

Abbreviations: CO, cardiac output; SVR, systemic vascular resistance; MAP, mean arterial pressure; PCWP, pulmonary capillary wedge pressure; HR, heart rate.

Precautions: Because of its potent alpha vasoconstrictor effects, dopamine should be administered through a central-line if possible, or through a large vein (antecubital or femoral). In the event of dopamine extravasation, phentolamine, an alpha-1 antagonist, should be infiltrated subcutaneously throughout the ischemic area. Other adverse effects associated with dopamine infusion include tachyarrhythmias, myocardial ischemia, increased pulmonary capillary wedge pressure (PCWP), pulmonary shunting, and impaired gastric motility.

Dosing: Low-infusion rates of dopamine (0.5–2 μg/kg per min) selectively act upon dopamine-1 and dopamine-2 receptors to cause dilation of the mesenteric and renal vasculature and an increase in urine output. This effect has led to the traditional use of "low-dose" or "renal-dose" dopamine to protect the kidney from nephrotoxins (e.g., contrast dye, vasopressors) or to treat acute renal failure. However, human studies have failed to confirm a consistent, substantial, and reproducible benefit of dopamine in preventing or treating acute renal failure.

In the medium dose range (∼3–8 μg/kg per min), beta-1 adrenergic stimulation is obtained in addition to the dopaminergic stimulation. This infusion range is used for treatment of heart failure. Cardiac output (CO) increases and further improvement in renal blood flow generally occurs. Systemic vascular resistance (SVR) decreases but PCWP usually does not change. Heart rate may increase, decrease, or remain unchanged. The variability seen in populations of patients is a consequence of an individual patient sensitivity to beta-1 chronotropic stimulation. Dopamine is commonly used in conjunction with vasodilators such as nitroprusside or nitroglycerin. The vasodilator enhances the hemodynamic effects of dopamine by reducing preload and afterload.

As doses of dopamine are increased beyond 8 μg/kg per min, the alpha-1 and alpha-2 receptors are recruited, in addition to the beta-1 effects. Stimulation of these receptors causes vasoconstriction and increases SVR and blood pressure. The range of doses for increasing blood pressure can be extremely variable. Rates of up to 50 μg/kg per min rarely have been used in patients with shock. Preload deficit must be corrected before starting dopamine in order to prevent excessive vasoconstriction necrosis and gangrene. Given the large doses required and the development of tachycardia and tachydysrhythmias, the routine use of dopamine as the initial vasopressor of choice in septic shock patients is being debated. Current studies have supported the early use of norepinephrine in supporting septic shock patients.

Summary: Dopamine, an agent with unique dose-related pharmacologic effects, remains one of the most commonly used agents for inotropic and hemodynamic support. Effects on heart rate are less pronounced than those of epinephrine, but are more common when compared with dobutamine and milrinone (11–15).

Dobutamine: Dobutamine mediates its effects by stimulation of beta-1, beta-2, and alpha receptors. Dobutamine does not cause release of endogenous norephinephrine as dopamine does.

The predominant effects of dobutamine are an increase in myocardial contractility, stroke volume, and CO without significant increases in heart rate and blood pressure. Because of competing peripheral alpha and beta-2 stimulation, pulmonary vascular resistance is also reduced. At doses of 5–15 μg/kg per min, dobutamine increases CO by 45–55%. Dobutamine increases myocardial oxygen consumption, while simultaneously increasing myocardial oxygen delivery. This augmented myocardial oxygen delivery arises from increased coronary blood flow as a result of decreased coronary vascular resistance.

Precautions: Use of dobutamine is contraindicated in patients with idiopathic hypertrophic cardiomyopathies. Dobutamine should be used with caution in patients with severe dysrhythmias because it can induce or exacerbate these conditions.

Dosing: Dobutamine is administered as a continuous IV infusion with a volumetric infusion pump. Unlike dopamine, dobutamine may be administered through a peripheral IV line. The starting dose is 3–5 µg/kg per min. The usual range is 3–20 µg/kg per min. Doses of 40 µg/kg per min or higher have been reported.

Summary: Dobutamine is a very effective inotropic agent that directly increases CO, decreases left ventricular filling pressure, and indirectly decreases SVR without significantly increasing heart rate or dysrhythmogenicity. The drug is useful in treating patients with acute ventricular dysfunction from myocardial infarction, ischemia, pulmonary embolism, sepsis, and chronic congestive heart failure (CHF) (11–13).

Milrinone: Unlike the other positive inotropic agents, milrinone's activity is not related to sympathomimetic stimulation. Milrinone is a phosphodiesterase III inhibitor that prevents the breakdown of cyclic adenosine monophosphate (c-AMP). The resultant increased levels of cellular c-AMP modulate intracellular calcium, causing enhanced myocardial contractility. In vascular smooth muscle, increased levels of c-AMP cause vasodilation with a resultant reduction in SVR, mean arterial pressure (MAP), and PCWP. Milrinone also improves diastolic function by increasing left ventricular diastolic relaxation. Milrinone mediated increases in CO usually are associated with unaltered or decreased myocardial oxygen consumption. The unique pharmacologic properties of positive inotropy and potent vasodilation have led milrinone to be termed an "inodilator." The primary role of milrinone has been in CHF. Milrinone has no benefit in distributive shock when compared with the catecholamine-type agents. By virtue of its potent vasodilation effect, milrinone may result in clinically significant hypotension.

Precautions: As is true with other inotropic agents, milrinone may worsen hemodynamics in patients with hypertrophic obstructive cardiomyopathy. Enhanced atrioventricular nodal conduction may lead to an increased ventricular response rate in patients with supraventricular tachyarrhythmias. Renal impairment significantly increases the terminal elimination of milrinone. Reduction in infusion rate may be necessary.

Dosing: The manufacturer recommends a loading dose of 50 µg/kg over 10 min to hasten the drug's onset of activity. However, to minimize the potential for severe hypotension, the loading dose can be given over a longer period of ~20 min. The maintenance dose ranges from 0.25 to 0.75 µg/kg per min. Administration is via an infusion pump. Hypotension increases with higher doses of the drug.

Summary: Milrinone is an effective alternative or adjunct to other inotropes in the treatment of severe CHF. The drug increases CO and reduces preload, afterload, and pulmonary vascular resistance. Tachyphylaxis does not occur short term with milrinone and the drug is minimally dysrhythmogenic (11–13).

Epinephrine: Epinephrine, a naturally occurring catecholamine, is used as an adjunct to dopamine or dobutamine for improvement of myocardial contractility. In the lower dosage range of 0.015–0.06 µg/kg per min or 1–4 µg/min, epinephrine acts on beta-1 and beta-2 receptors to increase CO, to increase heart rate, and to lower SVR. In the dosage range >0.06 µg/kg per min or 4 µg/min, the alpha-vasoconstrictive effects predominate and tachycardia can occur. Epinephrine is not used as a first-line inotrope because of the availability of dobutamine, dopamine, and milrinone, all of which have fewer chronotropic and vasoconstrictor effects.

Summary: Epinephrine is a useful second-line chronotrope/inotrope and vasopressor (11–13).

Isoproterenol: The pure beta-1 and beta-2 agonist isoproterenol has positive inotropic and chronotropic effects. It also has pulmonary and peripheral vasodilating properties. Its usefulness as an inotrope has been surpassed by the newer agents, which are less prone to increase heart rate, to increase myocardial oxygen consumption, and to cause ventricular dysrhythmias. Isoproterenol is currently used for its chronotropic effects in certain clinical situations, including atropine-refractory bradycardia. Dopamine and epinephrine should be tried as chronotropes before isoproterenol. In cardiac transplant patients, isoproterenol can stimulate the denervated heart and increase heart rate.

Precautions: Isoproterenol should not be used in cardiac arrest. Negative effects of isoproterenol include an increase in myocardial oxygen consumption and peripheral vasodilation.

Dosing: Isoproterenol is administered as a continuous IV infusion using an infusion pump, starting at a dose of 2 μg/min and titrating to the desired heart rate.

Summary: Isoproterenol is seldom used in the intensive care unit (ICU). It may be used as a second-line chronotrope after dopamine and epinephrine (11–13).

Vasopressors

Norepinephrine: Outcomes from retrospective and prospective studies using norepinephrine in patients with septic shock for hemodynamic support have shown a higher rate of achieving predetermined resuscitation end points and/or significant reduction in mortality compared with patients receiving dopamine and epinephrine. Norepinephrine should be considered a first-line vasopressor of choice in patients with distributive shock early in treatment as a consequence of its benefits on oxygen transport, regional blood flow, and vital organ perfusion pressure.

Precautions: Norepinephrine should be administered through a central-line to minimize extravasation and tissue injury. Infiltrated infusions of the drug may produce local skin necrosis and ulceration. Extravasation should be treated with local phentolamine (alpha-1 blocker) injection if recognized early. Careful monitoring of blood pressure, perfusion, and renal function is necessary to prevent organ ischemia and excessive increases in ventricular afterload.

Dosing: The usual starting IV infusion rate for norepinephrine is 0.03–0.06 μg/kg per min. The infusion is titrated to the desired blood pressure. In septic adults, high-infusion rates (up to 1.5 μg/kg per min) have been used.

Summary: Norepinephrine is a potent vasoconstrictor and should be considered a first-line vasopressor in septic shock patients (11–13).

Vasopressin: An old drug that has recently become significant in the management of septic shock is arginine vasopressin or antidiuretic hormone. Under normal physiologic conditions, vasopressin has no vasopressor effects. In the setting of hypotensive septic shock, vasopressin is one of the most potent vasopressors known. During shock states, serum concentrations of endogenous vasopressin are inappropriately low. Vasopressin binds to vascular vasopressin type 1 receptors and results in profound vasoconstriction. Several prospective studies have demonstrated a beneficial effect of vasopressin in restoring MAP in severely septic patients that were already receiving high doses of exogenous catecholamines. Vasopressin may also potentiate the pressor effects of catecholamines. Although not reported in clinical studies, the use of vasopressin may cause deleterious vasoconstriction of the renal, mesenteric, pulmonary, and coronary vasculature with resultant organ failure.

Precautions: Vasopressin should be infused via a central-line to avoid tissue damage from vasoconstriction and/or extravasation.

Dosing: Vasopressin is administered as a continuous IV infusion using a volumetric infusion pump. For treatment of hypotension associated with septic shock, the initial infusion rate is 1–4 units/h. An initial IV bolus dose of 2–4 units may be administered if a faster onset of activity is desired. The maintenance infusion can be titrated upward by 1–2 units per hour every 15 min until the desired blood pressure is achieved.

Summary: Vasopressin is an effective vasopressor useful in supporting blood pressure in patients with distributive shock who do not adequately respond to norepinephrine. Combinations of norepinephrine and vasopressin have been used (11–13,16,17).

Phenylephrine: Phenylephrine is a sympathomimetic agent with activity on alpha-1 receptors and no activity on beta receptors. Its use as a pressor agent in patients with shock syndromes is supported by a scant number of published studies. Phenylephrine produced a dose-related increase in MAP and SVR. In volume-resuscitated, hyperdynamic septic shock patients, phenylephrine did not impair CO or PCWP. Heart rate is usually unaffected or mildly decreased. Phenylephrine may have a role as a second-line vasopressor, after norepinephrine and vasopressin, in managing patients with distributive or hypovolemic shock after fluid resuscitation. It may be clinically advantageous in patients who develop tachycardia or clinical evidence of receptor desensitization with other catecholamines.

Precautions: As with norepinephrine, phenylephrine should be infused through a central-line to minimize the risk of extravasation and tissue injury. Phentolamine is an effective treatment of extravasation if recognized early. Phenylephrine should be used with caution, if at all, in patients with cardiogenic or obstructive shock.

Dosing: The usual starting IV infusion rate for phenylephrine is 0.5 μg/kg per min and titrated to blood pressure response. Doses as high as 3 μg/kg per min have been used.

Summary: Phenylephrine is a second-line vasopressor that may be useful when tachycardia is to be avoided (11–13).

Combination Therapy

There are many situations in clinical practice in which it is advantageous to use two or more inotropic/vasoactive agents concurrently. For instance, the combination of dopamine and dobutamine can be used in the setting of septic shock or cardiogenic shock. High-dose dopamine is used to support blood pressure via alpha vasoconstriction and dobutamine is used to increase CO via beta-1 agonist effects. Milrinone and dobutamine, which act through different pharmacologic mechanisms, can be used together to obtain a greater inotropic response that may be achieved with either of the agents alone. A combination of norepinephrine and vasopressin may be advantageous in a distributive shock patient in whom it is desirable to increase mean arterial pressure when the response to norepinephrine alone is not satisfactory. Inotropic agents may be combined with the vasodilators nitroprusside and nitroglycerin to obtain desired hemodynamic effects. In the management of CHF patients, dopamine in inotropic doses is commonly combined with nitroprusside to reduce systemic vascular resistance.

Antihypertensive Agents

The ideal drug for treating hypertension should have a rapid onset, a short elimination half-life in case of side effects, and a response that is titratable. Choice of agent requires a careful assessment of each patient's medical condition, the urgency of lowering blood pressure, and the hemodynamic and pharmacologic effects that may be troublesome for the patient. Tables 6 and 7 compare the pharmacodynamics of parenteral and oral antihypertensive agents, respectively.

Nitroprusside

Nitroprusside causes direct relaxation of arterial and venous smooth muscle. It is the classic balanced vasodilator with the capability to lower both pulmonary venous and systemic venous pressures and to increase stroke volume and CO in severe heart failure patients. Nitroprusside possesses characteristics that make it the vasodilator of choice in the critical care unit. Its onset of action is within seconds and its duration of action is 3–5 min.

Precautions: Hypotension is the major complication of nitroprusside therapy. The other major side effects are thiocyanate/cyanide toxicity and mild reductions in arterial oxygen tension as a result of inhibition of the pulmonary vasoconstrictor response. Nitroprusside is metabolized by red blood cells to hydrocyanic acid, which is further metabolized by the liver to thiocyanate and excreted by the kidneys. Both cyanide and thiocyanate have the potential for accumulating and causing toxicity under certain circumstances. In the presence of renal failure, thiocyanate can accumulate and cause toxic symptoms such as mental status changes, nausea, abdominal pain, tinnitus, hyperreflexia, and seizures. Thiocyanate toxicity is rare when infusion rates are kept below 3 μg/kg per min for periods of 72 h or less. Measurement of the serum thiocyanate concentration is advisable when high or prolonged dosage regimens are used or renal failure is present. Thiocyanate serum concentrations below 10 mg/dL indicate that continued use of nitroprusside is usually safe. Thiocyanate concentrations do not reflect cyanide toxicity. Toxic levels of thiocyanate can be managed by stopping the nitroprusside infusion, switching to a different antihypertensive agent, and using hemodialysis for removing thiocyanate.

Cyanide toxicity is a rare complication from nitroprusside that is potentially fatal. It occurs in patients with severe hepatic dysfunction, in sulfur-depleted patients, or in patients with excessive doses of nitroprusside. Signs of early cyanide toxicity include metabolic acidosis and increasing tolerance to the drug. Toxicity is associated with dyspnea, headache, vomiting, dizziness, and loss of consciousness. Other signs of cyanide poisoning are coma, imperceptible pulse, absent reflexes, widely dilated pupils, and a pink color. Oxygen therapy alone will not reverse the poisoning. If cyanide toxicity is suspected, the nitroprusside infusion is discontinued, a blood sample is obtained for determination of cyanide level, and treatment is instituted. Treatment consists of administering amyl nitrate inhalations for 15–30 s each minute until a 3% sodium nitrite solution can be prepared for IV administration. This solution is injected at a rate not exceeding 2.5–5 mL/min up to a total dose of 10–15 mL. Blood pressure is monitored for hypotension. Then sodium thiosulfate (12.5 g in 50 mL of 5% dextrose in water, infused IV over 10 min) is administered and the patient is observed for several hours. If signs of cyanide toxicity reappear, sodium nitrite and sodium thiosulfate injections are repeated using one half of the previous doses. Most hospital pharmacies have adopted the practice of adding sodium thiosulfate to the bag of nitroprusside at a ratio of 10:1 to protect against cyanide toxicity. Doses of nitroprusside should not exceed 8 μg/kg per min even in the presence of the antidote, sodium thiosulfate, in the infusion bag.

Table 6 Comparative Pharmacodynamics of Parenteral Antihypertensive Agents

Drug and usual dose	Mechanism of action	Onset	Duration	CO	SVR	MAP	PCWP	HR	Major side effects	Remarks
Nitroprusside (Nipride), initiate at 0.25–0.5 μg/kg per min IV, may titrate up to 8 μg/kg per min	Arteriolar and venous vasodilator	Seconds	3–5 min	+/−	−	−	−	+	Hypotension, nausea, cyanide toxicity, thiocyanate toxicity	Use cautiously in patients with liver and/or renal failure
Nitroglycerin (Tridil), 10–40 μg/min IV	Venous and arteriolar vasodilator	Seconds	Minutes	0	0	0	−	0	Hypotension, headache tachycardia	Less potent than nitroprusside as antihypertensive
Nitroglycerin (Tridil), 50–250 μg/min	Venous and arteriolar vasodilator	Seconds	Minutes	+	−	−	−	+	Hypotension, headache, tachycardia	Less potent than nitroprusside as antihypertensive
Hydralazine (Apresoline), 10–40 mg IV bolus repeated as needed	Arteriolar vasodilator	10–20 min	3–6 h	+	−	−	0	+	Tachycardia, headache	Avoid use or use with caution in patients with angina, myocardial infarction, and aortic dissection
Labetalol (Trandate, Normodyne), initial: 20 mg IV over 2 min, then 40–80 mg Q10–15 min until desired response	Alpha blockade and nonspecific beta blockade	5 min	3–6 h	0	−	−	0/−	−	Hypotension, nausea, vomiting	Avoid use in patients with asthma, CHF, bradycardia, and heart block greater than first degree

(*Continued*)

Table 6 Comparative Pharmacodynamics of Parenteral Antihypertensive Agents (*Continued*)

Drug and usual dose	Mechanism of action	Onset	Duration	CO	SVR	MAP	PCWP	HR	Major side effects	Remarks
Esmolol (Brevibloc), initial[a]: 0.25 mg/kg IV over 30 s, then 25–50 µg/kg per min infusion for 4 min. If necessary, increase infusion by increments of 50 µg/kg per min Q4 min up to maximum of 300 µg/kg per min.	Beta-1 specific beta blocker	Minutes	10–30 min	−	0	−	0	−	Hypotension, bradycardia	Contraindicated in patients with second or third degree heart block, sinus bradycardia, cardiogenic shock, or overt cardiac failure
Enalaprilat (Vasotec IV), 0.625–5 mg IV Q6h over 5 min	ACE inhibitor	15 min	6–8 h	0/+	−	−	−	0	Hypotension, dizziness, angioedema, rash, headache	Use lower dose for first dose in patients receiving diuretics to avoid hypotension
Fenoldopam (Corlopam), initial: 0.05–0.1 µg/kg per min. Titrate by 0.05–0.1 µg/kg per min every 15–20 min until blood pressure control or up to 1.6 µg/kg per min. For renal protective effect, goal rate is 0.3–0.5 µg/kg per min	Dopamine-1 Agonist	Minutes	15–30 min	0	−	−	0	0/+	Hypotension	Indicated for hypertensive crisis with concomitant renal injury

[a]The initial loading bolus of 0.25 mg/kg may be omitted; however, maximal response may be delayed.
Abbreviations: +, increase; −, decrease; 0, no change; CO, cardiac output; SVR, systemic vascular resistance; PCWP, pulmonary capillary wedge pressure; HR, heart rate.

Table 7 Comparative Dosing and Pharmacologic Effects of Oral Antihypertensive Agents

Drug	Initial oral dose	Maintenance oral dose[a]	Onset	Peak effect (h)	Duration (h)	RBF	PVR	CO	HR	Remarks
ACE inhibitors										Except for fosinopril, start with lower doses in patients receiving diuretics and in renal failure patients
Captopril (Capoten)	6.25–12.5 mg tid	25–50 mg tid	15–30 min	1–1.5	6–12	+	–	0/+	0	
Enalapril (Vasotec)	2.5–5 mg Qday	2.5–10 mg bid	60–120 min	4–8	12–24	+	–	0/+	0	
Lisinopril (Prinivil)	2.5–10 mg Qday	10–20 mg Qday	60 min	6–8	24	+	–	0	0	
Fosinopril (Monopril)	10 mg Qday	20–60 mg Qday	60–120 min	2–6	24	0	–	0	0	
Calcium channel blockers										Use verapamil and diltiazem cautiously in patients with poor left ventricular function. Avoid use in patients with second or third degree block or sick sinus syndrome
Verapamil (Calan)	40–80 mg tid	120 mg tid	30 min	1–2	2–6	0	–	–/+	–	
Amlodipine (Norvasc)	2.5–5 mg Qday	5–10 mg Qday	Gradual	6–12	24	+	–	0	0	
Diltiazem (Cardizem)	30 mg qid	90 mg tid or qid	30–60 min	3	6–10	0	–	0/+	–	
Beta blockers										Metoprolol and atenolol are beta-1 specific
Metoprolol (Lopressor)	50 mg bid or tid	100–200 mg bid	30 min	1–2	12–19	0/–	0/–	–	–	
Atenolol (Tenormin)	50 mg Qday	100 mg Qday	60 min	2–4	24	0/–	0	–	–	

(*Continued*)

Table 7 Comparative Dosing and Pharmacologic Effects of Oral Antihypertensive Agents (*Continued*)

Drug	Initial oral dose	Maintenance oral dose[a]	Onset	Peak effect (h)	Duration (h)	RBF	PVR	CO	HR	Remarks
Propranolol (Inderal)	40 mg bid	80 mg bid or tid	60 min	2–4 h	8–12 h	0/–	0/–	–	–	Avoid use in patients with asthma, CHF, bradycardia, and heart block greater than first degree
Alpha-1 blockers										Dizziness, headache, drowsiness, weakness, palpitations, and nausea occur frequently
Prazosin (Minipress)	1 mg bid or tid	2–5 mg tid	30–60 min	1–3	6–12	0	–	0/+	0	
Doxazosin (Cardura)	1 mg Qday	4–8 mg Qday	120 min	6	24	0	–	0/+	0	
Alpha-2 central agonists										Dry mouth, drowsiness, dizziness, fatigue and headache occur frequently. Avoid abrupt discontinuation
Clonidine (Catapres)	0.1 mg bid	0.1–0.3 mg bid or tid	30–60 min	2–4	6–12	0/–	–	0/–	–	
Guanfacine (Tenex)	1 mg Qday	1–3 mg Qday	60 min	1–4	24	0	–	0	–	
Alpha-1 and beta blocker										Beta-blocker activity is nonspecific. Follow same precautions as with other beta-blockers
Labetalol (Trandate)	100 mg bid	200–400 mg bid	30–60 min	1–3	8–12	0/+	–	0	–	

[a]Maintenance oral dose recommendations represent extended ranges. Dosages should be titrated to effect and to minimize side effects. Few patients are likely to require maximum maintenance dose.

Abbreviations: +, increase; –, decrease; 0, no change; RBF, renal blood flow; PVR, peripheral vascular resistance; CO, cardiac output; HR, heart rate.

Caution is advised when administering nitroprusside to patients with coronary ischemia and/or myocardial infarction. Nitroprusside may exacerbate cardiac ischemia by decreasing blood flow to ischemic areas.

Dosing: For patients with severe heart failure, a nitroprusside infusion is started at 0.2 μg/kg per min with a volumetric infusion pump. The infusion may be increased by 0.2 μg/kg per min increments every 5–15 min. Individual responses to nitroprusside are variable, but most patients with heart failure have a response at 1–2 μg/kg per min with a 20–25% decrease in PCWP and a 20–40% increase in CO. For patients with hypertension, nitroprusside is started at 0.25–0.5 μg/kg per min but is increased by increments of 0.5 μg/kg per min every 5–10 min until the desired blood pressure is achieved. Most patients have their blood pressure controlled with an average of 1.5–2 μg/kg per min. If adequate blood pressure reduction is not achieved within 10 min at an infusion rate of 10 μg/kg per min, the nitroprusside should be terminated and an alternative antihypertensive agent administered.

Summary: Nitroprusside is a potent parenteral vasodilator and has been used in the treatment of hypertensive emergencies, acute valvular insufficiency, low cardiac output states, and congestive myocardial failure (11,18,19).

Nitroglycerin

Nitroglycerin acts on smooth muscle to cause relaxation and vasodilation. It primarily dilates venous vessels but also dilates arterial vessels. Nitroglycerin is a less potent antihypertensive agent than nitroprusside, but it is useful in patients with hypertension associated with myocardial ischemia or infarction. The drug acts within seconds to lower systemic blood pressure, to lower pulmonary vascular resistance, and to increase CO. The drug also maintains or improves collateral coronary circulation. IV nitroglycerin has been shown to reduce infarct size and improve mortality in acute myocardial infarction. The drug is also useful for treating unstable angina. In patients with cardiogenic shock, IV nitroglycerin combined with inotropic agents (e.g., dopamine or dobutamine) or intra-aortic balloon counterpulsation can produce substantial hemodynamic improvement.

Precautions: Nitroglycerin is generally well tolerated, but side effects related to vasodilation do occur. They include hypotension, headache, and reflex tachycardia. Rare, but potentially dangerous, is paradoxical bradycardia. If administered continuously for longer than 24–48 h, many patients develop a tolerance to the hemodynamic and/or antianginal effects of nitroglycerin. Consideration should be given to provide a nitrate-free period of 6–8 h per 24 h period to prevent tolerance.

Dosing: Nitroglycerin is administered as a continuous IV infusion through a volumetric infusion pump. The starting dose is 0.25–0.5 μg/kg per min, with titration done every 5–10 min by 0.25–0.5 μg/kg per min increments to achieve the desired response. The normal therapeutic dosing range is 0.5–5 μg/kg per min.

Summary: Although not as effective an antihypertensive agent as nitroprusside, nitroglycerin is a useful agent for lowering blood pressure when cardiac ischemia is present (11,20,21).

Labetalol

Labetalol is a nonselective beta-receptor blocker that also has alpha-1 blocker activity. The potency for beta-receptor antagonism is five- to tenfold greater than that for alpha-1 blockade. This combination of alpha-1 and beta-receptor blockade makes it an ideal agent for lowering blood pressure and blunting reflex tachycardia acutely in the ICU.

Precautions: Hypotension and dizziness are dose-related, and the patient should remain in a supine position during administration. Other precautions with labetalol are related to its beta-blocking effects. The drug should not be used in patients with asthma, heart block greater than first degree, sinus bradycardia, or severe heart failure. The drug should be used with caution in patients with intermittent claudication or Raynaud's syndrome.

Dosing: The initial IV bolus dose is 5 mg slowly over 2 min, followed by repeated injections of 10, 20, 40, and 80 mg at 10 min intervals until a desired blood pressure is achieved or a total cumulative dose of 300 mg has been given. The peak effect of each bolus is usually seen in 10 min. The duration of effect with bolus administration is usually several hours. Labetalol may also be administered as a continuous IV infusion using an infusion pump starting at 2 mg/min. The dose can then be titrated to the blood pressure response. If an adequate response is obtained and oral administration is possible, oral labetalol can be instituted upon discontinuing parenteral labetalol. An initial oral dose is 200 mg followed by 200–400 mg, 6–12 h later, depending on blood pressure response. The usual maintenance dose is 200–400 orally two to three times daily.

Summary: Labetalol combines the advantages of alpha- and beta-blockers while lowering the unwanted effects of both types of agents. Many reports support its use in patients with severe hypertension and during hypertensive emergencies (11,20,22).

Fenoldopam

Fenoldopam is dopamine agonist that is selective for the dopamine-1 receptor. Unlike dopamine, fenoldopam has no dopamine-2, beta-1, or alpha-1 receptor activity. Fenoldopam has vasodilation effects in the renal and mesenteric beds and in higher doses lowers systemic blood pressure. Fenoldopam is indicated for in-hospital, short-term management of hypertensive emergency. Nitroprusside is generally the first-line agent for managing hypertensive emergency. Due to its high cost, fenoldopam is generally reserved for patients with malignant hypertension with deteriorating renal function.

Because of its selective dopamine-1 agonist effects on renal vasculature and the inconsistent effects of low-dose infusion of dopamine, great interest in using fenoldopam as a renal protective agent has arisen. A number of retrospective and prospective, nonrandomized trials have demonstrated some benefit for using fenoldopam in high-risk patients exposed to radiographic contrast. These high-risk patients include diabetics and/or patients with pre-existing renal failure. The results of future randomized, double blind, placebo-controlled trials are necessary to assess the efficacy, optimal dosing, and safety of fenoldopam as a renal protective agent.

Precautions: The most common adverse effect to fenoldopam is hypotension. Other side effects include headache and reflex tachycardia. Patients with a history of allergy to sulfites may develop an anaphylactic reaction to sodium metabisulfate in fenoldopam. Administer with caution to patients with glaucoma or intraocular hypertension because of possible increases in intraocular pressure.

Dosing: Fenoldopam is administered as a continuous IV infusion using an infusion pump. Do not administer as bolus doses. For prevention of radiographic contrast renal injury in high-risk patients, the following dosing schedule has been used. An infusion is initiated at a rate of 0.05–0.1 μg/kg per min, starting 2 h before the procedure. The infusion is titrated upward by increments of 0.05–0.1 μg/kg per min every 20 min until a goal infusion rate of 0.3–0.5 μg/kg per min is achieved. Blood pressure should be checked prior to each infusion rate change and systolic blood pressure should not be allowed to fall below 100 mm Hg. Usually the infusion is continued for 4–6 h postprocedure. Fenoldopam infusion may be discontinued abruptly without concern for postinfusion effects.

For the treatment of hypertensive emergency with ongoing renal injury, fenoldopam is initiated at 0.1 µg/kg per min and increased by 0.1 µg/kg per min every 15 min until the desired blood pressure is achieved. Dose up to 1.6 µg/kg per min have been studied.

Summary: Fenoldopam is a specific dopamine-1 agonist. It should be reserved for hypertensive emergency with concomitant ongoing renal injury (11,23–25).

Enalaprilat

Enalaprilat (Vasotec IV) is the active form of enalapril. It is currently the only angiotensin-converting enzyme (ACE) inhibitor available in the United States in a parenteral form. It is approved for the treatment of hypertension when oral therapy is not practical. Enalaprilat reduces blood pressure by supression of the renin–angiotensin–aldosterone system. The drug also lowers blood pressure in patients with low renin levels.

Precautions: Severe hypotension is the most common adverse effect of enalaprilat therapy, and patients should be closely monitored after starting therapy. Patients taking diuretics or those with renal failure should be started at an initial dose of 0.625 mg IV to avoid significant hypotension.

Dosing: The initial IV dose of enalaprilat is 1.25 mg IV over 5 min every 6 h. A clinical response is usually seen within 15 min. Peak effects may not occur for up to 4 h after administration.

Summary: Parenteral enalaprilat is a useful alternative antihypertensive agent. It is particularly useful in patients who have contraindications for using other agents or who have not had an adequate response (11,26).

Esmolol

Esmolol is a beta-1 selective beta-blocker having an ultra short duration of action. The drug has been used for prompt control of ventricular rate in patients with supraventricular tachycardias. Esmolol also has been used for the treatment of postoperative hypertension. The drug has a half-life of ~9 min. Upon discontinuation of esmolol, the drug's pharmacologic effects are reversed within 20–30 min.

Precautions: Severe hypotension is the most common adverse effect seen with esmolol. Hypotension will generally resolve with dose adjustments or termination of the infusion. As with other beta-1 selective blockers, esmolol should be used with caution in patients with bronchospastic disease. The drug is contraindicated in patients with heart block greater than first degree, sinus bradycardia, or severe heart failure.

Dosing: Esmolol is administered as an IV continuous infusion using an infusion pump. An IV loading bolus may be given to provide a quicker onset of activity. The loading dose is 0.25–0.5 µg/kg per min over 30–60 s. If too rapid a response in blood pressure is a concern, the loading dose can be eliminated. In that case, the normal maintenance continuous infusion is started at 25–50 µg/kg per min and titrated by increments of 25–50 µg/kg per min every 4 min to the desired response or a maximal dose of 300 µg/kg per min. When the bolus dose is eliminated, 20–30 min may be necessary to achieve the desired response, whereas the desired response may be seen in 5–10 min using the bolus dose. The continuous infusion has been used for up to 48 h.

Summary: Esmolol is an ultra short-acting beta-1 receptor blocker that has proved useful in controlling the rapid ventricular response in supraventricular tachycardias.

It may be a useful antihypertensive in postoperative patients with tachycardia and hypertension secondary to increased catecholamine release (11,20,27).

Sedative Agents

Many patients admitted to SICU will require sedative agents in addition to analgesia to allay anxiety and fear. Also, an amnestic effect is desirable. Among the drugs used for sedation are the benzodiazepines, propofol, and the newest agent, dexmedetomidine. Tables 8 and 9 summarize the pharmacokinetics and dosing of the IV sedatives and analgesics agents.

Propofol

The anesthetic/sedative agent propofol is a 2,6-diisopropylphenol, prepared as a 1% solution in a vehicle of 10% intralipid. The advantage of propofol is its fast onset and cessation of action. Most patients have return of consciousness within 15–20 min after stopping the drug. Propofol has also been used for treatment of status epilepticus. The drug can be titrated to a desired level of sedation.

Precautions: Propofol should generally be used only in intubated and ventilated patients, because it is a potent suppressor of respiratory function and can lead to respiratory arrest. Propofol can cause reductions in blood pressure, one of the principle side effects. Clinicians need to keep in mind that propofol is in 10% intralipid, and the fat calories need to be considered in determining nutritional intake. Patients receiving parenteral nutrition will require adjustments in the amount of intralipid they receive. With large doses of propofol (>75 μg/kg per min) patients can receive lipid doses >1 g/kg per day, which may impair cellular immune function and cause excessively high serum triglyceride levels. Propofol infusion syndrome (myocardial failure, metabolic acidosis, and rhabdomyolysis) has been reported with doses >90 μg/kg per min.

Dosing: Propofol is administered as a continuous IV infusion. Bolus dosing is not advised to reduce potential hypotensive effects. The starting dose for sedation is 5–10 μg/kg per min with incremental increases of 5–10 μg/kg per min every 10–15 min until the desired level of sedation is achieved. Much larger doses are necessary when propofol is used as an anesthetic. The clearance of propofol is reduced in elderly patients, who may respond to lower doses. To confirm that the patient is receiving the lowest effective dose of propofol, the infusion should be gradually weaned down on a daily basis to a dose that allows a reduction in the level of sedation consistent with a complete neurologic assessment. The patient can then be titrated to the level of sedation desired.

Propofol with its titratable sedation response and rapid clearance is an attractive sedative agent. For patients requiring sedation beyond 48–72 h, the use of a benzodiazepine such as lorazepam may be a more cost effective agent. With prolonged infusion, the rapid clearance of propofol loses importance. Also, if the patient no longer requires mechanical ventilation, but does require continued sedation, a drug like dexmedetomidine, which does not suppress respirations, is a better choice. When planning to stop the propofol therapy and extubate the patient, it is advisable not to stop the drug completely. Sudden withdrawal of the drug can cause the patient to awaken too quickly and become anxious and disoriented during the extubation process. A smoother transition can be accomplished by lightening the level of sedation to a degree where the patient can be reoriented and yet still be lightly sedated. After being oriented, the extubation process can proceed.

Summary: Propofol is advantageous when short-term sedation is required with extubation planned for the near future (11,28).

Table 8 IV Analgesic Comparison

Agent	Equivalent IV dose	Usual dose	Hepatic/renal elimination	Active metabolites	Comments
Morphine	1 mg	2–5 mg IV Q2–4 h, 0.5–6 mg/h IV infusion	90% hepatic 10% renal	Yes	Avoid in moderate to severe renal dysfunction because active metabolites may accumulate
Hydromorphone	0.15 mg	0.3–0.75 mg IV Q2–4 h, 0.1–0.9 mg/h IV infusion	100% hepatic	No	Useful agent for renal failure patients
Fentanyl	25 µg	50–125 µg IV Q0.5–2 h, 12.5–150 µg/h IV infusion	100% hepatic	No	Maybe used for morphine allergic patients and/or renal failure patients

Table 9 IV Sedative Comparison

Agent	Elimination half-life (h)	Usual dose	Hepatic/renal elimination	Active metabolites	Relative cost per day	Comments
Lorazepam (Ativan)	12	1–2 mg IV Q2–4 h	98% hepatic	No	$	Slower onset and longer duration than midazolam
Midazolam (Versed)	3	2–4 mg IV Q2–4 h	>95% hepatic	Yes	$	Active metabolites may accumulate after several days
Propofol (Diprivan)	0.5–1	10–50 µg/kg per min	hepatic	No	$$$$$$$	Vehicle is 10% intralipids. Should not be used in nonventilated patients
Dexmedetomidine (Precedex)	2	0.2–0.7 µg/kg per h	hepatic	No	$$$$$$$$$	Loading dose of 1 µg/kg over ten minutes is optional. Does not cause respiratory depression. Hepatic failure and elderly patients may require lower doses

Dexmedetomidine

Dexmedetomidine is a new, unique agent for sedation. The drug is an alpha-2 agonist that acts on the locus ceruleus and brain stem to produce sedation and analgesia. The sedation effect of this agent is different from that of benzodiazepines and propofol. Patients are sedated but easily arousable for neurological evaluation. Because the drug does not suppress respiratory function, it is not necessary for patients to be intubated and mechanically ventilated. Also, a patient can be extubated without prior discontinuation of the dexmedetomidine, a major advantage when compared with propofol.

Precautions: Hypotension is the most common side effect with dexmedetomidine via alpha-2 agonist effects in the brain decreasing sympathetic tone. If loading doses are used and given too rapidly to hasten onset of activity, hypertension can occur secondarily to alpha-1 agonist effects on blood vessels.

Dosing: A loading dose of 1 µg/kg IV over 20 min is used if a more rapid onset of action is desired. However, a higher incidence of hypertension or hypotension is associated with loading. Alternatively, the loading dose can be omitted and a starting dose of 0.1–0.7 µg/kg per h initiated. Sedation may take longer to achieve but may be safer. Maintenance doses can be titrated by 0.1–0.2 µg/kg per h until the desired effect is achieved. The manufacturer recommends a maximum maintenance infusion of 0.7 µg/kg per h. Some patients may require higher doses to see an effect. Doses up to 1.4 µg/kg per h can be used if the patient is monitored closely for side effects, such as hypotension. Elderly patients and those with liver dysfunction may have impaired drug clearance and require lower doses of the drug. The package insert limits the use of this agent to 24 h. Studies are currently ongoing to determine safety for longer periods.

Summary: Dexmedetomidine is a unique sedative agent without the risk of respiratory depression. The drug would be advantageous in patients requiring frequent neurological assessment. It can also be used in situations where sedation is required, but the patient does not require mechanical ventilatory support (11,28).

SUMMARY

- The correct dose of a drug is one that produces the desired therapeutic effect and minimal side effects.
- The dynamic course of critically ill patients affects absorption, distribution, metabolism, and excretion of drugs. These effects vary with time, and doses need revision as a patient's condition changes.
- Serum drug concentrations can help to guide therapy, especially for drugs with a narrow therapeutic index.
- Positive inotropic agents include dopamine, dobutamine, and epinephrine, which are beta agonists, and milrinone, which increases intracellular c-AMP, modulates intracellular calcium, and produces vasodilation.
- Antihypertensive agents include nitroprusside, nitroglycerin, labetalol, enalaprilat, and esmolol. Nitroprusside relaxes arteriolar and venous smooth muscle. Nitroglycerin primarily dilates venous vessels and is especially useful in patients with myocardial ischemia. Labetalol has both alpha- and beta-blocker activity. Enalaprilat is an ACE inhibitor. Esmolol is an ultra-short-acting beta-blocker.

- Propofol and dexmedetomidine are sedative agents. Propofol has a quick onset and offset of activity. Dexmedetomidine produces sedation but allows the patient to be arousable and does not cause respiratory depression.

REFERENCES

1. Williams RL. Drug administration in hepatic disease. N Engl J Med 1983; 309:1616.
2. Krueger KA, Garnett WR, Comstock TJ. Effect of two administration schedules of an enteral nutrient formula on phenytoin bioavailability. Epilepsia 1987; 28:706.
3. Hassan E, Ober JD. Predicted and measured aminoglycoside pharmacokinetic parameters in critically ill patients. Antimicrob Agents Chemother 1987; 31:1855.
4. Fuhs DW, Mann HJ, Kubajak CAM, Cerra FB. Inpatient variation of aminoglycoside pharmacokinetics in critically ill surgery patients. Clin Pharm 1988; 7:207.
5. Robert S, Zarowitz BJ. Is there a reliable index of glomerular filtration ratae in critically ill patients? DICP Ann Pharmcother 1991; 25:169.
6. Cockcroft DW, Gault MH. Prediction of creatinine clearance from serum creatinine. Nephron 1976; 16:31.
7. Jelliffe RW. Creatinine clearance: a bedside estimate. Ann Intern Med 1973; 79:604.
8. Jelliffe RW, Jelliffe SM. A computer program for estimation of creatinine clearance from unstable serum creatinine levels, age, sex, and weight. Math Biosci 1972; 14:17.
9. Szeto HH, Inturrisi CE, Houde R. Accumulation of normeperidine, an active metabolite of meperidine, in patients with renal failure or cancer. Ann Intern Med 1977; 86:738.
10. Drayer DE, Lowenthal DT, Woosley RL. Acccumulation of N-acetylprocainamide, an active metabolite of procainamide, in patients with impaired renal functions. Clin Pharmacol Ther 1977; 22:63.
11. Drug Facts and Comparisons. St. Louis: Wolters Kluwer, 2002.
12. Zaritsky, A. Catecholamines, Inotropic medications, and vasopressor agents. In: Chernow B, ed. The Pharmacologic Approach to the Critically Ill Patient. Baltimore: Williams and Wilkins, 1994:387–404.
13. Rudis MI, Wagner B, Dasta JF. Use of vasopressors and inotropes in the pharmacotherapy of shock. In: DiPiro JT, Talbert RL, Yee GC, Matzke GR, Wells BG, Posey LM, eds. Pharmacotherapy: A Pathophysiologic Approach, 4th ed. Stamford, Connecticut: Appleton and Lange, 1999:392–407.
14. Horan JL, Bobek MB, Arroliga AC. Acute renal failure: overview of current and potential therapies. Formulary 2000; 35:669–680.
15. Australian and New Zealand Intensive Care Society (ANZICS) Clinical Trials Group. Low-dose dopamine in patients with early renal dysfunction: a placebo-controlled randomized trial. Lancet 2000; 356:2139–2143.
16. Holmes, CL, Patel BM, Russell JA, Walley KR. Physiology of vasopressin relevant to management of septic shock. Chest 2001; 120:989–1002.
17. Tsuneyoshi I, Haruhiko Y, Kakihana Y, Nakamura M, Nakano Y, Boyle WA. Hemodynamic and metabolic effects of low-dose vasopressin infusions in vasodilatory shock. Crit Care Med 2001; 29:487–493.
18. Parrillo JE. Vasodilator therapy. In: Chernow B, ed. The Pharmacologic Approach to the Critically Ill Patient. Baltimore: Williams and Wilkins, 1994:470–483.
19. Hawkins DW, Bussey HI, Prisant LM. Hypertension. In: DiPiro JT, Talbert RL, Yee GC, Matzke GR, Wells BG, Posey LM, eds. Pharmacotherapy: A Pathophysiologic Approach, 4th ed. Stamford, Connecticut: Appleton and Lange, 1999:131–152.
20. Ziegler MG, Ruiz-Ramon PF. Antihypertensive therapy. In: Chernow B, ed. The Pharmacologic Approach to the Critically Ill Patient. Baltimore: Williams and Wilkins, 1994:405–428.

21. Johnson JA, Parker RB, Geraci SA. Heart failure. In: DiPiro JT, Talbert RL, Yee GC, Matzke GR, Wells BG, Posey LM, eds. Pharmacotherapy: A Pathophysiologic Approach, 4th ed. Stamford, Connecticut: Appleton and Lange, 1999:131–152.
22. Wilson DJ, Wallin JD, Vlachakis ND et al. Intravenous labetalol in the treatment of severe hypertension and hypertensive emergencies. Am J Med. 1983; 75:95.
23. Singer I, Epstein M. Potential of dopamine A-1 agonists in the management of acute renal failure. Am J Kidney Dis 1998; 31:743–755.
24. Mathur VS, Swan SK, Lambrecht LJ et al. The effects of fenoldopam, a selective dopamine receptor agonist, on systemic and renal hemodynamics in normotensive subjects. Crit Care Med 1999; 27:1832–1837.
25. Generali J, Cada DJ. Fenoldopam: prevention of contrast media nephrotoxicity. Hospital Pharm 2002; 37:287–294.
26. DeMarco T, Daly PA, Liu M et al. Enalaprilat, a new parenteral angiotensin converting enzyme inhibitor: rapid changes in systemic and coronary hemodynamics and humoral profile in chronic heart failure. J Am Coll Cardiol 1987; 9:1131.
27. Gary RJ, Bateman TM, Czer LSC et al. Comparison of esmolol and nitroprusside for acute post-cardiac surgical hypertension. Am J Cardiol 1987; 59:887.
28. Fraser GL, Riker R. Advances and controversies in adult ICU sedation, part 3: evolving pharmacological treatment issues. Hospital Pharmacy 2002; 37:362–368.

50
Adverse Drug Reactions and Drug Interactions in the Intensive Care Unit

Douglas DeCarolis
VA Medical Center, Minneapolis, Minnesota, USA

The critically ill patient presents the intensivist with the challenge of determining appropriate and effective pharmacotherapy. The combination of hemodynamic compromise, organ dysfunction, fluid and electrolyte imbalances, and central nervous system (CNS) dysfunction may profoundly affect the efficacy and safety of commonly used drugs. Even slight changes in pharmacokinetics and pharmacodynamics can produce unexpected responses to pharmaceutical agents in the critically ill patient. Medications routinely used outside the intensive care unit (ICU) and considered to have a wide margin between therapeutic and toxic effects may have a much narrower therapeutic window in the ICU. Some pharmacological effects may be seen with lower doses, while other pharmacological effects may be blunted in the critically ill patient, despite the use of the recommended doses. Clearly, medication use in the ICU requires careful consideration before prescribing and subsequent close monitoring of the patient to achieve intended therapeutic effects and avoid potential risks. Another important consideration in the pursuit of optimal medication use in the ICU is the potential of drugs to interact with each other.

This chapter will review the more commonly used drugs in the ICU. It will focus on the potential unintended effects of these medications, avoidance of unwanted effects, and monitoring patients for these complications. A brief review of drug interactions will increase awareness of their potential, provide methods to minimize their impact, and identify guidelines for monitoring their occurrence. The following discussion emphasizes some of the more common and clinically important potential adverse effects and drug interactions.

CARDIOVASCULAR AGENTS

Antiarrhythmic Drugs

Amiodarone
Use of amiodarone as an antiarrhythmic agent has increased dramatically in the ICU in the past years. This rise in frequency of administration is due to increased use in treating supraventricular arrhythmias such as atrial fibrillation, the most common arrhythmia encountered in the ICU. Amiodarone has replaced many of the older drugs that are less effective, have greater negative inotropic effects, and demonstrate more acute

proarrhythmia complications. Although amiodarone has shown improved success in maintaining normal sinus rhythm (NSR) when compared with other agents, evidence suggesting any superiority in chemically converting patients from atrial fibrillation to NSR is lacking (1). Amiodarone's neutral effects on contractility, absence of significant proarrhythmic risk, and availability in intravenous (IV) form have caused a marked increase in use. Amiodarone also blocks the atrioventricular (AV) node and slows the rapid ventricular response in many cases of atrial fibrillation. Potential adverse effects include symptomatic bradycardia or signs of heart block. Simultaneous use of other drugs with AV-blocking effects increases the potential for these side effects. These medications include the beta-blockers (e.g., metoprolol, atenolol, and propranolol), diltiazem, verapamil, and digoxin. When treating critically ill patients, one must be acutely aware of the potential additive effects of sinoatrial and AV node blockade and alter therapy, if necessary.

When administered intravenously, another adverse effect of amiodarone is hypotension. Amiodarone is a mild vasodilator, and blood pressure should be monitored during infusion. The oral form is associated with dose-related gastrointestinal effects such as nausea and vomiting. Avoiding single oral doses >400 mg will minimize these effects. When using oral loading doses of 800–1600 mg/day, the clinician should divide the daily dose to minimize adverse gastrointestinal effects. Although administering a drug with a very long half-life, such as amiodarone, in divided doses appears illogical, the gastrointestinal tolerance to this drug necessitates limiting each dose to ≤400 mg.

Amiodarone has other significant potential long-term adverse effects (hypothyroidism, hyperthyroidism, pulmonary fibrosis, corneal microdeposits, and photosensitivity) that typically do not affect ICU use. The potential complication of pulmonary fibrosis must be considered in patients with a history of fibrotic pulmonary disease or any acute pulmonary injury. Cases of acute pulmonary toxicity have been reported (2–4).

In addition to the additive AV-node-blocking effects of amiodarone and digoxin, a significant pharmacokinetic drug interaction between these two agents also occurs. Amiodarone will decrease the clearance of digoxin and double the serum digoxin concentration (5). As a consequence of this interaction, the usual maintenance dose of digoxin should be halved. Their concomitant use should not affect the loading dose. Serum concentrations of digoxin may be useful in determining appropriate maintenance-doses. As digoxin has a long half-life, treatment serum concentrations may be determined weekly. Once steady state is achieved and the digoxin serum concentration is stable (1–2 weeks), routine digoxin measurement is not necessary unless renal function changes, toxicity is suspected, or therapeutic effect is questioned.

Other significant drug interactions have consequences for critical care. Amiodarone can significantly increase the plasma concentrations of the following drugs: cyclosporine, phenytoin, procainamide, propafenone, quinidine, theophylline, and warfarin. These interactions may double the drug serum concentrations and increase toxic effects of these medications. Considering the toxicity of this group of drugs, very careful monitoring is mandatory. Empirically reducing the dose of these medications and obtaining serum concentration measurements are recommended. Amiodarone may have a significant effect on warfarin metabolism, and daily monitoring of the International Normalized Ratio (INR) is strongly recommended when both drugs are used.

Digoxin

Digoxin is used for control of rapid ventricular response in atrial arrhythmias and for chronic congestive heart failure therapy. As noted in the discussion of amiodarone, significant interactions between digoxin and amiodarone exist. Two other medications that significantly affect digoxin serum concentrations are verapamil and quinidine. When adding either of these agents to digoxin therapy, one can expect digoxin serum concentrations to rise 50–100% (6–8). To avoid the potential of digoxin toxicity, the clinician should empirically reduce the digoxin dose by half. Alternatively, one can use serum concentrations to guide further therapy. Practically, reducing the digoxin dose by half and following serum concentrations are preferable. The reader is referred to other drug information resources or drug interaction texts for additional discussion of other agents that interact with digoxin (9).

Angiotensin Converting Enzyme Inhibitors

Captopril, lisinopril, enalapril, enaliprilat, fosinopril, moexipril, quinapril, and trandolapril are widely used in ambulatory care for the treatment of hypertension, heart failure, and coronary artery disease. In diabetic patients, they are used to prevent nephropathy. In the ICU, angiotensin converting enzyme (ACE) inhibitors are usually administered for afterload reduction in patients sustaining myocardial infarction or other acute coronary syndromes, for treatment of hypertension, and for maintenance therapy. Although very safe as an outpatient medication, ACE inhibitors should be carefully monitored in the ICU, especially in patients who are hypovolemic. Individuals with inadequate intravascular volume may develop hypotension or acute renal failure (10–12). For these reasons, many clinicians use the shorter acting agent captopril when initiating ACE-inhibitor therapy in a critically ill patient. Available preparations of captopril allow more rapid onset of effect and a shorter duration of action. In addition, captopril is available in lower dosage equivalents, a feature that allows clinicians to titrate the dose more carefully. Once the patient has proven tolerance to an ACE inhibitor, and fluid deficits are replaced, a longer acting agent may be substituted for patient convenience. Although an IV form (enaliprilat) is available, it is not considered a first-line agent for hypertensive crisis or for afterload reduction in the ICU. Rather, agents with short half-lives, such as nitroprusside and nitroglycerin, are safer and much easier to titrate to effect. Once the blood pressure and condition of the patient are stabilized, conversion to an oral agent is usually uncomplicated.

Although ACE-inhibitors have been shown to be "renal protective," one must be aware of the potential for acute renal failure. In the presence of a significant fluid deficit or bilateral renal artery stenosis that results in decreased renal blood flow, the efferent renal arteriole will constrict in response to secretion of renin and angiotensin to counteract this decreased glomerular perfusion. This vasoconstriction is essential in maintaining glomerular capillary filtration pressure and nephron function. Administration of an ACE inhibitor at this time will block the effects of angiotensin II, dilate the efferent arteriole, and cause the intraglomerular pressure to fall precipitously. The result is an abrupt increase in serum creatinine and a decrease in urine output. Withholding the ACE inhibitor and providing fluid will promptly correct the renal insufficiency.

Another potential adverse effect of ACE-inhibitor therapy in acute care is hyperkalemia, especially in conjunction with vigorous potassium replacement (13). This complication can be minimized with proper monitoring and awareness. The incidence of angioedema is rare but should be considered in a patient recently started on ACE-inhibitor therapy who is admitted to the ICU for emergency endotracheal intubation.

A potential drug interaction may occur with exogenous potassium administration or use of potassium sparing diuretics such as triamterene or spironolactone. Combination of an ACE inhibitor with these drugs may increase the risk of hyperkalemia. The use of nonsteroidal anti-inflammatory drugs (NSAIDs) (e.g., ketorolac) may produce acute renal toxicity in susceptible patients.

Calcium Channel Blocking Agents

Nifedipine, amlodipine, felodipine, isradapine, diltiazem, and verapamil are examples of calcium channel blocking agents. The most common calcium channel blocking agent used in the ICU is IV diltiazem, which is indicated for the control of rapid ventricular rate in atrial fibrillation or flutter. Verapamil can also be used for this indication; however, its greater negative inotropic effect and less familiarity with its IV administration limit its use in the ICU. Orally, these two agents are used for maintenance of ventricular rate control, hypertension, and chronic stable angina. The dihydropyridine agents (nifedipine, amlodipine, felodipine, and isradapine) are used for treatment of hypertension and chronic stable angina. Because of the complications of hypotension, myocardial infarction, and exacerbation of myocardial ischemia, the rapid acting form of nifedipine is no longer used for acute therapy of hypertension.

The major adverse effects of diltiazem and verapamil are bradycardia, heart block, and hypotension. Concomitant use of calcium channel blockers with other medications that can block the AV node, for example, amiodarone, may result in increased incidence of bradycardia and heart block. The elderly are at higher risk for these complications, and the dose may require adjustment (15).

Another potential adverse effect of calcium channel blockers in the ICU, with the exception of amlodipine, is negative inotropy. Patients with a history of systolic heart failure, an ejection fraction of <40%, or acute decompensation of cardiac function may not tolerate calcium channel blockers (16). Patients sustaining myocardial infarction should have calcium channel blocker therapy carefully assessed.

Other Antiarrhythmic Agents

Lidocaine has rapid onset and is used for the treatment of ventricular arrhythmias. If selected for the treatment of life-threatening arrhythmias, lidocaine must be correctly administered. One bolus loading dose will achieve therapeutic concentrations quickly, but redistribution will cause a precipitous fall to subtherapeutic concentrations in 5–10 min. Simultaneous IV lidocaine infusion at the time of the initial bolus usually is not adequate to maintain plasma concentrations in a patient with life-threatening arrhythmias. Consequently, following the initial loading dose with another 1/2 bolus dose every 5 min for one to two additional doses, in addition to starting the continuous infusion, is recommended. Adverse effects of lidocaine include confusion, numbness, dizziness, paresthesia, agitation, disorientation, and hallucinations. They are more common in the elderly, patients with liver disease, or patients with heart failure. For these patients, the clinician should reduce the maintenance infusion. After 24 h of continuous infusion, lidocaine redistributes from tissues and enters the blood compartment. The subsequent increase in plasma concentration can produce adverse effects. If therapy is required for longer than 24 h, the maintenance dose can be reduced by half. Measurement of lidocaine serum concentrations can be useful if the infusion is continued longer than 24–48 h.

Procainamide is used for treatment of atrial and ventricular arrhythmias. Its slight negative inotropic effects, potential for QT prolongation, and preferential administration of amiodarone for treatment of arrhythmias have reduced its use. To avoid profound hypotension, procainamide should be administered slowly (no faster than 50 mg/min).

Monitoring the QT interval is necessary: procainamide administration should be discontinued if the QT interval is >500 ms or if it increases by >50% from baseline values. Procainamide administration in patients with renal insufficiency presents additional difficulties. An active metabolite, *n*-acetylprocainamide, can accumulate and cause toxicity. For patients with renal insufficiency, an alternate anti-arrhythmic agent is preferable. The oral form of procainamide frequently causes acute gastrointestinal upset and dyspepsia.

Administration of amiodarone to patients receiving procainamide will increase serum procainamide concentrations. Administration of cimetidine increases procainamide serum concentrations by decreasing clearance (17,18). Concomitant use with drugs that may increase the QT interval should be avoided, if possible. Ibutilide, another antiarrhythmic agent used for chemical conversion of atrial fibrillation/flutter, should not be administered within 4 h of procainamide therapy. An increased potential exists for QT prolongation and *torsades de pointes* (19). Other drugs that have potential to prolong the QT interval are listed in Table 1.

Vasoactive Drugs

Nitroprusside

Nitroprusside is the drug of choice for treatment of hypertensive emergencies or for rapid reduction of blood pressure. It also is used for afterload reduction for patients with acute heart failure. Close monitoring of the blood pressure is essential to prevent reduction of blood pressure that is too rapid. Reflex tachycardia may occur and may complicate myocardial ischemia by increasing myocardial oxygen demand. Nitroprusside produces vasodilation by release of nitric oxide from the parent compound. With metabolism of nitroprusside, cyanide ions are released, quickly scavenged by endogenous sulfhydryl groups, and converted to thiocyanate in the liver (20). This clearance mechanism minimizes cyanide accumulation and toxicity with lower doses. At higher doses (>3 µg/kg per min) or with prolonged use (>1–2 days), the endogenous sulfhydryl groups may become depleted, and free cyanide can accumulate in the blood. Cyanide toxicity may then develop. Tachyphylaxis (higher doses are required), metabolic acidosis, and CNS dysfunction herald cyanide toxicity. Measurement of serum concentrations of cyanide is not clinically useful in preventing cyanide toxicity. A more practical intervention is the

Table 1 Drugs That Prolong the QT Interval

Bepridil	Pentamidine
Cisapride	Pimozide
Desipramine	Probuchol
Disopyramide	Procainamide
Dofetilide	Quetiapine
Droperidol	Quinidine
Erythromycin	Risperidone
Flecainide	Sotalol
Gatifloxacin	Soarfloxacin
Haloperidol	Thioridazine
Ibutilide	Venlafaxine
Moxifloxacin	Ziprasidone

addition of exogenous sulfhydryl groups in the form of sodium thiosulfate to the nitroprusside infusion in 10 : 1 ratio (sodium thiosulfate : nitroprusside) (20). Some hospital pharmacies routinely add sodium thiosulfate to all nitroprusside infusions. If not standard practice, addition of sodium thiosulfate is recommended for patients receiving higher doses (>2 μg/kg/min) or therapy (>24 h).

The byproduct of cyanide scavenging by sulfhydryl groups is thiocyanate, a neurotoxin. Thiocyanate toxicity is rare and occurs only with prolonged infusion in patients with significant renal insufficiency. Monitoring of thiocyanate serum concentrations typically is reserved for patients (24) receiving prolonged infusions (>2 days) and with significant renal insufficiency. Many laboratories do not get results back for days, a feature that questions the value of monitoring the thiocyanate level.

Inotropic Agents

Dopamine, dobutamine, epinephrine, and milrinone may cause tachycardia, increased myocardial oxygen consumption, and tachyarrhythmias. In contrast to dopamine, dobutamine, and epinephrine, milrinone is not a catecholamine. Milrinone is a phosphodiesterase inhibitor, has a longer duration of action, and is cleared by the kidneys. Milrinone is a vasodilator. Its normal half-life of 1–3 h can be prolonged with renal insufficiency (21). When administered to patients with renal insufficiency, close monitoring for hypotension and tachyarrhythmias is warranted. A reduced dose, on the basis of renal function, is recommended.

Vasopressor Agents

Norepinephrine, phenylephrine, dopamine at infusion rates >10 μg/kg per min, and vasopressin are potent vasoconstrictors. As extravasation of these agents can cause significant tissue necrosis, administration through a central venous catheter is standard. If extravasation does occurs, 5–10 mg of phentolamine in 15 mL of saline is liberally infiltrated throughout the affected area within 12 h following extravasation (22).

Vasopressors may compromise mesenteric and renal blood flow with prolonged use. For patients with heart failure, use of these agents can increase afterload and, consequently, myocardial oxygen demand. To minimize myocardial ischemia, doses should be weaned to the lowest effective dose as soon as possible.

Sedative Agents

Benzodiazepines

Diazepam, midazolam, and lorazepam can cause respiratory depression and hypotension. Proper initial dose and IV rate of administration can minimize adverse effects. With careful monitoring, these medications have been used with a large margin of safety in the ICU (23). Benzodiazepines have long half-lives. When used for more than 24 h, accumulation may produce excessive sedation. Even midazolam, which has the shortest half-life, can accumulate in tissues and cause unwanted levels of sedation (24–26). Diazepam and midazolam have active metabolites that may persist in therapeutic concentrations after discontinuing the drugs. Lorazepam, although devoid of active metabolites, has a half-life of 10–20 h and can accumulate over time. The use of midazolam and lorazepam as continuous

IV infusions increases the potential for excessive sedation. As continuous sedation is often a goal for patients requiring mechanical ventilation, the use of continuous benzodiazepine infusions have become common in the ICU. A recent study showed value in a "daily wake-up" period. The sedative is withheld until the patient awakes and then resumed if needed at a minimal effective dose (27). This daily wake-up significantly reduced the duration of mechanical ventilation and the median length of stay in the ICU, and decreased diagnostic testing to assess changes in mental status.

High-dose continuous infusions of lorazepam recently have been cited as a cause of propylene glycol toxicity. When receiving high doses, patients can demonstrate hyperosmolality, metabolic acidosis, and hemolysis (28,29). Lorazepam has limited solubility in aqueous solutions; therefore, the injectable formulation uses propylene glycol and polyethylene glycol to enhance solubility. Although propylene glycol has been considered as an innocuous substance, recent reports have described toxicity associated with very high doses and prolonged use of lorazepam infusions. Typical lorazepam infusion doses used for ICU sedation (<10 mg/h) have not been associated with toxicity. Infusions of >20 mg/h for prolonged time periods produce a predictable dose dependant rise of serum osmolality. When the serum osmolality exceeds 350 mosm/L, metabolic acidosis may occur. Maintaining infusion rates at the lowest possible dose is essential to avoid this toxicity. If the dose exceeds 10 mg/h, the clinician should monitor the serum osmolality. The use of lorazepam in severe alcohol withdrawal presents a challenge, because symptoms of withdrawal can persist, despite high doses of lorazepam. Goals in treating withdrawal include use of minimum effective doses, rapid tapering once withdrawal symptoms are controlled, and frequent monitoring of serum chemistries and osmolality.

Midazolam is metabolized by the enzyme system CYP3A4. Inhibition of the enzyme activity may cause reduced clearance of the parent drug and prolonged sedation. Drugs that have been reported to cause this interaction include itraconazole, diltiazem, erythromycin, clarithromycin, and propofol (30–34). As lorazepam is metabolized by simple glucuronidation, drug interactions are less likely to alter its effects.

Propofol

Administration of propofol can produce profound respiratory depression. The use of propofol should be restricted to patients who are mechanically ventilated or can be intubated immediately. Propofol can cause vasodilation and induce hypotension in susceptible individuals (35,36). If vasopressors or inotropic agents are necessary to maintain blood pressure in patients receiving propofol, alternative sedative agents should be considered. Bradycardia has also been reported (37). As propofol is admixed in a lipid emulsion, hypertriglyceridemia is possible with long-term use or higher doses (26,38). When therapy continues for more than 3 days, measurement of serum triglycerides is recommended. The caloric contribution of a propofol emulsion must be included when prescribing nutritional formulations. As the lipid vehicle can be a source for bacterial contamination, manufacturer guidelines specify that infusion bottles and lines be changed within 12 h. When administered via a peripheral line, pain on injection is a common adverse effect, particularly when small veins are used (39).

Haloperidol

Haloperidol is used in the ICU for the treatment of delirium, fluctuating mental status, and disorganized thinking with or without agitation. Because of its long half-life, loading doses are often required for a timely response. A typical starting dose is 2 mg. If no effect is observed, the dose may be doubled every 20–30 min. The QT interval should be measured prior to initiation of haloperidol therapy. QT prolongation increases the risk of ventricular arrhythmias, particularly *torsades de pointes* (40–42). Haloperidol should be discontinued immediately, if QT prolongation occurs.

Haloperidol may cause extrapyramidal symptoms. It is also associated with neuroleptic malignant syndrome. This potentially severe adverse effect is rare but should be considered in critically ill patients, receiving haloperidol, who exhibit high fevers.

Droperidol

Droperidol is a related agent used for treatment of postoperative nausea and vomiting. Droperidol also can prolong the QT interval. Recent reports of fatal ventricular arrhythmias led to labeling changes. The package insert includes a black box warning and directions to obtain a baseline EKG to determine the QT interval prior to administration. Alternative drugs should be used whenever possible. If droperidol must be used, obtain a baseline EKG and avoid concomitant use with any agent known to prolong the QT interval (Table 1).

Analgesic Agents

Morphine, Fentanyl, Hydromorphone, and Meperidine

These agents are essential for the proper treatment and prevention of pain. Adverse effects include nausea, respiratory depression, oversedation, and diminished gastrointestinal motility. Frequent assessments of pain, level of alertness, respiratory rate, and nausea help determine the proper dose, interval, and route to minimize potential adverse effects. For treatment of acute pain in the ICU, the use of small IV bolus doses is preferred to other routes. This method of administration will provide rapid onset of action, accurate dose, and efficient titration to effect. Continuous infusions or scheduled doses are preferred when pain is continuous and predictable but require close monitoring of respiratory status, hemodynamic status, and level of alertness. Patient-controlled analgesia devices are effective in providing pain relief in patients who are able to understand and operate them. In contrast, the use of intramuscular (IM) or subcutaneous (SC) doses produce unpredictable absorption from the injection site and a delayed effect. Opiates given SC or IM often are prescribed in higher doses at less frequent intervals than those administered intravenously (e.g., morphine 10 mg IM q4 h). This practice may result in the larger bolus doses producing oversedation initially, and, with clearance of the drug, serum concentrations that fall below a therapeutic level prior to the next scheduled dose. This peak and valley variation in blood concentrations may cause the patient to experience initially high drug levels and side effects, a period of effective analgesia, and, finally, inadequate analgesia and pain prior to the next dose. Meperidine, with its short half-life, has a greater potential to demonstrate this sequence of events.

Morphine, with its familiar dose and duration of effect, is the most widely used analgesic in the ICU. Despite its widespread use, it may not be the best analgesic for all patients. It is known to release histamine and produce subsequent vasodilation to an extent greater than other opioids. Consequently, morphine may induce greater degrees of hypotension than fentanyl or hydromorphone (36). In hemodynamically unstable patients, fentanyl or hydromorphone are preferred. Morphine also may produce a vagal effect and should be used with caution in patients with significant bradycardia or heart block. In addition, caution is advised for patients with renal insufficiency, particularly if therapy is expected to continue for more than a few days. An active metabolite, morphine-6-glucuronide, may accumulate in renal failure (43). Alternative agents should be considered for patients at risk (36).

Fentanyl and hydromorphone may be substituted for morphine. Advantages of fentanyl include a more rapid onset and a shorter duration of effect. Prolonged administration leads to accumulation in adipose tissue. Following reduction of dose or discontinuation, fentanyl may diffuse into the blood and cause a marked prolongation of effect (44). Hydromorphone provides a similar duration of effect as morphine, has no active metabolites, and has less hemodynamic side effects. It is a good alternative when morphine cannot be used. Fentanyl and hydromorphone have largely replaced meperidine as alternative opioids for several reasons. The meperidine metabolite, normeperidine, accumulates in renal dysfunction and causes CNS excitation, agitation, and seizures. In addition, meperidine is associated with potentially fatal drug interactions with the monoamine oxidase (MAO) inhibitor class of antidepressants. For these reasons, its use is not recommended.

An underestimated adverse effect of opioid agents in the ICU is the development of physical dependence after continuous use of 1 week or more. Withdrawal symptoms, including tachycardia, diaphoresis, fever, hypertension, restlessness, irritability, and anxiety, can occur when opiates are abruptly stopped. Failure to identify these symptoms as opioid withdrawal will delay appropriate care. The weaning of daily doses by 25–50%, for patients receiving moderate to high doses of opioids for prolonged time periods can prevent withdrawal symptoms. Use of naloxone after prolonged analgesia may induce withdrawal symptoms and cardiac instability.

Non-opioid Agents

Nonsteroidal Anti-inflammatory Agents

Non-opioid analgesics have been shown to provide an opioid sparing effect, when combined with an opiate, for treatment of moderate to severe pain (45). The term opioid sparing refers to achieving the same degree of pain relief with lower doses of the opiate compared with the use of the opiate alone. Benefits of opiate sparing include reduction of adverse effects such as respiratory depression, sedation, and ileus, while maintaining adequate pain relief. The NSAIDs are useful as monotherapy for treatment of mild pain and may eliminate the need for opiate agents and their potential adverse effects. Although NSAID use is common outside the ICU and is considered safe in the ambulatory population, the critically ill patient requires more careful analysis of risks and benefits. The ICU patient is more susceptible to NSAID adverse effects, and the occurrence of these adverse effects may compromise overall outcome. For example, acute renal failure and gastrointestinal bleeding are potential NSAID adverse effects that can increase morbidity and mortality. Those at higher risk for adverse NSAID effects are the elderly, patients with renal insufficiency, hypovolemic patients, or patients with a history of prior gastrointestinal hemorrhage. As NSAIDs also inhibit platelet aggregation, they should be avoided in patients with overt bleeding or with high risk for bleeding. Their potential to cause acute renal failure is higher in patients with inadequate intravascular volume and in patients with low flow states, such as cardiogenic shock. In these situations, renal perfusion will depend on the vasodilatory properties of endogenous prostaglandins to maintain adequate renal perfusion. Inhibiting the production of these protective prostaglandins with the administration of NSAIDs can severely limit renal perfusion and cause acute renal failure.

Ketorolac is the only parenteral NSAID available for use in the ICU. Typically, it is used for treatment of acute, postoperative pain. Ketorolac has been shown to reduce morphine requirements and to be effective by itself for the treatment of mild to moderate pain (45). Its use has been associated with severe gastrointestinal bleeding. The major risk factors for adverse effects are advanced patient age ($>$65 years old), low body weight ($<$55 kg), renal insufficiency, history of gastrointestinal bleeding, magnitude of dose, and duration of therapy. Ketorolac administration should be avoided in patients with these risk factors. Although the manufacturer recommended dose for patients without contraindications is 30 mg IM/IV q6 h, serious consideration should be given to administering a lower dose of 15 mg to decrease risk. Limiting duration of therapy to a minimum number of days also decreases risk substantially. The labeling of this drug states that ketorolac may be used for a maximum 5-day course, but most clinicians limit therapy to 24–48 h. If patients can take oral medications, oral NSAID therapy has lower risk when compared with the risk of parenteral ketorolac. Patients receiving ketorolac should have the serum creatinine monitored and should be observed for signs of bleeding. Ketorolac should be discontinued with any deterioration of renal function or evidence of bleeding.

The new selective COX-2 inhibitors valdecoxib and celecoxib have a reduced risk of gastrointestinal side effects when compared with nonselective NSAIDs, and absence of platelet inhibition (46). Adverse renal effects are similar. Few data are available regarding their safety and comparative efficacy in the critically ill patient. They are available only as oral medications. Although COX-2 inhibitors are becoming popular anti-inflammatory and analgesic agents in ambulatory care, their use for analgesia in the critically ill patient requires further study. An increased incidence of myocardial infarction has caused the manufacturer to withdraw rofecoxib from the market.

Antimicrobials

Critically ill patients often are treated with antibiotics for infection. Accurate diagnosis of true infection in the critically ill patient is complicated. For example, leukocytosis, fever, and increased sputum production, common signs of respiratory infection in the ambulatory patient, are frequent in mechanically ventilated patients and may or may not be caused by infection. As sepsis can lead to hemodynamic instability or shock, infection must be identified and treated quickly. In addition, many antimicrobial agents are thought to have few adverse effects. Consequently, vast amounts of antimicrobials are used in the ICU. Despite a perceived low rate of adverse reactions, the high volume of antimicrobial use often makes antimicrobial agents a leading cause of reported adverse reactions in hospitalized patients.

Common adverse effects are typical allergic reactions, rashes, and hives. Anaphylaxis is an unusual complication. These adverse effects are often associated with beta-lactam antibiotics, penicillins, cephalosporins, and sulfonamides. Crampy abdominal pain and diarrhea may occur with antibiotic use. *Clostridium difficile* associated diarrhea is a common occurrence in the ICU and can cause significant morbidity and mortality. Aminoglycosides and amphotericin B are associated with acute renal failure. With prolonged use of these drugs, patients require close monitoring of renal function. Length of therapy is an important risk factor, and determination of blood concentrations of aminoglycosides is necessary to avoid complications. Many antimicrobials are renally excreted.

Adverse Drug Reactions and Interactions

Consequently, the clinician should match the dose of antimicrobial to the patient's renal function. For example, patients may experience seizures when penicillins or imipenem are used at normal doses in treating patients with impaired renal function.

Details about monitoring of commonly used antimicrobial agents are given in Table 2. Significant drug interactions that may occur with antimicrobials include:

1. *Concomitant use of oral quinolones with divalent cations*: Broad spectrum of activity and excellent absorption of oral forms make quinolones commonly used antimicrobials. Because of significantly lower costs of oral preparations, quinolones often are used enterally in the ICU. A significant interaction to avoid is the concomitant enteral administration of divalent ions within 2 h of administering these antibiotics. The cations chelate a significant amount of antibiotic and significantly reduce the amount available for absorption. Oral iron supplements, magnesium supplements, Maalox, Mylanta, milk of magnesia, aluminum hydroxide, and calcium supplements all significantly impair the absorption of these antibiotics. Providing a 2 h interval between quinolone administration and divalent ion administration will help ensure adequacy of dose.

Table 2 Monitoring of Antimicrobials

Acyclovir	Drug can crystallize in renal tubules and cause renal failure. Assure adequate hydration and give IV doses over at least 1 h. Monitor BUN/Cr. Adjust dose for renal impairment. Has caused encephalopathic changes in $\approx 1\%$.
Aminoglycosides	Nephrotoxicity, ototoxicity: monitor S. Cr., drug levels. Consider once daily administration. May deplete magnesium, potassium—monitor.
Amphotericin B	Nephrotoxicity: monitor S. Cr., sodium loading may help prevent (>100 mEq Na^+ per day). May cause fever, chills, infusion-related adverse effects (pre-treat with acetaminophen/diphenhydramine). May deplete magnesium, potassium.
Aztreonam	Adjust doses in renal insufficiency. Seizures with excessive dosing. Hypersensitivity (low cross-sensitivity with penicillins). Of note: aztreonam has minimal gram-positive coverage.
Cephalosporins	Monitor for signs of hypersensitivity. Cross-reactivity if penicillin allergic is 3–7%. May cause seizures in high doses. Adjust doses for renal insufficiency (exclude ceftriaxone). Monitor for pseudomembranous colitis. Rarely may have hematological effects (i.e., neutropenia).
Quinolones	Drug interactions include a significant decrease in oral absorption if coadministered within 2 h of divalent ions such as iron, calcium, and magnesium (antacids). Potential QT prolongation effects. Adjust doses in renal insufficiency. Ciprofloxacin significantly increases theophylline or cyclosporine levels.
Clindamycin	Monitor for antibiotic associated colitis. Dose unaffected by renal disease. Decrease dose in severe hepatic disease.
Cotrimoxazole	Monitor for hypersensitivity reactions, including hematological toxicity. Increased incidence of adverse effects in patients with AIDS. Maintain adequate fluid volume to prevent crystalluria and kidney stone formation. May significantly increase PT in patients receiving warfarin.

(Continued)

Table 2 Monitoring of Antimicrobials (*Continued*)

Erythromycin	Adjust doses for moderate to severe hepatic dysfunction. Uncommonly associated with hepatic dysfunction (erythromycin estolate). Most common adverse effect is abdominal cramping and discomfort that may occur with oral and IV forms. Venous irritation and phlebitis necessitates a slow infusion rate. Inhibits microsomal enzymes to produce significant drug interactions with terfenadine, astemizole, cisapride (cardiac arrhythmias/death), theophylline (↑levels), and warfarin (↑INR).
Fluconazole	Minimal adverse effects. Possible interaction with warfarin (↑INR). Comparable drug serum concentrations with oral vs. IV administration allows oral dose in most circumstances at significant cost savings. Adjust dose in renal impairment.
Foscarnet	Major toxicity is renal function impairment (occurs in most patients). Monitor BUN/Cr closely, maintain adequate hydration, and adjust doses on the basis of renal function. Electrolyte disorders include hypocalcemia, hypomagnesemia, hypokalemia, and hypo- or hyperphosphatemia. May predispose to seizures and cardiac abnormalities. Monitor electrolytes including "ionized" serum calcium (have patient report perioral numbness or parasthesias).
Gancyclovir	May cause granulocytopenia, anemia, and thrombocytopenia. Use with caution in patients with preexisting cytopenias and monitor closely. This effect may be increased when used with other drugs that inhibit the bone marrow (cytotoxic drugs, zidovudine). Adjust dose for renal impairment.
Imipenem/Cilastatin	Associated with seizures when dosing above recommended guidelines or in patients with CNS disorders. Concomitant therapy with gancyclovir increases seizure risk (use with caution). Adjust dose for renal impairment. Beware of hypersensitivity reaction. Cross-allergenicity with penicillin.
Linezolid	Monitor for myelosuppression: anemia, leukopenia, and thrombocytopenia.
Metronidazole	Seizures and peripheral neuropathy have occurred but incidence is low. Dose requires adjustment in moderate to severe liver dysfunction. May cause nausea, epigastric distress, and metallic taste in mouth. Neutropenia and thrombocytopenia are rare. May increase levels of warfarin, phenytoin, and lithium—monitor INR or drug levels closely.
Penicillins	Adjust dose for renal insufficiency, high doses may cause seizures. Monitor for signs of hypersensitivity (anaphylaxis, rash, and interstitial nephritis) and blood disorders (i.e., hemolytic anemia and thrombocytopenia).
Quinupristin/ Dalfopristin	Phlebitis, venous irritation. Central line preferred. Requires flushing with D5W before and after administration. Not compatible with NS.
Vancomycin	Red Man (Redneck) is a pseudo-allergic reaction characterized by a fall in blood pressure with or without a rash on the upper body. Caused by too rapid infusion and easily treated by stopping or slowing infusion rate or by administering diphenhydramine, if needed. Monitor renal function (BUN/Cr). Neutropenia may occur, but is rare.
Voriconazole	Avoid IV use in patients with renal insufficiency due to diluent. Oral use is acceptable. Most frequently reported adverse effect is visual disturbances. Review possible drug interactions before use.

2. *Interactions with warfarin*: Cotrimoxazole, metronidazole, and erythromycin inhibit warfarin metabolism, increase circulating warfarin concentration, and may produce an excessive degree of anticoagulation. A reduction in warfarin dose and a close monitoring of INR are necessary, if these antibiotics are administered to a patient receiving warfarin. Other antibiotics are thought to potentially increase the INR in patients receiving warfarin by reducing the population of vitamin-K-producing bacteria in the gastrointestinal tract.

Adverse reaction reporting of antimicrobials does not include the development of resistant organisms as a consequence of excessive antibiotic use. Infections from methicillin resistant *Staphylococcus aureus*, vancomycin resistant *Enterococcus*, and extended spectrum beta-lactamase-producing gram-negative organisms are all increasing and are thought to be correlated with antibiotic use. To reduce infections from such resistant organisms, the clinician should select the most appropriate agent with the narrowest spectrum necessary for suspected infection. Empirical therapy of infection is a necessity in the ICU, but should be reassessed every 48–72 h. In the absence of a definitive infection, serious consideration should be given to discontinuing antibiotic therapy.

REFERENCES

1. Hughes M, Binning A. Intravenous amiodarone in intensive care: time for reappraisal? Intensive Care Med 2000; 26:1730–1739.
2. Laprinsky SE, Mullen JB, Baller MS. Rapid pulmonary phospholipid accumulation induced by intravenous amiodarone. Can J Cardiol 1993; 9:322–324.
3. Donaldson L, Grant IS, Naysmith MR, Thomas JS. Amiodarone should be used with caution in patients in intensive care. Br Med J 1997; 314:1832.
4. Van Mieghem W, Coolen L, Malysse I, Lacquet LM, Deneffe GJD, Demedts MGP. Amiodarone and the development of ARDS after lung surgery. Chest 1994; 105:1642–1645.
5. Nademanee K, Kannan R, Hendrickson J, Ookhtens M, Kay I, Singh BN. Amiodarone–digoxin interaction, clinical significance, time course of development, potential mechanisms, and therapeutic implications. J Am Coll Cardiol 1984; 4:111–116.
6. Klein HO, Kaplinsky E. Verapamil and digoxin. Their respective effects on atrial fibrillation and their interaction. Am J Cardiol 1982; 50:894–902.
7. Bigger JT, Leahey EB. Quinidine and digoxin: an important interaction. Drugs 1982; 24:229–239.
8. Leahey EB Jr, Reiffel JA, Drusin RE, et al. Interaction between quinidine and digoxin. J Am Med Assoc 1978; 240:533–534.
9. Hansten PD, Horn JR. Drug interactions; Analysis and management facts and comparisons; 2002.
10. Squire IB, MacFayden RJ, Reid JL, et al. Differing early blood pressure and renin–angiotensin system responses to the first dose of angiotensin-converting enzyme inhibitors in congestive heart failure. Cardiovasc Pharmacol 1996; 27(5):657–666.
11. Manche A, Galea J, Busuttil W. Tolerance to ACE inhibitors after cardiac surgery. Eur J Cardiothorac Surg 1999; 15:55–60.
12. Wynckel A, Ebikili B, Melin J-P, et al. Long-term follow-up of acute renal failure caused by angiotensin converting enzyme inhibitors. Am J Hypertens 1998; 11:1080–1086.
13. Reardon LC, Macpherson DS. Hyperkalemia in outpatients using angiotensin-converting enzyme inhibitors. Arch Intern Med 1998; 158:26–32.
14. Grossman E, Messerli FH, Grodzicki T, Kowey P. Should a moratorium be placed on sublingual nifedipine capsules given for hypertensive emergencies and pseudoemergencies? J Am Med Assoc 1996; 276:1328–1331.

15. Pahor M, Manto A, Pedone C, et al. Age and severe adverse drug reactions caused by nifedipine and verapamil. J Clin Epidemiol 1996; 49:921–928.
16. Packer M, Kessler PD, Lee WH. Calcium-channel blockade in the management of severe chronic congestive heart failure: a bridge too far. Circulation 1987; 75(suppl V):V56–V64.
17. Saal AK, Werner JA, Greene HL, et al. Effect of amiodarone on serum quinidine and procainamide levels. Am J Cardiol 1984; 53:1264–1267.
18. Rodvold KA, Paloucek FP, Jung D, et al. Interaction of steady-state procainamide with H(2)-receptor antagonists cimetidine and ranitidine. Ther Drug Monit 1987; 9:378–383.
19. Product Information: Corvert(R), ibutilide fumarate injection. Upjohn Company, Kalamazoo, MI, 1998.
20. Hall VA, Guest JN. Sodium nitroprusside-induced cyanide intoxication and prevention with sodium thiosulfate prophylaxis. Am J Crit Care 1992; 2:19–27.
21. Product Information: Primacor(R) Injection, milrinone lactate. Sanofi-Synthelabo Inc, New York, NY, (PI revised 10/2000).
22. Product Information: Regitine(R), phentolamine mesylate. Physician's Desk Reference (electronic version), MICROMEDEX, Inc, Englewood, Colorado, 1998.
23. Kollef MH, Levy NT, Ahrens TS, Schaiff R, Prentice D, Sherman G. The use of continuous i.v. sedation is associated with prolongation of mechanical ventilation. Chest 1998; 114:541–548.
24. Malacrida R, Fritz ME, Suter P, et al. Pharmacokinetics of midazolam administered by continuous infusion to intensive care patients. Crit Care Med 1992; 20:1123.
25. Pohlman AS, Simpson KP, Hall JB. Continuous intravenous infusions of lorazepam versus midazolam for sedation during mechanical ventilatory support: a prospective, randomized study. Crit Care Med 1994; 22:1241–1247.
26. Carrasco G, Milina R, Costa J, Soler JM, Cabre L. Propofol vs. midazolam in short-, medium-, and long-term sedation of critically ill patients: a cost-benefit analysis. Chest 1993; 103:557–564.
27. Kress JP, Pohlman AS, O'Connor MF, Hall JB. Daily interruption of sedative infusions in critically ill patients undergoing mechanical ventilation. N Engl J Med 2000; 342:1471–1477.
28. Tayar J, Jabbour G, Saggi SJ. Severe hyperosmolar metabolic acidosis due to a large dose of intravenous lorazepam. N Engl J Med 2002; 346:1253–1254.
29. Crawley MJ. Short-term lorazepam infusion and concern for propylene glycol toxicity: case report and review. Pharmacotherapy 2001; 21:1140–1144.
30. Olkkola KT, Ahonen J, Neuvonen PJ. The effect of the systemic antimycotics, itraconazole and fluconazole, on the pharmacokinetics and pharmacodynamics of intravenous and oral midazolam. Anesth Analg 1996; 82:511–516.
31. Ahonen J, Olkkola KT, Salmenpera M, et al. Effect of diltiazem on midazolam and alfentanil disposition in patients undergoing coronary artery bypass grafting. Anesthesiology 1996; 85:1246–1252.
32. Olkkola KT, Aranko K, Luurila H, et al. A potentially hazardous interaction between erythromycin and midazolam. Clin Pharmacol Ther 1993; 53:298–305.
33. Gorski JC, Jones DR, Haehner-Daniels BD, et al. The contribution of intestinal and hepatic CYP3A to the interaction between midazolam and clarithromycin. Clin Pharmacol Ther 1998; 64:133–143.
34. Bailie GR, Cockshott ID, Douglas EJ, et al. Pharmacokinetics of propofol during and after long-term continuous infusion for maintenance of sedation in ICU patients. Br J Anaesth 1992; 68:486–491.
35. Product Information: Diprivan(R), propofol. AstraZeneca Pharmaceuticals, Wilmington, DE (PI revised 8/99) reviewed 5/2000.
36. Jacobi J, Fraser GL, Coursin DB, Riker RR, Fontaine D, Wittbrodt ET, Chalfin DB, Masica MF, Bjerke S, Coplin WM, Crippen DW, Fuchs BD, Kelleher RM, Marik PE, Nasraway SA Jr, Murray MJ, Peruzzi WT, Lumb PD. Clinical practice guidelines for the sustained use of sedatives and analgesics in the critically ill adult. Crit Care Med 2002; 30:119–141.

37. Hug CC Jr, McLeskey CH, Nahrwold ML, et al. Hemodynamic effects of propofol: data from over 25,000 patients. Anesth Analg 1993; 77:S21–S29.
38. Sanchez-Izquierdo-Riera JA, Caballero-Cubedo RE, Perez-Vela JL, et al. Propofol versus midazolam: safety and efficacy for sedating the severe trauma patient. Anest Analg 1998; 86:1219–1224.
39. Micromedex® Healthcare Series, Thomson Micrometex, Greenwood Village, Colorado (Edition express 12/2004).
40. Wilt JL, Minnema AM, Johnson RF, et al. *Torsades de pointes* associated with the use of intravenous haloperidol. Ann Inten Med 1993; 119:391–394.
41. Hunt N, Stern TA. The association between intravenous haloperidol and *torsades de pointes*. Psychosomatics 1995; 36:541–549.
42. Sharma ND, Rosman HS, Padhi D, et al. *Torsades de pointes* associated with intravenous haloperidol in critically ill patients. Am J Cardiol 1998; 81:238–240.
43. Portenoy RK, Foley KM, Stulman J, et al. Plasma morphine and morphine-6-glucuronide during chronic morphine therapy for cancer pain: plasma profiles, steady-state concentrations and the consequences of renal failure. Pain 1991; 47:13–19.
44. Nilsson C, Rosberg B. Recurrence of respiratory depression following neurolept analgesia. Acta Anaesthesiol Scand 1982; 26(3):240–241.
45. Parker RK, Holtmann B, Smith I, et al. Use of ketorolac after lower abdominal surgery. Anesthesiology 1994; 80:6–12.
46. Bombardier C, Laine L, Reicin A, et al. Comparison of upper gastrointestinal toxicity of rofecoxib and naproxen in patients with rheumatoid arthritis. N Engl J Med 2000; 343:1520–1528.

51
Anaphylaxis

Paul Druck
VA Medical Center, Minneapolis, Minnesota, USA

DEFINITIONS

Anaphylaxis, literally "reversal of protection," refers to an unpredictable, rapid, generalized, life-threatening reaction caused by exposure to an antigen to which the individual had been previously sensitized (Box 1). *Anaphylactoid reactions* are clinically similar but are not antigen–IgE mediated and do not require prior sensitization. *Idiopathic anaphylactic reactions* occur without an identifiable pharmcologic or physical stimulus. The more general term *allergic reaction* includes anaphylactic and anaphylactoid reactions, as well as less dramatic, localized responses such as urticaria and isolated bronchospasm. The term "anaphylaxis" will be used generically in this chapter to encompass all anaphylactic and anaphylactoid reactions, unless otherwise specified.

EPIDEMIOLOGY

Anaphylaxis is estimated to occur in 1 of 2700 hospital admissions (1), but the true incidence may be obscured by misdiagnosis. The two most common inciting agents, beta-lactam antibiotics and iodinated radiocontrast material (RCM), are each estimated to cause 500 deaths per year; iatrogenic anaphylaxis may thus account for more than 1000 deaths annually (1–3). In contrast, only 60–80 deaths are attributed to insect- or snake-venom-induced anaphylaxis each year (4).

No well-established risk factors for anaphylaxis exist other than a prior response to the agent in question. A history of atopy (a genetic predisposition to immediate hypersensitivity reactions, present in 10% of the population and typically manifest as allergic rhinitis, allergic asthma, or allergic dermatitis) does not clearly confer greater risk (5). However, some retrospective reviews have noted an increased incidence of idiopathic (6,7) and RCM-induced anaphylaxis (8) in patients with allergic asthma or atopy. Reexposure to inciting agents does not invariably cause repeat anaphylaxis. The risk is only 10–20% with penicillin (6) and 17–35% for iodinated RCM (9). However, these observations may reflect historical and diagnostic inaccuracy.

Box 1 Common Agents Capable of Causing Anaphylactic and Anaphylactoid Reactions

Antibiotics (especially beta-lactams and sulfa drugs)	Progesterone
	Protamine
Iodinated RCM	Quinidine
Latex rubber	Thiopental
Blood and plasma products	Thiazides
Peptide hormones and drugs [e.g., nonhuman insulin, pancreatic enzymes, streptokinase, Chymopapain (for discolysis)]	Seminal proteins
	Parenteral steroids
	Vitamin K (via IV route)
	Parasite-derived antigens (e.g., *Echinococcus*)
Local anesthetics	
Neuromuscular relaxing agents	Dialysis or pump oxygenator membranes
Opiates, salicylates, and NSAIDs	
Antineoplastic chemotherapeutic agents	Foods [especially seafood, milk and egg proteins, wheat, legumes (peanuts, soybeans), sunflower seeds, mangoes]
Complex polysaccharides (e.g., plasma expanders, iron–dextran complex)	
Acetylcysteine	Food and wine additives (especially sulfites, benzoates)
Albuterol	
Chlorpropamide	Insect and snake venoms
Ethylene oxide	Pollen, mold, animal dander
Fluorescein	Anaphylactoid syndrome of pregnancy ("amniotic fluid embolus")
Hydralazine	
Hydrocortisone	Vigorous exercise
Mannitol	Exposure to cold

INCITING AGENTS

By far the most common in-hospital causes of anaphylaxis are beta-lactam antibiotics (75% of reported cases) and iodinated radiocontrast dyes (1,3). The reported incidence of penicillin-related anaphylaxis ranges from 1 in 2500 to 1 in 25,000 courses, with a fatality rate of 1 per 100,000 courses (6,10). Of the newer penicillins, the monobactams (e.g., aztreonam) have demonstrated negligible cross-reactivity with older penicillins, whereas the carbipenims (e.g., imipenem) have shown significant cross-reactivity and should be avoided in penicillin-sensitive patients (6,11,12). Estimates of the cross-reactivity between penicillins and cephalosporins vary widely; 15% is a widely quoted but poorly documented figure. If minor reactions are excluded, most studies have demonstrated a very low incidence of cross-reactivity. Generally, cephalosporins exhibit less cross-reactivity among themselves than do the penicillins.

Because antibiotic metabolites are often responsible for allergic reactions, intradermal skin testing with the parent antibiotic in question is often falsely negative. If the clinical situation demands a potentially reactive antibiotic and time permits, consultation with allergy/immunology personnel for skin testing with a full panel of antibiotic "determinants" may offer a higher degree of test sensitivity (13).

Iodine-containing RCM causes adverse reactions in 4–12% of exposures, severe reactions in 1–2%, and fatal reactions in 0.002–0.009% (8,9,14). Nonionic contrast agents cause fewer adverse reactions overall than the older ionic media, but similar numbers of severe or fatal reactions (15,16). Iodinated contrast material reactions appear to be anaphylactoid (non-IgE dependent) in most cases; therefore, prior exposure is not a necessary precondition for the reaction. Evidence suggests that true anaphylactic reactions have very rarely occurred (17,18). Magnetic resonance imaging contrast media (chelated gadolinium preparations are the most common class in current use in the United States) have been reported to cause hives in 0.2–2% of cases (often with delayed presentation), but severe reactions have been extremely rare (19).

Latex allergy is emerging as a significant problem among both patients and health-care workers. A sensitivity rate between 10% and 17% among health-care workers, depending on testing methodology, has been noted, while latex allergy is present in fewer than 1% of the general population (20). Latex allergy is a true IgE-mediated reaction to various organic compounds that contaminate the plant-derived rubber polymer; it is not seen with synthetic rubber. Along with a history of atopy and hand dermatitis, frequency and intensity of exposure appear to be significant risk factors (21,22).

Other significant inciting agents include non-beta-lactam antiobiotics, peptide hormones (e.g., insulin, growth hormone), streptokinase, chymopapain, blood products and antisera, opiates, salicylates, nonsteroidal anti-inflammatory drugs (NSAIDs), neuromuscular blockers, barbiturates, some complex polysaccharides (e.g., plasma expanders, iron–dextran), and intravenous vitamin K (23). Ironically, reactions have been noted to certain parenteral steroid preparations and to albuterol, both potentially useful in the treatment of anaphylaxis. Foods (including food handled by latex-glove-wearing preparers and consumed by latex-allergic patients), food additives, and Hymenoptera stings (bees, wasps) may affect hospitalized patients as well. Nonpharmacologic stimuli, such as cold exposure and exercise, may induce anaphylactoid reactions (2,5,7,24).

Exposure to antigens may be effective by a variety of routes—intravenous, intramuscular, transcutaneous, or transmucosal (gastrointestinal, respiratory, genitourinary, or conjunctival). Prior exposure (sensitization) is necessary for true anaphylaxis but may not have been apparent. Anaphylactoid reactions may occur on the first exposure (e.g., contrast dyes, salicylates, opiates, NSAIDs) (Box 1).

PATHOPHYSIOLOGY

Mediators of Anaphylaxis

True anaphylaxis is initiated when antigen binds to membrane-bound IgE on circulating basophils and connective tissue mast cells. Stimulated cells release preformed, granule-stored histamine and eosinophil chemotactic factor (ECF-α). These cells then rapidly synthesize and release arachidonic acid metabolites such as leukotrienes B4, C4, D4, and E4 (slow-reacting substance of anaphylaxis, SRS-A) and prostaglandins (notably PGD2, PGE2, and PGF2α) as well as platelet-activating factor (PAF), heparin, chondroitin sulfate, and neutral proteases (chymase, tryptase). These primary mediators act on target tissues to produce the characteristic symptom complex of anaphylaxis and to stimulate release of secondary mediators such as lymphokines, interleukin-1, lysosomal enzymes, activated complement C3a, C5a (anaphylatoxins), activated coagulation and fibrinolytic factors, and kinins. Endogenous catecholamines (tertiary mediators?) may be released in response to developing physiologic derangements. Additional substances that may limit the response are released by migrating eosinophils and include histaminase, phospholipase D (inactivates PAF), aryl sulfatase B (inactivates leukotrienes), and membrane-stabilizing prostaglandins, which may prevent further mast cell degranulation (2,5,24).

Anaphylactoid reactions are not initiated by IgE–antigen binding; the agent in question acts on basophils and mast cells either directly or through activated intermediates such as complement, kallikrein, or plasmin. A syndrome clinically indistinguishable from true anaphylaxis is then produced by the similar spectrum of released mediators (2,24).

Idiopathic anaphylaxis may be initiated by the spontaneous release of histamine-releasing factor that is produced by neutrophils, lymphocytes, monocytes, and platelets. Elevated plasma and urine histamine levels have been documented during episodes, a finding that suggests typical mediators are involved (7).

Effects of the Principal Mediators

The H-1 receptor effects of histamine include vasodilation, increased capillary permeability, bronchial smooth muscle contraction, increased pulmonary secretion, and coronary vasoconstriction. H-2 receptor effects include increased gastric secretion and positive cardiac inotropy and chronotropy (2,9,24–27). The leukotrienes are by far the most potent bronchoconstrictors elaborated during anaphylaxis. Additional actions include increased pulmonary secretion, increased microvascular permeability, neutrophil chemotaxis, enhanced lysosomal enzyme release, coronary vasoconstriction, and depression of myocardial contractility (2). The prostaglandins have complex and often opposing effects. PGD2 and PGF2α cause bronchoconstriction, whereas PGE2 causes bronchorelaxation. The net effect is bronchospasm. Pulmonary hypertension, increased microvascular permeability, and vasodilation also are attributed to the prostaglandins (2). Activated kinins (especially bradykinin) have been implicated in vasodilation, increased microvascular permeability, and smooth muscle contraction as well. Activated complement also can cause increased capillary permeability and smooth muscle contraction, as well as stimulate chemotaxis and additional mediator release from mast cells and basophils (2,24). A significant negative inotrope, PAF decreases myocardial blood flow and may depress atrioventricular conduction (28).

CLINICAL MANIFESTATIONS

Manifestations of anaphylaxis may occur within seconds of exposure but generally occur within 15 min. In rare instances, the reaction is delayed for ≥ 1 h, particularly after oral or cutaneous exposure. In a significant proportion of cases, the reaction is biphasic or protracted (1). The cardinal manifestations of anaphylaxis are respiratory failure secondary to upper or lower airway obstruction, profound cardiovascular collapse (shock), and generalized cutaneous reactions (Box 2). Of patients dying from anaphylaxis, 70% succumb to respiratory complications and 24% to cardiovascular compromise (4).

Respiratory Effects

Nasal congestion, dysphonia, lingual or buccal swelling, a sensation of a "lump" in the throat, and dyspnea herald the onset of upper airway obstruction, which can progress

Box 2 Signs and Symptoms of Anaphylaxis

Respiratory
Stridor
Dysphonia
Lump in throat sensation
Swelling of tongue, buccal mucosa
Dyspnea, tightness in chest
Wheezing
Cyanosis
If already receiving mechanical ventilation: increased airway pressure, increased peak/plateau pressure gradient, and positive-end-expiratory pressure ("auto-PEEP")

Cardiovascular
Hypotension
Tachycardia
Tachyarrhythmias and conduction disturbances
Myocardial ischemia

If pulmonary artery catheter in place: decreased cardiac filling pressures, decreased systemic vascular resistance, variable changes in cardiac output (usually increased) and pulmonary artery pressures

Cutaneous
Urticaria
Angioedema
Pruritus
Flushing
Pilomotor erection
Diaphoresis

Miscellaneous
Anxiety
Headache
Mental status changes (confusion to syncope)
Seizures
Gastrointestinal and urinary-tract hypermotility
Uterine cramps

rapidly. Intense edema of oropharyngeal and glottic structures causing upper airway obstruction may be the most common cause of death (4,29).

Lower airway obstruction is primarily due to bronchospasm, perhaps aggravated by increased pulmonary secretions and small airway edema. Alveolar pulmonary edema is uncommon in the absence of *excessive* fluid resuscitation. Wheezing, coughing, dyspnea, and a sensation of tightness in the chest are early symptoms that can worsen rapidly.

Cardiovascular Effects

Hypotension is initially due to vasodilation, but is soon complicated by a reduction in circulating plasma volume as a result of increased capillary permeability. Decreased myocardial contractility and pulmonary hypertension may interfere with cardiac compensation. Myocardial ischemia, a result of coronary vasoconstriction, arterial hypotension, tachycardia, and hypoxia, can complicate both the diagnosis and the course of the episode. If a pulmonary artery catheter is in place, low cardiac filling pressures and low systemic vascular resistance are observed. Cardiac output may be elevated initially and then decrease as shock and ischemia supervene. Atrial and ventricular dysrhythmias and conduction disturbances may be observed. The most common electrocardiogram (ECG) abnormalities are sinus tachycardia, atrial fibrillation, ST–T wave changes consistent with ischemia, and ectopy. These ECG abnormalities may be caused or exacerbated by catecholamine treatment (see below) (2,5,24,30).

Mucocutaneous Manifestations

Mucocutaneous effects are common but not invariable. They may include pruritus, urticaria (hives: superficial, well-circumscribed, blanched, pruritic wheals with raised erythematous borders), angioedema (localized, deep cutaneous, and subcutaneous nonpitting edema), flushing, conjunctival edema, pilomotor erection, diaphoresis, and cyanosis (2,5).

Miscellaneous Manifestations

Other signs and symptoms may include severe anxiety, headache, mental status changes ranging from confusion to syncope, seizures, nausea, vomiting, diarrhea, colicky abdominal pain, urinary urgency, and uterine cramps (2,5).

TREATMENT

The occurrence of characteristic skin lesions with sudden hypotension and respiratory distress in a previously healthy individual should suggest anaphylaxis. The diagnosis may not be obvious in critically ill patients with cardiorespiratory instability, particularly if the syndrome is incomplete or if no temporal relation to administration of a suspicious agent is clear. The differential diagnosis is extensive (Box 3), but the most common alternatives are airway obstruction (secondary to asthma, chronic obstructive pulmonary disease, or mechanical obstruction), congestive heart failure, or hypovolemic or septic shock.

Initial Steps and Basic Support

With onset of symptoms, the patient should be returned to bed, given humidified oxygen by mask for respiratory distress, and placed in a supine position. Trendelenburg position may be used if significant hypotension exists. Continuous ECG and vital sign monitoring are essential; pulse oximetry is desirable. A medical, drug, and allergy history should be obtained, and adequate intravenous (IV) access should be assured. The ongoing administration of blood products or new drugs should be stopped. Arterial blood gases should be

Box 3 Differential Diagnosis of Anaphylaxis

Exacerbation of bronchospastic disease (asthma, chronic obstructive pulmonary disease)
Aspiration of foreign body
Hyperventilation syndrome
Globus hystericus
Vasovagal syncope
Septic or hypovolemic shock
Myocardial infarction, particularly if complicated by pulmonary edema or cardiogenic shock
Pulmonary embolus
Drug overdose
Hypoglycemia
Addisonian crisis
Seizure
Carcinoid syndrome
Pheochromocytoma
Systemic mastocytosis
Hereditary angioedema

Treatment of Respiratory Compromise

Upper Airway Obstruction

A patient showing signs of impending upper airway obstruction requires early endotracheal intubation once an upper airway foreign body has been ruled out. If advanced glottic edema has made intubation impossible, prolonged attempts at intubation or trials of aerosolized epinephrine should be abandoned and cricothyrotomy performed.

Bronchospasm

If anaphylaxis is suspected, epinephrine is the first-line therapy and may be given subcutaneously for mild reactions and intravenously for severe reactions, particularly if hypotension is compromising absorption (Box 4). If IV access is unavailable, intratracheal administration is effective (2,31). Doses may be repeated at 5–10 min intervals, but if frequent redosing is necessary to maintain a response, continuous infusion

Box 4 Pharmacologic Therapy of Anaphylaxis

Bronchospasm
Epinephrine: 4–10 μg/kg IM or SC q10 min if patient is stable (1:1000 @ 0.004–0.01 mL/kg or 1:100,000 10 mL slow IV injection if patient is unstable or hypotensive); administer intratracheally if IV access unavailable

If frequent redosing is necessary
Epinephrine: 1–4 μg/min continuous infusion

If ineffective
Metaproterenol: 5% solution, 0.2–0.5 mL + 2.5 mL normal saline via nebulizer or inhalation aerosol, two to three inhalations, or
Albuterol: 0.5% solution 0.5 mL + 2.5 mL normal saline via nebulizer or inhalation aerosol, two inhalations

Hypotension
Fluid resuscitation (colloid preferred), 10 mL/kg. Further fluid resuscitation as needed, or guided by pulmonary capillary wedge pressures, if appropriate

If ineffective
Epinephrine: 1–4 μg/min continuous infusion, titrate to mean arterial pressure ≥60 mm Hg

If ineffective, or patient has excessive tachycardia or myocardial ischemia
Phenylephrine: 20 μg/min continuous infusion, titrate upwards as needed to MAP ≥60 mm Hg, or
Norepinephrine: 1–4 μg/min continuous infusion, titrate to mean arterial pressure ≥60 mm Hg, or
Dopamine: 5 μg/kg per min continuous infusion, titrate upwards to mean arterial pressure ≥60 mm Hg

For refractory hypotension, consider
Glucagon: 1 mg IV bolus followed by continuous infusion at 5–15 μg/min
Diphenhydramine: 25–50 mg IV, or
Promethazine: 12.5–25 mg IV
Cimetidine: 300 mg IV

Ancillary therapy to shorten protracted reactions or limit relapses
Hydrocortisone: 100–200 mg IV q4–6 h, or
Prednisone: 25–50 mg PO QD

with intra-arterial pressure monitoring is indicated (2,32). If the response to epinephrine is inadequate, inhaled bronchodilators may be added. Methylxanthines such as aminophylline and theophylline have traditionally been advocated as adjunctive measures, but no evidence from controlled human trials indicates efficacy beyond that seen with beta-agonists (33). As for the safety of the combination of beta-agonists and methylxanthines, two small reviews failed to demonstrate increased adverse effects (34,35).

Patients receiving beta-blockers may not respond to epinephrine (32) and may require prompt doses of non-beta-agonist bronchodilators. If these are ineffective, a pure beta-agonist such as isoproterenol in sufficiently high doses may overcome the beta-blockade without incidental alpha side effects. The only contraindication to epinephrine or other beta-agonists is idiopathic hypertrophic subaortic stenosis. If the response, as assessed by clinical judgment, vital signs, and arterial blood gases, remains inadequate, intubation and mechanical ventilation are indicated. Respiratory rate, tidal volume, and inspiratory flow rate should be adjusted to provide adequate ventilation without excessive airway pressures (24). Steroids have no role in initial management (5), but a patient receiving long-term steroid therapy may require stress supplementation.

Hemodynamic Compromise

Hypotension should be treated with recumbency, fluid resuscitation, and, if necessary, pressors (Box 4). Resuscitation with colloid rather than crystalloid is recommended for the advantages of longer duration of action and lower effective volume (2). Failure to respond to judicious fluid loading, particularly in a patient with underlying cardiac disease, necessitates measuring cardiac filling pressures and cardiac performance with a pulmonary artery catheter. Primary myocardial dysfunction, as a result of ischemia or the negative inotropic effects of anaphylactic mediators, should be considered. Persistent hypotension (mean arterial pressure <60 mm Hg) requires the addition of pressors. If epinephrine administered for bronchospasm produces a favorable pressure response, continuous einephrine infusion with arterial pressure monitoring should be initiated. If epinephrine is ineffective or produces excessive tachycardia, or if the patient is receiving beta-blocking agents, phenylephrine or norepinephrine are alternatives (2,24). Glucagon, a nonadrenergic inotrope, may also be useful in the face of adrenergic blockade (2,5). Dopamine has been less effective for severe hypotension in this condition (24). Finally, if hypotension is unremitting (usually because of profound peripheral vascular collapse), cimetidine may be added to help oppose peripheral H-2-receptor-mediated vasodilation (2,36).

Adjunctive Measures and the Recovery Phase

Additional measures that may help limit the extent or duration of reaction, but are not considered urgent or first-line therapy, are parenteral antihistamines such as diphenhydramine, local subcutaneous injection of epinephrine at the antigen introduction site, or the intermittent application of a tourniquet at venous occlusion pressure to limit antigen absorption from an injection site (5,24).

Once the patient is stabilized, the principal considerations are preventing relapse (late-phase reaction), identifying the causative agent, and excluding complications such as myocardial infarction, pneumothorax, and aspiration. Late-phase reactions can be prevented by giving high-dose glucocorticoids for 24 h, followed by rapid taper. Patients should remain under observation for at least 24 h (1,5).

PREVENTION

Careful attention to patients' adverse reaction histories is critical to avoiding future reactions. Similarly, suspected anaphylactic reactions must be documented in the patient's medical record to prevent future exposures. Occasionally, intentional use of a known or suspected causative agent is strongly indicated. The two most common scenarios and their management are iodine-containing RCM and beta-lactam antibiotics.

Iodine-Containing RCM

New imaging modalities frequently offer alternatives to iodine-containing contrast studies in patients suspected of being radiocontrast-sensitive, i.e., those with a history of major anaphylactic reactions, unexplained hypotension, wheezing, oropharyngeal–laryngeal edema, angioedema, urticaria on previous exposure, or known iodine or seafood allergies. In those rare instances when the benefit is thought to outweigh the risk, pretreatment regimens (Box 5) can reduce the risk of recurrent anaphylaxis from the reported range of 17–35% to as low as 3% (vs. 1–2% for the general population) (37). One study observed an *increased* incidence of major reactions when an H-2 receptor antagonist was added to the pretreatment protocol. In view of this preliminary information, these agents should not be used prophylactically. It may be prudent to withold doses of H-2 receptor blockers from patients who are chronically receiving such drugs until the study is completed uneventfully (9).

Beta-Lactam Antibiotics

In those unusual circumstances when microbiologic sensitivity testing offers no alternative to a penicillin-family antibiotic for a life-threatening infection, desensitization protocols on the basis of lower antigenicity of enterally absorbed penicillins (38–40) may be followed (Box 6).

Box 5 Pretreatment Protocol: Emergency Administration of Radiocontrast Media in High-Risk Patients

---
Hydrocortisone: 100–200 mg IV q4 h until procedure completed (first dose administered at least 1 h before procedure)

Diphenhydramine: 50 mg IV 1 h before procedure

Ephedrine (optional): 25 mg PO 1 h before procedure; omit this step for patients with history of ischemic heart disease, history of tachyarrhythmias, significant hypertension, suspected coexistence of aortic dissection

Preliminary evidence suggests increased incidence of reactions with H-2 receptor antagonists; there may be potential benefit to holding last dose of a regularly scheduled H-2 blocker before procedure if risk does not outweigh potential benefit

Box 6 Beta-Lactam Antibiotic Desensitization

Contraindicated in patients with history of Stevens–Johnson syndrome or exfoliative dermatitis
Perform in consultation with allergy/immunology specialists
Obtain informed consent
Perform in monitored setting with IV access established and all materials necessary to treat full-scale anaphylaxis available
Antiallergic premedication is controversial
Hold beta-blockers if clinically advisable
 	
Specific procedures
Able to take PO: 100 U penicillin (or equivalent dose of other antibiotic)
   Administer successive double doses q15 min until 400,000 U achieved
      For mild cutaneous reaction, repeat dose
	For marked reaction, repeat lower dose after patient stabilizes
	   Administer 200,000, 400,000, 800,000, then 1,000,000 U IV at 15 min intervals, as tolerated
	Unable to take PO
	   Prepare series of 10-fold dilutions of antibiotic and determine lowest reactive concentration on scratch test (<4 mm wheal)
	   Administer 0.02 mL intradermally of next lower concentration; if no reaction occurs, proceed
	   Administer successive doubled doses sc q20 min until therapeutic concentration achieved; repeat dose if reaction occurs
	   Repeat challenge with therapeutic concentration IM, then IV

Once full therapy has begun, avoid lapses in treatment schedule; resensitization may occur rapidly.

SUMMARY

- Anaphylaxis is an unpredictable, rapidly progressive, life-threatening reaction that may occur without a clear allergic history.
- Common inciting agents are antibiotics (especially beta-lactams and sulfas), RCM, latex, foods, and insect venoms.
- Death may occur from upper airway edema and obstruction, intractable bronchospasm, or cardiovascular collapse.
- Associated clinical features are pruritus, urticaria, angioedema, tachyarrhythmias, cardiac conduction disturbances, and mental status changes.
- The differential diagnosis, depending on presenting features, includes exacerbation of a bronchospastic condition, aspiration of foreign body, septic or hypovolemic shock, myocardial infarction (especially if complicated by pulmonary edema or shock), pulmonary embolus, certain drug overdoses, and carcinoid syndrome.
- Bronchospasm is treated with epinephrine, inhaled bronchodilators, and, if necessary, mechanical ventilation. The role of methylxanthines is not well established.
- Hypotension is treated with fluid (preferably colloid) resuscitation, and, if necessary, pressor agents and inotropes. Patients receiving beta-blockers may not respond to conventional doses of beta-agonists.
- Adjunctive therapy includes steroids and antihistamines (H-1 and H-2 blockers may be helpful). The responsible agent must be identified, if possible, and complications such as myocardial infarction, pneumothorax and aspiration should be excluded.
- Pretreatment protocols can reduce the likelihood and severity of reactions to known offending agents when the use of those agents is potentially life-saving.

REFERENCES

1. Stark BJ, Sullivan TJ. Biphasic and protracted anaphylaxis. J Allergy Clin Immunol 1986; 78:7683.
2. Haupt MT, Carlson RW. Anaphylactic and anaphylactoid reactions. In: Shoemaker WC, Ayres S, et al., eds. Textbook of Critical Care Medicine. Philadelphia: WB Saunders, 1989:993–1002.
3. Lasser EC, Lang J, Sovak M. Steroids: theoretical and experimental basis for utilization in prevention of contrast media reactions. Radiology 1977; 125(1):1–9.
4. Barnard JH. Studies of 400 Hymenoptera sting deaths in the United States. J Allergy Clin Immunol 1973; 52(5):259–264.
5. Bochner BS, Lichtenstein LM. Anaphylaxis. N Engl J Med 1991; 32(25):1785–1790.
6. Weiss ME, Adkinson NF. Immediate hypersensitivity reactions to penicillin and related antibiotics. Clin Allergy 1988; 18:515–540.
7. Wiggins CA, Dykewicz MS, et al. Idiopathic anaphylaxis: a review. Ann Allergy 1989; 62:1–4.
8. Ansell G, Tweedie MCK, et al. The current status of reactions to intravenous contrast media. Invest Radiol 1980; 15(6):S32–S39.
9. Greenberger PA, Patterson R, et al. Prophylaxis against repeated radiocontrast media reactions in 857 cases. Adverse experience with cimetidine and safety of β-adrenergic antagonists. Arch Int Med 1985; 145:2197–2200.
10. Idsøe O, Guthe T, et al. Nature and extent of penicillin side-reactions with particular reference to fatalities from anaphylactic shock. Bull World Health Org 1968; 38:159–188.
11. Saxon A. Immediate hypersensitivity reactions to beta-lactam antibiotics. Ann Int Med 1987; 107:204–215.
12. Saxon A. Immediate hypersensitivity reactions to beta-lactam antibiotics. Rev Infect Dis 1983; 5:S368–S378.
13. Solley GO, Gleich GL, et al. Penicillin allergy: clinical experience with a battery of skin-test reagents. J Allergy Clin Immunol 1982; 69:238–244.
14. Shehadi WH. Adverse reactions to intravascularly administered contrast media. A comprehensive study based on a prospective survey. Am J Roentgenol Radium Ther Nucl Med 1975; 124:145–152.
15. Lasser EC, Lyon SG, et al. Reports on contrast media reactions: analysis of data from reports to the U.S. Food and Drug Administration. Radiology 1997; 203:605–610.
16. Wolf GL, Arenson RL, et al. A prospective trial of ionic vs. nonionic contrast agents in routine clinical practice: comparison of adverse effects. Am J Roentgenol 1989; 152:939–944.
17. Lieberman P. Anaphylactoid reactions to radiocontrast material. Immunol Allergy Clin N Am 1992; 12(3):649–670.
18. Stellato C, de Crescenzo G, et al. Human basophil/mast cell releasability. XI. Heterogeneity of the effects of contrast media on mediator release. J Allergy Clin Immunol 1996; 97:838–850.
19. Runge VM. Safety of magnetic resonance contrast media. Topics Magn Reson Imag 2001; 12(4):309–314.
20. Liss GM, Sussman GL. Latex sensitization: occupational versus general population prevalence rates. Am J Int Med 1999; 35:196–200.
21. Brehler R. Latex allergy. Comp Ther 2002; 28(4):244–249.
22. Turjanmaa K, Mäkinen-Kiljunen S. Latex allergy: prevalence, risk factors, and cross-reactivity. Methods 2002; 27:10–14.
23. Riegert-Johnson DL, Volcheck GW. The incidence of anaphylaxis following intravenous phytonadione (vitamin K_1): a 5-year retrospective review. Ann Allergy Asthma Immunol 2002; 89:400–406.
24. Carlson RW, Bowles AL, et al. Anaphylactic, anaphylactoid, and related forms of shock. Crit Care Clin 1986; 2(2):347–372.
25. Capurro N, Levi R. The heart as a target organ in systemic allergic reactions: comparison of cardiac anaphylaxis in vivo and in vitro. Circ Res 1975; 36(4):520–528.

26. Feigen GA, Prager DJ. Experimental cardiac anaphylaxis. Am J Cardiol 1969; 24:474–491.
27. Levi R, Allan G. Histamine-mediated cardiac effects. In: Bristow MR, ed. Drg Induced Heart Disease. Amsterdam: Elsevier-North Holland Biomedical Press, 1980:377.
28. Levi R, Burke JA. Acetyl glyceryl ether phosphorylcholine (AGEPC): a putative mediator of cardiac anaphylaxis in the guinea pig. Circ Res 1984; 54(2):117–124.
29. Delage C, Irey NS. Anaphylactic deaths: a clinicopathologic study of 43 cases. J Forensic Sci 1972; 17(4):525–540.
30. Moss J, Fahmy NR, et al. Hormonal and hemodynamic profile of an anaphylactic reaction in man. Circulation 1981; 63(1):210–213.
31. Heilborn H, Hjemdahl P, et al. Comparison of subcutaneous injection and high-dose inhalation of epinephrine—implications for self-treatment to prevent anaphylaxis. J Allergy Clin Immunol 1986; 78:1174–1179.
32. Barach EM, Nowak RM, et al. Epinephrine for treatment of anaphylactic shock. J Am Med Assoc 1984; 251(16):2118–2122.
33. Ernst ME, Graber MA. Methylxanthine use in anaphylaxis: what does the evidence tell us? Ann Pharmacother 1999; 33:1001–1004.
34. Josephson GW, Kennedy HL, et al. Cardiac dysrrhythmias during the treatment of acute asthma. Chest 1980; 78:429–435.
35. Fisher MM, Baldo BA. Acute anaphylactic reactions. Med J Aust 1988; 149:34–38.
36. Mayumi H, Kimura S, et al. Intravenous cimetidine as an effective treatment for systemic anaphylaxis and acute allergic skin reactions. Ann Allergy 1987; 58:447–450.
37. Greenberger PA, Halwig JM, et al. Emergency administration of radiocontrast media in high-risk patients. J Allergy Clin Immunol 1986; 77:630–634.
38. Sogn DD. Prevention of allergic reactions to penicillin. J Allergy Clin Immunol 1986; 78:1051–1052.
39. Sullivan TJ, Yecies LD, et al. Desensitization of patients allergic to penicillin using orally administered beta-lactam antibiotics. J Allergy Clin Immunol 1982; 69(3):275–282.
40. Wendel GD, Stark BJ, et al. Penicillin allergy and desensitization in serious infections during pregnancy. N Engl J Med 1985; 312(19):1229–1232.

dd
K. Coagulation and Transfusion

52
Disorders of Coagulation

Aneel A. Ashrani and Nigel S. Key
University of Minnesota, Minneapolis, Minnesota, USA

INTRODUCTION

Timely recognition and management of hemorrhage and thrombosis is fundamental to surgical critical care. Bleeding is a potential complication of almost every surgical procedure, and when appropriately anticipated, it can be managed with relative ease. The risk of venous thromboembolism is high postsurgery, but frequently can be reduced dramatically with appropriate prophylactic measures. This chapter reviews aspects of the pathophysiology of bleeding and thrombosis that are important to the critical care surgeon. By way of definition, the term "hemostasis" is used in reference to the normal physiologic (and usually desirable) blood clotting response to breaching of blood vessel integrity. Thrombosis is a term that refers to the pathologic (and therefore undesirable) response of the coagulation system to some form of insult, whether recognized or not.

PHYSIOLOGY OF HEMOSTASIS

Platelets, the blood vessel wall, and coagulation proteins all play a unique and cooperative role in achieving hemostasis. Incisional or traumatic disruption of the blood vessel wall exposes the vascular subintimal tissue and activates a sequence of catalytic events that culminates in clot formation. A severe abnormality of one component or a modest abnormality of two or more of these components may result in a hemostatic disorder postoperatively.

Role of Platelets

Primary hemostasis is initiated when circulating platelets are exposed to the vascular subendothelium and adhere specifically to it and its rich content of procoagulant proteins, such as von Willebrand factor, collagen, and fibronectin. Once adherent, platelets undergo an energy dependent shape change and release performed substances that serve several functions:

1. Vasoconstriction, mediated by thromboxane A_2, epinephrine, and serotonin, assists in the control of local hemorrhage.
2. Exposure of phosphatidyl serine on the platelet surface provides a template for local assembly of coagulation protein enzymatic complexes for further hemostatic events (see below).
3. Initiation of blood vessel wall repair by platelet-derived growth factor and angiogenic factors.

More platelets are recruited to the site of injury, and they aggregate to form a platelet plug, which is then stabilized by the insoluble fibrin meshwork (for details, see Ref. 1).

Role of the Coagulation Proteins: Secondary Hemostasis

The chief function of the coagulation pathway is to form a hemostatic plug, whereby soluble fibrinogen is converted to insoluble fibrin at the site of the injured vessel wall. Earlier "cascade" or "waterfall" theories of coagulation separated the coagulation pathway into "intrinsic" (contact pathway) and "extrinsic" [tissue factor (TF) pathway] systems. Evidence from the last two decades indicates with increasing clarity that, in vivo, probably only one pathway exists by which coagulation is initiated, namely the TF pathway. Evidence supports the concept that coagulation is initiated by the formation of a complex between TF, a protein which is expressed on certain cell surfaces (see below), and circulating activated factor VII (fVIIa) (Fig. 1).

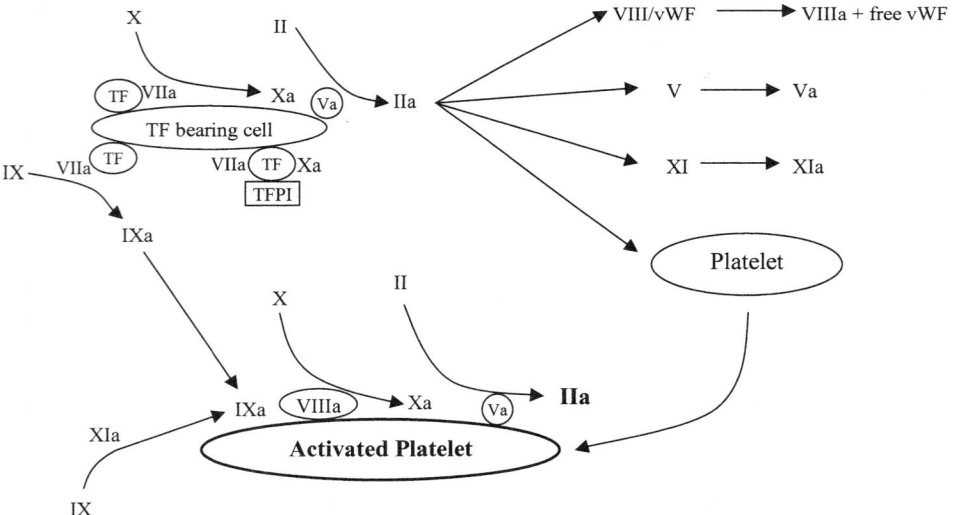

Figure 1 Cell-based model of coagulation cascade. The coagulation pathway is triggered by the TF/fVIIa complex, leading to the generation of sufficient amount of thrombin to activate platelets, factors V, VIII, and XI, before it is shut down by TFPI. The fVIIIa/fIXa complex then activates fX on the activated platelet surface, leading to a further "full thrombin burst." *Source*: Adapted from Hoffman, et al. Seminars in Hematology 2001; 38:4(suppl 12):6–9.

In order to preserve the essential hemostatic function of TF, while avoiding unwanted thrombosis, it is generally believed that TF is not normally exposed to the circulating blood, but is found on the surface of cells located in the outermost layers of vessel walls. Following injury to a vessel wall, TF is exposed to the circulating blood and forms complexes with fVIIa. Of the total factor VII protein $\sim 1\%$ normally is present in the circulation as the activated form (i.e., fVIIa). The TF–fVIIa complex activates factor X (fX), which then converts prothrombin (fII) to thrombin (fIIa). Thrombin then performs an amplification function by activating factors VIII and V, as well as platelets accumulated at the site of injury. This amplification phase is often referred to as the propagation phase of coagulation. These activated platelets expose phosphatidyl serine on their surfaces, thereby forming a template for the assembly of further hemostatic enzyme complexes.

The TF–fVIIa complex also activates factor IX (fIX) when it is bound to phosphatidyl serine on activated platelets. A complex is formed between fIXa and its cofactor, fVIIIa, which in turn activates fX to fXa. fXa complexes with fVa and converts additional fII to fIIa. All these processes occur on activated platelet surfaces and result in the generation of high concentrations of thrombin (full thrombin burst) necessary for formation of a solid fibrin hemostatic plug. Thrombin also activates (1) factor XIII, which acts as a fibrin stabilizing factor, and (2) thrombin activated fibrinolysis inhibitor (TAFI), which serves to render the fibrin plug more resistant to plasmin-mediated degradation.

Various mechanisms to limit the extent of clot progression are in place. These include:

1. Tissue factor pathway inhibitor (TFPI), which binds to fXa and then inhibits the TF–fVIIa complex.
2. Activated protein C (APC), which complexes with its cofactor (protein S) on the surface of platelets and endothelial cells to proteolytically inactivate fVa and fVIIIa, thus destroying their coagulant activity. Protein C in turn is activated by the thrombin–thrombomodulin complex (thrombomodulin is expressed on endothelial cells).
3. Antithrombin III, which rapidly inhibits free thrombin, and also factors IXa, Xa, XIa, and XIIa. Its inhibitory activity is greatly accelerated by the presence of exogenous heparin or heparin-like molecules expressed on endothelial cells.
4. Heparin cofactor II, which acts as a secondary inhibitor of thrombin. This effect is enhanced in the presence of endothelial dermatan sulfate and heparin.
5. Tissue plasminogen activator (t-PA) released from the endothelial cell, which converts plasminogen to plasmin. Plasmin is responsible for fibrinolysis, which reduces the size of the clot and initiates events that lead to vascular repair.

The reader is referred to References 2 and 3 for more details on the cell-based model of hemostasis.

Role of Vascular Endothelium

As implied in the previous section, the endothelium is far from being an inert lining layer on the inner surface of blood vessels. In fact, numerous substances synthesized by the vascular endothelium play a role in hemostasis, and these roles are summarized in Table 1.

Table 1 Endothelial Cell Regulation of Coagulation

Factor	Function
von Willebrand factor	Promotes platelet adhesion
Thrombomodulin	Binds thrombin and activates protein C
PAI-1	Inhibits fibrinolysis
t-PA	Promotes fibrinolysis
Tissue factor	Initiates coagulation
PGI_2 (prostacyclin)	Impairs platelet aggregation/vasodilator
Nitric oxide	Vasodilator
Endothelins (ET 1,2,3)	Vasoconstrictors

PATHOPHYSIOLOGY OF HEMORRHAGIC AND THROMBOTIC DIATHESES

Hemostasis results from a complex interaction of platelets, coagulation factors, blood vessel walls, and the inhibitory pathways. Potential dysregulation of any of these elements, either individually or collectively, may give rise to either excessive bleeding or thrombosis in the postoperative period. These perturbations can either be hereditary or acquired. Preoperative detection of these defects is the key to minimizing potential complications. A careful history and physical examination more often than not will offer clues to a patient's bleeding or thrombotic risk.

BLEEDING DISORDERS

Identification of a bleeding diathesis may portend a significant risk of intraoperative bleeding and its attendant complications (including wound infection, joint and muscle hematomas, and pressure necrosis). A working knowledge of the fundamental components of hemostasis helps identify potential defects, including

1. defects in platelet plug formation, due either to platelet or vessel wall defects;
2. defects in formation of a stable fibrin clot; and
3. excessive degradation/fibrinolysis of the thrombus.

The best preoperative screening test for a patient's bleeding risk is a careful bleeding history, including a history of bleeding with trauma, past surgical procedures (including tonsillectomy and circumcision, if performed), and dental procedures. A predilection for excessive mucocutaneous bleeding is suggestive of a primary hemostatic disorder, including platelet deficiency or dysfunction, vascular fragility disorders, and von Willebrand disease. A tendency for soft tissue/joint bleeding is more suggestive of coagulation protein deficiencies, including hemophilia A and B. Delayed bleeding after surgical procedures and poor wound healing may be indicative of factor XIII deficiency. A list of medications the patient is taking should also be sought, as a number of commonly used drugs can inhibit platelet function (Table 2). Although the likelihood of inducing serious bleeding with the use of aspirin and other NSAIDs by themselves is relatively low, their use may magnify other hemostatic defects (e.g., von Willebrand disease, mild hemophilia, uremia, or liver disease). A detailed family history provides clues to some of the hereditary forms of bleeding disorders (Table 3).

Table 2 Drugs Inhibiting Platelet Function

Nonsteroidal anti-inflammatory drugs	Psychotropic drugs	Cardiovascular drugs
Aspirin	Tricyclic antidepressants	Nitroglycerine
Sulfinpyrazone	Imipramine	Isosorbide dinitrate
Indomethacin	Amitriptyline	Propranolol
Ibuprofen	Notriptyline	Nitroprusside
Sulindac	Phenothiazines	Nifedipine
Naproxen	Chlorpromazine	Verapamil
Phenylbutazone	Promethazine	Diltiazem
Meclofenamic acid	Trifluoperazine	Quinidine
Mefenamic acid	Anesthetics	Miscellaneous
Diflunisal	Local	Ticlopidine
Piroxicam	Lidocaine	Clopidogrel
Tolmetin	Tetracaine	Clofibrate
Beta-lactam antibiotics	Butacaine	Ketanserin
Penicillins	Cyclaine	Radiographic contrast agents
Penicillin G	Nupercaine	Renographin-76
Carbenicillin	Procaine	Renovist II
Ticarcillin	Cocaine	Conray-60
Methicillin	Plaquenil	Antihistamines
Ampicillin	General	Diphenhydramine
Nafcillin	Halothane	Chlorpheniramine
Piperacillin	Narcotics	Mepyramine
Azlocillin	Heroin	Food and food additives
Mezlocillin	Oncologic drugs	Omega-3 fatty acids
Cephalosporins	Mithramycin	Ethanol
Cephalothin	Daunorubicin	Chinese black free fungus
Moxalactam	BCNU	Onion extract
Cefoxitin	Other drugs	Ajoene (garlic component)
Cefotaxime	Antibiotics	Cumin
Cefazolin	Nitrofurantoin	Turmeric
Glycoprotein IIb/IIIa inhibitors	Drugs that increase platelet cAMP	Clove
Abciximab	Prostacyclin	
Eptifibatide	Iloprost	
Tirofiban	Dipyrimidine	
Lamifiban	Anticoagulants	
	Heparin	
	Plasminogen activators	
	Plasma expanders	
	Dextran	
	Hydroxyethyl starch (hetastarch)	

Source: Adapted from George JN, Shattil SJ. Acquired disorders of platelet dysfunction. In: Hoffman R, et al. eds. From Hematology: Basic Principles and Practice, 3d ed. Churchill: Livingstone, 2000.

In combination with a good history and physical examination, screening laboratory tests have an important role in the preoperative evaluation. Given the variety of potential hemostatic defects, no single simple screening laboratory test exists. In general, routine assays offer a limited predictive value for perioperative bleeding. In

Table 3 Some Hereditary Bleeding Disorders

Disorder	Screening laboratory abnormality
Hemophilia A (factor VIII deficiency)	Prolonged PTT
Hemophilia B (factor IX deficiency)	Prolonged PTT
von Willebrand disease	Prolonged PFA-100 closure time, prolonged bleeding time, ±prolonged PTT
Hereditary hemorrhagic telangiectasia (Osler–Rendu–Weber syndrome)	None
Glanzmann's thrombasthenia	Prolonged PFA-100 closure time, prolonged bleeding time
Bernard Soulier syndrome	Prolonged PFA-100 closure time, prolonged bleeding time, low platelet count
Wiskott Aldrich syndrome	Prolonged PFA-100 closure time, prolonged bleeding time

patients undergoing surgical procedures with a low risk of bleeding (including surgery of nonvital organs, exposed surgical site, and limited dissection), no additional laboratory tests are required if the history is not suggestive of a bleeding tendency. For surgical procedures with moderate to high risk of bleeding (including surgery involving vital organs, deep or extensive dissection, bleeding likely to compromise surgical result, and frequent bleeding complications), screening tests may include a platelet count, platelet functional analysis with the Platelet Function Analyzer (PFA-100) collagen/epinephrine (Col/Epi) closure time, partial thromboplastin time (PTT), and international normalized ratio (INR), irrespective of bleeding history (Table 4). The bleeding time is not performed routinely for two reasons; it is very insensitive in predicting a patient's bleeding risk, and it is dependent on numerous variables. The PFA-100 device (see below) seems to offer more information on primary hemostasis (i.e., it is more sensitive and specific) than the bleeding time.

Table 4 Preoperative Screening for Bleeding Disorders

Bleeding risk	Bleeding history	Surgical procedure	Laboratory tests
Minimal	Negative	Low risk/minor (e.g., dental extraction and lymph node biopsy)	None
Moderate	Negative	Moderate risk/major (e.g., cholecystectomy, laparotomy, and bowel resection)	INR, PTT, platelet count
High	Questionable or negative	High risk (e.g., CNS surgery, cardiopulmonary bypass surgeries, and prostatectomy)	INR, PTT, platelet count, PFA-100 Col/Epi closure time
Very high	Positive	Minor or major	Same as "High" group. If screen normal, consider platelet aggregation studies, factor VIII and IX assays, TT, and screening for conditions mentioned in last column of Figure 2 (bleeding patients with normal INR and PTT)

Disorders of Coagulation

An approach to further evaluation of an abnormal coagulation profile is outlined in Figure 2. Thrombocytopenia or platelet dysfunction can lead to abnormal closure times measured by the PFA-100. A prolonged Col/Epi closure time also may be due to platelet dysfunction from aspirin ingestion. If one reading is abnormal, it should be repeated about 7 days after discontinuation of aspirin, along with the collagen/ADP (Col/ADP) closure time. Prolongation of one or the other closure times suggests an intrinsic platelet dysfunction. In patients with von Willebrand's disease, both Col/Epi and Col/ADP closure times are typically prolonged. For additional information, the reader is referred to References 4 and 5.

Preoperative and Postoperative Management of a Patient with a Hemostatic Defect

Determination of the type and severity of the hemostatic defect resulting in the hemorrhagic diathesis will direct the therapeutic approach. For example, if a specific coagulation

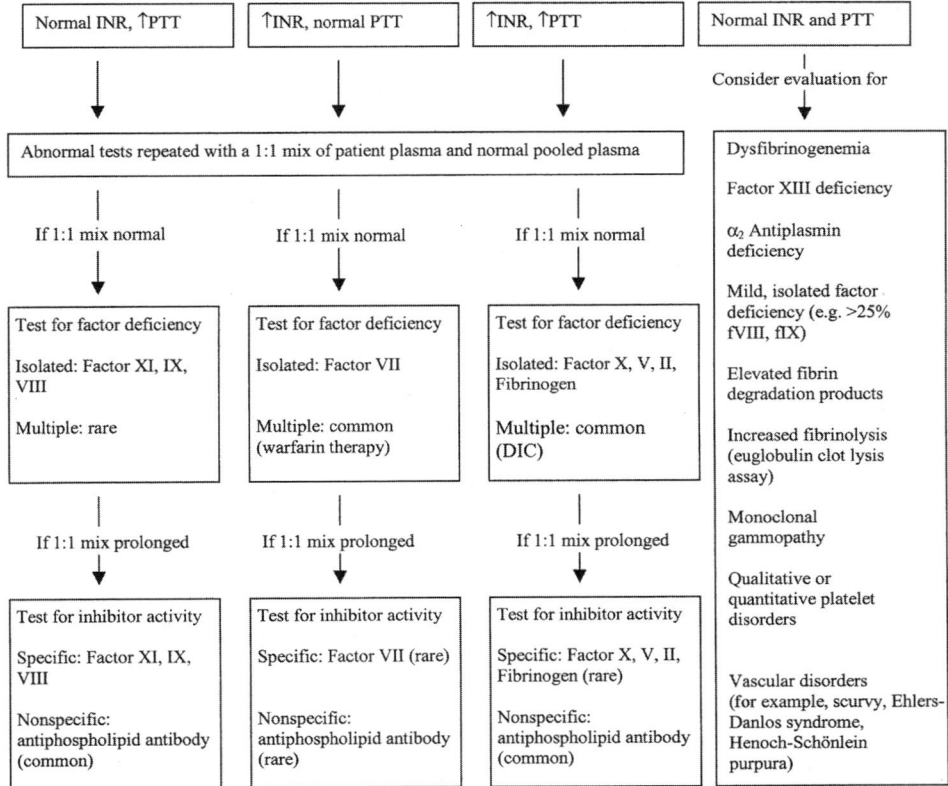

Figure 2 Approach to evaluation of the screening coagulation profile in the patient with an abnormal bleeding history. *Source*: Adapted from Santoro SA, Eby CS. Laboratory evaluation of hemostatic disorders. In: Hoffman R, et al. eds. From Hematology: Basic Principles and Practice, 3d ed. Churchill: Livingstone, 2000.

factor deficiency is identified, it can usually be corrected by replacing the deficient factor with specific factor concentrate, fresh frozen plasma, or cryoprecipitate to restore a level sufficient to achieve normal hemostasis (Table 5). For low-risk procedures, patients with mild hemophilia A (fVIII deficiency) and von Willebrand disease (types 1 and 2a) may benefit from preoperative use of deamino-8-D-arginine vasopressin (DDAVP), which promotes release of performed von Willebrand factor (vWF) and fVIII from vascular endothelial cells. Additionally, antifibrinolytic agents such as aminocaproic acid may be added postoperatively. DDAVP may also be used in patients with uremic platelet dysfunction, where it has been shown to improve hemostasis.

Intrinsic platelet functional defects (including Glanzmann's thrombasthenia, gray platelet syndrome, storage pool deficiency, Wiskott–Aldrich syndrome, and Bernard–Soulier syndrome) are managed with transfusion of platelets. Transfusion of 5 units of platelets preoperatively, with availability of an additional 5 units during the operative procedure, is usually adequate. Thrombocytopenia that is due to inadequate megakaryopoesis may also be treated with platelet transfusion. Transfusion is of limited value alone for the management of destructive idiopathic thrombocytopenic purpura or sequestrative thrombocytopenia (hypersplenism). In such cases, specific treatment of the underlying condition is imperative. Please refer to Table 6 for treatment options for common hemostatic problems prior to surgery.

Excessive bleeding in the intraoperative and postoperative periods can be potentially life threatening and requires prompt evaluation and institution of therapy. Determining whether the bleeding is due to hemostatic failure or a surgically correctable local cause is imperative. Failure to achieve adequate hemostasis at the operative site is the most frequent cause of postoperative bleeding. Excessive, rapid blood loss limited to the surgical site may be due to bleeding from a large vessel. In contrast, bleeding from a hemostatic defect is typically a more widespread "oozing" at the operative site, and may also involve

Table 5 Plasma Clotting Factors and Sources of Replacement

Factor	In vivo half-life	Minimum plasma level required for hemostasis[a]	Source of factor replacement
Fibrinogen	3–4 days	100 mg/dL	Cryoprecipitate
II	2–5 days	20–40%	FFP
V	15–36 h	25–30%	FFP
VII	4–7 h	10–20%	FFP or rf VIIa (NovoSeven®)
VIII	8–12 h	25–30%	Recombinant or plasma derived factor VIII concentrate
IX	20–24 h	25–30%	Recombinant or plasma derived factor IX concentrate
X	32–48 h	10–20%	FFP
XI	3 days	15–25%	FFP
XII	48–52 h	0%	(Correction not required)
XIII	12 days	<5%	FFP (or cryoprecipitate)
von Willebrand's	8–12 h	25–50%	Intermediate purity, plasma derived concentrate (Humate-P, Alphanate)

[a]Percentage values expressed as percentage of normal.
Abbreviation: FFP, fresh frozen plasma.

Table 6 Treatment Options for Common Hemostatic Problems Prior to Surgery

Problems	Value	Treatment
Thrombocytopenia		
Platelet count	$\geq 80,000/mm^3$	Bleeding unlikely
	<80,000 and >20,000/mm^3	Platelet transfusion may be needed
		Platelet transfusion may be needed
	<20,000/mm^3	Bleeding likely, platelet transfusion indicated
Acquired platelet dysfunction (bleeding history)		
PFA Col/Epi closure time	>180 s	DDAVP
Bleeding time	>15 min	Platelet transfusion if DDAVP ineffective
Liver disease		
Prothrombin time	≤3 s over control	Bleeding unlikely
	>3 s over control	FFP indicated, vitamin K may be helpful
Fibrinogen	<100 mg/dL	Cryoprecipitate indicated
Thrombocytopenia		As above
Accelerated fibrinolysis		Antifibrinolytic may be indicated

Source: Adapted from Francis CW, Kaplan KL. Hematologic problems in the surgical patient: bleeding and thrombosis. In: Hoffman R, et al. eds. From Hematology: Basic Principles and Practice, 3d ed. Churchill: Livingstone, 2000.

additional sites outside the surgical field. Consequently, when evaluating intraoperative and postoperative bleeding, the patient should be examined for petechiae, ecchymosis, gastrointestinal or genitourinary bleed, and bleeding from venipuncture and/or central venous catheter sites.

A strategy similar to that recommended for preoperative screening should be utilized in the postoperative evaluation and management of a bleeding diathesis. A preexisting hemostatic defect may not have been detected preoperatively, therefore, the patient's past medical and family history should be reviewed. Once again, the list of medications the patient is taking should be reviewed, and, if possible, medications that can potentially interfere with the coagulation system should be discontinued. It is noteworthy that many over-the-counter medications, including cold remedies, include aspirin. Furthermore, patients are at risk of developing vitamin K deficiency postoperatively, especially if oral intake has been poor and broad spectrum antibiotics have been employed. The bleeding diathesis in this case is due to an acquired deficiency of vitamin K dependent factors (factors II, VII, IX, and X). In addition to INR, PTT, thrombin time (TT), platelet count, and PFA-100 Col/Epi closure time, a peripheral blood smear, fibrinogen, and D-dimer (or fibrin degradation products) should be evaluated to rule out disseminated intravascular coagulation (DIC). Factors VIII, IX, and XI may be checked to rule out milder variants of congenital factor deficiencies that may not prolong the PTT. Many patients in the postoperative phase receive heparin, either via indwelling venous catheter flushes or as antithrombotic prophylactic or therapeutic strategies. Heparin administration complicates the laboratory evaluation of the coagulation system. A normal reptilase time, in combination with prolonged PTT and TT, is suggestive of heparin effect. Euglobulin clot lysis time, α_2-antiplasmin, and plasminogen activator inhibitor-1 levels may be checked if a defect in the fibrinolytic system is suspected. Massive blood transfusion (i.e., transfusion of more than one blood volume, ~5000 mL) may lead to dilutional thrombocytopenia and deficiencies of multiple coagulation factors, which may be compounded by an excessive build-up of citrate. These factors, along with other hemostatic abnormalities, may contribute to bleeding.

Therapy is dependent on the hemostatic defect identified, as discussed earlier in the section on preoperative evaluation.

SPECIAL HEMOSTATIC CHALLENGES

Certain medical and surgical conditions pose special hemostatic challenges. These include (1) cardiopulmonary bypass (CPB) surgery, (2) liver disease, and (3) renal disease.

Cardiopulmonary Bypass Surgery

The incidence of postoperative bleeding following CPB surgery is 0.8–5%. Bleeding may be profound and require reoperation. Perfusion of blood through the extracorporeal membrane oxygenator leads to hemostatic changes during CPB. The hemoglobin, platelet count, and serum concentration of coagulation and fibrinolytic factors are reduced to ~50% of baseline. Of special concern is factor V, which may have a serum concentration <20% baseline. Decrease in available factors may be due to:

1. exposure to artifical surfaces
2. tissue-factor-dependent coagulation related to the surgical trauma with resultant depletion of the factors

Furthermore, the bypass procedure leads to significant platelet dysfunction that is due to the release of α-granules and generation of platelet microparticles. This platelet dysfunction may be detectable as abnormal in vitro platelet aggregation tests and a prolonged bleeding time that usually corrects within 1 h postoperatively. Other factors, such as inadequate neutralization of heparin by protamine sulfate, may contribute to the bleeding disorder.

Management of the bleeding complications after CPB should include additional dose(s) of protamine sulfate, if heparin has been inadequately reversed, supportive care with cryoprecipitate fresh frozen plasma, and vitamin K for patients with acquired coagulation factor deficiencies. Studies have not demonstrated a beneficial effect of platelet transfusion. The administration of DDAVP may enhance coagulation and platelet function and decrease overall blood loss. Concerns regarding its potential to increase the rate of postoperative myocardial infarction have been raised. Antifibrinolytic agents such as aprotinin, epsilon-aminocaproic acid, and tranexamic acid have been shown to decrease both bleeding and transfusion requirements without apparently increasing the postoperative thrombosis risk. For additional details, the reader is referred to References 6 and 7.

Liver Disease

The liver plays a key role in hemostasis. Bleeding complications in patients with acute or chronic liver disease may arise from various causes.

1. *Clotting factor deficiencies.* These that are due to decreased production, vitamin K deficiency, or synthesis of abnormal forms of coagulation factors. All coagulation factors, with the exception of vWF and fVIII, are synthesized primarily

or exclusively by hepatocytes. Prolongation of the prothrombin time (PT/INR) is an indicator of the severity of liver disease and is used as a prognostic marker (in the Child–Pugh and Mayo indices of end-stage liver disease). A concomitant deficiency of vitamin K leads to further reduction of factors II, VII, IX, X, as well as proteins C and S, as vitamin K is required as a cofactor for hepatic γ-carboxylation of glutamic acid residues in the amino-terminal region of these proteins. The γ-carboxylated residues allow calcium ion binding, which is essential for binding to phospholipid membranes, the key to their functional activity. Dysfibrinogenemia is the most common qualitative factor defect in severe liver disease. An excessive number of sialic acid residues on fibrinogen interferes with its enzymatic cleavage by thrombin and results in abnormal polymerization of fibrin monomers. The result is a prolonged TT.

2. *Qualitative and quantitative platelet defects.* Thrombocytopenia is a common finding in patients with chronic liver disease, but is rarely below $30-40,000/mm^3$. Splenomegaly from portal hypertension is considered to be the main cause of a low platelet count in cirrhosis. Additionally, thrombopoietin (TPO) is a cytokine produced by the liver, which is responsible for the maturation of megakaryocytes and the production of platelets. Serum levels of TPO are reduced in patients with liver disease and thrombocytopenia. Furthermore, the platelet count may be reduced as a consequence of disseminated intravascular coagulation (discussed below). Alcohol abuse, a major cause of chronic liver disease, can result in thrombocytopenia either by directly inhibiting bone marrow synthesis or by associated nutritional deficiency of folic acid.

3. *Hyperfibrinolysis.* High circulating levels of t-PA, probably a result of decreased hepatic clearance, account for hyperfibrinolysis in end-stage liver disease. Moreover, progressive liver disease leads to low levels of α_2-antiplasmin and TAFI, which further accelerates fibrinolysis.

4. *Accelerated intravascular coagulation.* This phenomenon is seen in patients with advanced liver disease, and the coagulation abnormalities are similar to low-grade disseminated intravascular coagulation (discussed later).

Spontaneous bleeding is infrequent in patients with advanced liver disease, and often no therapy is required for the coagulation defect. Correction of the coagulation defect should be pursued if the patient has active bleeding, or is undergoing an invasive procedure. Administration of 10–20 mL/kg body weight of fresh frozen plasma usually shortens the PT/INR promptly. The effect is short-lived and generally lasts no more than 12–24 h. Cryoprecipitate may be administered in a bleeding patient when the fibrinogen level is <100 mg/dL. One unit of administered cryoprecipitate for every 10 kg body weight typically increases plasma fibrinogen by 50 mg/dL. Recombinant fVIIa is a promising agent for the correction of the hemostatic defect in patients with liver failure, and it may reduce blood product requirements during liver transplantation. However, further study is needed before its routine use can be endorsed. Platelet transfusions are required in patients with persistent bleeding if the platelet count is $<50,000/mm^3$. In that case, an attempt to maintain the count $>100,000/mm^3$ should be made. Prophylactic platelet transfusion is only indicated for patients undergoing invasive procedures or elective surgical procedures when the platelet count is $<60,000/mm^3$. Vitamin K deficiency is likely in a patient with cholestatic liver disease. Thus, a trial of 10 mg of vitamin K a day for 3 days (given orally or by slow intravenous administration) is a reasonable strategy to attempt normalization of the prolonged

PT/INR. Subcutaneous vitamin K has an inconsistent rate of absorption and has been demonstrated to be less efficacious than the oral or intravenous routes of administration. DDAVP has not been shown to benefit patients with bleeding esophageal varices. Antifibrinolytic agents such as aprotinin, epsilon-aminocaproic acid, and tranexamic acid have demonstrated benefit in controlling blood loss during orthotopic liver transplantation. However, care should be exercised in the use of these agents in patients with DIC, as they may increase the risk of thrombosis. For additional reading, please refer to Reference 8.

Renal Disease

Chronic renal insufficiency has a number of effects. Blood cell production, complement, and hemostatic systems, including qualitative and quantitative platelets, coagulation factor, and blood vessel wall, are all compromised by end-stage renal failure. These changes increase the risk of bleeding. It is noteworthy that with the advent and routine use of recombinant erythropoietin in patients with chronic renal insufficiency, bleeding complications have declined dramatically, a phenomenon illustrating an important role for the maintenance of a normal or near-normal hematocrit in these patients.

The retention of low-molecular-weight toxins (e.g., guanidinosuccinic acid and phenolic acid) decreases adenosine diphosphate (ADP)-induced platelet aggregation. In contrast, prostaglandins, which have a vasodilatory effect in chronic renal disease, activate platelets and induce activation of the coagulation cascade. In patients undergoing hemodialysis, the dialyzer membrane composition and flow design may also play a role in activating platelets. The decreased concentration of factors IX, XI, and XII reported is probably explained by their relatively low molecular weight, which facilitates glomerular filtration. In contrast, factors II, V, VII, VIII, X, and XIII are often increased.

A qualitative defect of vWF has also been noted in uremia. In patients with bleeding complications or those undergoing surgery, intravenous infusion of 0.3 μg/kg DDAVP may be tried, as it releases vWF from the α-granules of platelets. Dosing may be repeated every 24–48 h. More frequent administration of DDAVP is not effective and may lead to water retention with hyponatremia. Therefore, the patient's fluid intake should be restricted to 1 L/24 h after the administration of DDAVP. If DDAVP administration is not effective in controlling bleeding, cryoprecipitate may be considered. The clinician must realize that a small risk of transmission of blood borne pathogens exists. Intermediate purity factor VIII products (e.g., Humate-P and Alphanate) that have a high concentration of vWF may be tried, although adequate data are not available to support their routine use in this situation. Other potential therapeutic modalities include the use of conjugated estrogens. Their peak hemostatic effect is delayed, and the hemostatic benefit may not be observed for several days.

THROMBOTIC DISORDERS

Surgery is a major risk for thrombosis. Virchow's triad of flow disturbance, vessel wall injury, and excessive blood coagulability remain risk factors for deep vein thrombosis (DVT) after surgery. Surgery itself is thrombogenic for a variety of reasons: (1) release of tissue factor following incision and tissue injury, (2) use of general anesthesia, (3) bed rest and limb immobilization with consequent lack of calf muscle activity, and (4) decreased fibrinolytic activity postoperatively. Some thrombotic complications can be anticipated preoperatively through a careful medical history (including a personal and family history of arterial and venous thrombosis) and physical examination. Some of the known risk factors that predispose to venous thromboembolism (VTE) are listed in Table 7.

Postoperative VTE may appear as either acute symptomatic DVT or pulmonary embolism (PE). Apart from the short-term risk of death from PE, DVT is associated with significant long-term morbidity. The 8-year cumulative incidence of postthrombotic syndrome, the symptoms of which include chronic leg swelling, stasis dermatitis, skin ulceration, and pain, is ~30% (9). The risk of venous thrombosis varies with the type of surgery and patient characteristics; therefore, it is important to stratify the risk of VTE so that aggressive prophylactic measures can be instituted in high-risk patients (Table 8). This strategy also minimizes the potential adverse effects of anticoagulation in subgroups with a low risk of VTE (10).

Full anticoagulation with heparin is associated with a high incidence of postoperative bleeding complications and is inappropriate for prophylactic use, with the exception of patients with a recent history of VTE. Perioperative administration of low-dose unfractionated heparin (UFH) reduces the incidence of deep vein thrombosis by 60–80% in general surgery patients. The use of oral anticoagulation with warfarin is limited by the frequency of bleeding complications, the relative difficulty in achieving stable therapeutic values, and the delay in achieving sufficient anticoagulation. A target INR maintained between 2.0 and 3.0 is considered to provide adequate anticoagulation. Other agents like low-molecular-weight heparins (LMWH), heparinoids, and pentasaccharides (fondaparinux) have also been used successfully for prophylaxis (Table 9). Although the Sixth American College of Chest Physicians (ACCP) Consensus Conference recommends initiating prophylatic doses of anticoagulation 1–12 h prior to surgery (10), typically in the United States, the prophylactic therapy is started 6–12 h postoperatively, once adequate hemostasis is achieved.

Patients requiring long-term anticoagulation (e.g., prosthetic heart valves, chronic atrial fibrillation, antiphospholipid antibody syndrome, and history of recurrent VTE)

Table 7 Hypercoagulable States

Hereditary	Acquired
Factor V Leiden mutation (activated protein C resistance)	Anti-cardiolipin antibody and/or lupus anticoagulant
Protein C deficiency	Immobilization
Antithrombin III deficiency	Surgery/postoperative state
Dysfibrinogenemia	Pregnancy and postpartum period
Prothrombin 20210 G-A polymorphism	Nephrotic syndrome
Protein S deficiency	Paroxysmal nocturnal hemoglobinuria
Elevated factor VIII level	Hyperhomocysteinemia
Hyperhomocysteinemia	Therapeutic agents (L-asparaginase, mitomycin, tamoxifen, raloxifene, prothrombin complex concentrates)
	Trauma
	Estrogen use
	Malignancy
	Heparin-associated thrombocytopenia
	Myeloproliferative syndromes
	Congestive heart failure

Table 8 Guidelines for Prophylaxis of Deep Vein Thrombosis Based on Risk-Stratification

Category	Patients	Approximate risk (without prophylaxis) (%) Calf DVT	Prox. DVT	PE	Recommendations for prevention of venous thromboembolism
Low	Minor surgery in patients under age 40 with no additional risk factors, surgery lasting <30 min	2	0.4	0.2	Ambulation, leg exercises
Moderate	Nonmajor surgery in patients aged 40–60 years or major surgery in patients <40 years of age with no additional risk factors, minor surgery with additional risk factors	10–20	2–4	1–2	LDUH q12h, LMWH, graded compression elastic stocking, or intermittent pneumatic compression
High	Nonmajor surgery in patients >60 years, major surgery in patients above 40 or with additional risk factors	20–40	4–8	2–4	LDUH q8H, LMWH, or intermittent pneumatic compression
Highest	Major surgery in patients >40 years and with history of previous VTE, cancer, molecular hypercoagulable state, hip fracture surgery, hip or knee arthroplasty, major trauma	40–80	10–20	4–10	LMWH, warfarin, or intermittent pneumatic compression + LDUH/LMWH
Special situations	Neurosurgery or other patients with high bleeding risk				Intermittent pneumatic compression
	Open prostatectomy				Intermittent pneumatic compression

Abbreviations: LDUH, low-dose unfractionated heparin; LMWH, low molecular weight heparin.
Source: Adapted from The Sixth ACCP Consensus Conference on antithrombotic therapy. Chest 2001; 119(suppl 1).

Table 9 Regimens to Prevent Venous Thromboembolism

Class	Agent	Dose	Route and frequency
Unfractionated heparin	Heparin	5000 units	SC q8–12h
	Heparin	75–100 units/kg	SC q12h
LMWH	Enoxaparin	30 mg	SC q12h
	Enoxaparin	40 mg	SC qD
	Dalteparin	5000 units	SC qD
	Tinzaparin	75 units/kg	SC qD
	Tinzaparin	3500–4500 units	SC qD
Heparinoid	Danaparoid	750 units	SC q12h
Pentasaccharide (Xa inhibitor)	Fondaparinux	2.5 mg	SC qD
Vitamin K antagonist	Warfarin	5 mg	PO qD. Adjust dose to maintain INR between 2.0 and 3.0
Thrombin inhibitor	Desirudin (recombinant Hirudin)	15 mg	SC q12h

Abbreviation: LMWH, low molecular weight heparin.

need to be switched from oral warfarin to high-dose intravenous heparin or therapeutic doses of subcutaneous LMWH about 4–5 days prior to elective surgery. The dose of heparin/LMWH should be discontinued at least 12 h prior to the procedure and restarted 8–12 h after the surgery, once adequate hemostasis is achieved. Warfarin can be reinitiated once the patient resumes a normal diet, and heparin/LMWH overlapped with it for at least 2 days after the INR is above 2.0. For an emergency surgical procedure, the effect of warfarin is reversed by administering 1–2 mg of vitamin K orally or intravenously, along with infusion of fresh frozen plasma, to bring the INR below 1.4. High doses of vitamin K are usually unnecessary and may lead to prolonged resistance to subsequent re-anticoagulation with warfarin.

The threshold for screening patients manifesting symptoms consistent with DVT (e.g., leg swelling, pain, and tenderness on palpation of the calf muscles) or PE (e.g., pleuritic chest pain, shortness of breath, hemoptysis, and palpitations) should be low in the postsurgical setting. For ruling out DVT, a venous duplex ultrasound should be performed. A ventilation/perfusion lung scan or a high resolution chest computed tomography (CT) with pulmonary angiogram should be performed to confirm a diagnosis of PE. If DVT or PE is confirmed, patients should be treated with intravenous heparin after a baseline complete blood count (CBC), aPTT, and INR is obtained. A bolus of 80 units/kg heparin should be administered, and a continuous infusion at 18 units/kg per h initiated. The aPTT should be monitored every 6 h and maintained at 1.5–2.5 × the mean normal value. Additionally, a platelet count should be monitored at least every other day while a patient receives heparin to identify the possible development of heparin-associated thrombocytopenia (see later for details). Oral warfarin at a dose of 5 mg/day should be initiated along with heparin if the patient has resumed eating. Concomitant heparin and warfarin should be continued for at least 5 days. When the INR has been greater than 2.0 on two consecutive days, the heparin may be discontinued. Subcutaneous LMWH may be substituted for intravenous heparin if the creatinine clearance is within normal limits. When using

LMWH, the clinician should note that the half-life of these agents is longer than the half-life of unfractionated heparin and that protamine sulfate is not as effective an antidote for LMWH for bleeding complications. Usually, 3 months of therapy with warfarin is adequate for an episode of post-surgery DVT. For additional reading, please refer to Reference 11.

DISSEMINATED INTRAVASCULAR COAGULATION

By consensus, DIC is defined as "an acquired syndrome characterized by the intravascular activation of coagulation with loss of localization arising from different causes. It can originate from and cause damage to the microvasculature, which if sufficiently severe, can produce organ dysfunction" (12). The clinical manifestations can vary and range from laboratory abnormalities alone to hemorrhagic and/or thrombotic complications. Bleeding, the predominant clinical manifestation of DIC, is reported in 70–90% of patients. Commonly reported sites of bleeding include the skin, lungs, gastrointestinal and genitourinary tracts, surgical sites, and vascular access sites. Thromboembolic manifestations are less frequent (10–40%) and are seen more often in patients with underlying malignancies, pneumococcal sepsis, or meningococcal sepsis.

Numerous disorders are associated with the development of DIC, and these are listed in Table 10. Regardless of the underlying cause, the final common pathway in the pathogenesis of DIC is an unregulated and excessive generation of thrombin that results from the failure of the mechanisms that regulate thrombin generation (please refer to the section "Physiology of Hemostasis" for additional details; also see Table 11). The coagulation cascade is triggered by the exposure of blood to excessive amounts of TF (due to either mechanical tissue injury or endothelial and monocyte activation), which leads to thrombin generation. Thrombin converts fibrinogen to fibrin monomers. Additionally, thrombin is a potent agonist for platelet activation and aggregation. The above-mentioned processes produce either large-vessel thrombosis or, more commonly, microvessel fibrin

Table 10 Conditions Associated with DIC

Acute and subacute	Chronic
Infections	Malignancies (solid tumors)
Gram-negative bacteria	Obstetric complications
Encapsulated gram-positive bacteria	Dead fetus syndrome
Toxic shock syndrome	Localized intravascular coagulation
Viruses (e.g., Varicella)	Aortic aneurysm
Obstetric complications	Hemangiomas (Kasabach–Merritt syndrome)
Eclampsia/preeclampsia	Advanced liver disease
Abruptio placentae	LeVeen shunt
Amniotic fluid embolism	Fatty liver of pregnancy
Sepsis	
Saline-induced abortion	
Malignancies	
Leukemia, lymphoma	
Tissue injury/crush injury	
Burns	
Heat stroke	

Disorders of Coagulation

Table 11 Common Mediators of DIC

Mediators of DIC	Common examples
Increased tissue factor	Sepsis (endotoxin), malignancy, trauma, obstetric complications
Decreased AT III, PC, PS	Liver disease
Decreased PS	Pregnancy
Decreased TM, PC, AT III	Sepsis
Increased plasmin	APL, amniotic fluid embolism, prostate cancer, end-stage liver disease

Abbreviations: AT III, antithrombin III; PC, protein C; PS, protein S; TM, thrombomodulin; APL, acute promyelocytic leukemia (M3 subtype of AML).

deposition, which can result in tissue ischemia and organ dysfunction. Thrombin accelerates the proteolysis and depletion of coagulation factors, including fibrinogen, and factors II, V, VIII, and X. The depletion of these factors is a function of their relatively short plasma half-lives (Table 5) and the rate of synthesis by the liver. Furthermore, thrombin induces endothelial cells to release t-PA, which converts plasminogen to plasmin in the presence of the newly formed fibrin monomer. This production of plasmin results in fibrinolysis, which may lead to further consumption of coagulation factors, thus worsening bleeding. Finally, plasma levels of natural anticoagulants, including protein C and antithrombin III, are depleted during DIC. The laboratory abnormalities are enumerated in Table 12.

Therapy of DIC is aimed at prompt and aggressive management of the underlying condition. Other measures include initiation of basic support measures (e.g., correction of volume status, gas exchange, and electrolyte imbalance), replacement of platelets or clotting factors as necessary, and institution of anticoagulants to stem the progression of DIC, if needed.

Table 12 Laboratory Findings in DIC

Markers of thrombin generation	Prothrombin fragment 1.2 (↑)
	Fibrinopeptide A (↑)
	Thrombin–Antithrombin complex (↑)
	Assays for fibrin monomer (↑)
	D-Dimer (↑)
Screen for platelet and factor consumption	Platelet count (↓)
	PT/INR (↑)
	PTT (↑)
	Thrombin time (↑)
	Fibrinogen (↓)
Others	α_2-Antiplasmin (↓)
	Antithrombin III (↓)
	Factor V (↓)
	Euglobulin clot lysis time (↓)
	Fibrin/fibrinogen degradation products (↑)
	Microangiopathic hemolytic anemia
	Anemia, reticulocytosis, schistocytes on peripheral smear, LDH (↑), indirect bilirubin (↑), haptoglobin (↓)

Transfusion of platelets, fresh frozen plasma, and cryoprecipitate should be reserved for patients who have documented laboratory evidence of decompensated DIC and are bleeding, or for patients scheduled for an invasive procedure. Platelets should be maintained over 20,000–30,000/mm^3 in a bleeding patient, and >50,000/mm^3 in a patient undergoing a surgical procedure, or when there is significant blood loss. Cryoprecipitate should be administered to maintain a plasma fibrinogen >100 mg/dL. Fresh frozen plasma may be infused to correct prolonged PTT and INR in appropriate clinical circumstances. Replacement therapy may be required every 6–8 h while the underlying cause of DIC is being treated.

Heparin infusion should be considered in DIC if the patient has thromboembolic manifestations of DIC (e.g., purpura fulminans, dead fetus syndrome before induction of labor, aortic aneurysm, and malignancy-associated DIC). Heparin should be used with caution as it may exacerbate DIC-associated bleeding.

Antithrombin III concentrates have been used in the treatment of DIC associated with sepsis. A meta-analysis of randomized clinical trials demonstrated its benefit in preventing organ failure and death (13). However, a recent large, phase III trial of AT III in sepsis (KyberSept trial) did not demonstrate any difference in 28-day all-cause mortality between the AT III and placebo groups (14).

A recent randomized, doubled-blind, placebo controlled clinical trial using recombinant human activated protein C (rhAPC) in patients with sepsis demonstrated a 6.1% absolute risk reduction in the 28-day all-cause mortality ($P = 0.005$) (15). Remarkably, the most critically ill patients derived the maximal benefit. The primary safety concern was the increased risk of bleeding in the rhAPC group, and for this reason (as well as the high cost of the product) it should be used judiciously. For a review, please refer to References 16 and 17.

HEPARIN-ASSOCIATED THROMBOCYTOPENIA

The use of heparin is ubiquitous in the surgical intensive care unit. It is used as an anticoagulant for intra-arterial catheters, central venous access catheters, hemodialysis, and for perioperative prophylaxis against VTE.

Heparin associated thrombocytopenia (HAT) develops in 1–3% of patients treated with heparin. It is typically associated with mild to moderate thrombocytopenia (40,000–70,000/mm^3), although platelet counts may occasionally fall as low as 20,000/mm^3. Spontaneous bleeding is rare. Instead, disseminated or localized venous or arterial thrombosis may occur in 30–50% of patients with HAT. Thrombocytopenia, with or without thrombosis, typically appears 5–14 days after the initiation of heparin therapy (18,19).

HAT is caused by a heparin-dependent IgG antibody that recognizes a complex of heparin and platelet factor 4 (PF4). These immune complexes activate platelets via the platelet Fc receptors, and intravascular platelet aggregation, thrombocytopenia, and generation of thrombin occur (20). In addition, TF is expressed on endothelial cells that are activated by the HAT antibody, which may recognize PF4 bound to endothelial heparan sulfate. These processes may result in arterial or venous thrombosis. The immunogenicity and the platelet-activating effects of heparin are proportional to its molecular size and degree of sulfation; thus, unfractionated heparin is more likely to cause HAT when compared with LMWH. Other factors influencing the development of HAT include previous exposure to heparin and heparin from a bovine rather than porcine source. Only a minority of patients who generate HAT antibodies develop thrombocytopenia and thrombosis. Furthermore, clinical factors also play a role in determining the sequelae of HAT. For

Table 13 Therapy for Heparin-Associated Thrombocytopenia with Thrombosis

Agent	Half-life (h)	Excretion	Dose
Recombinant hirudin (lepirudin)	1–2	Renal	0.4 mg/kg IV bolus maintenance infusion 0.15 mg/kg per h[a,b]
Argatroban	0.5–1	Hepatic	2 μg/kg per min IV continuous infusion[b,c]
Danaparoid	18–28	Renal	2250 U IV bolus, followed by 400 U/h for 4 h, then 300 U/h for 4 h, maintenance 150–200 U/h[a,d]

[a]Adjust the dose for renal insufficiency.
[b]Maintain PTT 1.5–3.0× the median of the normal range.
[c]Adjust dose for hepatic insufficiency.
[d]Maintain the anti-Xa level between 0.5 and 0.8 anti-Xa U/mL.

example, postoperative orthopedic patients are at high risk for venous thrombosis, whereas postoperative cardiovascular patients are at relatively high risk for arterial thrombosis (21).

An enzyme-linked immunosorbent assay (ELISA) utilizing heparin/PF4 as the target antigen may be used to detect the pathogenic IgG in HAT. The assay for heparin-dependent platelet antibody detection by platelet aggregometry has high specificity, but low sensitivity. The clinical history—including the timing of onset of thrombocytopenia—is the most important clue to the diagnosis of HAT. The "gold standard" for diagnosis is the ^{14}C serotonin platelet release assay, which has >95% sensitivity and specificity, although it is available in relatively few institutions.

Once HAT is suspected, heparin from *all* possible sources should be discontinued. It is generally recommended that even in the absence of overt arterial or venous thrombosis, systemic anticoagulation with intravenous recombinant Hirudin (lepirudin), argatroban, or danaparoid should be considered (Table 13). Hirudin and argatroban are direct thrombin inhibitors and do not have any cross-reactivity with the HAT antibody. Danaparoid has 10–40% in vitro cross-reactivity with HAT antibody; however, clinically significant cross-reactivity is uncommon. LMWHs should not be substituted for unfractionated heparin when HAT is suspected, as there may be significant cross-reactivity between the antibody and LMWH. Warfarin should not be initiated in the absence of a rapid-acting systemic anticoagulant as warfarin depletes the regulatory protein C first (with its short half-life) and may exacerbate thrombosis.

To prevent the development of HAT, monitoring of the platelet count on alternate days (for at least 14 days) in all patients receiving heparin is recommended, regardless of the dose. Although LMWHs are less immunogenic when compared to unfractionated heparin, periodic checks on the platelet count are also recommended.

SUMMARY

- Primary hemostasis is initiated when circulating platelets are exposed to vascular subendothelium.
- In secondary hemostasis, the coagulation pathway leads to formation of a hemostatic plug. Tissue factor and circulating activated factor VII initiate the coagulation cascade.

- Substances released by adherent platelets induce vasoconstriction, provide a template for coagulation protein complexes, and initiate blood vessel wall repair.
- Tissue factor pathway inhibitor, activated protein C, antithrombin III, heparin cofactor II, and tissue plasminogen activator limit clot progression.
- The endothelium synthesizes many substances involved in hemostasis (Table 1).
- A careful history and physical examination will provide important clues to a patient's bleeding or thrombotic risk. The best screening test for bleeding risk is a careful bleeding history.
- Excessive mucocutaneous bleeding suggests a primary hemostatic disorder, including platelet deficiency or dysfunction, vascular fragility disorder, or von Willebrand disease.
- Tissue or joint bleeding suggests hemophilia A or B. Delayed bleeding after surgical procedures or poor wound healing suggests factor XIII deficiency.
- Routine laboratory assays have limited predictive value for perioperative bleeding. For moderate- to high-risk procedures, platelet count, platelet function analysis, PTT, and INR are useful.
- The therapeutic approach to a hemostatic deficit is determined by the type and severity of the defect. Factor deficiencies can be corrected by specific factor replacement, FFP, or cryoprecipitate.
- DDAVP may be used in patients with uremic platelet dysfunction and for patients with mild hemophilia A or von Willebrand disease undergoing minor procedures.
- Intrinsic platelet functional defects are managed with platelet transfusion.
- Failure to achieve local hemostasis is the most frequent cause of intraoperative and early postoperative bleeding.
- If inadequate local hemostasis at the surgical site is excluded as the cause of postoperative bleeding, consider medical and family history, medications, vitamin K deficiency, and postoperative administration of heparin.
- Following CPB, hemoglobin, platelet count, and coagulation factors are reduced in concentration by up to 50%. Platelet dysfunction also occurs.
- In management of bleeding complications after CPB, consider protamine sulfate, platelets, cryoprecipitate, fresh frozen plasma, vitamin K, DDAVP, and antifibrinolytic agents.
- Bleeding complications in patients with liver disease may arise from clotting factor deficiencies, qualitative and quantitative platelet defects, hyperfibrinolysis, and accelerated intravascular coagulation.
- If patients with liver disease have active bleeding or are to undergo an invasive procedure, fresh frozen plasma (10–20 mL/kg) and cryoprecipitate, if fibrinogen concentration is <100 mg/dL, are beneficial. Fresh frozen plasma correction of the INR usually lasts fewer than 24 hours. Vitamin K deficiency is likely and replacement should be considered. DDAVP is of no benefit in esophageal variceal bleeding.
- Chronic renal insufficiency adversely affects blood cell production, qualitative and quantitative platelet function, and blood vessel walls.
- In patients with uremia, a qualitative von Willebrand factor defect exists that may be counteracted by DDAVP.
- Surgery is thrombogenic as a result of release of tissue factor following incision and tissue injury, use of general anesthesia, immobilization, and decreased fibrinolytic activity.

- Careful medical history can suggest a high risk for venous thromboembolism postoperatively.
- Perioperative administration of low-dose UFH reduces DVT 60–80% in general surgery patients. LMWH is effective.
- Patients requiring long-term anticoagulation for prosthetic heart valves, antiphospholipid antibody syndrome, recurrent venous thromboembolism, or chronic atrial fibrillation should be switched from warfarin to IV UFH or therapeutic doses of LMWH 4–5 days prior to elective surgery. Anticoagulation with heparin should be stopped 12 h before surgery and restarted 8–12 h after surgery, in the absence of contraindications.
- High doses of vitamin K are usually unnecessary when correcting an elevated INR prior to surgery.
- The threshold for screening patients with suspected DVT or PE should be low. If DVT or PE is confirmed, and patients have no indication for a vena cava filter, they should be treated with IV heparin.
- Three months of warfarin therapy is usually adequate for postoperative DVT.
- Bleeding is the predominant clinical finding in DIC. The final common mechanism is unregulated and excessive generation of thrombin. Microthrombi can produce tissue ischemia and organ dysfunction.
- The main goal of therapy of DIC is treatment of the underlying disorder. Supportive measures are used as needed. Transfusion of platelets, fresh frozen plasma, and cryoprecipitate should be used in patients with laboratory evidence of DIC and bleeding, or the need for an invasive procedure.
- HAT develops in 1–3% of patients treated with heparin. Disseminated or localized venous thrombosis may occur in 30–50% of patients with HAT.
- UFH is more likely than LMWH to cause HAT.
- Once HAT is suspected, discontinue heparin from all sources. Therapy with IV hirudin, argatroban, or danaparoid should be considered, even in the absence of overt thrombosis.
- LMWH should not be substituted for UFH when HAT is suspected or confirmed.
- Monitor for HAT with frequent platelet count determination in patients receiving heparin.

REFERENCES

1. Plow EF, Ginsberg MH. The molecular basis of platelet function, In: Hoffman R, Benz EJ, Shattil SJ, Furie B, Cohen HJ, Silberstein LE, McGlave P, eds. Hematology: Basic Principles and Practice. Churchill: Livingstone, 2000:1741–1752.
2. Broze GJ Jr. Why do hemophiliacs bleed? Hosp Pract (Off Ed) 1992; 27(3):71–74, 79–82, 85–86.
3. Hoffman M, Monroe DM 3rd. A cell-based model of hemostasis. Thromb Haemost 2001; 85(6):958–965.
4. Coller BS, Schneiderman PI. Clinical evaluation of hemorrhagic disorders: the bleeding history and differential diagnosis of purpura. In: Hoffman R, Benz EJ, Shattil SJ, Furie B, Cohen HJ,

Silberstein LE, McGlave P, eds. Hematology: Basic Principles and Practice. Churchill Livingstone, 2000:1824–1840.
5. Santoro SA, Eby CS. Laboratory evaluation of hemostatic disorders, In: Hoffman R, Benz EJ, Shattil SJ, Furie B, Cohen HJ, Silberstein LE, McGlave P, eds. Hematology: Basic Principles and Practice, Churchill: Livingstone, 2000:1841–1850.
6. McCusker K, Lee S. Post cardiopulmonary bypass bleeding: an introductory review. J Extra Corpor Technol 1999; 31(1):23–36.
7. Despotis GJ, Goodnough LT. Management approaches to platelet-related microvascular bleeding in cardiothoracic surgery. Ann Thorac Surg 2000; 70(suppl 2):S20–32.
8. Amitrano L, Guardascione MA, Brancaccio V, Balzano A. Coagulation disorders in liver disease. Semin Liver Dis 2002; 22(1):83–96.
9. Prandoni P, Lensing AW, Cogo A, Cuppini S, Villalta S, Carta M, Cattelan AM, Polistena P, Bernardi E, Prins MH. The long-term clinical course of acute deep venous thrombosis [see comments]. Ann Intern Med 1996; 125(1):1–7.
10. Geerts WH, Heit JA, Clagett GP, Pineo GF, Colwell CW, Anderson FA Jr, Wheeler HB. Prevention of venous thromboembolism. Chest 2001; 119(suppl 1):132S–175S.
11. Hyers TM, Agnelli G, Hull RD, Morris TA, Samama M, Tapson V, Weg JG. Antithrombotic therapy for venous thromboembolic disease. Chest 2001; 119(suppl 1):176S–193S.
12. Taylor FB Jr, Toh CH, Hoots WK, Wada H, Levi M. Towards definition, clinical and laboratory criteria, and a scoring system for disseminated intravascular coagulation. Thromb Haemost 2001; 86(5):1327–1330.
13. Eisele B, Lamy M, Thijs LG, Keinecke HO, Schuster HP, Matthias FR, Fourrier F, Heinrichs H, Delvos U. Antithrombin III in patients with severe sepsis. A randomized, placebo-controlled, double-blind multicenter trial plus a meta-analysis on all randomized, placebo-controlled, double-blind trials with antithrombin III in severe sepsis. Intensive Care Med 1998; 24(7):663–672.
14. Warren BL, Eid A, Singer P, Pillay SS, Carl P, Novak I, Chalupa P, Atherstone A, Penzes I, Kubler A, Knaub S, Keinecke HO, Heinrichs H, Schindel F, Juers M, Bone RC, Opal SM. Caring for the critically ill patient. High-dose antithrombin III in severe sepsis: a randomized controlled trial J Am Med Assoc 2001; 286(15):1869–1878.
15. Bernard GR, Vincent JL, Laterre PF, LaRosa SP, Dhainaut JF, Lopez-Rodriquez A, Steingrub JS, Garber GE, Helterbrand JD, Ely EW, Fisher CJ Jr. Efficacy and safety of recombinant human activated protein C for severe sepsis. N Engl J Med 2001; 344(10):699–709.
16. Key NS, Ely EW, Coagulation inhibition for sepsis. Curr Opin Hematol 2002; 9(5):416–421.
17. Calverley DC, Liebman HA. Disseminated intravascular coagulation. In: Hoffman R, Benz EJ, Shattil SJ, Furie B, Cohen HJ, Silberstein LE, McGlave P, eds. Hematology: Basic Principles and Practice. Churchill Livingstone, 2000:1983–1995.
18. Warkentin TE, Levine MN, Hirsh J, Horsewood P, Roberts RS, Gent M, Kelton JG. Heparin-induced thrombocytopenia in patients treated with low-molecular-weight heparin or unfractionated heparin. N Engl J Med 1995; 332(20):1330–1335.
19. Warkentin TE, Kelton JG. Temporal aspects of heparin-induced thrombocytopenia, N Engl J Med 2001; 344(17):1286–1292.
20. Kelton JG, Sheridan D, Santos A, Smith J, Steeves K, Smith C, Brown C, Murphy WG. Heparin-induced thrombocytopenia: laboratory studies. Blood, 1988; 72(3):925–930.
21. Warkentin TE, Sheppard JA, Horsewood P, Simpson PJ, Moore JC, Kelton JG. Impact of the patient population on the risk for heparin-induced thrombocytopenia. Blood, 2000; 96(5):1703–1708.

53
Transfusion Therapy

James R. Stubbs
University of South Alabama Medical Center, Mobile, Alabama, USA

The decision to transfuse blood and blood components should be based on an assessment of the risks and benefits of such treatment, as well as on the availability and relative effectiveness of alternative therapies. Although a large amount of information regarding the known risks of transfusion is available, objective information about the indications and benefits of transfusion is not as extensive or as readily quantified. Because data on indications are not definitive, transfusion practice is not standardized. Consequently, patients may either be under-transfused or over-transfused. A number of "expert panel" and consensus conference guidelines on transfusion therapy have been published (1–4). Although these publications are useful aids, they should not serve as a substitute for clinical judgment in the transfusion decision-making process.

RED BLOOD CELL TRANSFUSION

Red blood cells (RBCs) are collected via apheresis or are prepared by removing 200–250 mL of plasma from donated whole blood. RBCs are stored at 1–6°C in specially designed bags that contain an anticoagulant-preservative solution. The type of anticoagulant-preservative solution used determines the hematocrit and the storage period for the RBCs. Examples of storage solutions for RBCs are citrate–phosphate–dextrose (CPD), citrate–phosphate–dextrose–adenine (CPDA-1), and additive solution (AS) (substances such as dextrose, adenine, mannitol, and sodium chloride added to the RBCs in anticoagulant-preservative solution after collection). RBCs stored in CPDA-1 have a hematocrit of 70–80% and a shelf life of 35 days (5–7). RBCs stored in CPD have a hematocrit similar to RBCs stored in CPDA-1 blood; however, their shelf life is 21 days. RBCs stored with AS have a shelf life of 42 days and a hematocrit of 52–60% (5–7). As a consequence of the lower hematocrit, effective rapid infusion is more easily achieved with AS RBCs. The final volume of AS RBC units (~330 mL) is higher than non-AS RBCs (~250 mL). In a nonbleeding, average-size adult, one unit of RBCs is expected to increase the hemoglobin concentration by ~1 g/dL and the hematocrit by ~3%.

RBCs are transfused to increase the oxygen carrying capacity of circulating blood. Because oxygen demand varies according to the type and severity of the underlying clinical condition, it may vary in different individuals or in a single individual over time. These differences in oxygen demand in various settings make standard guidelines based on laboratory values, such as threshold hemoglobin or hematocrit values for RBC transfusion, insufficient as the sole basis for transfusion decisions (3,8,9).

Principles of Oxygen Delivery and Oxygen Consumption

Oxygen delivery (DO_2) is the product of blood flow and arterial oxygen content (CaO_2). DO_2 can be calculated by the relation DO_2 = cardiac output × CaO_2. Perfusion pressure and the resistance of the vascular bed determine tissue blood flow. Blood becomes more viscous at lower flow rates; therefore, blood is least viscous in the aorta and most viscous in the venules. As RBC concentration is the primary determinant of viscosity, reduction of RBC concentration decreases both viscosity and resistance to flow. A reduction in red cell concentration eventually leads to an increase in cardiac output (10). In adults, the initial increase in cardiac output in response to anemia is usually the result of increased preload and decreased afterload, which are both influenced by decreased viscosity. Reduced blood viscosity leads to an increase in blood flow in the postcapillary venules, increased preload, a decrease in systemic vascular resistance, and decreased afterload.

Patients with anemia have a subnormal oxygen-carrying capacity. When the blood has decreased oxygen-carrying capacity, tissues adapt to maintain oxygen delivery. One adaptive mechanism is increasing tissue blood flow either by increasing the flow rate through existing capillaries or by increasing the number of capillaries receiving blood. Another mechanism is extracting more oxygen from the red cells as they pass through the vascular beds. An increase in oxygen extraction may be of greatest benefit in vascular beds that normally have lower extraction ratios. Some vascular beds, such as those of the heart, have very high levels of oxygen extraction under normal conditions and are often termed "supply dependent" from the perspective of oxygen delivery (11,12). Increased blood flow is an essential compensatory mechanism for decreased oxygen-carrying capacity in a supply-dependent vascular bed such as the coronary system. An inadequate compensatory increase in coronary blood flow can compromise ventricular function. Even with moderate coronary artery stenosis, coronary arterial blood flow may not be adequate to compensate for decreased oxygen-carrying capacity caused by modest reductions in red cell mass. Subjects with severe coronary artery stenosis or preexisting left ventricular dysfunction may not tolerate any decrease in red cell mass. A study of cardiovascular changes in patients following acute anemia with volume replacement showed electrocardiographic evidence of ischemia in 22% of subjects with preexisting left ventricular dysfunction and in no subjects with normal left ventricular function (13). Myocardial ischemia and infarction have been shown to be associated with low perioperative hemoglobin values (14).

The oxygen content of blood is dependent upon multiple factors: hemoglobin concentration (Hb), the binding coefficient of hemoglobin (β = 1.39 mL oxygen/g of hemoglobin), hemoglobin saturation (Sat), and dissolved oxygen. Dissolved oxygen is calculated by the relation PO_2 × 0.0031. Oxygen content is calculated by adding the product of the hemoglobin concentration, the binding coefficient of hemoglobin, and the hemoglobin saturation to the dissolved oxygen value [(Hb × β × Sat) + (0.0031 × PO_2)]. In practical application, the dissolved oxygen is usually omitted from the oxygen content calculation because the value is negligible with PO_2 values obtained in ambient air; therefore, hemoglobin concentration and saturation are the variables with the greatest influence on oxygen content. The extent of hemoglobin saturation with oxygen is dependent upon the oxygen affinity state of hemoglobin and the PO_2, but is independent of the hemoglobin concentration. The oxygen affinity state of hemoglobin is modeled by the sigmoidal hemoglobin–oxygen dissociation curve (Fig. 1). Oxygen affinity states are typically described as the oxygen tension at which the hemoglobin is 50% saturated, the P_{50} value. In human blood, the normal P_{50} value is 27 torr. When the affinity of hemoglobin for oxygen increases (i.e., oxygen becomes more tightly bound to hemoglobin), the hemoglobin–oxygen dissociation curve is shifted to the left of the normal curve. When the affinity of hemoglobin for oxygen decreases (i.e., oxygen becomes less tightly bound to hemoglobin), the hemoglobin–oxygen dissociation curve is shifted to the right of the normal curve. A decrease in the oxygen affinity of hemoglobin can be achieved through a decrease in the pH or an increase in the concentration of red cell 2,3-diphosphoglycerate (2,3-DPG). An increase in red cell 2,3-DPG, a compensatory response to a decrease in red cell mass, usually takes 12–36 h to occur. Because of the adaptive mechanisms that lead to decreased hemoglobin oxygen affinity, chronically anemic individuals with a 50% decrease in oxygen-carrying capacity have been shown to have a 25% decrease in oxygen availability (15).

Oxygen content, which is dependent on hemoglobin saturation and hemoglobin concentration, is also described graphically by a curve that has the same sigmoidal shape as the hemoglobin–oxygen dissociation curve. The height of the oxygen content curve is dependent upon the hemoglobin concentration. A right or left shift of the oxygen content curve is dependent upon the P_{50} value. The unloading of oxygen [i.e., $(CaO_2 - CvO_2)$] to the tissues can be derived from the oxygen content curve. The arterial PO_2 value (PaO_2) is the oxygen tension at which oxygen is loaded onto hemoglobin in the lungs. For a given PaO_2, the CaO_2 can be read off the y-axis of the oxygen content curve for a specific hemoglobin value. The mixed venous PO_2 value (PvO_2) is the oxygen tension of blood after it has unloaded oxygen to the tissues (i.e., PO_2 of pulmonary arterial blood). When the PvO_2

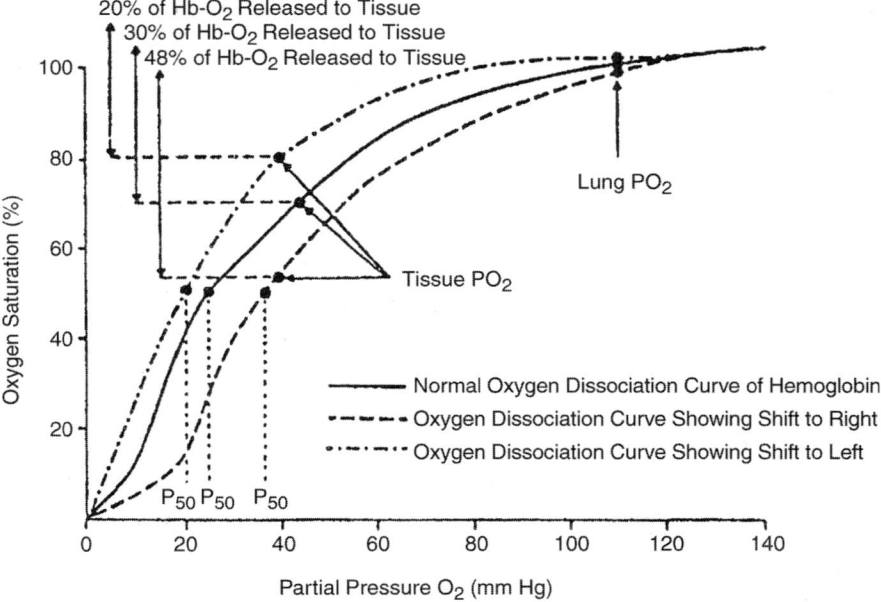

Figure 1 Oxygen dissociation curves under different conditions. *Source*: From Ref. 16.

and hemoglobin values are known, CvO_2 can also be derived from the oxygen content curve. Oxygen unloading to tissues ($CaO_2 - CvO_2$) can thus be obtained (Fig. 2).

Oxygen consumption (VO_2), the amount of oxygen used by tissues, is the product of blood flow and the difference in oxygen content between arterial and venous blood, ($CaO_2 - CvO_2$). VO_2 can be calculated using the Fick principle by the following relation:

$$VO_2 = \text{cardiac output} \times (CaO_2 - CvO_2)$$

In normal resting adults, oxygen delivery is much higher than oxygen consumption, a condition that provides a large reserve of oxygen available for delivery to the tissues.

The following are representative calculations for oxygen delivery and consumption in a normal resting adult:

$$\text{Cardiac output} = 5 \text{ L/min}$$
$$CaO_2 = 200 \text{ mL/L}$$
$$\text{Oxygen delivery } (DO_2) = \text{cardiac output} \times CaO_2 = 5 \text{ L/min} \times 200 \text{ mL/L}$$
$$= 1000 \text{ mL/min}$$
$$CvO_2 = 150 \text{ mL/L}$$
$$CaO_2 - CvO_2 = 200 \text{ mL/L} - 150 \text{ mL/L} = 50 \text{ mL/L}$$
$$\text{Oxygen consumption } (VO_2) = \text{cardiac output} \times (CaO_2 - CvO_2)$$
$$= 5 \text{ L/min} \times 50 \text{ mL/L} = 250 \text{ mL/min}$$

In this example, the normal resting adult's tissues extract 250 mL (25%) of the 1000 mL of oxygen delivered each minute. The oxygen extraction ratio, VO_2/DO_2 is 25%.

The volume of oxygen necessary for tissues to maintain aerobic function is the oxygen demand. When oxygen demand exceeds oxygen delivery, tissues attempt to

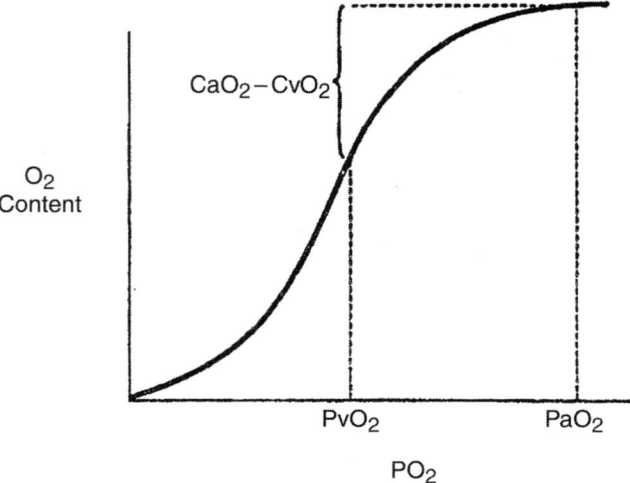

Figure 2 Oxygen content curve for whole blood, illustrating $CaO_2 - CvO_2$ and PvO_2. *Source*: From Ref. 17.

maintain function with anaerobic metabolism. A predominant state of anaerobic metabolism will not meet the tissue oxygen requirements of the critically ill patient. When patients suffer from conditions that disrupt oxygen equilibrium, red cell transfusion may became a therapeutic option. The optimum red cell mass, usually monitored with hemoglobin concentration or hematocrit, is the level at which the greatest amount of oxygen is delivered to the tissues at the lowest expense of energy for the organism. Some investigators have concluded that the optimum hemoglobin value for whole body oxygen delivery is 10 g/dL (hematocrit 30%) (18,19). In euvolemic subjects, a decrease in hemoglobin from 15 to 10 g/dL resulted in decreased blood viscosity, increased blood flow, and increased systemic oxygen transport. When the hemoglobin reached 9 g/dL, oxygen delivery was at or below baseline values (20). Because oxygen delivery was documented to remain acceptable in euvolemic subjects over the hemoglobin range of 9–15 g/dL, many clinicians consider red cell transfusions as unnecessary under these conditions. Clinical trials support the concept that, for most patients with hemoglobin values ranging from 9 to 15 g/dL, red cell transfusions are of little or no benefit (21–23).

Although defining the optimum hemoglobin/hematocrit for oxygen delivery may be valuable, defining the minimum tolerable values may have more relevance. In a review article on the clinical experience with Jehovah's Witnesses, 54 publications involving 134 patients with hemoglobin values ≤ 8 g/dL (hematocrit $\leq 24\%$) were evaluated (24). The overall fatality rate was 37%. Except for three patients who died after cardiac surgery, all subjects determined to have died as a direct result of anemia (23 total deaths) had a hemoglobin concentration <5 g/dL at the time of death. Twenty-seven patients, with hemoglobin concentrations ≤ 5 g/dL survived. The age was known in 23 of 27 survivors, and 15 of 23 were <50 years of age. In contrast, of the 15 subjects of known age who died as a result of anemia, 9 were >50 years of age. No fatalities attributable to anemia were observed in subjects with hemoglobin concentrations between 5 and 8 g/dL. These findings indicate that patients, especially younger individuals, can survive low hemoglobin concentrations. Avoidance of mortality, however, is not the only goal of red cell transfusion therapy. It is important to note that much of the information pertaining to tolerable reductions in red cell mass was obtained from studies where factors other than anemia, including blood volume, were controlled. In clinical practice, such carefully controlled conditions are rarely encountered. Patients, especially those receiving critical care, typically have concurrent, multiple medical problems, which may adversely influence their ability to tolerate anemia. These factors must be taken into account in red cell transfusion decisions. Unfortunately, information on how to adjust such decisions for all possible concurrent diseases or abnormalities is lacking.

Individuals who sustain blood loss, and have their blood volume maintained with nonsanguineous solutions such as crystalloid, eventually can reduce their red cell mass to a state where compensatory mechanisms must function to maintain adequate oxygen delivery. Otherwise healthy individuals compensate by increasing cardiac output. Studies of acute normovolemic hemodilution performed in healthy subjects show that adequate oxygen delivery can be maintained during anemia by cardiac compensation (25,26). In a study performed on eight healthy adult subjects ranging from 19 to 25 years of age, DO_2 was reduced by acute normovolemic hemodilution followed by the infusion of the beta-adrenergic antagonist esmolol. The goal of this investigation was determination of the critical level below which DO_2 fails to meet metabolic oxygen needs (25). The subjects' hemoglobin concentrations decreased from a baseline of 12.5 ± 0.8

to 4.8 ± 0.2 g/dL at the end of hemodilution and to 4.7 ± 0.2 g/dL after esmolol infusion. Oxygen delivery values decreased from a baseline of 14.0 ± 2.9 to 9.9 ± 2.0 mL/kg per min at the end of hemodilution and to 7.3 ± 1.4 mL/kg per min after esmolol infusion. Oxygen consumption values showed an increase from a baseline of 3.0 ± 0.5 to 3.4 ± 0.6 mL/kg per min at the end of hemodilution and to 3.2 ± 0.6 mL/kg per min after esmolol infusion (Fig. 3). Plasma lactate concentrations increased from a baseline of 0.5 ± 0.10 to 0.62 ± 0.16 mM at the end of hemodilution and to 0.66 ± 0.14 mM after esmolol infusion. The authors concluded that, despite an ∼50% reduction in DO_2 from baseline, inadequate oxygenation could not be demonstrated either by VO_2, which did not decrease appreciably, or by plasma lactate concentrations, which stayed within the upper limit of normal, <2 mM. Furthermore, the reduction of DO_2 to 7.3 ± 1.4 mL/kg per min in resting healthy young adults does not result in inadequate systemic oxygenation. Studies such as this support the notion that decisions regarding red cell transfusion therapy should not be based solely on hemoglobin concentration or hematocrit. Rather, decisions to transfuse red cells should include information about the status of oxygen delivery and oxygen consumption. Therapeutic measures to preserve aerobic metabolism should be taken when oxygen equilibrium is altered, and evidence of diminished oxygen reserve is present.

Low hemoglobin concentrations are not as well tolerated in older patients. Elderly individuals have limited ability to increase stroke volume and heart rate with exercise (27). Many normovolemic elderly patients with anemia have decreased oxygen delivery, because compensation via increased cardiac output is inadequate. Such patients maintain oxygen consumption through increased oxygen extraction. Compensation with increased oxygen extraction has been observed in the elderly with coronary artery disease and noncardiac medical conditions, as well as in healthy subjects (28–30). Although some elderly individuals may have excellent compensatory mechanisms for oxygen delivery, in general, the elderly are less able to preserve oxygen delivery when red cell mass is decreased. In addition to having decreased physiologic compensation, the elderly often exhibit decreased tolerance of anemia, which is likely related to a higher incidence of coronary artery disease (13).

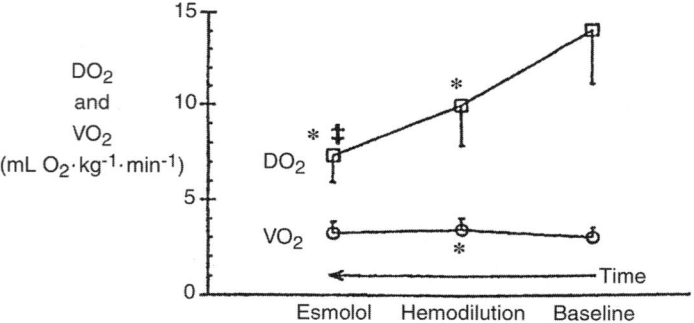

Figure 3 Oxygen delivery (DO_2) and oxygen consumption (VO_2) in eight healthy adults before isovolemic hemodilution (hemoglobin concentration, 12.5 ± 0.8 g/dL) and after (hemoglobin concentration, 4.8 ± 0.2 g/dL), and during intravenous infusion of a β-adrenergic antagonist, esmolol (with hemoglobin concentration of 4.7 ± 0.2 g/dL). *Indicates $p < 0.05$ vs. baseline; ‡indicates $p < 0.05$ vs. hemodilution without esmolol. *Source*: From Ref. 25.

The PvO_2 is considered an important variable for assessment of the adequacy of oxygen transport. The typical PvO_2 value in normal resting adults is 40 torr. A decrease in PvO_2 can result from a decreased DO_2, an increased VO_2, or both. Alterations in cardiac output, oxygen saturation of arterial blood, hemoglobin, and P_{50} influence DO_2; therefore, they also influence PvO_2. When a decreased PvO_2 is encountered, more than one of the variables influencing DO_2 likely has changed. Additionally, VO_2 may be significantly altered. When the PvO_2 is decreased, a careful assessment of all variables influencing DO_2 and VO_2 may help delineate the cause and influence the approach to patient management.

When oxygen delivery to the heart becomes inadequate, the heart, which is normally a site of lactate uptake, starts to produce lactate, an indicator of myocardial conversion to anaerobic metabolism. In healthy primates, myocardial lactate production is observed when the oxygen extraction ratio exceeds 50%, an event that occurs when the hematocrit is <10% (9). A study of 14 anesthetized dogs evaluated the effect of critical stenosis of the left anterior descending coronary artery (LAD) when combined with anemia from acute blood loss (31). Seven control dogs and seven dogs with critical LAD stenosis (LAD dogs) sustained isovolemic hemodilution. Baseline hematocrit and systemic oxygen extraction values were similar in all study animals. To compensate for acute anemia, control dogs increased their cardiac output, coronary blood flow, and oxygen extraction. LAD dogs were able to increase only oxygen extraction. Significant increases in the systemic oxygen extraction ratio occurred when the hematocrit reached values of $\leq30\%$ in LAD dogs and $\leq20\%$ in control dogs. The difference in the systemic oxygen extraction ratio between LAD and control dogs reached statistical significance at hematocrit values of $\leq30\%$. A systemic oxygen extraction ratio of >50% occurred at a higher hematocrit in LAD dogs (~20%) than in control dogs (~10%). Myocardial lactate production occurred in all dogs when the oxygen extraction ratio exceeded 50% and preceded hemodynamic instability in both groups. In control dogs, cardiac failure occurred at a hematocrit of $8.6 \pm 0.4\%$. In LAD dogs, cardiac failure occurred at a hematocrit of $17.0 \pm 0.5\%$. The authors concluded that a systemic oxygen extraction ratio of >50% is a valid indicator of myocardial anaerobic metabolism in anemic patients with limited coronary vascular reserve and may prove to be a useful guide for transfusion therapy.

The preceding animal studies support the concept that critical values for oxygen reserve exist and are identified by monitoring variables that reflect oxygen delivery and oxygen consumption. On the basis of these studies, the critical values indicating a marginal oxygen reserve requiring therapy are

$PvO_2 < 25$ torr

$VO_2 < 50\%$ of baseline value

Oxygen extraction ratio $(VO_2/DO_2) > 50\%$

[Chapter 3 explores the additional information provided by the use of the (lactate)/(pyruvate) ratio as an indicator of mitochondrial function.]

An underlying clinical condition (e.g., coronary artery disease) may influence the hemoglobin/hematocrit values at which anaerobic metabolism occurs. In these studies, the systemic oxygen extraction ratio may provide a valuable clue that a patient is near, at, or above the anaerobic metabolic threshold and requires red cell transfusion therapy.

Note that no single variable or derived quantity (e.g., threshold hemoglobin or systemic oxygen extraction ratio values) can be considered an absolute indication for red cell transfusion. The use of such information in addition to careful clinical assessment may allow for more effective prevention of tissue hypoxia or ischemia with red cell transfusion therapy (32).

In a study designed to assess the safety and efficacy of the synthetic oxygen-carrying solution Fluosol DA (Alpha Therapeutics, Los Angeles, California) in patients with acute anemia and religious objections to blood transfusions, the critical values obtained from the animal studies served as the basis for infusions of the solution (33). Fifteen patients did not receive Fluosol DA. The mean hemoglobin value in the noninfused group was 7.2 ± 0.5 g/dL (i.e., moderate anemia). Fourteen of these patients survived. Eight patients received Fluosol DA. The mean hemoglobin value in the infused group was 3.0 ± 0.4 g/dL (i.e., severe anemia). Six of these eight patients died. The authors concluded that Fluosol DA was unnecessary in moderate anemia and ineffective in severe anemia. Nevertheless, oxygen transport variables performed well in identifying subjects destined for good or poor outcomes, a finding that lends support for their use in transfusion decisions. The goal of red cell transfusion therapy should be to increase oxygen delivery in patients who demonstrate a physiologic need. Red cell transfusions should not be administered in the absence of apparent physiologic need. An understanding of the abnormalities responsible for deficits in oxygen delivery aids decision making with respect to the benefits of red cell transfusion therapy.

The heart, a primary compensatory organ when red cell mass is decreased, is at risk during acute blood loss. In a retrospective study of 1958 patients ≥ 18 years of age, the natural history of anemic patients who underwent surgery without transfusions was evaluated (34). The patients declined blood transfusion for religious reasons. The overall 30-day mortality was 3.2%. The 30-day mortality for patients with a preoperative hemoglobin of 12.0 g/dL or more was 1.3%. The 30-day mortality for patients with a preoperative hemoglobin <6.0 g/dL was 33.3%. The impact of blood loss on mortality was greater in patients with lower preoperative hemoglobin. The presence of cardiovascular disease further increased the risk of death associated with low preoperative hemoglobin. According to the authors, the risk of perioperative death was higher in patients with cardiovascular disease when the preoperative hemoglobin was ≤ 10 g/dL. Cardiovascular disease and operative blood loss had the same pattern of influence on in-hospital morbidity. This study revealed that a low preoperative hemoglobin concentration or considerable blood loss during an operative procedure increased the risk of death or serious morbidity, and this risk was even greater in patients with cardiovascular disease. The authors recommended that cardiovascular status and operative blood loss be considered, in addition to hemoglobin concentration, in making transfusion decisions. One could infer that transfusion therapy may have a positive impact on survival in selected surgical patients, especially those with low preoperative hemoglobin levels, cardiovascular disease, significant operative blood loss, and, especially, some combination of these factors.

Hemodynamic and oxygen transport variables were utilized in a study designed to evaluate the consequences of reduced red cell mass in critically ill patients (22). The study involved five male patients ranging in age from 19 to 65 years with severe burns ($\geq 50\%$ of total body surface area). All patients had good cardiac, pulmonary, and renal function during the study period, and all were managed with similar fluid resuscitation. None of the patients had evidence of sepsis at the time of study. The study subjects received three units of red cells 36–48 h after undergoing total burn wound excision

Transfusion Therapy

and skin grafting. The subjects did not receive red cell transfusion prior to this procedure. The study patients' pretransfusion hemoglobin was 7.5 ± 0.2 g/dL. Their posttransfusion hemoglobin was 10.5 ± 0.4 g/dL ($p < 0.01$). Posttransfusion, cardiac index dropped to 7.2 ± 0.8 L/min per m^2 from a pretransfusion value of 8.2 ± 0.8 L/min per m^2 ($p < 0.05$). The pretransfusion and posttransfusion stroke volume indices were 66.4 ± 6.5 and 60.2 ± 6.5 mL/m^2, respectively ($p < 0.05$). Oxygen delivery increased to 1060 ± 116 mL/min per m^2 posttransfusion from a pretransfusion value of 882 ± 91 mL/min per m^2 ($p < 0.05$). The oxygen extraction ration decreased to 20.1 ± 3.1% posttransfusion from a pretransfusion value of 24.0 ± 0.06% ($p < 0.05$). The posttransfusion oxygen consumption value of 206 ± 27 mL/min per m^2 was not found to be significantly different from the pretransfusion value of 199 ± 26 mL/min per m^2. In addition, no significant pre- to posttransfusion differences in mean arterial pressure, pulmonary capillary wedge pressure, heart rate, or blood viscosity were observed. Red cell transfusions in these study patients, whose burn injury stimulated the systemic inflammatory response, significantly lowered the cardiac index, stroke volume, and oxygen extraction ratio and significantly increased oxygen delivery. Oxygen consumption, which was elevated pre- and posttransfusion, remained comparable. The pretransfusion oxygen extraction ratio was not markedly abnormal, a finding that suggests adequate compensation for decreased red cell mass with cardiac mechanisms. Red cell transfusions resulted in a nonsignificant change in oxygen consumption and were, in all likelihood, of little or no benefit. The authors suggested that cardiac reserve should be a major factor in blood transfusion decisions and that maintenance of the hematocrit in the 30–33% range may reduce cardiac risk in certain critically ill patients.

Babineau et al. (23) studied the impact of red cell transfusion on oxygen consumption in critically ill surgical patients. Thirty-three consecutive red cell transfusions were evaluated in 30 surgical intensive care unit (ICU) patients. Twenty-five of 30 patients required mechanical ventilation. The average age of the patients was 63 ± 8 years with an age range of 33–86 years. Eleven transfusions were given to patients >63 years of age. Eighteen transfusions were given to patients classified as having septicemia. All study transfusions were administered more than 48 hours after surgery. All patients were considered euvolemic and hemodynamically stable at the time of transfusion. The red cells were administered according to a traditional transfusion criterion (i.e., hemoglobin <10 g/dL). Posttransfusion, the subjects' hemoglobin value rose to 10.4 ± 0.3 from a pretransfusion value of 9.4 ± 0.2 ($p < 0.001$). Oxygen delivery increased from a pretransfusion value of 401 ± 20 to 433 ± 21 mL/min per m^2 posttransfusion ($p = 0.01$). A significant pre- to posttransfusion increase was also observed for SvO_2 (pretransfusion 67 ± 1%, posttransfusion 70 ± 1%, $p = 0.005$). Significant pre- to posttransfusion decreases were observed for SaO_2 (pretransfusion 96 ± 1%, posttransfusion 95 ± 1%, $p = 0.005$) and systemic oxygen extraction ratio (pretransfusion 31 ± 1%, posttransfusion 28 ± 1%, $p = 0.003$). The pretransfusion and posttransfusion oxygen consumption values, however, did not change significantly (pretransfusion 117 ± 4 mL/min per m^2, posttransfusion 115 ± 5 mL/min per m^2, $p =$ NS). The observed change in oxygen consumption was <10% in 19 (58%), 10–20% in 6 (18%), and >20% in 8 (24%) of the 33 transfusions. Of the 11 transfusions administered to patients >63 years old, the change in oxygen consumption was <10% in 7 (63%), 10–20% in 2 (18%), and >20% in 2 (18%). Oxygen consumption increased in 16 (88%) of 18 patients with septicemia and in 2 (13%) of 15 patients without septicemia. The mean change in oxygen consumption in patients with septicemia was +7.2 ± 10% (range: +28% to −9%) compared with a mean change of $-9.1 \pm 20\%$ (range: $+52\%$ to -33%) in those individuals without septicemia. The changes in oxygen consumption in patients with and without septicemia were not statistically significant. An increase in oxygen consumption was observed in only three of the eight patients with $>20\%$ change (five patients had a $>20\%$ decrease in oxygen consumption). Therefore, a $>20\%$ increase in oxygen consumption was documented in 3 (9%) of 33 transfusions. Lactic acid, measured pretransfusion in 10 patients, was within the reference range in all cases (1–2 mM/L). Nonsignificant pretransfusion to posttransfusion changes were documented for cardiac index, heart rate, mean arterial pressure, and systemic vascular resistance. The authors concluded that red cell transfusions administered to critically ill but hemodynamically stable patients, based on a hemoglobin concentration <10 g/dL, did not significantly affect oxygen consumption. In the majority of patients (58%), red cell transfusions resulted in a change in oxygen consumption of $<10\%$; therefore, the benefit of red cell transfusion was questionable. No pretransfusion marker (e.g., heart rate, cardiac index, mean arterial pressure, or systemic oxygen extraction ratio) reliably predicted an increase in oxygen consumption of $>20\%$. Because lactic acid serum concentrations were normal in all patients measured, the study subjects likely lacked an oxygen debt sufficient to exhibit an increase in oxygen consumption following red cell transfusion. The study does, however, reinforce the point that multiple variables, not just hemoglobin concentrations, must be taken into account in red cell transfusion decisions. Achieving an increase in red cell mass does not always equate to benefit in the critically ill patient.

Although laboratory variables such as hemoglobin concentration or hematocrit can be measured, the correlation of a desired clinical effect to red cell transfusion is often difficult, especially in patients with complex medical conditions. Some insight has come from studies of patients who have declined blood transfusion. In one review, 16 reports involving a series of at least nine nontransfused Jehovah's Witness patients undergoing major surgery were evaluated (total number of operative procedures = 1404) (35). A total of 20 (1.4% of patients) deaths were reported. In eight cases (0.6% of patients), death was directly attributed to a lack of blood. In 12 instances (0.8% of patients), lack of blood was considered a factor contributing to death. Of the 20 deaths, 19 occurred in patients undergoing cardiovascular surgery (18 adults and 1 pediatric patient). The author posed the question, "Are transfusions overrated?" The data suggested that the lack of transfusion resulted in little extra morbidity and mortality.

A recent randomized trial evaluated red cell transfusion in patients with hip fracture (36). In this study, patients with hip fracture who had undergone surgical repair were eligible for the trial if their hemoglobin concentration was <10 g/dL during the first three postoperative days. Patients were randomly assigned to one of two transfusion groups. In group one (symptomatic transfusion group), red cells were transfused for symptoms of anemia or for a hemoglobin concentration <8 g/dL. Symptomatic anemia was defined as chest pain thought to be cardiac in origin; myocardial infarction; congestive heart failure; unexplained tachycardia, hypotension, or decreased urine output unresponsive to fluid replacement; and poor rehabilitation, defined as inability to get out of bed for rehabilitation on the third postoperative day. In group two (threshold transfusion group), patients received one unit of red cells at the time of random assignment and as many red cell transfusions as necessary to maintain the hemoglobin concentration >10 g/dL. Eighty-four patients were enrolled in the trial. The mean hemoglobin concentration prior to randomization was 9.1 ± 0.6 g/dL. The mean age of the study population was 82.3 ± 9.5 years. Cardiovascular disease was present in 45.2%. The median number of red cell units transfused to group one was 0 (maximum number of red cell units transfused: 6). Nineteen (45.2%) patients in group one received red cell transfusions. The median number of red cell units transfused to group two was 2 (maximum number of red cell units transfused: 4, $p < 0.001$). The hemoglobin ranges after randomization were 5.6–11.4 g/dL in group one and 8.6–14.0 g/dL in group two. The mean daily hemoglobin concentrations from the time of randomization until hospital discharge was $\sim$1 g/dL higher in group two. Five group one patients (11.9%) and two group two patients (4.8%) were dead by 60 days after randomization ($p = 0.43$). Sixteen patients in group one (39%) and 19 patients in group two (45.2%) met the criteria for the combined outcome measure of death or the inability to walk without assistance (either 10 feet or across the room) at 60 days ($p = 0.57$). No other significant differences were observed between the groups for other outcome measures (i.e., morbidity, place of residence, and length of stay). The authors concluded that the symptomatic transfusion approach, although providing a lower number of red cell transfusions and maintaining lower mean hemoglobin values, might be effective. The small number of study subjects made the study inadequately powered to reach definitive conclusions regarding mortality, morbidity, and functional status.

A large multi-institutional study involving 20 hospitals in the United States evaluated the effect of perioperative red cell transfusion in 8787 consecutive patients $\geq$60 years of age who underwent surgery due to hip fracture (37). The primary and secondary outcome measures were death within 30 days and death within 90 days of the operative procedure, respectively. Red cell transfusions were given to 3699 (42%) patients within the 7-day period following their surgical procedure. The "transfusion trigger" was defined as the lowest hemoglobin value obtained prior to the first red cell transfusion. Red cell transfusions were given to 1014 (90.5%) of 1120 patients with a hemoglobin concentration <8.0 g/dL, to 2474 (55.6%) of 4452 patients with a hemoglobin concentration between 8.0 and 9.9 g/dL, and to 211 (6.6%) of 3195 patients with a hemoglobin concentration >10 g/dL. Preoperative red cell transfusions were given to 682 (7.2%) of 9474 patients included in the preoperative transfusion analysis. At 30 days, the overall mortality was 4.6% (402 patients), whereas the 90-day mortality rate was 9.0% (788 patients). Death at 30 days occurred in 5.3% of postoperatively transfused patients and 4.0% of non-postoperatively transfused patients. The authors were unable to demonstrate an overall association between perioperative red cell transfusion and a reduction of postoperative mortality at 30 days and 90 days. The adjusted odds ratio (adjusted for trigger hemoglobin, cardiovascular disease, and other risk factors for death) for 30-day mortality in postoperatively transfused patients was 0.96 [95% cardiac index (CI), 0.74–1.26], whereas the adjusted hazard ratio for 90-day mortality was 1.08 (95% CI, 0.90–1.29). No difference in 30-day mortality was observed between patients who received and who did not receive preoperative red cell transfusions (adjusted odds ratio 1.24; 95% CI, 0.81–1.90). The authors concluded that, in this elderly population, red cell replacement in patients with hemoglobin concentrations $\geq$8.0 g/dL did not influence the risk of death at 30 and 90 days following surgery. Because 90.5% of patients with a hemoglobin concentration <8.0 g/dL received red cell replacement, the relative benefit of red cell transfusion, as it relates to mortality, could not be determined for this group.

A recent multicenter, randomized trial from Canada, known as the Transfusion in Critical Care (TRICC) trial, was designed to clarify the potential risks and benefits of red cell transfusion in critically ill patients (38). The major question addressed was whether a *restrictive* approach to red cell transfusion, maintenance of hemoglobin between 7.0 and 9.0 g/dL, was equivalent to a *liberal* approach, maintenance of hemoglobin between 10.0 and 12.0 g/dL, in euvolemic, critically ill patients. Subjects were eligible if their expected stay in the ICU was more than 24 h, their hemoglobin was ≤9.0 g/dL within 72 h of ICU admission, and they were considered euvolemic. Subjects assigned to the restrictive transfusion group received red cell transfusion when their hemoglobin concentration dropped to <7.0 g/dL. Subjects assigned to the liberal transfusion group received red cell transfusion when their hemoglobin concentration dropped to 10.0 g/dL. The primary outcome measure was death from all causes in the 30-day period following randomization. Secondary outcome measures were the 60-day rate of death from all causes, the mortality rate in the ICU, the mortality rate during hospitalization, survival time for the first 30 days following randomization, organ failure, multiple organ dysfunction score, length of stay in the ICU, and length of hospitalization.

In the TRICC trial 838 subjects were enrolled, with 418 and 420 subjects assigned to the restrictive and liberal transfusion groups, respectively. The average daily hemoglobin concentration in the restrictive group, 8.5 ± 0.7 g/dL, was significantly lower than the average daily value for the liberal group, 10.7 ± 0.7 g/dL ($p < 0.01$). Subjects in the restrictive group received an average of 2.6 ± 4.1 red cell units compared with an average of 5.6 ± 5.3 red cell units in the liberal group ($p < 0.01$). Overall, a relative 54% decrease in the number of red cell transfusions was achieved in the restrictive group. Furthermore, 33% of subjects in the restrictive group received no red cell transfusions after randomization compared with 0% of subjects in the liberal group ($p < 0.01$). The rate of death from all causes in the 30-day period following randomization, the primary outcome measure, was 18.7% in the restrictive group and 23.3% in the liberal group ($p = 0.11$). When 30-day mortality was assessed in subgroups, no significant differences were seen in subjects with a primary or secondary diagnosis of cardiac disease, in subjects with severe infections and septic shock, or in trauma patients. However, for patients <55 years of age and for patients with an APACHE II score of 20 or less, 30-day mortality was significantly lower in the restrictive transfusion group (p values of 0.02 and 0.03, respectively). The overall mortality rate during hospitalization was 22.2% in the restrictive group and 28.1% in the liberal group ($p = 0.05$). No significant differences were observed for the other mortality-related outcome measures evaluated. The number of subjects with multiorgan failure, defined as the failure of more than three organs, was not significantly different in the study groups, whereas the mean multiple organ dysfunction score was marginally lower (lower score indicates less severe organ dysfunction) in the restrictive group ($p = 0.10$). However, similar to the pattern seen with 30-day mortality, patients <55 years of age and patients with an APACHE II score of 20 or less had adjusted multiple organ dysfunction scores that were significantly lower in the restrictive transfusion group (p values of 0.03 and 0.01, respectively).

The authors of the TRICC study concluded that, in normovolemic critically ill patients, a red cell transfusion threshold as low as 7.0 g/dL, combined with the maintenance of hemoglobin concentrations between 7.0 and 9.0 g/dL, was at least as effective and possibly superior to a liberal transfusion threshold of 10.0 g/dL, with maintenance of hemoglobin values between 10.0 and 12.0 g/dL. The authors observed that the use of red cell transfusion to augment oxygen delivery did not provide a survival advantage in normovolemic subjects when the hemoglobin concentration was >7.0 g/dL. Although other studies have raised concerns about the harmful effects of anemia in patients with ischemic heart disease, the TRICC study showed that the restrictive transfusion approach was equally safe in subjects with and without cardiac disease (34,39). From these data, the authors concluded that the restrictive strategy can be used in patients with coronary artery disease but should be implemented with careful consideration in the setting of acute myocardial infarction or unstable angina. Because of the diversity of subjects enrolled in the TRICC study, the authors indicated that the conclusions drawn from the trial were generalizable to most critically ill patients, with the possible exception of patients with active coronary ischemic syndromes. Therefore, the authors recommended that critically ill patients receive red cell transfusion for hemoglobin concentration <7.0 g/dL and the hemoglobin concentration should be maintained between 7.0 and 9.0 g/dL.

What can be concluded from all of this information? The foregoing data support the idea that euvolemic, clinically stable patients without coronary artery disease most likely benefit from red cell transfusion when the hemoglobin concentration is <7 g/dL. Benefit is unlikely when the hemoglobin concentration is >9 g/dL. In addition to decreased physiologic compensation, the decreased tolerance of anemia in the elderly is likely related to a higher incidence of coronary artery disease, which reduces the ability to adequately increase coronary blood flow (4). Elderly patients, especially those with coronary artery disease, are less likely to tolerate decreases in red cell mass. Such individuals will likely benefit from red cell transfusion to maintain the hemoglobin at a higher concentration. Data about oxygen delivery and consumption can be useful in making red cell transfusion decisions. Frequently, transfusion decisions must be made in the absence of such data and rely on patient attributes (age, presence of cardiovascular disease, and other factors affecting the ability to tolerate decreased red cell mass), stability (e.g., no blood loss vs. mild blood loss vs. massive blood loss), and vital signs.

In acute blood loss, the accuracy of hemoglobin concentration as a "surrogate" for the circulating red cell mass may be poor, because it is dependent on the rapidity and extent of blood loss and the status and degree of fluid resuscitation efforts. Hemoglobin concentration interpretation in acute blood loss is a "snapshot" of a continuous process: By the time a hemoglobin value is received for interpretation, the patient's oxygen-carrying capacity could be markedly different. Because many variables affect the correlation of hemoglobin concentration with red cell mass in an actively bleeding patient, the concept of a globally applicable transfusion threshold based on a single hemoglobin "trigger" is not supportable (1,40). The decision to transfuse red cells in acute blood loss is dependent upon multiple factors in addition to the hemoglobin concentration. The rate and extent of blood loss, the likelihood of continued blood loss, the presence of other medical conditions, evidence of organ dysfunction, acid–base status, other laboratory variables, and vital signs are all important contributors to the transfusion decision. The goals in the management of acute blood loss are the restoration of intravascular volume, cessation of blood loss, and maintenance of adequate oxygen-carrying capacity. When available, the management of acute blood loss in association with elective surgery may include intraoperative and postoperative blood salvage, acute normovolemic hemodilution, and the use of autologous units of blood collected and stored in anticipation of surgery. These measures help provide a ready supply of compatible blood and decrease the need for allogeneic blood.

Important differences between chronic anemia and acute blood loss exist that influence management with red cell transfusion. Often, in acute blood loss, the initial concern is the management of hypovolemia. Patients with chronic anemia are typically normovolemic or even hypervolemic. Transfusion decisions related to chronic anemia usually allow more time to consider the risks, benefits, and alternatives. The cause of chronic anemia may make non-transfusion-based therapy more appropriate. For example, iron deficiency anemia or anemia from deficiencies of vitamin B_{12} or folic acid can often be managed without transfusion.

When the hemoglobin concentration is >7–8 g/dL, otherwise healthy people may experience dyspnea on exertion but are usually without signs or symptoms of anemia at rest. At a hemoglobin concentration of 6 g/dL, most individuals complain of weakness. When the hemoglobin concentration is 3 g/dL, most suffer from dyspnea at rest. Congestive heart failure is frequent at hemoglobin concentrations of 2–2.5 g/dL (41).

Interpretation of symptoms related to chronic anemia is often difficult. A study of subjects with iron deficiency anemia demonstrated no correlation between symptoms such as breathlessness, dizziness, fatigue, headache, irritability, and palpitations and hemoglobin concentration in the range of 8–12 g/dL (42). Subjects treated with iron replacement had an average hemoglobin increase of 2.3 g/dL; however, no symptomatic improvement was observed when compared with subjects who received placebo. A study of 118 anemic, dialysis-dependent, chronic renal failure patients with hemoglobin <9 g/dL evaluated the effect of anemia on quality of life and exercise capacity (43). In this randomized, placebo-controlled trial, subjects were divided into three groups: placebo (mean hemoglobin 7.4 g/dL), low-dose erythropoietin (mean hemoglobin 10.2 g/dL), and high-dose erythropoietin (mean hemoglobin 11.7 g/dL). Compared with placebo-treated individuals, kidney disease questionnaire results in erythropoietin-treated subjects showed better scores for fatigue, physical symptoms, relationships, and depression. Erythropoietin-treated subjects also had better global and physical scores on a sickness impact profile. No significant difference in quality of life or exercise capacity was detected between the two erythropoietin-treated groups. Erythropoietin-treated patients walked a farther distance in a stress test; however, no difference was noted between placebo- and erythropoietin-treated groups in the 6 min walk test or in variables that assessed overall quality of life.

When red cell transfusion therapy is necessary for the acute management of chronic anemia, the goal is increasing the red cell mass to a level that will prevent cardiac failure or other consequences of inadequate oxygen delivery. Achieving a normal hemoglobin is not necessary. When red cell transfusion therapy is considered for the long-term management of chronic anemia, certain questions should be addressed:

1. What are the important anemia-related signs and symptoms for a particular patient?
2. Can these signs and symptoms realistically be prevented or lessened with red cell transfusion?
3. What is the minimum hemoglobin concentration that needs to be maintained to avoid these signs and symptoms?
4. Does the potential benefit of red cell transfusion therapy outweigh the risks?

Factors to consider when answering these questions include degree of expected activity, the projected duration of anemia, the presence of other medical conditions, for example, congestive heart failure, and the overall prognosis. Once a decision to proceed with chronic red cell transfusion therapy is made, a treatment schedule should be established, for example, 2 red cell units transfused every 2 weeks. Evaluation of risks and benefits should be ongoing to allow adjustments in or cessation of the treatment protocol.

PLASMA TRANSFUSION

Plasma components available for transfusion include fresh frozen plasma (FFP), donor retested plasma (DRP), and thawed plasma (TP). DRP is plasma withheld from availability as a transfusable component until the blood donor returns to donate on a second occasion at least 112 days later. If infectious disease testing at the time of the second donation is negative, the first donated plasma unit is made available for transfusion. FFP and DRP are prepared by separating plasma from whole blood or by collecting units via plasmapheresis. FFP and DRP are stored $\leq -18°C$ within 8 h of collection. The defined storage period for FFP and DRP is 12 months when maintained at $\leq -18°C$. FFP and DRP contain all noncellular components of human blood, including all of the circulating coagulation factors and naturally occurring coagulation inhibitors. By definition, FFP and DRP contain one unit of coagulation factor activity per milliliter of component. For example, the factor VIII activity considered present in a 225 mL bag of FFP is 225 units. TP is thawed FFP or DRP stored at refrigerated temperatures (1–6°C) for 4 days beyond the expiration date of FFP or DRP. With the exception of the labile procoagulant factors, factors V and VIII, the concentration of coagulation factors in TP is similar to FFP or DRP. The volume of FFP, DRP, or TP components obtained from whole blood donations is $\sim$200–250 mL. The volume of FFP or DRP collected via plasmapheresis typically ranges from 400 to 600 mL. With the exception of viruses transmitted by leukocytes, such as cytomegalovirus (CMV) and the human T-cell lymphotropic viruses, the risk of transfusion-transmitted viral disease associated with FFP and TP derived from FFP is similar to other blood components. A quarantine period that encompasses the "window period" of the test negativity for the known transfusion-transmissible viruses makes DRP and TP derived from DRP a decreased risk for the transmission of human immunodeficiency virus-1 and -2; hepatitis B and C viruses; and human T-lymphotropic virus-I and -II. Currently, many specific virus-inactivated or recombinant coagulation factor concentrates are available for clinical use. For the correction of deficiencies of specific coagulation factors or other proteins, such concentrates have been shown to be more effective and safe than plasma components.

Indications

1. Vitamin K deficiency or correction of oral anticoagulation
2. Severe liver disease
3. Disseminated intravascular coagulation
4. Massive transfusion
5. Cardiopulmonary bypass
6. Thrombotic thrombocytopenic purpura (TTP): In normal individuals, unusually large von Willebrand factor (UL-vWF) multimers are cleaved by a protease into circulating von Willebrand factor (vWF) multimers of normal size and distribution. In TTP, this physiologic process is disturbed by excessive release of UL-vWF or interference with the proteolytic cleavage of UL-vWF (44). The circulating UL-vWF binds to platelets, causes platelet activation, and potentiates intravascular deposition of platelet aggregates. The platelet aggregates cause ischemia or infarction in various organs, including the brain or kidneys. Plasma components are used in the management of TTP, often as part of plasma exchange procedures. Plasma exchange accomplishes two objectives in TTP. First, the removal of patient plasma reduces the concentration of circulating UL-vWF. The use of normal plasma as replacement provides UL-vWF cleaving protease to the patient. The amount of plasma used in plasma exchange procedures is typically in the range of 3–4 L. FFP is the most common plasma component used in plasma exchange for TTP. The efficacy of cryo-poor plasma as a potentially superior replacement alternative in TTP is being investigated in a large randomized clinical trial (45).

Contraindications

In general, plasma transfusion should not be used when a safer and equally (or more) effective treatment is available (3,46–50). The following list summarizes situations where products other than plasma components are recommended:

1. Crystalloids, synthetic colloids, or purified human albumin solutions are the recommended products for intravascular volume repletion or expansion.
2. Crystalloids, synthetic colloids, or purified human albumin solutions are the recommended products for therapeutic plasma exchange in most conditions (plasma components are the replacement solution of choice in selected situations, such as TTP).
3. Purified human albumin or synthetic amino acid solutions are the recommended products for the correction of hypoalbuminemia or protein malnutrition.
4. Purified human immunoglobulin concentrates are recommended for the correction of hypogammaglobulinemia.
5. Desmopressin (DDAVP), virus-inactivated concentrates, or recombinant concentrates are recommended for the treatment of hemophilia A or von Willebrand disease (vWD).
6. When available, virus-inactivated concentrates or recombinant concentrates are recommended for the treatment of other isolated, inherited protein deficiencies, for example, recombinant factor VIIa or antithrombin concentrate.

PLATELETS

Platelets are prepared from donated whole blood. An individual unit of platelets should contain a minimum of 5.5×10^{10} platelets in 50–70 mL of plasma. In adults, multiple units are usually pooled for transfusion. A common dose in adults is 1 unit/10 kg of body weight. Platelets pheresis is a blood component collected from a donor via a 1–3 h cytapheresis procedure. A unit of platelets pheresis should contain a minimum of 3.0×10^{11} platelets in 200–400 mL of plasma. Recently developed apheresis equipment allows for the collection of platelets pheresis that can be labeled as leukocyte reduced without the need for further leukocyte reduction techniques. A unit of platelets pheresis or six-unit dose of platelets is expected to increase the platelet count of a 70 kg adult by 30,000–60,000 μL^{-1}. Platelet components are transfused therapeutically to treat and prophylactically to prevent platelet-related bleeding.

Platelet Selection

ABO antigens are present on the surface of platelets. Platelet recovery is decreased with major ABO incompatibility, for example, when group A platelets are transfused to group O recipients (51). Although not optimal, transfusion of platelets across ABO groups may sometimes be necessary if platelet inventory is limited. Augmentation of platelet count is usually comparable with that found with ABO compatible transfusion. A decrease in expected platelet count increments and very rare episodes of hemolysis have been observed in recipients of platelets containing ABO-incompatible plasma, for example, minor ABO incompatibility, such as group O platelets to a group A recipient (52). Patients requiring long-term support with platelet transfusion derive significant benefit from the receipt of

ABO-identical platelets (53,54). Patients who received ABO-identical platelets had higher posttransfusion platelet counts, received approximately half the number of platelet transfusions early in their clinical course, did not have an increase in existing human leukocyte antigens (HLA) antibody titers, and had delayed onset of refractoriness to platelet transfusion compared with subjects transfused with ABO-unmatched platelets. From the standpoint of posttransfusion platelet increments, the least effective combination was the transfusion of group O platelets to non-group O recipients. This finding suggests that incompatible plasma was a major contributor to less-than-optimal platelet transfusion outcomes (53,55). Studies of patients with acute leukemia and of bone marrow transplant recipients have provided evidence that recipients of minor ABO-incompatible or ABO-identical plasma-containing products had superior survival over patients not exclusively receiving such products (56,57). Increased amounts of immune complexes, for example, A antigen/anti-A complex, are present in the blood of subjects who receive ABO-unmatched platelets (52). These immune complexes can result in rapid clearance of platelets from the circulation and, quite possibly, impairment of cellular immunity against infection and malignancy (58–66). The use of ABO-matched platelets is advisable whenever possible, especially for patients expected to receive multiple platelet transfusions. If the need for platelet transfusion is urgent, the provision of platelets should not be delayed until ABO-matched platelets are located.

Because the D antigen is not present on platelets, the posttransfusion survival of platelets obtained from D-positive donors is normal in recipients with anti-D. The D antigen is problematic in platelet transfusion therapy, because even with proper manufacturing technique, platelets and platelets pheresis may contain a small amount of red cells. Consequently, the transfusion of platelets from a D-positive donor to a D-negative recipient can lead to anti-D formation. The transfusion of D-positive platelets into D-negative women of childbearing potential has to be avoided to decrease the chance of hemolytic disease of the newborn in the future. If the transfusion of D-positive platelets to such patients is necessary, Rh immune globulin [RhIg; intravenous (IV) and intramuscular (IM) preparations are available] should be administered. A full dose of RhIg (300 μg) is considered to be protective against up to 15 mL of D-positive red cells; therefore, it should protect against at least 30 units of platelets or 7 units of platelets pheresis.

Prophylactic Platelet Transfusion

General

Although prophylactic platelet transfusions are common in a wide variety of clinical situations, little scientific evidence supports this practice. In a study that attempted to determine indications for platelet transfusion in patients with thrombocytopenia, 56 children were randomized to either prophylactic or therapeutic transfusion groups (68). Subjects in the prophylactic group received platelet transfusion for a platelet count below 20,000 μL^{-1}. Subjects in the therapeutic group were given platelets whenever significant bleeding occurred and not according to a predetermined threshold platelet count. The prophylactic group demonstrated a significantly longer interval until their first bleeding episode and a significantly lower number of bleeding episodes. No significant difference was observed between the groups in overall survival or bleeding-related deaths. Overall, subjects in the prophylactic group received twice as many platelet transfusions. Interestingly, prior to the last month of life, subjects in the prophylactic group had a significantly lower number of days with bleeding; however, in the last month of life, the prophylactic group had bleeding episodes that were significantly longer in duration. The longer bleeding episodes in the prophylactic group during the last month of life were postulated to be a consequence of a higher incidence of immune refractoriness to platelet transfusion. This observation raises the question of whether prophylactic platelet transfusions should be reserved for patients with thrombocytopenia that is expected to be temporary (69). For patients in whom a prolonged course of thrombocytopenia or platelet dysfunction is expected, prophylactic platelet therapy ultimately may be detrimental and potentiate the development of a refractory state. Caution in platelet transfusion may be of particular importance in patients with intact immune function, such as those with aplastic anemia or some of the inherited platelet function defects.

Bone Marrow Hypoplasia

Prophylactic platelet transfusions are often administered to patients with thrombocytopenia from bone marrow hypoplasia, such as occurs as a result of tumor invasion, primary aplasia, radiation therapy, or chemotherapy. Many stable patients with thrombocytopenia due to marrow hypoplasia can have platelet counts as low as 5000 μL^{-1} without serious bleeding (70). When the platelet count drops below 5000 μL^{-1}, the likelihood of spontaneous hemorrhage increases (71). Bleeding also is likely with invasive procedures, trauma, or ulceration. Platelet transfusion is recommended for patients with a platelet count below 5000 μL^{-1}, even in the absence of bleeding. When the platelet count is between 5000 and 10,000 μL^{-1} spontaneous hemorrhage does occur, and the likelihood of bleeding in association with invasive procedures, trauma, or ulceration is high. When the platelet count is between 10,000 and 50,000 μL^{-1}, the likelihood of bleeding in association with invasive procedures, trauma, or ulceration is variable. Prospective randomized trials have demonstrated that a platelet count of 10,000 μL^{-1} for platelet transfusion is safe as an acceptable prophylactic platelet transfusion threshold for thrombocytopenia from marrow hypoplasia (70,72,73). When other factors or conditions are present, such as fever, sepsis, rapid platelet consumption, additional hemostatic abnormalities, an elevated white blood cell count that poses a risk of cerebral leukostasis, or an intracranial lesion, a higher platelet count (20,000–50,000 μL^{-1}) is commonly chosen as the prophylactic platelet transfusion threshold (74). Other factors that may indicate increased bleeding risk with thrombocytopenia and lead to more liberal platelet transfusion thresholds include confluent petechiae, significant gastrointestinal (GI) blood loss, continuous bleeding from a wound or other location, or a complaint of headache. Central nervous system and GI hemorrhage typically pose the most serious bleeding risks in patients with thrombocytopenia or platelet dysfunction. Retinal hemorrhage is a significant finding and is an indication for platelet transfusion. A more liberal platelet transfusion threshold is not necessarily required in patients with scattered petechiae, minor mouth bleeding, minor nose bleeding, or evidence of trace amounts of blood in the urine or stool.

Invasive Procedures

Although common practice, prophylactic platelet transfusions prior to surgery or other invasive procedures in patients with thrombocytopenia or platelet dysfunction have little experimental data for support. A review of blood utilization guidelines reveals that the prophylactic platelet transfusion threshold for patients prior to invasive procedures is usually somewhere between 50,000 and 100,000 μL^{-1} (3). Two studies of prophylactic platelet transfusions administered to subjects who were expected to develop intraoperative thrombocytopenia, from cardiopulmonary bypass in one study and hemodilution in the other, demonstrated that such an approach was ineffective (75,76). The NIH consensus panel on platelet transfusion therapy proposed that prophylactic platelet transfusions prior to invasive procedures were most beneficial when the possiblility for hemorrhage that could not be observed was present, or if a small volume of hemorrhage could have devastating results, such as bleeding into the central nervous system (69). Despite the lack of scientifically proven efficacy, guidelines have been published with a recommended prophylactic platelet transfusion threshold of 50,000 μL^{-1} for most major surgical procedures and a threshold of 100,000 μL^{-1} for neurosurgery and ophthalmology procedures (3,48).

Platelet Destruction

Prophylactic platelet transfusions have been shown to be of limited value in thrombocytopenia from consumption in TTP, from drug-induced antibodies, from antibodies related to autoimmune or lymphoproliferative disorders, or from idiopathic antiplatelet antibodies.

Therapeutic Platelet Transfusion

Platelet transfusion is indicated when significant bleeding occurs in association with thrombocytopenia or platelet dysfunction (77). Factors influencing the decision to transfuse platelets include the site and severity of bleeding, the patient's underlying clinical condition, the cause of bleeding, the platelet count, and platelet function (3,48,69,74). Platelet transfusion will be most effective when the cause of bleeding is directly attributable to a platelet function defect or thrombocytopenia. Bleeding associated with certain acquired platelet function defects respond well to platelet transfusion, such as aspirin-induced or cardiopulmonary bypass (CPB)-related defects. Other platelet function defects, such as those associated with uremia, are not as readily corrected with platelet transfusion. Transfused platelets have a propensity to acquire the functional defect associated with uremia. When bleeding patients have multiple hemostatic defects, the transfusion of other blood components, in addition to platelets, may be necessary. Drugs affecting platelet function are listed in Table 1.

When major surgery is performed on patients who are considered hemostatically competent prior to surgery, platelet transfusion is recommended when microvascular bleeding, such as small vessel bleeding in the surgical field, occurs and the platelet count is below 50,000 μL^{-1} (48). Platelet transfusion has been shown to be effective for post-CPB bleeding related to acquired platelet dysfunction. Some have recommended that platelets should be transfused post-CPB to patients with major unexplained bleeding, normal prothrombin time (PT) and partial thromboplastin time (PTT), and a platelet count below 100,000 μL^{-1} (79).

Platelet Refractoriness

Of thrombocytopenic patients who receive multiple transfusions, 20–27% develop less than expected posttransfusion platelet count increments (80). Platelet refractoriness is a particular problem in patients undergoing treatment for malignant hematologic diseases. Platelet refractoriness has been variably defined. Definitions of platelet refractoriness include unsatisfactory platelet count increments following two consecutive platelet transfusions, or following a total of three platelet transfusions given over a 2-week period (81,82). Calculation of the corrected count increment (CCI) or the predicted platelet count increment (PPCI) can be used to help determine the presence of a refractory state (Table 2).

Table 1 Drugs That Affect Platelet Function

Drugs that inhibit thromboxane synthesis	Quinidine
Cyclo-oxygenase inhibitors	Angiotensin converting enzyme inhibitors
Aspirin	Anticoagulants
Nonsteroidal anti-inflammatory agents	Heparin
Indomethacin, phenylbutazone, ibuprofen, sulfinpyrazone, sulindac, meclofenamic acid	Thrombolytic agents
	Streptokinase, tissue plasminogen activator, urokinase
ADP receptor antagonists	Psychotropics and anesthetics
Ticlopidine, clopidogrel	Tricyclic antidepressants
GPIIb-IIIa receptor antagonists	Imipramine, amitryptyline, nortriptyline
c7E3 (abciximab), tirofiban, eptifibatide	Phenothiazines
Drugs that increase platelet cyclic AMP or cyclic GMP	Chlorpromazine, promethazine, trifluoperazine
Adenylate cyclase activators	Local anesthetics
Prostaglandins I_2, D_2, E_1 and analogs	General anesthesia (halothane)
Phosphodiesterase inhibitors	Chemotherapeutic agents
Dipyridamole	Mithramycin
Cilostazol	BCNU
Methyl xanthines	Daunorubicin
Caffeine, theophylline, aminophylline	Miscellaneous agents
Nitric oxide and nitric oxide donors	Dextrans
Antimicrobials	Lipid lowering agents (clofibrate, halofenate)
Pencillins	ε-Aminocaproic acid
Cephalosporins	Antihistaminics
Nitrofurantoin	Ethanol
Hydroxychloroquine	Vitamin E
Cardiovascular drugs	Radiographic contrast agents
β-Adrenergic blockers (propranolol)	Food items and alternative medications
Vasodilators (nitroprusside, nitroglycerin)	(onions, garlic, ginger, cumin, turmeric, clove, black tree fungus)
Diuretics (furosemide)	
Calcium channel blockers	

For most of the drugs, there is little evidence that their impact on platelet aggregation responses or on the bleeding time is associated with a clinically significant hemostatic defect.
Source: From Ref. 315.

In addition to alloimmunization, multiple conditions or processes can lead to suboptimal posttransfusion platelet counts. These conditions include fever, sepsis, massive bleeding, disseminated intravascular coagulation (DIC), TTP, immune thrombocytopenic purpura (ITP), splenomegaly, IV amphotericin B, other medications via immune mechanisms, or inappropriate platelet storage (Table 3). Other clinical features may also influence the outcome of platelet transfusion. A study designed to identify factors that independently influence platelet transfusion efficacy in patients following hematopoietic progenitor cell transplantation identified high total bilirubin, total body irradiation, high serum tacrolimus concentration, and high serum cyclosporine A concentration as major factors that independently predicted a low CCI (84). Of note, refractoriness to platelet transfusion is often the result of multiple factors, for example, sepsis in an alloimmunized patient. Approaches to platelet transfusion that address one source of refractoriness in the presence of multiple causes often achieve less than satisfactory results.

Table 2 Determination of Response to Transfused Platelets

Calculation of the corrected count increment (CCI)

$$\text{CCI} = \frac{\text{PI} \times \text{SA} \times 10^{11}}{N}$$

PI = platelet count increment (Posttransfusion platelet count − pretransfusion platelet count)
SA = body surface area in m^2
N = number of platelets transfused (no. of platelet units × 10^{11})

Example: If 4×10^{11} platelets are transfused to a patient whose body surface area (BSA) is 1.8 m^2 and the increase in platelet count posttransfusion is 25,000, then:

$$\text{CCI} = \frac{25,000 \times 1.8 \times 10^{11}}{4 \times 10^{11}} = 11,250 \text{ platelets}$$

Calculation of the predicted platelet count increment (PPCI)

$$\text{PPCI} = \frac{N \times 0.67}{1000 \times \text{Blood volume in mL}}$$

N = number of platelets transfused (no. of platelet units × 10^{11})
0.67 = correction factor for splenic uptake
Blood volume = 70 mL/kg body weight × actual weight in kg

Example: If 4×10^{11} platelets are transfused to a 70 kg person (blood volume = 4900 mL), then:

$$\text{PPCI} = \frac{4 \times 10^{11} \times 0.67}{1000 \times 4900} = 54,700 \text{ platelets}$$

If the observed platelet count increase posttransfusion is 25,000, then:

$$\%\text{PPCI} = \frac{25,000}{54,700} = 46\%$$

Table 3 Common Critical-Care Drugs Implicated in Thrombocytopenia

Antiarrythmics	Histamine H$_2$ blockers
Procainamide	Cimetidine
Quinidine	Ranitidine
Anti-GPllb/Illa agents	Acetaminophen
Abciximab	Amrinone
Eplifibalide	Carbamazepine
Tirofiban	Gold
Antimicrobial agents	Heparin
Amphotericin B	Hydrochlorothiazide
Linezolid	Nonsteroidal anti-inflammatory agents
Rifampin	Quinine
Trimethoprim-sulfamethoxazole	
Vancomycin	

Source: From Ref. 317.

HLA antibodies, ABO antibodies, drug-dependent antibodies, platelet-specific alloantibodies, and platelet-reactive autoantibodies can all cause immune-mediated refractoriness to platelet transfusion. HLA antibodies are responsible for the most common immune-mediated type of platelet refractoriness. Interestingly, HLA antibodies and platelet-specific antibodies can disappear in some patients who receive continued transfusion therapy (85).

The approach to platelet transfusion therapy in refractory patients with HLA antibodies typically involves the selection of HLA-matched or crossmatch-compatible components. HLA-matched platelets pheresis are commonly used and are frequently effective in this context (86). The term HLA-matched is not synonymous with HLA-identical. HLA-matched platelets vary with regard to the extent of match present. They are graded from best (i.e., grade A—all four donor antigens are identical to the recipient antigens) to worst (i.e., grade D—two antigens of the donor are not present in the recipient, and the antigens are not cross-reactive with the recipient antigens) (Table 4). The most successful outcomes with HLA-matched platelets, as documented by the largest increases in CCI, occur when grade A or B matches are used. When an order for HLA-matched platelets is received, the platelets provided are typically the best match available relative to factors such as donor availability and time considerations for delivery of the platelets. As a result, less-than-ideal HLA-matched platelets are often provided to refractory patients. For example, one study documented that 43% of HLA-matched platelets provided to subjects were in the suboptimal grade B or C categories (87). To prevent transfusion-associated graft-vs.-host disease (TA-GVHD), HLA-matched platelets should be gamma-irradiated.

When a decision is made to provide HLA-matched platelets, an investigation should be performed for platelet-specific antibodies that would limit the potential success of transfusion of HLA-matched platelets. If platelet-specific antibodies are present, more successful platelet transfusions may be achieved if family members, who are statistically more likely to share the recipient's platelet antigen phenotype, or individuals matching the recipient's phenotype are used as donors.

An alternative HLA-based approach to the management of platelet refractoriness is called the antibody specificity prediction (ASP) method (81). In the ASP method, the specificities of a recipient's anti-HLA antibodies are determined, and individuals lacking the corresponding HLA antigens are selected as donors. A study comparing platelet transfusion outcomes in refractory patients documented that platelets selected via the ASP

Table 4 Degree of Matching for HLA-Matched Platelets

Match grade	Description	Examples of donor phenotypes for a recipient who is A1,3;B8,27
A	4-antigen match	A1,3;B8,27
B	No mismatched antigens present	
B1U	1 antigen unknown or blank	A1,—;B8,27
B1X	1 cross-reactive group	A1,3;B8,7
B2UX	1 antigen blank and 1 cross-reactive	A1,—;B8,7
C	1 mismatched antigen present	A1,3;B8,35
D	2 or more mismatched antigens present	A1,32;B8,35
R	Random	A2,28;B7,35

Source: From Ref. 67.

method were superior to random donor selection and equivalent to donor selection by HLA-matching or platelet cross-matching (81). Compared with the HLA-matching criteria, many more potential donors were available in the same directory of HLA-typed donors when the ASP method was applied. The ASP method may be a more efficient method of identifying potentially successful platelet donors for refractory patients.

A viable alternative to HLA-matched platelets, platelet cross-matching is another approach used to address platelet refractoriness. One study documented that cross-match-compatible platelets, even in the absence of an HLA-match, provided posttransfusion platelet count increments similar to HLA-matched platelets (88). Furthermore, an inadequate platelet count increment was observed in all 31 cross-match-incompatible platelet transfusions, including 13 cross-match-incompatible HLA-matched platelet transfusions. The authors concluded that HLA-matched platelets for refractory patients are of no benefit when cross-match-compatible platelets are available. Platelet cross-matching, therefore, avoids the exclusion of HLA-mismatched donors that could provide successful platelet transfusion outcomes. In addition, platelet cross-matching aids in the selection of potentially beneficial platelet products when platelet-specific antibodies are present. The technique is most useful in identifying donor-recipient pairs to avoid, because pretransfusion incompatibility had been found to be predictive of an unsuccessful platelet transfusion (89). A major drawback of platelet cross-matching is the limited supply of compatible donors. In a study of 41 subjects refractory to platelet transfusion, cross-matches were performed using two different techniques [33 with a microenzyme-linked immunosorbent assay (microELISA) and 8 with a solid-phase assay (SPA)] (90). The microELISA yielded incompatible results in 733 (74%) of 944 cross-matches, whereas the SPA yielded incompatible results in 352 (85%) of 417 cross-matches. The authors concluded that identifying compatible units for heavily alloimmunized patients with these techniques is difficult. Some authors have recommended that HLA-matched platelets may be more practical when 70% or more of donors are found to be cross-match-incompatible for a patient (67).

Platelet Alloimmunization—Prevention

Patients who receive platelet transfusions generally develop HLA antibodies 21–28 days following primary antigenic exposure; however, primary alloimmunization can occur in as few as 10 days (91). Previously transfused or pregnant individuals can form HLA antibodies 4 days after secondary exposure to antigens via platelet transfusion (91). The estimates of primary HLA alloimmunization from transfusion vary from 18% to 50% (92). Primary alloimmunization to HLA antigens (including HLA Class I antigens) requires exposure to HLA Class II antigens, which are present on leukocytes but absent on platelets. Platelets express HLA Class I antigens; therefore, HLA alloimmunization to platelets is due primarily to exposure to HLA Class II antigen-bearing leukocytes from transfusion or pregnancy. Consequently, the risk of primary HLA alloimmunization to platelets is decreased when HLA Class II antigen exposure is minimized or rendered ineffective. Methods to prevent transfusion-related alloimmunization from HLA Class II antigen exposure include ultraviolet B (UVB) irradiation or leukocyte reduction of blood components. The results of the Trial to Reduce Alloimmunization to Platelets (TRAP) study showed that the use of UVB-irradiated or leukocyte-reduced (leukocyte filtration) blood components was associated with an incidence of HLA antibody formation of 17–21% compared to an incidence of 45% in subjects not receiving these components (93). Compared with 16% of subjects in the comparison group, refractoriness to platelet transfusion was observed in 7–10% of subjects receiving UVB-irradiated or leukocyte-reduced blood components (93). Some investigators have reported that alloimmunization is related to the number of donor exposures (94). Others have not observed a relationship between the number of donor exposures and alloimmunization (95). The findings of the TRAP study support the concept that leukocyte reduction, rather than the limitation of donor exposures, was the principal factor in the prevention of platelet alloimmunization (93). From the standpoint of prevention of alloimmunization, a pool of leukocyte-reduced platelets is equivalent to a unit of leukocyte-reduced platelets pheresis (96).

Contraindications

The transfusion of platelets is relatively contraindicated when the probability of therapeutic benefit is low. Platelet transfusion in such cases would waste a precious blood component that may benefit another patient. Example of such relative contraindications include prophylactic transfusions to stable refractory patients or stable patients with ITP (97). When splenectomy is performed on patients with ITP, platelet transfusion should be withheld until the vascular pedicle is clamped. Unless severe, potentially life-threatening bleeding is present, platelet transfusion is not recommended for patients with heparin-induced thrombocytopenia (HIT) or TTP. The likelihood of benefit is low, and because platelet thrombi are an integral component of the pathophysiology of these processes, platelet transfusion may worsen these conditions (98).

CRYOPRECIPITATE TRANSFUSION

Cryoprecipitate (CRYO) is a concentrated source of some, but not all, plasma proteins. CRYO is prepared by thawing a unit of FFP at 1–6°C, which leads to precipitation of certain protein constituents. All but 10–15 mL of the supernatant is then removed. The precipitate plus the 10–15 mL of remaining supernatant is then refrozen and stored at $-18°C$ or colder within 1 h of preparation. CRYO stored at $-18°C$ or colder has a shelf life of 1 year. Important constituents of CRYO include factor VIIIc, vWF, factor XIII, and fibrinogen. Currently, CRYO is the only concentrated fibrinogen product available for transfusion in the United States. One bag of CRYO contains approximately 80–120 units of factor VIII and at least 150 mg of fibrinogen (99). The average amount of fibrinogen in one bag of CRYO is ~250 mg. CRYO also contains ~20–30% of the factor XIII and ~40–70% of the vWF in the parent unit of FFP. ABO antibodies are present in CRYO.

Indications

The major indication for the transfusion of CRYO is the replacement of fibrinogen in patients with hypofibrinogenemia or dysfibrinogenemia. For fibrinogen replacement, the following can be used to calculate the dose (100):

1. Patient weight (kg) × 70 mL/kg = patient blood volume (mL)
2. Patient blood volume (mL) × (1.0 − hematocrit) = patient plasma volume (mL)

3. Mg of fibrinogen required = [desired fibrinogen level (mg/dL) − initial fibrinogen level (mg/dL) × patient plasma volume (mL)/(100 mL/dL)]
4. Number of CRYO bags required = fibrinogen required (mg)/(250 mg/CRYO bag)

In the past, a major indicaton for CRYO was the treatment of vWD. The current availability of virus-inactivated factor VIII concentrates with proven effectiveness against vWD, such as Humate P, has replaced therapy with CRYO for this indication. Virus-safe factor VIII concentrates are also preferred over CRYO for the treatment of hemophilia A. CRYO is a treatment option for vWD or hemophilia A when immediate therapy is necessary, and the preferred therapeutic products are not readily available (48).

Other indications for CRYO include the treatment of uremia-associated platelet dysfunction and isolated factor XIII deficiency. CRYO, as a source of fibrinogen, can be used to form a topical fibrin sealant (101). To make the fibrin sealant, topical thrombin, with or without calcium, is drawn into one syringe and one to two units of CRYO, which may be autologous, are drawn into a second syringe. When the two syringes are sprayed simultaneously on a surface, the fibrinogen from CRYO is converted to fibrin by topical thrombin. The use of topical bovine thrombin has been associated with antibody formation, including antibodies with specificity for thrombin and factor V (102,103). The anti-bovine thrombin and anti-bovine factor V antibodies occasionally cross-react with human thrombin and factor V. Patients with these antibodies typically have abnormal PT and activated partial thromboplastin time (aPTT), and some develop a bleeding diathesis. Virus-inactivated fibrin sealants containing human thrombin, higher amounts of fibrinogen, and bovine aprotinin to decrease fibrinolysis are now available. These fibrin sealants have been licensed for use in cardiac surgery, splenic trauma, and colostomy closure (104). Fibrin sealants are also used for other purposes, such as eardrum or dura mater repair procedures.

LEUKOREDUCED BLOOD COMPONENTS

Leukocytes or the cytokines they produce are associated with a number of transfusion-related adverse effects. Examples include febrile nonhemolytic transfusion reactions (FNHTR), alloimmunization to HLA or leukocyte-specific antigens, TA-GVHD, and the transmission of leukocyte-associated viruses (e.g., CMV). Another proposed but not universally agreed upon effect attributed to leukocyte exposure is immune modulation that may confer an increased risk of postoperative infection and tumor recurrence following surgical resection.

Febrile Nonhemolytic Transfusion Reactions

Fever is estimated to occur in association with ∼1% of red cell transfusions and up to 30% of platelet transfusions (105–107). FNHTR, a diagnosis of exclusion, is defined as a transfusion-associated rise in recipient temperature of $\geq 1°C$, with or without chills or rigors, not attributable to hemolysis, infection, or other cause (108). Leukocytes in blood products have been implicated in the pathogenesis of transfusion-associated fever (80). FNHTR can occur via at least three different processes. In the first, alloantibodies in the recipient react with donor leukocyte HLA or non-HLA antigens to cause the release of inflammatory cytokines, for example, interleukin-1, from donor white cells. Inflammatory cytokines such as interleukin-1, interleukin-6, and tumor necrosis factor induce the synthesis of fever-producing prostaglandins by the hypothalamus (109). In the second, complement activation occurs as a result of antigen–antibody complex formation, for example, recipient antibody–donor antigen complex. The C5a produced during complement activation causes the release of inflammatory cytokines from recipient monocytes (110–112). The third process involves inflammatory cytokines that have accumulated in the blood component during storage (113–115). A number of observations support the contention that this third mechanism plays a prominent role in the incidence of FNHTRs (107,113): (1) FNHTRs occur in patients with no documented previous alloimmune exposure (e.g., allogeneic transfusions or pregnancies) (106,113); (2) the provision of leukocyte-reduced blood components does not prevent all FNHTRs; and (3) the incidence of FNHTRs is positively correlated with the age of transfused blood components (107,113–116).

Although red cell components stored at 1–6°C are known to contain a higher number of leukocytes, FNHTRs occur more frequently in association with the transfusion of platelets, which are stored at 20–24°C (106,107,117). A study published in 1994 evaluated the role of plasma in reactions associated with platelet transfusion (113). The investigators separated platelet concentrates into their plasma and cellular portions and transfused them into study subjects in random order. Twelve subjects were transfused with 64 component pairs. The plasma and cellular portions were associated with 20 and 6 transfusion reactions, respectively ($p = 0.009$). More severe reactions were observed with the plasma portions. The plasma reactions were positively correlated with the concentrations of interleukin-1 beta and interleukin-6 in the components. Interleukin-1 beta and interleukin-6 concentrations rose progressively in platelets during storage and were related to the leukocyte content of the platelet components. Other investigators have confirmed the occurrence of cytokine accumulation during blood storage (107,114,118–121). The initial leukocyte count, length of storage, storage temperature, and interleukin-6 concentrations have all been correlated with the incidence of FNHTRs (107,113–115). Cytokine accumulation in blood components can be effectively minimized with prestorage leukocyte reduction.

Leukocyte-reduced red cell components are effective in decreasing the incidence of FNHTRs. A reduction in the leukocyte content in red cell units to less than 5×10^8 has been shown to effectively prevent such reactions in subjects with a history of recurrent FNHTRs (107,110,118,119,121–127). Prestorage leukocyte reduction is probably better than bedside filtration for the prevention of FNHTRs associated with red cell transfusions. In a study designed to evaluate prestorage vs. bedside leukocyte reduction, recipients of 4726 units of prestorage leukoyte-reduced red cells were compared with recipients of 6447 units of bedside-filtered leukocyte-reduced red cells (107,122). The incidences of FNHTRs were 1.1% and 2.15% in the prestorage and bedside-filtered recipients, respectively ($p = 0.0045$).

The data supporting the use of leukocyte-reduced platelets for the prevention of FNHTRs is less consistent. Several reports, mainly from the 1980s, which involved small numbers of patients, provided evidence supporting a reduced incidence of febrile reactions with leukocyte-reduced platelet components (128–133). In a 1991 study, 36 patients who had febrile reactions associated with unmodified platelets were evaluated for their response to leukocyte-reduced platelets (107,117). Prior to being treated with poststorage leukocyte-reduced platelets, the patients received a total of 409 transfusions of unmodified platelets and experienced 84 febrile reactions, an overall febrile reaction rate of 20.5%. The febrile reaction rates associated with pooled concentrates, non-HLA-matched apheresis platelets, and HLA-matched apheresis platelets were 27.2%, 14.0% ($p < 0.01$ when compared with pooled concentrates), and 6.5% ($p < 0.001$ when compared with pooled concentrates), respectively. A febrile reaction was documented in 84 (13.5%) of 623 total leukocyte-reduced platelet transfusions ($p < 0.02$). The febrile reaction rate associated with pooled concentrates dropped to 17%, and the rate associated with non-HLA-matched apheresis platelets dropped to 7%. Unfortunately, febrile reactions to platelets persisted in 28 of 36 patients, and only two patients achieved a significant decrease in their reaction rate with poststorage leukocyte-reduced platelets. The results of this study suggest that the overall benefit of poststorage leukocyte reduction is questionable. In another study, reactions to platelet transfusions were evaluated 6 months before and after the use of bedside leukocyte filters in hematology/oncology patients (107,134). Transfusion reaction evaluations were conducted on 32 (1.7%) of 1901 transfusions of pooled platelet concentrates prior to leukocyte reduction and on 90 (5.3%) of 1704 pooled platelet transfusions following leukocyte reduction ($p < 0.001$). Bedside leukocyte filtration of platelets provided no benefit in this study population.

Given the advent of prestorage leukocyte reduction of platelet components, a reevaluation of leukocyte reduction for the prevention of FNHTRs to platelets appears justified. In a study of apheresis platelet transfusions administered over a 32-month period to hematology/oncology patients who had two prior febrile reactions, the incidence of additional febrile reaction in association with prestorage or poststorage leukocyte-reduced platelets was documented (135). Twenty-two subjects received both prestorage and poststorage leukocyte-reduced apheresis platelets. Ten subjects had reactions during the study period. Nine of the ten subjects had a lower reaction rate with prestorage leukocyte-reduced apheresis platelets. The overall reaction rate for prestorage leukocyte-reduced apheresis platelets was $0.78 \pm 2.1\%$ when compared with a reaction rate of $4.8 \pm 9.1\%$ for poststorage leukocyte-reduced apheresis platelets. The authors concluded that prestorage leukocyte reduction was more effective than poststorage leukocyte reduction for the prevention of subsequent febrile reactions to platelets.

Apheresis machines in current use are capable of collecting a therapeutic dose of platelets with fewer than 1×10^6 contaminating leukocytes. Platelets pheresis, collected with these apheresis machines, can be labeled as leukocyte reduced without additional manipulation. These components are prestorage leukocyte-reduced platelets pheresis and are a therapeutic option when leukocyte-reduced blood components are deemed necessary.

Cytomegalovirus

CMV, a member of the herpes virus family, is a leukocyte-associated DNA virus that is transfusion transmissible (136). In the United States, 50–80% of blood donors are seropositive for CMV. Although serological testing documents a large percentage of blood donors with evidence of CMV exposure, <1% of blood components prepared from known seropositive donations are postulated to transmit the virus (137). Transfusion-transmitted CMV infection is usually of no clinical significance in immunocompetent recipients. For many transfusion recipients, the provision of blood components known to be of reduced risk for CMV is not necessary. However, CMV infection can cause serious adverse sequelae (e.g., retinitis, gastroenteritis, or interstitial pneumonitis) in susceptible individuals. Certain transfusion recipients identified to be susceptible to the serious consequences of CMV should be protected from transfusion-transmitted CMV (137). The provision of CMV-seronegative blood components is one strategy to minimize the risk of transfusion-transmitted CMV. As an example of the success of this strategy, studies evaluating seronegative marrow transplant patients documented incidences of CMV infection of 1–4% in subjects transfused with CMV-seronegative blood components and 23–37% in recipients of CMV-unscreened blood (138–141). Unfortunately, seronegative blood does not eradicate transfusion-transmitted CMV. Explanations for the failure to totally eliminate transfusion-transmitted CMV infection include (1) the intrinsic false-negative rate of the serologic test for anti-CMV, (2) a decrease in antibody titer in the blood donor to below the threshold of detection of the anti-CMV assay, (3) the possibility of transient viremia with binding of virus to circulating antibody, which blocks detection of antibody with the anti-CMV assay, or (4) some healthy individuals who test negative for anti-CMV still harbor the virus (142,143).

A second strategy is the use of leukocyte-reduced blood components. This option is appealing because the high seroprevalence of anti-CMV in the donor population limits the availability of CMV-seronegative blood components (142). Many studies have evaluated the effectiveness of leukocyte-reduction for the prevention of transfusion-transmitted CMV (141,144–153). One such trial was a multicenter study involving 502 marrow transplant patients (141). Prior to transplant, the subjects were randomized to receive CMV-seronegative or leukocyte-reduced blood components. CMV infections occurring more than 21 days after transplant were considered to be transfusion related. Subjects were monitored for evidence of CMV infection between days 21 and 100 posttransplant. In the primary analysis of all identified infections, no significant differences were observed between the two groups for probability of CMV infection (1.3% for recipients of seronegative blood, 2.4% for recipients of leukocyte-reduced blood, $p = 1.0$), CMV disease (0% in the seronegative group, 2.4% in the leukocyte-reduced group, $p = 1.0$), or probability of surivival ($p = 0.6$). In the secondary analysis of all infections from day 0 to day 100 posttransplant, infection rates were observed to be similar; however, the difference in the incidence of CMV disease between the treatment groups achieved statistical significance (0% in the seronegative group, 2.4% in the leukocyte-reduced group, $p = 0.03$). Even though a higher rate of CMV disease in subjects receiving leukocyte-reduced blood components was observed, the actual rate of CMV disease was <5%. An acceptable rate was defined by the investigators as ≤5%. The authors concluded that leukocyte reduction, poststorage leukocyte reduction via white cell filtration, was an effective alternative to seronegative blood components for the prevention of transfusion-associated CMV infection in marrow transplant patients. Whether prestorage leukocyte-reduction provides different efficacy in the prevention of transfusion-transmitted CMV is not known.

The types of patients in whom CMV-safe blood components should be considered include the following (142):

1. Patients receiving chemotherapy intended to produce severe neutropenia, such as individuals undergoing treatment for certain forms of leukemia or lymphoma. If such patients are CMV seronegative, the use of CMV-seronegative or leukocyte-reduced blood components is indicated.
2. Pregnant patients. If such patients are CMV seronegative, the use of CMV-seronegative or leukocyte-reduced blood components is indicated.
3. Patients infected with HIV. If such patients are CMV seronegative, the use of CMV-seronegative or leukocyte-reduced blood components is indicated.

4. Solid organ allograft recipients not requiring massive transfusion support. If such patients are CMV seronegative, and they receive an organ from a CMV-seronegative donor, the use of CMV-seronegative of leukocyte-reduced blood components is indicated.
5. Allogeneic or autologous hematopoietic progenitor cell transplant recipients. If such patients are CMV seronegative, the use of CMV-seronegative or leukocyte-reduced blood components is indicated.
6. Low-birth-weight (<1200 g) premature infants. The use of CMV-seronegative or leukocyte-reduced blood components is indicated. In a CMV-seronegative recipient, the use of leukocyte-reduced blood components may be slightly preferred because of the potential for the transfusion of anti-CMV antibody.

Immunomodulation

In 1973, Opelz et al. (154) published a report on the beneficial immunosuppressive effect of allogeneic blood transfusion on allograft survival in kidney transplant recipients. Allogeneic blood has been associated with a reduction in the recurrence rate in individuals with Crohn's disease, and it has shown efficacy in patients with recurrent spontaneous abortions (155,156). Concern exists that immunosuppression associated with allogeneic blood may also have harmful effects, such as increasing the risk of postoperative infections and tumor recurrence. Proposed mediators of allogeneic transfusion-associated immunosuppression include donor leukocytes, soluble HLA molecules, and plasma factors, for example, transforming growth factor β (157). The role of leukocyte-reduced blood components for the prevention or minimization of immunosuppression is not firmly established. In 1981, Gantt proposed that the transfusion of allogeneic blood in the perioperative period could be associated with an increased recurrence rate for resected malignancies (158). Subsequently, numerous reports of randomized trials and observation studies evaluating the effect of allogeneic transfusion on cancer recurrence have been published. Approximately two-thirds of the observational studies report an association of allogeneic transfusion with an increased rate of cancer recurrence (159). A meta-analysis of 20 papers published between 1982 and 1990 evaluated the impact of perioperative allogeneic blood transfusion in 5236 patients who underwent surgery for colorectal carcinoma (160). The odds ratios for disease recurrence, death from cancer, and death from any cause for recipients of perioperative blood transfusions were 1.8 (95% CI, 1.30–2.51), 1.76 (95% CI, 1.15–2.66), and 1.63 (95% CI, 1.12–2.38), respectively. The authors concluded that perioperative blood transfusion was associated with increased risk of colorectal carcinoma recurrence and death from colorectal carcinoma.

A randomized trial published in 1993 evaluated whether prognosis in colorectal cancer patients was improved in recipients of autologous blood transfusions compared with recipients of allogeneic blood (161). Subjects in the autologous group donated two units prior to surgery. A total of 475 subjects, 236 subjects in the allogeneic group and 239 subjects in the autologous group, were enrolled in the trial. The overall colorectal-cancer-specific survival rates at 4 years were 67% in the allogeneic group and 62% in the autologous group ($p = 0.39$). Of the 423 subjects who underwent curative surgery, no recurrence of colorectal cancer at 4 years was documented in 66% of the allogeneic group and 63% of the autologous group ($p = 0.93$). The authors observed that the relative recurrence rate in transfused subjects was significantly higher than nontransfused subjects (relative recurrence rates: allogeneic recipients 2.1, $p = 0.01$; autologous recipients 1.8,

$p = 0.04$). The authors concluded that autologous blood does not improve prognosis in patients with colorectal cancer; however, transfusions in general are associated with a poorer prognosis. This finding likely was due to conditions requiring transfusion. In contrast, another randomized trial of subjects with colorectal cancer documented allogeneic blood as an independent predictor of tumor recurrence. In this trial, autologous blood was not an independent predictor of tumor recurrence (162). Autologous blood is not inert with respect to immune effects on the recipient (163). Consequently, autologous arms of studies are not equivalent to negative controls. If autologous blood has immunosuppressive effects, studies utilizing such blood may complicate the interpretation of the overall immunomodulatory effect of allogeneic blood.

The impact of leukocyte-depletion on tumor recurrence and postoperative infection also has been studied. In one multicenter trial, surgical patients with colorectal cancer were randomized to receive either leukocyte-reduced red cells or red cells prepared with buffy coat removal (164). No differences between the two transfusion groups were detected for survival, disease-free survival, cancer recurrence, or overall infection rates after an average follow-up period of 36 months. Subjects undergoing curative resection and red cell transfusion of any sort had a lower 3-year survival than nontransfused subjects (69% vs. 81%, $p = 0.001$) and a higher infection rate (39% vs. 24%, $p < 0.001$). Because standard red cells in the United States are not prepared by buffy coat removal, the relevance of this study is questionable for transfusions administered in the United States. Lack of clinical data with blood components routinely used in the United States makes the impact of leukocyte-reduction of allogeneic blood on tumor recurrence uncertain.

The majority of observational studies have shown an association of perioperative transfusion with an increased incidence of postoperative infection (165). A number of randomized trials evaluated the impact of allogeneic, autologous, and leukocyte-reduced blood on postoperative infection (161,164,166–169).

In a study evaluating autologous compared to allogeneic blood, 120 surgical patients with colorectal cancer were randomized to receive allogeneic (62 subjects) or autologous (58 subjects) blood transfusions (166). A significant difference in the rate of postoperative infections was detected: 17 (27%) in the allogeneic group and 7 (12%) in the autologous group ($p < 0.05$). Following multivariate regression analysis, the odds ratio for postoperative infection with allogeneic blood compared with autologous blood was 2.84. In contrast, another randomized trial found nearly indentical postoperative infection rates in association with allogeneic and autologous blood transfusions (25% and 27%, respectively) in subjects with colorectal cancer (161).

A small number of randomized trials suggest that leukocyte depletion reduces the risk of postoperative infection (167–169). In a study of 197 individuals undergoing elective colorectal surgery, subjects were randomized to receive whole blood or filtered blood "free from leukocytes and platelets" (167). In total, 56 subjects received whole blood and 48 received filtered blood. Postoperative infections were documented in 13 (23%) whole blood recipients, 1 (2%) filtered blood recipient, and 2 (2%) nontransfused subjects ($p < 0.01$ for whole blood vs. other groups). In another trial, patients undergoing colorectal surgery were randomized to receive leukocyte-reduced (118 recipients) or buffy coat poor red cells (142 recipients) (168). The rates of wound infection, intra-abdominal abscess, and postoperative pneumonia were significantly higher in subjects receiving buffy coat poor red cells (12%, 5%, and 23%, respectively) than in subjects receiving leukocyte-reduced red cells (0%, 5%, and 3%, respectively). The authors concluded that the association between allogeneic blood transfusion and postoperative infection is limited to components not adequately depleted of leukocytes. A meta-analysis of four randomized clinical trials disclosed a relative risk of 1.03 for postoperative infection associated with buffy coat poor allogeneic red cells compared with autologous or leukocyte-reduced red cells (170). This meta-analysis was designed to detect a difference of ≥33% in the risk of postoperative infection. Any difference of <33% was not detected by the analysis. Similar to the investigations of tumor recurrence, the impact of leukocyte reduction of allogeneic blood on the incidence of postoperative infection awaits clarification.

RECOMBINANT FACTOR VIIa

Recombinant factor VIIa (rFVIIa) is a product originally developed for the treatment of bleeding in hemophilia A or B patients with inhibitors to factor VIII or factor IX. The successful use of rFVIIa has been documented in nonhemophiliacs with acquired inhibitors to factor VIII. Studies support a hemostatic effect of rFVIIa in patients with thrombocytopenia, platelet function defects, liver function abnormalities, and in other bleeding patients with less well-defined hemostatic problems (171–177).

rFVIIa is an appealing therapeutic option. Factor VIIa does not activate factor X unless it has formed a complex with tissue factor (TF). TF is not normally exposed to circulating blood; therefore, infusion of rFVIIa should not induce systemic activation of coagulation. Circulating factor VIIa is not directly inactivated by naturally occurring anticoagulants, such as antithrombin. Theoretically, infused rFVIIa travels, without inhibition by circulating natural anticoagulants, to sites of injury where TF is expressed, and initiates hemostasis without activation of coagulation elsewhere (179). In animal studies, rFVIIa administration has not been shown to cause systemic activation of coagulation (180,181).

rFVIIa has been used to treat patients with specific coagulation factor deficiencies or inhibitors, including hemophilia A or B patients with and without inhibitors, patients with acquired inhibitors to factor VII or factor IX, and factor VII deficient patients. The clinical indications for rFVIIa in such patients include muscle hemorrhage, joint hemorrhage, mucocutaneous hemorrhage, surgical prophylaxis, intracerebral hemorrhage, and other emergency situations. A randomized, multicenter trial published in 1998 compared the efficacy of two dosage regimens of rFVIIa for the treatment of joint, muscle, and mucocutaneous hemorrhage in subjects with hemophilia A or B, with or without inhibitors (182). Subjects received either 35 or 70 µg/kg at intervals of 2.5 ± 0.5 h. The total number of bleeding episodes treated was 179; 145 episodes of acute hemarthrosis occurred. The results showed that rFVIIa in doses of 35 or 70 µg/kg were safe and effective for the treatment of joint and muscle hemorrhages. For joint hemorrhage, both doses of rFVIIa showed equivalent efficacy. Seventy-one percent of the episodes in both groups were categorized as having an effective or excellent response within 12 h. When subjects with only inhibitors were evaluated, an effective or excellent response within 12 h was documented in 78% of patients treated with 35 µg/kg and in 68% treated with 70 µg/kg. The authors concluded that the appropriate dose for the treatment of joint and peripheral muscle hemorrhage in hemophiliac patients with inhibitors is 35–70 µg/kg given every 2–3 h until hemostasis is achieved. Because small numbers of subjects were treated for mucocutaneous hemorrhage, the authors arrived at no conclusions for the treatment of mucocutaneous hemorrhage with rFVIIa. The authors did acknowledge that the prior compassionate use experience with rFVIIa for the treatment of serious hemorrhages revealed excellent results with higher doses (e.g., 90 μg/kg every 2–3 h); therefore, a higher dose than evaluated in their trial may be even more effective (182–185). Another study evaluated the safety and efficacy of a 90 μg/kg does of rFVIIa administered at home to hemophilia A or B patients with inhibitors who experienced mild to moderately severe joint, muscle, or mucocutaneous hemorrhage (186). Subjects received up to three 90 μg/kg doses, initiated within 8 h of the onset of hemorrhage, at 3 h intervals. Effective hemostasis was achieved in 566 (92%) of 614 evaluable hemorrhagic episodes after a mean of 2.2 doses of rFVIIa. Maintenance of hemostasis 24 h following an initial effective response to rFVIIa was documented 95% of the time. Overall efficacy for joint, muscle, and mucocutaneous hemorrhages was comparable. The authors concluded that rFVIIa administered at this dosing regimen was effective and well-tolerated at home when used to treat mild to moderate bleeding episodes in patients with hemophilia A or B with inhibitors.

Successful major surgery in rFVIIa-treated hemophilia A and B patients with inhibitors has been reported (184,185,187,188). In these reports, surgical procedures performed included total hip replacement and bilateral total knee replacement. The dosing schedule was 90–120 μg/kg every 2 h for the first 24 h. Subsequent treatment decisions were made according to type of surgery and clinical response. Most subjects were also treated with tranexamic acid, a lysine analog antifibrinolytic agent. A recent prospective, randomized double-blind trial evaluated two does of rFVIIa (35 and 90 μg/kg) during and after elective surgery in 28 male patients with factor inhibitors (25 hemophilia A, 2 hemophilia B, 1 nonhemophiliac with an acquired factor VIII inhibitor) (189). Eleven major surgical procedures were performed and included two hip arthroplasties, five synovectomies, two knee procedures, one bone graft, and one laparoscopic renal biopsy. Eighteen surgical procedures were considered minor, including placement of central venous catheters, placement of other venous access devices, and the removal of a Port-a-Cath. Subjects received rFVIIa immediately prior to incision and then intraoperatively every 2 h and as necessary. Subjects received rFVIIa every 2 h for the first 48 h after wound closure and every 2–6 h for the next 3 days (total length of double-blind period was 5 days). The dose of 90 μg/kg was effective for subjects undergoing major or minor surgical procedures throughout the double-blind period (83% and 100% satisfactory hemostasis, respectively). The 35 μg/kg dose provided satisfactory hemostasis in virtually all minor procedures. A drop in efficacy was noted near the end of the double-blind period (40% satisfactory hemostasis) in subjects undergoing major procedures. The investigators concluded that 35 μg/kg was probably inadequate for postoperative management, and 90 μg/kg was more effective for both minor and major surgical procedures.

rFVIIa has been used in patients without hemophilia or specific factor inhibitors. Some promising results with rFVIIa have been obtained in trauma patients and in other situations where extensive bleeding has been encountered, such as GI bleeding (173,174,190–192). rFVIIa has been administered with success in a patient with profuse bleeding from an intra-abdominal gunshot wound (174). Prior to rFVIIa therapy, the patient was losing 300 mL of blood a minute despite antifibrinolytic therapy and aggressive transfusion therapy with red cells, FFP, platelets, and CRYO. Following a 60 μg/kg dose of rFVIIa, the rate of bleeding decreased to 10–15 mL/min. Bleeding stopped when a second 60 μg/kg dose was given 1 h after the first dose. Surgical exploration was performed, and no further significant blood loss was encountered. These investigators subsequently reported on their experience with rFVIIa in nine more trauma victims (175). The causes of injuries were stabbing, high velocity bullets, motor vehicle accidents, and falls. Uncontrolled hemorrhage occurred in all subjects despite surgical intervention and massive transfusion therapy with red cells, FFP, platelets, and CRYO.

The doses of rFVIIa administered ranged from 40 to 120 µg/kg. Four patients received more than one dose, and the median dose for all patients was two. The mean red cell requirement prior to rFVIIa administration was 36.5 units of RBCs (range 20–70 units of RBCs). The mean red cell requirement after rFVIIa administration was 2 units of RBCs (range 1–2 units of RBCs). Three of nine patients died. One patient, hypothermic, acidotic, and in shock for 14 h prior to rFVIIa administration, died during surgery. The other two fatalities occurred 4 weeks following rFVIIa treatment from sepsis and liver failure.

Additional reports of the successful use of rFVIIa for extensive bleeding continue to accumulate. rFVIIa had a successful impact in a patient with massive bleeding after cesarean section (185). Patient management included massive transfusion (40 units of RBCs), emergency hysterectomy, ligation of the iliac arteries, and packing of the pelvis. A decrease in bleeding was observed within minutes of administration of 90 µg/kg of rFVIIa. A second 90 µg/kg dose of rFVIIa was given 1 hour later, and no further blood loss was encountered.

rFVIIa has been reported to be successful in a stab wound victim (single 90 µg/kg dose), two Crohn's disease patients with profuse postsurgical lower GI bleeding (one or two 90 µg/kg doses), one patient with a bleeding duodenal ulcer (90 µg/kg every 2 h for 21 h), one patient with extensive abdominal bleeding associated with chronic myeloid leukemia in blast crisis, and a patient with cervical cancer who experienced significant postoperative bleeding (173,190,192).

In summary, anecdotal and case report evidence support rFVIIa use in trauma and other settings with extensive bleeding. Successful hemostasis has been achieved with one to two doses in the range of 60–120 µg/kg.

rFVIIa has been used in inherited factor VII deficiency (173,190,194–197). In a study of 17 subjects with inherited factor VII deficiency, rFVIIa was used to treat 27 spontaneous bleeding episodes, and to minimize bleeding in 7 major and 13 minor surgical procedures (197). The doses ranged from 8.08 to 70.5 µg/kg. Single doses of rFVIIa were effective in 13 of 15 episodes of hemarthosis. rFVIIa therapy was considered effective or excellent in 5 of 6 bleeding episodes not involving joints. Effective hemostasis was obtained in all surgical procedures, although more than one dose was necessary for all major surgical and nine minor surgical cases. One subject, a 2-week-old infant, developed antibodies directed at factor VII ~5 weeks after therapy.

rFVIIa has been used to reverse the effect of vitamin K antagonists. In a randomized, placebo-controlled trial performed on 28 volunteers, subjects were administered acenocoumarol to achieve a therapeutic INR value (198). The subjects' assayed factor VII activity levels at INR values more than 2.0 ranged from 4% to 17%. The INR returned to normal in subjects given one dose of rFVIIa in doses ranging from 5 to 320 µg/kg. The INR stayed within the reference range for 12 h when doses of more than 120 µg/kg were given. Clinically, seven adult patients, three of whom required surgery, with INR values ranging from 3.2 to 13.9 had their INR values rapidly corrected with rFVIIa (doses ranging from 20 to 90 µg/kg) (199). In a case report, two 80 µg/kg doses of rFVIIa were used to successfully achieve hemostatic control in a warfarin-treated patient with an INR of 2.9 and spontaneous epistaxis (200). It appears that rFVIIa can effectively reverse the anticoagulant effect of vitamin K antagonists.

Liver disease is another setting where rFVIIa may provide benefit. In a study of subjects with cirrhosis, individuals with a PT >2 s above the upper limit of the reference range were given IM vitamin K (201). In 10 subjects, vitamin K failed to correct the PT to <2 s above the upper limit of the reference range. Nonresponding subjects were given three doses of rFVIIa (5, 20, and 80 µg/kg) over 3 weeks. In all subjects, the PT temporarily returned to the reference range following all three rFVIIa doses. No adverse effects were reported. In a study of cirrhotic patients undergoing laparoscopic liver biopsy, 65 subjects were given rFVIIa in doses ranging from 5 to 80 µg/kg in association with the procedure (202). Thirteen subjects received an additional 80 µg/kg dose of rFVIIa. None of the subjects required transfusion or surgical intervention after the biopsy procedure. The authors concluded that rFVIIa could be used to successfully perform laparoscopic liver biopsy in patients with coagulopathy from liver disease for whom the risk of hemorrhage could be a contraindication.

rFVIIa has been used to treat children with liver failure and DIC (176). In this report, two children were in prolonged shock from Dengue fever. A third child, with hepatoblastoma, had 60% of his liver resected. Active bleeding was present in all three children. The two children with Dengue fever received rFVIIa in addition to other blood components. rFVIIa was the only hemostatic agent given to the child with hepatoblastoma. Bolus doses ranging from 40 to 180 µg/kg were followed by continuous rFVIIa infusions of 16.5–33 µg/kg per h. rFVIIa therapy resulted in a shortening of the PT, a significant increase in factor VII activity, and control of bleeding.

rFVIIa has been evaluated in cirrhotic patients undergoing orthotopic liver transplantation (OLT) (203). In this single-center pilot study designed to assess the efficacy and safety of rFVIIa, six subjects received a single 80 µg/kg dose within 10 min of the start of the OLT procedure. Compared with a set of matched control subjects, the number of transfused allogeneic red cell, autologous red cell, total red cell, and FFP units was significantly lower in rFVIIa-treated subjects. The authors concluded that a single 80 µg/kg dose of rFVIIa significantly reduced transfusion requirements during OLT.

rFVIIa has been used in patients with thrombocytopenia. One study was designed to evaluate whether rFVIIa infusion caused a shortening of the bleeding time (171). A decrease in the bleeding time was observed in 55 (52%) of 105 instances. The reduction in bleeding time was significantly greater in subjects with a platelet count $>20,000$ μL^{-1}. Eight subjects received nine rFVIIa infusions to treat bleeding. Bleeding slowed in all and stopped in six subjects. A successful hemostatic effect with rFVIIa was reported in another patient with a platelet count <5000 μL^{-1} (204). rFVIIa has been reported to have positive hemosatic effects in patients with Glanzmann thrombasthenia and Bernard–Soulier disease (172,205–207).

The total number of reported adverse events associated with rFVIIa therapy is small. After more than 170,000 standard rFVIIa doses, a total of five thromboembolic events had been reported. Two thromboembolic episodes were reported in hemophilia patients, and one episode each occurred in patients with acquired hemophilia, Glanzmann thrombasthenia, and vWD.

Acute myocardial infarction has been reported in at least six rFVIIa-treated patients (193). Three of six patients had hemophilia, two had acquired hemophilia, and one had uremia. Five of six were >70 years of age, and two hemophilia patients and one patient with acquired hemophilia had a history of cardiovascular disease.

Cerebrovascular abnormalities have been reported in at least four rFVIIa-treated patients, of whom three were >55 years of age (193). Three patients had acquired hemophilia, and one had hemophilia.

These findings indicate that the overall risk of arterial and venous thromboembolism associated with rFVIIa therapy is low. Case reports suggest that the thrombotic risk may be higher in subjects with other risk factors for thrombotic events, such as a history of cardiovascular disease or advanced age.

Massive Transfusion

The replacement of at least one blood volume with blood components over a period of minutes to 24 h is considered massive transfusion. In a 70 kg adult, one blood volume replacement is ~5000 mL of blood. Massive transfusion is often associated with multiple complications, including metabolic, coagulation, and respiratory abnormalities. These abnormalities are primarily the result of hypoperfusion and tissue injury related to trauma or hemorrhage (208,209). Hypothermia and the infusion of large volumes of blood products or asanguinous solutions also contribute to abnormalities that arise during massive transfusion. Blood warming devices and filters may minimize some of the adverse effects related to the infusion of large volumes of fluids.

One complication of massive transfusion is the development of abnormal hemostasis (76,210,211). The degree of hemostatic derangement is related to the extent of tissue injury and duration of hypotension, factors that also determine the degree of hemostatic support necessary (212). Laboratory tests of hemostasis are abnormal in up to 90% of massively transfused patients, and abnormal bleeding or bleeding from noninjured or non-operative sites occurs in one-third to more than one-half (213). Abnormal bleeding does not correlate well with laboratory test results or the volume of transfusion (209). Patients who require massive transfusion may have hypotension, hypothermia, systemic acidosis, sepsis, brain injury, lung injury, hepatic ischemia, underlying liver or renal disease, and various levels of activation of their procoagulant and fibrinolytic systems (214). Consequently, hemostatic defects arising during massive transfusion are often due to a complex interaction of multiple conditions that influence the platelet count, platelet function, coagulation status, and fibrinolytic status. In addition, dilutional effects are often present. The conditions influencing the development of abnormal bleeding during massive transfusion can be present in numerous different combinations. A standardized approach to the prevention, management, and correction of abnormal bleeding associated with massive transfusion is difficult (48).

Thrombocytopenia is the most frequently encountered hemostatic abnormality with massive transfusion. When crystalloids, colloids, red cells, and plasma components are used for resuscitation, platelet losses from hemorrhage and consumption often exceed endogenous platelet production and release. The platelet count may fall as much as 50% for each blood volume replaced. Platelet release from the bone marrow and spleen provides partial compensation for the loss of platelets. Because of this mechanism, the massive transfusion-associated decrease in platelet count is less than that predicted from dilution alone (76). Patients surviving massive transfusion tend to develop a subsequent drop in platelet count 2–3 days after the event. The proposed explanation for this finding is that the circulating platelets share a similar, short intravascular lifespan (213). The association of abnormal bleeding with thrombocytopenia (platelet count $<100,000\ \mu L^{-1}$) varies in massive transfusion. Some patients do not bleed abnormally even when the platelet count approaches $50,000\ \mu L^{-1}$, whereas others show evidence of a bleeding diathesis at higher platelet counts. The variability of thrombocytopenia-associated bleeding is thought to be associated upon the level of concurrent platelet dysfunction.

Platelet function defects can arise during massive transfusion. The causes of platelet dysfunction include hypothermia, systemic acidosis, dilution of vWF, changes in platelet membrane receptors, and the presence of circulating, transfused platelets with compromised hemostatic function (215).

The dilution and consumption of coagulation factors during massive transfusion also may contribute to the hemostatic deficit (216). Inadequate concentrations of coagulation factors necessary for hemostasis are not accurately predicted by mild to moderate elevations of the PT and aPTT. There is a wide variety of PT and aPTT reagents commercially available. These reagents exhibit varied sensitivity to decreases in functional concentrations of coagulation factors. Truly accurate transfusion decision-making based on PT and aPTT values requires an understanding of the sensitivity of the reagent-coagulation instrument combinations in use. Some authors believe that microvascular bleeding from decreased concentrations of coagulation factors is unlikely unless PT or aPTT values are more than 1.5 times normal (217). Generally, the likelihood of microvascular bleeding increases in association with the degree of abnormality of coagulation tests (217,218).

Although the complex interactions of the factors causing abnormal bleeding in massive transfusion are poorly characterized by routine laboratory methods, such testing can be used to aid the transfusion decision-making process. Despite its limitations, laboratory testing during massive transfusion results in better use of blood products and an improved patient outcome (219). The major purpose of laboratory monitoring is to avoid the development of a significant deficit of platelets and coagulation factors.

In the management of massive transfusion, one approach is the administration of prophylactic component therapy to avoid the development of hemostatic defects. The other approach is the administration of blood components on the basis of clinical findings and laboratory test results. In one study of massively transfused patients, the empiric transfusion of FFP or platelets did not reduce the incidence of abnormal bleeding and did not decrease overall transfusion requirements (209). In another study, massively transfused patients failed to develop abnormal bleeding, despite the presence of platelet dysfunction and marked reductions in platelet count (220). These findings suggest that platelet transfusions are not required unless abnormal bleeding occurs. In the opinion of other investigators and practitioners, evidence of high mortality in massively transfused patients who develop abnormal bleeding justifies the routine inclusion of platelet and plasma transfusions in the resuscitative effort (221). With empiric approaches, the clinician must remember that the replacement of FFP or platelets according to preset rules may result in insufficient replacement of hemostatic elements in patients needing additional transfusion therapy, such as is required for consumptive coagulopathy. In other situations, replacement therapy according to preset criteria may lead to unnecessary transfusions.

The following is an approach based on recommendations from the Puget Sound Blood Center (213):

>   Start Point of the algorithm

Is generalized microvascular oozing present? If not, one should consider whether the bleeding could be corrected surgically. If generalized microvascular oozing is present, blood samples should be sent to the clinical laboratory for the performance of a platelet count, fibrinogen, and PT.

Patients with generalized microvascular oozing are divided into two groups on the basis of whether they have received 10 or more red cell transfusions.

Algorithm 1: If the patient has received 10 or more red cell transfusions

   I. Transfuse 4–6 units of platelet concentrates (or a single apheresis platelet unit) immediately and send a blood sample for a posttransfusion platelet count.
  II. If generalized microvascular oozing is controlled in association with the platelet transfusion, check the platelet count, fibrinogen, and PT after every 6–10 units of red cells or every 30–45 min.

III. If generalized oozing is not controlled with platelet transfusion, is the fibrinogen <100 mg/dL?
   A. If the fibrinogen is ≥100 mg/dL, is the INR 1.6 or more?
      1. If the INR is less than 1.6, consider whether bleeding is due to a surgically correctable cause or platelet dysfunction and return to the Start Point.
      2. If the INR is 1.6 or more, transfuse 3–5 units of plasma immediately, check posttransfusion platelet count, fibrinogen, and PT, and return to the Start Point.
   B. If the fibrinogen is <100 mg/dL, transfuse 10–15 units of CRYO immediately and check posttransfusion platelet count, fibrinogen, and PT.
      1. If the bleeding is controlled, check the platelet count, fibrinogen, and PT after every 6–10 units of red cells or every 30–45 min.
      2. If the bleeding is not controlled, is the INR 1.6 or more?
         a. If the INR is less than 1.6, consider whether bleeding is due to a surgically correctable cause or platelet dysfunction and return to the Start Point.
         b. If the INR is 1.6 or more, transfuse 3–5 units of plasma immediately, check posttransfusion platelet count, fibrinogen, and PT, and return to the Start Point.

Algorithm 2: If a patient received fewer than 10 red cell transfusions

I. If the platelet count is <100,000 μL^{-1}, return to step I of Algorithm 1 and continue.
II. If the platelet count is ≥100,000 μL^{-1} or more, is the fibrinogen <100 mg/dL?
   A. If yes, return to step IIIB of Algorithm 1 and continue.
   B. If no, return to step IIIA of Algorithm 1 and continue.

Although an algorithmic approach can be helpful, decisions regarding the management of massive transfusion should also depend upon specific case-related factors such as the site, severity, and control of the underlying abnormality or injury; associated medical conditions; and the anticipated transfusion requirement. For example, if the primary source of bleeding has been controlled and the patient has been stabilized, monitoring the hemostatic status of the patient with PT, aPTT, fibrinogen, platelet count, and, if available, thromboelastography, and withholding transfusions of plasma, platelets, and CRYO until evidence of abnormal bleeding occurs may be prudent. If, on the other hand, the patient is unstable, the bleeding is uncontrolled, abnormal bleeding is present, and the underlying abnormality or injury is extensive or difficult to manage, transfusions may need to be given empirically until an opportunity exists to obtain the laboratory data to guide subsequent transfusion decisions. One empiric approach is the transfusion of 6 platelet concentrates or 1 apheresis platelet unit, and 2–4 plasma units for every 10–12 transfused red cell units (213).

TRANSFUSION-ASSOCIATED GRAFT-vs.-HOST DISEASE

TA-GVHD, an often fatal complication of transfusion, is caused by the infusion of viable T lymphocytes into a susceptible recipient. In susceptible hosts, donor T lymphocytes are not cleared by the recipient's immune system. The donor T lymphocytes undergo clonal expansion and orchestrate the immune destruction of host tissues. In 1955, a case of postoperative erythroderma in a transfused patient was described in Japan (222). In 1965, erythroderma, hepatomegaly, and fatal aplastic anemia were described in two infants who received multiple transfusions of fresh blood (223). Subsequently, many more cases have been reported and TA-GVHD is now recognized as a distinct pathological process.

The signs and symptoms of TA-GVHD typically appear 2–50 days following an implicated transfusion (224). Manifestations include fever, anorexia, nausea, vomiting, a maculopapular exanthem, hepatitis, enterocolitis, and pancytopenia. The maculopapular exanthem often starts centrally and proceeds to the extremities. Severe skin manifestations include generalized erythroderma, edema, and bullae formation. Enterocolitis is characterized by severe, watery diarrhea with passage of up to 3–4 L/day. Laboratory tests of liver function often show markedly elevated aspartate transaminase, alanine transaminase, alkaline phosphatase, and bilirubin values. Bone marrow examination typically shows a reduction of all cellular elements. Pancytopenia renders TA-GVHD victims vulnerable to hemorrhagic and infectious complications. The overall mortality rate of TA-GVHD is ~90% (225–227). Death usually occurs 1–3 weeks following the onset of clinical signs and symptoms, usually as a result of overwhelming infection (224). TA-GVHD has been treated with an assortment of immunosuppressive agents, including steroids, antithymocyte globulin, and cyclophosphamide. No therapy has been shown to be effective. Successful recovery from milder cases of TA-GVHD has been reported; however, whether survival is directly attributable to a specific therapeutic approach is uncertain (227). Clearly, prevention of TA-GVHD is the most important consideration.

A number of clinical situations are associated with an increased risk for TA-GVHD. Factors influencing TA-GVHD risk include recipient immune status, the number of donor lymphocytes transfused, and the degree of HLA similarity between donor and recipient (228). TA-GVHD has been reported in patients with Hodgkin's disease, non-Hodgkin's lymphoma, acute myeloid leukemia, acute lymphoblastic leukemia, chronic lymphocytic leukemia, severe combined immunodeficiency syndrome, Wiskott–Aldrich syndrome, and in newborns with erythroblastosis fetalis (229). Individuals with these conditions are considered to be at risk, and measures should be taken to prevent TA-GVHD by using gamma irradiated blood components.

TA-GVHD has been reported in premature infants receiving nonirradiated blood components and in patients treated with radiation therapy or cytotoxic drugs (230–232). Some of the premature infants were thought to have sepsis, and some had hyaline-membrane disease or respiratory distress syndrome. None had erythroblastosis fetalis or were suspected to have a congenital immundeficiency syndrome. TA-GVHD in patients with solid tumors was first reported in children who received intensive therapy for neuroblastoma (233,234). A study of 34 subjects with solid tumors who were treated with ablative chemotherapy followed by autologous bone marrow transplant identified four cases of TA-GVHD associated with the use of nonirradiated blood components (235). TA-GVHD has been reported in patients with bladder, cervical, esophageal, lung, prostate, and renal carcinoma in the absence of intensive chemotherapy (236). This finding suggests that intensive chemotherapy is not a prerequisite for TA-GVHD in some patients with solid tumors.

TA-GVHD has occurred in seemingly immunocompetent individuals. In many cases, the blood donor was homozygous for an HLA haplotype shared with a heterozygous recipient. Thaler et al. (237) provided a detailed description of this phenomenon in 1989.

The authors reported two cases of fatal TA-GVHD in immunocompetent adult patients after cardiac surgery. Both recipients were transfused with fresh, nonirradiated whole blood donated by their children. In both cases, one of the blood donors was homozygous for an HLA haplotype shared with the heterozygous recipient. In this case, the recipient recognizes the donor T lymphocytes as "self," and they are not removed. The donor T lymphocytes recognize the nonshared haplotype of the recipient as foreign, and an immune response culminating in TA-GVHD ensues. A review of the English language literature on TA-GVHD revealed that 87% of cases were associated with blood collected <96 h before transfusion, 56% of cases involved unrelated donors and recipients, and 87% of cases involved donors homozygous for a shared haplotype in a heterozygous recipient (238). The greatest probability of a "homozygote to heterozygote" transfusion exists between parents and children (239). The second highest probability is between grandparents and grandchildren or aunts/uncles and nephews/nieces, and the third highest probability is between siblings (239). These data provide support for the practice of gamma irradiation of all cellular blood components collected from blood relatives of transfusion recipients.

Implicated Blood Components

Any blood component that contains a sufficient number of viable T cells has the potential to cause TA-GVHD. Whole blood (fresh and stored), platelets, granulocytes, and fresh plasma have been documented to cause TA-GVHD (240–243). Frozen blood components, including FFP, CRYO, and frozen red cells, have not been implicated.

Prevention

The standard of practice for the prevention of TA-GVHD is gamma irradiation of blood components. Gamma irradiation currently is not performed on all blood components in the United States for many reasons, including cost; decreased shelf life of irradiated red cells; problems with timely provision of components in emergency, rural, or small clinic settings; and the low incidence of TA-GVHD in immunocompetent recipients of blood collected from unrelated donors (244–246). In accord with Food and Drug Administration (FDA) directive, the dose of gamma irradiation for the prevention of TA-GVHD must be a minimum of 2500 cGy delivered to the midline of the blood container and a minimum dose of 1500 cGy delivered to the remaining portions of the blood component (247). This dose of gamma irradiation abolishes the replication ability of T lymphocytes with minimal detrimental effects on red cells, platelets, and granulocytes. Leukocyte reduction is not considered to be an adequate or acceptable alternative to gamma irradiation for the prevention of TA-GVHD (248,249).

Gamma Irradiation Guidelines

Guidelines for gamma-irradiated blood components can be divided into definite (unequivocal), probable (equivocal, but strong data to support practice), and possible (data in support of practice nondefinitive) indications.

Definite indications for gamma-irradiated cellular blood components include:

1. Patients with congenital cellular immune deficiency(223,240,250–254)
2. Recipients of allogeneic hematopoietic stem cell transplants (255)
3. Recipients of autologous hematopoietic stem cell transplants (235)

4. Patients with Hodgkin's disease (229,232,256–263)
5. Recipients of granulocyte transfusions (257,264–267)
6. Recipients of intrauterine transfusions (268–271)
7. Neonates previously receiving intrauterine transfusions (269)
8. Recipients of blood components donated by blood relatives (237,317,238, 239,272,273)

Probable indications for gamma-irradiated cellular blood components include:

1. Premature infants (<1500 g) (230,274–277)
2. Patients with hematologic malignancies other than Hodgkin's disease receiving cytotoxic therapy (264–267,278–285)
3. Any patient receiving high-dose chemotherapy, radiation therapy, and/or aggressive immunosuppressive therapy (233,234,257,286–288)
4. Recipients of HLA-matched or cross-match-compatible platelets (289–291)

Possible indications for gamma-irradiated cellular blood components include:

1. Recipients of solid organ transplants (292,293)
2. Exchange or large volume transfusions in term neonates without prior intrauterine transfusions (294)
3. Term neonates on extracorporeal membrane oxygenation (295)
4. Patients with aplastic anemia not receiving aggressive immunosuppressive therapy (296)

TA-GVHD has not been reported in subjects with human immunodeficiency virus (HIV), although many such patients have received nonirradiated cellular blood components. HIV infection is not currently considered an indication for gamma-irradiated cellular blood components. Gamma irradiation is not indicated for term neonates, elderly patients, patients with autoimmune disease, immunocompetent surgical patients, pregnant patients, hemophilia patients, or patients with red-cell-membrane, red-cell-metabolism, or hemoglobin disorders (294,295).

NONINFECTIOUS RISKS OF TRANSFUSION (297)

Acute

1. *Hemolytic*. Incidence—1 : 38,000 to 1 : 70,000; cause—red cell incompatibility; presentation—chills/rigors, fever, hemoglobinuria, hypotension, renal failure with oliguria, DIC, back pain, pain of the vein used for infusion, and anxiety; therapeutic/prophylactic approach—keep urine output >100 mL/h with fluids and IV diuretic (furosemide), analgesics (may need morphine), pressor for hypotension (low-dose dopamine), hemostatic components (platelets, cryo, FFP) for bleeding.
2. *Fever/chill nonhemolytic*. Incidence RBCs—1 : 17 to 1 : 200; incidence platelets—1 : 3 to 1 : 100; cause—antibody to donor white blood cells, complement activation from antigen–antibody complex formation, and accumulated cytokines in blood bag; presentation—chills/rigors, fever, headache, and vomiting; therapeutic/prophylactic approach—antipyretic premedication or treatment (acetaminophen, no aspirin), leukocyte-reduced blood (prestorage leukocyte-reduced blood minimizes cytokine accumulation).

3. *Urticarial.* Incidence—1 : 33 to 1 : 100; cause—antibody to donor plasma proteins; presentation—urticaria, pruritis, flushing; therapeutic/prophylactic approach—antihistamine premedication or treatment (orally or intravenously), if urticaria are localized, one can restart the implicated unit slowly after antihistamine if symptoms completely resolve.
4. *Anaphylactic.* Incidence—1 : 20,000 to 1 : 50,000; cause—antibody to donor plasma proteins (includes IgA and C4); presentation—hypotension, urticaria, bronchospasm (wheezing, respiratory distress), edema (including laryngeal edema), anxiety; therapeutic/prophylactic approach—Trendelenberg position, fluid therapy, epinephrine (adult dose: 0.3–0.5 mL of 1 : 1000 solution subcutaneously or intramuscularly; in severe cases 10 mL of 1 : 10,000 IV), antihistamines, corticosteroids, beta-2 agonist, IgA-deficient blood components (see Chapter 51).
5. *Transfusion-related acute lung injury (TRALI).* Incidence—1 : 5000 to 1 : 190,000; cause—antibodies to white blood cells present in blood component (antibodies occasionally present in the recipient), other white blood cell activating agents in blood component; presentation—hypoxemia, fever, hypotension, respiratory failure; therapeutic/prophylactic approach—supportive care until recovery, defer implicated blood donors (see Chapter 27).
6. *Circulatory overload.* Incidence— < 1 : 100; cause—volume overload; presentation—dyspnea, orthopnea, cough, tachycardia, hypertension, headache; therapeutic/prophylactic approach—upright posture, oxygen, IV diuretic (furosemide), phlebotomy (250 mL increments).
7. *Nonimmune hemolysis.* Incidence—rare; cause—physical or chemical destruction of blood (heating, freezing, hemolytic drug or solution added to blood); presentation—hemoglobinuria; therapeutic/prophylactic approach—identify and eliminate cause.
8. *Hypotension associated with angiotensin converting enzyme (ACE) inhibitors.* Incidence—unknown, probably rare; cause—inhibited metabolism of bradykinin with infusion of bradykinin (negatively charged blood filters) or activators of prekallikrein; presentation—flushing, hypotension; therapeutic/prophylactic approach—withdraw ACE inhibition, use of nonalbumin volume replacement for plasmapheresis, avoid bedside leukocyte filtration.
9. *Hypothermia.* Incidence—dependent on clinical situation (e.g., encountered in massively transfused patients); cause—rapid infusion of cold blood components; presentation—cardiac conduction abnormalities, hemostatic dysfunction; therapeutic/prophylactic approach—warming of patient and blood components (i.e., employ use of blood warmer).
10. *Hypocalcemia.* Incidence—dependent on clinical situation (e.g., encountered in massively transfused patients and patients undergoing apheresis procedures); cause—rapid infusion of citrate; presentation—paresthesias, tetany, cardiac arrhythmia (may manifest as a prolonged QT interval on an electrocardiogram); therapeutic/prophylactic approach—in severe cases, slow calcium infusion with careful monitoring of ionized calcium levels, for milder cases, oral calcium supplementation may suffice (e.g., during an apheresis procedure).
11. *Air embolus.* Incidence—rare; cause—infusion of air into vascular system; presentation—sudden shortness of breath, acute cyanosis, pain, cough, hypotension, cardiac arrhythmia; therapeutic/prophylactic approach—lay patient on his/her left side and elevate the legs above the chest and head.

Delayed

1. *Alloimmunization to red cell antigens.* Estimated risk—1–1.6% per transfused RBC unit; cause—immune response to foreign antigens on red cells; presentation—positive red cell antibody screen, delayed hemolytic transfusion reaction, hemolytic disease of the newborn; therapeutic/prophylactic approach—avoid unnecessary red cell transfusion, provision of red cell components for transfusion negative for the offending red cell antigen.
2. *Alloimmunization to platelets (discussed elsewhere).*
3. *Hemolytic.* Incidence—1 : 5000 to 1 : 11,000; cause—anamnestic immune response to red cell antigens; presentation—fever, jaundice, decreasing hemoglobin unexplained by other causes, new positive direct antiglobulin test, new red cell antibody identified; therapeutic/prophylactic approach—supportive care as needed (see section on acute hemolysis; however, delayed hemolytic reactions are rarely of similar severity), identify antibody, provision of red cell components for transfusion negative for the offending red cell antigen.
4. *TA-GVHD (discussed elsewhere).*
5. *Posttransfusion purpura.* Incidence—rare; cause—apparent antiplatelet alloantibodies (usually anti-HPA-1a) present in the recipient that destroy autologous platelets; presentation—thrombocytopenic purpura, bleeding, onset is usually 8–10 days following transfusion; therapeutic/prophylactic approach—plasmapheresis, IV IgG, provision of platelet components for transfusion negative for the offending platelet antigen.
6. *Immunomodulation (discussed elsewhere).*
7. *Iron overload.* Incidence—invariable after >100 units of RBCs; cause—multiple transfusions of red cell components; presentation—cardiomyopathy, cirrhosis, diabetes; therapeutic/prophylactic approach—iron chelation therapy (deferoxamine).

INFECTIOUS RISKS OF BLOOD TRANSFUSION

Ongoing improvements and advances in the screening and testing of blood donors continue to improve the safety of the blood supply. Unfortunately, the blood supply has not achieved zero risk status. Viral, bacterial, and parasitic diseases can still be transmitted by transfusion. The following is a brief risk overview of certain important transfusion-transmitted diseases.

The American Red Cross, which collects approximately one-half of the blood used for transfusion in the United States, recently published data on the incidence and prevalence of infectious disease markers on the basis of a comprehensive database of their voluntary blood donors compiled from 1995 through 2001 (298). From these data, the authors calculated the residual risk of collecting an infectious donation during the window period (i.e., the risk of collecting an infectious unit in the face of negative testing for infectious disease markers). The data will be presented here as a representative estimate of current infectious disease risk for the blood supply in the United States. The residual risk estimate for hepatitis B was calculated with and without an adjustment that compensates for the transient expression of hepatitis B surface antigen (HBsAg) in some acute infections (i.e., 70% of acutely infected individuals have transient antigenemia and 53% of those individuals are identified with the HBsAg test) (299,300). The residual risk estimates generated by the American Red Cross investigators are as follows (298):

1. Hepatitis B virus (without adjustment)—1 : 488,000
2. Hepatitis B virus (with adjustment)—1 : 205,000
3. Hepatitis C virus (antibody test only)—1 : 276,000
4. Hepatitis C virus (plus nucleic acid testing)—1 : 1,935,000
5. Human immunodeficiency virus (antibody plus p24 antigen testing)—1 : 1,468,000
6. Human immunodeficiency virus (plus nucleic acid testing)—1 : 2,135,000
7. Human T cell lymphotropic virus (years 2000 and 2001)—1 : 2,993,000

The estimated risks for other transfusion-transmitted diseases are as follows:

1. Parvovirus B19 (estimated risk per unit transfused)—1 : 3300 to 1 : 40,000 (301).
2. Babesia and malaria (estimated risk per unit transfused)—<1 : 1,000,000 (629).
3. *Trypanosoma cruzi* (estimated risk per unit transfused)—1 : 42,000 (302).
4. CMV—discussed elsewhere
5. Creutzfeldt–Jacob disease (CJD) and variant Creutzfeldt–Jacob disease (vCJD)—although there is concern about the possibility of transmission and donor screening/deferral measures have been implemented to minimize risk, no cases of transfusion-transmitted CJD or vCJD have been reported in the United States.

West Nile Virus

West Nile Virus (WNV) belongs to the Japanese encephalitis complex of flaviviridae. The virus, which is arthropod-borne, is primarily transmitted via mosquito bites. The majority of WNV infections in humans (~80%) are asymptomatic. Approximately 20% of WNV-infected humans develop mild symptoms that may include body aches, eye pain, fever, gastrointestinal symptoms, headache, a generalized rash, or swollen lymph nodes. Severe disease occurs in 0.5–0.75% of WNV-infected humans. Individuals with severe illness may experience acute flaccid paralysis, encephalitis, meningitis, or meningoencephalitis singly or in any combination. Fatal encephalitis occurs in about 1 in 1000 WNV infections. The fatality rate for individuals hospitalized with severe WNV infection in the United States has been estimated to be 10–14%.

Between August 28, 2002, and March 1, 2003, 61 cases of possible transfusion-transmitted WNV infection were reported to the Centers for Disease control (CDC) (303). Epidemiological investigations and testing of retained donor samples revealed transfusion as the likely source of WNV infection in 21 of these cases. Fourteen donors were implicated in the 21 cases. Symptoms compatible with WNV were reported by 9 of 14 donors before or after blood donation. In one investigation, WNV was isolated from a unit of frozen plasma quarantined after a suspected donation, a finding that proves WNV survives in frozen blood components. WNV-related illness started between 2 and 21 days (median 11 days) following the implicated transfusions.

In May 2003, the FDA issued a revised final guidance for industry to safeguard the blood supply against WNV (303). The document contains recommendations for deferral of blood donors that could potentially harbor WNV. In the summer of 2003, blood centers across the United States began testing donor blood for WNV genetic material under an Investigation New Drug Application from the FDA (304).

Bacteria

Transfusion-transmitted bacterial infection, one of the earliest known complications of blood transfusion, continues to be a significant concern. Sepsis from bacterially contaminated platelets is the most common transfusion-transmitted disease. Since platelet components are stored at 20–24°C, bacterial growth during storage can occur. Skin commensal organisms are the most common platelet contaminants (e.g., *Bacillus cereus, Staphylococcus epidermidis*) (305,306). Both gram-positive and gram-negative bacteria have been implicated in fatal reactions to contaminated platelets. Fifty-one transfusion-related fatalities from bacterial contamination of platelets were reported to the U.S. FDA between 1976 and 1998 (307). The contamination rates for single units of platelets and platelets pheresis are approximately 1 in 2000. Because platelets are usually pooled prior to transfusion (e.g., in pools of 6–10 units), the risk of transfusion-transmitted bacterial infection is typically 6–10× more than the risk with platelets pheresis (307). Approximately 150 platelet recipients experience significant morbidity or mortality as a consequence of transfusion-transmitted bacterial infection in the United States annually (308).

The clinical outcomes from the transfusion of bacterially contaminated platelets are wide ranging. They are often less severe than the sequelae of bacterially contaminated RBC transfusions (309). Some subjects have no transfusion-related signs or symptoms. Others may have mild fever, which appears similar to an FNHTR. More serious sequelae include hypotension, sepsis syndrome, and death. The mortality rate for platelet transfusion-associated sepsis has been reported as 26% (310). Some authors recommend that broad-spectrum antibiotic therapy be considered for any patient who develops fever within 6 h of platelet transfusion (311,312).

In May 2003, the American Association of Blood Banks (AABB) issued a document on the implementation of a new standard for bacteria reduction and detection (313). This document describes new AABB standards that were implemented in November 2003 and March 2004. The new standards describe requirements for methods to limit and detect bacterial contamination in all platelet components.

Transfusion-transmitted bacterial infection is less commonly encountered with RBC transfusions. Twenty-six fatalities attributed to transfusion-transmitted bacterial infection via whole blood or red cells were reported to the U.S. FDA between 1976 and September 1998 (307). The estimated number of whole blood and RBC transfusions administered annually over this time period was 10–12 million. On the basis of FDA data, one death from bacterial infection occurred for every 10 million transfused RBC or whole blood units (314,315). The risk of death from bacterially contaminated red cell components is likely underestimated and underreported in the United States. In contrast to the low number of cases reported in the United States, data from New Zealand document one case of transfusion-transmitted *Yersinia enterocolitica* for every 65,000 RBC transfusions and one fatal case of transfusion-transmitted *Y. enterocolitica* for every 104,000 RBC transfusions (314,315). Gram-negative bacteria typically cause RBC transfusion-related sepsis, and *Y. enterocolitica* is the most commonly implicated organism. Characteristically, RBC-related gram-negative sepsis has a rapid onset and is clinically severe. Between 1987 and 1996, 20 cases of RBC transfusion-transmitted *Y. enterocolitica* infection were reported to the CDC (316). Death occurred in 12 of 20 cases in 37 days or fewer after transfusion. The median time from transfusion to death was 25 h.

Severe septic reactions can be characterized by fever, shock, and DIC. As soon as bacterial contamination is suspected, the transfusion must be stopped. Samples should be obtained directly from the blood component, not from attached segments, for microbial culture and Gram-stain analysis. The identification of bacteria with the Gram stain confirms the presence of contamination. A negative Gram-stain result does not exclude contamination. Microbial culture results are necessary to exclude contamination when Gram-stain findings are negative.

Because of the life-threatening nature of some septic reactions, therapy should be started promptly; it should not be delayed pending laboratory confirmation. Treatment should include IV broad-spectrum antibiotics and the management of shock, DIC, renal failure, respiratory failure, or other complications that may arise.

SUMMARY

- The decision to transfuse blood and blood components requires careful analysis of risks and benefits of transfusion and availability and efficacy of alternative therapies.
- RBCs are transfused to increase the oxygen-carrying capacity of circulating blood.
- Depending on the anticoagulant-preservative solution used, RBCs have a hematocrit from 52% to 80% and a shelf life of 21–42 days.
- The oxygen content of blood (CaO_2) depends upon hemoglobin concentration (Hb), binding coefficient of hemoglobin (β), hemoglobin oxygen saturation (Sat), and partial pressure of oxygen dissolved in the blood (PO_2). $CaO_2 = (Hb \times \beta \times Sat) + (0.0031 \times PO_2)$
- Optimum red cell mass is the level at which the greatest amount of oxygen is delivered to tissues at the lowest energy expenditure for the individual. For most patients, when the hemoglobin ranges from 9 to 15 g/dL, transfusions are probably not beneficial.
- Elderly patients do not tolerate anemia as well as younger individuals do. Compensation with increased stroke volume and heart rate is limited.
- Critical values that indicate marginal oxygen reserve that will most likely require therapy include $PvO_2 < 25$ torr, $VO_2 < 50\%$ of baseline value, $VO_2/DO_2 > 50\%$.
- Normovolemic clinically stable patients without significant coronary artery disease most likely benefit from red cell transfusion when the hemoglobin concentration <7 g/dL. Benefit is unlikely when the hemoglobin concentration >9 g/dL. Elderly patients with coronary artery disease may benefit from maintaining higher hemoglobin concentrations.
- Because many variables affect the correlation of hemoglobin concentration with red cell mass in an actively bleeding patient, the accuracy of hemoglobin concentration as an indicator of red cell mass may be poor.
- While patients with acute blood loss may be hypovolemic, individuals with chronic anemia are usually normovolemic or hypervolemic. Decisions regarding transfusion in patients with chronic anemia may be more deliberate.
- Fresh frozen plasma and donor retested plasma contain all circulating coagulation factors and naturally occurring coagulation inhibitors.
- For the correction of specific coagulation deficiencies, virus inactivated or recombinant coagulation factor concentrates, if available, are more effective and safer.

- Indications for plasma transfusion include vitamin K deficiency, correction of oral anticoagulation, severe liver disease, disseminated intravascular coagulation, massive transfusion, cardiopulmonary bypass, and thrombotic thrombocytopenic purpura.
- Agents other than plasma are recommended for intravascular volume repletion, most conditions requiring plasma exchange, hypoalbuminemia, hypogammaglobulinemia, hemophilia A, von Willebrand disease, and isolated or inherited protein deficiencies.
- A six-unit dose of platelets or a unit of platelets pheresis usually increases the platelet count by 30,000–60,000 μL^{-1}.
- Platelet count recovery is reduced with transfusion of ABO-incompatible platelets. Use of ABO-matched platelets is recommended, but urgent platelet transfusion should not be delayed until ABO-matched platelets are available.
- Avoid transfusing D-positive platelets to D-negative women of childbearing potential.
- Patients with bone marrow hypoplasia may be stable with platelet counts as low as 5000 μL^{-1}. An acceptable prophylactic platelet transfusion threshold for thrombocytopenia from marrow hypoplasia is 10,000 μL^{-1}.
- Platelet transfusion is indicated with retinal hemorrhage associated with thrombocytopenia.
- Guidelines recommend prophylactic platelet transfusion thresholds of 50,000 μL^{-1} for major surgical procedures and 100,000 μL^{-1} for neurosurgery and ophthalmology procedures.
- Platelet transfusion is indicated for significant bleeding associated with thrombocytopenia or platelet dysfunction. Platelet transfusion is effective for cardiopulmonary-bypass-related bleeding.
- Prevention of platelet alloimmunization relies principally on leukocyte reduction.
- Unless severe bleeding is present, platelet transfusion is not recommended for patients with heparin-induced thrombocytopenia or TTP.
- The major indication for cryoprecipitate administration is replacement of fibrinogen in patients with hypofibrinogenemia or dysfibrinogenemia. Other indications include uremia-associated platelet dysfunction and isolated factor XIII deficiency.
- Febrile non-hemolytic transfusion reactions (FNHTR) are defined as a transfusion-related rise in temperature of 1°C or more, with or without chills or rigors, not caused by hemolysis, infection, or other cause. FNHTRs occur more frequently with platelet transfusion than with RBC transfusion. Transfused leukocytes are thought to be a cause of FNHTR, and leukocyte-reduced red cell components are effective in reducing their incidence.
- Cytomegalovirus (CMV) is a leukocyte-associated DNA virus that may be transmitted by transfusion. Transfusion-related CMV infection is usually of no clinical significance in immunocompetent individuals. Patients for whom CMV-safe blood components should be considered include patients receiving chemotherapy intended to produce severe neutropenia, pregnant patients, patients infected with HIV, solid organ allograft recipients not requiring massive transfusion support, allogeneic or autologous hematopoietic progenitor cell transplant patients, and low-birth-weight premature infants.
- Recombinant factor VIIa (rFVIIa) is used to treat patients with hemophilia A, hemophilia B, factor VII deficiency, and acquired inhibitors to factor VIII or factor IX. Promising results with rFVIIa administration have been observed in trauma, massive gastrointestinal hemorrhage, post-cesarean-section bleeding, reversal of Vitamin K antagonists, liver disease, and thrombocytopenia.

- Thrombocytopenia is the most frequently encountered hemostatic abnormality with massive transfusion.
- Causes of platelet dysfunction during massive transfusion include hypothermia, systemic acidosis, dilution of von Willebrand factor, changes in platelet membrane receptors, and presence of circulating transfused platelets with impaired hemostatic function.
- Dilution and consumption of coagulation factors during massive transfusion contribute to hemostatic defects.
- In massive transfusion, the major purpose of laboratory monitoring is avoiding the development of significant thrombocytopenia and coagulation factor deficiency.
- An algorithmic approach may be helpful in managing massive transfusion (see Puget Sound Blood Center algorithm).
- Transfusion-associated graft-vs.-host disease (TA-GVHD) is caused by infusion of viable T lymphocytes into a susceptible patient. It can be a fatal complication.
- The standard of practice for the prevention of TA-GVHD is gamma irradiation of blood components.
- Noninfectious risks of transfusion include hemolysis, fevers, chills, urticaria, anaphylaxis, acute lung injury, circulatory overload, nonimmune hemolysis, hypotension with ACE inhibitors, hypothermia, hypocalcemia, air embolus, alloimmunization, TA-GVHD, posttransfusion purpura, iron overload, and immunomodulation.
- Infectious risk of blood transfusion include hepatitis B, hepatitis C, HIV, human T cell lymphotropic virus, parvovirus B19, babesia, malaria, trypansoma cruzi, CMV, Creutzfeldt–Jacob disease, variant Creutzfeldt–Jacob disease, and West Nile Virus (see text for incidence).

REFERENCES

1. Consensus Conference (National Institute of Health). Perioperative red blood cell transfusion. J Am Med Assoc 1988; 2700–2703.
2. American College of Physicians. Practice strategies for elective red blood cell transfusion. Ann Intern Med 1992; 116:403–406.
3. American Society of Anesthesiologists Task Force on Blood Component Therapy. Practice guidelines for blood component therapy. Anesthesiology 1996; 84:732–747.
4. Expert Working Group. Guidelines for red blood cell and plasma transfusions for adults and children. CMAJ 1997; 156(suppl 11):S1–S24.
5. Moore GL, Ledford ME, Peck CC. The in vitro evaluation of modifications in CPD-adenine anticoagulated-preserved blood at various hematocrits. Transfusion 1980; 20:419–426.
6. Heaton A, Miripol J, Aster R, et al. Use of Adsol preservative solution for prolonged storage of low viscosity AS-1 red blood cells. Br J Haematol 1984; 57:467–478.
7. Simon TL, Marcus CS, Myhre BA, Nelson, EJ. Effects of AS-3 nutrient-additive solution on 42 and 49 days of storage of red cells. Transfusion 1987; 27:178–182.
8. Welch HG, Meehan KR, Goodnough LT. Prudent strategies for elective red blood cell transfusion. Ann Intern Med 1992; 116:393–402.

9. Wilkerson DK, Rosen AL, Gould SA, et al. Oxygen extraction ratio: a valid indicator of myocardial metabolism in anemia. J Surg Res 1987; 42:629–634.
10. Priebe HJ. Hemodilution and oxygenation. Int Anesthesiol Clin 1981; 19:237–255.
11. Allen JB, Allen FB. The minimum acceptable level of hemoglobin. Int Anesthesiol Clin 1981; 19:1–21.
12. Tuman KJ. Tissue oxygen delivery: the physiology of anemia. Anesthesiol Clin North Am 1990; 9:451–469.
13. Rao TL. Montoya A. Cardiovascular, electrocardiographic, and respiratory changes following acute anaemia with volume replacement in patients with coronary artery disease. Anaesthesiol Rev 1985; 12:49–54.
14. Nelson AH, Fleischer LA, Rosenbaum SH. Relationship between postoperative anemia and cardiac morbidity in high-risk vascular patients in the intensive care unit. Crit Care Med 1993; 21:860–866.
15. Moroff G, Dende D. Characterization of biochemical changes occurring during storage of red cells: comparative studies with CPD and CPDA-1 anticogulant-preservative solutions. Transfusion 1983; 23:484–489.
16. Preparation, storage, and distribution of components from whole blood donations. In: Brecher ME, ed. Technical Manual. Bethesda, MD: American Association on Blood Banks, 2002:161–187.
17. Goodnough LT. Red blood cell support in the perioperative setting. In: Simon TL, Dzik WN, Snyder EL, Stowell CP, Strauss RG, eds. Rossi's Principles of Tranfusion Medicine. Philadelphia, PA: Lippincott William and Wilkins, 2002: 590–601.
18. Messmer K. Hemodilution–possibilities and safety aspects. Acta Anaesthesiol Scand 1988; 32:49–53.
19. Messmer K, Lewis DH, Sunder-Plassmann L, Klovekorn WP, Mendler N, Holper K. Acute normovolemic hemodilution. Changes of central hemodynamics and microcirculatory flow in skeletal muscle. Eur Surg Res 1972; 4:55–70.
20. Duruble M, Martin JL, Duvelleroy M. Effects theoriques, experimentaux et cliniques des variations de l'hematocrite au cours de l'hemodilution. Ann Anesthesiol Fr 1979; 9:805–814.
21. Shah DM, Gottlieb ME, Rahm RL, et al. Failure of red blood cell transfusion to increase oxygen transport or mixed venous PO_2 in injured patients. J Trauma 1982; 22:741–746.
22. Gore DC, Demaria EJ, Reines HD. Elevations in red blood cell mass reduce cardiac index without altering the oxygen consumption in severely burned patients. Surg Forum 1992; 43:721–723.
23. Babineau TJ, Dzik WH, Borlase BC, Baxter JK, Bistrian D, Benotti PN. Reevaluation of current transfusion practices in patients in surgical intensive care units. Am J Surg 1992; 164:22–25.
24. Viele MK, Weiskopf RB. What can we learn about the need for transfusion from patients who refuse blood? The experience with Jehovah's Witnesses. Transfusion 1994; 43:396–401.
25. Lieberman JA, Weiskopf RB, Kelley SD, et al. Critical oxygen delivery in conscious humans is less than 7.3 mL $O_2 \times kg^{-1} \times min^{-1}$. Anesthesiology 2000; 92:407–412.
26. Messmer K, Sunder-Plassman L, Jesch F, et al. Oxygen supply to the tissues during limited normovolemic hemodilution. Res Exp Med 1973; 159:152–166.
27. Smith JJ, Kampine JP. Physiology of exercise and the effect of aging. In: Smith JJ, Kampine JP, eds. Circulatory Physiology: The Essentials. Baltimore, MD: William & Wilkins, 1984:219–246.
28. Vara-Thorbeck R, Guerrero-Fernandez Marcotte JA. Hemodynamic response of elderly patients undergoing major surgery under moderate normovolemic hemodilution. Eur Surg Res 1985; 17:372–376.
29. Spahn DR, Zollinger A, Schlumpf RB, et al. Hemodilution tolerance in elderly patients without known cardiac disease. Anesth Analg 1996; 82:681–686.

30. Spahn DR, Schmid ER, Seifert B, Pasch T. Hemodilution tolerance in patients with coronary artery disease who are receiving chronic β-adrenergic blocker therapy. Anesth Analg 1996; 82:687–694.
31. Woodson RD, Willis RE, Lenfant C. Effect of acute and established anemia on O_2 transport at rest, submaximal, and maximal work. J Appl Physiol 1978; 44:36–43.
32. Goodnough LT, Despotis GJ, Hogue CW. On the need for improved transfusion indications in cardiac surgery. Ann Thorac Surg 1995; 60:473–480.
33. Gould SA, Rosen AL, Sehgal LR, et al. Fluosol DA as a red cell substitute in acute anemia. N Engl J Med 1986; 314:1653–1656.
34. Carson JL, Duff A, Poses RM, et al. Effect of anemia and cardiovascular disease on surgical mortality and morbidity. Lancet 1996; 348:1055–1060.
35. Kitchens CS. Are transfusions overrated? Surgical outcome of Jehovah's Witness (Editorial). Am J Med 1993; 94:117–119.
36. Carson JL, Terrin ML, Barton FB, et al. A pilot randomized trial comparing symptomatic vs hemoglobin-level driven red blood cell transfusions following hip fractures. Transfusion 1998; 38:522–529.
37. Carson JL, Duff A, Berlin JA, et al. Perioperative blood transfusion and postoperative mortality. J Am Med Assoc 1998; 279:199–205.
38. Hebert PC, Wells G, Blajchman MA, Marshall J, Martin C, Pagliarello G, Tweeddale M, Schweitzer I, Yetisir E. A multicenter, randomized, controlled clinical trial of transfusion requirements in critical care. N Engl J Med 1999; 340:409–417.
39. Hebert PC, Wells G, Tweeddale M, et al. Does transfusion practice affect mortality in critically ill patients? Am J Respir Crit Care Med 1997; 155:1618–1623.
40. Zauder HL. Preoperative hemoglobin requirement. Anesthesiol Clin N Am 1990; 8:471–480.
41. Linman J. Physiologic and pathophysiologic effects of anemia. New Engl J Med 1968; 279:812–818.
42. Elwood PC, Waters WE, Greene WJ, Sweetnam P, Wood MM. Symptoms and circulating haemoglobin level. J Chronic Dis 1969; 21:615–628.
43. Canadian Erythropoietin Study Group. Association between recombinant human erythropoietin and quality of life and exercise capacity of patients receiving hemodialysis. Br Med J 1990; 300:573–578.
44. Moake HL. Studies on the pathophysiology of thrombotic thrombocytopenic purpura. Semin Hematol 1997; 34:83–89.
45. Rock G, Porta C, Bobbio-Pallavicini E. Thrombotic thrombocytopenic purpura treatment in the year 2000. Haematologica 2000; 85:410–419
46. British Committee for Standards in Haematology, Working Party of the Blood Transfusion Task Force. Guidelines for the use of fresh frozen plasma. Transfus Med 1992; 2:57–63.
47. Consensus Development Panel (United States National Institutes of Health). Fresh-frozen plasma: indications and risks. J Am Med Assoc 1985; 253:551–553.
48. Development Task Force of the College of American Pathologists. Practice parameter for the use of fresh-frozen plasma, cryoprecipitate, and platelets: fresh-frozen plasma, cryoprecipitate, and platelets administration practice guidelines. J Am Med Assoc 1994; 271:777–781.
49. British Committee for Standards in Haematology, Blood Transfusion Task Force. Guidelines for administration of blood products: transfusion of infants and neonates. Transfus Med 1994; 4:63–69.
50. Association of Hemophilia Clinic Directors of Canada. Hemophilia and von Willebrand's disease: 1. Diagnosis, comprehensive care, and assessment. Can Med Assoc J 1995; 153:19–25.
51. Aster RH. Effect of anticoagulant and ABO incompatibility on recovery of transfused human platelets. Blood 1965; 26:732–743.
52. Heal JM, Masel D, Rowe JM, Blumberg N. Circulating immune complexes involving the ABO system after platelet transfusion. Br J Haematol 1993; 85:566–572.

53. Heal JM, Rowe JM, McMican A, Masel D, Finke C, Blumberg N. The role of ABO matching in platelet transfusion. Eur J Haematol 1993; 50:110–117.
54. Carr R, Hutton JL, Jenkins JA, Lucas GF, Amphlett NW. Transfusion of ABO-mismatched platelets leads to early platelet refractoriness. Br J Haematol 1990; 75:408–413.
55. Heal JM, Rowe JM, Blumberg N. ABO and platelet transfusion revisited. Ann Hematol 1993; 66:309–314.
56. Benjamin RB, Antin JH. ABO-incompatible bone marrow transplantation: The transfusion of incompatible plasma may exacerbate regimen-related toxicity. Transfusion 1993; 39:1273–1274.
57. Heal JM, Kenmotsu N, Rowe JM, Blumberg N. A possible survival advantage in adults with acute leukemia receiving ABO-identical platelet transfusions. Am J Hematol 1994; 45:189–190.
58. Peerschke EI, Ghebrehiwet B. C1q augments platelet activation in response to aggregated Ig. J Immunol 1997; 159:5594–5598.
59. Birmingham DJ, Hebert LA, Shen XP, Higgins P, Yeh CG, Creasey AA. Effects of immune complex formation and complement activation on circulating platelets in the primate. Clin Immunol 1999; 91:99–105.
60. Virgin HW, Kurt-Jones EA, Wittenberg GF; Unanue ER. Immune complex effects on murine macrophages. II. Immune complex effects on activated macrophages cytotoxicity, membrane IL 1, and antigen presentation. J Immunol 1985; 135:3744–3749.
61. Tripp CS, Beckerman KP, Unanue ER. Immune complexes inhibit antimicrobial responses through interleukin-10 production. Effects in severe combined immunodeficient mice during Listeria infection. J Clin Invest 1995; 95:1628–1634.
62. Gamberale R, Giordano M, Trevani AS, et al. Modulation of human neutrophil apotosis by immune complexes. J Immunol 1998; 161:3666–3674.
63. Berger S, Chandra R, Ballo H, et al. Immune complexes are potent inhibitors of interleukin-12 secretion by human monocytes. Eur J Immunol 1997; 27:2994–3000.
64. Waymack JP, Gallon L, Barcelli U, Alexander JW. Effect of blood transfusions on macrophage function in a burned animal model. Curr Surg 1986; 43:305–307.
65. Babcock GF, Alexander JW. The effects of blood transfusion on cytokine production by TH1 and TH2 lymphocytes in the mouse. Transplantation 1996; 61:465–468.
66. Carpentier NA, Fiere DM, Schuh D, et al. Circulating immune complexes and the prognosis of acute myeloid leukemia. N Engl J Med 1982; 307:1174–1180.
67. American Association of Blood Banks. Platelet and granulocyte antigens and antibodies. In: Brecher ME, ed. Technical Manual. Bethesda, 2002:341–359.
68. Murphy S, Litwin S, Herring LM, et al. Indications for platelet transfusion in children with acute leukemia. Am J Hematol 1982; 12:347–356.
69. National Institute of Health Consensus Development Conference. Platelet transfusion therapy. Transfus Med Rev 1987; 1:195–200.
70. Gmür J, Burger J, Schanz U, et al. Safety of stringent prophylactic platelet transfusion policy for patients with acute leukemia. Lancet 1991; 338:1224–1226.
71. Slichter SJ. Controversies in platelet transfusion therapy. Annu Rev Med 1980; 31:509–540.
72. Rebulla P, Finazzi G, Marangoni F, et al. The threshold for prophylactic platelet transfusions in adults with acute myeloid leukemia. N Engl J Med 1997; 337:1870–1875.
73. Wandt H, Frank M, Ehninger G, et al., Safety and cost effectiveness of a $10 \times 10(9)/L$ trigger for prophylactic compared with the traditional $20 \times 10(9)/L$ trigger: a prospective comparative trial in 105 patients with acute myeloid leukemia. Blood 1998; 91:3601–3606.
74. Friedburg RC, Gaupp B. Platelet transfusion: indications, considerations, and specific clinical settings. In: Kickler TS, Herman VH, eds. Current Issues in Platelet Transfusions and Platelet Alloimmunity. Bethesda, MD: AABB Press, 1999:1–32.
75. Simon TL, Akl BF, Murphy W. Controlled trial of routine adminstration of platelet concentrates in cardiopulmonary bypass surgery. Ann Thorac Surg 1984; 37:359–364.

76. Reed RL, Ciavarella D, Heimbach DM, et al. Prophylactic platelet administration during massive transfusion; a prospective, randomized, double-blind clinical study. Ann Surg 1986; 203:40–48.
77. Norfolk DR, Ancliffe PJ, Contreras M, et al. Synopsis of background papers (Consensus Conference on Platelet Transfusion). Br J Haematol 1998; 101:609–614.
78. Rao AK. Disorders of platelet function. In: Kitchens CS, Alving BM, Kessler CM, eds. Consultative Hemostasis and Thrombosis. Philadelphia, PA: Saunders, 2002:133–148.
79. Goodnough LT, Johnston MF, Ramsey G, et al. Guidelines for transfusion support in patients undergoing coronary artery bypass grafting. Ann Thorac Surg 1990; 50:675–683.
80. Dzik WH. Leukoreduced blood components: laboratory and clinical aspects. In: Rossi EC, Simon TL, Moss GS, Gould SA, eds. Principles of Transfusion Medicine. Baltimore, MD: Williams and Wilkins, 1996:353–373.
81. Petz LD, Garratty G, Calhoun L, et al. Selecting donors of platelets for refractory patients on the basis of HLA antibody specificity. Transfusion 2000; 40:1446–1456.
82. Koerner TAW, Vo TL, Wacker KE, Strauss RG. The predictive value of three definitions of platelet transfusion refractoriness. Transfusion 1988; 28:33S.
83. DeLoughery TG. Hemorrhagic and thrombotic disorders in the intensive care setting. In: Kitchens CS, Alving BM, Kessler CM, eds. Consultative Hemostasis and Thrombosis. Philadelphia, PA: Saunders, 2002:493–513.
84. Ishida A, Handa M, Wakui M, et al. Clinical factors influencing post-transfusion platelet increment in patients undergoing hematopoietic progenitor cell transplantation—a prospective analysis. Transfusion 1998; 38:839–847.
85. Murphy MF, Metcalfe P, Ord J, et al. Disappearance of HLA and platelet-specific antibodies in acute leukemia patients alloimmunized by multiple transfusions. Br J Haematol 1987; 67:255–260.
86. Moroff G, Garratty G, Heal JM, et al. Selection of platelets for refractory patients by HLA matching and prospective crossmatching. Transfusion 1992; 32:633–640.
87. Dahlke MB, Weiss KL. Platelet transfusions from donors mismatched for 83 crossreactive HLA antigens. Transfusion 1984; 24:299–302.
88. Friedberg RC, Donnelly SF, Mintz PD. Independent roles for platelet crossmatching and HLA in the selection of platelets for alloimmunized patients. Transfusion 1994; 34:215–220.
89. Rachel JM, Summers TC, Sinor LT, et al. Use of a solid phase red blood cell adherence method for pretransfusion platelet compatibility testing. Am J Clin Pathol 1988; 90:63–68.
90. O'Connell BA, Schiffer CA. Donor selection for alloimmunized patients by platelet crossmatching of random-donor platelet concentrates. Transfusion 1990; 20:314–317.
91. Howard JA, Perkins HA. The natural history of alloimmunization to platelets. Transfusion 1978; 18:496–503.
92. Godeau B, Foromont P, Seror T, et al. Platelet alloimmunization after multiple transfusions: a prospective study of 50 patients. Br J Haematol 1992; 81:395–400.
93. The Trial to Reduce Alloimmunization to Platelets Study Group. Leukocyte reduction and ultraviolet B irradiation of platelets to prevent alloimmunization and refractoriness to platelet transfusions. N Engl J Med 1997; 337:1861–1869.
94. Gmür J, von Felton A, Osterwalder B, et al. Delayed alloimmunization using random single donor platelet transfusions: a prospective study of thrombocytopenic patients with acute leukemia. Blood 1983; 62:473–479.
95. Dutcher JP, Schiffer CA, Aisner J, Wiernik PH. Alloimmunization following platelet transfusion: the absence of a dose-response relationship. Blood 1981; 57:395–398.
96. Kruskall MS. The perils of platelet transfusions (editorial). N Engl J Med 1997; 337:1914–1915.
97. Warkentin TE, Kelton JG. Immune thrombocytopenia and its management. In: Rossi EC, Simon TL, Moss GS, Gould SA, eds. Principles of Transfusion Medicine. Baltimore, MD: Williams and Wilkins, 1995:275–295.

98. Gordon LI, Kwaan HC, Rossi EC. Deleterious effects of platelet transfusions and recovery thrombocytosis in patients with thrombotic microangiopathy. Semin Hematol 1987; 24:194–201.
99. Gorlin JB, ed. Standards for blood banks and transfusion services. Bethesda, MD: American Association of Blood Banks, 2002.
100. Blood transfusion practice. In: Brecher ME, ed. Technical Manual. Bethesda, MD: American Association of Blood Banks, 2002:451–483.
101. Reiss RF, Oz MC. Autologous fibrin glue: production and clinical use. Transfus Med Rev 1996; 10:85–92.
102. Rapaport SI, Zivclin A, Minow RA. Clinical significance of antibodies to bovine and human thrombin and factor V after surgical use of bovine thrombin. Am J Clin Path 1992; 97:84–91.
103. Zehnder JL, Leung LK. Development of antibodies to thrombin and factor V with recurrent bleeding in a patient exposed to topical bovine thrombin. Blood 1990; 76:2011–2016.
104. Rousou J, Levitsky S, Gonzalez-Levin J, et al. Randomized clinical trial of fibrin sealant in patients undergoing resternotomy or reoperation after cardiac operations. J Thorac Cardiovasc Surg 1989; 97:194–203.
105. Menitove JE, McElligott MC, Aster RH. Febrile transfusion reaction: what component should be given next? Vox Sang 1982; 42:318–321.
106. Chambers LA, Donovan LM, Pacini DG, Kruskall MS. Febrile reactions after platelet transfusion: the effect of single versus multiple donors. Transfusion 1990; 30:219–221.
107. Heddle NM, Klama LN, Griffith L, et al. A prospective study to identify the risk factors associated with acute reactions to platelet and red cell transfusions. Transfusion 1993; 33:794–797.
108. Heddle NM, Kelton JG. Febrile nonhemolytic transfusion reactions. In: Popovsky MA, ed. Transfusion Reactions. Bethesda, MD: AABB Press, 2001:45–82.
109. Dinarello CA, Wolff SM. Molecular basis of fever in humans. Am J Med 1982; 72:799–819.
110. Mintz PD. Febrile reactions to platelet transfusions. Am J Clin Pathol 1991; 95:609–612.
111. Dzik WH. Is the febrile response to transfusion due to donor or recipient cytokine? (letter) Transfusion 1992; 32:594.
112. Okusawa S, Dianrella CA, Endres S, et al. C5a induction of interleukin-1: synergistic effect with endotoxin or interferon-gamma. J Immunol 1987; 139:2635–2640.
113. Heddle NM, Klama L, Singer J, et al. The role of the plasma from platelet concentrates in transfusion reactions. N Engl J Med 1994; 331:625–628.
114. Muylle L, Wouters E, Peetermans ME. Febrile reactions to platelet transfusion: the effect of increased interleukin 6 levels in concentrates prepared by platelet-rich plasma method. Transfusion 1996; 36:886–890.
115. Riccardi D, Raspollini E, Rebulla P, et al. Relationship of the time of storage and transfusion reactions to platelet concentrates from buffy coats. Transfusion 1997; 37:528–530.
116. Muylle L, Wouters E, DeBock R, et al. Reactions to platelet transfusion: the effect of the storage time of the concentrate. Transfus Med 1992; 2:289–293.
117. Mangano MM, Chambers LA, Kruskall MS. Limited efficacy of leukopoor platelets for prevention of febrile transfusion reactions. Am J Clin Pathol 1991; 95:733–738.
118. Aye MT. Production of cytokines in platelet concentrates. Canadian Red Cross Society Symposium on Leukodepletion: Report of Proceedings. Transfus Med Rev 1994; 8:8–9.
119. Stack G, Baril L, Napychanck P, Snyder EL. Cytokine generation in stored, white cell-reduced, and bacterially contaminated units of red calls. Transfusion 1995; 35:199–203.
120. Currie LM, Harper JR, Allan H, Connor J. Inhibition of cytokine accumulation and bacterial growth during storage of platelet concentrates at 4°C with retention of in vitro functional activity. Transfusion 1997; 37:18–24.
121. Shanwell A, Kristiansson M, Remberger M, Ringdén O. Generation of cytokines in red cell concentrates during storage is prevented by prestorage white cell reduction. Transfusion 1997; 37:678–684.

122. Federowicz I, Barrett BB, Anderson JW, et al. Characterization of reactions after transfusion of cellular blood components that are white cell reduced before storage. Transfusion 1996; 36:21–28.
123. Muylle L. Peetermans ME. Effect of prestorage leukocyte removal on the cytokine levels in stored platelet concentrates. Vox Sang 1994; 6:14–17.
124. Dzieczkowski JS, Barrett BB, Nester D, et al. Characterization of reactions after exclusive transfusion of white cell-reduced cellular blood components. Transfusion 1995; 35:20–25.
125. Sirchia G, Rebulla P, Parravicini A, et al. Leukocyte depletion of red cell units at the bedside by transfusion through a new filter. Transfusion 1987; 27:402–405.
126. Sirchia G, Wenz B, Rebulla P, et al. Removal of white cells from red cells by transfusion through a new filter. Transfusion 1990; 30:30–33.
127. Wenz B. Microaggregate blood filtration and the febrile transfusion reaction, a comparative study. Transfusion 1983; 23:95–98.
128. Dan ME, Stewart S. Prevention of recurrent febrile transfusion reactions using leukocyte poor platelet concentrates prepared by the "leukotrap" centrifugation method (abstract). Transfusion 1986; 26:569.
129. Kalmin ND, Orell JE, Villarreal IG. An effective method for the preparation of leukocyte-poor platelets. Transfusion 1987; 27:281–283.
130. Schiffer CA. Prevention of alloimmunization against platelets (editorial). Blood 1991; 77:1–4.
131. Slichter SJ, O'Donnell MR, Weiden PL, et al. Canine platelet alloimmunzation: the role of donor selection. Br J Haematol 1986; 63:713–727.
132. Stec N, Kickler TS, Ness PM, et al. Effectiveness of leukocyte (WBC) depleted platelets in preventing febrile reactions in multi-transfused oncology patients (abstract). Transfusion 1986; 26:569.
133. Sternbach M, Champagne J, Rybka W, et al. Leukotrap, a device for white cell poor platelets. Quality control studies in vitro and in vivo. Transfus Sci 1989; 10:57–62.
134. Goodnough LT, Riddell J, Lazarus H, et al. Prevalence of platelet transfusion reactions before and after implementation of leukocyte-depleted platelet concentrates by filtration. Vox Sang 1993; 65:103–107.
135. Muir JC, Herschel L, Pickard C, AuBuchon JP. Prestorage leukocyte reduction decreases the risk of febrile reactions in sensitized platelet recipients (abstract). Transfusion 1995; 35(suppl):45S.
136. Tegtmeier GE. Transfusion-transmitted cytomegalovirus infections: significance and control. Vox Sang 1986; 51(suppl 1):22–30.
137. Sayers M. Cytomegalovirus and other herpes-viruses. In: Petz LD, Swisher SN, Kleinman S, et al., eds. Clinical Practice of Transfusion Medicine. New York: Churchill Livingstone, 1996: 875–889.
138. Bowden RA, Sayers M, Flournoy N, et al. Cytomegalovirus immune globulin and seronegative blood products to prevent primary cytomegalovirus inflection after marrow transplantation. N Engl J Med 1986; 314:1006–1010.
139. Miller WJ, McCullough J, Balfour HH Jr, et al. Prevention of cytomegalovirus infection following bone marrow transplanation: a randomized trial of blood product screening. Bone Marrow Transplant 1991; 7:227–234.
140. Bowden RA, Sayers M, Gleaves CA, et al. Cytomegalovirus-seronegative blood components for the prevention of primary cytomegalovirus infection after marrow transplantation: consideration for blood banks. Transfusion 1987; 27:478–481.
141. Bowden RA, Slichter SJ, Sayers M, et al. A comparison of filtered leukocyte-reduced and cytomegalovirus (CMV) seronegative blood products for the prevention of transfusion-associated CMV infection after marrow transplant. Blood 1995; 86:3598–3603.
142. Leukocyte reduction for the prevention of transfusion-transmitted cytomegalovirus (TT-CMV). Association Bulletin 97-2, Bethesda, MD: American Association of Blood Banks, 1997.

143. Murphy MF, Grint PC, Hardiman AE, et al. Use of leukocycte-poor blood components to prevent primary cytomegalovirus (CMV) infection in patients with acute leukemia (letter). Br J Haematol 1988; 70:253.

144. Verdonck LF, de Graan-Hentzen YC, Dekker AW, et al. Cytomegalovirus seronegative platelets and leukocyte-poor red blood cells from random donors can prevent primary cytomegalovirus infection after bone marrow transplantation. Bone Marrow Transplant 1987; 2:73–78.

145. Murphy MF, Grint PC, Hardiman AE, et al. Use of leukocyte-poor blood components to prevent primary cytomegalovirus (CMV) infection in patients with acute leukemia. Br J Haematol 1988; 70:253–255.

146. Gilbert GL, Hayes K, Husdon IL, et al. Prevention of transfusion-acquired cytomegalovirus infection in infants by blood filtration to remove leucocytes. Lancet 1989; 1:1228–1231.

147. Degraan-Hentzen YC, Gratama JW, Mudde GC, et al. Prevention of primary cytomegalovirus infection in patients with hematologic malignancies by intensive white cell depletion of blood products. Transfusion 1989; 29:757–760.

148. Bowden RA, Sayers MH, Cays M, et al. The role of blood product filtration in the prevention of transfusion associated cytomegalovirus (CMV) infection after marrow transplant. Transfusion 1989; 29(suppl):57S.

149. De Witte T, Schattenberg A, van Dijk BA, et al. Prevention of primary cytomegalovirus infection after allogeneic bone marrow transplanation by using leukocyte-poor random blood products from cytomegalovirus-unscreened blood-bank donors. Transplantation 1990; 964–968.

150. Bowden RA, Slichter SJ, Sayers MH, et al. Use of leukocyte-depleted platelets and cytomegalovirus-seronegative red blood cells for the prevention of primary cytomegalovirus infection after marrow transplant. Blood 1991; 78:246–250.

151. Eisenfeld L, Silver H, Mclaughlin J, et al. Prevention of transfusion-associated cytomegalovirus infection in neonatal patients by the removal of white cells from blood. Transfusion 1992; 32:205–209.

152. van Prooijien HC, Visser JJ, van Oostendorp WR, et al. Prevention of primary transfusion-associated cytomegalovirus infection in bone marrow transplant recipients by the removal of white cells from blood components with high affinity filters. Br J Haematol 1994; 87:114–117.

153. Xu D, Yonetani M, Uetani Y, Nakamura H. Acquired cytomegalovirus infection and blood transfusion in preterm infants. Acta Paediatr Jpn 1995; 37:444–449.

154. Opelz G, Senger DP. Mickey MR, et al. Effect of blood transfusion on subsequent kidney transplants. Tranplant Proc 1973; 5:253–259.

155. Peters WR, Fry RD, Fleshman JW, et al. Multiple blood transfusions reduce the recurrence rate of Crohn's disease. Dis Colon Rectum 1989; 32:749–753.

156. Clark DA, Gunby J, Daya S. The use of allogeneic leukocytes or IV IgG for the treatment of patients with recurrent spontaneous abortions. Transfus Med Rev 1997; 11:85–94.

157. Dzik WH. Mechanisms for the immunomodulatory effect of transfusion. In: Vamvakas EC, Blajchman MA, eds. Immunomodulatory Effects of Blood Transfusion. Bethesda, MD: AABB Press, 1999:73–88.

158. Gantt CL. Red blood cells for cancer patients. Lancet 1981; 2:363.

159. Blumberg N. Allogeneic transfusion and infection: economic and clinical implications. Semin Hematol 1997; 34(3 suppl 2):34–40.

160. Chung M, Steinmetz OK, Gordon PH. Perioperative blood transfusion and outcome after resection for colorectal carcinoma. Br J Surg 1993; 80:427–432.

161. Busch OR, Hop WC, van Papendrecht, et al. Blood transfusions and prognosis in colorectal cancer. N Engl J Med 1993; 328:1372–1376.

162. Heiss MM, Mempel W, Delanoff C, et al. Blood transfusion-modulated tumor recurrence: first results of randomized study of autologous versus allogeneic blood transfusion in colorectal cancer surgery. J Clin Oncol 1994; 12:1859–1867.

163. Heiss MM, Fraunberger P, Delanoff C, et al. Modulation of immune response by blood transfusion: evidence for a different effect of allogeneic and autologous blood in colorectal cancer surgery. Shock 1997; 8:402–408.
164. Houbiers JG, Brand A, van de Watering LM, et al. Randomised controlled trial comparing transfusion of leucocyte-depleted or buffy-coat-depleted blood in surgery for colorectal cancer. Lancet 1994; 344:573–578.
165. Vamvakas EC, Carven JH, Hibberd PL. Blood transfusion and infection after colorectal cancer surgery. Transfusion 1996; 36:1000–1008.
166. Heiss MM. Mempel W, Jauch KW, et al. Beneficial effect of autologous blood transfusion infections complications after colorectal cancer surgery. Lancet 1993; 342:1328–1333.
167. Jensen LS, Andersen AJ, Christiansen PM, et al. Postoperative infection and natural killer cell function following blood transfusion in patients undergoing elective colorectal surgery. Br J Surg 1992; 79:513–516.
168. Jensen LS, Kissmeyer-Neilson P, Wolff B, Qvist N. Randomised comparison of leucocyte-depleted versus buffy-coat-poor blood transfusion and complications after colorectal surgery. Lancet 1996; 348:841–845.
169. van de Watering LM. Beneficial effects of leukocyte depletion of transfused blood on postoperative complications in patients undergoing cardiac surgery: a randomized clinical trial. Circulation 1998; 97:562–568.
170. Vamvakas EC. Transfusion-associated cancer recurrence and postoperative infection: meta-analysis of randomized, controlled clinical trials. Transfusion 1996; 36:175–186.
171. Kristensen J, Killander A, Hippe E, et al. Clinical experience with recombinant factor VIIa in patients with thrombocytopenia. Haemostasis 1996; 26(suppl 1): 159–164.
172. Poon MC, Demers C, Jobin F, Wu JW. Recombinant factor VIIa is effective for bleeding and surgery in patients with Glanzmann thrombasthenia. Blood 1999; 94:3951–3953.
173. White B, McHale J, Ravi N, et al. Successful use of recombinant FVIIa (Novoseven) in the management of intractable post-surgical intra-abdominal haemorrhage. Br J Haematol 1999; 107:677–678.
174. Kenet G, Walden R, Eldad A, Martinowitz U. Treatment of traumatic bleeding with recombinant factor VIIa. Lancet 1999; 354:1879.
175. Martinowitz U, Kenet G, Onaca N, et al. New treatment of uncontrolled hemorrhage in trauma/surgical patients: induction of local hypercoagulation. 60th Annual Meeting of the American Association for the Surgery of Trauma, October 12–14, 2000, San Antonio, Texas.
176. Chuansumrit A, Chantarojanasiri T, Isarangkura P, Teeraratkul S, Hongeng S, Hathirat P. Recombinant activated factor VII in children with acute bleeding resulting from liver failure and disseminated intravascular coagulation. Blood Coagul Fibrinolysis 2000; 11(suppl 1):S101–S105.
177. Papatheodoridis G, Chung S, Keshev S, et al. Recombinant factor VIIa is used in a Jehovah's Witness with liver cirrhosis to correct prothrombin time, bleeding time, and thromboelastographic parameters, enabling safe percutaneous injection of hepatocellular carcinoma. Thromb Haemost 1999; 82(abstract suppl):620.
178. Bolan CD, Klein HG. Transfusion medicine and pharmacologic aspects of hemostasis. In: Kitchens CS, Alving BM, Kessler CM, eds. Consultative Hemostasis and Thrombosis. Philadelphia, PA: Saunders, 2002:395–417.
179. Hedner U, Kisiel W. Use of human factor VIIa in the treatment of two hemophila A patients with high-titer inhibitors. J Clin Invest 1983; 71:1836–1841.
180. Hedner U. Ljungberg J, Lund-Hansen T. Comparison of the effect of plasma-derived and recombinant human FVIIa in vitro and in a rabbit model. Blood Coagul Fibrinolysis 1990; 1:145–151.
181. Diness V, Bregengaard C, Erhardsten E, Hedner U. Recombinant human factor VIIa (rFVIIa) in a rabbit stasis model. Thromb Res 1992; 67:233–241.

182. Lusher JM, Roberts HR, Davignon G, et al. A randomized, double-blind comparison of two dosage levels of recombinant factor VIIa in the treatment of joint, muscle and mucocutaneous haemorrhages in persons with haemophilia A and B, with and without inhibitors. RFVIIa Study Group. Haemophilia 1998; 4:790–798.
183. Lisman T, Nieuwenhuis HK, Meihers JC, de Groot PG. Recombinant factor VIIa prevents premature fibrinolysis in plasmas of some but not all patients with severe haemophilia A. Thromb Haemost 1999; 82(abstract suppl):504.
184. Hedner U, Glazer S, Pingel K, et al. Successful use of recombinant factor VIIa in patient with severe haemophilia A during synovectomy. Lancet 1988; 2:1193
185. Lusher J, Ingerslev J, Roberts H, Hedner U. Clinical experience with recombinant factor VIIa. Blood Coagul Fibrinolysis 1998; 9:119–128.
186. Key NS, Aledort LM, Beardsley D, et al. Home treatment of mild to moderate bleeding episodes using recombinant factor VIIa (Novoseven) in haemophiliacs with inhibitors. Thromb Haemost 1998; 80:912–918.
187. Ingerslev J, Freidman D, Gastineau D, et al. Major surgery in haemophilic patients with inhibitors using recombinant factor VIIa. Haemostasis 1996; 26(suppl 1):118–123.
188. Hedner U, Ingerslev J. Clinical use of recombinant FVIIa (rFVIIa). Transfus Sci 1998; 19:163–176.
189. Shapiro AD, Gilchrist GS, Keith Hoots WK, et al. Prospective, randomised trial of two doses of rFVIIa (NovoSeven) in haemophilia patients with inhibitors undergoing surgery. Thromb Haemost 1998; 80:773–778.
190. Essex D, Bluth M, Glostre E, et al. Successful use of recombinant factor VIIa (rFVIIa) for trauma-associated massive hemorrhage. Blood 2000; 96:268a.
191. Vlot AJ, Ton E, Mackaay AJ, Kramer MH, Gaillard CA. Treatment of a severely bleeding patient without preexisting coagulopathy with activated recombinant factor VII. Am J Med 2000; 108:421–423.
192. Laffan MA, Cummins M. Recombinant factor VIIa for intractable surgical bleeding. Blood 2000; 96:85b.
193. Hedner U, Erhardtsen E. Potential role for rFVIIa in transfusion medicine. Transfusion 2002; 42:114–124.
194. Mariani G, Mannucci PM, Massucconi MG, Capitantio A. Treatment of congenital factor VII deficiency with a new concentrate. Thromb Haemost 1978; 39:675–682.
195. Bech R, Nicolaisen EM, Anderson PM, et al. Recombinant factor VIIa for the treatment of congenital factor VII deficient patients. Thromb Haemost 1989; 62:55.
196. Ingerslev J, Knudsen L, Hvid I, et al. Use of recombinant factor VIIa in surgery in factor-VII-deficient patients. Haemophilia 1997; 3:215–218.
197. Mariani G, Testa MG, Di Paolantonio T, et al. Use of recombinant, activated Factor VII in the treatment of congenital factor VII deficiencies. Vox Sang 1999; 77:131–136.
198. Erhardtsen E, Nony P, Dechavanne M, et al. The effect of recombinant factor VIIa (NovoSeven) in healthy volunteers receiving acenocoumarol to an International Normalized Ratio above 2.0. Blood Coagul Fibrinolysis 1998; 9:741–748.
199. Deveras RA, Kessler CM, Recombinant factor VIIa (rFVIIa) successfully and rapidly corrects the excessively high international normalized ratios (INR) and prothrombin times induced by warfarin. Blood 2000; 96:638a.
200. Berntorp E, Stigenda L, Lethagan S, et al. NovoSeven in warfarin-treated patients. Blood Coagul Fibrinolysis 2000; 11(suppl 1): S113–S115.
201. Bernstein DE, Jeffers L, Erhardsten E, et al. Recombinant factor VIIa corrects prothrombin time in cirrhotic patients: a preliminary study. Gastroenterology 1997; 113:1930–1937.
202. Jeffers L, Balart L, Erhardsten E, et al. Efficacy and safety of rFVIIa in patients with severe coagulopathy undergoing laparoscopic liver biopsy. Blood 1999; 10:A236.
203. Hendriks HG, Meijer K, de Wolf JT, et al. Reduced transfusion requirements by recombinant factor VIIa in orthotopic liver transplantation. Transplantation 2001; 71:402–405.

204. Vidarsson B, Onundarson PT. Recombinant factor VIIa for bleeding in refractory thrombocytopenia. Thromb Haemost 2000; 83:634–635.
205. Tengborn L, Petruson B. A Patient with Glanzmann thrombasthenia and epistaxis succuessfully treated with recombinant factor VIIa. Thromb Haemost 1996; 75:981–982.
206. Chuansumrit A, Sangkapreecha C, Hathirat P. Successful epistaxis control in a patient with Glanzmann thrombasthenia by increased bolus injection dose of recombinant factor VIIa. Thromb Haemost 1999; 82:1778.
207. Peters M, Heijboer H. Treatment of a patient with Bernard-Soulier syndrome and recurrent nosebleeds with recombinant factor VIIa. Thromb Haemost 1998; 80:352.
208. Collins JA. Massive blood transfusions. Clin Haematol 1976; 5:201–222.
209. Mannucci PM, Federici AB, Sirchia G. Hemostasis testing during massive blood replacement: a study of 172 cases. Vox Sang 1982; 42:113–123.
210. Rutledge R, Sheldon GF, Collins ML, Massive transfusion. Crit Care Clin 1986; 2:791–805.
211. Ham JM, Transfusion reactions. In: Condon RE, DeCosses JJ, eds. Surgical Care: A Physiologic Approach to Clinical Management. Philadelphia, PA: Lea & Febriger, 1980: 178–186.
212. Collins JA. Recent developments in the area of massive transfusion. World J Surg 1987; 11:75–81.
213. Crookston KP, Spiess BD. Coagulation support in the perioperative setting. In: Simon TL, Dzik WN, Snyder EL, Stowell CP, Strauss RG, eds. Rossi's Principles of Transfusion Medicine. Philadelphia, PA: Lippincott, Williams & Wilkins, 2002:602–621.
214. Martin DJ, Lucas CE, Ledgerwood AM, et al. Fresh frozen plasma supplement to massive red blood cell transfusion. Ann Surg 1985; 205:505–511.
215. Ferrara A, MacArthur JD, Wright HK, et al. Hypothermia and acidosis worsen coagulopathy in the patient requiring massive transfusion. Am J Surg 1990; 160:515–518.
216. Murray DJ, Pennell BJ, Weinstein SL, Olson DJ. Packed red cells in acute blood loss: dilutional coagulopathy as a cause of surgical bleeding. Anesth Analg 1995; 80:336–342.
217. Murray DJ, Olson J, Strauss R, Tinker JH. Coagulation changes during packed red cell replacement of major blood loss. Anethesiology 1988; 69:839–845.
218. Ciavarella D, Reed RL, Counts RB, Baron L, Pavlin EG, Heimbach E, et al. Clotting factor levels and the risk of diffuse microvascular bleeding in the massively transfused patient. Br J Haematol 1987; 67:365–368.
219. Reiss RF. Hemostatic defects in massive transfusion: rapid diagnosis and management. Am J Crit Care 2000; 9:158–165.
220. Harrigan C, Lucas CE, Ledgerwood AM, et al. Serial changes in primary hemostasis after massive transfusion. Surgery 1985; 99:836–844.
221. Phillips TF, Soulier G, Wilson RF. Outcome of massive transfusion exceeding two blood volumes in trauma and emergency surgery. J Trauma 1987; 27:903–910.
222. Shimoda T. The case report of post-operative erythroderma. Geka 1955; 17:487.
223. Hathaway WE, Githens JH, Blackburn WR, et al. Aplastic anemia, histiocytosis and erythroderma in immunologically deficient children. N Engl J Med 1965; 273:953–958.
224. Suzuki K, Akiyama H, Takamoto S, et al. Transfusion-associated graft-versus-host disease in a presumably immunocompetent patient after transfusion of stored packed red cells. Transfusion 1992; 32:358–360.
225. Anderson KC. Clinical indications for blood component irradiation. In: Baldwin ML, Jeffries LC, eds. Irradiation of Blood Components. Bethesda, MD: American Association of Blood Banks, 1992:31–49.
226. Andersen CB, Ladefoged SD, Taaning E. Transfusion-associated graft-vs-graft and potential graft-versus-host disease in a renal allotransplanted patient. Hum Pathol 1992; 23:831–834.
227. Mori S, Matsushita H, Ozaki K, et al. Spontaneous resolution of transfusion-associated graft-versus-host disease. Transfusion 1995; 35:431–435.

228. Sazama K, Holland P. Transfusion-induced graft-vesus-host disease. In: Garratty G, ed. Immunobiology of Transfusion Medicine. New York: Marcel Dekker, 1994:631–656.
229. von Fliedner V, Higby DJ, Kim U. Graft-versus-host reaction following blood product transfusion. Am J Med 1982; 72:951–961.
230. Ohto H, Anderson KC. Posttransfusion graft-versus-host disease in Japanese newborns. Transfusion 1996; 36:117–123.
231. Berger RS, Dixon SL. Fulminant transfusion-associated graft-versus-host disease in a premature infant. J Am Acad Dermatol 1989; 20:945–950.
232. Kessinger A, Armitage JO, Klassen LW, et al. Graft vs host disease following transfusion of normal blood products to patients with malignancies. J Surg Oncol 1987; 36:206–209.
233. Woods WG, Lubin BH, Fatal graft-versus-host disease following a blood transfusion in a child with neuroblastoma. Pediatrics 1981; 67:217–221.
234. Kennedy JS, Ricketts RR. Fatal graft-versus-host disease in a child with neuroblastoma following a blood transfusion. J Pediatr Surg 1986; 21:1108–1109.
235. Postmus PE, Mulder NH, Elema JD. Graft vs host disease after transfusions of non-irradiated blood cells in patients having received autologous bone marrow: a report of 4 cases following ablative chemotherapy for solid tumors. Eur J Cancer Clin Oncol 1988; 24:889–894.
236. Webb IJ, Anderson KC. Transfusion-associated graft-vs-host disease. In: Popovsky MA, ed. Transfusion Reactions. Bethesda, MD: AABB Press, 2001:171–186.
237. Thaler M, Shamiss A, Orgad S, et al. The role of blood from HLA-homozygous donors in fatal transfusion-associated graft-versus-host disease after open-heart surgery. N Engl J Med 1989; 321:25–28.
238. Petz LD, Calhoun L, Yam P, et al. Transfusion-associated graft-versus-host disease in immunocompetent patients: report of a fatal case associated with transfusion of blood from a second-degree relative, and a survey of predisposing factors. Transfusion 1993; 33:742–750.
239. Kanter MH. Transfusion-associated graft-versus-host disease: do transfusions from second-degree relatives pose a greater risk than those from first-degree relatives? Transfusion 1992; 32:323–327.
240. Douglas SD, Fudeberg HH. Graft-versus-host reaction in Wiscott-Aldrich syndrome: antemortem diagnosis of human GvH in an immunologic deficiency disease. Vox Sang 1969; 16:172–178.
241. Rubinstein A, Radl J, Cottier H, et al. Unusual combined immunodeficiency syndrome exhibiting kappa-IgD paraproteinemia, residual gut-immunity and graft-versus-host reaction after plasma infusion. Acta Paediatr Scand 1973; 62:365–372.
242. Park BH, Good RA, Gate J, Burke B. Fatal graft-vs.-host reaction following transfusion of allogeneic blood and plasma in infants with combined immunodeficiency disease. Transplant Proc 1974; 6:385–387.
243. Roberts GT, Sacher RA. Transfusion-associated graft-versus-host disease. In: Rossi EC, Simon TL, Moss GS, Gould SA, eds. Principles of Transfusion Medicine. Baltimore, MD: Williams and Wilkins, 1996:785–801.
244. Lind SE. Has the case for irradiating blood products been made? Am J Med 1985; 78:543–544.
245. Perkins H. Should all blood from related donors be irradiated? Transfusion 1992; 32:302–303.
246. Anand AJ, Dzik WH, Imam A, Sadrazadeh SM. Radiation-induced red cell damage: role of reactive oxygen species. Transfusion 1997; 37:160–165.
247. Food and Drug Administration. Guidance for industry. Gamma irradiation of blood and blood components. A pilot program of licensing. (February 2000). Rockville, MD: CBER Office of Communication, Training, and Manufacturers Assistance, 2000.
248. Akahoshi M, Takanashi M, Masuda M, et al. A case of transfusion-associated graft-versus-host disease not prevented by white cell-reduction filters. Transfusion 1992; 32:169–172.

249. Hayashi H, Nishiuchi T, Tamura H, Takeda K. Transfusion-associated graft-versus-host disease caused by leukocyte-filtered stored blood. Anesthesiology 1993; 79:1419–1421.
250. Hong R, Kay EM, Cooper MD, et al. Immunological reconstitution in lymphopenic immunological deficiency syndrome. Lancet 1968; 1:503–506.
251. Jacobs JC, De Capoa A, McGilvray E, et al. Complement deficiency and chromosomal breaks in case of Swiss-type agammaglobulinaemia. Lancet 1968; 1:499–503.
252. Gatti RA, Platt N, Pomerance H, et al. Hereditary lymphopenic agammaglobulinemia associated with distinctive form of short-linked dwarfism and ectodermal dysplasia. J Pediatr 1969; 75:675–684.
253. McCarty JR, Raimer SS, Jarratt M. Toxic epidermal necrolysis from graft-versus-host disease. Occurrence in a patient with thymic hypoplasia. Am J Dis Child 1978; 132:282–284.
254. Walker MW, Lovell MA, Kelly TE, et al. Multiple areas of intestinal atresia associated with immunodeficiency and posttransfusion graft-versus-host disease. J Pediatr 1993; 123:93–95.
255. Fagiolo E, D'Addosio AM. Post-transfusion graft-versus-host disease (GVHD): immunopathology and prevention. Haematologica 1985; 70:62–74.
256. Kunstmann E, Bocker T, Roewer L, et al. Diagnosis of transfusion-associated graft-versus-host disease by genetic fingerprinting and polymerase chain reaction. Transfusion 1992; 32:766–770.
257. Schmidmeir W, Feil W, Gebhart W, et al. Fatal graft-versus-host reaction following granulocyte transfusions. Blut 1982; 45:115–119.
258. Dinsmore RE, Straus DJ, Pollack MS, et al. Fatal graft-versus-host disease following blood transfusion in Hodgkin's disease documented by HLA typing. Blood 1980; 55:831–834.
259. Burns LJ, Wesbury MW, Burns CP, et al. Acute graft versus host disease resulting from normal donor blood transfusion. Acta Haematol 1984; 71:270–276.
260. Spitzer TR, Cahill R, Cotler-Fox M, et al. Transfusion induced graft-versus-host disease in patients with malignant lymphoma: a case report and review of the literature. Cancer 1990; 66:2346–2349.
261. Groff P, Torhorst J, Speck B, et al. Die graft-versus-host-krankheit, eine wening bekannte komplikation der bluttransfusion. Schweiz Med Wochenschr 1976; 106:634–639.
262. Stutzman L, Nisce L, Friedman M. Increased toxicity of total nodal irradiation (TNI) following combination chemotherapy (abstract). Proc Am Soc Clin Oncol 1979; 20:391.
263. Mathe G, Schwartzenberg L, deVries MJ, et al. Les divers aspects du syndrome secondaire comliquant les transfusions allogeniques du moelle osseuse ou de leukocytes chez des sujets atteints d'hemopathies malignes. Eur J Cancer 1965; 1:75–113.
264. DeDobbeleer GP, Ledoux-Corbusier MH, Achten GA. Graft versus host reaction. An ultrastructural study. Arch Dermatol 1975; 3:1597–1602.
265. Ford JM, Lucey JJ, Cullen MH, et al. Fatal graft-versus-host disease following transfusion of granulocytes from normal donors. Lancet 1976; 2:1167–1169.
266. Weiden PL, Zuckerman N, Hansen JA, et al. Fatal graft-versus-host disease in a patient with lymphoblastic leukemia following normal granulocyte transfusions. Blood 1981; 57:328–332.
267. Tolbert B, Kaufman CE Jr, Burgdorf WH, Brubaker D. Graft versus host disease from leukocyte transfusions. J Am Acad Dermatol 1983; 9:416–419.
268. Naiman JL, Punnett HH, Lischner HW, et al. Possible graft-versus-host reaction after intrauterine transfusion for Rh erythroblastosis fetalis. N Engl J Med 1969; 281:697–701.
269. Parkman R, Mosier D, Umansky I, et al. Graft-versus-host disease after intrauterine and exchange transfusions for hemolytic disease of the newborn. N Engl J Med 1974; 290:359–363.
270. Bohm N, Kleine W, Enzel U. Graft-versus-host disease in two newborns after repeated blood transfusions because of rhesus incompatibility. Beitr Pathol 1977; 160:381–400.
271. Hentschel R, Broecker EB, Kolde G, et al. Intact survival with transfusion-associated graft-versus-host disease proved by human leukocyte antigen typing of lymphocytes in skin biopsy specimens. J Pediatr 1995; 126:61–64.

272. Ito K, Yoshida H, Yanagibashi K, et al. Change of HLA phenotype in postoperative erythroderma. Lancet 1988; 1:413–414.
273. Wagner FF, Flegel WA. Transfusion-associated graft-versus-host disease: risk due to homozygous HLA haplotypes. Transfusion 1995; 35:284–291.
274. Pahwa S, Sia C, Harper R, Pahwa R. T-lymphocyte subpopulations in high-risk infants: influence of age and blood transfusions. Pediatrics 1985; 76:914–917.
275. Sanders MR, Graeber JE. Posttransfusion graft-versus-host disease in infancy. J Pediatr 1990; 117:159–163.
276. Flidel O, Barak Y, Lifschitz-Mercer B, et al. Graft versus host disease in extremely low birth weight neonates. Pediatrics 1992; 89:689–690.
277. Anderson KC, Goodnough LT, Sayers M, et al. Variation in blood component irradiation practice: implications for prevention of transfusion-associated graft-versus-host disease. Blood 1991; 77:2096–2102.
278. Szaley F, Buki B, Kalouics I, Keleman E. Post transfusion GVHR in an adult with acute leukemia and aplastic anemia. Orv Hetil 1972; 113:1275–1280.
279. Rosen RC, Heustis DW, Corrigan JJ Jr. Acute leukemia and granulocyte transfusion: fatal graft versus host reaction following transfusion of cells obtained from normal donors. J Pediatr 1978; 93:268–270.
280. Lowenthal RM, Menon C, Challis DR. Graft-versus-host disease in consecutive patients with acute myeloid leukemia treated with blood cells from normal donors. Aust N Z J Med 1981; 11:179–183.
281. Nikoskelainen J, Soderstrom K-O, Rajamaki A, et al. Graft versus host reaction in 3 adult leukemia patients after transfusion of blood cell products. Scand J Haematol 1983; 31:403–409.
282. Schmitz N, Kayser W, Gassman W, et al. Ten cases of graft-versus-host disease following transfusion of irradiated blood products. Blut 1982; 44:83–88.
283. Siimes MA, Koskimies S. Chronic graft versus host disease after blood transfusions by incompatible HLA antigens in bone marrow (letter). Lancet 1982; 1:42–43.
284. Pflieger H. Graft-versus-host disease following blood transfusions. Blut 1983; 46:61–66.
285. Gossi U, Bucher U, Brun del Re G, et al. Acute graft versus host disease following a single transfusion of erythrocytes. Schweiz Wochenschr 1985; 115:34–40.
286. Remlinger K, Buckner CD, Clift RA, et al. Fatal graft versus host disease and probable graft versus host reaction due to an unradiated granulocyte transfusion after allogeneic bone marrow transplant. Transplant Proc 1983; 15:1725–1728.
287. Labotka RJ, Radvany R. Graft vs host disease in rhabdomyosarcoma following transfusion with nonirradiated blood products. Med Pediatr Oncol 1985; 13:101–104.
288. Capon SM, DePond WD, Tyan DB, et al. Transfusion-associated graft-versus-host disease in an immunocompetent patient. Ann Intern Med 1991; 114:1025–1026.
289. Grishaber JE, Birney SM, Strauss RG. Potential for transfusion-associated graft-versus-host disease due to apheresis platelets matched for HLA Class I antigens. Transfusion 1993; 33:910–914.
290. Benson K, Marks AR, Marshall MJ, Goldstein JD. Fatal graft-versus-host disease associated with transfusions of HLA-matched, HLA-homozygous platelets from unrelated donors. Transfusion 1994; 34:432–437.
291. Takanashi M, Nishimura M, Tadokoro K, Juji T. Graft-versus-host disease associated with transfusions of HLA-matched, HLA-homozygous platelets. Transfusion 1995; 35:276–277.
292. Wisecarver JL, Cattral MS, Langnas AN, et al. Transfusion-induced graft-versus-host disease after liver transplantation. Transplantation 1994; 58:269–271.
293. Klein HG. Transfusion in transplant patients: the good, the bad, and the ugly. J Heart Lung Transplant 1993; 12:S7-S12.
294. Gorlin JB, Mintz PD. Transfusion-associated graft-vs-host disease. In: Mintz PD, ed. Transfusion Therapy: Clinical Principles and Practice. Bethesda, MD: AABB Press, 1999:341–357.
295. Hatley RM, Reyolds M, Paller AS, Chou P. Graft-versus-host disease following ECMO. J Pediatr Surg 1991; 26:317–319.

296. Lowenthal RM, Grossman L, Goldman JM, et al. Granulocyte transfusions in treatment of infection in patients with acute leukemia and aplastic anemia. Lancet 1975; 1:353–358.
297. American Association of Blood Banks. Noninfectious complications of blood transfusion. In: Brecher ME, ed. Technical Manual. Bethesda: MD, 2002:585–612.
298. Dodd RY, Notari IV, Stramer SL. Current prevalence and incidence of infectious disease markers and estimated window-period risk in the American Red Cross blood donor population. Transfusion 2002; 42; 975–979.
299. Couroucé AM, Pillonel J. Transfusion-transmitted viral infections. The Retrovirus and Viral Hepatitis Working Groups of the French Society of Blood Transfusion. N Engl J Med 1996; 335:1609–1610.
300. Barrera JM, Francis B, Ercilla G, et al. Improved detection of anti-HCV in post-transfusion hepatitis by a third-generation ELISA. Vox Sang 1995; 68:15–18.
301. Prowse C, Ludlam CA, Yap PL. Human parvovirus B19 and blood products. Vox Sang 1997; 72:1–10.
302. US General Accounting Office. Blood supply: transfusion-associated risks. GAO/PEMD-97-1. Washington DC: US Government Printing Office, 1997.
303. Food and Drug Administration. Guidance for industry: revised recommendations for the assessment of donor suitability and blood and blood product safety in cases of known or suspected West Nile Virus infection. Final guidance. (May 2003) Rockville, MD: CBER Office of Communication, Training, and Manufacturers Assistance, 2003.
304. American Association of Blood Banks. Statement of the American Association of Blood Banks, America's Blood Centers, the American Red Cross and the Armed Services Blood Program: update on national testing of blood for West Nile Virus. (April 18, 2003) Bethesda, MD: American Association of Blood Banks, 2003.
305. Klein HG, Dodd RY, Ness PM, et al. Current status of microbial contamination of blood components: summary of a conference. Transfusion 1997; 37:95–101.
306. Halpin TJ, Kilker S, Epstein J, et al. Bacterial contamination of platelet pools—Ohio, 1991. Morb Mortal Wkly Rep 1992; 41:36–37.
307. Lee J, United States Food and Drug Administration. Presented at the FDA/CBER Bacterial Contamination of Platelets Workshop; September 1999, Bethesda, MD.
308. Bacterial contamination of blood components. Bulletin 96-6. AABB Faxnet 294. Bethesda, MD: American Association of Blood Banks, 1996.
309. Morro JF, Braine HG, Kickler TS, et al. Septic reactions to platelet transfusions. A persistent problem. J Am Med Assoc 1991; 266:555–558.
310. Goldman M, Blajchman MA. Blood product-associated bacterial sepsis. Transfus Med Rev 1991; 5:73–83.
311. Chiu EKW, Yuien KY, Lie AKW, et al. A prospective study of symptomatic bacteremia following platelet transfusion and its management. Transfusion 1994; 34:950–954.
312. Krishnan LS, Brecher ME. Transfusion transmitted bacterial infection. Hematol Oncol Clin North Am 1995; 9:167–185.
313. Guidance on implementation of new bacteria reduction and detection standard. Bulletin 03-7. Bethesda, MD: American Association of Blood Banks, 2003.
314. Wallace EL, Churchill WH, Surgenor DM, et al. Collection and transfusion of blood and blood components in the United States, 1994. Transfusion 1998; 38:625–636.
315. Goodnough LT, Brecher ME, Kanter MH, et al. Medical progress: transfusion medicine, part I. Blood transfusion. New Engl J Med 1999; 340:438–447.
316. Cookston St, Arduino MJ, Aguero SM, et al. Yersinia enterocolitica-contaminated red blood cells (RBCs): an emerging threat to blood safety. In: Program and Abstracts of the 36th Interscience Conference on Antimicrobial Agents and Chemotherapy, September 15–18, 1996, New Orleans, Louisiana. Washington DC: American Society for Microbiology, 1996:237(abstract).
317. Ohto H, Anderson KC. Survey of transfusion-associated graft-versus-host disease in immunocompetent recipients. Transfus Med Rev 1996; 10:31–43.

54

Agents Used for Anticoagulation

James R. Stubbs
University of South Alabama Medical Center, Mobile, Alabama, USA

WARFARIN

The plasma half-life of warfarin ranges from 0.5 to 3 days (average 44 h) with wide individual variations (1). Intravenously administered vitamin K_1 has a terminal half-life of 1.7 h (2,3). The difference in the half-lives of warfarin and vitamin K_1 must be considered in the management of warfarin overdose. Multiple, frequent doses of vitamin K_1 may be necessary in some cases to restore adequate coagulation factor activity.

An INR of >5.0 is considered a critical value. Warfarin should be stopped in such cases. When evaluating the cause of an elevated international normalized ratio (INR), a review of the patient's diet, alcohol intake, and medications is necessary. Any recent changes should be noted and documented. In many cases, stopping warfarin for 1–2 days will allow the INR to return to the desired therapeutic range. The interval required for changes in the INR is dependent upon vitamin K stores and dietary intake.

The method of correcting the INR will be dictated by the indication for warfarin therapy and the concurrent risk of bleeding. If intestinal fat absorption is intact, vitamin K_1 can be administered orally. In the absence of significant bleeding, and for a concurrent condition requiring anticoagulant therapy, full correction of an elevated INR may not be necessary. In such cases, normalization of the prothrombin time (PT) INR may place a patient at risk for thrombosis. In these cases, a more conservative approach using low doses of vitamin K_1 is recommended. Low doses provide adequate amounts of vitamin K_1 and minimize the difficulty of achieving a therapeutic INR when anticoagulation may be resumed safely. Vitamin K_1 can be administered in repeated small doses orally, by subcutaneous injection, or by slow intravenous injection (>10 min for doses of 1 mg or more). For example, a nonbleeding patient with an elevated INR can receive 0.2–0.5 mg of vitamin K_1 once or twice daily. The INR should be monitored at 6–12 h intervals. This strategy can return the INR values to within the therapeutic range without overcorrection. A dose of 0.5–1.0 mg of vitamin K_1, administered intravenously or subcutaneously, can correct markedly prolonged PT values from warfarin therapy within 8 h (4). Because the half-life of vitamin K is significantly shorter than that of warfarin, multiple doses of vitamin K_1 may be necessary to achieve the desired INR correction. As the INR approaches the upper limit of the therapeutic range, warfarin can be started again with a new maintenance dose. The INR can fall below the therapeutic range if resumption of warfarin therapy is delayed too long. If overcorrection of the INR occurs, heparin or low-molecular-weight heparin (LMWH) therapy may be necessary for anticoagulation until a therapeutic effect is achieved with warfarin.

An oral vitamin K_1 dose of 5 mg/day for 5–10 days will provide full restoration of vitamin-K-dependent coagulation factor activity and will replenish vitamin K stores. Depending on the clinical situation, supplemental oral vitamin K_1 therapy may not be necessary for hemostatic correction in patients capable of eating and absorbing fat from a well-balanced diet. When liver function is adequate, the PT/INR may return to the "reference range" within 1–2 days. Despite a normal PT/INR, certain coagulation factors, such as prothrombin, will take several days before full restoration of activity is achieved.

If significant warfarin-related bleeding is present, infusions of products containing vitamin-K-dependent factors, for example, fresh frozen plasma (FFP) or prothrombin complex concentrates, may be necessary. Transfusion of 15 mL/kg of FFP rapidly restores effective hemostatic function in warfarin-treated patients experiencing serious bleeding. Duration of the beneficial effect of FFP is limited by the half-lives of the transfused vitamin-K-dependent factors, particularly factor VII. Some patients may require multiple infusions of FFP to control bleeding. The most important aspect of warfarin-related bleeding treatment is the restoration of adequate concentration of functional prothrombin (factor II).

Because patients require warfarin for the prevention or the treatment of thrombosis, concern exists that the transfusion of FFP will make them vulnerable to thromboembolic complications. In some cases, bleeding can be controlled and the thrombotic risk minimized with correction limited to decreasing the PT/INR values to within the desired therapeutic range. More severe bleeding will require replacement therapy with the goal of normalizing the PT/INR and the aPTT. Although the risk of thromboembolism following reversal of warfarin therapy is increased, it does not appear to be an immediate danger. However, the duration of minimal thrombotic risk is unpredictable. Patients with prosthetic cardiac valves who stop taking warfarin and achieve correction of their PT/INR through diet alone probably have several days before thrombotic risk increases. This finding may reflect a slow return of prothrombin activity to >20–25%. Once warfarin effects are corrected and hemostasis has been achieved, anticoagulant therapy should be resumed in those individuals with an ongoing need for anti-thrombotic protection.

Other measures to control bleeding may be necessary in certain patients with warfarin-related bleeding. In some patients, for example those with bleeding gastric ulcer, surgery or other invasive procedures may be necessary in addition to the replacement of vitamin-K-dependent factors to control bleeding. Patients who are hypervolemic, such as individuals with severe liver disease, may not tolerate the volume of FFP needed to correct the warfarin effect. In these patients, the infusion of prothrombin concentrate may be preferable.

Reagents used for the performance of the PT/INR vary greatly in their sensitivity to reductions in factor activities and may yield normal results before full factor activity is restored. The laboratory analysis may indicate a normal PT/INR in a patient without adequate hemostatic function. Inadequate restoration of hemostatic function may result in unexpected or excessive bleeding in patients who are considered satisfactory candidates for surgery or invasive procedures on the basis of rapid PT/INR correction alone (5). When restoring hemostatic function following oral anticoagulation, the clinician should monitor the aPTT, as well as the PT/INR.

For patients who have received a significant overdose of warfarin, intravenous administration of 15–30 mg of vitamin K_1 may be necessary to achieve hemostatic correction. Multiple doses may be required. Vitamin K_1 can also be administered subcutaneously; however, intramuscular injections should be avoided because local intramuscular injections have risk of significant local bleeding.

Rapid intravenous infusion of vitamin K_1 may result in serious hypotension, cardiovascular collapse, and death (6). Such reactions may occur with initial intravenous exposure to vitamin K_1. The first case of cardiovascular collapse associated with intravenous vitamin K_1 administration was reported in 1976 (7). Two more cases of severe complications, including one death, associated with IV vitamin K_1 were reported in 1982 (8). The authors recommended that an oral administration of vitamin K_1 be used whenever possible. When vitamin K_1 is given intravenously, it should be given at a rate considerably slower than 1 mg/min (8). Intravenous vitamin K_1 doses <1 mg should also be injected very slowly. When a decision is made to administer vitamin K_1 intravenously, a small test dose prior to delivery of the therapeutic dose is advisable.

UNFRACTIONATED HEPARIN AND LMWH

Bleeding is the principle adverse effect of unfractionated heparin (UFH) administered in therapeutic doses. The estimated risks of fatal bleeding, major bleeding, and all bleeding associated with UFH are 0.05%, 0.8%, and 1.0–2.0% per day of therapy, respectively (9,10). The overall incidence of UFH-related fatal hemorrhage was estimated at 0.4%.

Landefeld and Ibrahim conducted an analysis designed to identify patient characteristics associated with an increased risk of bleeding with UFH (10). They identified four:

1. Heart disease, liver disease, renal disease, poor physical condition, or any combination thereof
2. An aPTT >80 s
3. Age over 80 years
4. Liver dysfunction that worsens during the course of care

Another study also documented an association of advancing age and bleeding risk (11). Higher heparin serum concentrations for any given dose were found in older patients, and the heparin concentration best correlated with bleeding incidence. The investigators concluded that higher concentration per given heparin dose observed in the aged population was not simply a consequence of decreased muscle mass. Rather, they proposed that heparin metabolism changes as a consequence of aging. Other investigators found that the best predictor of bleeding was the overall physical condition of the patient (12). Other predictors of bleeding were a history of bleeding, recent surgery, or recent trauma. Age, anemia, gender, and cancer were not found to be predictors of bleeding. In this study, 12% of heparin-treated subjects experienced bleeding during therapy. When stratified according to the World Health Organization (WHO) functional categories, the bleeding incidences for categories I and II (normal and slightly ill), III (severely ill), and IV (totally bedridden) were 2%, 25%, and 29%, respectively. These incidences reflected bleeding in association with both UFH and LMWH.

Other medications can influence bleeding in heparin-treated patients. For example, the risk of bleeding is increased in patients also receiving aspirin or other nonsteroidal anti-inflammatory drugs (NSAIDs) (13,14). The sites of heparin-associated bleeding are associated with the indication for treatment. In a study of LMWH prophylaxis for subjects undergoing hip or knee replacement, the great majority of bleeding episodes occurred in the wound or soft tissue located at the operative site (15). On the other hand, the gastrointestinal (GI) tract was the most common location for bleeding in an analysis that included primarily medical patients (16). Although the retroperitoneum and the central nervous system are the most common sites for fatal bleeding, when considered together, these locations are involved in only ~5% of all heparin-related bleeding episodes.

When bleeding occurs in heparin-treated patients, several considerations deserve emphasis. First, the likelihood that bleeding is heparin related or from other causes should be assessed. The clinician should consider the possibility of localized bleeding from a specific anatomic site, such as an ulcer, tumor, friable tissue, or a specific vessel. Bleeding from an anatomic lesion is a common explanation for bleeding occurring in patients who receive appropriately managed therapeutic heparin (17). Frequently, postoperative bleeding encountered in heparin-treated patients can be traced to a vessel that was inadequately cauterized or ligated during surgery (18).

Second, is the amount of heparin administered to the patient adequate to cause the type and the degree of bleeding encountered? The amount and time of the last dose of heparin should be reviewed. The plasma half-life of UFH is dose dependent. With increasing doses, the strength and duration of the anticoagulant effect increases. For example, when IV bolus doses increase from 25 to 100 U/kg to 400 U/kg, the corresponding plasma half-lives of UFH are 30, 60, and 150 minutes, respectively (19–21). Because UFH has a relatively short half-life, an effective, commonly used approach to UFH-related bleeding is discontinuation of therapy. When therapeutic doses of UFH have been discontinued, the anticoagulant effect is typically no longer present within 2 h. When very large doses of UFH have been given, for example, during cardiopulmonary bypass, or when major bleeding is present, UFH neutralization with protamine sulfate is indicated.

Two dosing schedules for the reversal of UFH with protamine sulfate are:

Protocol 1 (22)

1. If the last dose of UFH was administered <30 min previously, the protamine dose is 1.0 mg/100 U UFH.
2. If the last dose of UFH was administered 30–60 min previously, the protamine dose is 0.5–0.75 mg/100 U UFH.
3. If the last dose of UFH was administered 60–120 min previously, the protamine dose is 0.375–0.5 mg/100 U UFH.
4. If the last dose of UFH was administered >120 min previously, the protamine dose is 0.25–0.375 mg/100 U UFH.

Protocol 2 (23)

One milligram of protamine sulfate is recommended for every 100 U of heparin that remain in the patient. The amount of heparin in the patient can be calculated assuming a 60-min half-life for UFH. The calculation should incorporate 3 h of therapy.

For example, if a patient has been receiving 1000 U of UFH per hour, the infusion should be stopped. The dose of protamine should be based on the amount of heparin calculated to be present in the patient on the basis of the past 3 h. For the most recent hour (0–1 h time period), 1000 U of UFH are assumed to be present in the patient. For the time periods of 1–2 and 2–3 h prior to cessation of therapy, 500 and 250 U of UFH are assumed to be present in the patient, respectively. The total amount of heparin present is calculated at 1750 U. A 1.0 mg protamine sulfate per 100 U of UFH dose calculates to a total dose of 17.5 mg.

The maximum intravenous (IV) protamine sulfate dose is 50 mg. The infusion rate for a 10 mg/mL solution should be ≤5 mg/min. Patients who have previously received protamine therapy, protamine-containing insulin, or have known hypersensitivity to fish may experience hypersensitivity reactions to protamine sulfate. Although plasma components are often used for heparin-related bleeding, they are not indicated (24). Plasma does not act directly on heparin to reverse its activity, transfused procoagulant factors are subject to heparin's anticoagulant effects, and transfused antithrombin could be the target of additional heparin activity (10,17).

A third decision point is the possibility of potentiating factors (10,25). A number of other medications can contribute to bleeding in heparin-treated patients. Examples include aspirin, other NSAIDs, thrombolytic agents, anti-GP IIb–IIIa agents, oral anticoagulants, or acquired vitamin K deficiency. Some patients may have thrombocytopenia from underlying disease, sepsis, disseminated intravascular coagulation (DIC), or drugs. Desmopressin (DDAVP) may benefit patients who have received anti-platelet agents. Platelet transfusion may be required for extensive bleeding or severe thrombocytopenia. When bleeding occurs with thrombolytic therapy, the thrombolytic agent should be stopped. If hypofibrinogenemia is present, usually fibrinogen <100 mg/dL, replacement with cryoprecipitate (CRYO) should be considered. Acquired platelet dysfunction from thrombolytic therapy, for example, fibrinogen degradation product (FDP) coating of platelets, may be treated with platelet transfusion. Bleeding patients receiving concomitant oral anticoagulants may benefit from measures directed at correcting defects associated with such therapy.

A fourth point to consider is whether the need for anticoagulation is more important for the overall welfare of the patient than the bleeding encountered or the potential risk of bleeding. Bleeding itself is not an absolute contraindication to heparin therapy. Decreasing the dose of heparin to minimize bleeding, while maintaining an anti-thrombotic effect, may be possible. Support with blood components, for example, red cell transfusion, can be provided, if necessary. When possible, alternative forms of thromboembolic protection, including vena caval filters, intermittent pneumatic compression devices, and alternative anti-thrombotic medications, should be considered in patients who are bleeding or are at risk for significant heparin-related bleeding. Serial lower extremity venous ultrasound examinations can provide surveillance for significant venous thrombosis in the high-risk patient.

Major bleeding is a potential complication of LMWH therapy. Clinical trials evaluating the use of the LMWH for the prevention or treatment of venous thromboembolism or unstable angina demonstrated bleeding rates similar to those observed with UFH (22). LMWH has a half-life that is two to four times longer than UFH. The longer half-life of LMWH does provide many therapeutic advantages; however, it is a disadvantage with bleeding. Another disadvantage is incomplete neutralization with protamine sulfate. Although protamine sulfate effectively neutralizes LMWH's anti-thrombin activity, the neutralization of LMWH's anti-factor Xa activity is incomplete (26–33). The efficacy of protamine sulfate for LMWH-related bleeding is unknown. Although bleeding rates associated with UFH and LMWH may be similar, LMWH-related bleeding may be more difficult to control. On the basis of package insert instructions, not clinical trials (22), the recommended dose of protamine sulfate for reversal of LMWH administered within 8 h is 1 mg/100 anti-Xa units. If bleeding continues following the initial protamine dose, a second dose of 0.5 mg/100 anti-Xa units is recommended.

SUMMARY

- Because the half-lives of warfarin (average 44 h), and vitamin K_1 (average 1.7 h after IV infusion) are different, multiple frequent doses of vitamin K_1 may be necessary to restore coagulation activity.
- An INR >5.0 is a critical value. Warfarin therapy should be discontinued.
- Low-dose vitamin K_1 therapy can provide adequate correction of the INR and minimize the difficulty of achieving a therapeutic INR, if the need for anticoagulation remains.
- Vitamin K_1 should be administered orally whenever possible.
- Despite a normal INR, certain coagulation factors, especially prothrombin, may not have full activity.
- Bleeding is the major complication of UFH therapy. Major bleeding is estimated to occur in 0.8% of patients per day of therapy, and fatal bleeding is estimated to occur in 0.4% of patients overall.
- Heart disease, liver disease, renal disease, poor physical condition, aPTT >80 s, age >80 years, and liver dysfunction that worsens during the course of care confer increased risk of bleeding with UFH therapy.

When bleeding complicates heparin therapy, consider the following:

- Is localized bleeding from a specific anatomic site, such as an ulcer, tumor, or specific vessel?
- Is the amount of heparin administered adequate to explain the type and the degree of bleeding observed?
- Are other factors contributing to bleeding? These factors could include aspirin therapy, NSAID therapy, administration of thrombolytic agents, anti-GP IIb–IIIa therapy, oral anticoagulation, acquired vitamin K deficiency, or thrombocytopenia.
- Is the need for anticoagulation more important for the overall welfare of the patient than the bleeding encountered or the potential risk of bleeding?
- Bleeding rates complicating LMWH therapy are comparable with those observed with UFH therapy.

REFERENCES

1. Breckenridge AM. Oral anticoagulant drugs: pharmacokinetic aspects. Semin Hematol 1978; 15:19–26.
2. Park BK, Scott AK, Wilson AC, Haynes BP, Breckenridge AM. Plasma disposition of vitamin K_1 in relation to anticoagulant poisoning. Br J Clin Pharmacol 1984; 18:655–662.
3. Bjornsson TD, Meffin PJ, Swezey SEB, T.F. Disposition and turnover of vitamin K_1 in man. In: Suttie JW, ed. Vitamin K Metabolism and Vitamin K-dependent proteins. Baltimore, MD: University Park Press, 1979:328–332.
4. Hirsh J, Dalen JE, Deykin D, Poller L, Bussey H. Oral anticoagulants. Mechanisms of action, clinical effectiveness, and optimal therapeutic range. Chest 1995; 108:231S–246S.
5. Robinson GA, Nylander A. Warfarin and cataract extraction. Br J Ophthalmol 1986; 73:702–703.
6. Hirsh J. Substandard monitoring of warfarin in North America: time for a change (editorial). Arch Intern Med 1992; 152:257–258.

7. Hirsh J, Poller L. The international normalized ratio: a guide to understanding and correcting its problems. Arch Intern Med 1994; 154:282–288.
8. Critchfield GC, Bennett ST, Swaim WR. Calibration verification of the international normalized ratio. Am J Clin Pathol 1996; 106:786–794.
9. Landefeld CS, Beyth RJ. Anticoagulant-related bleeding: clinical epidemiology, prediction, and prevention. Am J Med 1993; 95:315–328.
10. Ibrahim SA, Landefeld CS. Bleeding and unfractionated heparin. In: Ginsberg J, Kearon C, Hirsh J, eds. Clinical Decisions in Thrombosis and Hemostatis. Hamilton: BC Decker, 1998:154–160.
11. Campbell NR, Hull RD, Brant R, et al. Aging and heparin-related bleeding. Arch Intern Med 1996; 156:857–860.
12. Nieuwenhuis HK, Albada J, Banga JD, Sixma JJ. Identification of risk factors for bleeding during treatment of acute venous thromboembolism with heparin or low molecular weight heparin. Blood 1991; 78:2337–2343.
13. Levine M, Raskob GE, Landefeld CS, Kearon C. Complications of anticoagulant treatment. Chest 1998; 114:511S–523S.
14. Mahaffey KW, Granger CB, Collins R, et al. Overview of randomized trials of intravenous heparin in patients with acute myocardial infarction treated with thrombolytic therapy. Am J Cardiol 1996; 77:551–556.
15. Leclerc JR, Gent M, Hirsh, et al. The incidence of symptomatic venous thromboembolism during and after prophylaxis with enoxaparin. Arch Intern Med 1998; 158:873–878.
16. Landefeld CS, Anderson PA. Guideline-based consultation to prevent anticoagulant-related bleeding. Ann Intern Med 1992; 116:829–837.
17. Landefeld CS, Rosenblatt MW, Goldman L. Bleeding in outpatients treated with warfarin: relation to the prothrombin time and important remedial lesions. Am J Med 1989; 87:153–159.
18. Kitchens CS. Surgery and hemostasis: the influence of one on the other. In: Ratnoff OD, Forbes CD, eds. Disorders of Hemostasis. Philadelphia, PA: Saunders, 1996:346–382.
19. de Swart CAM, Nijmeyer B, Roelofs JMM, et al. Kinetics of intravenously administered heparin in normal humans. Blood 1982; 60:1251–1258.
20. Olsson P, Lagergren H, Ek S. The elimination from plasma of intravenous heparin: an experimental study on dogs and humans. Acta Med Scand 1963; 173:619–630.
21. Bjornsson TO, Wolfram BS, Kitchell BB. Heparin kinetics determined by three assay methods. Clin Pharmacol Ther 1982; 31:104–113.
22. Hirsh J, Warkentin TE, Shaughnessy SG, Anand SS, Halperin JL, Raschke R, Granger C, Ohman EM, Dalen JE. Heparin and low-molecular-weight heparin: mechanisms of action, pharmacokinetics, dosing, monitoring, efficacy, and safety. Chest 2001; 119:64S–94S.
23. Kitchens CS. Evaluation and treatment of bleeding associated with heparin and low-molecular-weight heparin administration. In: Alving BM, ed. Blood Components and Pharmacologic Agents. Bethesda, MD: AABB Press, 2000:167–184.
24. Development Task Force of the College of American Pathologists. Practice parameter for the use of fresh-frozen plasma, cryoprecipitate, and platelets: fresh-frozen plasma, cryoporecipitate, and platelets administration practice guidelines. J Am Med Assoc 1994; 271:777–781.
25. Penner JA. Managing the hemorrhagic complications of heparin therapy. Hematol Oncol Clin North Am 1993; 7:1281–1289.
26. Racanelli A, Farred J, Walenga JM, et al. Biochemical and pharmacologic studies on the protamine interactions with heparin: its fractions and fragments. Semin Thromb Hemost 1985; 11:176–189.
27. Lindblad B, Borgstrom A, Wakefield TW, et al. Protamine reversal of anticoagulation achieved with a low molecular weight heparin: the effects on eicosanoids, clotting and complement factors. Thromb Res 1987; 48:31–40.
28. Massonnet-Castel S, Pelissier E, Bara L, et al. Partial reversal of low molecular weight heparin (PK 10169) anti-Xa activity by protamine sulfate: *in vitro* and *in vivo* study during cardiac surgery with extracorporeal circulation. Haemostasis 1986; 16:139–146.

29. Hirsh J, Buchanan MR. Comparative effects of heparin and LMW heparin on hemostasis. Thromb Res 1991; 14:11–17.
30. Woltz M, Weltermann A, Nieszpaur-Los M, et al. Studies on the neutralizing effects of protamine on unfractionated and low molecular weight heparin (Fragmin) at the site of activation of the coagulation system in man. Thromb Haemost 1995; 73:439–443.
31. Gram J, Mercker S, Bruhn HD. Does protamine chloride neutralize low molecular weight heparin sufficiently? Thromb Res 1988; 52:353–359.
32. Sugiyama T, Itoh M, Ohtawa M, et al. Study on neutralization of low molecular weight heparin by protamine sulfate and its neutralization characteristics. Thromb Res 1992; 68:119–129.
33. Harenberg J, Gnasso A, de Vries JX, et al. Inhibition of low molecular weight heparin by protamine chloride *in vivo*. Thromb Res 1985; 38:11–20.

Part V
Common SICU Procedures

55
Bronchoscopy

Marshall I. Hertz and Paul Gustafson
University of Minnesota, Minneapolis, Minnesota, USA

Flexible fiberoptic bronchoscopy (FFB) is an important tool in the diagnostic and therapeutic armamentarium of the critical care practitioner. In this chapter the indications, contraindications, and complications of FFB are discussed. FFB requires specialized training and should be performed only by experienced individuals; therefore, a detailed review of the technique of the procedure is beyond the scope of this chapter. A brief description of the method of performing FFB and bronchoalveolar lavage (BAL) in critically ill patients is included to assist critical care physicians in the management of patients during and after these procedures.

OVERVIEW

FFB allows direct visualization of the central airways (i.e., lobar, segmental, and subsegmental bronchi) and biopsy of central and peripheral respiratory tract structures. It is also of therapeutic use in patients with mucus plugging, hemoptysis, and foreign bodies. In the SICU, FFB most commonly is used to sample the respiratory tract secretions of patients with suspected pneumonia (1–3).

Several approaches are used to obtain bronchial secretions through FFB. Sputum may simply be suctioned through the FFB. "Bronchial washings" are obtained by instilling saline solution in small amounts (5–10 mL) into the distal bronchi and suctioning through the bronchoscopic channel. "Bronchial brushings" are obtained by use of small plastic bristle brushes passed through the FFB channel. A modified bronchial brush, the "protected brush catheter," uses a telescoping catheter system through which the brush is passed. This device enables the bronchoscopist to obtain bronchial secretions uncontaminated by upper respiratory or endotracheal tube micro-organisms carried to the lower respiratory tract by the FFB. To increase the specificity of protected brush catheter specimens, quantitative cultures have also been used (3).

Because FFB usually is performed to evaluate pneumonia in immunocompetent or immunocompromised patients, sampling the alveolar contents is the ultimate goal of the procedure. The initial application of FFB that enabled alveolar sampling was the transbronchial biopsy (TBB). TBB is performed by passing a small forceps through the bronchoscopic channel and obtaining small (~1 mm diameter) biopsies of lung parenchyma under fluoroscopic control. TBB is unique among transbronchoscopic procedures in that it alone can provide specimens for histologic examination. As some pneumonic processes, particularly granulomatous infections, may not result in shedding of organisms in bronchial or alveolar secretions, TBB remains a useful procedure in selected patients. However, several features of TBB limit its use in most critically ill patients. First, the patient must be transported to the fluoroscopy suite, a requirement that entails risks in unstable patients. Further, major complications, including hemorrhage and pneumothorax, occur after TBB in up to 3% of patients (4). Many immunocompromised patients are thrombocytopenic. They often are not candidates for TBB, because they have a prohibitive risk of hemorrhage. Finally, TBB samples approximately 100 alveoli per biopsy; with a total of 150 million alveoli per lung, the sampling error may be very significant.

In recent years, BAL has become an important technique for the diagnosis of suspected lower respiratory tract infection (5,6). This procedure involves instilling relatively large volumes of saline solution (~100 mL) into the alveolar spaces, while the bronchoscope is wedged in a segmental or subsegmental bronchus to prevent spillage of the solution throughout the airways. The saline solution, mixed with alveolar and distal bronchial contents, is recovered by suction through the bronchoscope channel and is sent for cultures and analytic studies. BAL avoids many of the drawbacks of other transbronchoscopic procedures, for BAL can be performed at the bedside. The procedure does not result in bleeding or pneumothorax and thus can be offered to many patients in whom TBB is contraindicated. Finally, each lavage samples approximately 1 million alveloli, and consequently, reduces the magnitude of the sampling error.

INDICATIONS

FFB is used in critically ill patients for both diagnostic and therapeutic indications (Table 1).

Suspected Pneumonia

The need for bronchoscopically collected lower respiratory tract culture material must be evaluated on a patient-by-patient basis. In general, patients with post-operative pulmonary infiltrates who are producing sputum containing a predominant organism do not require

Table 1 Indications for Flexible Fiberoptic Bronchoscopy in Critically Ill Patients

	Diagnostic	Therapeutic
Suspected pneumonia	×	
Atelectasis	×	×
Hemoptysis	×	×
Foreign body	×	×
Suspected tracheobronchial disruption	×	×
Smoke inhalation	×	
Difficult intubation		×

FFB. However, for patients from whose sputum a likely pathogen cannot be obtained or those not producing sputum despite clinical and radiographic deterioration, FFB with protected brush catheter sampling or BAL is indicated. In immunocompromised hosts, the spectrum of infectious microorganisms causing pneumonia is much broader; BAL and cultures for detecting bacteria (including *Legionella*), fungi, viruses, and mycobacteria are indicated in most of these patients. In patients with suspected fungal pneumonia, TBB may also be helpful.

Atelectasis

FFB is often of therapeutic benefit in patients with postoperative atelectasis. When major atelectasis occurs (e.g., total atelectasis of a lobe or lung), the chest X-ray film should be examined first for improper endotracheal tube placement. Assuming that the tube is properly positioned, FFB can be therapeutic if an endobronchial mucous plug is seen and evacuated. Bronchoscopy is *not* of benefit if mucous obstruction of the bronchus is not present. The physical examination is of help in determining the need for bronchoscopy; that is, FFB usually is useful only when breath sounds in the atelectatic area are decreased. This is of particular relevance to postcoronary artery bypass patients who frequently develop left lower lobe atelectasis. In most cases this is "open bronchus atelectasis" with preserved breath sounds, and the condition will not be improved by bronchoscopy.

In patients who develop minor degrees of atelectasis without physiologic compromise, chest physical therapy with percussion and postural drainage, encouragement of upright posture, and cough and deep breathing are indicated before FFB and frequently result in radiographic and clinical improvement (7).

FFB also is indicated in patients who have undergone thoracic surgical procedures, including lobectomy and pneumectomy, and who develop major atelectasis with or without pneumothorax. FFB is used in these patients to identify an endobronchial blood clot, mucous plugging, or disruption of the bronchial stump.

Hemoptysis

In SICU patients with normal platelet counts and coagulation tests, hemoptysis is due most commonly to local trauma from the end of the tracheostomy or endotracheal tube or from vigorous suctioning efforts. In such cases FFB allows identification of the bleeding site and leads to appropriate corrective actions. Hemoptysis in patients with tracheostomies may also result from erosion through the trachea into the innominate artery. This complication generally results in massive hemoptysis, and the source is seldom seen with the FFB. Hemoptysis in postoperative patients may also result from other bronchoscopically diagnosable conditions, including endobronchial lesions of the major airways, such as bronchogenic carcinoma and less common tumors. In patients with negative bronchoscopic evaluations for hemoptysis, many other causes must be considered, including pulmonary embolus. Pneumonia, especially in patients with coagulopathy, may produce parenchymal bleeding.

FFB also is useful therapeutically in SICU patients with hemoptysis. Hemostatic medications, including epinephrine (3–5 mL of 1:10,000 solution), and topically applied thrombin can be applied directly to bleeding endobronchial lesions. When blood is emanating from a distal airway site, these medications can be instilled while the bronchoscope is wedged in a proximal airway. When bleeding is not controlled with medications, but can be localized to a bronchopulmonary segment, a 4 or 5 Fr balloon-tipped catheter, passed through the channel of the instrument and inflated in the bronchus, may tamponade the bleeding enroute to more definitive diagnostic and therapeutic efforts (e.g., arteriography, bronchial artery embolization, or surgery as indicated).

Foreign Body

Foreign body aspiration in the SICU is unusual but occasionally occurs. Most aspirated foreign bodies can be visualized with the FFB, and, in many cases, retrieval of the foreign body with a forceps is possible. Large foreign bodies may require use of a rigid bronchoscope for removal.

Suspected Tracheobronchial Disruption

In patients who have sustained major chest trauma, particularly when it is associated with first and second rib fractures, partial or complete disruption of the bronchial tree at the level of the trachea or main bronchi is not uncommon (8). In trauma patients with pneumothorax, accompanied by a major air leak after chest tube placement, FFB is indicated to evaluate the integrity of the trachea and main bronchi. Nontraumatic bronchopleural fistulas also can be identified by observing bubbling at the bronchial orifice after saline solution instillation. Successful closure of bronchopleural fistulas has been reported after instillation of "fibrin glue," which consists of fibrinogen and thrombin (9).

Smoke Inhalation

Patients rescued from closed-space fires, particularly those with burns of the nose and mouth, have a very high incidence of laryngeal and tracheal burns (10). Such patients should be evaluated by FFB immediately to identify laryngeal and tracheal edema and to place an endotracheal tube prophylactically when indicated.

Difficult Intubation

FFB can be used for difficult nasotracheal or orotracheal intubations. The endotracheal tube is placed over the FFB, and the tip is visually guided past the glottic aperture. Once the bronchoscope is in the trachea, the endotracheal tube can be advanced through the glottis, using the FFB as a stylette.

CONTRAINDICATIONS

A thorough prebronchoscopy evaluation is necessary to identify factors contraindicating the procedure (see Box 1). Thrombocytopenic patients (i.e., with a platelet count $<80,000-100,000/mm^3$) and those in whom a pneumothorax would not be tolerated, even if recognized and treated immediately, should not undergo transbronchial biopsies.

Less traumatic procedures that are performed through the FFB, including BAL, are contraindicated in many critically ill patients unless endotracheal intubation is done before the procedure. Such patients include those with rapidly deteriorating respiratory status, those in whom an arterial partial pressure of oxygen (PaO_2) of at least 70 mm Hg

Box 1 Contraindications to FFB

Factors mandating endotracheal intubation before bronchoscopy
    Severe respiratory distress (e.g., respiratory rate >30/min, use of accessory muscles)
    Inability to achieve partial pressure of oxygen in arterial blood (PaO_2) ≥70 mm Hg (9.3 kPa)
      with supplemental oxygen by mask
    Abnormal mental status precluding cooperation with the procedure
Factors contraindicating bronchoscopy in intubated patients unless corrected
    Cardiovascular instability (e.g., hypotension, significant dysrrhythmias) despite pharmacologic
      intervention
    Inability to acheive $PaO_2 > 70$ mm Hg (9.3 kPa) on fraction of inspired oxygen (FIO_2) of 1
    Severe electrolyte or metabolic disturbance (e.g., pH < 7.3, potassium level >5.3 meq/L)

---

cannot be achieved with supplemental oxygen by mask, and those with abnormal mental status (e.g., agitation, somnolence) that would preclude cooperation with the procedure or contraindicate the administration of sedating medications.

Previously intubated patients are evaluated to identify factors contraindicating FFB unless corrected. These factors include cardiovascular instability despite pharmacologic intervention. Patients whose blood pressure can be maintained above 100 mm Hg systolic with moderate doses of pressor medications and those with nonthreatening cardiac dysrhythmias (e.g., with occasional premature ventricular contractions) are not prohibited from undergoing FFB. Patients in whom a $PaO_2 > 70$ mm Hg cannot be achieved despite a fraction of inspired oxygen (FIO_2) of 1 are excluded, because the risk of developing refractory hypoxemia during the procedure is high. Severe electrolyte or metabolic disturbances are corrected before FFB.

BRONCHOSCOPY AND BRONCHOALVEOLAR LAVAGE WITH INTUBATION

Once the need for BAL is established and the prebronchoscopy evaluation (including obtaining informed consent) is completed, this protocol is followed:

Supplemental Oxygen

Fifteen minutes before the procedure, the FIO_2 is increased to 1, and it is continued at that level throughout the procedure. An FIO_2 of 1 is necessary, because even healthy individuals and stable patients undergoing bronchoscopy experience significant decreases in PaO_2 during the procedure (11,12). After BAL, the FIO_2 gradually is weaned to the lowest FIO_2 required to maintain arterial oxyhemoglobin saturation ≥92%.

Bronchoscope

The FFB consists of optical fiber bundles, flexion–extension cables, and a hollow channel for suction and instrument passage, all packaged in a durable plastic sheath. Instruments commonly used in the critical care setting have outside diameters of 4–5 mm. The FFB can be passed transnasally or transorally in awake, unintubated patients. In intubated patients an instrument is chosen that can be passed through the endotracheal tube with adequate clearance to allow ventilation. In general, the endotracheal tube's diameter must be at least 2.5 mm larger than the bronchoscope's diameter. Because the pediatric bronchoscope (outside diameter of 4 mm) provides suboptimal BAL fluid returns, an 8 or 9 mm endotracheal tube, which will permit passage of a 5 mm diameter instrument, should be placed if possible. When changing to a larger endotracheal tube is not feasible, the smaller bronchoscope is used. A small glottic aperture or a requirement for uninterrupted positive end-expiratory pressure may preclude changing to a larger endotracheal tube.

Ventilator Management

The goal is to provide the patient with a minute ventilation during the procedure that is equivalent to that which the patient was receiving before the procedure. The ventilator pressure limit alarm is set at 40 cm H_2O or 10 cm H_2O above the prebronchoscopy baseline level, whichever is higher. The tidal volume is decreased by $\sim$33%, the respiratory rate is increased by an equal proportion, and the inspiratory flow rate is decreased. In this manner, a constant minute ventilation is provided at a lower peak airway pressure. After the bronchoscope has been inserted into the airway, the exhaled minute volume is monitored. The inspired tidal volume is increased to compensate for the volume lost when air leak occurs at the site of bronchoscopic insertion.

Monitors

All patients are monitored with continuous ECG and continuous pulse oximetery. Many patients have indwelling arterial catheters for blood pressure monitoring. Intermittent automated blood pressure monitoring is generally used for patients who do not have indwelling arterial catheters.

Medications

Analgesics and tranquilizers (opiates and benzodiazepines, respectively) are used to ensure patient comfort during the procedure. In most cases, a nondepolarizing muscle relaxant is required to maintain optimal control of the procedure (i.e., to eliminate cough and agitation). In patients judged not to require muscle relaxation, 1% lidocaine (Xylocaine) is applied topically to the airways as needed to control cough.

Bronchoalveolar Lavage Technique

After the administration of medications, the bronchoscope is passed into the endotracheal tube through a plastic adapter with a rubber diaphragm designed to minimize air leakage. The bronchoscope is attached to tubing with a three-way stopcock between the suction port and the collection traps (Fig. 1). The bronchoscopist wedges the bronchoscope in the optimal position while an assistant performs the lavage. Use of two persons minimizes the likelihood of dislodging the bronchoscope and spilling saline solution throughout the airways. The bronchoscopic channel is flushed with saline solution and gently wedged in a segmental or subsegmental bronchus in the area of abnormality observed on chest X-ray film. In patients with diffuse pulmonary infiltrates, two to three nondependent segments, usually the right middle lobe and the lingula of the left upper lobe, are lavaged, because lavage of nondependent segments results in a higher percent recovery of the instilled fluid.

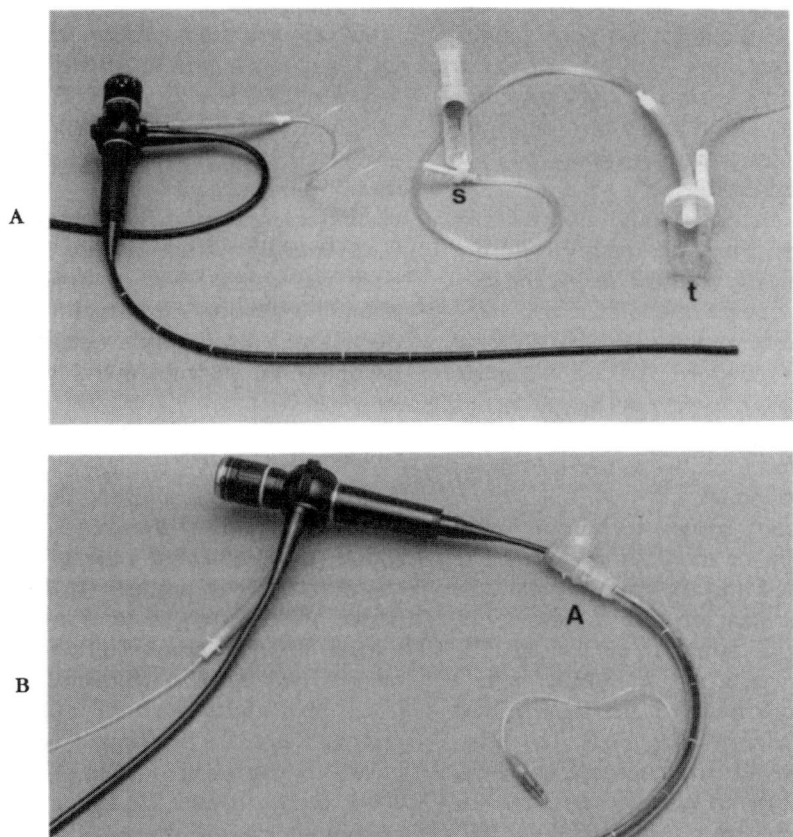

Figure 1 A, Bronchoscope is modified by interposition of three-way stopcock (s) in suction tubing to allow instillation and withdrawal of lavage fluid by an assistant, leaving both hands of bronchoscopist free to manipulate bronchoscope. Collection traps (t) are introduced into suction tubing circuit after local anesthetic has been administered, upper airway secretions are cleared, and bronchoscope is wedged in segmental or subsegmental bronchus. B, Bronchoscope is passed into endotracheal tube through plastic adapter (A) with a rubber diaphragm. [From Ref. (13).]

Lavage is carried out in each anatomic location by instilling 100 mL of sterile isotonic saline solution (at 37°C) in five 20 mL aliquots, with each aliquot gently suctioned before administration of the next aliquot. In general, 50–75% of the instilled saline solution is recovered in the lavage effluent. A lavage is considered acceptable after $\geq 40\%$ of the volume of instilled saline solution is returned. The lavage effluent from all sites is usually pooled and treated as a single specimen.

At our institution, lavage effluent from all SICU patients is sent for the following studies: RBC and WBC counts and WBC differential; cytologic examination; cultures for bacteria, mycobacteria, *Legionella*, fungi and viruses; and direct fluorescent antibody for *Legionella*. In immunocompromised patients additional rapid shell vial culture with monoclonal antibody staining to identify cytomegalovirus ("rapid antigen") and respiratory syncytial virus antigen detection by enzyme-linked immunosorbent assay are performed.

COMPLICATIONS

Complications are unusual during FFB performed to visualize the airways, but laryngospasm (in unintubated patients) and bronchospasm may occur, particularly in asthmatic patients. Arterial oxygen tension regularly falls during FFB (11,12). Administering supplemental oxygen will correct hypoxemia. When additional procedures, such as transbronchial biopsy and BAL are performed, additional complications may ensue (Table 2). Transbronchial biopsy poses a 1–3% risk of pneumothorax, and a similar incidence of severe bleeding, even in patients with normal platelet count and coagulation parameters. In patients who are uremic, thrombocytopenic, or coagulopathic, the risk or major bleeding increases dramatically (4).

Complications of BAL include hypoxemia, fever, and pneumonia. Hypoxemia begins during or soon after the procedure and persists until residual fluid is absorbed from the alveoli into the vascular space. Therefore, patients are given supplemental oxygen for 2 h after BAL. Approximately 5% of patients develop fever after BAL. Although shaking chills may accompany the fever, blood cultures are usually sterile, and the fever resolves promptly with symptomatic treatment. Prolonged fever should raise the suspicion of BAL-induced pnemonia, which occurs after <1% of such procedures. Pneumonia as a result of BAL may be difficult to diagnose, as the procedure usually is performed in patients who already have pulmonary unfiltrates. In addition, the BAL itself will cause a pulmonary infiltrate that may not resolve for 24 h, even when pneumonia is not present. Therefore, our practice has been to administer antibiotics empirically if post-BAL fever has not resolved within 12–24 h.

In addition to fever and pneumonia, BAL can adversely affect respiratory function in critically ill, mechanically ventilated patients. We recently analyzed 99 consecutive BAL procedures performed in 81 such patients (13), including 46 men and 35 women, with ages ranging from 18–80 years (median, 47 years). All BAL procedures were performed to evaluate suspected lower respiratory tract infection. Both immunocompromised ($n = 44$) and nonimmunocompromised ($n = 37$) patients underwent BAL. Variables of airflow resistance (peak inspiratory airway pressure) and lung mechanics (static lung

Table 2 Complications of Transbronchoscopic Procedures

	Transbronchial biopsy	Bronchoalveolar lavage
Major hemorrhage	<1%[a]	
Pneumothorax	1–3%	
Decreased arterial oxygenation	Common	Common
Fever		~5%
Pneumonia		~1%

[a]Risk markedly increased in patients with uremia, thrombocytopenia, or other coagulopathy.
Source: Modified from Ref. (4).

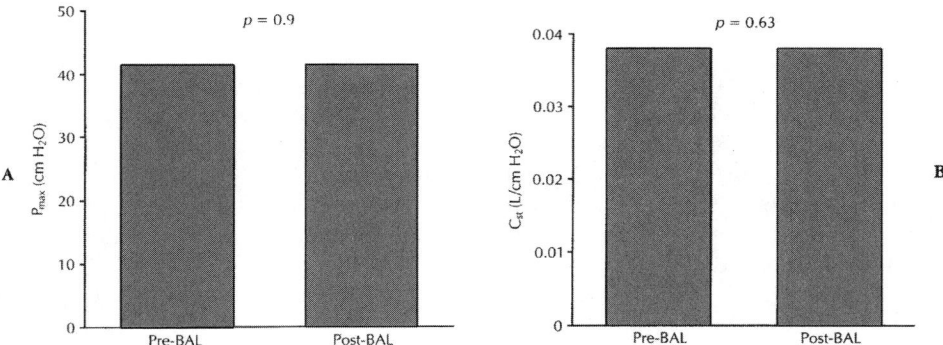

Figure 2 Variables reflecting lung mechanics before and after bronchoalveolar lavage. **A,** No significant change occured in maximal inspiratory airway pressure (P_{max}) after BAL (41.45 ± 2.98 cm H_2O pre-BAL vs. 41.58 ± 2.76 cm H_2O post-BAL; $p = 0.90$). **B,** No significant change occurred in static lung compliance (C_{st}) after BAL (0.0378 ± 0.004 L/cm H_2O pre-BAL vs. 0.0384 ± 0.004 L/cm H_2O post-BAL; $p = 0.63$).

compliance) showed no significant change after BAL (Fig. 2). Two variables reflecting the efficiency of arterial oxygenation were examined: the alveolar to arterial oxygen gradient (A-aDO_2) and the PaO_2 to FIO_2 ratio (PaO_2/FIO_2) (Fig. 3). For the patient group as a whole, no statistically significant change in these variables occured after BAL. However, 13 of 67 patients (19%) experienced widening of the A-aDO_2 by more than 100 mm Hg. On review of the medical charts, the deterioration seen in these patients could not have been predicted by assessment of readily available clinical characteristics, including sex, age, and number of days on the ventilator before BAL. Therefore, the oxygenation status of all patients must be carefully monitored after BAL to identify those who deteriorate after the procedure.

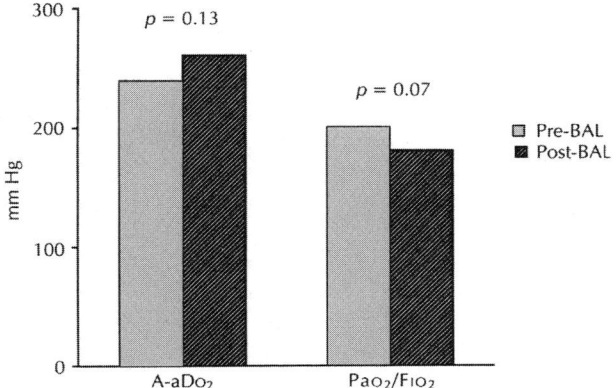

Figure 3 Comparison of A-aDO_2 and PaO_2/FIO_2 before and after BAL. No significant change occurred in A-aDO_2 (240.55 ± 36.68 mm Hg pre-BAL vs. 261.63 ± 31.29 mm Hg post-BAL; $p = 0.13$) or PaO_2/FIO_2 ratio (201.08 ± 26.49 pre-BAL vs. 180.77 ± 20.20 post-BAL; $p = 0.07$).

SUMMARY

- FFB allows direct visualization of central airways, biopsy of respiratory tract structures, and suctioning of bronchial secretions.
- FFB permits treatment of mucus plugging, hemoptysis, and foreign bodies.
- Indicators for FFB include suspected pneumonia, atelectasis, hemoptysis, presence of foreign bodies; suspected tracheobronchial disruption, smoke inhalation, and difficult intubation.
- FFB must not be performed in hemodynamically unstable patients, severely hypoxemic patients ($PaO_2 < 70$ mm Hg on FIO_2 of 1), or patients with severe metabolic disturbances.
- The use of diagnostic FFB should be considered when sputum culture fails to reveal a pathogen and for immunocompromised patients.

REFERENCES

1. Olopade CO, Prakash UBS. Bronchoscopy in the critical-care unit. Mayo Clin Proc 1989; 64:1255.
2. Saito H, Anaissie EJ, Morice RC, et al. Bronchoalveolar lavage in the diagnosis of pulmonary infiltrates in patients with acute leukemia. Chest 1988; 94:745.
3. Ognibene FP, Shelhamer J, Gill V, et al. The diagnosis of *Pneumocystis carinii* pneumonia in patients with the acquired immunodeficiency syndrome using subsegmental bronchoalveolar lavage. Am Rev Respir Dis 1984; 129:929.
4. Fulkerson WJ. Current concepts: fiberoptic bronchoscopy. N Engl J Med 1984; 311:511–516.
5. Chastre J, Fagon J-Y, Soler P, et al. Diagnosis of nosocomial bacterial pneumonia in intubated patients undergoing ventilation: comparison of the usefulness of bronchoalveolar lavage and the projected specimen brush. Am J Med 1988; 85:499.
6. Torres A, de la Bellacasa JP, Xaubet A, et al. Diagnostic value of quantitative cultures of bronchoalvelolar lavage and teleshopping plugged catheters in mechanically ventilated patients with bacterial pneumonia. Am Rev Respir Dis 1989; 140:306.
7. Kirilloff LF, Owens GR, Rogers RM, Mazzocco MC. Does chest physical therapy work? Chest 1985; 88:436.
8. Hood RM. Injury to the trachea and major bronchi. In: Hood RM, Boyd AD, Culliford AT, eds. Thoracic trauma. Philadelphia, PA: WB Saunders, 1989.
9. Baumann MH, Sahn SA. Techniques for managing bronchopleural fistuals: how to maximize ventilation and resolve fistulas medically. J Crit Illness 1990; 5:627.
10. Crapo RO. Smoke-inhalation injuries. J Am Med Assoc 1981; 246:1694.
11. Albertini RE, Harrell JH, Kurihara N, et al. Arterial hypoxemia induced by fiberoptic bronchoscopy. J Am Med Assoc 1974; 230:1666.
12. Karetsky MS, Garvey JW, Brandstetter RD. Effect of fiberoptic bronchoscopy of arterial oxygen tension. NY State J Med 1974; 1:62.
13. Hertz M, Woodward ME, Gross CR, Swart M, Marcy TW, Bitterman PB. Safety of bronchoalveolar lavage in the critically ill, mechanically ventilated patient. Crit Care Med 1991; 19:1526–1532.

56
Vascular Access

Thomas Wozniak
Cardiothoracic and Vascular Surgery, Indianapolis, Indiana, USA

Larry Micon[*]
Tower Surgical, Indianapolis, Indiana, USA

Access to the central venous and arterial circulation is frequently required in surgical patients. Numerous methods and routes for central venipuncture exist, each with inherent advantages and risks. The most frequently used sites are the subclavian, internal jugular, and femoral veins. Central venous access also may be achieved via the axillary, external jugular, and antecubital veins. Potential sites for arterial access include radial, femoral, dorsalis pedis, axillary, and brachial arteries. This chapter discusses the indications, contraindications, placement techniques, and complications of vascular access procedures.

CENTRAL VENOUS ACCESS
Indications for Catheterization

Indications for central venous catheterization can be grouped into four major categories: hemodynamic monitoring, fluid or medication infusion, parenteral nutrition, and other invasive maneuvers (see Box 1). Many SICU patients require careful assessment and ongoing monitoring of their circulation, aided by a pulmonary artery or central venous catheter. Some medications require central administration. Patients needing parenteral nutrition require central venous access.

A number of less commonly performed procedures, including hemodialysis, plasmapheresis, transvenous cardiac pacing, vena caval filter placement, and transvenous pulmonary embolectomy, necessitate central venipuncture. Once the need for such access is established, a consideration of available sites should follow.

Maintenance of a sterile field is essential. An adequate area including and surrounding the venipuncture location should be clipped or shaved, scrubbed with antiseptic, and isolated with sterile drapes. We use sterile gloves and sterile gowns. Institutions variably require masks, head and shoe covers, and protective eyewear. Sufficient personnel to aid in line placement should be present before beginning the procedure.

---

[*]Deceased. Dr. Micon's contributions to this chapter have been updated by Dr. Abrams.

Box 1 Indications for Central Venous Catheterization

Hemodynamic assessment
   Central venous pressure monitoring
   Pulmonary artery pressure monitoring
   Thermodilution cardiac output monitoring
Fluid or medication administration
   Intravenous fluid administration (when peripheral access is unavailable)
   Continuous vasoactive medication administration
   Administration of sclerosing medications (e.g., KCL, amphotericin B)
   Chronic medication administration and blood sampling (e.g., chemotherapy, opiates)
Parenteral nutrition
Other procedures
   Acute hemodialysis
   Plasmapheresis
   Transvenous cardiac pacing
   Diagnostic radiology
   Vena caval filter placement
   Transvenous pulmonary embolectomy

Source: From Micon LT. Internal jugular venous cannulation. Perspect Crit Care 1990; 3(2):75.

Subclavian Vein Catheterization

Successful cannulation of the subclavian vein occurs in over 95% of attempts. The only absolute contraindications to this approach is known preexisting thrombosis of the vessel. Relative contraindications are listed in Box 2.

Proper positioning of the patient is important to ensure successful venipuncture. The patient should be supine with the head turned to the contralateral side. The bed is then placed in the Trendelenburg (head-down) position to distend the upper central venous system. A rolled-up towel or sheet may be placed longitudinally between the scapulae to abduct the shoulders. After preparation and draping, the skin puncture site is anesthetized. The subcutaneous tissue and, most importantly, the periosteum of the clavicle are infiltrated with local anesthetic. The skin puncture site is placed 1 cm below the clavicle, at the point of maximal

Box 2 Contraindications to Subclavian Vein Catheterization

Absolute
   Thrombosed vessel
Relative
   Coagulopathy
   Transvenous pacemaker
   Axillary-femoral bypass
   Mastectomy
   Distal hemodialysis access
   Tenuous pulmonary reserve

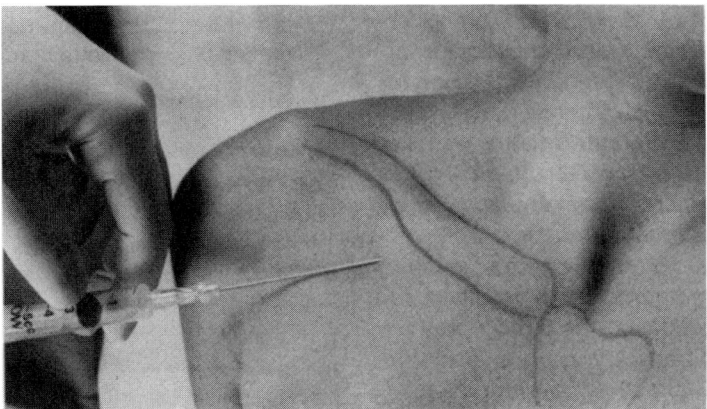

Figure 1 Infraclavicular approach to subclavian vein. Clavicle and manubrium are outlined.

"bend" as the clavicle passes laterally from the sternoclavicular joint (Fig. 1). This site is in proximity to the junction of the medial and middle thirds of the clavicle, which may also be used to identify an appropriate site. The needle is directed toward the sternal notch at approximately a 30° posterior angle to the skin until it contacts the clavicle. The needle should be "walked down" the clavicle by carefully redirecting the needle to a steeper angle of entry. As the needle passes under the clavicle, constant subatmospheric pressure is maintained on the attached syringe. Abrupt return of blood into the syringe signals successful venipuncture. To prevent an air embolus, a finger should be placed over the open end of the introducer needle when inserting the guidewire. Catheterization is then completed by passing first a guidewire, then the catheter into the vein. The catheter tip should come to rest in the superior vena cava, ~15 cm from a skin puncture on the right side or 17 cm from the left side in the average-size adult. Intravenous placement is confirmed by aspiration of blood from the catheter. The procedure is completed by securing the catheter with sutures and applying a sterile dressing. A CXR should be obtained promptly to verify appropriate positioning and to exclude a pneumothorax.

The most frequently encountered complications with subclavian venipuncture are pneumothorax, arterial puncture, and malpositioning of the catheter tip (1–6). Other less frequently encountered complications are listed in Box 3.

Box 3 Complications of Percutaneous Central Venous Catheterization

Pneumothorax	Subclavian artery pseudoaneurysm
Hemothorax	Vertebral artery pseudoaneurysm
Arterial puncture	Guidewire embolus
Chylothorax	Thoracic duct injury
Air embolus	Dysrhythmia
Catheter embolus	Cardiac tamponade
Brachial plexus injury	Thromboembolism
Horner's syndrome	Tracheal perforation
Catheter tip malposition	Right atrial perforation

Internal Jugular Approach

Internal Jugular vein cannulation is a second means of accessing central venous circulation. Absolute contraindications are known thrombosis or absence (from previous surgery) of the vessel. Relative contraindicates are few (see Box 4). Advantages of the internal jugular route include decreased likelihood of pneumothorax and only local hematoma (rather than hemothorax) should bleeding occur.

Proper positioning for internal jugular line placement includes rotation of the head away from the side of cannulation, and the Trendelenburg position. The neck is prepared with antiseptic and the field isolated with sterile drapes. The anterior and posterior borders of the sternal and clavicular heads of the sternocleidomastoid muscle are carefully delineated. Anterior, central, and posterior approaches to internal jugular venipuncture have been described. The right side is preferable, because the internal jugular and innominate veins are more directly aligned with the right atrium. In addition, the left side carries a greater risk of potential for thoracic duct injury.

In the anterior approach, the skin is punctured along the anterior border of the sternocleidomastoid muscle ~5 cm above the clavicle (Fig. 2). The needle is advanced toward the ipsilateral nipple with a 45° posterior angle to the skin. Suction is maintained on the attached syringe, and prompt venous return signals successful venipuncture. The guidewire and then the catheter are introduced. Intravascular placement is confirmed by aspiration of blood from the catheter.

The procedure is completed by securing the catheter with sutures and applying a sterile dressing. Correct catheter tip position is in the superior vena cava should be verified by CXR examination before use. The atriocaval junction is ~15 cm from a rightsided venipuncture in an average adult (slightly further from the left).

The central technique uses a puncture site at the apex of the triangle created by the sternal and clavicular heads of the sternocleidomastoid muscle and the clavicle (see Fig. 2). The needle is introduced at a 30–45° posterior angle to the skin and directed toward the ipsilateral nipple. The posterior technique is performed by inserting the needle along the posterior border of the sternocleidomastoid muscle, 5 cm above the clavicle, and directing the needle toward the suprasternal notch (see Fig. 2). Similar success rates (~85%) will be achieved for all three methods.

Complications of internal jugular catheterization are similar to subclavian line placement (7). Pneumothorax is still possible but should occur less frequently with the internal jugular approach. Arterial puncture and catheter tip malpositioning occur with similar frequency. The less common complications listed in Box 3 apply to both routes. Hemothorax and hydrothorax should occur less frequency with internal jugular lines (8).

Box 4 Contraindications to Internal Jugular Vein Catheterization

Absolute
  Thrombosed vessel
  Surgical absence of vessel
Relative
  Coagulopathy
  Carotid-subclavian artery bypass

Vascular Access

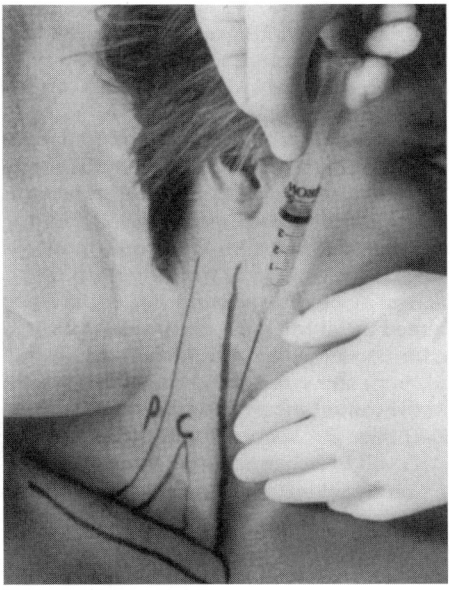

Figure 2 Anterior approach to internal jugular vein. Sternocleidomastoid muscle and clavicle are outlined. Central (C) and posterior (P) puncture sites are shown.

Horner's syndrome resulting from stellate ganglion injury or compression and phrenic nerve paralysis have been reported after catheterization (9).

Femoral Vein Cannulation

The femoral vein is another commonly used portal to the central venous circulation. Femoral vein cannulation may be necessary if the other sites are thrombosed, already cannulated, or difficult to access, as during closed cardiac massage.

The technique for femoral vein cannulation relies on the ability to palpate the femoral artery just below the inguinal ligament. The site of venipuncture is then just medial to the physician's fingers on the femoral artery.

After infiltration of the skin and deeper tissues with local anesthetic at the selected site, the needle is introduced at approximately a 30° posterior angle to the skin (Fig. 3). Suction is maintained on the attached syringe. Successful venipuncture is indicated by prompt return of venous blood. A guidewire is passed into the femoral vein. The catheter is then fully inserted (20 cm) and sutured in place.

Femoral line placement does not entail many of the hazards associated with subclavian or internal jugular venipuncture, such as pneumothorax or hemothorax. It still, however, carries risks of arterial puncture, nerve injury, and catheter or guidewire embolus.

A common belief is that femoral lines are at higher risk for line-related sepsis. However, with careful preparation, strict sterile insertion technique, and proper line care, the infection rate is acceptable and, in many studies, is no higher than for other routes of central venous access (10,11). The main drawback to femoral catheters is that of impaired mobility in otherwise ambulatory patients.

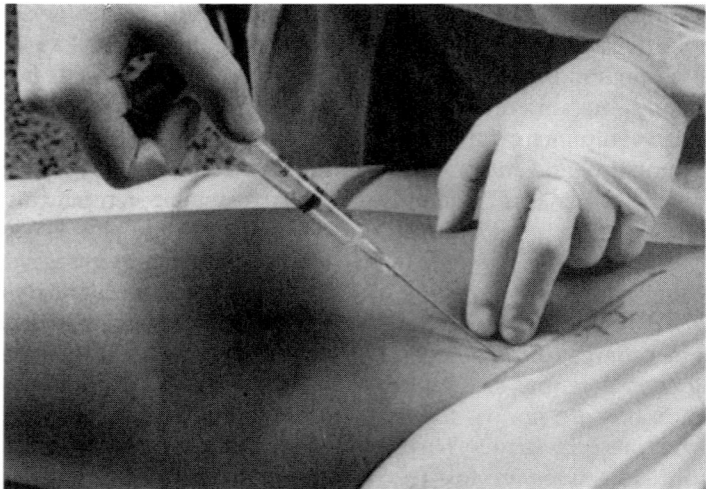

Figure 3 Femoral vein cannulation. Femoral artery (physician's fingers) and vein (introducer needle) are outlined. IL, inguinal ligament.

PULMONARY ARTERIAL ACCESS

Catheterization of the right side of the heart has allowed a window through which the clinician can objectively monitor the balance of oxygen supply and demand over time (12,13). Chapters 2 and 61 discuss use of oxygen transport variables and the controversies surrounding this approach to critically ill patients. Patients with complicated illnesses may be significantly aided by PA catheter monitoring. Examples include patients with impaired cardiac function after myocardial infarction or valvular disease, patients with hyperlacticacidemia during critical illness, and patients requiring high levels of positive end expiratory pressure for the treatment of respiratory failure. The differentiation of cardiogenic from noncardiogenic pulmonary edema may require PA measurements.

A unique relative contraindication to PA catheter placement is a preexisting left bundle branch block (LBBB). The development of a new right bundle branch block (RBBB) has been described with PA catheterization, and in patients with an existing LBBB, complete heart block can result. Although it is a potentially hazardous complication, the incidence of complete heart block is low. Nonetheless, external or transvenous cardiac pacing should be ready before attempting right-side heart catheterization (14).

Technique

PA catheters are passed through introducer sheaths placed in a central vein (usually the subclavian or internal jugular vein) using the methods previously described. Once the sheath has been sutured in place, the PA catheter is brought into the sterile field and calibrated at the patient's fourth intercostal space in the mid-axillary line (15,16). The balloon is tested, and if an eccentric (asymmetric) balloon is noted, a new catheter should be used. Eccentric balloon tips have a higher incidence of PA perforation. The catheter is threaded through the introducer sheath to a distance of 20 cm, and the balloon is inflated.

Vascular Access

To decrease the risk of atrial, ventricular, or PA perforation, the catheter should not be advanced without the balloon inflated. The catheter should never be withdrawn with the balloon inflated. The catheter is then advanced or "floated" through the right side of the heart into the pulmonary artery with the aid of waveform monitoring. Fluoroscopy may occasionally be necessary in cases of anomalous venous anatomy or low output states. As the catheter tip passes through the right atrium, right ventricle, and pulmonary artery and ultimately into the wedge position, the monitor displays the respective pressures. A characteristic waveform is illustrated in Fig. 4. The normal right-sided heart pressures (mm Hg) for each location are:

- Right atrium, 0–8
- Right ventricle, 20–30/0–7
- Pulmonary artery, 15–30/5–15
- Pulmonary capillary wedge, 5–12

The approximate distances (cm) from the insertion site to each location are:

- Right atrium, 20
- Right ventricle, 30–40
- Pulmonary capillary wedge, 45–60

Once the catheter is "wedged," the balloon is deflated to display the PA waveform. If a "wedge" waveform persists, the catheter has been advanced too far and should be withdrawn (with the balloon deflated) until a PA waveform is observed.

Complications

The complications associated with PA catheter placement may be considered the same as those from accessing the central venous circulation and those unique to the longer, balloon-tipped device. The former have already been discussed in this chapter. Other complications directly related to PA catheterization are listed in Box 5. Preexisting LBBB entails a risk of complete heart block and necessitates immediate availability of cardiac pacing. Ventricular dysrhythmias are common but only occasionally require treatment. Patients with preexisting ventricular dysrhythmia may be given prophylactic lidocaine.

Puncture of the right ventricle can occur if the catheter tip lodges in the trabeculae during insertion. The resulting cardiac tamponade is indicated by PA catheter readings. Prompt evacuation of the pericardial sac and surgical closure of the puncture are required for successful management.

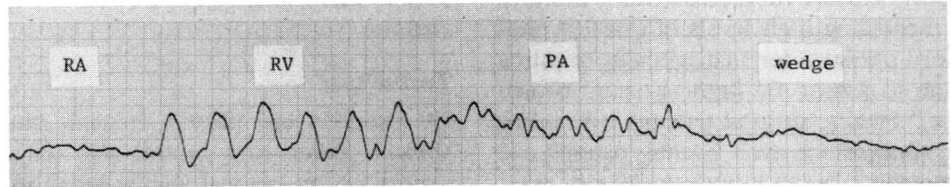

Figure 4 Actual PA catheter waveform as balloon tip passes from right atrium to wedge position in pulmonary vasculature. Note differences in right atrial (RA), right ventricular (RV), pulmonary artery (PA), and wedge waveforms.

Box 5 Complications of PA Catheterization

Complications of central venipuncture
Complications unique to PA catheter
Dysrhythmia
Heart block
Catheter knotting
Catheter tip malposition
Cardiac tamponade
Valvular injury
PA perforation
Pulmonary infarction

Source: Data from Horst MH, et al. The risks of pulmonary arterial catheterization. Surg Gynecol Obset 1984; 159:229–232; Elliot C, et al. Complications of pulmonary artery catheterization in the care of critically ill patients. Chest 1979; 76:647–652.

Pulmonary infarction results from excessively distal placement or migration of the catheter tip and can be recognized by bloody sputum, changes in oxygenation, or a wedge-shaped deformity on chest X-ray examination. PA perforation can be recognized by the abrupt onset of hemoptysis or suctioning of blood from the lungs. It can be caused by migration of the tip, overinflation of the balloon, or the use of an eccentric balloon (17–19). The catheter should be pulled back immediately and the balloon reinflated; if the hemorrhage does not subside, prompt surgical therapy may be required.

Cardiac valvular injury is rare but results from traumatic passage or withdrawal of the catheter through the pulmonic or tricuspid valve with the balloon inflated. Intracardiac knotting is likewise rare and usually occurs during insertion. Manipulation under fluoroscopy, occasionally with a guidewire, may resolve the problem. If not, surgical cutdown is necessary for withdrawal.

"Wedge" Pressure Interpretation

The pulmonary capillary wedge pressure (PCWP) is used to estimate left ventricular preload. A fundamental assumption is that PCWP, left atrial pressure (LAP), and left ventricular end-diastolic pressure (LVEDP) are equivalent and accurately reflect left ventricular end-diastolic volume (LVEDV), the most reliable clinical measure of the left ventricular preload.

Circumstances in which these assumptions are not true are relatively common and make accurate interpretation of the wedge pressure difficult. The wedge pressure will not correlate with the LAP if the catheter is malpositioned or the monitoring system is not properly calibrated, contains air bubbles, or is excessively affected by overdamping or underdamping (20,21). Other situations in which pulmonary artery diastolic (PAD) pressure may not equal PCWP include chronic obstructive pulmonary disease, increased pulmonary arteriolar resistance, a heart rate >125 beats/min, wedge position other than a zone III portion of the lung, increased pulmonary interstitial pressure, and constriction of pulmonary veins. In addition, overwedging or an eccentric balloon may affect the accuracy with which the PCWP correlates with the LAP (22).

The PCWP and the LAP may not reflect the LVEDP in instances of aortic or mitral valvular disease or altered left ventricular compliance. Finally, the relationship between LVEDP and LVEDV may be distorted. Alterations of pericardial pressure, right ventricle volume, and ventricular stiffness have significant influence on the pressure–volume relationship of the left ventricle (23).

Thus a measure of clinical expertise is required to assess the accuracy of the PCWP value and to interpret its clinical significance. In combination with other data obtained from the PA catheter (e.g., cardiac output, oxygen delivery, and oxygen consumption), the wedge pressure provides essential information about the hemodynamic state of a critically ill patient.

SYSTEMIC ARTERIAL CATHETERIZATION

Indications for arterial catheterization include continuous blood pressure monitoring, frequent sampling of blood, especially for arterial blood gas determination, and blood pressure monitoring of patients in shock when indirect methods are unreliable. The usual sites of catheterization in order of preference are the (1) radial, (2) dorsalis pedis, (3) femoral, and (4) axillary arteries. Note that brachial artery lines are rarely used. In some patients, a brachial arterial line may cause ischemic injury to the hand and resulting loss of tissue and function. Patients at risk include those with small-vessel disease of the upper extremity, such as those with diabetes mellitus.

The radial artery is the most commonly cannulated artery and consequently the most familiar. It is in a superficial location, which makes it easier to cannulate. The ulnar artery usually provides abundant collateral circulation. The modified Allen's test is designed to assess the collateral circulation of the hand and should be done on all patients before insertion of a radial artery catheter. Patients elevate their hand, and the examiner occludes both the radial and ulnar arteries. The patient is asked to make a fist to empty the hand of blood. The hand is lowered and opened. The wrist should not be hyperextended to prevent a false positive interpretation. Pressure over the ulnar artery is then released and the time to return of flush to the hand noted. The flush should occur in fewer than 6 sec. Both ulnar and radial arteries should be tested. Doppler flow studies should be added in cases of questionable flow (24).

Some problems exist with radial catheterization. Catheter malfunction, which occurs in 13–38% of the cases, may be related to the length and caliber of the catheter (25). Arterial flow can be obstructed and again relates to catheter size. Ischemia and tissue loss occur far less frequently than thrombosis (26). Inaccurate blood pressure readings may be produced when vessels lose elasticity or are involved with atherosclerosis. Additional information about arterial blood pressure measurement is found in Chapter 60.

Dorsalis Pedis Artery

Like the hand, the foot has good collateral circulation. In the foot, collateral blood flow arises from the posterior tibial artery. A similar test of collateral flow can be performed. The dorsalis pedis and the posterior tibial arteries are occluded, producing blanching in the great toe. The posterior tribal artery is released and flow should return to the toe within 5 s.

Again blood pressure accuracy may be a problem in the face of atherosclerotic vascular disease This artery is congenitally absent in 12% of the population (26).

Femoral Artery

The femoral artery is often the only palpable pulse in a patient with shock. Larger vessels have a lower incidence of thrombosis and embolism. The femoral artery provides reliable blood pressure monitoring. Care should be exercised when using this vessel in patients with peripheral vascular disease. The overall catheter complication rate for this location is 8% (27).

Axillary Artery

As with the femoral artery, the axillary artery is a large blood vessel that has a lower incidence of thrombosis and provides reliable blood pressure monitoring. It is deeper, however, and therefore more difficult to cannulate. If the right side is chosen, a risk of air embolus to the cerebral circulation exists (28).

Brachial Artery

The brachial artery is often easier to palpate than the radial artery. It does not have collateral circulation, so thrombosis or embolization results in greater ischemia and tissue loss. Safe short-term use has been documented, but this artery is not recommended if other sites are available (29).

Technique

1. The skin of the chosen site is cleansed with antiseptic solution and a sterile field prepared.
2. Sterile gloves are worn and the pulse palpated. The areas overlying and on either side of the artery are infiltrated with 1% lidocaine.
3. For small vessels a 20 gauge catheter should be used. Larger vessels will accommodate an 18- or 16 gauge catheter.
4. If the radial site is chosen, the wrist should be hyperextended with the thumb abducted. If the dorsalis pedis artery is chosen, the ankle should be plantarflexed as much as possible. When the axillary artery is chosen, the arm is abducted and the elbow flexed.
5. The artery is punctured at an approximately 45° angle. When blood return is observed, the needle is inserted a few millimeters farther. The guidewire is then passed through the needle into the artery. The needle is removed carefully to prevent dislodging the guidewire from the cannulated artery. The catheter is then carefully advanced into the vessel over the guidewire. The guidewire is removed and free return of blood is noted. The catheter can be capped to prevent further spillage of blood. The catheter is secured with 2-0 or 3-0 suture, and the transducer is connected.

Complications

1. *Thrombosis.* The incidence of thrombosis is increased with multiple arterial punctures, atherosclerosis, increased duration of catheterization, and low cardiac output. Catheters larger than 20 gauge and those made of polypropylene have a higher incidence of thrombosis. Catheters left longer than 4 days have a

higher incidence of thrombosis. Rates vary from 11% to 29% (30). Distal embolization may occur and produces ischemic necrosis. Examination of the patient for blanching when the artery is flushed may identify patients at risk and allow intervention before thrombosis.
2. *Infection.* The risk of infection is increased for catheters left longer than 4 days. There may be no local signs of inflammation. The reported incidence of infection is 1–2% (31).
3. *Other complications.* Neuropathies secondary to prolonged hyperextension, median nerve injury, or hematomas around the brachial artery are other complications of arterial catheterization. Pseudoaneurysms can occur in any location.

Doppler-Guided Catheterization

A needle is now available that contains an internal Doppler probe. This device can be helpful in patients who have poorly palpable pulses (edematous patients or patients who have had multiple catheters). Once the vessel has been located with needle and probe, the probe is withdrawn, a wire is inserted, and a catheter is threaded over the wire.

SUMMARY

- Use central venous catheterization for hemodynamic monitoring, fluid or medication infusion, parenteral nutrition, acute hemodialysis, plasmapheresis, transvenous cardiac pacing, and vena caval filter placement.
- Strict sterile technique of insertion reduces incidence of catheter infection.
- Common access sites include the subclavian, internal jugular, and femoral veins. Similar complications occur for subclavian and internal jugular approaches. With proper line care, femoral catheterization does not have a higher infection rate.
- When placing a PA catheter in patients with LBBB, have external or transvenous cardiac pacing device ready.
- Use arterial catheterization for continuous blood pressure monitoring, frequent sampling of ABGs, monitoring for patients in shock, and when other methods are unreliable.
- Arterial cannulation sites in order of preference are radial, dorsalis pedis, femoral, and axillary.
- Perform Allen's test before attempting radial artery cannulation.

REFERENCES

1. Feliciano DV, Mattox KL, Graham JM, et al. Major complications of percutaneous subclavian vein catheters. Am J Surg 1979; 138:869–874.
2. Edwards H, King T. Cardiac tamponade from central venous catheters. Arch Surg 1982; 117:965–967.

3. Maschke S, Rogove H. Cardiac tamponade associated with a multilumen central venous catheter. Crit Care Med 1984; 12:611–613.
4. Conces D, Holden R. Aberrant locations and complications in initial placement of subclavian vein catheters. Arch Surg 1984; 119:293–295.
5. Zavall J, Taha A, Thomford N. Cardiac tamponade from central venous catheterization. Hosp Phys 1989; 25(12):16–19.
6. Amaral JF, Grigoriev VE, Dorfman GS, et al. Vertebral artery pseudoaneurysm. A rare complication of subclavian artery catheterization. Arch Surg 1990; 125:546–547.
7. Krespi YP, Komisar A, Lucente FE. Complications of internal jugular vein catheterization. Arch Otolaryngol 1981; 107:310–312.
8. Khalil KG, parker FB Jr, Mukherjee N, et al. Thoracic duct injury: a complication of internal jugular vein catheterization. J Am Med Assoc 1972; 221:908–909.
9. Parikh RK. Horner's syndrome. A complication of percutaneous catheterization of the internal jugular vein. Anesthesia 1972; 27:327–329.
10. Williams JF, Seneff MG, Friedman BC, et al. Use of femoral venous catheters in critically ill adults: Prospective study. Crit Care Med 1991; 19:550–553.
11. Getzen LC, Pollak EW. Short-term femoral vein catheterization: a safe alternative venous access? Am J Surg 1979; 138:875–878.
12. Nelson LD. Continuous venous oximetry in surgical patients. Ann Surg 1986; 20:329–333.
13. Vaughn S, Puri V. Cardiac output changes and continuous mixed venous oxygen saturation measurement in the critically ill. Crit Care Med 1988; 16:495–498.
14. Sprung CL, Elser B, Schein RM, et al. Risk of right bundle-branch block and complete heart block during pulmonary artery catheterization. Crit Care Med 1989; 17:1–3.
15. Amin DK, Shah PK, Swan HJC. The Swan-Ganz catheter: tips on interpreting results. J Crit Ill 1986; 1(4): 24–25.
16. Swan HBL, Shah PK. The rationale for bedside hemodynamic monitoring. J Crit Ill 1989; 1(5):40–61.
17. Khan AH, Taha AM, Thomford NR, et al. Perforation of the pulmonary artery secondary to Swan–Gnaz catheters. Contemp Surg 1989; 34:53–56.
18. Barash PG, Nardi D, Hammond G, et al. Catheter-induced pulmonary artery perforation. Mechanisms, management, and modifications. J Thorac Cardiovasc Surg 1981; 82:5–12.
19. Pape LA, Nardi D, Hammond G, et al. Fatal pulmonary hemorrhage after use of the flow-directed balloon-tipped catheter. Ann Intern Med 1979; 90:344–347.
20. Raper R, Sibbald WJ. Misled by the wedge? The Swan–Ganz catheter and left ventricular preload. Chest 1986; 89:427–434.
21. Abrams JH, Olson ML, Marino JA, et al. Use of a needle valve variable resistor to improve invasive blood pressure monitoring. Crit Care Med 1984; 12:978–982.
22. Calvin JE, Driedger AA, Sibbald WJ. Does the pulmonary capillary wedge pressure predict left ventricular preload in critically ill patients? Crit Care Med 1981; 9:437–443.
23. Rajacich N, Burchard KW, Hasan FM, et al. Central venous pressure and pulmonary capillary wedge pressure as estimates of left artrial pressure: effects of positive end-expiratory pressure and catheter tip malposition. Crit Care Med 1989; 17:7–11.
24. Ejrup B, Fischer B, Wright IS, et al. Clinical evaluation of blood flow to the hand: the false positive Allen test. Circulation 1966; 33:778–780.
25. Weis BM, Gattiker RI. Complications during and following radial artery cannulation: a prospective study. Intensive Care Med 1986; 12:424–428.
26. Clark CA, Harman EM. Hemodynamic monitoring: Arterial catheters. In: Taylor RW, Civetta JM, Kirby RR, eds. Techniques and Procedures in Critical Care. Philadelphia, PA: JB Lippincott, 1990:218–231.
27. Gurman GM, Kriermerman S. Cannulation of big arteries in critically ill patients. Crit Care Med 1985; 13:217–220.

28. Bryan-Brown CW, Kwun KB, Lumb PD, et al. The axillary artery catheter. Heart Lung 1983; 12:492–497.
29. Barnes RW, Foster EJ, Janssen GA, et al. Safety of brachial artery catheters as monitors in the intensive care unit—prospective evaluation with the Doppler ultrasonic velocity detector. Anesthesiology 1976; 44:260–264.
30. Sladen A. Compilations of invasive hemodynamic monitoring in the intensive care unit. Curr Probl Surg 1988; 25(2):75–145.
31. Band JD, Maki DG. Infections caused by arterial catheters used for hemodynamic monitoring. Am J Med 1979; 67:735–741.

57
Care of Central Lines

Steven D. Eyer
St. Mary's Medical Center, Duluth, Minnesota, USA

Central lines are important in the management of many surgical patients. They reduce patient discomfort and interventions when long-term or multiple IV access is needed. They are essential for hemodynamic monitoring, parenteral nutrition, and acute dialysis. Two principal complications of their use relating to line care are thrombosis and infection. The purpose of this chapter is to provide an understanding of and to prevent central line thrombosis, colonization, and sepsis.

CATHETER-RELATED SEPSIS

Incidence

The incidence of infectious complication from central lines varies with patient population. It is near 0% in nonstressed patients requiring central catheters for <72 h, 1.5–5% in mixed SICU patients, 3–15% in various parenteral nutrition groups, and as high as 23% in patients receiving parenteral nutrition in bone-marrow transplant units. Because catheters are used so frequently, catheter-related sepsis affects thousands of patients annually and increases their morbidity, length of stay, and hospital costs.

Causes

The accepted causes of catheter infection are multiple. Implicated causes are infusate contamination, endogenous seeding, hub colonization with internal migration down the catheter, and skin colonization with external migration to the subcutaneous tract followed by migration down the catheter. Infusate contamination is uncommon and of such small inoculum that when it does occur, it rarely produces clinical infection. It is least likely to occur when IV medications are formulated by pharmacists under sterile conditions and in laminar flow hoods. To minimize this complication, parenteral nutrition formulas should be prepared under similar conditions and discarded after 24 h.

Endogenous infection preceding catheter colonization or sepsis is of particular concern in surgical patients with complications. A distant abscess or recurrent isolation of a sputum pathogen from a patient with pneumonia may be followed by bacteremia and secondary growth on the catheter. Although unsupported by data, a reasonable assumption is that patients with recurrent bacteremia from other sources are at higher risk for catheter colonization and sepsis.

Hub colonization has been well documented. This source is correlated to the number of infusions through the hub for multiple interventions and poor adherence to aseptic technique. The importance of swabbing hubs before disconnecting and reconnecting cannot be overemphasized.

The skin site is the most common source of catheter colonization in nearly all study populations reported, and *Staphylococcus epidermidis* is the most common organism. Antiseptic skin preparation at the time of line placement, use of antibiotic ointment or an antibiotic or antiseptic-impregnated cuff or catheter, provision of an antiseptic dressing change every 48 h, and prompt line removal when skin site infection is suspected are clinically important aspects of care. Infrequent catheter manipulation may minimize subcutaneous tract colonization.

A number of factors have been recognized that affect the incidence of catheter-related sepsis including aseptic technique, frequent line manipulations, number of lumens, insertion site, catheter longevity, severity of underlying disease, repeated catheterizations, presence of an infection elsewhere, absence of antimicrobial therapy, bacteremia, type of catheter material used, and physician experience. Frequency of line manipulations and use of multilumen catheters are factors associated with the severity of underlying disease and need for interventions.

Triple-lumen catheters clearly are more likely to become colonized and develop subsequent sepsis than single-lumen central lines, but less clear is whether this observation is a result of increased portals of entry, manipulations, or patient illness. Nonrandomized studies suggest less infection risk for subclavian catheters than for internal jugular catheters. This reduction in risk must be balanced by a higher risk of mechanical complications with subclavian insertions. Use of bedside ultrasound to assist placement reduces the incidence of mechanical complications and may favor subclavian placement.

Although steel is the least infection-prone material, it is impractical for central line construction. Many other synthetic catheters are available for clinical use. Although there are differences among nonsteel catheters, thrombus and fibrin sheath formation commonly occur with all synthetic catheters including Teflon, silicone, polyurethane, and polyvinyl chloride. The perfect material is still being sought. Physician experience is more important with regard to mechanical complications than to infections. Catheter sepsis rates are directly related to catheter longevity but not to frequency of catheter changes. Careful consideration should be given before placing central lines, and reconsideration of their continued use should be made on a daily basis. Pulmonary artery catheters and dialysis access catheters have the highest risk of colonization and sepsis. They should be removed at the earliest possible time when no longer needed. Pulmonary artery catheter sepsis is particularly hazardous, because increased risk exists for endocarditis of the right side of the heart and for pulmonary arteritis. Maintenance of stringent asepsis is the most important and the easiest way of reducing risk of infection.

ASEPTIC TECHNIQUE

An institutional infection control program with policy and procedure and surveillance for nosocomial infections is the single most effective means of decreasing catheter-related blood stream infection. All central lines should be placed under strict aseptic technique.

The operator should wear a mask, sterile gown, and sterile gloves. The placement site should be widely prepared with an antiseptic (povidone-iodine or chlorhexidine) scrub and solution. In randomized studies, 2% chlorhexidine is the superior agent. The use of large sterile drapes minimizes catheter contamination during placement. A full-time nurse epidemiologist, central line team, or monitoring service should supervise all catheter placements. This surveillance not only helps ensure preparation according to protocol and adherence to sterile technique, but is of proven effectiveness in reducing catheter sepsis. Because sepsis is less stringent under emergency conditions, lines placed for emergency resuscitation should be replaced electively by guidewire exchange as soon as patient stability permits.

Adherence to aseptic principles extends the life of a catheter. Infection-free use of the central catheter requires protocols for catheter care. Occlusive dressings and IV tubing should be changed routinely; change in less than 72 hours is recommended. Soiled dressings should be changed immediately. Gloves are used to remove old dressings. The skin puncture site is inspected for local infection. If no local skin infection is present, the nurse should sterilely reglove, apply antiseptic solution to the skin site and catheter; cleanse, disconnect, and swab the hub with antiseptic solution, and perform the tubing change. Antiseptic ointment may be applied to the line entrance site, and a new sterile occlusive dressing is placed. Any suspected skin-site infection is called to the attention of the responsible physician. Injection sites are swabbed with an antiseptic before use. Hyperalimentation should be administered only through dedicated catheter ports.

Antibiotic prophylaxis is of no proven benefit. Though IV vancomycin has been shown to reduce the incidence of catheter sepsis, it does so at the cost of increased antimicrobial resistance and hence is not recommended. Antibiotic-impregnated cuffs can reduce catheter sepsis rates by preventing cutaneous migration of bacteria. Antiseptic hubs can prevent intraluminal bacterial migration. Antibiotic- or antiseptic-impregnated catheters on internal and external surfaces decrease migration by both routes. The use of above-mentioned devices may not be necessary to decrease infection complications. In my experience, overgrowth of bacteria on skin is not a significant problem with good skin site aseptic protocols. Antibiotic- and antiseptic-impregnated catheters offer significant promise. For optimum effect, both internal and external surfaces should be impregnated. Potential disadvantages of antibiotic-impregnated catheters include emergence of antibiotic resistant organisms and interference with catheter *in vitro* culture. Rare cases of anaphylaxis have been reported.

The site of percutaneous puncture is considered infected if purulent drainage from the site, expanding erythema and cellulitis (tenderness and edema), or erythema and a positive qualitative skin culture from a moist swab of the site after 24 h are present. The nursing staff should contact the physician if a skin-site infection is suspected. In all cases, a saline solution moistened sterile swab is applied onto the site using sterile gloves. With purulence or cellulitis, the catheter should be removed and replaced at a new site by percutaneous technique. For erythema alone, the catheter may be left in place. If after 24 h the skin culture is positive, the catheter should be removed and a new line placed at a different site.

CATHETER REMOVAL OR EXCHANGE

Central Venous Catheters

Central venous catheters and the surrounding skin should be prepared thoroughly with antiseptic scrub and solution. The patient should be supine. This preparation should include all aspects of catheter system within the draped sterile field, including the entire catheter, the hub, and a portion of the attached IV tubing, if necessary. The field is defined with sterile drapes, and the tubing is disconnected and the hub wiped with an antiseptic solution. If desired, a drawback blood culture may be obtained. If the line is to be exchanged, the central venous line is cut into two with sterile scissors and the dominant lumen of the indwelling cut catheter is threaded with a sterile guidewire. The catheter is then removed and suspended by its tip with sterile forceps. The distal 3 cm is cut with a second sterile scissors, placed into a sterile cup properly labeled, and submitted for semiquantitative culture. If a tunnel segment is also desired, the originally suspended line, once withdrawn, is cut 0.5 cm distal to the junction of antiseptic staining (brown) and catheter slime (clear). With sterile scissors, 3-cm segments are cut from the tunnel and catheter-tip ends, placed into sterile containers, labeled appropriately (catheter tip or catheter tunnel), and sent immediately to the microbiology laboratory for culture. Some centers prefer one culture site over the other, but both sites are not always synchronously involved in documented catheter sepsis. Culturing only tips is recommended. Concomitant tunnel cultures increase the positive culture yield only slightly but at a considerable increase in expense. If there is no clinical suspicion of catheter infection and that another line will not be exchanged through the guidewire at the same site, culture of the catheter is not necessary.

Pulmonary Artery Catheters

Pulmonary artery catheters must be managed in a different manner. Because of their length and attached contamination shield, the latter must be disconnected and retracted and a sufficient length of exposed catheter prepared with antiseptic scrub and solution. Specific attention should be paid to antiseptic preparation of the introducer valve where the pulmonary artery catheter enters with the patient supine. The catheter is withdrawn to 10-cm distance marker and grasped firmly to prevent whipping while it is completely withdrawn. Cutting the catheter into two facilitates its handling; the tip is then cut as for a central venous line. Pulmonary artery catheters are inserted through introducers. If a tunnel segment is desired, it should be taken from the introducer on its subsequent removal and not from the pulmonary artery catheter. When pulmonary artery catheters are exchanged for central lines, the pulmonary artery catheter is removed and the introducer is threaded with a guidewire before its removal.

Samples for Culture

Catheter samples for culture should be transferred to the microbiology laboratory as quickly as possible. The catheters are first rolled onto blood and chocolate agar plates in four quadrants. Sonication increases positive culture results. The plates are incubated at 35°C in 5% carbon dioxide and are examined at 24 and 48 h. Positive cultures are reported when more than 15 colony-forming units are detected during this period of time.

Replacement of Lines

Central lines should be removed at the earliest possible time they are no longer needed. Multiple studies have demonstrated no utility to a frequent line replacement strategy. Lines should remain in place until they are no longer needed or a clear indication exists for line change. A no change policy decreases costs, mechanical complications, and line colonization. Guidewire exchange of central lines is controversial when catheter sepsis is suspected.

Clinical Reasons for Replacement

Catheters do require changing under certain clinical circumstances (Box 1). Lines should be removed and replaced at a new site in the presence of skin-site infection. The site is considered infected if purulent drainage from the site or expanding erythema and cellulitis (tenderness and edema) are present. For erythema alone, any positive qualitative skin culture from a moist swab of the site should be considered infected. Lines placed under emergency conditions for the purpose of resuscitation should be replaced under strict aseptic conditions once the patient is stable and time allows. Less stringent attention is paid to sterile technique when placing vascular catheters under emergency conditions. Leaking, malpositioned, and thrombosed catheters usually must be replaced, although thrombolytic infusion may be useful in some cases of catheter thrombosis.

If the ports of a triple-lumen catheter or pulmonary artery catheter are needed for patient care, discontinuing or adding a pulmonary artery catheter requires either changing one for the other (interconversion) or adding an extra catheter. Interconversion is preferred for reduction in mechanical and infectious risks.

Positive blood cultures necessitate central line changes. Because the positive blood culture could be secondary to a catheter source, removal of the catheter is the only way to determine catheter sepsis (positive blood culture and catheter segment culture with the same organism). All indwelling venous and arterial lines should be changed and sent for culture, the only exception being lines that have changed in the interval between the time of obtaining the blood specimen that now demonstrates organisms and its reporting.

Hyperalimentation should be administered through dedicated lumens not previously used for other purposes. No medications should be administered through this lumen, nor should blood be drawn from it. When central lines are placed and hyperalimentation is

Box 1   Catheter Management Guidelines

- Lines will be left in place and not changed unless otherwise indicated.
- Lines will be changed by guidewire exchange for the following:
  1. All central lines placed under emergency conditions within 24 h of admission to the SICU
  2. Line malfunction
  3. Central lines exchanged for pulmonary artery catheters and vice versa
  4. Any positive blood culture obtained since the line was last changed
  5. For a septic clinical pattern when there is no other likely source of sepsis
  6. To provide an unused port for delivery of hyperalimentation.
- Lines will be removed and replaced at a new site when:
  1. Skin-site infection is determined by the following criteria:
     a. Purulent drainage at the skin puncture site (culture site)
     b. Cellulitis (erythema, tenderness, and edema) at the skin puncture site (culture site)
     c. Erythema at the skin puncture site and a skin organism at 24 h by qualitative culture.
  2. A guidewire exchanged catheter culture returns positive (catheter colonization).

anticipated, a port should be capped and labeled "for total parenteral nutrition (TPN) only."

Although all patients with a fever do not have line sepsis, an appropriate strategy is catheter replacement to rule out a catheter source for any septic clinical pattern when no other obvious cause is identified. However, the patient with an isolated head injury who has a persistent high fever and extensive but nondiagnostic evaluation for infection, including line change and culture, does not need repeated line changes. Similarly, the newly septic patient with clinical and X-ray film evidence of acute pneumonia does not need line change and culture unless the process does not respond to appropriate therapy.

Guidewire Exchange

When catheters do require change, available data are less clear on the practice of guidewire exchange. The advantages of this practice include minimal placement complications, ease, and patient comfort. Guidewire exchange can be considered for central lines placed under emergency conditions; for catheter malfunction, thrombosis or leaking; for interconversion with pulmonary artery catheters; for positive blood cultures since the line was last changed; for a septic clinical pattern when there is no likely source; to provide an unused port for hyperalimentation. Microorganisms can reside in the subcutaneous portion of the catheter tract, and guidewire exchange of culture-positive catheters has the theoretic disadvantage of transferring microbes to the new catheter and increasing the risk of sepsis. Culture-negative guidewire exchange can be repeated indefinitely. My practice currently is to remove guidewire exchanged lines when the prior catheter culture returns positive (catheter colonization).

CATHETER-RELATED THROMBOSIS

Catheter-related thrombosis has been studied far less than catheter infection. Indwelling catheters develop a thrombus sheath within hours of their placement. Heparin bonding effectively averts this problem for at least 15–30 h but at an increased cost. At this time, no prospective, randomized data on the effectiveness of heparin flushing of central lines in preventing line thrombosis exists, although unpublished data on radial artery lines suggest this practice might be helpful. Peripheral lines used for 48–72 h have equal patency rates with heparin and saline solution flushes. Until more convincing evidence is available, saline solution flushing of central lines is currently recommended to avoid the problem of heparin antibody-induced thrombocytopenia.

SUMMARY

- Major complication of central venous catheter use are thrombosis and infection.
- Sources of catheter infections include skin colonization with migration of organisms to the catheter, catheter hub colonization from frequent use, endogenous seeding from distant sites of infection, or infusate contamination.

- Poor adherence to aseptic technique, increased number of catheter manipulations, increased number of lumens per catheter, increased time of use, increased severity of underlying disease, repeated catheterizations, presence of an infection elsewhere, absence of antimicrobial therapy, bacteremia, inappropriate catheter material and physician inexperience are associated with increased infectious or mechanical complications.
- Site of percutaneous catheter puncture is infected if purulent drainage from the site, expanding erythema and cellulitis (tenderness and edema), or erythema and a positive qualitative skin culture are present.
- Guidelines for changing central venous catheters are listed in Box 1.
- Hyperalimentation (TPN) should be administered through a dedicated port not previously used. The TPN port subsequently should not be used for other IV infusion.
- Saline solution flushes of central venous catheters achieve comparable patency of ports as heparin flushes without the risk of heparin-induced thrombocytopenia.

SUGGESTED READING

Cook D, Randolph A, Kernerman P, Cupido C, King D, Soukup C, Brun-Buisson C. Central venous catheter replacement strategies: a systemic review of the literature. Crit Care Med 1997; 25(8):1417–1424.

Farr BM. Preventing vascular catheter-related infections: current controversies. Clin Infect Dis 2001; 33(1):173–178.

Pearson ML. Guideline for the prevention of intravascular-device-related infections. Infect Control and Hosp Epidemiology 1996; 17(8):438–473.

58
Percutaneous Tracheostomy

Jeffrey G. Chipman
VA Medical Center, Minneapolis, Minnesota, USA

INTRODUCTION

Tracheostomy is one of the most commonly performed surgical procedures to provide long-term ventilator access and to facilitate tracheal function in critically ill patients; it has traditionally been performed in the operating room. For many reasons, including facilitating surgery in a timely manner and avoiding the risks of transporting critically ill, ventilator-dependent patients, surgeons have sought ways to perform tracheostomies at the bedside. Such bedside procedures can be performed successfully but may be limited by personnel, poor space, inadequate lighting, and lack of necessary equipment.

Percutaneous tracheostomy has emerged over the last decade as a safe procedure. Without arguing the merits of one technique over another, this chapter will briefly follow the acceptance of percutaneous tracheostomy from experiment to mainstream, present the accepted indications and contraindications, outline the procedure's steps, and discuss potential complications.

BACKGROUND

Tracheostomy was performed in ancient times. The beginning of the twentieth century marks the modern history of open tracheostomy, when the first formal report of the procedure was published.

Since tracheostomy was accepted as a surgical technique, many efforts have been made to create an instrument that could cut and dilate tissue to quickly gain access to the trachea. None of the original products was successful enough to enjoy widespread use, and some actually created more harm than benefit (1). In 1985, Ciaglia proposed using percutaneous nephrostomy instruments to dilate the trachea and place a tracheostomy tube (2). What has evolved is the dilational percutaneous tracheostomy procedure that employs a small skin incision and sequential dilation of the subcutaneous and pretracheal tissues, as well as the tracheal wall. A guide wire, placed into the tracheal lumen, guides all of these steps. Though the procedure can be done percutaneously with only a small skin incision, most practitioners follow the procedure suggested by Griggs to dissect and separate the underlying tissue before the trachea is accessed by the "percutaneous" instruments (3).

Several kits, complete with the necessary needles, wires, dilators, and tracheostomy tubes, are available. The components have evolved since the appearance of the first kits to make the procedure easier, safer, and potentially less costly than an open procedure. Another proposed advantage concerns timeliness of the procedure. Because operating room scheduling difficulties can be avoided, percutaneous tracheostomy may facilitate tracheostomy in a timely manner, once the decision to operate has been made. However, if the procedure is performed in the operating room, the cost benefits may not be realized (4).

The safety of the percutaneous tracheostomy has been debated since its origins. Critics have argued that a limited operative field would hinder efforts to control bleeding, ensure inappropriate location of the tracheotomy, and prevent absolute control of the airway. Inclusion of bronchoscopy in the procedure has eliminated some of these arguments. Several prospective comparison trials have demonstrated that its safety is similar to that of the open technique, especially if performed by surgeons (1,4–12). Moreover, two meta-analyses of prospective trials demonstrate that the percutaneous procedure has advantages over the open procedure in a lower overall postoperative complication rate, a lower incidence of perioperative and postoperative bleeding, and fewer postoperative infections (13,14).

INDICATIONS AND CONTRAINDICATIONS

Percutaneous tracheostomy is a reasonable choice for most patients requiring tracheostomy who are already intubated. Relatively few contraindications to performing percutaneous tracheostomy exist. One contraindication is the inability to intubate a patient transorally if control of the airway were lost; replacement of the endotracheal tube via the mouth is the method of choice to secure the airway if the percutaneous method is unsuccessful. Some have argued that coagulopathy is a contraindication because the surgeon has reduced ability to control bleeding in the small operative field. In fact, several studies suggest that postoperative bleeding is decreased with the percutaneous approach, presumably because the tracheostomy tube tamponades bleeding in the small incision and dissection area (13,14). Obesity or large neck size is another relative contraindication. If transoral intubation is possible in these patients and an appropriately sized tracheostomy tube is available, some argue that the percutaneous method is easier, less dissection is required, and a large incision in an obese person may be avoided.

One absolute contraindication is the need for emergency control of the airway. Cricothyrotomy remains the procedure of choice, though a method for percutaneous cricothyrotomy using a Seldinger technique has been developed that may prove useful after further evaluation (15). Additional contraindications are a neck mass and pediatric patient.

TECHNIQUE

Location

Whether the procedure is performed at the bedside or in the operating room depends on the experience of the personnel and the resources of the institution. Percutaneous tracheostomy has been performed safely in the intensive care unit (ICU) at the bedside, as well as in the operating room. More important than the location are the ability of personnel and the accessibility of equipment to handle potential complications.

Personnel

Successful percutaneous tracheostomy requires several people. First is the surgeon. Although many nonsurgeons have performed the procedure, there is evidence that improved outcome is achieved when performed by surgeons familiar with the anatomy of the neck (5).

Equally important is the person responsible for managing the airway. This person must be capable of transoral intubation if the endotracheal tube were prematurely removed before the trachea is intubated by the tracheostomy tube. This person can often be the same person who performs the intraoperative bronchoscopy. Bronchoscopy has been adopted to ensure that the catheter used to access to the trachea is placed in the midline of the anterior tracheal wall and not through the posterior wall. In addition, bronchoscopic visualization can determine if the needle is placed caudal to the end of the endotracheal tube, that dilation occurs transtracheally and not paratracheally, and that the guide wire is directed distally in the trachea. Additionally, with the bronchoscope in place in the trachea, if the endotracheal tube is removed too far, it can be replaced using the bronchoscope as a guiding stent (16).

Other helpful personnel may include a surgical assistant, who can help load catheters onto wires and provide other needed assistance. An additional individual, not involved in the actual placement, should provide anesthetics, analgesics, and sedatives as well as assist with bronchoscopy.

Equipment

Commercially prepared kits are available and may include only the catheter, dilators, and guide wire. Other kits add scalpels, local anesthesia, tracheostomy tubes, sterile drapes, and surgical instruments. Equipment necessary to perform a standard surgical airway should be available in case an emergency arises. Additionally, equipment for bag-mask ventilation and endotracheal intubation including a direct laryngoscope, suction, and endotracheal tubes, should be at hand. Endotracheal intubation is the first route to re-establish a controlled airway in case of tracheostomy failure and loss of airway.

As mentioned previously, bronchoscopy has been advocated as an adjunct to performing a percutaneous tracheostomy to ensure an appropriate location of the tracheostomy and proper placement of tracheostomy tube. Many consider it a necessity (12,16).

The procedure can be performed either in the operating room or in the ICU. In the ICU, adequate overhead lighting, instrument access, and personnel positioning are important considerations.

Method

The patient is preoxygenated with 100% oxygen, and the ventilator is set to provide an adequate minute ventilation. Several methods to sedate the patient are available. A combination of narcotic and benzodiazepine is adequate. Propofol is another option. A long acting muscle relaxant is often employed to keep the patient from moving during the operation. Manipulation of the airway can cause reflex movement that can hinder the procedure. If a muscle relaxant is used, the patient must be adequately sedated prior to its administration.

Positioning is aided with a shoulder roll to allow maximal extension of the neck. Neck extension elevates the trachea out of the mediastinum and displaces the chin to allow greater access to the anterior neck. Intravenous catheters, electrocardiogram leads, ventilator tubing, and oral or nasal tubes should be positioned away from the operative field. Disposable sheets keep the bed clean and reduce nursing care. The exposed neck can then be washed with a standard surgical scrub. The surgeon wears appropriate eye protection, hair cover, mask, a sterile gown, and sterile gloves. A sterile field is then created with towels and drapes.

A point midway between the cricoid cartilage and the sternal notch is palpated and marked. Local anesthesia is then infiltrated in the skin, subcutaneous tissues, and into the trachea. A vertical or transverse incision may be used. It should be large enough to contain the tracheostomy tube. Of importance, the incision should be symmetric in relation to the midline of the trachea to aid subsequent orientation. A clamp is then used to separate the underlying tissue. Dissection proceeds to the level of the anterior tracheal fascia. The surgeon is careful to avoid dissecting to the side of the trachea.

At this point the bronchoscope is passed. The surgeon uses a finger to palpate the trachea while the endotracheal tube is slowly withdrawn with the cuff deflated if possible. The surgeon can usually feel the tip of the endotracheal tube slide as it reaches a point superior to the tracheotomy location. In averaged-sized adults, the tube can be withdrawn to ~ 18 cm mark at the teeth. If the endotracheal tube is retracted too far, or if it is removed prematurely, it can be replaced over the bronchoscope. Occasionally, if palpating the endotracheal tube is difficult, the bronchoscope tip can be placed at the end of the endotracheal tube, and the light can be observed through the incision. The bronchoscope can also show indentation of the trachea with palpation, another guide to locating the tracheotomy site.

Once assured that the endotracheal tube is cephalad to the tracheotomy site, a needle and catheter are placed into the trachea. Aspirating an attached syringe containing a small amount of water will indicate, when air bubbles through the water, that the tracheal wall has been punctured. Puncture of the trachea is observed through the bronchoscope to ensure the needle traverses the trachea in the midline. The catheter is then left in the trachea. The guide wire is then passed into the trachea through the catheter in view of the bronchoscope to verify that the wire passes caudally in the trachea (Fig. 1). A mark on the wire indicates the appropriate depth. A wire placed too deep in the trachea can potentially cause bronchoconstriction or lung injury.

The first dilator is placed over the wire followed by the guiding catheter (Fig. 2). Again, the marks on the wire guide the operator in maintaining constant position of the wire. The mark on the guiding catheter is kept at the level of the skin. The dilator(s) are then lubricated and sequentially placed over the guiding catheter and into the trachea sequentially to enlarge the tracheotomy (Fig. 3). The tracheostomy tube is then placed over a lubricated dilator of the correct size for the tube, and together they are placed into the trachea over the guiding catheter (Fig. 4). Passing the tracheostomy tube cuff through the dilated tract requires some force. The dilator guiding catheter and wire are removed, leaving the tracheostomy tube in place. The cuff is inflated, the inner canula is inserted, and the ventilator tubing is attached. Placement is confirmed by auscultation of both lung fields, return of a full tidal volume on the ventilator, and bronchoscopy.

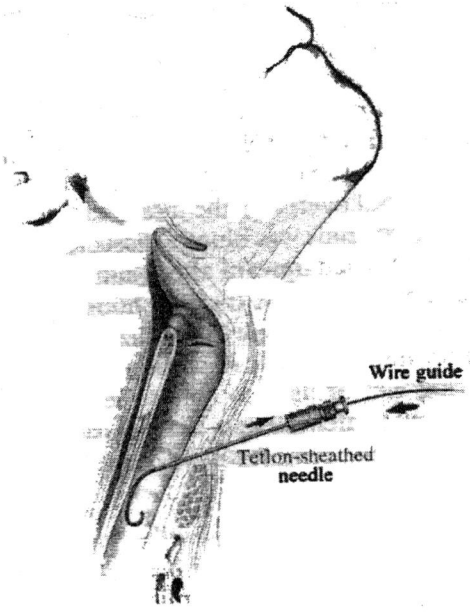

Figure 1 The trachea is accessed by a catheter and a guide wire placed into the trachea through the catheter. [Adapted from Ref. (5).]

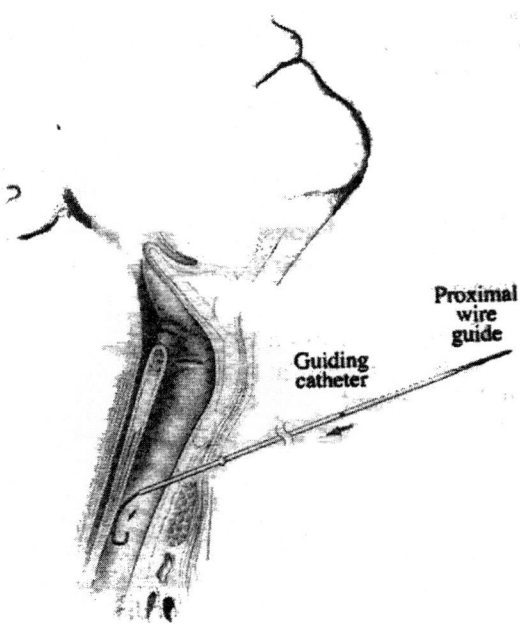

Figure 2 The first dilator is placed over the guide wire followed by the guiding catheter. Note the flange on the guiding catheter placed at skin level. Subsequent dilators are placed over the guiding catheter and must abut the flange. [Adapted from Ref. (5).]

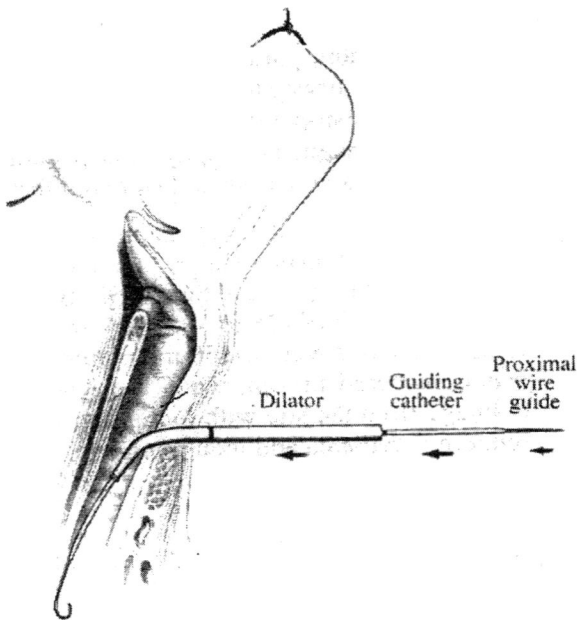

Figure 3 Sequential dilation is performed with one tapering or several sequentially larger diameter dilators placed over the guiding catheter depending on the system used. [Adapted from Ref. (5).]

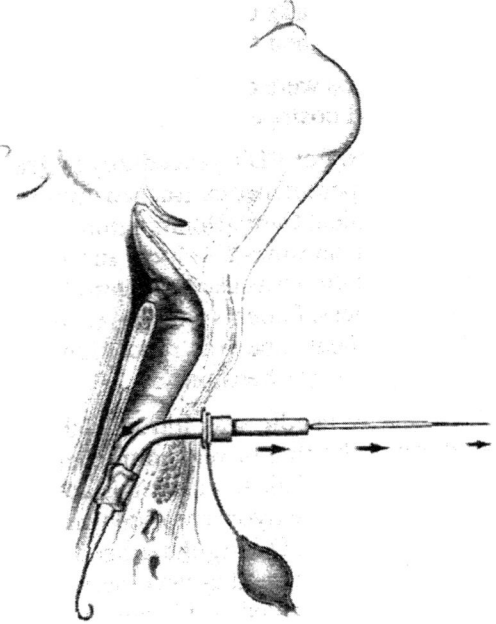

Figure 4 The tracheostomy tube is loaded onto the appropriate-sized dilator and then placed into the trachea over the guiding catheter and guide wire. [Adapted from Ref. (5).]

The endotracheal tube is then removed. The tracheostomy tube is then secured to the skin with suture and a tie around the neck. A postprocedural chest radiograph is then obtained.

PITFALLS

The most common complication is premature extubation (17). Use of bronchoscopy minimizes the consequences during the procedure, because the endotracheal tube can be replaced over the scope. Bleeding is another potential complication but can be minimized with care during the dissection. Crossing veins can be ligated and larger vessels can be avoided. Studies suggest that bleeding is less with the percutaneous technique, because the tracheostomy tube in the small operative field tamponades bleeding.

The devastating complications of paratracheal insertion and tracheoesophageal fistula have been virtually eliminated with the use of bronchoscopy (1). Another potentially serious complication is bronchospasm. Bronchospasm can occur if the guide wire is passed deep into the tracheobroncheal tree and spasm is triggered. Keeping the wire in the appropriate location indicated by the guiding marks and pretreating patients with known reactive airway disease with steroids can limit this complication.

Other complications of percutaneous tracheostomy are similar to the open procedure. Tracheal stenosis may result because of the tracheal dilation. Theoretically, dilation could produce a larger tear of the trachea compared to a controlled incision done during an open procedure. The tear might result in a higher incidence of tracheal stenosis, but has not been observed clinically (18). Tracheoinnominate fistula has been described following percutaneous tracheostomy, but it occurs no more frequently than with the open procedure. Parastomal infection has an incidence equal to the open procedure (13,14).

CONCLUSIONS

Percutaneous dilational tracheostomy is an effective method to electively provide long-term airway control for the intubated patient in whom tracheostomy is required. Experienced practitioners can safely perform it at the bedside in the ICU and may produce time and cost savings. Overall complications are similar to open tracheostomy, and those unique to the percutaneous technique can be minimized with bronchoscopic surveillance.

SUMMARY

- Tracheostomy provides long-term ventilator access and facilitates tracheal suctioning.
- Percutaneous tracheostomy can be performed safely.
- Contraindications to percutaneous tracheostomy include inability to intubate a patient transorally, coagulopathy, obesity, a neck mass, and young age.

- An absolute contraindication to percutaneous tracheostomy is the need for emergency airway control. Cricothyrotomy is the procedure of choice for an emergency airway.
- Safe percutaneous tracheostomy requires a surgeon, an individual capable of transoral intubation and who may perform bronchoscopy. Helpful additional personnel include a surgical assistant and an individual to administer pharmacologic agents.
- Percutaneous tracheostomy can be performed at the bedside or in the operating room.
- The most common complication is premature extubation. Paratracheal insertion, tracheoesophageal fistula, and bronchospasm are additional complications.
- Overall complications are similar to those of open tracheostomy.
- Complications of percutaneous tracheostomy can be minimized with bronchoscopic surveillance.

REFERENCES

1. Moe KS, Stoeckli SJ, Schmid S, Weymuller EA Jr. Percutaneous tracheostomy: a comprehensive evaluation. Ann Otol Rhinol Laryngol 1999; 108:384–391.
2. Ciaglia P, Firsching R, Syniec C. Elective percutaneous dilational tracheostomy. Chest 1985; 87:715–719.
3. Griggs WM, Worthly LI, Gilligan JE, Thomas PD, Myburg JA. A simple percutaneous tracheostomy technique. Surg Gynecol Obstet 1990; 170:543–545.
4. Freeman BD, Isabella K, Cobb JP, Boyle WA III, Schmieg RE Jr, Kolleff MH, Lin N, Saak T, Thompson EC, Buchman TG. A prospective, randomized study comparing percutaneous with surgical tracheostomy in critically ill patients. Crit Care Med 2001; 29:926–930.
5. Lim JW, Friedman M, Tanyeri H, Lazar A, Caldarelli DD. Experience with percutaneous dilational tracheostomy. Ann Otol Rhinol Laryngol 2000; 109:791–796.
6. Gysin C, Dulguerov P, Guyot J-P, Perneger TV, Abajo B, Chevrolet J-C. Percutaneous versus surgical tracheostomy: a double-blind randomized trial. Ann Surg 1999; 230:708–714.
7. Porter JM, Ivatury RR. Preferred route of tracheostomy-percutaneous versus open at the bedside: a randomized, prospective study in the surgical intensive care unit. Am Surg 1999; 2:142–146.
8. Hazard P, Jones C, Benitone J. Comparative clinical trial of standard operative tracheostomy with percutaneous tracheostomy. Crit Care Med 1991; 19:1018–1024.
9. Friedman Y, Fildes J, Mizock B, Samuel J, Patel S, Appavu S, Roberts R. Comparison of percutaneous and surgical tracheostomies. Chest 1996; 110:480–485.
10. Crofts SL, Alzeer A, McGuire GP, Wong DT, Charles D. A comparison of percutaneous and operative tracheostomies in intensive care patients. Can J Anaesth 1995; 42:775–779.
11. Holdgaard HO, Pedersen J, Paaske PB, Jensen RH, Outzen KE, Nielsen PH, Juhl B. Percutaneous dilational tracheostomy versus conventional surgical tracheostomy. A clinical randomized study. Acta Anaesthesiol Scand 1998; 42:545–550.
12. Barba CA, Angood PB, Kauder DR, Latenser B, Martin K, McGonigal MD, Phillips GR, Rotondo MF, Schwab CW. Bronchoscopic guidance makes percutaneous tracheostomy a safe, cost-effective, and easy-to-teach procedure. Surgery 1995; 118:879–883.
13. Freeman BD, Isabella K, Lin N, Buchman TG. A meta-analysis of prospective trials comparing percutaneous and surgical tracheostomy in critical ill patients. Chest 2000; 118:1412–1418.
14. Cheng E, Fee WE Jr. Dilational versus standard tracheostomy: a meta-analysis. Ann Otol Rhinol Laryngol 2000; 109:803–807.

15. Eisenburger P, Laczika K, List M, Wilfing A, Losert H, Hofbauer R, Burgmann H, Bankl H, Pikula B, Benumof JL, Frass M. Comparison of conventional surgical versus Seldinger technique emergency cricothyrotomy performed by inexperienced clinicians. Anesthesiology 2000; 92:687–690.
16. Byhahn C, Wilke H, Halbig S, Lischke V, Westphal K. Percutaneous tracheostomy: ciaglia blue rhino versus the basis ciaglia technique of percutaneous dilational tracheostomy. Anesth Analg 2000; 91:882–886.
17. Kearney PA, Griffen MM, Ochoa JB, Boulanger BR, Tseui BJ, Mentzer RM Jr. A single-center 8-year experience with percutaneous dilational tracheostomy. Ann Surg 2000; 231:701–709.
18. Norwood S, Vallina VL, Short K, Saigusa M, Fernandez LG, McLarty JW. Incidence of tracheal stenosis and other late complications after percutaneous tracheostomy. Ann Surg 2000; 232:233–241.

59

Lumbar Puncture, Thoracentesis, Thoracostomy, and Paracentesis

Sharon Henry
University of Maryland, College Park, Maryland, USA

LUMBAR PUNCTURE

The usual indications for lumbar puncture, that is, tapping of the subarachnoid space in the lumbar region, include the following: to diagnose suspected CNS infection; to diagnose subarachnoid hemorrhage (if CT scan is normal); to diagnose certain demyelinating neurologic diseases (e.g., multiple sclerosis); to treat pseudotumor cerebri; and to administer antibiotics, analgesics, and chemotherapy.

The major contraindication to lumbar puncture is increased intracranial pressure (ICP). Decreasing lumbar pressure with the removal of CSF can result in tonsillar herniation. Coagulopathy or thrombocytopenia increases the risk of intraspinal hemorrhage, and local skin infections increase the risk of secondary CSF infection.

Anatomy

In the adult's spinal column, the spinal cord terminates between L1 and L2. Each vertebra is composed of the body, laminae, pedicles and transverse and spinous processes. The vertebral ligaments include the supraspinous, the interspinous, and the ligamentum flavum (1) (Fig. 1).

Positioning

Patients are placed in the lateral decubitus position with knees and hips flexed while attempting to touch their chin to the knees. The back should be at right angles to the bed. In critically ill patients the position indicated in Fig. 2A is normally the only possible approach. Alternatively, the patient is seated and leans forward against a table or an assistant, with their feet supported on a stool (Fig. 2B).

Procedure

An imaginary line is drawn between the iliac crests. This line represents the L3–4 interspace. (The L4–5 interspace may also be used.) The area is prepared with antiseptic solution and is draped. Sterile gloves are worn by the clinician. The landmarks are

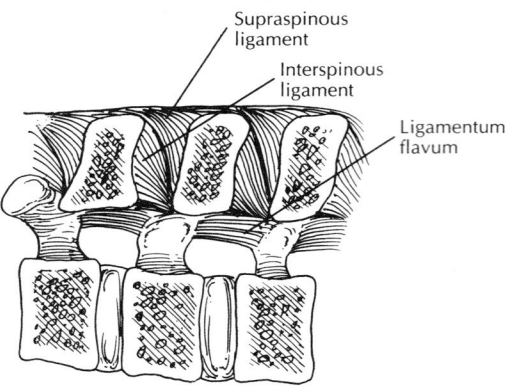

Figure 1 Vertebral ligaments. (Redrawn from Taylor RW, Civetta JM, Kirby RR, eds. Techniques and Procedures in Critical Care. Philadelphia: JB Lippincott, 1990:390.)

reestablished and the spinous process of L3–4 palpated with the thumb. Using 1% lidocaine and a 25-gauge needle, the clinician anesthetizes the skin overlying the site. Then a 20-gauge or smaller spinal needle with stylet in place is advanced perpendicular to the axis of the spine, with the bevel oriented horizontally. Once through the skin, the needle is advanced with a firm steady pressure to allow the needle to pass beneath the spinous process (2). A sensation of a "give" or "pop" is experienced once the ligamentum flavum is passed. The obturator is removed, and the clinician checks for flow of fluid. The needle may be rotated 90° or 180° if no fluid flow occurs. The obturator is replaced before further respositioning of the needle. If hard resistance is met, bone most likely has been encountered, and the needle should be repositioned. Once spinal fluid has returned, pressures can be measured. A manometer is attached to the needle by way of a stopcock. Readings in excess of 20 cm H_2O are abnormal. Measurements made with the patient in the upright position are less reliable (2).

Paramedian Approach

The paramedian approach is used on patients who are unable to flex the lumbar spine adequately or who have ligamentous calcification. The skin is infiltrated slightly lateral to and below the spinous process. The needle is advanced to the lamina. The needle is removed and then reinserted after being angled medially. The needle can then be slipped into the ligamentum flavum (1).

CSF Analysis

A cell count of the CSF >5 WBC/mm^3 is abnormal. Normal glucose level is 50–75 mg/dL; whereas, the normal protein level is 15–45 mg/dL. CSF to serum glucose concentration ratios range from 0.6 to 0.7. Protein electrophoresis is performed on the CSF, as are assays for bacterial antigens and for myelin base protein. Bacterial, fungal, viral, and tuberculin cultures are obtained, as are Gram's acid-fast bacillus, and cytologic stains. Cytology is performed. Any xanthochromic appearance is noted. India ink is used to evaluate the possibility of cryptococcal infection.

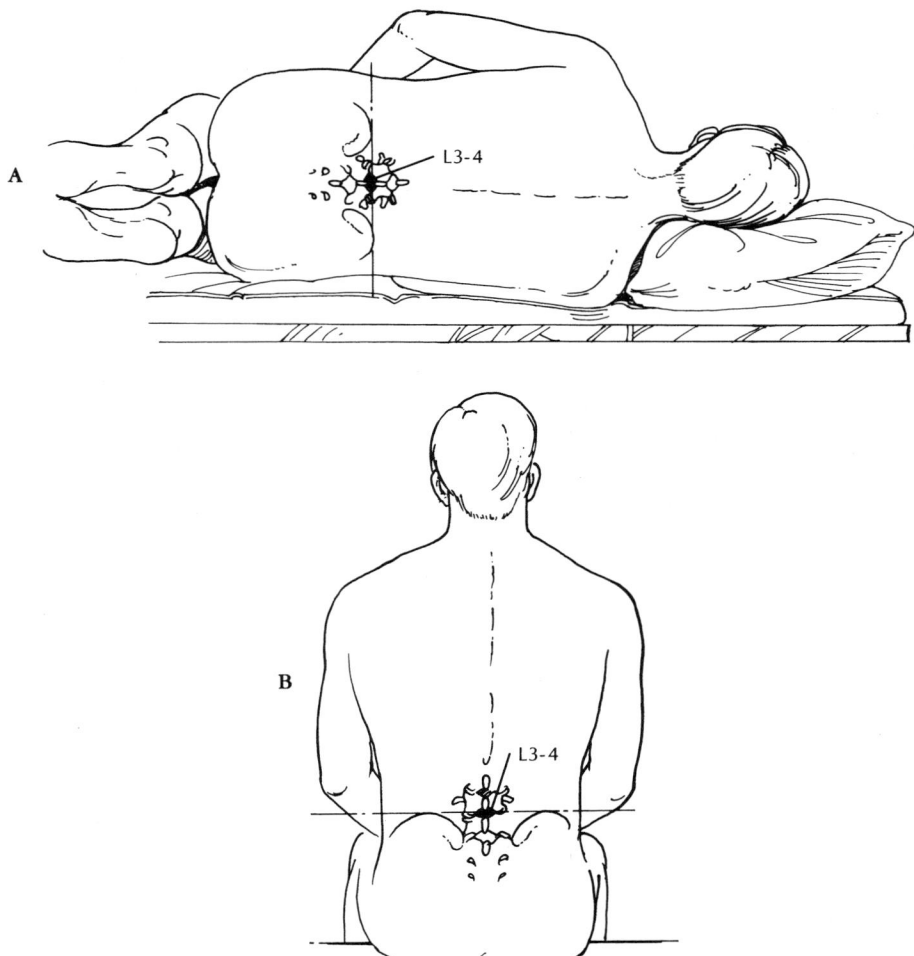

Figure 2 Lumbar puncture positions. (A) Usual position, especially for critically ill patients. (B) Alternative position. (Redrawn from Taylor RW, Civetta JM, Kriby RR, eds. Techniques and Procedures in Critical Care. Philadelphia: JB Lippincott, 1990:391.)

Complications

Headache occurs as a complication of lumbar puncture in 10–25% of patients (2). This incidence is decreased by using a smaller gauge needle and possibly by having the patient lie prone after the procedure.

Painful and persistent paresthesias that resolved within 1 year occurred in 0.2–0.7% of patients. Persistent or disabling complications occurred in 0.19–0.43% of patients undergoing spinal anesthesia (3).

Local bleeding as a result of a traumatic tap occurs in up to 20% of patients. Coagulopathic or thrombocytopenic patients are at increased risk and may develop spinal epidural or sub-dural hematomas (4). Spinal subdural or epidural hematomas are rarely reported but are more common in patients with coagulopathy (4).

Infection occurs uncommonly, even in bacteremic patients, and tonsillar herniation may occur in patients with increased ICP.

THORACENTESIS

Thoracentesis, puncture of the chest wall to enter the pleural cavity to aspirate fluids, is indicated either to diagnose or to treat pleural effusion. Localization with CT scan or ultrasound may be necessary if loculated effusions are present.

Procedure

The patient may be supine or in the lateral decubitus position. Alternatively, the patient may be seated, and lean over a stand or table (Fig. 3). The level of the fluid is identified by percussion; if indicated, ultrasound or CT localization is used. One or two interspaces below the fluid location is chosen as the site for the thoracentesis, but it should generally be performed at or above the eighth intercostal space.

The skin is prepared with antiseptic solution and sterilely draped. At the midportion of the rib, 1–2% lidocaine is infiltrated to the skin and subcutaneous tissue. A 20-gauge or larger angiocatheter, with syringe attached, is used to enter the skin at the midportion of the rib and then is "walked" up the rib. The syringe is used for aspiration, and the angiocatheter is advanced. The pleural cavity is entered above the rib. The pleural cavity must not be entered at the inferior edge of the next superior rib. In that location, risk of injury to intercostal vessels in high.

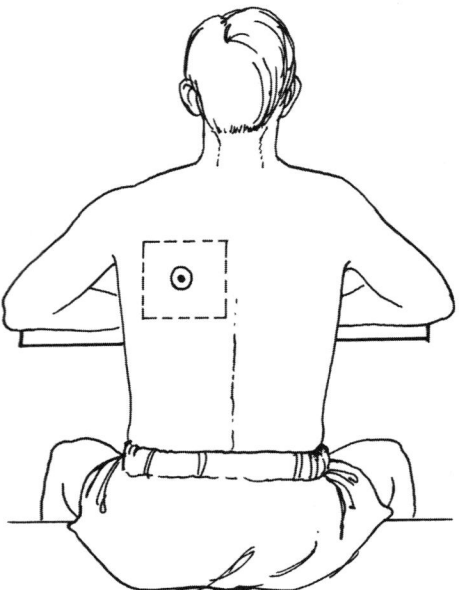

Figure 3 Seated position for thoracentesis. (Redrawn from Taylor RW, Civetta JM, Kirby RR, eds. Techniques and Procedures in Critical Care. Philadelphia: JB Lippincott, 1990:296.)

When fluid returns, the catheter is advanced into the pleural cavity. A stopcock can be attached. It is connected to a drainage bag with extension tubing. With the use of a stopcock, risk of introducing air into the thoracic cavity is reduced, and chance of spillage of the fluid is decreased. Specimens for analysis are taken. Then the needle is removed, and a dressing is applied.

Complications

Complications of thoracentesis include pneumothorax, bleeding, and visceral punctures.

Fluid Analysis

Analysis of fluids aspirated from the pleural cavity reveals the following: cell count, protein content, lactate dehydrogenase (LDH) values, pH, cultures (bacterial and fungal), and stains (Gram's and acid-fast bacillus).

THORACOSTOMY

Thoracostomy, the creation of an opening in the chest wall to allow drainage, is done because of trauma (i.e., for pneumothorax, hemothorax, pneumohemothorax, or chylothorax) or in patients with certain nontraumatic conditions (i.e., spontaneous pneumothorax, pleural effusion, empyema, or chylothorax).

Precautions must be observed in patients with a previous thoracotomy, multiple adhesions, clotting disorders, or a massive hemothorax with hypovolemia. Care should be exercised when considering tube thoracostomy in patients with bullous emphysema. Placement of a chest tube into a bleb can produce bleeding or a bronchopleural fistula. A CT scan may be necessary to distinguish a large bleb from a loculated pneumothorax.

Procedure

The procedure begins with tube selection. Small-caliber tubes (18–22 Fr) are used to remove air, and large-caliber tubes (36–40 Fr) are used to drain fluid. An anterior site (the second intercostal space, midclavicular line) or a posterolateral site (intercostal space 4–8) is used. Standard practice when selecting a posterolateral site is to use the fifth or sixth intercostal space between the anterior and midaxillary lines. The patient is either supine or in the lateral decubitus position with the elbow bent. Except for emergencies, the procedure must be explained to the patients and their informed consent obtained. The area for thoracostomy is prepared with antiseptic solution and is draped with sterile towels. Many institutions provide thoracostomy trays, which contain two large kelly clamps, a scalpel, a needle holder, forceps, 0 sutures, a cup for local anesthetic, 22- and 18-gage needles, 10 and 20 mL syringes, and gauze pads. Adequate local anesthetic must be administered. The proposed area of insertion and an interspace above and below it should be liberally injected with 1% or 2% lidocaine (20–25 mL).

The skin incision is made parallel to the long axis of the rib, overlying the rib an interspace below the proposed site of insertion (Fig. 4A). A large Kelly clamp is used to dissect the area for a tunnel up to the superior border of the rib (Fig. 4B). The intercostal muscles are bluntly dissected at the superior margin of the rib. Entering the pleural space at

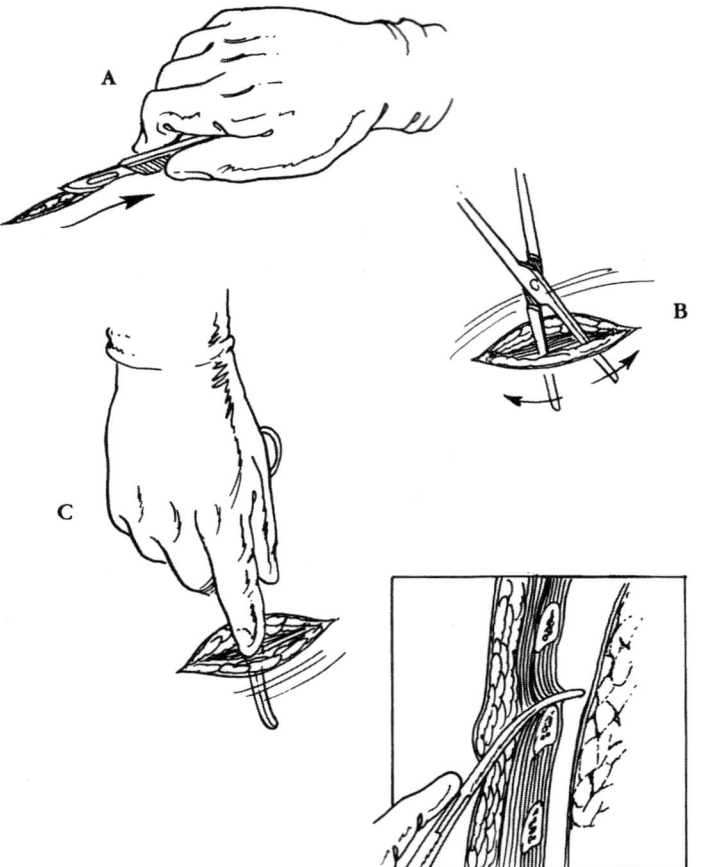

Figure 4 Thoracostomy. (A) Skin incision, (B) Kelly clamp used for dissection, and (C) Insertion of finger into pleural space. Inset: Insertion of clamp into pleural space. (Redrawn from Taylor RW, Civetta JM, Kirby RR, eds. Techniques and Procedures in Critical Care Philadelphia: JB Lippincott, 1990:303.)

the superior margin of the rib avoids injury to the intercostal neurovascular bundle. The jaws of the clamp then are closed and placed over the superior margin of the rib, and the pleural space is entered. A finger is inserted into the pleural space and rotated 360° to ensure that the lung is not adherent to the chest wall (Fig. 4C).

The chest tube is then inserted, using a Kelly clamp to guide it into the apex, if air is being drained, or it is inserted posteriorly if fluid is being drained. A second clamp should be placed on the end of the tube to prevent spillage. A 0 silk purse-string suture is placed in the skin surrounding the tube. A single knot is thrown, and the remaining length of the suture is wrapped around the tube and tied. This suture can be used to close the skin opening when the tube is removed. Another suture can be used to close the skin around the tube if a large incision has been made. The tube is connected to a closed drainage system.

Petrolatum gauze and a dressing are applied and securely taped. All connections should be secured with tape or chest tube bands. If the patients is in extremis with a tension pneumothorax, a 14-gauge IV catheter should be placed in the second intercostal space at the midclavicular line. This maneuver relieves the tension and allows more controlled placement of the chest tube.

Complications

Malpositioning of Tube

A tube inserted too far can injure mediastinal structures. One not inserted far enough can lead to persistent air leak or incomplete drainage of the pneumothorax. The tube also may be positioned completely outside the thoracic cavity. Intra-abdominal insertions may occur if too low an interspace is chosen. The insertion site should be carefully chosen in patients with elevated diaphragms. Malpositioned tubes should be removed, and a new tube inserted through a new incision (5).

Bleeding

Intercostal vascular injury may occur during insertion. Pulmonary vessels may be injured when the trocar technique is used (use of a trocar is not recommended). Adhesions can be very vascular and, if disrupted, can cause bleeding. If digital examination reveals extensive adhesions, an alternate site is chosen.

Abdominal Visceral Injury

Such an injury can occur during this procedure, especially if too low an insertion site is chosen. The liver and spleen are at greatest risk. Extreme caution must be used in patients with elevated hemidiaphragms in order to avoid this complication.

Mechanical Problems Associated with Collection System

Such problems include tubing constrictions, clotting of the tube (if an air leak persists, the patient could develop a tension pneumothorax); and disconnection of the chest tube from the collecting system.

Reexpansion Pulmonary Edema

Reexpansion pulmonary edema usually occurs hours after reexpansion of the lung after evacuation of a long-standing pneumothorax or drainage of a massive effusion. The mechanism is thought to involve increased capillary permeability in the collapsed lung. This phenomenon can be avoided by using gradual reexpansion and drainage. Large collections should be allowed to drain to a water seal, rather than being placed initially to suction.

Infection

Local infections at the insertion site can occur. Attention to skin care can prevent this complication. Pneumonias and empyemas are rarer events (3%) (6).

Lung Injury

Lung injury occurs more often when the trocar technique is used or when patients have decreased lung compliance or adhesions (7).

Drainage Systems

Modern drainage systems use a variation of the three-bottle system (Fig. 5). The chest tube is connected to the apparatus by rubber tubing that is usually 0.5 in. in internal diameter, allows flow of 50–60 mL/min, and is 6 ft in length (8). The tubing from the patient is connected to the collection chamber or bottle, which is in turn connected to the water seal bottle. In the water seal bottle the water level will move in synchrony with respiration if the tube is not occluded. If an air leak is present air will bubble through this chamber.

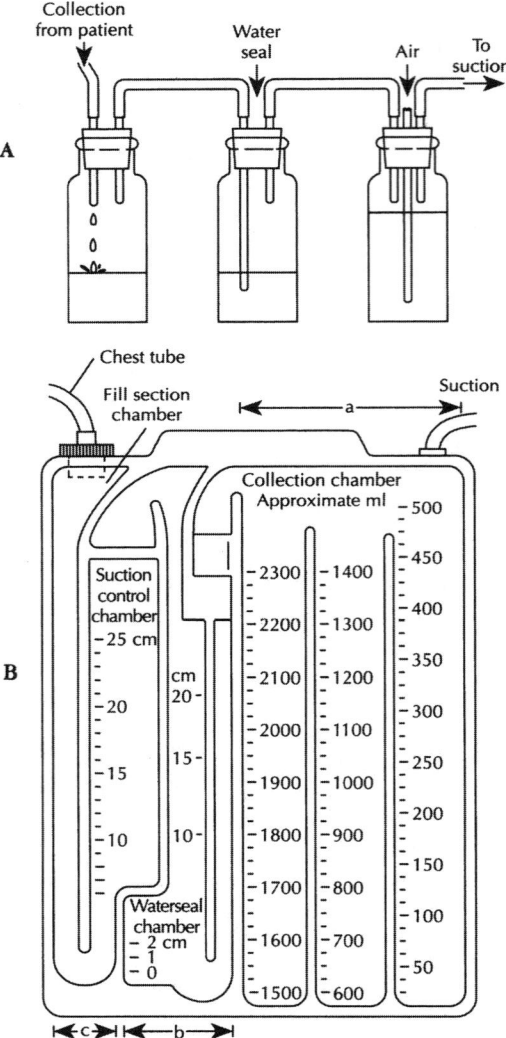

Figure 5 Drainage systems. (A) Three-bottle system. (B) Variation of three-bottle system; (a) collection chamber; (b) water seal chamber; (c) suction control chamber. (Redrawn from Taylor RW, Civetta JM, Kirby RR, eds. Techniques and Procedures in Critical Care. Philadelphia: JB Lippincott, 1990:311.)

Connected to this bottle is the suction control bottle, which is connected to a vacuum. This bottle determines the amount of subatmospheric pressure exerted on the pleural cavity; 20 cm of H_2O is standard.

Chest Tube Removal

The tube is removed when no air leak is noted for 24 h. A CXR with the patient on water seal alone ("clamped"), without suction, is usually obtained. If no pneumothorax is observed, the chest tube can be removed. If the tube has been placed to drain fluid, it can be removed when the drainage is <100 mL/day.

Procedure

To perform chest tube removal the dressings are removed and sutures cut. The patient is asked to inspire deeply and perform a Valsalva maneuver (9), which increases intrathoracic pressure and discourages air from entering the thorax. The tube is removed rapidly, and the sutures are tied. Petrolatum gauze and gauze pads are applied.

Sclerosis

Pleural sclerosis can be used to treat recurrent effusion or malignant effusions. When the lung is completely reexpanded, no air leak persists, and fluid drainage is <100 mL/day, the following procedure is used.

- 1 g of tetracycline is instilled into the thorax through the chest tube.
- The tube is clamped for 4–6 h (procedure is painful, and adequate analgesia must be provided).

Maintaining Chest Tube Patency

Chest tube patency is maintained by using the following methods: (1) stripping, (2) irrigation, (3) instillation of urokinase, or (4) mechanical dislodgment of obstructing matter using an endotracheal suction catheter (10).

PARACENTESIS

Paracentesis, puncture of the abdominal cavity to aspirate peritoneal fluid, is used for the diagnostic evaluation of ascites, treatment of disabling ascites, and diagnosis of intraabdominal sepsis. Its use is contraindicated in patients who have had multiple previous abdominal operations, those who currently have massive bowel distention or abdominal wall cellulitis, or women who are pregnant.

Procedure

A useful site for performing paracentesis is lateral to the rectus muscle at the level of the umbilicus or 1 cm below or above the umbilicus (Fig. 6). Sonography or a CT scan can be used to guide the appropriate choice of site.

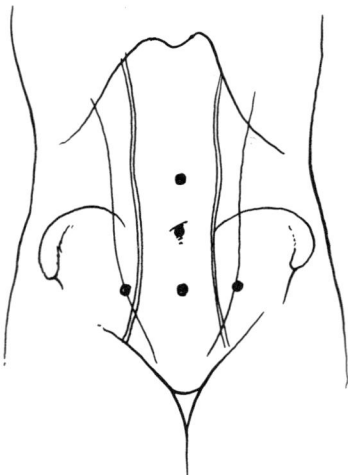

Figure 6 Sites for paracentesis. (Redrawn from Taylor RW, Civetta JM, Krby RR, eds. Techniques and Procedures in Critical Care. Philadelphia: JB Lippincott, 1990:312.)

The skin is prepared with antiseptic solution, and the sterile field is draped. A 25-gauge needle is used to administer local anesthetic with epinephrine. A 21-gauge IV catheter (larger gauge may be used) with syringe attached is passed through the skin perpendicularly and then is angled to create a Z tract. As the needle is advanced, the syringe is aspirated. A pop or give is felt as the needle passes through the fascia and peritoneum. When fluid is aspirated, the catheter is advanced, and the needle is removed. A larger syringe then is attached to collect fluid for diagnostic study. Alternatively, a stopcock can be attached to the catheter, which is connected to extension tubing and a drainage bag, and the desired amount of fluid removed through a closed system. The catheter is removed and the area covered with a dressing.

Diagnostic Tests

Diagnostic tests of the peritoneal fluid include the following:

- Specific gravity
- Protein content
- Cell count
- Cytology
- Gram's stain
- Bacterial and fungal cultures
- Acid-fast bacillus stain
- Amylase
- Bilirubin

Complications

Complications of paracentesis include bowel or bladder perforation, infection, persistent ascitic leak, and hypotension, if too much volume is removed (6).

OPEN AND CLOSED PERITONEAL TAP AND LAVAGE

Diagnostic peritoneal lavage (DPL) is used to evaluate both blunt and penetrating trauma. It is also useful for evaluating peritonitis in patients with altered mental status, patients with altered sensation, and critically ill patients in whom transport represents a major risk (11).

Caution must be used in performing this procedure in a patient with multiple abdominal scars. The procedure is absolutely contraindicated only if there is a definite indication for laparotomy.

Closed Procedure

The closed peritoneal tap (Fig. 7) is usually performed at the infraumbilical midline. If the patient has pelvic fractures, the supraumbilical midline is used. The area is prepared with

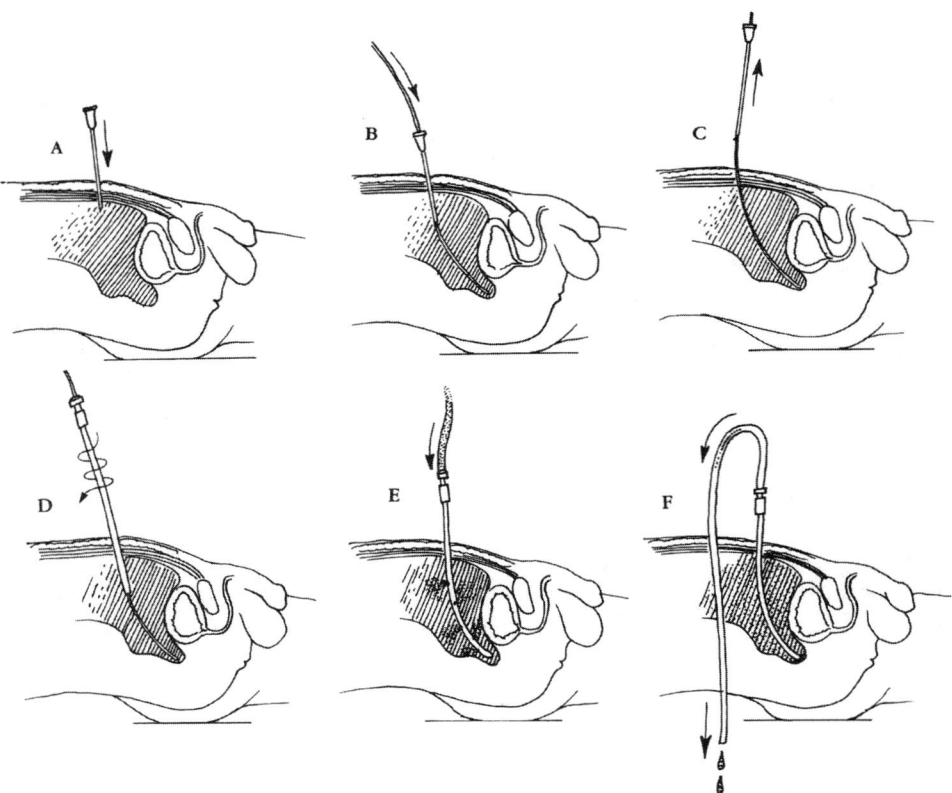

Figure 7 Closed peritoneal tap and lavage. (A) Needle is inserted into peritoneal cavity. (B) Flexible guidewire is passed through needle. (C) Needle is withdrawn with guidewire left in place. (D) Teflon catheter is advanced over wire. (E) Wire is withdrawn and salt solution is infused through catheter. (F) Seal on intravenous solution is broken and fluid is allowed to drain into infusion container. (Redrawn from Danto L. Paracentesis and diagnostic peritoneal lavage. In: Blaisdell FW, Traukey DD, eds. Trauma Management, Vol. 1. Abdominal Trauma. New York: Thieme Medical, 1982:45–57.)

antiseptic solution and is sterilely draped. The skin is puntured with a No. 11 blade, and pressure is held with a gauze pad until the bleeding stops. Kits are available that contain an 18-gauge needle, a guidewire, and a 14 Fr catheter with multiple side holes. The needle is passed through the rectus fascia and peritoneum. A characteristic pop or give is felt, the guidewire is passed through the needle, and the needle is withdrawn. The catheter is passed over the wire into the peritoneal cavity. A 10 mL syringe is used to aspirate the catheter. If ≤ 5 mL of blood is obtained, lavage is performed, and 1L of normal saline solution or lactated Ringer's solution is infused and allowed to return by gravity. At least 200 mL should return. The fluid is sent for cell count and amylase and bilirubin concentrations.

Open Procedure

After the patient has been scrubbed with antiseptic solution, draped, and anesthetized, an incision is made in the skin. The soft tissues are dissected and the rectus fascia identified. Rectus fascia is divided in the midline, and stay sutures are placed on either side. The peritoneum is grasped, and a purse-string suture is placed. The peritoneum is then incised, and a dialysis catheter is inserted and directed to the pelvis. If ≤ 5 mL of blood are aspirated, lavage is performed. The catheter is removed after the fluid is recovered, and the purse-string suture is tied. The rectus fascia is repaired with No. 0 or 1 suture and the skin is closed with 3-0 or 4-0 nylon.

Semi-open Procedure

This procedure involves visualizing the fascia and then passing a peritoneal lavage catheter through the fascia blindly. The procedure is useful in the obese patient.

Results

Results of peritoneal tap and lavage are 97% accurate, with a false positive rate of 1% (12). The red cell count in a patient with blunt trauma is considered positive with $>100,000$ RBC/mm^3 and equivocal with 50,000–100,000 RBC/mm^3. In a patient with penetrating trauma, $>20,000$ RBC/mm^3 is considered positive; whereas, 10,000–20,000 RBC/mm^3 is considered equivocal. A WBC count >500 WBC/mm^3 is positive, and one of 100–500 WBC/mm^3 is equivocal. A positive DPL is indicated by the presence of stool or particulate matter, bile, bacteria on a Gram's stain, or an amylase concentration >175 U/dL (13).

SUMMARY

- Use lumbar puncture to diagnose CNS infection, subarachnoid hemorrhage, or demyelination.
- Use lumbar puncture to administer antibiotics, analgesics, or chemotherapy.
- Do not perform lumbar puncture in patients with elevated ICP, coagulopathy, or local skin infection.

- Perform lumbar puncture at the L3–4 or the L4–5 interspace.
- Perform thoracentesis for diagnosis or treatment of pleural effusion. Loculated effusions may require ultrasound or CT localization.
- When performing thoracentesis or thoracostomy, enter the pleural cavity over the superior edge of the rib that defines the lower border of the selected intercostal space.
- Perform thoracostomy for pneumothorax, hemothoax, pneumohemothorax, chylothorax, or empyema.
- Use large-caliber tubes (36–40 Fr) for drainage of hemothorax.
- Perform paracentesis for diagnosis of ascites, diagnosis of abdominal sepsis, or treatment of refractory ascites.
- Avoid performing paracentesis in patients with multiple previous operations, massive bowel distention, abdominal wall cellulitis, or pregnancy.
- Perform peritoneal lavage in evaluation of blunt trauma or penetrating trauma. Consider peritoneal lavage in diagnosing abdominal pathology in high-risk patients with equivocal signs and symptoms.
- Use caution in patients with previous abdominal surgery.
- Do not perform peritoneal lavage in patients with a definite indication for laparotomy.

REFERENCES

1. Brown DL, Flynn JF. Lumbar punture and epidural analgesia in the ICU. In: Taylor RW, Civetta JM, Kirby RR, eds. Techniques and Procedures in Critical Care. Philadelphia: JB Lippincott, 1990:388–399.
2. Gorelick PE, Biller J. Lumbar puncture: technique, indications, and complications. Postgrad Med 1986; 79(8):257–266.
3. Marton KI, Gean AD. The spinal tap: a new look at an old test. Ann Intern Med 1986; 104:840–848.
4. Edelson RN, Chernick NL, Posnen JB, et al. Spinal subdural hematomas complicating lumbar puncture: occurrence in thrombocytopenic patients. Arch Neurol 1974; 31:134–137.
5. Dalbec DL, Krome RL. Thoracostomy. Emerg Med Clin North Am 1986; 4:441–457.
6. Yeston NS, Niehoff JM. Important procedures in the intensive care unit. In: Taylor RW, Civetta JM, Kirby RR, eds. Techniques and Procedures in Critical Care. Philadelphia: JB Lippincott, 1990:295–345.
7. Fraser RS. Lung perforation complicating tube thoracostomy: pathologic description of three cases. Hum Pathol 1988; 19:518–523.
8. Miller KS, Sahn S. Chest tubes: indications, techniques, management and complications. Chest 1987; 91:258–264.
9. Daly RC, Mucha P, Pairolero PC, et al. The risk of percutaneous chest tube thoracostomy of blunt thoracic trauma. Ann Emerg Med 1985; 14:865–870.
10. Halejian BA, Badach MJ, Trilles F, et al. Maintaining chest tube patency. Surg Gynecol Obstet 1988; 167:521–522.
11. Richardson JD, Flint LM, Polk HC, et al. Peritoneal lavage: a useful diagnostic adjunct for peritonitis. Surgery 1983; 94:826–829.
12. Powell DC, Bivins BA, Bell RM, et al. Diagonostic peritoneal lavage. Surg Gynecol Obstet 1982; 155:257–264.
13. Danto L. Paracentesis and diagnostic peritoneal lavage. In: Blaisdell FW, Traukey DD, eds. Trauma Management, Vol. 1. Abdominal Trauma. New York: Thieme-Medical, 1982:45–57.

Part VI

Measurement and Interpretation of Data

60
Blood Pressure Monitoring

Jerome H. Abrams
VA Medical Center, Minneapolis, Minnesota, USA

The use of indwelling pressure monitoring catheters is widespread in the SICU. Clinicians rely on accurate blood pressure measurements from the arteries and the heart to support oxygen delivery and organ function. Although blood pressure measurements alone do not provide information about blood flow, optimum outcome requires combined blood pressure, blood volume, and blood flow information (1–3).

Invasive pressure monitoring presents certain problems to the clinician. Most clinicians can recall instances when the blood pressure measured by the arterial line disagreed by 15 mm Hg or more with the value obtained by a blood pressure cuff. Which is the correct value? Are all indwelling catheters accurate? The answers to these questions require familiarity with resonance and damping.

DAMPED OSCILLATING SYSTEMS: RESONANCE

The phenomenon of resonance can be very important: one need only ask the designers of the Tacoma Narrows Bridge, which was destroyed when the wind excited its resonance frequencies and caused high-amplitude vibrations of the bridge roadway (4,5) (Fig. 1). Any damped system that oscillates can demonstrate resonance—the production of large-amplitude vibrations in response to a succession of small impulses applied at the proper time. The frequency at which the forced oscillations have their maximum amplitude is termed the resonance frequency (Fig. 2). Resonance can occur in clinical practice, for example, in peripheral and pulmonary artery blood pressure monitoring systems. In such situations, resonance can produce artificially high blood pressure peaks. Commercial electronic monitors cannot detect the presence of resonance and may give elevated readings, 15 mm Hg or above the correct reading (6).

The peripheral and pulmonary arterial pressure measuring systems may be described as a damped harmonic oscillator. An oscillating system of mass (m) with a sinusoidal driving force $F(t)$, a linear restoring force (kx) or spring constant, and a damping force (cx) conforms to the following equation (7):

$$m\ddot{x} + c\dot{x} + kx = F(t)$$

From this relationship, a plot of amplitude ratio vs. frequency ratio may be obtained. The amplitude ratio is the amplitude of the damped system divided by that of an undamped

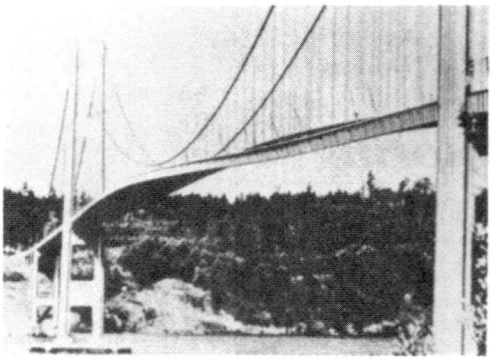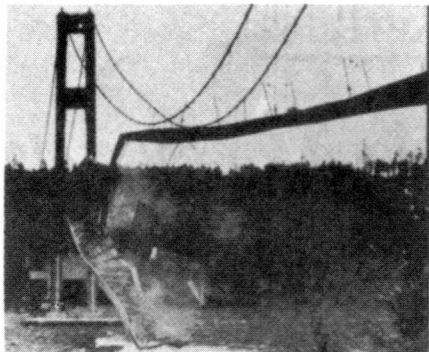

Figure 1 On July 1, 1940, the Tacoma Narrows Bridge at Puget sound, Washington, was completed and opened to traffic. Just 4 months later, a mild gale set the bridge oscillating until the main span broke up, ripping loose from the cables and crashing into the water below. The wind produced a fluctuating resultant force in resonance with a natural frequency of the structure. This caused a steady increase in amplitude until the bridge was destroyed. Many other bridges were later redesigned to make them aerodynamically stable. [From Ref. (4).]

reference system, and the frequency ratio is the driving frequency divided by the resonance frequency of the system. The family of curves obtained, which can be verified experimentally (8), is shown in Fig. 3. Several features should be noted. First, the damping coefficient (h) can be determined by varying the frequency over a sufficiently wide range and examining the amplitude of a test system compared to a reference system. Second, if the resonance frequency is sufficiently large, its effect on the system may be small. In other words, if the resonance frequency is far from the frequency to be measured, little effect of resonance will be seen. Third, no increase in the amplitude ratio will occur at

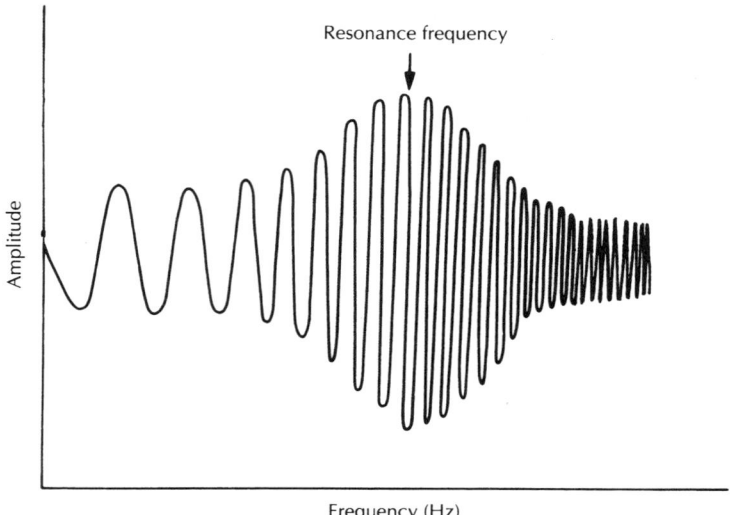

Figure 2 Amplitude vs. frequency of driving force. [From Ref. (11).]

Blood Pressure Monitoring

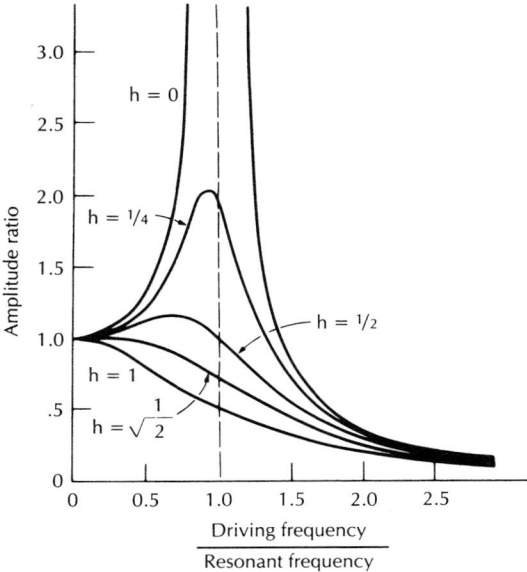

Figure 3 Amplitude ratio vs. frequency ratio. [From Ref. (11).]

any frequency if the value of the damping coefficient is $1/\sqrt{2}$, approximately 0.707, or greater. With these considerations, if one wishes to measure a quantity whose frequency falls in the range of the resonance frequency of the measuring system, the situation can be improved by increasing the damping of the measuring system. The resonance frequency of the patient's catheter monitoring system is fixed by the length, diameter, and compliance of the connecting tubing and by the nature of the pressure transducer. Do the commonly found pressure measuring systems in clinical use have favorable frequency characteristics? To answer this question, one needs to know both their resonance frequencies and their damping coefficients.

MEASURING DAMPING COEFFICIENT

Theory

How might the resonance frequencies and the damping coefficients be obtained? The frequency–amplitude response curves in Fig. 3 show one method of evaluating these two variables. The resonance frequency can be determined from the amplitude maximum as the system is driven over an appropriate frequency range. A damping coefficient (h) can be obtained from:

$$h = \left(\frac{1 - w_r^2/w_u^2}{2}\right)^{1/2}$$

where w_r is the resonance frequency of the damped system and w_u is the frequency at which the phase lag is 90°. Generally, a frequency range of 10× the fundamental

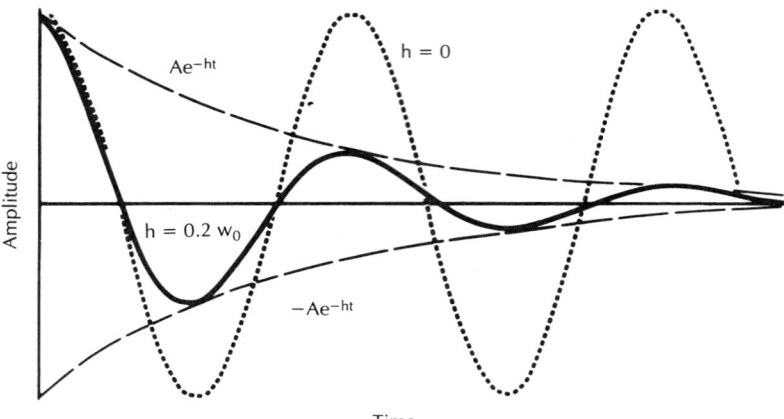

Figure 4 Amplitude vs. time for decay of a free vibration: h, damping coefficient; w_0, natural frequency in absence of damping. [From Ref. (11).]

frequency allows for reasonable approximations of the blood pressure waveform (9). Since the fundamental frequency is heart rate, ~2 Hz, a frequency range of 0–20 Hz should be adequate. Another method is the decay of the step impulse or the square-wave impulse (10), the clinical analog of which is the snap test (Fig. 4). It can be noted the rate of decay of the impulse falls within an envelope that may be modeled as an exponential. The damping coefficient (h) may be obtained from:

$$h = \left[\frac{[\ln(x_2/x_1)]^2}{\pi^2 + [\ln(x_2/x_1)]^2} \right]^{1/2}$$

where x_1 is the amplitude of the first peak above the amplitude of the square-wave impulse, and x_2 the amplitude of the second peak above the amplitude of the square-wave impulse.

Clinical Application

Do the usual blood pressure monitoring configurations in common use have adequate frequency characteristics? If not, can their measuring performance be improved? Damping coefficients have been measured by the two methods described here in systems used in actual clinical practice for blood pressure measurement (11). A snap test was used to adjust damping. In the snap test, a shunt positioned around the capillary device that allows for continuous flushing of the arterial line is quickly opened and suddenly occluded. A variable-resistance damping device (Fig. 5), one method for adding damping, was then manipulated to allow for ~5–7% overshoot with respect to the steady-state response to the step impulse. The variable resistor was adjusted without any knowledge of patient's blood pressure. This device can be easily placed in the monitoring system and readily adjusted to produce a satisfactory step-impulse response, or square-wave test (Fig. 6), of the pressure monitoring system. Measurement of the damping coefficient and the resonance frequency both before and after adding auxiliary damping allowed evaluation of the increase in damping that was caused by the variable resistance.

Blood Pressure Monitoring

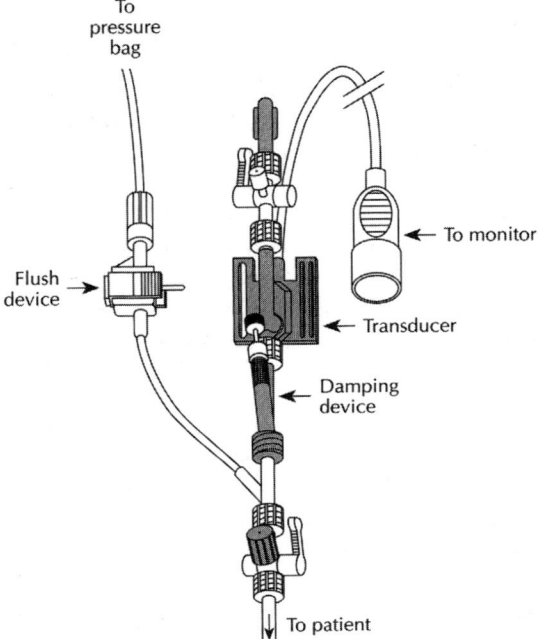

Figure 5 Location of variable resistor in monitoring system. (Courtesy of Cardiorespiratory Services, University of Minnesota, MN.)

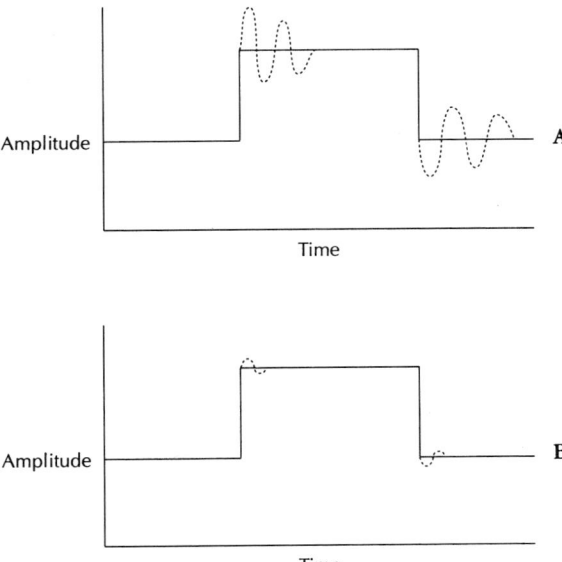

Figure 6 Square-wave test: (A) no auxiliary damping; and (B) auxiliary damping added.

In commonly used arterial blood pressure monitoring systems without additional damping, arterial line pressure was often higher than cuff blood pressure. After adjustment of the variable resistor to more closely approximate a square-wave without knowledge of the patient's blood pressure, the arterial line and cuff blood pressures agreed well. Without additional damping, the resonance frequency of the measuring system was in some cases only twice the fundamental frequency, the heart rate. In nearly all cases, an increase in damping was required to approximate a square-wave without excessive ringing. An example of a pressure waveform from the pulmonary artery, before and after the addition of damping, is shown in Fig. 7. An example of a radial artery pressure waveform, also before and after additional damping, is shown in Fig. 8.

What should a damping coefficient be in clinical practice? Probably everyone agrees that a pressure measuring system is functioning properly if the input of a square-wave results in the output, by the measure system, of an identical square-wave. Such a result

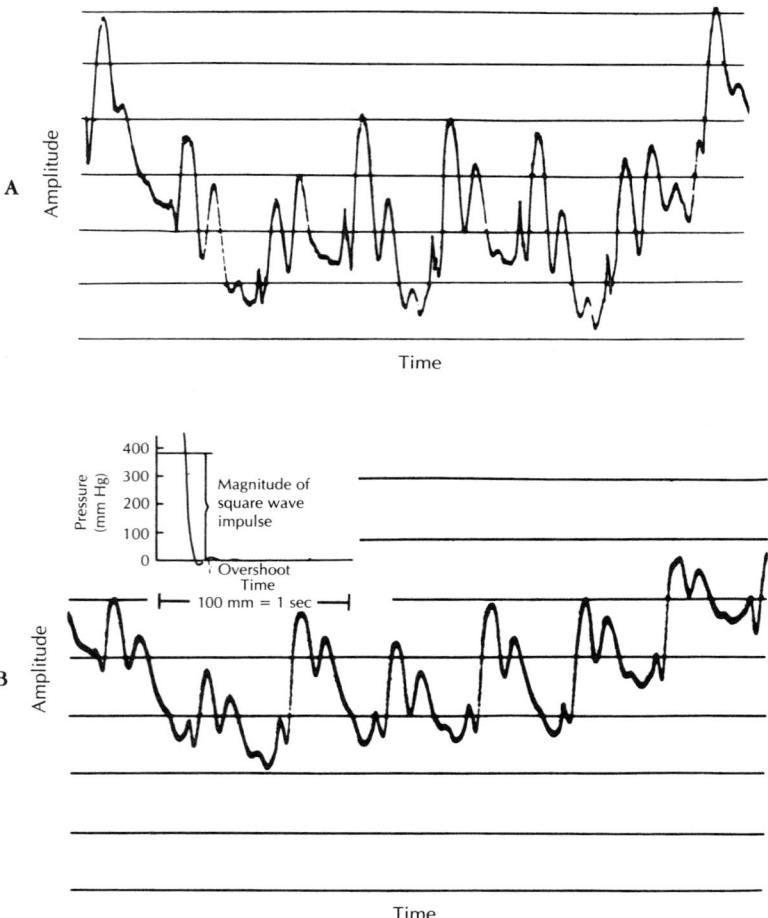

Figure 7 (A) Uncorrected pulmonary artery tracing; resonance frequency, 5 Hz; damping coefficient, 0.38. (B) Corrected pulmonary artery tracing; damping coefficient, 0.67. Inset shows bedside snap test. [From Ref. (11).]

Blood Pressure Monitoring

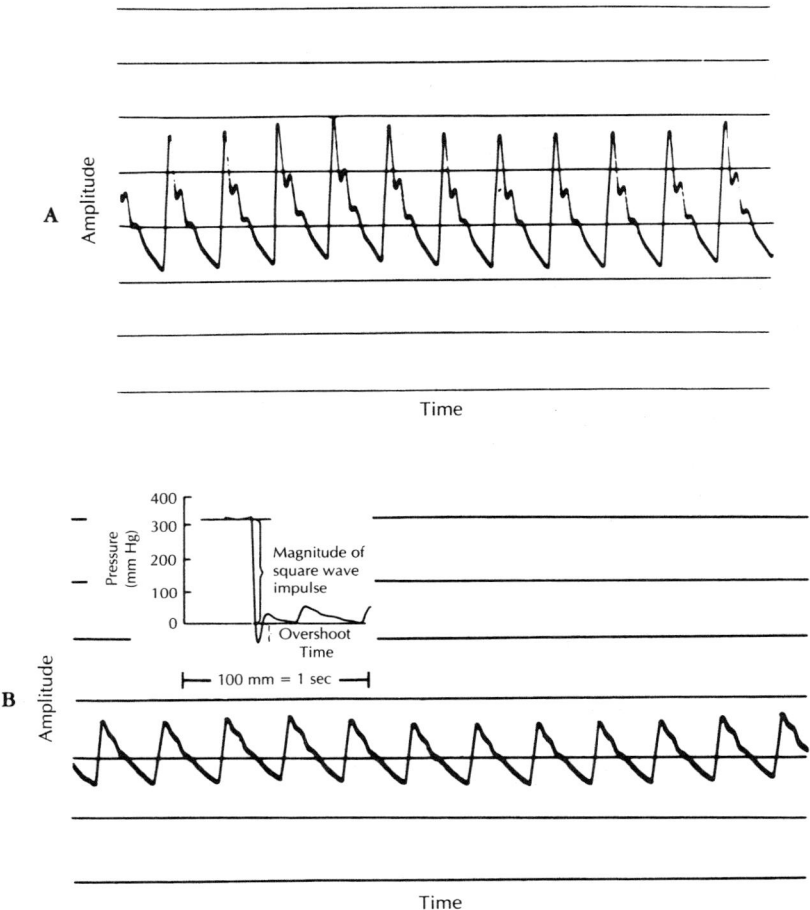

Figure 8 (A) Uncorrected radial artery tracing; resonance frequency, 12.7 Hz; damping coefficient, 0.15. (B) Corrected radial artery tracing; damping coefficient, 0.49. Inset shows bedside snap test. [From Ref. (11).]

is impossible in a damped oscillator. If the system is underdamped, the amount of overshoot will be unacceptably high. If the system is overdamped, it will take an unacceptably long time to reach the amplitude of the input pressure. Therefore, a compromise must be reached.

As the damping coefficient is increased, the time response also increases (Fig. 9). The optimum compromise between damping and time response depends on the context. In clinical practice, decisions are nearly always made on the basis of the pressure magnitude averaged over several hundred heartbeats. Few clinical decisions are made that require fractional-second time response in the blood pressure measurement. In clinical practice, a reasonable compromise is minimizing overshoot rather than minimizing response time. A damping coefficient in the range 0.5–0.75 has proved satisfactory. This seemingly wide range is related to the wide range of resonance frequency in the

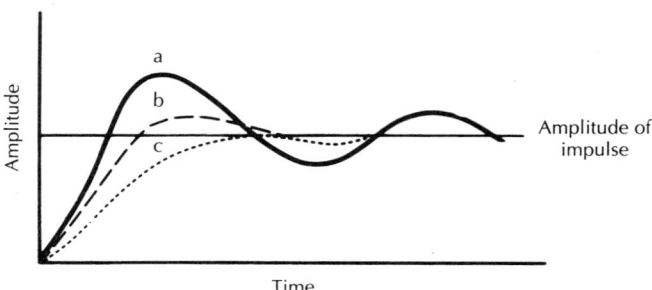

Figure 9 Amplitude vs. time. Damping coefficient is such that damping for system $a < b < c$. [From Ref. (11).]

tubing configurations in common use: the higher the resonance frequency of the tubing configuration, the lower the damping coefficient may be.

If an auxiliary damping device is not available, an alternative is the return-to-flow systolic pressure measurement. In this procedure, a manual inflation blood pressure cuff is placed on the extremity with the arterial line. The blood pressure cuff is inflated until the arterial pressure waveform is flattened. The cuff is then slowly deflated. The pressure that appears on the manual blood pressure cuff when the first evidence of arterial pulsation appears on the monitor is taken as the correct systolic blood pressure (12).

SUMMARY

- Standard pressure measurement systems are frequently underdamped; as a result, pressure values may be artificially high.
- Resonance frequency of these pressure monitoring systems is often in the range of physiologic interest.
- A variable resistor or other damping device improves accuracy of blood-pressure amplitude measurement when invasive blood-pressure monitoring is used.
- Improved amplitude transmission is obtained by degrading time response, but the results are clinically useful.
- Damping may be successfully added in actual clinical practice with simple devices.
- Calibration of the pressure monitoring system using a step-impulse test can be done easily at the patient's bedside. In the absence of an auxiliary damping device, return-to-flow systolic blood pressure measurement may be used for calibration.

REFERENCES

1. Shoemaker WC, Appel PL, Bland RD. Use of physiologic monitoring to predict outcome and to assist in clinical decisions in critically ill postoperative patients. Am J Surg 1983; 146:43–50.
2. Shoemaker WC. Hemodynamic and oxygen transport patterns is septic shock: physiologic mechanisms and therapeutic implications. In: Sibbald WJ, Sprung CL, eds. Perspectives on Sepsis and Septic Shock. Fullerton, CA: Society of Critical Care Medicine, 1986:203–234.

3. Abrams JH, Brake RA, Cerra FB. Quantitative evaluation of the clinical course of septic patients: the data conform to catastrophe theory. J Trauma 1984; 24:1028–1037.
4. Resnick R, Halliday D. Physics, Part I. New York: John Wiley, 1967:372.
5. Braun M. Differential Equations and Their Applications, 3rd ed. New York: Springer-Verlag, 1983:167–173.
6. Gardner RM. Direct blood pressure measurement—dynamic response requirements. Anesthesiology 1981; 54:227–236.
7. Fry DL. Physiologic recordings by modern instruments with particular reference to pressure recording. Physiol Rev 1960; 40:753–788.
8. Wylie CR. Advanced Engineering Mathematics. New York: McGraw-Hill, 1975:186.
9. Shinozaki T, Deane RS, Mazuzan JE. The dynamic responses of liquid-filled catheter systems for direct measurement of blood pressure. Anesthesiology 1980; 53:498–504.
10. Marion JB. Classical Dynamics of Particles and Systems. New York: Academic Press, 1970:287.
11. Abrams JH, Olson MI, Marino JA, Cerra FB. Use of a needle valve variable resistor to improve invasive blood pressure monitoring. Crit Care Med 1984; 12:978–982.
12. Zimmerman JL, Taylor RW, Dellinger RP, Farmer JC. Basic Hemodynamic Monitoring. Fundamental Critical Care Support. Anaheim: Society of Critical Care Medicine, 1996:58.

61
Cardiac Output

Jerome H. Abrams
VA Medical Center, Minneapolis, Minnesota, USA

The use of invasive hemodynamic monitoring in the SICU remains controversial. Singer, in an insightful review of cardiac output determination and significance, recalls the statement of Karl Ludwig: "The fundamental problems in the circulation derive from the fact that the supply of adequate amounts of blood to the organs of the body is the main purpose of the circulation while the pressures that are necessary to achieve it are of secondary importance; but the measurement of flow is difficult while that of pressure is easy so that our knowledge of flow is usually derivatory (1)." Although the technology for measuring flow exists, the value of measuring flow in improving outcomes continues to be contentious. In several studies of high-risk surgery patients, increasing oxygen transport preoperatively by manipulating cardiac output resulted in significantly better outcomes (2–4). In the critically ill patient, data are contradictory. Chapter 63 provides a review and analysis of flow manipulation in the critically ill patient.

In our practice, the use of invasive hemodynamic monitoring falls into three general categories: restoration of oxygen transport, optimization of specific organ function, and preoperative cardiac evaluation. Restoration of oxygen transport, described in Chapter 2, requires measurement of cardiac output to determine both oxygen consumption and oxygen delivery. Optimization of specific organ function is a theme of several chapters in this book. For example, the presence of pulmonary edema in the patient with renal insufficiency and known congestive heart failure who sustains a septic insult provides a challenging problem. Is the extravascular lung water a consequence of intravascular volume excess or the systemic inflammatory response? Is the renal insufficiency a result of intravascular volume depletion or acute tubular necrosis? Is systemic perfusion adequate? Should treatment include diuresis to decrease extravascular lung water or should preload be replaced to correct renal failure from prerenal causes? In the setting of the conflicting demands of the different major organ systems, invasive hemodynamic monitoring can help to answer these questions. Preoperatively, knowledge of left-ventricular function is refined by measuring cardiac output and correlating it with the pressures necessary to produce that flow. Information about systolic function, diastolic function, and systemic response to stress is obtainable, in part, through measurement of cardiac output. The use of invasive hemodynamic monitoring preoperatively to reduce perioperative cardiac morbidity is discussed in Chapter 8.

In the SICU, the most commonly used procedure for clinical measurement of cardiac output is thermodilution. Thermodilution measurements are an extension of the Fick principle. This chapter considers the Fick principle, thermodilution cardiac output, and other procedures, which may enjoy wider use in the future. As thermodilution measurements are an extension of the Fick principle, an understanding of this principle is important for a better appreciation of the foundations of thermodilution measurements.

THE FICK PRINCIPLE

The Fick principle states that the total uptake or release of a substance by an organ is the product of blood flow to the organ and the arteriovenous concentration difference of the substance (5).

In the direct Fick method, oxygen consumption ($\dot{V}O_2$) and the arteriovenous oxygen content difference ($CaO_2 - C\bar{v}O_2$) determine cardiac output from the relation (6):

$$CO = \frac{\dot{V}O_2}{CaO_2 - C\bar{v}O_2} \times 10$$

The factor of 10 is necessary to maintain consistent units.

In the absence of intracardiac shunt, and if pulmonary blood flow equals systemic blood flow, the direct Fick method can be used to measure cardiac output. The measurement requires determination of oxygen consumption, arterial oxygen content, and mixed venous oxygen content. Methods for direct determination of oxygen consumption include collection of expired gas using a Douglas bag or analysis of oxygen consumption by the metabolic rate cart. Arterial oxygen content measurement is routinely done in most hospitals. Measurement of mixed venous oxygen content requires catheterization of the pulmonary artery. Under steady-state conditions, the Fick method provides reproducible cardiac outputs with a standard error of ~7% of the average value (7–9).

Sources of error are largely a result of technical problems in expired gas sampling, expired gas collection, or the inability to achieve a steady state. If the Douglas bag method of expired gas sampling is used, incomplete collection will produce a measured cardiac output that is lower than the actual cardiac output. Another source of error arises from the absence of stable pulmonary volume during the measurement interval. Both the Douglas bag and the metabolic rate cart measure uptake of oxygen by the lungs. If the lung, acting as a reservoir, were to trap gas during the measurement, uptake of oxygen by the circulation might not equal that of the lung. Another source of error arises from the respiratory quotient. As the volume of expired carbon dioxide does not equal the volume of oxygen consumed in the same interval, failure to use the respiratory quotient introduces some error into the cardiac output determination (5).

An extension of the Fick principle is the indicator dilution procedure. In the direct Fick method, the indicator is oxygen and the injection site is the lung. A continuous infusion of oxygen is the injection procedure. In the indicator dilution methods, an appropriate indicator is chosen, the injection site is usually a proximal vessel or chamber of the heart, and either continuous or bolus injection is done.

The most widely used indicator in clinical practice is temperature, and the bolus injection procedure is the norm. The use of indocyanine green, another indicator, involves a continuous infusion procedure. For indicator dilution procedures to be successful, certain requirements must be met (5):

1. The indicator is nontoxic, mixed completely with blood, and can be measured with sufficient accuracy.
2. The indicator substance, once injected, is not lost or metabolized before it reaches the detector.
3. The indicator flows past the detector before recirculation begins.
4. The indicator substance mixes thoroughly.

To perform thermodilution measurements, the clinician most commonly places a thermistor-equipped pulmonary artery catheter (Fig. 1). A thermal indicator, usually iced or room temperature saline, is injected into the right atrial port. The thermal indicator mixes and is detected downstream by the thermistor. Hamilton et al. (10) observed that the amount of an appropriate indicator detected downstream from the site of injection is equal to the product of cardiac output and the integrated change in concentration for the duration of the measurement. Cardiac output can be calculated from:

$$I = \text{CO} \int_0^\infty C(t)\,dt$$

Rearranging as:

$$\text{CO} = \frac{I}{\int_0^\infty C(t)\,dt}$$

where CO is the cardiac output; I, the amount of indicator; and $C(t)$, the concentration of indicator as a function of time. An example of an indicator dilution curve is shown in Fig. 2.

A bolus of cold solution produces a time–temperature curve that is similar to the time–concentration curve of, for example, indocyanine green dye (11). For measurement

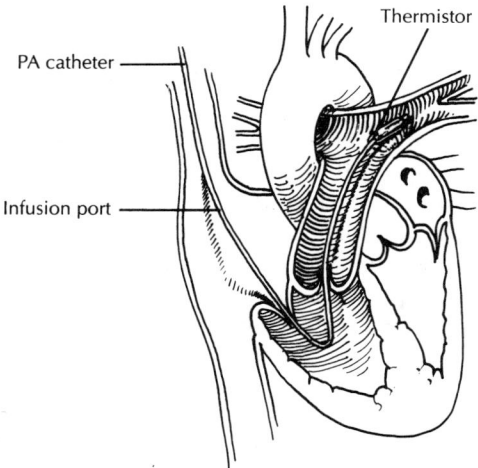

Figure 1 Position of pulmonary artery catheter for measurement of cardiac output.

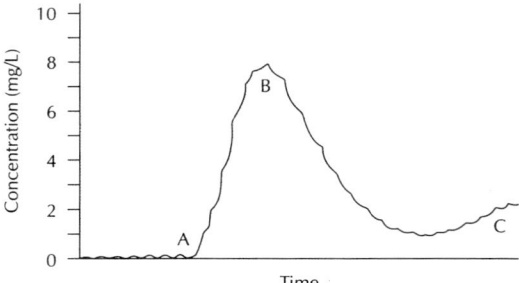

Figure 2 Indicator dilution concentration curve in a patient with normal cardiac output: 1 mL of indocyanine green dye solution (5.0 mg/mL) was injected into pulmonary artery at time zero. Blood was withdrawn continuously from brachial artery through a densitometer cuvette, and a time–concentration curve from densitometer was recorded. First appearance (A) is followed by a steep rise to peak concentration (B), and subsequent gradual decline of indicator curve, which is interrupted by a secondary rise (C) due to recirculation of indicator substance. [From Ref. (5), p. 114. Reprinted with permission.]

of cardiac output by thermodilution, the relation described by Hamilton and colleagues needs modification. As a thermal indicator is used, the volume of injectate (V), the initial blood temperature (T_B), the initial injectate temperature (T_I), a density factor (K_1), and a computation constant (K_2) are used. Then the cardiac output may be calculated as:

$$CO = \frac{V(T_B - T_I)K_1 K_2}{\int_0^\infty \Delta T_B(t)\, dt}$$

The denominator is the integral of temperature change of blood (6). Accuracy of thermodilution, when compared with that of calibrated mechanical pumps, is 7–13% (12,13). For single injections of thermal indicators, differences from calibrated flow were as high as 15–25% (13). Correlation coefficients of 0.96 and 0.91 have been obtained for thermodilution cardiac outputs compared with the direct Fick and indocyanine green methods, respectively (14).

In clinical practice, the error of measurement, when commercially available equipment is used, makes a 12–15% change in cardiac output necessary to be of clinical significance (15). Other clinical variables may affect cardiac output determination by thermodilution. Injection of the thermal indicator at different phases of the respiratory cycle can result in significant variation of the cardiac output (16,17). Errors in the cardiac output determination during rapid intravenous volume infusion have been reported (18). Slowing of the heart rate after injection of iced saline as a thermal indicator also has been reported (19,20).

Careful technique is necessary for minimizing the error with thermodilution. The commercially available cardiac output computers use carefully specified volumes and temperatures of thermal indicator. If the amount of indicator injected is less than that programmed, the cardiac output value will be falsely elevated. Further, if the temperature of the indicator is higher than that programmed, the amount of indicator will appear to the cardiac output computer to be less than that expected. The calculated cardiac output will be similarly elevated. Use of iced saline is more likely to produce the latter type of error. Underestimation of cardiac output occurs when a greater volume of indicator is injected than was programmed (6). In view of these considerations, multiple injections of thermal indicator should be used. With three injections, the probability that the thermodilution cardiac output is within 10% of the true value is 89%. With five injections, a 98% probability exists that the cardiac output is within 10% of the true value (21).

OTHER METHODS OF MEASUREMENT

The error in measurement and the capability of obtaining only intermittent cardiac output measurements with thermal dilution present limitations. Other methods for measuring cardiac output attempt to address these limitations. Thoracic electrical impedance has been used for clinical determination of cardiac output. Using pairs of electrodes placed on the neck, thorax, and the upper abdomen, changes in impedance that result from pulsatile flow in the thoracic aorta are measured (22,23). Stroke volume is determined from several equations, which include correction factors to the relation described by Kubicek in 1966:

$$SV = \rho * \frac{L^2}{Z_0^2} * \left(\frac{dZ}{dt}\right)_{max} * LVET$$

where SV, is the stroke volume; ρ, the resistivity of blood; L, the distance between electrodes, $(dZ/dt)_{max}$, the maximum of first derivative of the impedance signal; and LVET, the left ventricular ejection time.

Ultrasound methods have the potential to provide continuous (beat-to-beat) cardiac outputs and are noninvasive. Cardiac output is the product of blood velocity ($\bar{v}$) and aortic cross-sectional area (A):

$$CO = \bar{v} * A$$

Both $\bar{v}$ and A may be obtained from ultrasound by using both the Doppler principle and ultrasound range gating, respectively. The Doppler principle can evaluate blood velocity ($\bar{v}$) from the velocity of ultrasound in tissue (c), the Doppler shift (Δf), the ultrasound carrier frequency (f_0), and the angle of the ultrasound beam with respect to flow (ϑ) (24–26).

$$\bar{v} = \frac{c\Delta f}{2f_0 \cos \vartheta}$$

Ultrasound range gating can provide a blood vessel diameter. If a circular cross section (A) is assumed, the cross-sectional area required for calculation of cardiac can be found. Different anatomic windows have been used for ultrasound measurements. Cardiac outputs have been obtained transesophageally (27), transtracheally (28,29), and from the suprasternal notch (30). Potential advantages of the transtracheal Doppler procedure include (1) accuracy over a wide range of cardiac outputs, (2) ability to detect changes in flow sensitively, (3) absence of effect on cardiac output by the measurement procedure, (4) ability to measure continuous cardiac output, and (5) low risk.

SUMMARY

- Cardiac output measurements are necessary for restoration of oxygen transport, optimization of specific organ function, and preoperative cardiac evaluation.
- Thermodilution is the most widely used clinical method of determining cardiac output.
- Thermodilution evolved from the Fick principle. Indicator dilution methods estimate cardiac output from the general relationship:

$$CO = \frac{I}{\int_0^\infty C(t)\,dt}$$

- For accurate thermodilution measurements, careful technique, with precise volume and temperature of injectate, is necessary. Five injections per cardiac output determination produce a 90% chance of being with 10% of the true cardiac output value.
- A 12–15% change in cardiac output is necessary to have clinical significance when thermodilution is used in clinical settings.
- Variations in respiration or intravenous volume infusion can introduce error in thermal dilution cardiac output determination.
- Ultrasonic and electrobioimpedance methods show promise for use in continuous noninvasive cardiac output determination.

REFERENCES

1. Singer M. Cardiac output in 1998. Heart 1998; 79:425–428.
2. Shoemaker WC, Appel PL, Kram HB. Prospective trial of supranormal values of survivors as therapeutic goals in high-risk surgical patients. Chest 1988; 94:1176–1186.
3. Boyd O, Grounds RM, Bennet ED. A randomized clinical trial of the effect of deliberate perioperative increase of oxygen delivery on mortality in high-risk surgical patients. J Am Med Assoc 1993; 270:2699–2707.
4. Berlauk JF, Abrams JH, Gilmour IJ, O'Connor R, Knighton DR, Cerra FB. Preoperative optimization of cardiovascular hemodynamics improves outcome in peripheral vascular surgery. Ann Surg 1991; 214:289–299.
5. Grossman W. Blood flow measurement: the cardiac output. In: Grossman W, ed. Cardiac Catherization and Angiography. Philadelphia, PA: Lea & Febiger, 1986:101–117.
6. Thys DM. Cardiac output. Anesthesiol Clin North Am 1998; 6:803–824.
7. Selzer A, Sudrann RB. Reliability of the determination of cardiac output in man by means of the Fick principle. Circ Res 1958; 6:485–490.
8. Thomasson B. Cardiac output in normal subjects under standard basal conditions. Scand J Clin Lab Invest 1957; 9:365–376.
9. Howell CD, Horvath SM. Reproducibility of cardiac output measurements in the dog. J Appl Physiol 1959; 14:421–423.
10. Hamilton WF, Moore JW, Kinsman JM, Spurling RG. Studies on the circulation IV. Further analysis of the injection method, and changes in hemodynamics under physiological and pathological conditions. Am J Physiol 1932; 99:534–551.
11. Fegler G. Measurement of cardiac output in anesthetized animals by a thermodilution method. Q J Exp Physiol 1954; 39:153–164.

12. Salgado CR, Galleti PM. *In vitro* evaluation of the thermodilution technique for the measurement of ventricular stroke volume and end-diastolic volume. Cardiologia 1966; 49:65–78.
13. Bilfinger TV, Lin C-Y, Anagnostopoulos CE. *In vitro* determination of accuracy of cardiac output measurements by thermal dilution. J Surg Res 1982; 33:409–414.
14. Goodyer AVN, Huvos A, Eckhardt WF, Osterberg RH. Thermodilution curves in the intact animal. Circ Res 1959; 7:432–441.
15. Stetz CW, Miller RG, Kelly GE. Reliability of the thermodilution method in the determination of cardiac output in clinical practice. Am Rev Respir Dis 1982; 126:1001–1004.
16. Snyder JF, Powner DJ. Effects of mechanical ventilaion on the measurement of cardiac output by thermodilution. Crit Care Med 1982; 10:677–682.
17. Stevens JH, Raffin TA, Mihm FG. Thermodilution cardiac output measurements. J Am Med Assoc 1985; 253:2240–2242.
18. Wetzel RC, Latson TW. Major errors in thermodilution cardiac output measurement during rapid volume infusion. Anesthesiology 1985; 62:684–687.
19. Nisikawa T, Dohi S. Slowing of heart rate during cardiac output measurement by thermodilution. Anesthesiology 1932; 57:538–539.
20. Harris AP, Miller CF, Battie C. The slowing of sinus rhythm during thermodilution cardiac output determination and the effect of altering injectate temperature. Anesthesiology 1985; 63:540–541.
21. Hoel BL. Some aspects of the clinical use of thermodilution in measuring cardiac output. Scand J Clin Lab Invest 1978; 38:383–388.
22. Kubicek WG, Karegis JN, Patterson RP, Witsoe DA, Mattson RH. Development and evaluation of an impedance cardiac output system. Aerospace Med 1966; 37:1208.
23. Bernstein DP. Continuous non-invasive real-time monitoring of stroke volume and cardiac output by thoracic electrical bio-impedance. Crit Care Med 1986; 14:898–901.
24. Baker DW. Pulsed ultrasonic Doppler blood-flow sensing. IEEE Trans Sonic Ultrasonics. 1970; SU 17:170–185.
25. Hartley CJ, Cole JS. An ultrasonic pulsed Doppler system for measuring blood flow in small vessels. J. Appl Physiol 1974; 37:626–629.
26. Blair AK, Lucas CL, Hsia HS. A removable ultrasound Doppler probe for continuous monitoring of changes in cardiac output. J Ultrasound Med 1983; 2:357–362.
27. Kamal GD, Symreng T, Stan J. Inconsistent esophageal Doppler cardiac output during acute blood loss. Anesthesiology 1990; 72:95–99.
28. Abrams JH, Weber RE, Holmen KD. Transtracheal Doppler: a new procedure for continuous cardiac output measurement. Anesthesiology 1989; 70:134–138.
29. Abrams HJ, Weber RE, Holmen KD. Continuous cardiac output determination using transtracheal Doppler: initial results in humans. Anesthesiology 1989; 71:11–15.
30. Hunstman LL, Stewart DK, Barnes SR. Noninvasive Doppler determination of cardiac output in man. Circulation 1983; 67:593–602.

62

Respiratory Monitoring

Ian J. Gilmour
Anesthesia Associates of Martinsville, Inc., Martinsville, Virginia, USA

In the SICU, gas movement and gas exchange are the determinants of respiratory function. Although performing formal pulmonary function tests before the onset of acute lung injury might be valuable, formal pulmonary function testing is generally not possible in the SICU. As optimal patient management requires information about current lung function, the remaining discussion considers monitoring of gas flow and then gas exchange in the SICU patient. Table 1 lists definitions and gives explanation of acronyms.

Pressure (P), gas flow, and lung volumes are all related. For example, an inverse relationship between lung volume and resistance to flow has been identified Fig. 1. For constant flow, airway resistance is a hyperbolic function of lung volume.

Inspiratory airway resistance to flow in mechanically ventilated patients can be assessed by the following relationship:

$$R = \frac{\Delta P}{V} \tag{1}$$

where R is resistance, ΔP is $P_{AO} - P_{ALV}$, and V is flow.

Direct measurement of R requires measurement of both pressure gradient and gas flow. Measurement of both P_{ALV} and gas flow is extremely difficult. P_{ALV} is usually estimated by interrupting flow and measuring airway pressure at zero flow; if flow is truly zero, airway pressure will be the same as P_{ALV}.

In patients with severe obstructive lung disease (OLD), the zero flow requirement probably will not be met, and airway pressure does not represent P_{ALV}. Because of these limitations, calculation of actual inspiratory resistance is not commonly undertaken in clinical medicine. Measurement of expiratory resistance is more difficult, because flow rate during expiration is not constant: lung elastic recoil, the driving force, is a nonlinear function of lung volume.

If it is assumed that flow is constant during inspiration, R can be estimated using pressures obtained from the ventilator's manometer. Two of these pressures are the pressure at which inspiration is initiated [positive end-expiratory pressure (PEEP)] and P_{max}. The difference between P_{max} and PEEP is the pressure required to overcome resistance in the airway and to inflate the lungs. End-inspiratory pressure (P_{ei}) can also be obtained easily. The difference between P_{max} and P_{ei} (ΔP) approximates the pressure required to overcome resistance in the system (i.e., ventilator circuit, endotracheal tube, and

Table 1 Glossary of Respiratory Terms

Term or abbreviation	Definition
Restrictive lung disease (RLD)	Abnormality of lung parenchyma or chest wall that results in a decrease in TLC
Obstructive lung disease (OLD)	Lung disease resulting from increased resistance to flow in the tracheobronchial tree
Static lung volume	Lung volume that does not change during ventilation (e.g., functional residual capacity, residual volume)
Dynamic lung volume	Lung volume that changes with ventilation (e.g., IC, VT, VC)
Resistance (R)	Application of Ohm's law; pressure drop per unit flow
Compliance (C)	Change in volume per unit change in pressure
P_{max}	Peak airway pressure achieved on inspiration during positive pressure ventilation; reflects both resistance and compliance
P_{ei}	End-inspiratory pressure; pressure at end inspiration with no gas flow; reflects elastic recoil of the respiratory system (i.e., compliance); also called plateau pressure
Auto-PEEP	Intrinsic positive end-expiratory pressure (PEEP); an increase in airway pressure that occurs because emptying of the lung is incomplete; thought to reflect P_{ALV}
P_{ALV}	Alveolar pressure: driving pressure for exhalation
P_{PL}	Pleural pressure; most commonly measured indirectly by esophogeal balloon
CCO_2	Oxygen content of blood in pulmonary capillaries
CaO_2	Oxygen content of arterial blood
$C\bar{V}O_2$	Oxygen content of mixed venous blood
PAO	Pressure at the airway opening (i.e., endotracheal tube, mouth)
V_T	Tidal volume (see Fig. 4)
IC	Inspiratory capacity (see Fig. 4)
VC	Vital capacity (see Fig. 4)
TLC	Total lung capacity (see Fig. 4)
C_L	Lung compliance
C_{CW}	Chest wall compliance
C_{RS}	Compliance of respiratory system
V	Flow
$\dot{V}_A$	Alveolar ventilation per minute
$\dot{V}_E$	Total minute ventilation (respiratory rate × V_T)
A-aDO_2	Difference between alveolar oxygen tension (PAO_2) and arterial oxygen tension (PaO_2)
FIO_2	Fraction of inspired oxygen
PIO_2	Partial pressure of inspired oxygen

tracheobronchial tree). Although not identical to $P_{AO} - P_{ALV}$ [Eq. (1)], ΔP is suitable for clinical use. As the contribution of the ventilator circuit and the endotracheal tube remains constant, changes in ΔP at constant inspiratory flow and volume represent changes in R within the tracheobronchial tree; thus ΔP can be used as an approximation of resistance, and changes in P represent changes in R. For example, the effect of bronchodilators can be assessed by noting ΔP before and after their administration. For these comparisons to be meaningful, inspiratory flow rate must be kept constant, because flow changes will affect ΔP (1).

Respiratory Monitoring

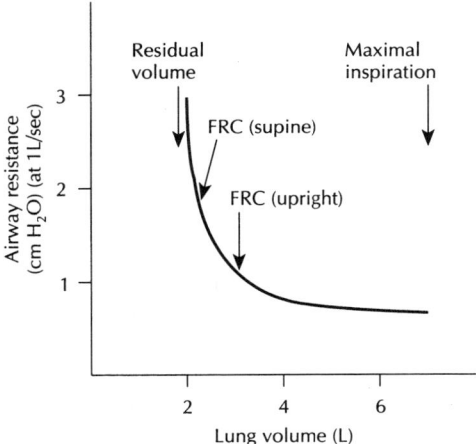

Figure 1 Airway resistance is an increasing hyperbolic function of decreasing lung volume. Functional residual capacity (FRC) decreases with changing from upright to supine position. (From Nunn JF. Applied Respiratory Physiology, 3rd ed. London: Butterworth-Heinemann Limited, 1987:64.)

Most modern ventilators offer a choice of flow patterns. Assuming that flow actually is constant for a square-wave flow pattern, square-wave flow patterns, if available, should be used for R estimates. With a square-wave flow of 40–60 L/min in patients with endotracheal tubes of reasonable size (7–7.5 mm in adult females; 8–8.5 mm in adult males), a ΔP of <5 cm H_2O can be expected. ΔP greater than this value suggests that resistance to flow pattern is not available, ΔP will not correlate well with R, but changes in ΔP from one situation to the next, assuming constant flow and volume, will correspond to changes in R. As P_{max} represents all the work required to inflate the lung, ventilatory efforts by the patient may either exaggerate or cause underestimation of ΔP.

Auto-PEEP is usually defined as airway pressure higher than preset machine PEEP at end expiration and is thought to reflect an elevated P_{ALV} caused by incomplete emptying of the lung (Fig. 2). The presence of intrinsic PEEP or auto-PEEP is thought to reflect

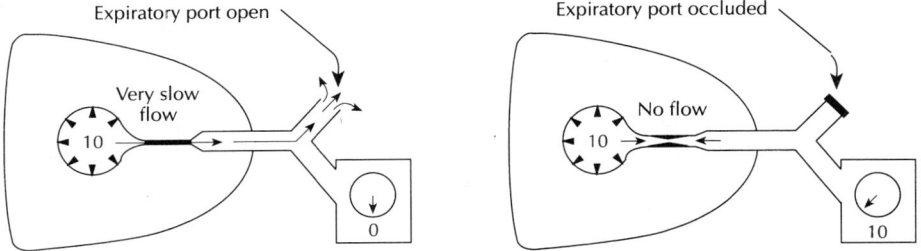

Figure 2 Auto-PEEP effect and its measurement. In presence of severe airflow obstruction and high ventilation requirements, alveolar pressure at end exhalation remains elevated as flow continues throughout expiration, driven by recoil pressure of hyperexpanded lung (left). Transiently stopping flow at end exhalation allows equilibration of pressure throughout circuit. Occult alveolar pressure is then detectable on ventilator manometer. (From Marini JJ, Wheeler AD. Respiratory Monitoring in Critical Care Medicine: The Essentials. Baltimore: Williams & Wilkins, 1989:47–60.)

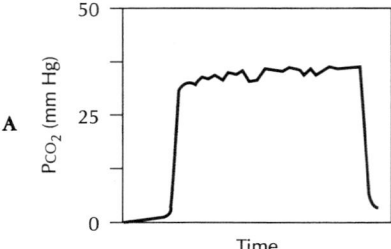 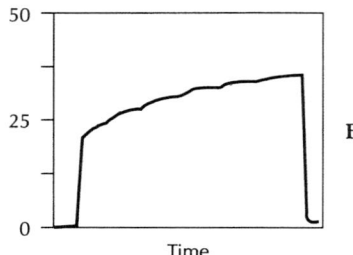

Figure 3 Examples of capnograph waveforms. (A) Normal tracing. (B) Increased slope of phase III, usually representing uneven gas mixing within lung. See also Fig. 8. (From Moon RE, Camporesi EM. Respiratory monitoring in anesthesia. In: Miller RD, ed. Anesthesia, 3rd ed. New York: Churchill Livingstone, 1990:1146.)

increased resistance (2). Auto-PEEP is most often seen in patients with OLD but can be caused by anything that increases resistance, such as a pinched or obstructed endotracheal tube, or by an excessive respiratory rate.

A capnograph, if available, may indicate abnormal airway resistance. An increased slope, coupled with a large gradient between partial pressure of end-tidal carbon dioxide ($PetCO_2$) and partial pressure of carbon dioxide ($PaCO_2$) is often seen with OLD (3) (Fig. 3).

Pressure measurements can also be useful during weaning. Maximum inspiratory pressure (MIP; also called negative inspiratory force) has long been used to assess the instantaneous strength of inspiratory muscles. To determine MIP, the airway is occluded for 20–25 s at end expiration to insure maximal effort. A pressure more negative than -30 cm H_2O (in this case the more negative, the better) is a favorable indication for weaning. Note that a satisfactory MIP does not guarantee that the patient will be able to sustain adequate ventilation.

MONITORING LUNG VOLUMES

Most acute pulmonary dysfunction is restrictive and usually associated with decreases of both static and dynamic lung volumes (Fig. 4). In most instances, restrictive lung disease (RLD) is caused by lung parenchymal disease [adult respiratory distress syndrome (ARDS), atelectasis]. RLD may also arise from problems in the pleural space (hemothorax, pneumothorax), the chest wall (ascites, obesity), or neuromuscular disease (Guillain-Barré). Preexisting pulmonary disease compounds and confuses the problem.

Ventilator spirometers can be used to measure spontaneous IC or VC, measurements that are useful in weaning. Note that inspiratory capacity (IC) or vital capacity (VC) cannot be measured in the sedated, unconscious, or paralyzed SICU patient, and attempts to do so are potentially dangerous. Ventilator spirometers can also provide a reasonably accurate estimate of tidal volume (V_T) which may be used to calculate total minute ventilation ($\dot{V}_E$). $\dot{V}_E$ is affected by both metabolic rate and lung function: increases in either metabolic rate or dead space demand a greater $\dot{V}_E$ to maintain normal $PaCO_2$. $\dot{V}_E$ also can be used to assess the probability of weaning a patient from mechanical ventilation. Many patients are unable to maintain the level of respiratory work required when spontaneous $\dot{V}_E > 10$ L/min.

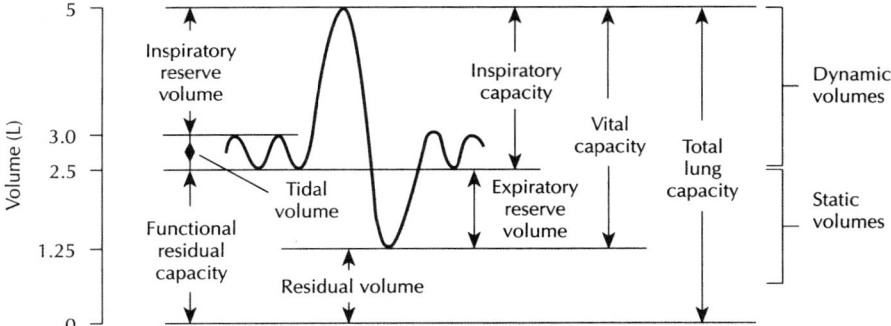

Figure 4 Dynamic lung volumes that can be measured by simple spirometry are tidal volume, inspiratory reserve volume, expiratory reserve volume, inspiratory capacity, and vital capacity. Static lung volumes are residual volume, FRC, and total lung capacity. Static lung volumes cannot be measured by observation of a spirometer trace and require separate methods of measurement. (From Benumof JL. Respiratory physiology and respiratory function during anesthesia. In: Miller RD, ed. Anesthesia, 3rd ed. New York: Churchill Livingstone, 1990:519.)

Ventilator-recorded V_T also can be used for compliance measurements. Compliance measures the stiffness of the lung and/or chest wall. Generally, the lower the lung compliance (C_L) the more severe is the degree of dysfunction.

$$C_{RS} = \frac{\Delta V}{\Delta P} \qquad (2)$$

where C_{RS} is the compliance of the respiratory system, ΔV is V_T, and ΔP is P_{ei} − PEEP.

Compliance is measured in L/cm H_2O or mL/cm H_2O. When C_{RS} is <40 mL/cm H_2O, respiratory work is markedly increased, and mechanical ventilation is often required. To use V_T in compliance measurements, it must be recalled that a portion of each V_T distends and is compressed within the ventilator circuitry. Although this volume is measured by the spirometer, it is not delivered to the patient. Volume lost this way is called machine compliance volume (MCV). MCV is a function of both the ventilator circuit and the pressures achieved; therefore Eq. (2) should be modified as follows:

$$C_{eff} = \frac{V_T - C_{cf}[\Delta P]}{\Delta P} \qquad (3)$$

where C_{cf} is the compliance factor of the ventilator and ΔP is the pressure change.

Dynamic compliance (C_{dyn}) considers the volume change resulting from the total pressure change (P_{max} − PEEP) and includes the pressure necessary to overcome airway resistance (see discussion on resistance at beginning of chapter). Static compliance (C_{st}) takes into account only the pressure required to inflate the lung and chest wall (i.e., P_{ei} − PEEP). In this section, static lung compliance is discussed:

$$C_{st} = \frac{V_T - C_{cf}(P_{ei} - \text{PEEP})}{P_{ei} - \text{PEEP}} \qquad (4)$$

As shown in Fig. 5, the compliance curves of the lung and chest wall do not coincide (3). In clinical practice, compliance is commonly calculated for the respiratory system as a whole. In the presence of massive ascites or other chest wall diseases, the shape and slope of the chest wall compliance curve may change enough that it would be necessary to consider chest wall mechanics separately (2).

$$C_L = \frac{\Delta V}{\Delta(P_{ALV} - P_{PL})} \tag{5}$$

$$C_{CW} = \frac{\Delta V}{\Delta P_{PL}} \tag{6}$$

To separate C_L or C_{CW} from C_{RS}, one must be able to measure pleural pressure (P_{PL}). Direct measurement of P_{PL} is technically difficult and seldom performed. Indirect measurement, using esophageal balloon manometry, is more readily available, but requires experience. Although gas exchange frequently improves as lung volumes (and compliance) improve, the relationship between C_L and gas exchange is complex. The interaction between intrathoracic pressure and cardiorespiratory function is not fully explained by compliance.

Static lung volumes (most commonly FRC) can be measured by a variety of techniques in mechanically ventilated patients, including open and closed circuit techniques and planimetry of CXRs or CT scans. Body plethysmography is not practical in mechanically ventilated patients. These methods share technical problems, require sophisticated

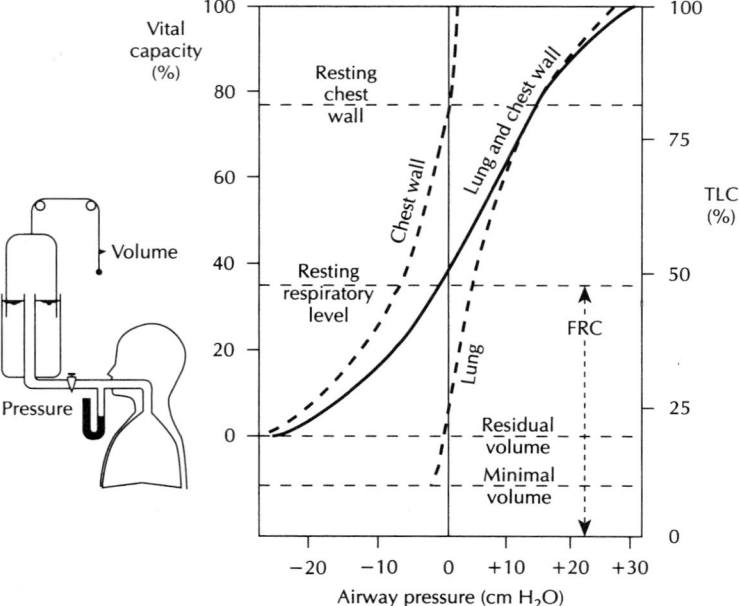

Figure 5 Relaxation pressure–volume curve of lung and chest wall. Patient inspires (or expires) to a certain volume from spirometer, tap is closed, and he/she relaxes respiratory muscles. Curve for lung and chest wall can be explained by addition of individual lung and chest wall curves. (Modified from West JB. Respiratory Physiology—The Essentials, 4th ed. Baltimore: Williams & Wilkins, 1990:100.)

technology, and are difficult to perform. Their usefulness in clinical care is limited. Respiratory impedance (inductance) plethysmography can be used to detect changes in FRC that result from various therapeutic maneuvers. It has become a popular clinical tool for measuring volume and breathing pattern. Wide elastic bands enclosing Teflon-insulated electrical coils are placed around the chest and abdomen. Expansion of the rib cage and abdomen alters inductance and changes the oscillator-generated frequency of the electrical current coursing through the coils. Of the available nonairway-dependent monitoring methods, respiratory impedance plethysmography is least affected by changes in body position, provided that the bands fit snugly and are not displaced (1). Although generally available, this type of plethysmography requires training and experience before it is useful (4).

MONITORING GAS EXCHANGE

Over the last decade, intensivists have been assessing partial pressure of oxygen (PaO_2) in the light of tissue oxygen delivery (Chapter 2). In this chapter, however, the use of arterial blood gas (ABG) data to estimate lung efficiency is emphasized.

A common method of assessing the efficiency of oxygenation is calculating the shunt fraction (Q_S/Q_T):

$$\frac{Q_S}{Q_T} = \frac{CCO_2 - CaO_2}{CCO_2 - C\bar{v}O_2} \tag{7}$$

where CCO_2 is oxygen content of blood in pulmonary capillaries, CaO_2 is oxygen content of arterial blood, and $C\bar{v}O_2$ is oxygen content of mixed venous blood.

This equation assumes the three-compartment lung model [i.e., all alveoli are either ideal (functioning perfectly), shunting ($V_A/Q_T = 0$), or functioning as dead space ($V_A/Q_T = \infty$)] (5). The normal $Q_S/Q_T < 5\%$ is caused by anatomic shunts (e.g., thebesian veins) (2). Using Q_S/Q_T to assess oxygenation is cumbersome, requires extensive laboratory data and calculations for each measurement, and is an oversimplification of ventilation/perfusion relationships. Abnormalities in the average SICU patient occur at many points on the continuum between shunt and dead space.

For these reasons several other methods of assessing the efficiency of oxygenation have been used, most commonly the difference between alveolar oxygen tension and arterial oxygen tension, (A-aDO_2). Alveolar oxygen tension PAO_2 is calculated using the alveolar gas equation:

$$PAO_2 = (P_B - PH_2O)FIO_2 - \frac{PACO_2}{R} + F \tag{8}$$

where F is ($PACO_2$) (FIO_2) $[(1 - R)/R]$, R is respiratory quotient, P_B is barometric pressure, and PH_2O is water vapor pressure.

For clinical purposes, this equation can be simplified to:

$$PAO_2 = PIO_2 - 1.25(PaCO_2) \tag{9}$$

The A-aDO_2 is limited by its dependence on the fraction of inspired oxygen (FIO_2). In other words, an A-aDO_2 of 100 is not necessarily worse than an A-aDO_2 of 50 (Fig. 6).

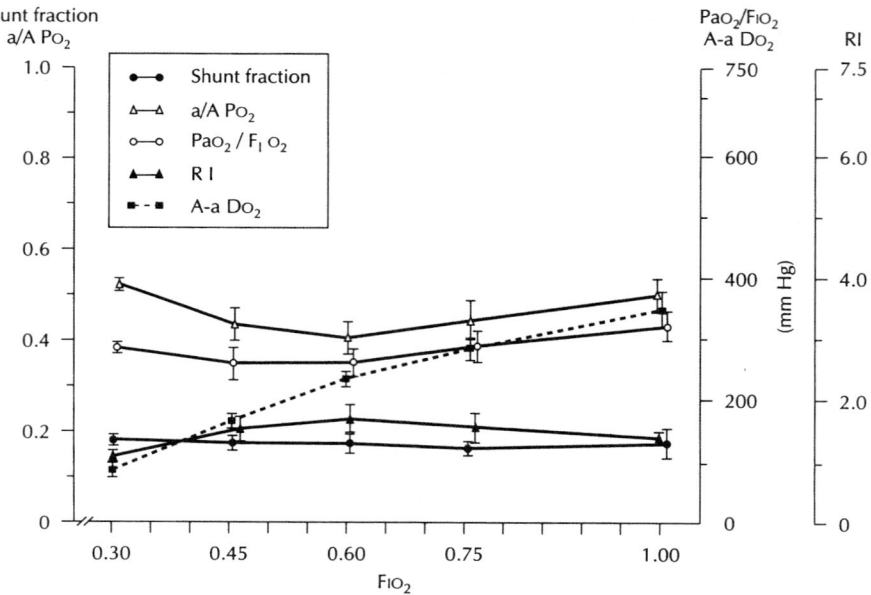

Figure 6 Mean value for each index and for shunt fraction at each level of FIO_2. Bars represent standard error of mean ($n = 8$ at $FIO_2 = 0.30$; $n = 10$ at all other levels of FIO_2). For visual clarity, some data points have been adjusted laterally at each level of FIO_2. (From Herrick IA, Champion LK, Froese AB. A clinical comparison of indices of pulmonary gas exchange with changes in inspired oxygen concentration. Can J Anaesth 1990; 37:69–76.)

The discrepancy results from the dependence of this type of index on changes in PaO_2; whereas, shunt fraction depends on changes in oxygen content, a much more accurate reflection of how efficiently the lungs are oxygenating blood (6). Shunt (or A-aDO_2) is not necessarily increased in patients whose hypoxia arises from alveolar hypoventilation; in these patients, PaO_2 falls as partial pressure of carbon dioxide in the alveoli ($PACO_2$) rises. As an illustration, the alveolar gas equation is used to calculate PAO_2 in a patient breathing room air, assuming a $PACO_2$ of 80 mm Hg:

$$PAO_2 = (P_B - PH_2O)FIO_2 - \frac{PACO_2}{R} + F$$

$$= (760 - 47)(0.21) - \frac{80}{0.8} + (80)(0.21)\left(\frac{1 - 0.8}{0.8}\right)$$

$$= 150 - 100 + 4.2$$

$$= 54.2 \text{ mm Hg}$$

Alternatives to using intermittent ABG values for monitoring oxygenation have important limitations. Transcutaneous oximetery and pulse oximetry do not allow differentiation between ischemic hypoxia (tissue hypoxia resulting from inadequate blood flow) and hypoxemic hypoxia (tissue hypoxia from inadequate arterial oxygen content) (7). Nonetheless, these techniques are available and can provide very useful information if

Respiratory Monitoring

their limitations are recognized. Pulse oximetry has become a very popular tool to monitor changes in oxygenation. Because of its limitations, transcutaneous monitoring is seldom used in adults; accordingly, it is not discussed.

PULSE OXIMETRY

For details of pulse oximetry design and function, see the articles by Kemper (7) and Kemper and Barker (8). Pulse oximeters have become popular, because they are easy to use. No calibration is necessary, and probes are easily placed and are noninvasive. They were designed to assess oxygenation during airway procedures (e.g., intubation, bronchoscopy), to monitor unstable patients (e.g., those with changing FIO_2, respiratory distress), or for use in any situation in which trending information is useful to alleviate patient safety concerns.

However, pulse oximeters do have several drawbacks that limit their usefulness as diagnostic tools:

- Pulse oximeters reveal nothing about alveolar ventilation. It is quite possible for a patient with perfectly acceptable pulmonary oxygen saturation (SPO_2) and percent oxygen saturation in arterial blood (SAO_2) to have a severe respiratory acidosis.
- Pulse oximeters are unreliable in vasoconstricted patients, because they depend on pulsatile flow to calculate saturation. Data from a pulse oximeter in which the pulse rate is inaccurate should be viewed with suspicion.
- Pulse oximeters are accurate only to within $\pm 2-3\%$ and only at $SPO_2 > 85\%$ (7). As demonstrated in Fig. 7, a wide variation in PaO_2 within the range of $\pm 3\%$ saturation on the steep part of the oxhemoglobin dissociation curve can occur. As diffusion of oxygen to the tissues depends on PaO_2, a low PaO_2 may have an adverse effect on tissue oxygenation. Thus pulse oximetry data

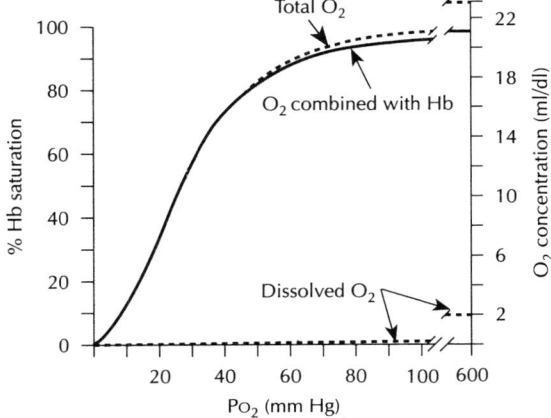

Figure 7 Oxygen dissociation curve (solid line) for pH 7.4, PCO_2, 40 mm Hg, and 37°C. Total blood oxygen concentration also is shown for hemoglobin concentration of 15 g/dL of blood. (From West JB. Respiratory Physiology—The Essentials, 4th ed. Baltimore: Williams & Wilkins, 1990:70.)

should be confirmed by obtaining blood gas values at low saturations ($SPO_2 \leq 93\%$), and the SPO_2 should be used only as trending data.
- Substances such as methylene blue, indocyanine green, methemoglobin, and carboxyhemoglobin, which interfere with light absorption at red and infrared frequencies, will cause erroneous readings (7,9). Normal tissue pigments or hyperbilirubinemia do not appear to cause clinically significant variability.
- Other sources of light, particularly fluorescent light, can interfere with the photodiode and cause inaccurate readings. For this reason, pulse oximetric probes usually should be covered with an opaque dressing.
- Long-term placement of probes, particularly if the probe is from a manufacturer different from that of the electronic monitor, can result in patient burns (10).
- Pulse oximeters cannot detect changes in oxygenation reliably until saturation drops below 97% ($PaO_2 \approx 80$ mm Hg), because hemoglobin (Hb) is 100% saturated as long as PaO_2 is above 154 mm Hg (see Fig. 7) and pulse oximeters are accurate only to $\pm 3\%$. The pulse oximeter cannot be used to detect endobronchial intubation reliably. With endobronchial intubation, enough desaturation may not occur (7).
- SPO_2 reflects events in the pulmonary circulation at a place in the peripheral circulation. The inherent delay must be recognized during intubations and ventilator changes.

MONITORING CARBON DIOXIDE REMOVAL

Most of the carbon dioxide produced by normal metabolic processes ($\dot{V}CO_2$) is excreted through the lungs. The efficiency of that process is usually assessed intermittently by measuring partial pressure of carbon dioxide (PCO_2) in a sample of arterial blood with a Severinghaus electrode. The clinician obtains "snapshots" of carbon dioxide excretion. In critical situations, continuous on-line measurement of partial pressure of carbon dioxide ($PaCO_2$) would be preferred. The use of end-tidal PCO_2 ($PetCO_2$) as a reflection of $PaCO_2$, may be of benefit.

The amount of carbon dioxide in arterial blood, as reflected by $PaCO_2$, is inversely proportional to alveolar ventilation ($\dot{V}_A$). The lower the $\dot{V}_A$, the higher $PaCO_2$ will be:

$$PACO_2 = \frac{\dot{V}CO_2}{\dot{V}_A} K \quad (10)$$

where K is a constant.

Equation (10) is valid for any reason that causes a change in $\dot{V}_A$. $\dot{V}_A$ may fall because of a decrease in total minute ventilation ($\dot{V}_E$), such as might occur after administration of morphine sulfate, or if the dead space (V_D) increases, as in emphysema.

To understand the limitations of capnometry, as the measurement of expired carbon dioxide is called, review of the concept of V_D is necessary. The portion of V_T that does not participate in gas exchange is referred to as V_D. In healthy people, V_D approximates the volume of the tracheobronchial tree and is called anatomic dead space. In pathologic high V/Q situations, when perfusion to ventilated alveoli is relatively diminished, V_D will consume an increasing portion of each V_T, and $\dot{V}_A$ will fall unless $\dot{V}_E$ increases.

Using the Bohr equation, V_D relative to V_T can be calculated, if an assumption that all alveoli are "ideal," "shunt," or "dead space is made."

$$\frac{V_D}{V_T} = \frac{PaCO_2 - PeCO_2}{PaCO_2} \qquad (11)$$

where $PeCO_2$ = mixed expired PCO_2.

High V_D/V_T supports V/Q mismatch as the cause of elevated $PaCO_2$ as opposed to problems such as hypoventilation (caused by an excess of narcotics) or increased carbon dioxide production (e.g., caused by an abnormal respiratory quotient or increased metabolic rate). In healthy people V_D and anatomic dead space are nearly equal, and $PaCO_2 \approx PeCO_2$. In patients with pulmonary dysfunction, expired gas comes from alveoli with a myriad of V/Q's. $PetCO_2$ will be significantly lower than $PaCO_2$; the difference between the two is an indirect measure of the increase in V_D as a result of V/Q mismatch (Table 2).

Commonly, capnometers use infrared technology, but other systems are available. Regardless of the technology used, expired gas is sampled as close to the patient as possible, and expired carbon dioxide is plotted as a function of time to provide a waveform or capnogram. A normal capnogram can be seen in Fig. 8. Causes of variation from the normal capnogram can be found in Table 3.

Table 2 Arterial End-Tidal Carbon Dioxide Tension ($PaCO_2 - PetCO_2$) Gradient During General Anesthesia

Investigator	Year	$PaCO_2 - PeCO_2$ (mm Hg) Mean	Range	Comments
Nunn	1960			No cardiac or pulmonary disease
		4.5 ± 2.5	−0.4 to 7.7	Spontaneous respiration
		4.7 ± 2.5	1.7 to 9.1	Artificial respiration
Askrog	1964	3.6	1.5 to 6.1	After induction (halothane group)
		5.5	2.6 to 10	After 90–150 min of halothane anesthesia
		0.9	0.6 to 1.9	Unanesthetized controls
Takki	1972	3.5 ± 0.5		
Whitesell	1981	0.8 ± 0.3		No lung disease
		3.3 ± 0.6		Lung disease
				Stable gradient on repeated measurements
Valentin	1982	5	−4 to 13	Pediatric patients Spontaneous respiration
Raemer	1983	4.1	0.8 to 13	Varying gradient on repeated measurements
Fletcher	1984	4.6	1.5 to 10.1	Small tidal volumes
		2.3	−0.8 to 8.5	Large tidal volumes
Shanker	1986	5.3 ± 2.9	3.5 to 7.1	Nonpregnant patients
		0.8 ± 0.7	−4 to 6.8	Pregnant patients; 50% had negative gradients

Source: From Good ML. Capnography: uses, interpretations, and pitfalls. In: Barash PG, ed. Refresher Courses in Anesthesiology. Philadelphia: JB Lippincott, 1990:184.

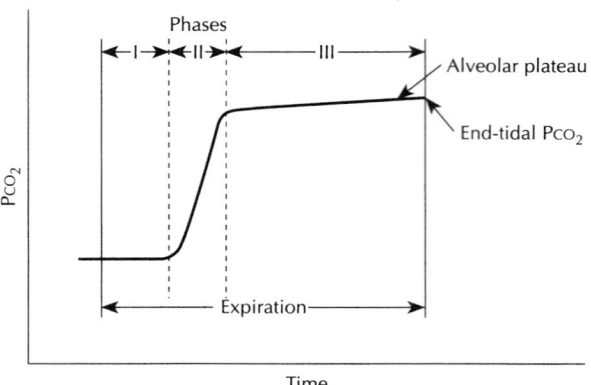

Figure 8 Three phases of normal capnogram. Phase I is series dead space, length of which depends on amount of apparatus and anatomic dead space. Phase II is mixture of anatomic series and alveolar parallel gas. Phase III (alveolar plateau) is produced by mixture of ideal alveolar gas from well-perfused alveoli and alveolar dead space gas from unperfused alveoli. (From Kemper KK. Interpretation of noninvasive oxygen and carbon dioxide data. Can J Anaesth 1990; 37:S27–S32.)

Table 3 Untoward Situations Detected with Capnography

Problem	Causes
No (or little) exhaled carbon dioxide	Esophageal intubation, tracheal extubation, disconnection, complete obstruction, apnea, cardiac arrest, pulmonary embolism
Elevated inspiratory baseline (phase I)	Incompetent expiratory valve
Prolonged expiratory upstroke (phase II)	Obstruction (equipment, pulmonary disease), slow gas sampling or instrument response time
Upward sloping expiratory plateau (phase III)	Obstruction (equipment, pulmonary disease)
Prolonged inspiratory downstroke (phase IV)	Incompetent inspiratory valve, slow gas sampling or instrument response time
Elevated $PetCO_2$	Hypoventilation (leak, obstruction, inadequate ventilator settings), carbon dioxide rebreathing, increased carbon dioxide production or delivery (malignant hyperthermia, febrile illness, carbon dioxide insufflation, bicarbonate administration)
Decreased $PetCO_2$	Hyperventilation, decreased carbon dioxide production or delivery (hypothermia, decreased cardiac output), increased arterial to end-tidal carbon dioxide gradient [ventilation/perfusion mismatching, hypotension, endobronchial intubation, pulmonary embolism (air, fat, thrombus, amniotic fluid), shallow or rapid breathing, instrument or sampling problems, sampling leak, miscalibration]

Source: Modified from Good ML. Capnography: uses, interpretations, and pitfalls. In: Barash PG, ed. Refresher Courses in Anesthesiology. Philadelphia: JB Lippincott, 1990:190.

Box 1 Comparison of Mainstream vs. Sidestream Capnometers

Mainstream	Sidestream
Fast	Sampling delay
No problem with condensation	Apparatus dead space
	Limited sampling rate
Very heavy	Problems with condensation
High cost	Potential for multiple gas analysis

Most currently used capnometers are sidestream samplers, which means they sample only a portion of the expired gas. Some infrared spectrometers, however, are capable of mainstream sampling (Box 1).

Although capnometry is a useful monitor of $\dot{V}_A$, several simple rules must be followed (11):

- Rely on the capnogram rather than digitally reported $PetCO_2$.
- Consider the possibility of equipment malfunction such as sampling leaks.
- Remember that changes in $PetCO_2$ often do not parallel changes in $PaCO_2$.

After pulmonary embolism, although $PetCO_2$ has decreased precipitously, $PaCO_2$ may well be rising unless $\dot{V}_A$ is increased. $PetCO_2$ and $PaCO_2$ may diverge without any obvious clinical signs. For this reason, $PetCO_2$ alone is an unreliable monitor for such purposes as weaning from mechanical ventilation, and $PetCO_2$ data should periodically be confirmed by ABG values (12,13).

SUMMARY

- P_{max} − PEEP is pressure required to overcome airway resistance and to inflate the lungs.
- $P_{max} - P_{ei}$ is pressure required to overcome total airway resistance.
- Changes in $P_{max} - P_{ei}$ at constant flow and volume approximate changes in tracheobronchial resistance.
- Auto-PEEP is increase in airway pressure above preset PEEP at end expiration.
- Most acute pulmonary dysfunction is restrictive.
- Static lung compliance:

$$C_{st} = \frac{V_T - C_{cf}(P_{ei} - \text{PEEP})}{P_{ei} - \text{PEEP}}$$

-
$$Q_S/Q_T = \frac{CCO_2 - CaO_2}{CCO_2 - C\bar{V}O_2}$$

- For clinical use $PAO_2 = PIO_2 - 1.25\ (PaCO_2)$.
- $PaCO_2$ varies inversely with alveolar ventilation.
- Capnometry despite limitations, has clinical use in monitoring carbon dioxide excretion.

REFERENCES

1. Marini JJ. Lung mechanics determinations at the bedside: Instrumentation and clinical application. Respir Care 1990; 35:669–693.
2. Marini JJ, Wheeler AD. Respiratory Monitoring in Critical Care Medicine: The Essentials. Baltimore: Williams & Willkins, 1989:47–60.
3. Moon RE, Camporesi EM. Repiratory monitoring in anesthesia. In: Miller RD, ed. Anesthesia, 3rd ed. 1989:1129–1165.
4. Pearson DJ. Measuring and monitoring lung volume outside the pulmonary function laboratory. Respir Care 1990; 35:660–667.
5. West JB. Respiratory Physiology—The Essentials, 4th ed. Baltimore: Williams & Wilkins, 1990:100.
6. Herrick IA, Champion LK, Froese AB. A clinical comparison of indices of pulmonary gas exchange with changes in the inspired oxygen concentration. Can J Anaesth 1990; 37:69–76.
7. Kemper KK. Interpretation of noninvasive oxygen and carbon dioxide data. Can J Anaesth 1990; 37:S27–S32.
8. Kemper KK, Barker SJ. Fundamental principles of monitoring instrumentation. In: Miller RD, ed. Anesthesia, 3rd ed. 1989:957–999.
9. Schweitzer SA. Spurious pulse oximeter desaturation due to methemeglobinemia. Anaesth Intens Care 1991; 19:269–271.
10. Murphy KG, Secunda JA, Rockoff MA. Severe burns from a pulse oximeter. Anesthesiology 1990; 76:350–352.
11. Good ML. Capnography: uses, interpretations and pitfalls. In: Barash PG, ed. Refresher Courses in Anesthesiology. Philadelphia: JB Lippincott, 1990;175–193.
12. Russell GB, Graybeal JM, Strout JC. Stability of arterial to end tidal carbon dioxide gradients during postoperative cardiorespiratory support. Can J Anaesth 1990; 37:560–566.
13. Hess D, Schlottag A, Levon B, et al. An evaluation of the usefulness of end tidal PCO_2 to aid weaning from mechanical ventilation following cardiac surgery. Respir Care 1991; 36:837–843.

SUGGESTED READING

Gravenstein JS. Gas monitoring and pulse oximetry. London: Butterworth-Heinemann, 1990.
Kemper KK, Barker SJ. Pulse oximetry. Anesthesiology 1989; 20:98–108.
Szaflarski NL, Cohen NH. Use of capnography in critically ill adults. Heart Lung 1991; 20:363–374.
Tobin MJ. Respiratory monitoring in the intensive care unit. Am Rev Respir Dis 1988; 138:1625–1642.
Truwit JD, Marini JJ. Evaluation of thoracic mechanics in the ventilated patient. Part I: Primary measurements. J Crit Care 1988; 3:133–150.
Truwit JD, Marini JJ. Evaluation of thoracic mechanics in the ventilated patient. Part II: Applied mechanics. J Crit Care 1988; 3:199–213.

Part VII
Approaches to Complex Problems

63
Responding to Uncertainty in the Intensive Care Unit: Some Unanswered Questions in Critical Care and How They Got That Way

Jerome H. Abrams
VA Medical Center, Minneapolis, Minnesota, USA

The long day of caring for the ICU patients and their families has ended. Along with the satisfaction from progress in some patients, sadness at the loss of some patients, frustration with documentation requirements, and muscular aches from standing for untold hours comes a profound sense of exhaustion. Did this exhaustion arise simply from the long hours? Is another source the culprit? Perhaps the endless battle with uncertainty is the reason. The care of patients in the ICU requires decisions to be made, often with urgency and with far reaching consequences, with, at best, incomplete information. The burden is daunting, and the toll may be severe.

The source of the uncertainty is plain; the response to it is not. If one tries to imagine the number of variables that contribute to the state of a patient at any moment, a large number, probably a larger number than one could count in a lifetime, comes to mind. Of that large number of variables, collectively we can name a number of variables of order 100,000. Of those hundreds of thousands of variables, we measure a number of order 10 routinely in the ICU. To add to the difficulties, comparable magnitudes can have markedly different meanings. For example, a bilirubin of 4.0 mg/dL in one patient may be associated with life-threatening cholangitis; whereas, a bilirubin of 4.0 mg/dL in another patient may demonstrate resolving cholestasis. One patient is on a path to increasing severity of illness; whereas, the other is recovering. In that sense, the variables exhibit degeneracy. From that small number of variables, we are expected to understand the course of complex illness and to provide care that will eliminate the morbidity and mortality of disease. Unfortunately, the problems that confront us are high dimensional, dynamic, and nonlinear. We attempt to solve them with sparse, static information that typically receives linear analysis that cannot resolve the degeneracy. No wonder we are exhausted.

The foregoing chapters present an expert view of clinical problems in the face of uncertainly. The present chapter identifies some additional useful tools, which include evidence-based evaluation of clinical data, resolving degeneracy-distinguishing response variables from control variables, dynamical systems, joint probabilities, and statistical ensembles. The use of evidence-based medicine to evaluate clinical data is well described by the group at McMaster University. Their landmark work has sharpened our appreciation of the strength of conclusions reached in clinical trials and will continue to inform us. Regrettably, not all problems will allow themselves to be solved by prospective randomized trails. An historical example is dialysis: dialysis was never subjected to a prospective randomized trial and will never be studied in that fashion. Nontheless, dialysis remains a mainstay in the support of the critically ill. The remaining discussion will consider resolving degeneracy-distinguishing response variables from control variables in the context of oxygen transport, dynamical systems applied to the construction of the ventricular pressure volume (PV) loop, joint probabilities in the diagnosis of ventilator-associated pneumonitis, and the hidden variable problem using statistical ensembles in the optimization of ventilator support. The menu approach is necessary in the absence of understanding the organizing principles at an appropriate level.

Caring for the critically ill requires clear understanding of the nature of the critical illness and the possibilities for treatment. Dispelling the cloud of uncertainty is certainly consistent with that goal. The present chapter does not pretend to eliminate uncertainty. It will be remarkable more for its failings than for its successes. But if its failings are described clearly, and if its failings stimulate additional ideas to bring clarity, it will have accomplished an essential task.

RESOLVING DEGENERACY-DISTINGUISHING RESPONSE VARIABLES FROM CONTROL VARIABLES

A review of the literature describing the effects of increasing oxygen delivery leads to several disparate conclusions. Some investigators report that increasing oxygen delivery leads to increased oxygen consumption and produces improved survival in high risk surgery patients (1,2). Others identify an improvement in survival if oxygen delivery is increased, and the improvement in survival occurs in the absence of demonstrating increased oxygen consumption (3,4). Several studies suggest that the increase in oxygen consumption observed with increase in oxygen delivery is an artifact of the method used to calculate the oxygen consumption. Coupling of variables results in spurious correlation (5,6). Finally, a clinical study indicates that oxygen delivery can be augmented in the critically ill patient, oxygen consumption does not increase, and efforts to increase oxygen consumption in these patients result in increased mortality (7). Clearly, these conclusions are markedly different. How could they result from examination of what is thought to be the same phenomenon? In an effort to resolve these different points of view, the remaining discussion will review data about oxygen transport, consider the appropriate dimensionality to describe the problem, and propose a model for evaluating oxygen transport.

Interest in the relationship between oxygen delivery and oxygen consumption was stimulated by Cain in 1977 (8). In dogs made anemic or hypoxemic, an increase in oxygen consumption was seen as oxygen delivery was increased. Shibutani and colleagues demonstrated a similar effect in human patients. In their study, patients on cardiac bypass were observed to increase oxygen consumption as the bypass pump was used to increase oxygen delivery (9). In neither of these two studies was an inflammatory state present. Natanson et al. (10) used a canine model of septic shock and demonstrated that the combination of antibiotic treatment coupled with fluid resuscitation was superior to either antibiotics alone or fluid resuscitation alone. Although not directly measured, the use of fluid resuscitation is inferred to increase oxygen delivery.

Bihari and colleagues examined the role of increased oxygen delivery and consumption in the septic patient. Oxygen delivery was augmented in this group of patients with the use of a vasodilator, prostacyclin. These investigators observed an increase in oxygen consumption in the nonsurvivors; whereas, the survivors failed to demonstrate an increase in oxygen consumption. They concluded that nonsurvivors have poorly perfused vascular beds that are unmasked by the administration of prostacyclin. Further, these poorly perfused areas contribute to overall mortality (11).

Further data about humans in the setting of the inflammatory state were described by Abraham et al. (1). In their 1984 publication, the authors retrospectively examined several physiologic variables that distinguished survivors from non-survivors in 8 h prior to the onset of septic shock. They identified cardiac index, oxygen delivery, and oxygen consumption as important discriminators of survival. Retrospectively, survivors demonstrated higher cardiac index, higher oxygen delivery, and higher oxygen consumption than nonsurvivors. When tested prospectively in a cohort of high risk surgical patients, the augmentation of oxygen delivery, oxygen consumption, and cardiac index was associated with a marked improvement in mortality. Although the study has several design flaws, the results sparked active investigation into the dependence of mortality on oxygen transport in the critically ill patient.

Tuchschmidt et al. (3) examined this issue in septic patients. In their study, the primary outcome variable was an increase in cardiac index. In this study, mortality was lower in the group that achieved a cardiac index in excess of 4.5 L/min per m^2. Approximately half the patients in the control group spontaneously achieved a cardiac index of 4.5 L/min per m^2; whereas, approximately half of the patients in the treatment group failed to achieve the target cardiac index. Mortality in the control group was 72%, and mortality in the treatment group was 50%. One would expect the large degree of crossover between groups to diminish the difference between the groups. The mortality benefit was observed in the absence of demonstrable increase in oxygen consumption. Another aspect of this study that deserves emphasis is the use of serum lactate concentration as an inclusion criterion. A study by Yu et al. (12) found that patients with an oxygen delivery >600 mL/min per m^2 had improved survival. This improvement was observed if the augmented oxygen delivery occurred spontaneously or pharmacologically. Again, the survival benefit was observed despite no significant increase in oxygen consumption.

Boyd et al. (4) studied a high risk group of surgical patients. The patients received dopexamine to augment oxygen delivery in the preoperative period. A statically significant improvement in mortality was observed in this experimental group. The improvement occurred in the absence of increased oxygen consumption. Another preoperative study of augmented oxygen delivery is that of Berlauk et al. (13). A high risk group of patients undergoing distal lower extremity bypass for limb salvage was studied. The experimental group was monitored with a pulmonary artery catheter. With augmentation of preload and afterload reduction, the study patients met clinical targets for pulmonary capillary wedge pressure and for systemic vascular resistance. If needed, congestive failure was treated, and inotropes were used. With these interventions, cardiac index and consequently oxygen delivery were increased in the majority of the experimental patients. Although the primary outcome variable of this study was not increased oxygen delivery, perioperative complications were reduced in the experimental group. These patients had decreased perioperative cardiac morbidity and decreased early graft thrombosis.

The foregoing studies indicate an advantage of augmenting oxygen delivery. Not all investigators agree. The study of Hayes et al. (7) examined the effects of augmenting oxygen delivery in a group of patients who failed fluid resuscitation. This cohort of patients was then managed with inotropes and vasoconstrictors, sometimes at high doses. The requirement that the patients fail fluid resuscitation allowed delay in the use of inotropes or vasoconstrictors and provided a bias in the selection of patients for study. These investigators demonstrated that oxygen delivery could be augmented; whereas, oxygen consumption could not. Further, the group treated with increasing oxygen delivery had a higher mortality. A study by Gattinoni et al. (14) looked at mortality in patients in whom the cardiac index was augmented. In this study, the control population had a normal cardiac index. The experimental group failed to achieve the study target of a cardiac index of 4.5 L/min per m^2 in 55%. No significant difference in mortality was observed in the two groups. These investigators concluded that augmenting cardiac index produced no survival advantage. The inability to achieve the study target for cardiac index in over half of the patients raises the important question of whether the conclusion is based on the inability to attain the cardiac index under investigation.

In their meta-analysis, Heyland et al. (15) combined the data in these studies, with the exclusion of the Berlauk et al. study, in which the primary endpoint was not oxygen delivery, and observed that only two studies demonstrated a risk reduction, the studies of Shoemaker et al. and Boyd et al., respectively. As noted in this meta-analysis, these two studies augmented oxygen delivery prior to a general surgical procedure. Timing may be of great importance. In the study of Hayes et al., delay in starting the protocol may have contributed to the adverse effect observed.

Early goal-directed therapy in patients with sepsis and septic shock was studied by Rivers et al. (16). Cardiac preload, afterload, and contractility were manipulated to balance oxygen delivery with oxygen demand. Mortality was reduced in the experimental group.

The controversy extends to another issue. Archie (6) argued that the observation of delivery-dependent oxygen consumption occurs as a result of coupling of data, when the oxygen consumption is calculated from the product of cardiac index and arteriovenous oxygen content difference. Ronco et al. (5) argued that oxygen consumption, when measured in expiratory gas, is not increased when oxygen delivery is augmented. They further argued that the delivery-dependent oxygen consumption observed by others is a result of coupling of data, when the oxygen consumption is calculated by the Fick method.

This review of the oxygen transport literature illustrates the varied conclusions reached by various investigators about the benefit of augmented oxygen delivery. One consistent area of controversy is the existence of the oxygen consumption–oxygen delivery curve that is shown in Fig. 1. An attempt to resolve these controversial viewpoints requires critical analysis of this relationship. In an intuitive sense, the requirement that patients be oxygen-transport-deficient prior to randomization to an increased oxygen delivery protocol is not clearly defined in the literature reviewed. Do the patients studied demonstrate oxygen transport deficiency prior to augmenting oxygen delivery? Are the coordinates appropriate, and are they orthogonal? Is the problem adequately described in two dimensions? The remaining discussion will develop a response surface that describes oxygen transport. The response surface will address the question of how many dimensions are necessary to describe the problem and how the values of the control parameters affect the observed responses to increased oxygen delivery.

An approach to this problem can begin with an analysis of clinical variables that are used to assess patients in shock. One such set of variables consists of: cardiac index, mean arterial pressure, central venous pressure, heart rate, mixed venous oxygen tension, mixed venous carbon dioxide tension, mixed venous pH, and arterial − mixed venous oxygen

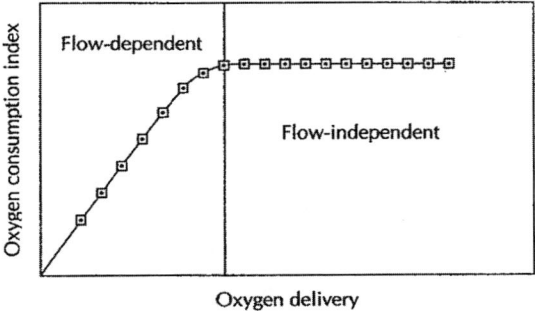

Figure 1 Idealization of flow-dependent oxygen consumption. (From Abrams JH. Indications for hemodynamic monitoring. In Najarian JS, Delaney JP, eds. Progress in Trauma and Critical Care Surgery. St. Louis: Mosby–Year Book, 1992, p. 275.)

content difference. In addition, three values derived from a dye-dilution cardiac output determination are included. These are the mixing time, the dispersive time, and the ejection time (17). Inspection of these variables indicates that they are not all independent. If they are not independent, are all 11 variables necessary to describe the state of the patient? To answer this question, these variables were subjected to a principal components analysis (18). The principal components algorithm provides a statistical weighting for each of the variables and describes a new coordinate that is a linear combination of the variables. The greater the absolute value of the coefficient, the greater the variance accounted for by that variable. The results are shown in Table 1. The first four principal components accounted

Table 1 First Four Principal Components

	P1	P2	P3	P4
CI	−0.408	−0.077	0.200	−0.135
tm	0.408	0.104	0.094	0.124
td	0.446	0.114	0.048	0.125
ET	−0.254	0.401	0.352	0.288
MAP	−0.086	0.067	−0.469	0.823
CVP	0.120	−0.067	0.527	0.245
HR	0.089	−0.536	−0.361	−0.075
P_vO_2	−0.371	−0.285	0.061	0.206
P_vCO_2	0.146	−0.336	0.383	0.235
V_{pH}	−0.098	0.559	−0.213	−0.163
DvO_2	0.452	0.082	−0.031	−0.032
Eigenvalue	4.03	1.86	1.19	0.98

Note: P1, P2, P3, P4, principal components; CI, cardiac index; tm, mixing time; td, dispersive time; ET, ejection time; MAP, mean arterial pressure; CVP, central venous pressure; HR, heart rate; P_vO_2, mixed venous oxygen partial pressure; P_vCO_2, mixed venous carbon dioxide pressure; V_{pH}, mixed venous pH; and DvO_2, arterial − mixed venous oxygen content difference.

for ~89% of the variance. This result suggests that not all 11 dimensions are necessary to describe the state of the patient. Although the reduction in dimensionality is encouraging, the result of the principal component's calculation has two significant limitations. First, the coefficients may not be unique. Second, a description of the state of the system is not coordinate-specific. Transformation of the coordinates would not change the mathematical object being described. By inspecting the results of the principal components calculation, we find those variables that are related to oxygen consumption are heavily weighted. We, then, postulated: (1) the state of the patient is determined by energy use, (2) the state can be identified by variables that reflect energy use, both aerobic and anaerobic, and (3) the state variables are independent of time although an individual's path through the state space may be time-dependent.

With these postulates, one can describe the state of the patient as

$$F = a_1 VO_2 + a_2(L/P)$$

where F is the patient state, a_1 is the constant converting oxygen consumption to energy units, a_2 is the constant converting (L/P) to energy units, and L/P is the the ratio of serum lactate concentration to serum pyruvate concentration.

With this assumption,

$$F = F(CI, DvO_2, L/P)$$

where CI is the cardiac index and DvO_2 is the arterial − mixed venous oxygen content difference.

Examination of ordered triples revealed the following empirical relationship:

$$DvO_2 = \frac{k(L/P)}{CI}, \quad k = \text{empirical constant} = 0.58$$

With this relationship, only two of the variables need to be considered independent.
Let

$$CI = f_1(DvO_2, F)$$
$$L/P = g_1(DvO_2, F)$$

Solve simultaneously

$$DvO_2 = f_2(CI, L/P)$$
$$F = g_2(CI, L/P)$$

Let A = aerobic energy use.

Responding to Uncertainty in ICU

Then

$$A = a_1(\text{CI})(D\text{vO}_2)$$

$$dA = \frac{\partial A}{\partial \text{CI}} d\text{CI} + \frac{\partial A}{\partial D\text{vO}_2} d(D\text{vO}_2)$$

$$= a_1(D\text{vO}_2)\, d\text{CI} + a_1 \text{CI}\, d(D\text{vO}_2)$$

Since $D\text{vO}_2 = f(\text{CI}, L/P)$

$$d(D\text{vO}_2) = \frac{\partial(D\text{vO}_2)}{\partial \text{CI}} d\text{CI} + \frac{\partial(D\text{vO}_2)}{\partial(L/P)} d(L/P)$$

$$= \frac{k}{\text{CI}} d(L/P) - \frac{k}{\text{CI}^2}(L/P)\, d\text{CI}$$

Substitute for $d(D\text{vO}_2)$

$$dA = \frac{k}{\text{CI}} d(L/P) - \frac{k(L/P)}{\text{CI}^2} d\text{CI}$$

$$= a_1 D\text{vO}_2\, d\text{CI} + a_1 k\, d(L/P) - \frac{a_1 k(L/P)}{\text{CI}} d\text{CI}$$

Since $F = F(\text{CI}, L/P)$

$$dF = \frac{\partial F}{\partial \text{CI}} d\text{CI} + \frac{\partial F}{\partial(L/P)} d(L/P)$$

$$= a_1(D\text{vO}_2)\, d\text{CI} + \frac{\partial F}{\partial(L/P)} d(L/P)$$

The anaerobic energy utilization is the total energy utilization minus the aerobic component.

Let

$$dB = \text{the anaerobic energy utilization} = dF - dA$$

$$= (a_2 - a_1 k)\, d(L/P) + \frac{a_1 k(L/P)}{\text{CI}} d\text{CI}$$

Observe that $dB/(L/P)$ is an exact differential. Define

$$d\sigma = \frac{dB}{(L/P)}$$

then

$$d\sigma = \frac{(a_2 - a_1 k)\,d(L/P)}{(L/P)} + \frac{a_1 k\,dCI}{CI}$$

and

$$\Delta\sigma = (a_2 - a_1 k)\ln\left(\frac{L/P_{\text{final}}}{L/P_{\text{ref}}}\right) + a_2 k\left(\frac{CI_{\text{final}}}{CI_{\text{ref}}}\right) + \text{const}$$

Then

$$dF = (L/P)d\sigma + dA$$

By application of Stokes' theorem to the vector field generated by this equation, one can demonstrate that the curl is zero. Consequently, dF is independent of path.

When the points are plotted in ΔF, $\Delta\sigma$, DvO_2 space, a response surface topologically equivalent to a cusp catastrophe manifold is found (18).

An example illustrates the clinical application. Consider a patient involved in a motor vehicle crash. He sustained multiple injuries, including a liver laceration, colon injury, spleen injury, and pelvic fracture. After treatment of his injuries in the operating room, he is admitted to the surgical intensive care unit. His admission cardiac index, DvO_2, and L/P are indicated in Table 2. His position on the response surface is indicated in Fig. 2. On postoperative day 5, the patient developed pancreatitis and became markedly volume depleted. The values of CI, DvO_2, and L/P are shown in Table 2. Plotting his position on the response surface reveals a position in the area of cardiac insufficiency (Fig. 3). Resuscitation produced new values for CI, DvO_2, and L/P that are again shown in Table 2. The position of the patient on the response surface has changed to the area of the systemic inflammatory response (Fig. 4). At the time of discharge from the intensive care unit, the patient was in the area of compensation (Fig. 5). Please note that the benefit of augmenting oxygen delivery would be very different if studied when the patient's state is the point shown in Fig. 3 compared with the effect when the patient's state is that shown in Fig. 4. In the context of this model, the control parameters are at different values in the two figures. Much of the controversy in understanding the benefit of augmenting oxygen transport may arise from the values of the control parameters at the time the intervention of augmenting oxygen transport begins. Since the literature does not describe the value for the control parameters at the time of the intervention, disparate conclusions about

Table 2

CI	DvO_2	L/P	Refer to:
5.2	3.0	16.5	Fig. 2 (ICU admission)
1.4	5.7	41.0	Fig. 3 (Hypovolemia)
11.2	2.8	5.6	Fig. 4 (SIRs)
4.7	4.1	20.3	Fig. 5 (Discharge)

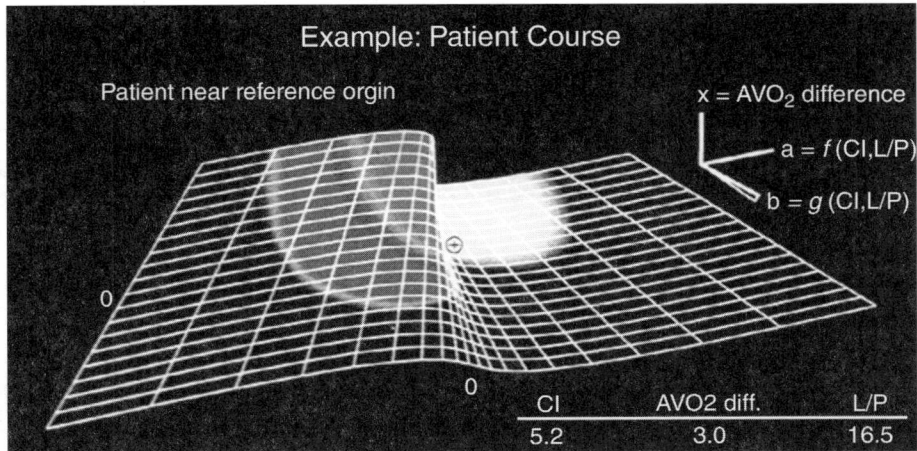

Figure 2 Patient's state as described by cusp catastrophe model at time of admission to the ICU.

the efficacy of restoration of oxygen transport may be explained by different values for the control parameters at the time of intervention.

USE OF DYNAMICAL SYSTEMS

A commonly observed response to the stress of illness is augmented cardiac output. In the process of resuscitating patients, the clinician is often faced with the need to increase

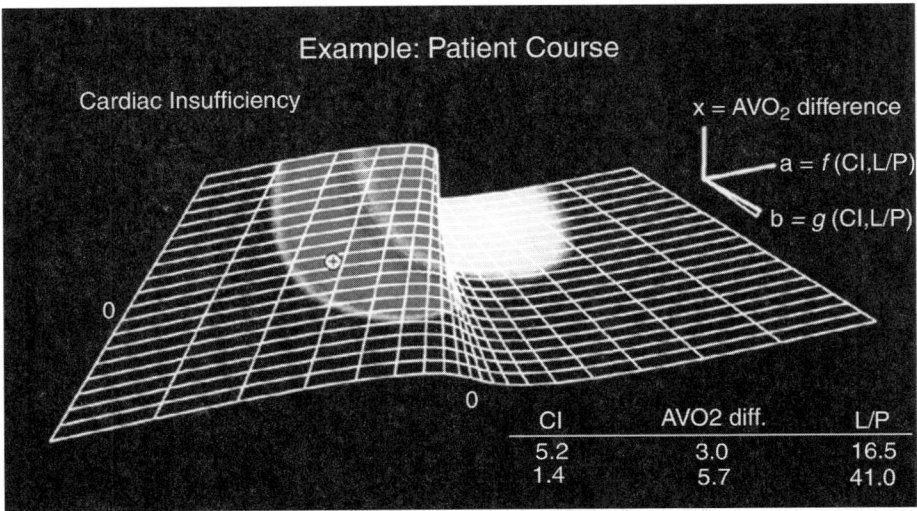

Figure 3 Patient's state as described by cusp catastrophe model during hypovolemia.

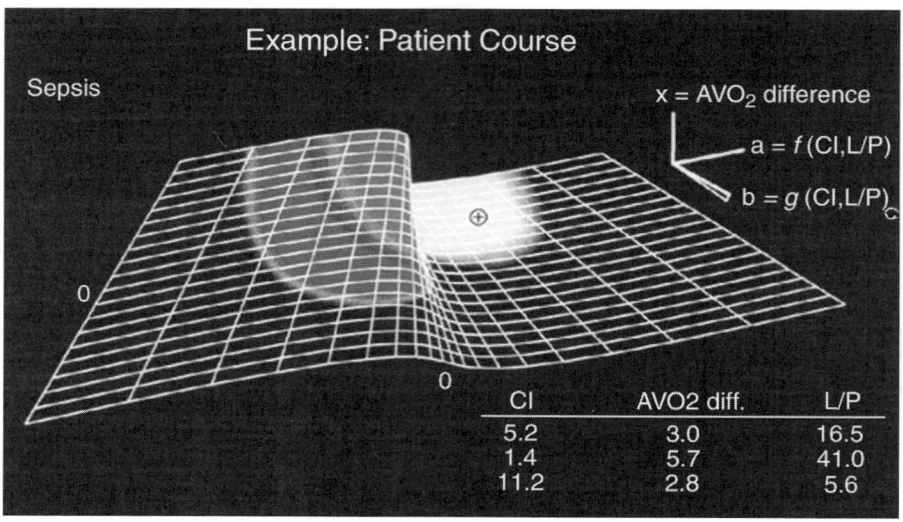

Figure 4 Patient's state as described by cusp catastrophe model during episode of acute pancreatitis.

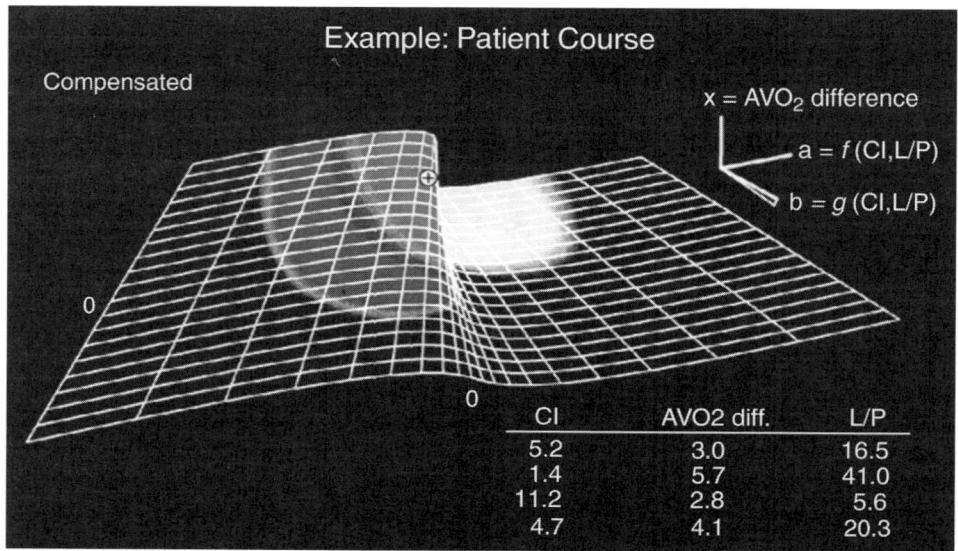

Figure 5 Patient's state as described by cusp catastrophe model demonstrating physiologic compensation.

cardiac output. Ideally, clinical strategies should increase cardiac output in the most efficient manner: increased cardiac output with the minimum increase in myocardial oxygen consumption. Presumably, increase in stroke volume with the minimum increase in heart rate and myocardial wall tension would satisfy that criterion. Achieving this clinical goal requires a detailed understanding of ventricular mechanics.

The standard representation of ventricular mechanics is the ventricular PV loop. The PV loop provides much useful information. The area within the PV loop is the left ventricular stroke work. Suga (19) has demonstrated that the PV loop can be used to estimate myocardial oxygen consumption. Rankin has demonstrated a linear relationship between LVSW and left ventricular end diastolic volume. In his analysis, the cardiac cycle could be represented as a slope, the contractility coefficient, and an intercept, the unstressed end diastolic volume (20). Although useful in research applications, the PV loop is not practically measured in the ICU. Can we construct the PV loop from clinically measured variables and increase our understanding of ventricular function?

The cardiac cycle is similar to the behavior of a triode circuit (21). In the case of the cardiac cycle, energy is imparted during diastole and dissipated during systole. van der Pol formulated an equation to describe such behavior in a triode circuit. As adapted to the performance of the ventricle, van der Pol's oscillator can be restated as:

$$\frac{dP}{dt} = \mu \left[V - \left(\frac{P^3}{3} - \alpha P \right) \right]$$

$$\frac{dV}{dt} = \frac{-P}{\mu}$$

where P is the left ventricular pressure, V is the left ventricular volume, and α, μ are the phenomenological coefficients.

When van der Pol's oscillator is numerically integrated, the ventricular PV loop may be simulated. Figure 6 shows the numerical integration compared with a ventricular PV loop obtained by direct measurement of LV pressure with an intraventricular pressure transducer and LV volume with ultrasound crystals placed on and within the left ventricular myocardium. Numerical fitting of the two parameters, α and μ, provides a close fit of the experimentally obtained PV loop.

If one could measure cardiac output with a beat to beat measurement, then integration of the volume flow rate would provide a measure of the change in left ventricular volume as a function of time. With an estimate of left ventricular pressure, half of the PV loop could be determined. Figure 7 shows the half of the of the PV loop obtained for systole with a measure of cardiac output and a measure of left ventricular pressure. If the values obtained by numerically fitting α and μ to the portion of the PV loop obtained in systole were applied to diastole, then the entire PV loop could be derived. Figure 8 shows the PV loop obtained by such a numerical procedure and compares it with an experimentally obtained PV loop. As one can see, the fit is close. If the technology to measure continuous cardiac output becomes routine, and, if calculation of change in cardiac volume coupled with an estimate of LV pressure derived from peripheral pressure is satisfactory, the possibility of construction of the ventricular PV loop in the critically ill patient may be a reality (22).

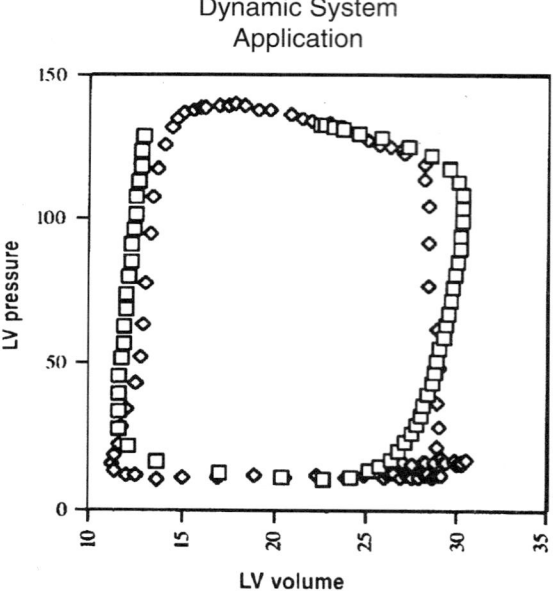

Figure 6 Comparison of numerical integration of van der Pol oscillator and measured ventricular PV loop. Squares indicate numerical integration. Diamonds are experimentally measured pressure–volume ordered pairs.

JOINT PROBABILITIES

Nosocomial bacterial pneumonia is the second most common hospital acquired infection and carries the highest mortality of any nosocomial infection. Unfortunately, the clinical

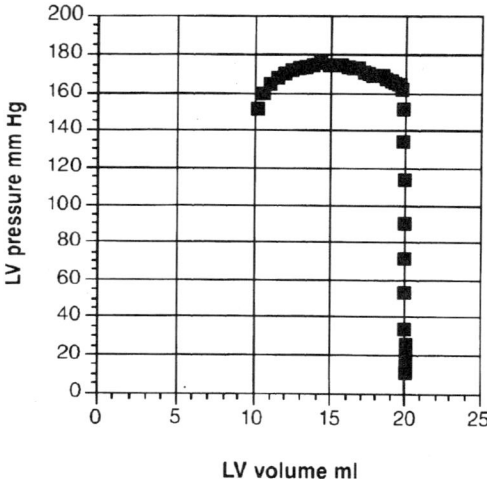

Figure 7 Portion of PV loop obtained by integrating change in cardiac output during systole with simultaneous measures of LV pressure.

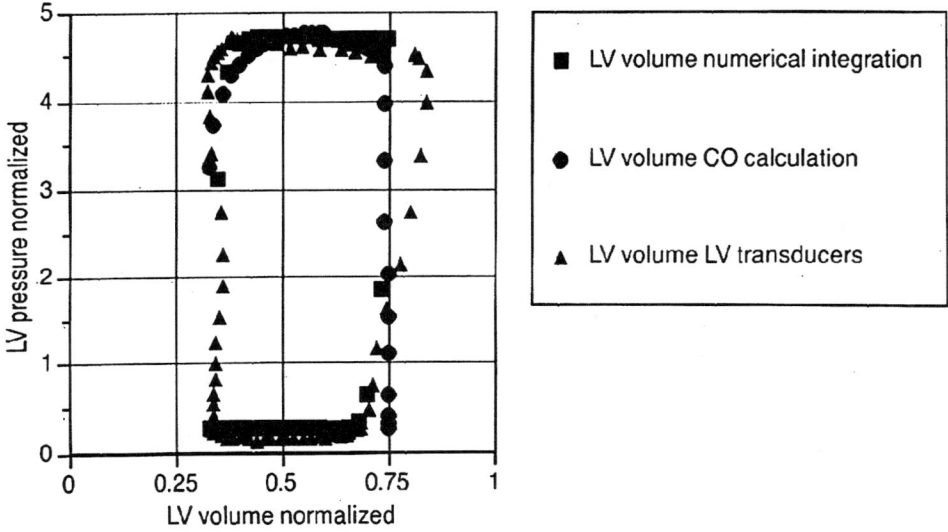

Figure 8 Comparison of PV loops obtained by integrating change in cardiac output during systole with simultaneous measure of LV pressure as in Fig. 7 (circles), numerically fitting μ and α to complete the loop as in Fig. 6 (squares), and comparing the numerically integrated loop with the experimentally measured loop using transducers attached to the LV to measure LV volume (triangles).

and microbiologic criteria that indicate pneumonia in the non-intubated patient cannot be extrapolated to the intubated patient.

Intubated patients can manifest symptoms of systemic illness as a consequence of their underlying illness. In addition, these patients are susceptible to colonization of the tracheobronchial tree as result of intubation. Although delayed diagnosis and treatment may have untoward consequences, the unnecessary use of antibiotics may also lead to unwanted complications of superinfection with resistant strains of organisms.

The usual criteria of pneumonia include infiltration of neutrophils in the terminal bronchioles, which are surrounded by alveoli that are partially filled with neutrophils, fibrinous exudate, and cellular debris. Neutrophils that have phagocytosed gram–negative bacteria may produce a proteolytic response that results in lung necrosis. Accurate diagnosis of pneumonia depends upon the combination of microbiologic and inflammatory data (23).

The suspicion of pneumonia usually begins with a clinical assessment. Leukocytosis, fever, hypoxemia, increased tracheobronchial secretions, and infiltrate on the chest radiograph raise concern that a pulmonary infection exists. In one prospective study to determine the accuracy of clinical judgment in diagnosing VAP, careful consideration of these clinical variables resulted in accurate diagnosis in 62% of patients. Sixteen percent of patients were started on antibiotics unnecessarily, and 67% of the antibiotic regimens chosen were inappropriate for the organisms that were present and their patterns of sensitivity. These findings support the impression that these clinical variables are not sufficient for accurate diagnosis of VAP (24).

In an effort to identify reliable microbiologic criteria, investigators evaluated several sampling methods, including endotracheal tube aspiration, bronchoalveolar lavage (BAL), and protected specimen brush. Endotracheal tube aspirates are easily obtained and subject to contamination by heavily colonized proximal airways. When simultaneous culture of the deep trachea and open lung biopsies were performed, only 40% of the paired cultures agreed (25). ETA may be highly sensitive but probably suffers from low specificity. The use of quantitative ETA cultures, using a diagnostic threshold ≥1 million colony forming units/mL led to a false negative rate of approximately one-third (26). The sensitivity was 68%; whereas, the specificity was 84%. These findings stimulated interest in bronchoscopic sampling of secretions in the distal airways.

Although bronchoscopy is usually well tolerated, the procedure should provide a significant diagnostic advantage to justify the added risk and cost. Routine bronchoscopic aspirates have no advantage over ETA. BAL uses infiltrates on chest radiograph or the location of purulent secretions to sample a segmental or subsegmental bronchus. Sensitivity ranges from 72% to 100%, and specificity range 69% to 100%. An advantage of BAL is the sampling of approximately one million alveoli. A significant limitation is the possibility of contamination of the sampling channel by organisms in the upper airway (27). False positive cultures may be found in up to 30% of cultures. The protected specimen brush employs a sampling brush that is protected from upper airway contamination, until it is deployed in the lower airways. A small volume of secretions is sampled, diluted, and cultured. Using a quantitative threshold, the PSB procedure has a mean sensitivity of 82% and mean specificity of 92%. PSB appears to have somewhat greater specificity than sensitivity (28).

Do these more intensive approaches reduce uncertainty enough to justify their routine use? Would alternate interpretation of simpler tests equally increase the certainty of diagnosis? Consider the use of Bayes' theorem to include conditional probabilities in the analysis of the possible VAP. Bayes' theorem recognizes that any diagnostic test supports or refutes a disease state only in the context of the likelihood of disease before the test was performed. Few, if any, tests in clinical use have 100% accuracy. The power of a test to discriminate the presence of disease from the absence of disease depends on the test's sensitivity and specificity. In one formulation of Bayes' theorem, the probability of a disease state being present $p[D_{post}]$ is given by:

$$p[D_{post}] = \frac{p[D_{prior}] \times \text{sensitivity}}{(p[D_{prior}] \times \text{sensitivity}) + ((1 - p[D_{prior}]) \times (1 - \text{specificity}))}$$

The probability of disease in the case of negative test may be expressed:

$$p[D_{post}] = \frac{(p[D_{prior}] \times (1 - \text{sensitivity}))}{(p[D_{prior}] \times (1 - \text{sensitivity})) + ((1 - p[D_{prior}]) \times \text{specificity})}$$

When the prior probability of a disease is extremely low or extremely high, additional confirmatory tests will do little to change the existing probability. If an intermediate probability of disease exists, and the clinician is comfortable neither with dismissing the diagnosis nor with subjecting the patient to the risks of potential treatment, then a diagnostic test may significantly reduce uncertainty. Use of Bayes' theorem illustrates that the higher the specificity of a given diagnostic test, the higher the post-test probability of a disease when the result is affirmative. In contrast, the higher the sensitivity of a given diagnostic test, the lower the post-test probability of disease when the result is negative. Tests of high sensitivity are most useful for withholding therapy, while tests of high specificity decrease uncertainty for initiating treatment.

To apply these ideas to the question of treating an intubated patient with a positive sputum culture, we must first ask what the probability of VAP was prior to obtaining the culture. Assume that a post-test probability of 75% for the presence of VAP is high enough to warrant treatment. What pre-test probability is high enough to produce a post-test probability of 75% using the least invasive and expensive of the tests described, the quantitative ETA? Recall that the quantitative ETA has a sensitivity of 68% and a specificity of 84%. Using the first of the two formulations of Bayes' theorem, we find that the pretest probability of 41% yields a post-test probability of 75%. Table (3) lists probabilities of VAP being present for different pretest probabilities.

The appearance of a new infiltrate on chest radiograph, increased tracheal secretions, fever, and leukocytosis provides a pretest probability of at least 40%. A positive quantitative ETA would then serve as a reasonable indication for treatment. In situations where the prior probability for VAP is low-intermediate, a test of greater sensitivity and specificity, such as BAL with microanalysis, would aid in making the appropriate decision. If the results of the bronchoscopic procedure were negative, this finding would lower the probability of disease further and would support the withholding of antibiotic treatment. If the results of the procedure were positive, the additional high specificity of the test would raise the probability of VAP and support the decision to initiate antibiotic therapy (23).

USE OF STATISTICAL ENSEMBLES

The state of a patient in the ICU is the result of an enormous number of interacting variables. The number of variables is likely to be uncountably large. We can name a number of variables of order 10^5, and we routinely measure a number of variables that is much smaller, of order 10. Although unnamed and unmeasured, the hidden variables influence the outcomes of therapy. Can we account for them in some way?

A model problem concerns the optimization of support of patients on ventilators. A large number of variables affect the gas exchange in the acutely injured lung. If one asks what combination of ventilator settings, including tidal volume, PEEP, respiratory rate, pressure wave form, and flow characteristics, is optimal, the answer clearly depends on the criterion that is being optimized. The remaining discussion addresses this problem using statistical ensembles to define a quantity to be optimized. The approach allows the hidden variables affecting gas exchange in the lung to be embedded in clearly defined independent states of the system.

Table 3 Probability of VAP for Different Pretest Probabilities

Test	Sensitivity	Specificity	Prior probability of VAP (%)	Probability of VAP if test positive (%)
Quantitative ETA	0.68	0.84	7	25
Quantitative ETA	0.68	0.84	19	50
Quantitative ETA	0.68	0.84	41	75
Quantitative ETA	0.68	0.84	68	90

To develop the ensemble, we note that alveoli have both ventilation and perfusion. We model each alveolus as a two-bit object. The first bit represents ventilation, and the second bit represents perfusion. If ventilation is present, the first bit is 1; if absent, the first bit is 0. Similarly, if perfusion is present, the second bit is 1; if perfusion is absent, the second bit is 0. Four possible configurations are possible:

	Perfusion present	Perfusion absent
Ventilation present	{1,1}	{1,0}
Ventilation absent	{0,1}	{0,0}

The lung is then represented as a sequence of 1s and 0s. Model alveoli are allowed to combine, three alveoli at a time, in all possible ways. The choices of a one-dimensional model and combination of three individual units at a time were made to reduce computational time.

The initial strings, both for ventilation and for perfusion, are chosen randomly. Cellular automata rules then operate independently on each of the strings for ventilation and for perfusion, respectively (29). We illustrate the operation of the cellular automata for three-bit words, each word representing the aggregate function of three alveoli in the initial step. Iteration of the cellular automata rule determines the next level of function in subsequent steps. For three-bit words with two states per bit, 0 and 1, eight possible words exist: {000}, {001}, {010}, {011}, {100}, {101}, {110}, and {111}. If each three-bit word can assume the value of 0 or 1, then 2^8, 256, possible rules or independent states exist. A rule table can be constructed in the following manner:

Word	Rule 0	Rule 1	Rule 2	...	Rule 90	...	Rule 255
000	0	0	0	...	0	...	1
001	0	0	0	...	1	...	1
010	0	0	0	...	0	...	1
011	0	0	0	...	1	...	1
100	0	0	0	...	1	...	1
101	0	0	0	...	0	...	1
110	0	0	1	...	1	...	1
111	0	1	0	...	0	...	1

As an illustration, we demonstrate a single one of the 256 possible rules, designated in the rule table as rule 90. Consider each of the eight possible states of three adjacent sites, depicted in the upper line, and the bit to which it maps, depicted in the lower line:

000	001	010	011	100	101	110	111
0	1	0	1	1	0	1	0

The lower line then specifies a rule for the iterative evolution of the cellular automaton by giving the value to be taken by the central site of the three on the next step. The rule

Responding to Uncertainty in ICU

chosen for this example is one of 256 possibilities and was not chosen for special physiologic significance.

Continuing with the example, we begin with an initial random string for ventilation, designated s_0. We then apply rule 90 to generate the next string s_1. Rule 90 may be applied in succession to produce additional strings, for example s_2:

Initial string	s_0	010110110110101...
Apply rule 90 once	s_1	0011011011000...
Apply rule 90 again	s_2	11101101110...

Any of the remaining 255 rules could be chosen, as well. In the complete calculation, all of the possible rules are tested. Note that any possible sequence of eight binary digits specifies a cellular automaton. After n iterations, the ventilatory state is computed by adding the number of 1s that remain in the string.

A similar procedure is performed to determine all possible states of perfusion. The initial string is chosen randomly, and rules of combination are applied using the rule table. The perfusion state at the end of the iteration is computed by adding the number of 1s that remain in the string. A computed V/Q ratio is obtained by dividing the total number of 1s in the last string for ventilation by the total number of 1s in the last string for perfusion. By this procedure, each rule for perfusion is tested with each rule for ventilation. Each iteration may be thought of as representing the next branch of the tracheobronchial tree (Fig. 9). Although the rule that maps each of the 8 three-bit words to 0 produces a model lung with no function, that rule is completely determined and represents a possible state of the system. Then, $256 \times 256 = 65{,}536$ possible ratios, or independent states, of the system exist.

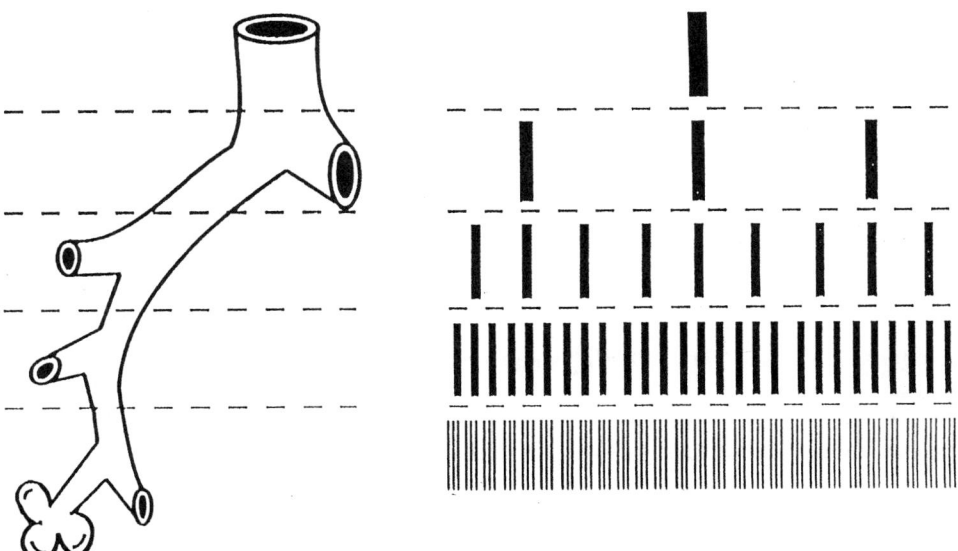

Figure 9 Iterations of cellular automata and relationship to branches of the bronchial tree.

To model the retentions R and excretions E, we employ the relations described by Farhi for R and E in steady-state for a gas of solubility λ (30). In a steady-state,

$$R = \frac{\lambda}{(\lambda + V_A/Q)}$$

For a homogeneous lung, retention equals excretion, but an actual lung is not homogeneous, and R is greater than E. As defined in the foregoing discussion, V_A is the density of 1s in the last string for ventilation. Similarly, Q is the density of 1s in the last string for perfusion. Then, V_A/Q will be given by

$$\frac{V_A}{Q} = \frac{\text{1s in last string for ventilation}}{\text{1s in last string for perfusion}}$$

The retention is defined as

$$R = \frac{\lambda}{\lambda + \text{1s in last string for ventilation}/\text{1s in last string for perfusion}}$$

Similarly excretion is defined by

$$E = \frac{\lambda}{\lambda + \text{1s in last string for ventilation}/\text{1s in last string for perfusion}}$$

We then apply constraints in the form of the experimentally measured retentions and excretions. If R is predicted by the foregoing calculation to within 5% of the experimentally measured R, we define that rule as an accessible state. Let α be the number of rules that predict R to within 5%. Let β equal the total number of rules. We define the retention ratio g_R as $g_R = \log(\alpha/\beta)$. For gases of different solubilities, we can then define the sum of the retention ratios as $\sum g_R = \sum \log(\alpha_i/\beta_i)$. A similar calculation can be performed for E. Let γ be the number of rules that predict E to within 5%. The excretion ratio is defined as $g_E = \log(\gamma/\beta)$. For gases of different solubilities, the sum would be $\sum g_E = \sum \log(\gamma_i/\beta_i)$.

Using smooth changes of coordinates, the calculated and measured curves are superimposable, a result indicating topological equivalence between the experimentally obtained data of Ratner and Wagner and g_R computed from iterating the cellular automata relations (32) (Figs. 10 and 11). With smooth changes of coordinates, the calculated g_E and measured excretion curves for excretion are superimposable. (Figs. 10 and 11). These results indicate that both retentions and excretions may be interpreted as the log of the ratio of accessible states of the system to total states of the system. Please note the similarity of these ratios to the definition of entropy in thermal physics.

These relations permit an approach to the problem defining optimum ventilator support. Let Γ be the sum of the retention ratio and excretion ratio, g_R and g_E, respectively. Since changing the ventilator pressure and volume settings affects retentions and excretions (Lim and Abrams, unpublished data), we expect a change in Γ for each change in P and V.

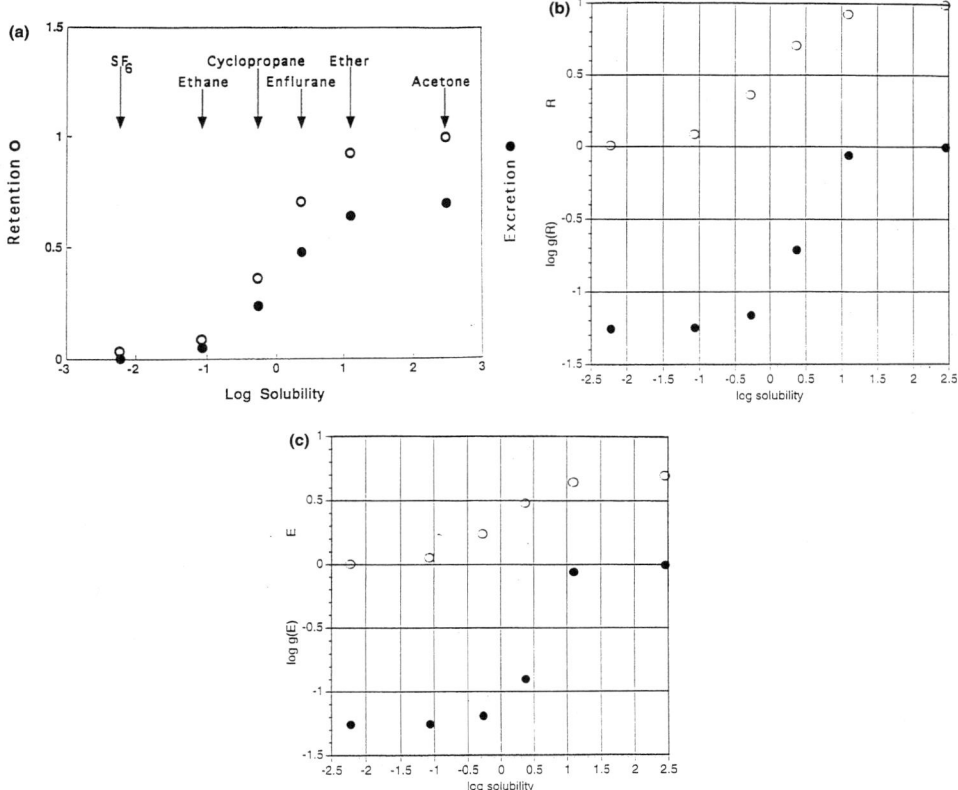

Figure 10 (a) Experimentally measured retentions and excretions as a function of log solubility for six inert gases, adapted from Ref. (32). (b) Retentions and log g_R as a function of log solubility. Open circles are measured retentions, and closed circles are log g_R. (c) Excretions and log g_E as a function of log solubility. Open circles are measured excretions, and closed circles are log g_E.

Then Γ will be a function of λ, P, and V or $\Gamma = (\lambda, P, V)$. At constant λ,

$$\Gamma_{\lambda\,\text{const}} = \Gamma(P, V)$$
$$d\Gamma_{\lambda\,\text{const}} = \frac{\partial \Gamma}{\partial P}\, dP + \frac{\partial \Gamma}{\partial V}\, dV$$
$$d\Gamma_{\lambda\,\text{const}} = f_1(P, V)\, dP + f_2(P, V)\, dV$$
$$\Delta\Gamma = \int_{P_1}^{P_2} f_1(P, V)\, dP + \int_{V_1}^{V_2} f_2(P, V)\, dV + \text{const} \tag{1}$$

By measuring retentions and excretions at two different pressures and two different volumes, we can obtain values for each term on the right hand side of Eq. (1). The quantity Γ can provide an answer to the question of optimizing ventilator support. The healthy lung has a minimal mismatch of V_A and Q and exhibits efficient gas exchange. For the patient on the ventilator, the optimum combination of adjustable ventilator variables, including pressure and volume, depends on the quantity optimized. We propose that the adjustable ventilator variables be arranged at the combination of settings that minimizes the difference between

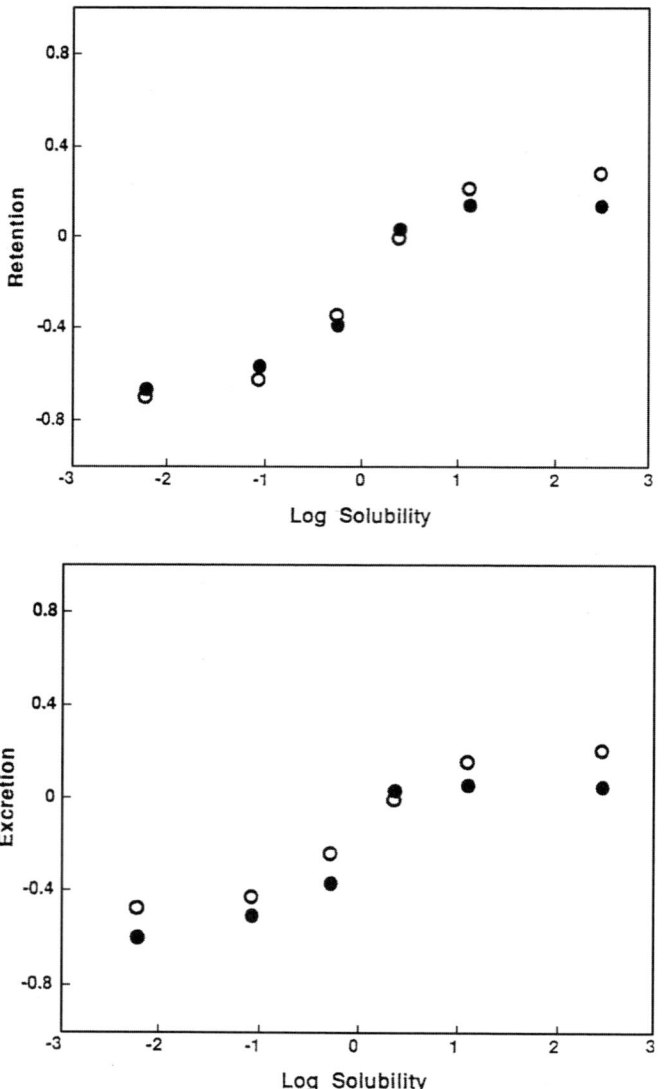

Figure 11 (top) Experimentally measured retentions (○) and calculated retention (g_R) (●) as function of log solubility of six inert gases. g_R has been transformed by a smooth change of coordinates to demonstrate topologic equivalence. (bottom) Experimentally measured excretions (○) and calculated excretion g_E (●) as a function of log solubility of six inert gases. g_E has been transformed by a smooth change of coordinates to demonstrate topologic equivalence.

Γ for the general population of spontaneously breathing people and Γ for the ventilator-dependent patient. Additional constraints on the optimization problem may include minimizing peak and mean airway pressures and keeping the inspired tidal volume within a specified range. The foregoing example uses only two adjustable variables, P and V, in the calculation. The argument could be extended to include additional variables that may be adjusted on the ventilator (31).

SUMMARY

- The problems presented by critically ill patients are high dimensional, dynamic, and non-linear.
- Evidence-based medicine, distinguishing response variables from control variables, dynamical systems, joint probabilities, and statistical ensembles are responses to these challenges.
- Controversy in understanding the role of oxygen transport in the care of the critically ill may be resolved by defining control parameters and their values in a cusp catastrophe model.
- Use of a two parameter non-linear van der Pol oscillator allows ventricular function to be modeled without using a specific geometric shape for the ventricle. In principle, the ventricular PV relationship could be constructed from continuous cardiac output measurements and measurement of ventricular pressure.
- Bayes analysis of pretest probability and the sensitivities and specificities of clinical tests improves the value of the tests in making clinical decisions.
- Unnamed and unmeasured variables that affect the state of patients may be modeled as independent states with the use of cellular automata. With this model, the unnamed, unmeasured variables are embedded in rules of computation. A quantity analogous to entropy in thermal physics can be defined. Its behavior when the system is perturbed can be quantified. With this method, optimum mechanical ventilator support of patients can be defined.

REFERENCES

1. Abraham E, Bland RD, Cobo JC, Shoemaker WC. Sequential cardiorespiratory patterns associated with outcome in septic shock. Chest 1984; 85:75–80.
2. Shoemaker WC, Appeal PL, Kram HB, Waxman K, Lee T-S. Prospective trial of supranormal values of survivors as therpeutic goals in high-risk surgical patients. Chest 1988; 94:1176–1186.
3. Tuchschmidt J, Fried J, Astiz M, Rackow E. Elevation of cardiac output and oxygen delivery improves outcome in septic shock. Chest 1992; 102:216–220.
4. Boyd O, Grounds RM, Bennett ED. A randomized clinical trial of the effect of deliberate perioperative increase of oxygen delivery on mortality in high-risk surgical patients. JAMA 1993; 270:2699–2707.
5. Ronco JJ, Phang PT, Walley KR, Wiggs B, Fenwick JC, Russell JA. Oxygen consumption is independent of changes in oxygen delivery in severe adult respiratory distress syndrome. Am Rev Respir Dis 1991; 143:1267–1273.
6. Archie JP. Mathematic coupling of data. Ann Surg 1981; 193:296–303.
7. Hayes MA, Timmins AC, Yau EHS, Palazzoni M, Hinds CJ, Watson D. Elevation of systemic oxygen delivery in the treatment of critically ill patients. N Engl J Med 1994; 330:1717–1722.
8. Cain SM. Oxygen delivery and uptake in dogs during anemia and hypoxic hypoxia. J Appl Physiol 1997; 42:228–234.
9. Shibutani K, Komatsu T, Kubal K, Sanchala V, Kumar V, Bizzari D. Critical level of oxygen delivery in anesthetized man. Crit Care Med 1983; 11:640–643.
10. Natanson C, Danner RL, Reily JM, Doerfler ML, Hoffman WD, Akin GL, Hosseini JM, Banks SM, Elin RJ, MacVittie TJ, Parrillo JE. Antibiotics versus cardiovascular support in a canine model of human septic shock. Am J Physiol 1990; 259:H1440–1447.

11. Bihari D, Smithies M, Gimson A, Tinker J. The effects of vasodilation with prostacyclin in oxygen delivery and uptake in critically ill patients. N Engl J Med 1987; 317:397–403.
12. Yu M, Levy MM, Smith P, Takiguchi SA, Miyasaki A, Myers SA. Effect of maximizing oxygen delivery on morbidity and mortality rates in critically ill patients: a prospective randomized trial. Crit Care Med 1993; 21:830–838.
13. Berlauk JF, Abrams JH, Gilmour IJ, O'Connor R, Knighton DR, Cerra FB. Preoperative optimization of cardiovascular hemodynamics improves outcome in peripheral vascular surgery. Ann Surg 1991; 214:289–299.
14. Gattinoni L, Brazzi L, Pelosi P, Latini R, Tognoni G, Pesenti A, Fumagalli R. A trial of goal oriented hemodynamic therapy in critically ill patients. N Engl J Med 1995; 333:1025–1032.
15. Heyland DK, Cook DJ, King D, Kernerman P, Brun-Buisson C. Maximizing oxygen delivery in critically ill patients: a methodologic appraisal of the evidence. Crit Care Med 1996; 24:517–524.
16. Rivers E, Nguyen B, Havstad S, Ressler J, Muzzin A, Knoblich B, Peterson E, Tomlanovich M. Early goal-directed therapy in the treatment of severe sepsis and septic shock. N Engl J Med 2001; 345:1368–1377.
17. Siegel JH, Farrell EJ, Miller M, Goldwyn RM, Friedman HP. Cardiorespiratory interactions as determinants of survival and the need of respiratory support in human shock states. J Trauma 1973; 13:602–619.
18. Abrams JH, Barke RA, Cerra FB. Quantitative evaluation of clinical course in surgical ICU patients: the data conform to catastrophe theory. J Trauma 1984; 24:1028–1037.
19. Suga H, Sagawa K, Shoukas AA. Load independence of the instantaneous pressure–volume ratio of the canine left ventricle and effects of epinephrine and heart rate on the ratio. Circ Res 1973; 32:314–322.
20. Rankin JS, Hemodynamic management. In: Wilmore D, Brenner M, Hacker A (eds). Care of the Surgical Patient, vol 1. New York, NY: Scientific American, 1989:II2–3.
21. Beltrami E. Mathematics for Dynamic Modeling (ed 1). Boston, MA: Academic Press, 1987:182.
22. Abrams JH, Irwin ED, Walvatne CS, Segar LK, Foker JE, Cerra FB. Use of a modified van der Pol's oscillator to construct ventricular pressure–volume relations. J cardiothorac Vasc Anesthe 1993; 7:195–199.
23. Farber MS, Abrams JH. A positive sputum culture in an intubated patient is an indication for treatment. Surg Infect Forum 1997; 1:2–7.
24. Fagon J-Y, Chastre J, Hance AJ, Domart Y, Trouillet J-L, Gibert C. Evaluation of clinical judgment in the identification and treatment of nosocomial pneumonia in ventilated patients. Chest 1993; 103:547–553.
25. Hill JD, Ratliff JL, Parrott JCW, Lamy M, Fallat RJ, Koeniger E, Yaeger EM, Whitmer G. Pulmonary pathology in acute respiratory insufficiency: lung biopsy as a diagnostic tool. J Thorac Cardiovasc surgery 1976; 71:64–71.
26. Jourdain B, Novara A, Joly-Guillan M-L, Dombret M-C, Calvat S, Trouillet J-L, Gibert C, Chasture J. Role of quantitative cultures of endotracheal aspirates in the diagnosis of nonocomial pneumonia. Am J Respir Crit Care Med 1995; 152:241–246.
27. Pingleton SK, Fagon JY, Leeper KV Jr. Patient selection for clinical invesitigation of ventilator-associated pneumonia. Criteria for evaluating diagnostic techniques Chest 1992; 102(5 Suppl 1):553s–556s.
28. Chastre J, Fagon JY, Trouillet JL. Diagnosis and treatment of nosocomial pneumonia in patients in intensive care units. Clin Infect Dis 1995; 21(suppl 3):S226–237.
29. Wolfram S. Statistical mechanics of cellular automata. Rev Mod Phys 1983; 55:601–643.
30. Farhi LE. Advances in Respiratory Physiology, Caro CG ed. Baltimore MD, 1966:Chapter 5.
31. Abrams JH, Slovut DP, Lim J P-K, Bugedo G. Modeling inert pulmonary gas exchange using cellular automata. Complexity 2000; 5:36–45.
32. Ratner ER and Wagner PN. Resolution of the multiple inert gas method for estimating VA/Q maldistribution. Respir Physiol 1982; 49:293–313.

Index

AABB. *See* American Association of Blood Banks
Abacavir, for HIV, 709
Abciximab, in myocardial infarction, 372
Abdomen, 591–604
   acalculous cholecystitis, 599
   diagnosis, 595–601
   examination of, 69–70
   with HIV/AIDS, 711
   immunosuppression, 601
   laboratory tests, 595–596
   mesenteric ischemia, 599–601
   monitoring, 594–595
   nonsurgical causes, 600
   pancreatitis, 601
   patient history, 591–594
   physical examination, 591–594
   radiologic tests, 596–597
   resuscitation, 594–595
   treatment, 597–599
Abdominal aortic aneurysm surgery, renal failure with, 140
Abdominal cavity, anatomy, 693
Abdominal CT scan, in trauma patient, 74–75
Abdominal injury
   abdominal CT scan, 74–75
   Focused Assessment for Sonographic Examination of Trauma Patient, 74–76
   initial approach to, 74–76
   peritoneal lavage, 74–75, 75t
   in trauma patient, 74–76
   ultrasonography, 74–76

Abdominal pain
   with HIV/AIDS, 711
   nonsurgical causes of, 600
Abscess
   intra-abdominal, 698–699
      antibiotic therapy, 697t
      bacteria causing, 696
      diagnosis, 698–699
      management, 699
   of lung, 484
   pyogenic, 208
Absence seizures, 210
Absorption of medications, 745–746. *See also under specific medication*
Acalculous, in cholecystitis, 583–584, 599
ACE inhibitors. *See* Angiotensin-converting enzyme inhibitors
Acetaminophen
   hepatic failure with, 607
   lactic acidosis, 36
   overdose of, 36, 608
   thrombocytopenia with, 853
   toxicity of, hepatic failure, 607
Acetazolamide, with metabolic acidosis, 518
Acid–base homeostasis, 511–526
   abnormalities, precipitating factors, 323
   anion gap
      in metabolic acidosis, 517
      in metabolic alkalosis, 518
   arterial blood gas chemistries, 511
   bicarbonate, 511
   conjugate acid–base pairs, 511
   disturbances of, 511–526
      as indication for dialysis, 536

Acid–base homeostasis (*Contd.*)
　Henderson–Hasselbalch relationship, 515
　　bicarbonate buffer system, 513–514
　　　respiratory acidosis, 521–522
　　interpretation, 511–516
　　intracellular hemoglobin buffer
　　　system, 512–513
　　metabolic acid–base disorders, 516–519
　　metabolic acidosis, 514, 516–518
　　metabolic alkalosis, 514, 518–519
　　　classification of, 520
　　　factors contributing to, 520
　　partial pressure of carbon dioxide, 511
　　partial pressure of oxygen, 511
　　renal tubular cell, 513
　　respiratory acid–base disorders, 519–524
　　respiratory acidosis, 521–522
　　　causes of, 523
　　respiratory alkalosis, 514, 522–524
　　　causes of, 524
　　Winter's formula, metabolic acidosis, 517
Acidemia, respiratory, in discontinuation of
　　mechanical ventilation, 508
Acidosis. *See also* Ketoacidosis
　lactic, 33–42
　metabolic, 514, 518
　respiratory, 521–523
Acinetobacter baumannii
　control/prevention, 686
　epidemiology, 686
　therapy, 686
ACLS. *See* American Heart Association
　　Advanced Cardiac Life Support
Acquired immune deficiency syndrome (AIDS)
　antiretroviral therapy, 712–717
　clinical presentation, 711t
　epidemiology, 704–705
　ethical issues, 718–719
　legal issues, 718–719
　needle stick, 706–707
　postexposure prophylaxis, 708–710
　risk to surgeon, 703–724
Acromegaly, airway management with, 477
ACTH stimulation test, 631–632
Activated protein C, with acute respiratory
　　distress syndrome, 429
Acute abdomen. *See* Abdomen
Acute lung injury, 7, 421–432
　acute respiratory distress syndrome, 421
　alternative ventilator strategies, 428–429
　chest x-ray, ground-glass appearance, 425
　clinical course, 425–426

　criteria for, 422t
　defined, 421
　diuresis, 427
　early nutritional support, 426
　fibrotic phase III, 424–425
　fluid resuscitation, 426
　hemoglobin, 426
　hypoxia, 427
　incidence, 422
　inspiratory time, prolongation of, 428
　lung stretch, 428
　management, 426–427
　mechanical ventilation, 427–428
　mediators of, 422–423
　over-inflated alveoli, 428
　pathophysiology, 424–425
　PEEP, 426–427
　pharmacologic therapies, 429–429t
　proliferative phase, 424–425
　prone positioning, 428
　pulmonary function, 421–432
　pulmonary sequelae, 426
　respiratory distress syndrome risk, 423t
　risk factors, 422
　sepsis syndrome, 422
　shunt fraction, 425
　static lung compliance, 425
　subacute phase, 424–425
　tracheal gas insufflation, 428
　veno-arterial extracorporeal membrane
　　oxygenation, 429
　veno-venous low frequency positive
　　pressure ventilation, 429
　ventilator-associated complications, 427
　volume status, 426
Acute myocardial infarction, 327, 367–383
　anatomy, 367–368
　angioplasty, 374–375
　angiotensin-converting enzyme
　　inhibitors, 377
　antiarrhythmics, 378
　antiplatelet therapy, fibrinolytic therapy,
　　combination, 371–372
　aspirin, 375
　β-blockers, 377
　calcium antagonists, 378
　cardiogenic shock, 380
　　abciximab, 372
　　reteplase, 370
　　streptokinase, 370
　　tenecteplase, 371
　　tirofiban, 372

Index

tissue plasminogen activator, 370
complications, 379–380
coronary arteries, distributions of, 368
coronary stenting, 373–374
defined, 367
diagnosis, 368–369
glycoprotein IIb/IIIa antagonists, 372–374
heparin, 376
medical therapy, 375–378
mitral regurgitation, 379
nitrates, 376–377
in nonparoxysmal junctional tachycardia, 347
pathogenesis, 367–368
percutaneous intervention, vs. thrombolytic therapy, 374t
postinfarction angina, infarct extension, 379
primary PCI in, 372–375
right ventricular infarction, 379–380
thienopyridines, 375–376
thrombolytic therapy, 369–372, 370t
transfusion therapy and, 866
ventricular free wall rupture, 379
ventricular septal rupture, 379
Acute-on-chronic liver failure, 605–607
Acute renal failure, 139–150, 527–538
acidosis, as complication, 535
acute tubular necrosis, contrasted, 531, 531t
bladder catheterization, 532–533
bleeding, 536
causes, 532
complications of, 534t
course of, 536–537
diagnosis, 532–533
dialysis, 536
indications for, 536t
differential diagnosis, 527–533, 529t
dopamine, 534
drug dosing, 536
evaluation of patient with, 530t
fluid balance, 534
hyperkalemia
as complication, 535
therapy of, 535t
hyperphosphatemia, as complication, 535
hypocalcemia, as complication, 535
hyponatremia, as complication, 535
intrinsic, 531–532
acute tubular necrosis, 531
causes, 531–532
nephrotoxicity, 531–533
prolonged renal hypoperfusion, 531

loop diuretics, 533–534
management, 534–536
mannitol, 533–534
nutrition, 536
poor prognosis in, 537t
prerenal, 527–531
acute tubular necrosis, 527
causes, 527–530
central pressure, monitoring, 530
diagnosis, 530–531
differential diagnosis, 529t
glomerular filtration rate, 527
patient evaluation, 530t
treatment, 531
vs. acute tubular necrosis, 531, 531t
prevention, 533–534
prognosis, 536–537, 537t
radiocontrast medium-induced, 145t, 532
prevention of, 146t
treatment, 532–533
Acute respiratory distress syndrome, 421
as cause of hypoxemia, 506
as cause of respiratory acidosis, 523
criteria, 422t
nursing care, 178
pancreatitis and, 577
pharmacologic therapies, 429t
risk categories, 423t
with spinal cord injury, 259
Acute tubular necrosis, 139, 527, 531
acute renal failure, contrasted, 531
defined, 529
prerenal acute renal failure, contrasted, 531, 531t
Acyclovir, 793
Addisonian crisis, with anaphylaxis, 804
Addison's disease, 629
abdominal pain with, 600
Adenosine, with atrioventricular nodal re-entry, 349
Adenovirus, as cause of fulminant hepatic failure, 608
Adrenal crisis, 629–630. See also Hypoadrenalism
Adrenal function, biochemical tests of, 631
Adrenal insufficiency, 629–634, 641
adrenal crisis, treatment of, 631–632
adrenal function, biochemical tests of, 631
clinical features, 630
diagnosis, 630–631

Adrenal insufficiency (*Contd.*)
  etiology of, 629-630
  glucocorticoid potencies, 630t
  prior steroid therapy, 630-631
Adrenergic agonists, in bronchospasm, 436t
Advanced Trauma Life Support, American College of Surgeons, course recommendations, 66
Adverse drug reactions, 783-798. *See also under specific drug*
  analgesic therapy, 790-791
    fentanyl, 790-791
    hydromorphone, 790-791
    meperidine, 790-791
    morphine, 790-791
  antiarrhythmic drugs, 783-786
    amiodarone, 783-784
    angiotensin-converting enzyme inhibitors, 785-786
    antiarrhythmic therapy, 786-787
    calcium channel blocking therapy, 786
    digoxin, 784-785
  cardiovascular therapy, 783-795
  inotropic therapy, 788
  non-opioid therapy, 791-795
    antimicrobials, 792-795
    nonsteroidal anti-inflammatory therapy, 791-792
  QT interval, drugs prolonging, 787t
  sedative therapy, 788-790
    benzodiazepines, 788-789
    droperidol, 790
    haloperidol, 789-790
    propofol, 789
  vasoactive drugs, 787-788
    nitroprusside, 787-788
  vasopressor therapy, 788
Aerobic glycolysis, in oxygen transport, 27
Aerobic gram-negative gut bacteria, elimination of, 553
AFFIRM. *See* Atrial Fibrillation Follow-up Investigation of Rhythm Management
Afterload, cardiac, 313
  defined, 313
  pulmonary vascular resistance, 313
  systemic vascular resistance, 313
Aggrastat, in myocardial infarction, 372
AIDS. *See* Acquired immune deficiency syndrome
Air embolus
  with catheter use, 51
  as complication of percutaneous central venous catheterization, 917
  transfusion therapy and, 873
Air trapping, in bronchospasm, 434, 439
Airway evaluation, in burns, 88
Airway management, 63-65, 113-114, 469-488, 471t. *See also* Breathing; Ventilation
  blind nasotracheal intubation, 64
  in cardiac arrest, 113-114
  chin-lift maneuvers, 113
  cricothyroidotomy, 64
  difficult airway, 473-474
  endotracheal intubation, 114, 469
    complications of, 472
    congential syndromes associated with difficulty in, 475t
    head position for, 474
    indications for, 469
    route of, 469-471
    standard approaches, 471-473
    successful, confirmation of, 474-477
  endotracheal tube, 469
    blind, 473
    confirmation of placement, 478t
    construction, 481
    cuffed vs. noncuffed, 480-481
    inner cannula, 481
    misplaced, 479t
    position, 479t
    selection, 480-481
    shape, 481
    size, 479t
  epiglottis, 476
  esophageal-tracheal Combitube, 64
  extubation, 477-479
  initial approach, 63-64
  intubating laryngeal mask airway, 64
  jaw-thrust, 113
  laryngeal mask airway, 64
  nasotracheal intubation, orotracheal intubation, compared, 471t
  nursing care, 176-178
  oropharyngeal airway, 114
  orotracheal intubation, 64, 114
  orotracheal tube, changing of, 477
  pathologic states, 476-477t
  pulmonary hemorrhage/massive hemoptysis, 484-486
    angiography/embolization, 485
    balloon tamponade, 485
    bronchoscopy, 485

Index

radionuclear scanning, 485
surgery, 485–486
respiratory failure, clinical signs of, 63
rubber nasopharyngeal airway, 114
tracheostomy, 64, 479–484
   recent, 481–482
tracheostomy tube, 469
   changing, 482–484
   changing over suction catheter, 483
   indications for tube change, 482
   procedure, 482–484
in trauma patient, 65t
unstable cervical spine, methods of intubation for, 478t
Airway pressure release ventilation, 497
Alanine aminotransferase, increases in, hepatic function and, 130
Albumin, hepatic function and, 131–132
Albumin dialysis, as liver assist device, 621
Albuminuria, 141t
   defined, 141t
   renal failure and, 141t
Albuterol, allergic reaction, 801
Alcoholic cirrhosis, 605
Alcohol-induced anion gap acidosis, 518
Alcoholism
   as cause of seizure, 209
   hepatic function and, 131
Alcohol withdrawal seizures, 215
Aldosteronism, primary, 520
Alertness, in head injury, anatomic substrates of, 230
ALI. *See* Acute lung injury
Alkali therapy, lactic acidosis, 39
Alkalosis, hypokalemia and, 670
Allergic reaction, 799–810. *See also* Anaphylaxis
Allogeneic blood transfusion, transfusion therapy and, 861
Alloimmunization to red cell antigens, transfusion therapy and, 874
α-2-agonist, withdrawal of, as cause of hypertensive crisis, 386
α blockers, pharmacodynamics of, 772
α-hemolytic streptococcus, tertiary peritonitis, 700
α hydroxylase deficiency, 520
α vasopressor effects, 118–119
Altered cardiac physiology
   diastolic dysfunction, treatment of, 317t
   septic shock, 320

Altered mental status, in bronchospasm, 438
Altered microbial flora, in immunocompromised patient, 732–733
Altitude, as cause of respiratory disorder, 524
Alveolar gas equation, in respiratory monitoring, 987–988
American Association of Blood Banks, standards, 876
American College of Surgeons, Advanced Trauma Life Support, course recommendations, 66
American Disabilities Act of 1990, 719
American Heart Association Advanced Cardiac Life Support, guidelines, 357
American Medical Association and American college of Physicians, guidelines, 719
Amikacin
   antibiotic resistance, 684
   serum concentration monitoring, 755
Aminoglycosides, 793
Amiodarone, 121, 378
   as antiarrhythmic, 337–338
   in cardiac arrest, 121
   with multifocal atrial tachycardia, 345
   with sustained ventricular tachycardia, 357
Ammonium chloride, with metabolic acidosis, 518
Amphotericin B, 793
Ampicillin
   antibiotic resistance, 686
   as cause of fulminant hepatic failure, 608
   in pancreatitis, 576
Amplitude ratio, in blood pressure monitoring, 963–965
Amputation, with frostbite, 95
Amrinone, thrombocytopenia with, 853
Amylase, in pancreatitis, 573
Amyloidosis, with atrial fibrillation, 330
Amyotrophic lateral sclerosis, respiratory acidosis with, 523
Anaerobic microflora, gut, preservation of, 553
Analgesic therapy
   adverse reactions, 790–791
   intravenous delivery, 777t
Anaphylaxis, 434, 799–810
   basic support with, 804–805
   β-lactam antibiotic desensitization, 808
   bronchospasm, 805
   cardiovascular effects, 803
   clinical manifestations, 802–804

Anaphylaxis (*Contd.*)
  differential diagnosis, 804
  drugs causing, 800
  effects of, 802
  epidemiology, 799–800
  hemodynamic compromise, 806
  inciting therapy, 800–801
  manifestations of, 804
  mediators of, 801–802
  mucocutaneous manifestations, 803–804
  pathophysiology, 801–802
  pharmacologic therapy, 805
  pretreatment protocol, 807
  prevention, 807–808
    β-lactam antibiotics, 807–808
    iodine-contained RCM, 807
  recovery phase, 806–807
  respiratory compromise,
      treatment of, 805–806
  respiratory effects, 802–803
  therapy causing, 800
  treatment, 804–807
  upper airway obstruction, 805
Anasarca, with malnutrition, 44
Ancrod, with stroke, 282
Anemia
  with chronic renal failure, 148
  lactic acidosis, 36
  with malnutrition, 44
  transfusion therapy and, 845–846
Anesthesia
  arterial end-tidal carbon dioxide tension
      during, 991t
  as cause of respiratory acidosis, 523
  with chronic renal failure, 147–148
  effect on hepatic function, 129–130
  pulmonary complications with, 154–155
Angina
  abdominal pain with, 600
  after myocardial infarction, 379
  postoperative ischemic event risk, 103
  with sustained ventricular
      tachycardia, 355
Angioedema
  airway management with, 476
  with anaphylaxis, 804
Angiography
  with sustained ventricular tachycardia, 357
  in trauma patient, 76–78
Angioplasty
  in myocardial infarction, 374–375
  with stroke, 282

Angiotensin-converting enzyme inhibitors
  in myocardial infarction, 377
  pharmacodynamics of, 771
  with stroke, 280–281
  systolic dysfunction, 316
Anion gap
  in metabolic acidosis, 517
  in metabolic alkalosis, 518
Ankylosing spondylitis, airway management
    with, 476
Ankylosis, airway management with, 476
Anorectal disease, with HIV/AIDS, 711
Anoxia
  as cause of seizure, 208
  coma with, 189
Anoxic encephalopathy, prognosis, 199–200
Antabuse, as cause of fulminant hepatic
    failure, 608
Antacids, gastrointestinal hemorrhage
    and, 561
Anterior cord syndrome, 254
Anteroposterior cervical spine radiograph,
    spinal cord injury, 250
Antero-septal myocardial infarction, 328
Antiarrhythmic therapy, 337t
  adverse reactions, 783–786
  with atrial fibrillation, 337t
    classification of, 335t
  with atrioventricular nodal re-entry, 349
  classification of, 335t
  with myocardial infarction, 378
  thrombocytopenia with, 853
Antibiotic resistance, 675–692
  Acinetobacter baumannii, 686
    control/prevention, 686
    epidemiology, 686
    therapy, 686
  antibiotic class, scheduled
      changes of, 678–679
  β-lactamase-producing *Klebsiella
      pneumoniae*, extended-spectrum,
      685–686
    control/prevention, 685–686
    epidemiology, 685
  broad-spectrum antibiotics, use of, 676
  contact precautions, 681
  cycling of antibiotics, 679–680
  enterobacter species, 684–685
    control/prevention, 685
    epidemiology, 684
    therapy, 685
  epidemiology of, 675–681

antibiotic utilization, 676–680
hand hygiene, 680
infection control, role of, 680–681
infection treatment guidelines, 677–678
infectious disease specialists, 680
methicillin-resistant *Staphylococcus aureus*, 681–682
    control/prevention, 681–682
    epidemiology, 681
    therapy, 681
monitoring, 677
prevalence, ICU, non-ICU isolates compared, 677t
Pseudomonas aeruginosa, 683–684
    control/prevention, 684
    epidemiology, 683
    therapy, 683
rates of, 676t
vancomycin-resistant enterococci, 682–683
    control/prevention, 683
    epidemiology, 682
    therapy, 682–683
Antibiotics. *See also under specific antibiotic*
class, scheduled changes of, 678–679
effect on platelet function, 815
Antibody deficiency, in immunocompromised patient, 733
Antibody specificity prediction, transfusion therapy and, 854–855
Anti-cardiolipin antibody, 823
Anticoagulation, 895–902
aspirin, 897
with atrial fibrillation, 339
with atrial flutter, 344
effect on platelet function, 815
fresh frozen plasma, warfarin-related bleeding, 896
low molecular weight heparin, 897–899
molecular weight heparin, 896
NSAIDs, 897
procoagulant, homeostatic balance, 13
protamine sulfate, dosing schedules, 897
prothrombin complex concentrate, warfarin-related bleeding, 896
with stroke, 282–283
therapy used for, 895–902
transfusion therapy and, 847–848
unfractionated heparin, 897–899
vitamin K, nonbleeding patient, 895–896
warfarin, 895–897
    overdose, 895–897
    vitamin K, differences in half-lives, 895–897

Antidepressants
with bradyarrhythmias, 325
as cause of fulminant hepatic failure, 608
Antidiuretic hormone, 662–663
Antiepileptic drugs, 215–217
in acute setting, 216
long-term management, 217
pharmacologic considerations, 216–217
Antifungal therapy. *See also under specific antifungal*
in pancreatitis, 576–577
Antigen-antibody complex formation, transfusion therapy and, 858
Antihistamines, effect on platelet function, 815
Antihypertensive therapy, 767–776
dosing, 767–776
fenoldopam, 389
fentanyl, 388
in hypertensive emergencies, 388–391
midazolam, 388
nitroprusside, 389
pharmacodynamics of, 769–770t
sodium nitroprusside, 389
Anti-inflammatory therapy,
in bronchospasm, 433, 437
Antimicrobial therapy. *See also under specific antimicrobial*
in immunocompromised patient, 728–729
for intra-abdominal infection, 696–700
with liver failure, 614
monitoring of, 793–795t
thrombocytopenia with, 853
Antiplatelet therapy
fibrinolytic therapy, combination, ST-segment elevation myocardial infarction, 371–372
with spinal cord injury, 260
Antiretroviral therapy
complications of, 713–716t
interactions with medications, 713–716t
lactic acidosis and, 36
Antisecretory support in pancreatitis, 578–579
Antisera, allergic reaction to, 801
Anti-shock garment, for trauma patient, 76
Antitachycardia, 358
Antithrombin, transfusion therapy and, 848
Antithrombin III deficiency, 823
Anton syndrome, 276
Anxiety
as cause of respiratory disorder, 524
perioperative hypertension with, 386

Aortic dissection, in hypertensive
  emergencies, 392–393
Aortic injury, in trauma patient, 73–73t
Aortic procedures, vascular
  complications, 416
  perioperative bleeding, 416
Aortic surgery, renal failure and, 147
Apathetic hyperthyroidism, in thyroid
  dysfunction, 635
Aphasia
  in differential diagnosis of seizure, 212
  with stroke, 275
Apheresis platelet transfusions, transfusion
  therapy and, 859
Apnea, 202
  in bronchospasm, 438
Apneustic respiration, in coma, 232
Apprehension, with pulmonary embolism, 446
ARAS. *See* Ascending reticular activating
  system
Arch aortogram, in trauma patient, 73
ARDS. *See* Acute respiratory distress
  syndrome
ARF. *See* Acute renal failure
Argatroban, in pulmonary embolism, 459–460
Arginine chloride, with metabolic
  acidosis, 518
Arrested heart, 115–117
  pulseless electrical activity,
    guidelines for, 117
Arrhythmia. *See* Cardiac arrhythmia
Arsenic, abdominal pain with, 600
ART. *See* Antiretroviral therapy
Arterial blood gas
  bronchospasm and, 435
  in cardiac arrest, 123–124
  chemistries, 511
  in mechanical ventilation, 490t, 503
Arterial catheterization, systemic, 923–925
Arterial end-tidal carbon dioxide tension,
  during general anesthesia, 991t
Arterial injury, with catheter use, 51
Arterial insufficiency, 411–413
  lower extremity ischemia, 411–413
    arterial thromboembolism, 412
    arterial thrombosis, 412
    clinical presentation, 411–412
    differential diagnosis, 412
    medical, surgical treatment, 412–413
    non-occlusive ischemia, 412
  upper extremity ischemia, 413
    arterial thromboembolism, 413

    arterial thrombosis, 413
    clinical presentation, 413
    differential diagnosis, 413
    medical, surgical treatment, 413
    vasospasm or non-occlusive
      ischemia, 413
Arterial oxygen
  tension, alveolar oxygen tension,
    differences between, 987–988
  transfusion therapy and, 834
Arterial oxygenation decrease, as
  complication of transbronchoscopic
  procedure, 912
Arterial pressure, intracranial pressure,
  relationship between, 83
Arterial puncture, as complication of
  percutaneous central venous
  catheterization, 917
Arterial thromboembolism, with upper
  extremity ischemia, 413
Arteriography, complications of,
  as source of cerebral
  ischemia, 272
Arteriovenous malformation, as cause of
  hemoptysis, 484
Arthritis, abdominal pain with, 600
Artificial liver, 622–623
  biologic component, 622–623
  mechanical obstruction, 609–610
  nitric oxide, role of, 610
  pathologic supply dependency, 610–611
  synthetic substrate, 622
  trials, 622t
Ascending reticular activating system,
  with coma, 187–188
Ascites, hepatic function and, 131–132, 135
Aspartate aminotransferase, increases in,
  hepatic function and, 130
Aspergillus, in immunocompromised
  patient, 728, 732
Aspiration
  with acute respiratory distress
    syndrome, 423
  during enteral feed, 50
  with spinal cord injury, 259
Aspirin, 897
  with atrial fibrillation, 339
  in myocardial infarction, 375
  with stroke, 282
Asplenia, in immunocompromised
  patient, 730
Assist-control ventilation, 493–494

Index

Asthma
   bronchospasm, 434
   as cause of respiratory disorder, 524
   defined, 433
   with lactic acidosis, 36
Asystole, guidelines for, 118
Ataxic respiration, in coma, 232
Atelectasis, 152
   bronchoscopy with, 907
   as cause of hypoxemia, 506
   in spinal cord injury, 259
Atherosclerosis, as source of cerebral ischemia, 272
ATLS. *See* American College of Surgeons, Advanced Trauma Life Support
ATN. *See* Acute tubular necrosis
Atracurium, 757–758
Atrial arrhythmias, 330–347
Atrial fibrillation, 330–340
   amyloidosis, 330
   antiarrhythmic therapy, 337t
     classification of, 335t
   anticoagulation, 339
   aspirin, 339
   Atrial Fibrillation Follow-up Investigation of Rhythm Management, 336–338
   atrial maze operation, 339
   β-adrenergic blocking drugs, 334
   β-blocker therapy, 332
   calcium channel blockers, 334
   cardiomyopathy, 330
   cardioversion, 334–336, 340
   catheter-based ablation procedures, 338–339
   chronic therapy, 336–339
   clinical presentation, 332–334
   coronary artery diseases, 330
   digoxin, 334
   dofetilide, 340
   esmolol, 335
   etiology of, 330–331
   fibrillatory waves, 332
   hypertension, 330
   hyperthyroidism, 330
   ibutilide, 340
   incidence of, 330–331
   intravenous diltiazem, 335
   lidocaine, 335–336
   mitral valve replacement, 339
   tachycardia, 331
   transesophageal echocardiography, 340
   treatment, 334–336
   valvular heart diseases, 330
   warfarin, 340
   warfarin therapy, 339
   wide complex tachycardia, 332
   Wolff-Parkinson-White syndrome, 335
Atrial Fibrillation Follow-up Investigation of Rhythm Management, 336–338
Atrial flutter, 340–344
   acute therapy, 342–343
   anticoagulation, 344
   atrial overdrive pacing, 342–343
   cardioversion, 343
   catheter ablation, 344
   chronic therapy, 343–344
   clinical presentation, 340–342
   ECG, 341–342
   embolic risk, 342
   etiology of, 340
   flutter rate, 340–341
   intravenous esmolol therapy, 343
   QRS synchronized DC cardioversion, 342–343
   suppressive drug therapy, 343
   transesophageal echocardiogram, 344
Atrial maze operation, with atrial fibrillation, 339
Atrial overdrive pacing, with atrial flutter, 342–343
Atrial pacing, in nonparoxysmal junctional tachycardia, 347
Atrial perforation, as complication of percutaneous central venous catheterization, 917
Atrioventricular nodal reentry, 347–349
   acute therapy, 349
   antiarrhythmic drugs, 349
   β-adrenergic blockers, 349
   breath holding, 349
   calcium channel blockers, 349
   carotid massage, 349
   catheter modification, 349
   chronic therapy, 349
   clinical presentation, 348–349
   etiology of, 347–348
   intravenous adenosine, 349
   narrow QRS complex, 348
   premature atrial impulse, 347
   syncope, 348
   twelve-lead ECG, 348
   Valsalva maneuver, 349

Atrioventricular re-entry tachycardia, 349–352
  acute therapy, 351
  adenosine, 351
  anti-arrhythmic drugs, 351–352
  antidromic reciprocating tachycardia, 351
  β-adrenergic blockers, 351
  calcium channel blockers, 351
    avoidance of, 351
  cardioversion, 351
  carotid massage, 351
  catheter ablation, 352
  chronic therapy, 351–352
  clinical presentation, 349–351
  digoxin, 351
    avoidance of, 351
  etiology of, 349
  orthodromic reciprocating tachycardia, 349–350
  twelve-lead ECG
    tachycardia, 350
    ventricular pre-excitation, 350
  Valsalva maneuver, 351
  verapamil, 351
Atrium, perforation of, with catheter use, 51
Atropine, 120
  in cardiac arrest, 120
Autointoxication, gut, 550
Autonomic dysreflexia with spinal injury, 261
Autonomic nervous system, activation in multiple organ failure, 8–13
Auto-positive end-expiratory pressure, 398, 401
Axillary artery catheterization, 415, 924
  complications associated with, 415
Axillary-femoral bypass, as contraindication to subclavian vein catheterization, 916
Axonal injury, as cause of seizure, 208
AZT, with HIV/AIDS, 712
Aztreonam, 793

Babesia, with transfusion therapy, 875
Babesiosis, in immunocompromised patient, 730
Bachmann's bundle pacing, 338
Bacillus cereus, transfusion therapy and, 876
Bacteremia, defined, 4
Bacteria, with transfusions, 876–877
Bacteroides species, as cause of peritonitis/abscess, 696
Balloon tamponade, gastrointestinal hemorrhage with, 559

Barbiturate coma, 285
Barbiturates, allergic reaction, 801
Bariatric surgery, hepatic function and, 133
Barotrauma prevention in mechanical ventilator support, 496
Barriers, for infection control, 684
Barter's syndrome, 520
Basilar skull injury, 233–234
  airway management with, 476
  seizure with, 233–234
Battle's sign
  in head injury, 233–234
Bayes' theorem, 1010
BCAAs. *See* Branched-chain amino acids
Bedside abdominal ultrasound, 586
Benedickt syndrome, 276
Bepridil, 787
Bernard Soulier syndrome, 816, 818
Best interest standard, informed consent, 163
β-blockers, 324
  with atrial fibrillation, 332, 334
  with atrioventricular nodal re-entry, 349
  with bradyarrhythmias, 324
  in myocardial infarction, 377
  pharmacodynamics of, 771
β-human chorionic gonadotropin levels, 595
β hydroxylase deficiency, 520
β-lactam antibiotics
  allergic reaction, 800–801
  anaphylaxis prevention, 807–808
  desensitization, 808
    anaphylaxis, 808
  effect on platelet function, 815
  inciting therapy, 799
Bicarbonate buffer system, Henderson-Hasselbalch equation, 513–514
Biguanides, lactic acidosis, 36
Bilateral cerebral hemispheric lesions, 230
Bile secretion, 662
Biliary cirrhosis, hepatic function and, 131
Biliary complications, 583–590
  bedside abdominal ultrasound, 586
  bilirubin fractionation, 586
  cholangiography, 586
  cholecystectomy, 586
  cholecystitis, 583–586
    acalculous, 583–584
    biliary complications, 585
    calculous, 583
    diagnosis, 584–585

epidemiology of, 583
pathogenesis of, 583–584
radionuclide cholescintigraphy, 584
TPN-associated cholecystitis, 583
treatment, 586
cholestasis, 586
Crigler-Najjar syndrome, 588
during critical illness, 583–590
Dubin-Johnson syndrome, 588
Gilbert's syndrome, 588
hepatitic ischemia, 588
hyperbilirubinemia, 586
jaundice, initial evaluation, 586
Kupffer cell-attracted neutrophils, 588
liver enzyme profiles, 586
nonobstructive jaundice, 587–589
cholangitis, 586–589
hemolysis, 588–589
hepatocellular dysfunction, 587–588
obstructive jaundice, cholangitis, 586–589
Charcot's triad, 587
endoscopic retrograde cholangiography, 587
endoscopic transpapillary sphincterotomy, 587
percutaneous transhepatic cholangiography, 587
Rotor syndrome, 588
viral hepatitis, 588
Bilirubin
fractionation, 586
hepatic function and, 131
Bioartificial liver, 622–623
biologic component, 622–623
mechanical obstruction, 609–610
nitric oxide, role of, 610
pathologic supply dependency, 610–611
synthetic substrate, 622
trials, 622t
Bioavailability, defined, 745
Biotin deficiency, in lactic acidosis, 36
Bivalirudin, in pulmonary embolism, 459–460
Biventricular diastolic compliance, 397
Bladder
catheterization, with renal failure, 532–533
distention, in spinal cord injury, 261
Bleeding disorders, 814–820
with chronic renal failure, 148
hereditary, 816t
preoperative screening for, 816t
Blind endotracheal tube, 473
Blind intestinal loop syndrome, 36

Blind nasal intubation, 471–472
Blind nasotracheal intubation, 64
Blind oral intubation, 471–472
Blood alcohol concentration, in coma evaluation, 195
Blood flow in oxygen transport, 22–24
Blood pressure monitoring, 963–972
amplitude ratio, 963–965
clinical application, 966–970
damped oscillating systems, 963–965
damping, time response, compromise between, 969–970
damping coefficient, 964
measuring, 965–970
frequency ratio, 963–964
pulmonary artery tracing, 968
resonance, 963–965
frequency of, 964–966
snap test, 966
square-wave, 967–969
theory, 965–966
time response, damping, compromise between, 969–970
variable resistor location, 967
Blood pressure reduction, in hypertensive emergencies, 388
Blood products, allergic reaction to, 801
Blood samples, in trauma patient, 68
Blood sugar control, in multiple organ failure, 15
Blood transfusion in trauma patient, indications for, 66
Blood urea nitrogen
dialysis adequacy and, 540
factors affecting value, 542t
Blunt multiple trauma, fractures in, 81–86, 82t
cerebral perfusion pressure, 93
coagulopathy, 84
diagnostic tests, 81
early fracture stabilization, advantages of, 82
femur fractures, plates, 83t
fracture management, 84–85
hemothorax, 93
hypothermia, 84
initial survey, 81
intracranial pressure, 93
mean arterial pressure, intracranial pressure, relationship between, 83
multi-disciplinarian nature of, 84–85
plates for femur fractures, 83t
pulmonary contusion, treatment of, 82–83

Blunt multiple trauma, fractures in (Contd.)
  resuscitation, 81
  severe pelvic injury, 84
  treatment, 84-85
Bohr equation, in respiratory
    monitoring, 991
Bolus injection procedure,
    cardiac output, 974-976
Bone marrow hypoplasia,
    transfusion, 850
Brachial artery
  catheterization, 924
  complications associated with, 415
Brachial plexus injury
  with catheter use, 51
  as complication of percutaneous central
    venous catheterization, 917
Bradyarrhythmias, 324-330
  abnormalities of atrioventricular
    conduction, 326-327
  acute myocardial infarction, 327
  antero-septal myocardial infarction, 328
  antiarrhythmic therapy, 324
  antidepressants, 325
  approach to, 325
  atrial sensing, 329
  atrioventricular conduction
    abnormalities, 326-327
  β-adrenergic blockers, 324
  calcium channel blockers, 324
  cimetidine, 325
  digoxin, 324
  dual chamber pacing, 329
  ECG lead II demonstrating, 327
  electrical pacing, 326
  etiology of, 324, 327-329
    permanent pacing, 329
    temporary pacing, 328-329
  inferior myocardial infarction, 327
  Inter-Society Commission on Heart Disease
    Resources, three-position
    letter code, 329
  Lev-Lenegre's disease, 327
  lithium carbonate, 325
  pacemaker code, 329-330
    general considerations, 329
  pacemaker selection, 329-330
  pacemaker syndrome, 329
  pain management, 324
  permanent pacing, 329
  sick sinus syndrome, 329
  sinus node dysfunction, 324

  sympatholytic antihypertensive
    therapy, 324
  tachycardia-bradycardia syndrome, 324
  temporary pacing, 328-329
  three-position ICHD code, 329t
  tracheal stimulation, limiting
    duration of, 324
  transcutaneous, 328
  treatment, 324-326
  valvular heart disease, 328
Bradycardia with spinal cord
    injury, 257-258
Brain death, 201-202, 201t
  determination of, 201t
Brainstem infarct, as cause of respiratory
    acidosis, 523
Brainstem reflexes, lack of, 202
Brainstem syndromes, 276t
Brain tumor, as cause of seizure, 209
Branched-chain amino acids, 48
  hepatic function and, 133-134
Breath holding, with atrioventricular nodal
    re-entry, 349
Breathing
  in critically ill patient, 64-65
    airway management in, 65t
    intracranial pressure
      reduction, 64-65
  evaluation, in burns, 88
  in injured patient, initial
      approach, 64-65
Bromide intoxication, 518
Bronchial adenoma, as cause of
    hemoptysis, 484
Bronchiectasis
  as cause of hemoptysis, 484
  as cause of respiratory acidosis, 523
Bronchitis, airway management with, 476
Bronchoalveolar lavage, 910-912,
    1009-1010
  with intubation, 909-912
Bronchodilators
  in bronchospasm, 435-436
  inhaled, 806
  with pulmonary complications, 156
Bronchogenic carcinoma, as cause of
    hemoptysis, 484
Broncholithiasis, as cause of
    hemoptysis, 484
Bronchopneumonia, as cause of
    hemoptysis, 484
Bronchoscope, 909-910

Bronchoscopy, 905–914
  atelectasis, 907
  bronchoalveolar lavage
    with intubation, 909–912
    technique, 910–912
  bronchoscope, 909–910
  complications, 912–912t
  contraindications, 908–909
  difficult intubation, 908
  flexible fiberoptic bronchoscopy,
    indications for, 906t
  with foreign body aspiration, 908
  hemoptysis, 907–908
  indications for, 906–908
  with intubation, 909–912
  medications, 910
  monitors, 910
  pneumonia, suspected, 906–907
  smoke inhalation, 908
  in spinal cord injury, 255
  supplemental oxygen, 909
  suspected tracheobronchial disruption, 908
  ventilator management, 910
Bronchospasm, 433–442
  adrenergic agonists, 436t
  adrenergic agonists for, 436t
  with anaphylaxis, 805
  anti-inflammatory therapy, 437
  bronchodilator therapy, 435–436
  as cause of hypoxemia, 506
  as cause of respiratory acidosis, 523
  clinical findings, 434–435
  intubation, 438–440
  laboratory data, 435
  mechanically ventilated patient, 438–440
  medical therapies, 437–440
  pathophysiology, 433–434
  with percutaneous tracheostomy, 943
  physical examination, 434–435
  traditional medical therapy, 435–436
Bronchospastic disease, with anaphylaxis, 804
Brown-Sequard syndrome, 251–254
Budd-Chiari syndrome, 608
  as cause of fulminant hepatic failure, 608
  with liver failure, 616
Bulbar poliomyelitis, respiratory acidosis
    with, 523
BUN. *See* Blood urea nitrogen
Buprenorphine, 759–760
Burns, 87–93
  airway, evaluation of, 88
  breathing evaluation, 88
  calculation of burn size, methods for, 88
  as cause of hypertensive crisis, 386
  chemical, 87
  circulation evaluation, 88
  debridement, 91
  depth of burn, 88
  dressing, 91
  early excision, 92–93
  electrical, 87
  endotracheal intubation, 90
  enteral feedings, preference of, 92
  escharotomy, 91
    placement, 92
  facial edema, 91
  first-degree burn, 87
  fluid resuscitation, 89–90
  Foley catheter, 89
  grafting, 92–93
  head-to-toe examination, secondary, 88
  initial laboratory evaluation for, 88
  itching, 93
  late management, 93
  Lund and Browder chart, burn size, 88–89
  metabolic support, 92
  nasogastric tube, 90
  Parkland formula, 90
  patient preparation for treatment, 90
  psychologic effects, 93
  radiation, 87
  rule of nines, 88
    inaccuracy in children, 89
  rule of palm, 88
  second-degree
    deep, 87
    superficial, 87
  silver sulfadiazine, 90
  skin dryness, 93
  skin hyperpigmentation, 93
  third-degree burn, 87
  topical antibiotic, 90
  total body surface area, 87
  treatment, 90–92

Calcium, 121, 647–651
  in cardiac arrest, 121
  with chronic renal failure, 148–149
  homeostasis, 648
  hypercalcemia, 650–651, 657
  hypocalcemia, 648–650, 657
  serum concentration, ionized calcium
    concentration, relationship
    between, 647

Calcium antagonists, in myocardial
    infarction, 378
Calcium channel blockers
    with atrial fibrillation, 334
    with atrioventricular nodal re-entry, 349
    with bradyarrhythmias, 324
    with multifocal atrial tachycardia, 345
    pharmacodynamics of, 771
Calcium gluconate, with hyperkalemia, 535
Calcium sensing receptor, 648
Calculation of burn size, methods for, 88
Calculous, in cholecystitis, 583
Caloric requirements
    in nutritional support, 46–47
Candida
    antibiotic resistance, 676
    in immunocompromised patient, 728, 732
    tertiary peritonitis, 700
Cannon A waves, 347, 352
Capnocytophaga canimorsus, in
    immunocompromised patient, 730
Capnogram, normal, phases of, 992
Capnography, 992t
    untoward situations detected with, 992t
    waveform examples, 984
Capnometer, mainstream, sidestream,
    comparison of, 993
Captopril, with hypertensive emergencies, 391
Carbamazepine
    with epilepsy, 217
    serum concentration monitoring, 755
    thrombocytopenia with, 853
Carbapenems
    antibiotic resistance, 685–686
    in pancreatitis, 576
Carbenoxolone, 520
Carbon dioxide
    excretory failure, as cause of respiratory
        acidosis, 523
    partial pressure of, 511
    removal
        in mechanical ventilator
            support, 489–490
        monitoring, 990–993
Carbonic anhydrase inhibitors, 518
Carbon monoxide poisoning,
    lactic acidosis, 36
Carcinoid syndrome, with anaphylaxis, 804
Carcinomatous meningitis, as cause
    of seizure, 209
Cardiac arrest, 123–124
    airway management, 113–114
    amiodarone, 121
    arrested heart, 115–117
    arterial blood gases, 123–124
    atropine, 120
    calcium, 121
    care setting, 123
    as cause of respiratory acidosis, 523
    circulation, 114–115
    do-not-resuscitate orders, 124–125
    dopamine, 120
    duration of resuscitation, 123
    epinephrine, 117–119
    initial cardiac rhythm, 123
    isoproterenol, 120
    lidocaine, 121–122
    life support, 113–128
    norepinephrine, 119–120
    patient outcome, 124
    pharmacologic approach, 117–122
    prearrest factors, 123
        age, 123
        associated disease, 123
        sex, 123
    procainamide, 122
    recurrent arrest, 123
    resuscitation, 122–124
    sodium bicarbonate, 120–121
    vasopressin, 119
    ventilation, 114
Cardiac arrhythmias, 323–366
    antitachycardia, 358
    atrial, 330–347
    atrioventricular nodal reentry, 347–349
    atrioventricular re-entrant arrhythmias,
        349–352
    bradyarrhythmias, 324–328
    with catheter use, 51
    defibrillator devices, 358
    in differential diagnosis of seizure, 212
    from electrical injury, 93
    tachyarrhythmias, 330–347
    ventricular arrhythmias, 352–358
Cardiac Arrhythmia Suppression Study, 353
Cardiac index in oxygen transport, 25
Cardiac mass reduction, with malnutrition, 43
Cardiac morbidity, perioperative, 97
    reduction of, 97–112
Cardiac output, 309, 973–980
    bolus injection procedure, 974–976
    dilution concentration curve,
        normal cardiac output, 976
    expired gas sampling, 974

Index

Fick principle, 974–977, 1000
  indicator dilution procedure, 974
  measurement error, 975–976
  organ function, optimization of, 963
  in oxygen transport, determinants of, 23t
  perioperative cardiac morbidity, reduction of, 973
  pulmonary artery catheter placement, 975
    thermistor-equipped, 975
  thermodilution, 973–974
  thoracic electrical impedance, 977
  time-concentration curve, indocyanine green dye, 974–976
  ultrasound measurement, 977
Cardiac physiology, 309–322
  afterload, 313
    defined, 313
      pulmonary vascular resistance, 313
      systemic vascular resistance, 313
  angiotensin-converting enzyme inhibitors, systolic dysfunction, 316
  cardiac output, 309
  contractility, 314
    ejection fraction, estimation of, 314
  diastolic dysfunction, 317–318
  digoxin, systolic dysfunction, 315
  dilated cardiomyopathy, 314–317
  diuretics, systolic dysfunction, 315
  elevated filling pressures, 314
  heart failure
    clinical features present in, 316t
    pathophysiology of, 314–318
  heart rate, 309–310
    dysrhythmias, 309
    sinus tachycardia, 309–310
  hemodynamic variables, normal ranges, 313t
  hypertensive heart disease, 314–317
  inotropic therapy, systolic dysfunction, 315
  ischemic heart disease, 314–317
  left ventricular hypertrophy, 317
  nitrates, systolic dysfunction, 315
  nitroprusside, systolic dysfunction, 315
  normal physiology, 309–314
  pericardial tamponade, 318–320
    form of diastolic dysfunction, 319
    pericardial effusions, 319
  preload, 310–312
    carbon monoxide, relationship, 310
    central venous pressure, 310–312
    compliance, 310
    defined, 310
    Frank-Starling principle, 310–312
    left ventricular pressure–volume loops, 311
    pulmonary artery occlusion pressure, 311
    right atrial pressure, 310
  pure diastolic dysfunction, pure systolic dysfunction, contrasted, 318
  sepsis, 320
    antibiotic therapy, 320
    closed space infections, drainage of, 320
    decreased contractility, 320
    ejection fraction, 320
    left ventricular dilation, 320
  systolic dysfunction, 314–317
    diastolic dysfunction, distinguished, 317–318
    treatment of, 317t
  valvular heart disease, 314–317
Cardiac pump theory, 115
Cardiac risk factors with stroke, 271
Cardiac tamponade
  with percutaneous central venous catheterization, 917
  with pulmonary artery catheterization, 922
  in trauma patient, 73
Cardioembolism, 271
Cardiogenic shock, 380
Cardiomyopathy, 314–317, 330
Cardiopulmonary arrest, in trauma patient, 70
Cardiopulmonary bypass
  with acute respiratory distress syndrome, 423
  coagulation disorders, 820
  pancreatitis and, 569
  renal failure, 140
  transfusion therapy and, 847
Cardiopulmonary exercise testing, preoperative, 153
Cardiopulmonary interactions, 395–410
  auto-PEEP, 401
  biventricular diastolic compliance, 397
  clinical applications, 399–402
  to diagnose cardiovascular insufficiency, 402–403
  functional residual capacity, 396
  heart failure patients, 401
  intrapulmonary gas exchange, 395
  intrathoracic pressure, 397
    changes in, 397–399
  intrinsic hyperinflation, 398
  Kussmaul's sign, 402

Cardiopulmonary interactions (*Contd.*)
  lung volume, 395–397
    changes in, 395–397
  occult mesenteric ischemia, 400–401
  positive end-expiratory pressure (PEEP), 396–397, 401–402
  positive-pressure inspiration, 398–399
  pulmonary vascular resistance, 396–397
  right ventricular ejection pressure load, 396
  spontaneous inspiration, 397–398
  systolic pressure variation, 402–403
  transmural LV ejection pressure, defined, 398
  venous return, 398
  ventilation
    effect on cardiac function, 396t
    hemodynamic effects of, 397t
    weaning from, 399–400
  ventricular interdependence, 399
Cardiopulmonary resuscitation, 66
  principles of, 113
Cardiopulmonary risk assessment, preoperative, 154
Cardiorespiratory arrest, defined, 113
Cardiorespiratory function, intrathoracic pressure, interaction between, 986–987
Cardiovascular disease, 97–112
  angina, postoperative ischemic event risk, 103
  congestive heart failure, 97
  coronary artery disease, 97
  diabetes with, 103
  dipyridamole thallium scan, 102
  dobutamine stress echo, 102–104
  functional status, clinical assessment of, 101–104
  intermediate clinical predictors, approach to patient with, 105
  intravascular volume, 108
  ischemic heart disease, 103
    multivariate predictors, 103t
  left ventricular dysfunction, 108
  low risk index, 102t
  low risk variables, evaluation of, 102
  minor clinical predictors, approach to patient with, 106
  myocardial infarction, 97, 99t
    alveolar pulmonary edema, 100
    cardiac risk index, 100
    chronic stable angina, 100
    ischemia, 100

    multivariate analysis, 100
    stepwise logistic regression, 100
  perioperative cardiac morbidity, 97
  perioperative cardiovascular evaluation, for non-cardiac surgery, 105
  physiology assessment, 106
  preoperative cardiovascular tune-up, 107
  pulmonary artery catheter, preoperative placement of, 104–109
  pulmonary capillary wedge pressure, 108
  in renal failure, 140
  risk factors, 97–100
  surgical risks, historical predictors of, 98
  thallium imaging, 103
  vascular surgery, candidates for, 102
  ventricular ectopy, postoperative ischemic event risk, 103
Cardiovascular function, 309–420
  acute myocardial infarction, 367–383
  altered cardiac physiology, 309–322
  cardiac arrhythmias, 323–366
  cardiopulmonary interactions, 395–410
  hypertensive emergencies, 385–394
  perioperative evaluation, 105
  vascular emergencies, 411–420
Cardiovascular risk, 97–112
  assessing, guidelines for, 100–109
  managing, guidelines for, 100–109
  risk factors, 97–100
Cardiovascular surgery, renal failure and, 146–147
Cardioversion
  with atrial fibrillation, 340
  with atrial flutter, 343
Carotid endarterectomy, 416–417
  cervical hematoma, 417
  hyperperfusion syndrome, 417
  hypotension/hypertension, 417
Carotid massage, with atrioventricular nodal re-entry, 349
Carotid-subclavian artery bypass, with internal jugular vein catheterization, 918
CaSR. *See* Calcium sensing receptor
CAST. *See* Cardiac Arrhythmia Suppression Study
Cataplexy, in differential diagnosis of seizure, 212
Cathacholamine excess states, as cause of hypertensive crisis, 386
Catheter. *See also* Catheterization
  ablation, with atrial flutter, 344
  central venous, removal, 931–932

Index

embolus, as complication of percutaneous central venous catheterization, 917
Foley
  in burn patient, 89
  in trauma patient, 68
knotting, with pulmonary artery catheterization, 922
management guidelines, 933
modification, with atrioventricular nodal re-entry, 349
pulmonary artery
  monitoring oxygen delivery, 27–29
  placement, 104–109, 975
removal, 931–934
  central venous catheters, 931–932
  clinical reasons for replacement, 933–934
  pulmonary artery catheters, 932
  replacement of lines, 932–933
  samples for culture, 932
sepsis, 929–930
  causes, 929–930
  incidence, 929
suction, changing tracheostomy tube over, 483
thermistor-equipped pulmonary artery, 975
tip malposition
  as complication of percutaneous central venous catheterization, 917
  with pulmonary artery catheterization, 922
urinary, 739
vascular, 739
ventriculostomy, 240
Catheter-based ablation procedures, with atrial fibrillation, 338–339
Catheterization
  bladder, with renal failure, 532–533
  central venous, indications for, 916
  Doppler-guided, 925
  internal jugular vein, contraindications to, 918
  percutaneous central venous, complications of, 917
  pulmonary artery, complications of, 922
  radial artery, 415
  subclavian vein, contraindications to, 916
  systemic arterial, 923–925
Cation-exchange resin, with hyperkalemia, 535
Cefepime, antibiotic resistance, 685

Cellular automata, bronchial tree branches, relationship, 1013
Cellular automata rule, 1012–1013
Cellular hypoxia, lactic acidosis, 33
Cellular procoagulants, in peritoneal response to infection, 694
Central cord syndrome, 254
Central diabetes insipidus, 666–667
Central lines, 929–936
  aseptic technique, 930–931
  catheter management guidelines, 933
  catheter-related sepsis, 929–930
    causes, 929–930
    incidence, 929
  catheter removal, 931–934
    central venous catheters, 931–932
    clinical reasons for replacement, 933–934
    pulmonary artery catheters, 932
    replacement of lines, 932–933
    samples for culture, 932
  guidewire exchange, 934
  sepsis, catheter-related, 929–930
  thrombosis, catheter-related, 934
Central nervous system function, 187–308
  coma, 187–206
  encephalopathy, 297–308
  head injury, 229–245
  seizures, 207–228
  spinal cord injury, 245–268
  stroke, 269–296
Central sleep apnea, respiratory acidosis with, 523
Central vein thrombosis, with catheter use, 51
Central venipuncture, complications of, 922
Central venous access, 915–920
  femoral vein cannulation, 919–920
  indications for catheterization, 915–916
  internal jugular approach, 918–919
  subclavian vein catheterization, 916–917
Central venous catheterization
  indications for, 916
  removal of catheter, 931–932
Central venous pressure monitoring, hepatic function and, 135
Cephalosporins, 793
  cephalosporin cefepime, antibiotic resistance, 683
  cephalosporin ceftazidime, antibiotic resistance, 683
  effect on platelet function, 815
Cerebellar hemorrhage, coma with, 189–190

Cerebral arterio-venous malformation, as cause of seizure, 209
Cerebral autoregulation
  during ischemia, 272
  stroke and, 273-274
Cerebral blood flow, 188t, 273
  autoregulation of, 274
  with coma, 187-188, 188t
  stroke and, 273
Cerebral contusion, as cause of seizure, 208
Cerebral dysfunction, nursing care, 181
Cerebral edema
  barbiturate coma, 285
  in hypertensive emergencies, 393
  hypertonic saline, 285
  hyperventilation, 284
  with liver failure, 618
  management, 284-285
  osmotic therapy, 284
  steroids, 284
Cerebral hemorrhage, 271
Cerebral infarction, as cause of seizure, 208
Cerebral ischemia, 271
  physiology of, 272-273
  sources of, 272t
Cerebral perfusion pressure
  formula to determine, 238
  in fracture management, 93
Cerebrovascular abnormalities, transfusion therapy and, 866
Cerebrovascular accident
  as cause of respiratory disorder, 524
  encephalopathy and, 298-299
Certified enterostomal nurses, 178-179
Cervical cord trauma, as cause of respiratory acidosis, 523
Cervical hematoma, with carotid endarterectomy, 417
Cervical spinal cord anatomy, 248
Cervical spine
  injury, airway management with, 476
  unstable
    intubation, 478t
    methods of intubation for, 478t
Cesarean section, transfusion therapy and, 865
Changes in mental status, 299-300
  cardiovascular causes, 303-304
    dysrhythmias, 303
    myocardial infarction, 303
    on-pump CAB, 303-304
  endocrine causes, 303
    Addison's disease, 303

Cushing's syndrome, 303
diabetes mellitus, 303
hypothyroidism, 303
hemorrhagic stroke, 300
hepatic causes, 304-305
  cirrhosis, 304
  liver failure, 304
  portal hypertension, 304
  portal-systemic bypass, 304
iatrogenic causes, 304
  anesthetics, 304
  lights, 304
  narcotics, 304
  sedatives, 304
  sleep deprivation, 304
  steroids, 304
ischemic stroke, 299-300
meningitis, 300
metabolic/electrolyte causes, 300-303
  hypercalcemia, 302
  hypernatremia, 302
  hypocalcemia, 302
  hyponatremia, 300-301
  osmolar abnormalities, 302-303
  thiamine deficiency, 303
septic encephalopathy, 305-306
  mental status, 305
  respiratory alkalosis, 305
  tachypnea, 305
uremic encephalopathy, 306
  aluminum neurotoxicity, 306
  asterixis, 306
  diagnosis of exclusion, 306
  dialysis disequilibrium syndrome, 306
Charcoal hemoperfusion, as liver assist device, 621
Chemical burns, 87
Chemical homeostasis, 661-674
  body compartments, 661-662
  colloid solutions, 664t
  crystalloid solutions, 664t
  electrolytes, distribution of, 661-662
  fluid and electrolyte therapy, goal of, 664
  fluid balance, normal state, 662t
  gastrointestinal secretions, composition of, 662t
  hormonal response, 663-664
  hypernatremia, 664-672
  causes, treatment of, 668t
  hyperosmolality, 664-672
  hypertonicity, 664-672
  hyponatremia, 668-669

cause, treatment of, 669t
hypo-osmolality, 668–669
potassium, 670–672
stress of surgery, effect of, 662–664
trauma, effect of, 662–664
water, distribution of, 661–662
Chemoreceptor trigger zone, vomiting control, 593
Chemotherapy
as cause of fulminant hepatic failure, 608
transfusion therapy and, 860
Chest injury, 72–73
aorta injury, 73
chest radiograph, 73t
arch aortogram, 73
cardiac tamponade, 73
CT angiography, 73
echocardiography, 73
examination of, 69
great vessel injury, 73
chest radiograph, 73t
initial approach to, 72–73
myocardial contusion, 73
pulmonary contusion, 73
septal injury, 73
sucking chest wound, 72–73
transesophageal echocardiography, 73
valvular injuries, 73
Chest tube removal, 955
Chest X-ray, ground-glass appearance, 425
Ceyne–Stokes respiration, in coma, 232
Child–Pugh classification, hepatic function, 131
Child–Pugh class A cirrhosis, 559
Child–Pugh class C cirrhosis, 559
Child's classification, hepatic function, 131–132
Child–Turcotte–Pugh system, hepatic function, 131–132
Chloramphenicol
with hepatic failure, 748
serum concentration monitoring, 755
Cholangiography, 586
Cholangiopancreatography, endoscopic, retrograde, pancreatitis and, 569
Cholangitis, obstructive jaundice, 586–589
Cholecystectomy, 586
Cholecystitis, 583–586
acalculous, 583–584
biliary complications, 585
calculous, 583
diagnosis, 584–585

epidemiology of, 583
pathogenesis of, 583–584
radionuclide cholescintigraphy, 584
TPN-associated cholecystitis, 583
treatment, 586
Cholestasis, 586
Chorionic gonadotropin levels, 595
Chronic health evaluation, nursing care in, 175
Chronic obstructive pulmonary disease, 434
bronchospasm, 433
as cause of respiratory acidosis, 523
Chronic renal failure, 139, 147–149. *See also* Renal failure
anemia, 148
anesthesia, 147–148
with anion gap acidosis, 518
bleeding disorders, 148
calcium, 148–149
deamino-arginine vasopressin, preoperative administration of, 148
dialysis, 147
magnesium levels, 148–149
phosphorus, 148–149
r-HuEPO therapy, 148
Chvostek's sign, 649
Chylothorax, as complication of percutaneous central venous catheterization, 917
Chymopapain, allergic reaction, 801
Cimetidine
as antiarrhythmic, 337
with bradyarrhythmias, 325
Ciprofloxacin
antibiotic resistance, 684
as cause of fulminant hepatic failure, 608
Circulation in critically ill patient, 65–67, 114–115
American College of Surgeons, Advanced Trauma Life Support, course recommendations, 66
blood transfusion, indications for, 66
cardiac arrest, 114–115
cardiopulmonary resuscitation, 66
clotting factors, 66
extremity fracture, 66
flail chest, 67
fluid resuscitation, 66
Focused Assessment for Sonographic Examination of Trauma Patient, 67
intractable shock, cause of, 66
intravenous access, 65–66
pelvic fracture, 66
pericardial tamponade, 67

Circulation in critically ill patient (Contd.)
    platelets, replacement of, 66
    tension hemothorax, 67
    tension pneumothorax, 67
    vasopressors, 66
Circulatory overload, transfusion
        therapy and, 873
Cirrhosis
    alcoholic, 605
    as cause of respiratory disorder, 524
    Child–Pugh class A, 559
    Child–Pugh class C, 559
    in encephalopathy, 304
    hepatic function and, 130–133, 131t
        surgical mortality, 132t
Cisapride, 787
    gut motility enhancement, 552
Cisatracurium, 757–758
Citrate-phosphate-dextrose,
        additive solution, 833
Citrate-phosphate-dextrose-adenine,
        storage, 833
CJD. *See* Creutzfeldt-Jacob disease
Classic stress response, 663
Claude syndrome, 276
Clavulanate, antibiotic resistance, 683
Clindamycin, 793
    with hepatic failure, 748
Clinical judgment, made by physician, 161
Clonidine, with hypertensive
        emergencies, 391
Clopidogrel, in myocardial infarction,
        375–376
Closed peritoneal tap and lavage, 957–958
Closed space infections drainage, with cardiac
        sepsis, 320
Clostridium clostridiiforme, tertiary
        peritonitis, 700
Clostridium difficile
    colitis, 549–550
    diarrhea associated with, 553
    in immunocompromised patient, 732–733
Clostridium perfringens
    peritonitis, 700
    tertiary peritonitis, 700
Clostridium species, as cause of
        peritonitis/abscess, 696
Clot lysis, in pulmonary embolism, 460
Clotting factor deficiencies, 820–821
Cluster respiration, in coma, 232
Coagulation
    anticoagulation therapy, 895–902

    endothelial cell regulation of, 814t
Coagulation cascade, 825–827
    in multiple organ failure, 12–13
Coagulation disorders, 811–832
    bleeding disorders, 814–820
        hereditary, 816t
        preoperative screening for, 816t
    cardiopulmonary bypass surgery, 820
    coagulation proteins, role of, 812–813
    deep vein thrombosis, prophylaxis
        guidelines, 824t
    disseminated intravascular coagulation,
        826–828
        conditions associated with, 826t
        laboratory findings, 827t
        mediators of, 827t
    drugs inhibiting platelet function, 815t
    endothelial cell regulation, 814t
    hemorrhagic diatheses,
        pathophysiology of, 814
    hemostasis, physiology of, 811–814
    hemostatic defect, patient
        management, 817–820
    heparin-associated thrombocytopenia,
        828–829, 829t
    hypercoagulable states, 823t
    liver disease, 820–822
    plasma clotting factors, 818t
    platelets, role of, 811–812
    renal disease, 822
    thrombotic diatheses,
        pathophysiology of, 814
    thrombotic disorders, 822–826
    treatment options, 819t
    vascular endothelium,
        role of, 813–814
    venous thromboembolism, regimens to
        prevent, 825t
Coagulation factors, transfusion
        therapy and, 867–868
Coagulation proteins, role of, 812–813
Coagulopathy, 619–620
    as contraindication to subclavian vein
        catheterization, 916
    with internal jugular vein
        catheterization, 918
    with liver failure, 619–620
    in multiple blunt trauma, 84
Cockcroft-Gault equation, 142
Cognition impairment, nursing care, 181
Cold exposure, allergic reaction, 801
Colistin, antibiotic resistance, 686

Index

Collagen-vascular diseases, as cause of hemoptysis, 484
Colloid solutions, 664t
Colon cancer, lower gastrointestinal hemorrhage with, 563
Colonic polyps, lower gastrointestinal hemorrhage with, 563
Colon ischemia, following abdominal aneurysm repair, 416
Colonization resistance, gut mucosa, 549
Colony-stimulating factors, in immunocompromised patient, 729
Coma, 187–206
  with acute renal failure, 537
  barbiturate, 285
  causes of, 189t
  diagnosis, 199
  differential diagnosis, 188–191, 190t
    aids to, 190t
  etiology of, 199
  examination of patient, 192–195
  general examination of patient, 192
  Glasgow Coma Scale, 192–193t
  Glasgow Outcome Scale, 199–199t
  history of patient, 191–192
  as indication for dialysis, 536
  laboratory evaluation of, 195t
  nonstructural pathologies, 191
  patient approach, 191–198
  respiratory patterns in, 232t
  structural pathologies, 191
  talk and deteriorate syndrome, 189
Competency, legal term, made by judge, 161
Complement deficiency, in immunocompromised patient, 730
Complex problems, approaches to, 995–1018
Complications associated with, access complications, 416
Compression fractures, cervical vertebrae, 251
Confusion, in differential diagnosis of seizure, 212
Congestive heart failure, 97, 434, 823
  as cause of respiratory disorder, 524
  modification of nutritional regimen with, 52
  radiocontrast medium-induced acute renal failure, risk factor, 145
  surgical risks with, 98
  in thyroid dysfunction, 634
  volume overload with, precipitating factors, 323
Conjugate acid–base pairs, 511
Conjunctival edema, with anaphylaxis, 804
Connective tissue disorders, abdominal pain with, 600
Contact precautions, 681, 685–686
  gloves, 681
Continuously oscillating beds, with spinal cord injury, 260
Continuous positive airway pressure, mechanical ventilator support and, 490
Continuous venovenous hemofiltration, 543
  with dialysis, 543
  hemodialysis, comparison, 543–544, 544t
Contractility, cardiac, 314
  ejection fraction, estimation of, 314
  with sepsis, 320
Contraction alkalosis, 520
Contralateral neglect, with stroke, 275
Contralateral weakness, with stroke, 275
Contrast material, radiocontrast medium-induced acute renal failure, risk factors, 145
Contrast nephropathy, in renal failure, 145
Control mode ventilation, 493
Control variables, response variables, distinguished, 998–1005
Convulsive seizures, 209–210
COPD. *See* Chronic obstructive pulmonary disease
Cori cycle, lactic acidosis, glyconeogenesis, 34
Corneal reflexes in coma, 194
Coronary arteries, distributions of, 368
Coronary artery disease, 97
  with atrial fibrillation, 330
Coronary atherosclerotic plaque, rupture of, 367–368
Coronary bypass surgery
  in hypertensive emergencies, 393
  pancreatitis, 569
Coronary stenting, in myocardial infarction, 373–374
  glycoprotein IIb/IIIa antagonists, 373–374
Cortical necrosis, defined, 529
Corticosteroids
  bronchospasm, 437
  with liver failure, 619
  in multiple organ failure, 15
Cotrimoxazole, 793
Cough, with pulmonary embolism, 446
Coumadin, with stroke, 283
Counahan-Barratt equation, use with children, 143

Council of Ethical and Judicial Affairs, guidelines of, 124
CPDA-1. *See* Citrate-phosphate-dextrose-adenine
CPP. *See* Cerebral perfusion pressure
Cranial nerve dysfunction, in head injury, 234
Cranial nerve examination in coma, 193–194
Cranial nerve palsies, 276
Creatine kinase, in coma evaluation, 195
Creatine phosphokinase, elevation of, in myocardial infarction, 369
Creatinine
　clearance of, 747–748
　in coma evaluation, 195
　in electrical injury, 93
　　total muscle damage, indicator of, 93
　factors affecting, 542t
　hemodialysis and, 542t
　increased, 142t
　measurement of, 141–142
Creatinine concentrations, dialysis adequacy and, 540
Creutzfeldt-Jacob disease, transfusion therapy and, 875
Cricothyroidotomy
　with spinal cord injury, 255
　in trauma patient, 64
Crigler-Najjar syndrome, 588
Crixivan, for HIV, 709
Crohn's disease, transfusion therapy and, 861
Croup, airway management with, 476
CRYO. *See* Cryoprecipitate
Cryoprecipitate transfusion, 856–857
　indications for, 856–857
Cryptogenic seizures, 207
CSFs. *See* Colony-stimulating factors
Cushing's syndrome, 520
Cusp catastrophe model, 1004–1006
CVA. *See* Cerebrovascular accident
CVP. *See* Central venous pressure
CXR. *See* Chest x-ray
Cyanide toxicity, 768
　lactic acidosis, 36
Cyanosis
　with anaphylaxis, 804
　with bronchospasm, 438
Cycling of antibiotics, 679–680
Cyclo-oxygenase inhibitors, 852
Cyclosporine, serum concentration monitoring, 755
Cysticercosis, as cause of seizure, 209
Cystic fibrosis, as cause of hemoptysis, 484

Cystitis, abdominal pain with, 600
Cytokines, in peritoneal response to infection, 694t
Cytomegalovirus
　as cause of fulminant hepatic failure, 608
　in immunocompromised patient, 734
　transfusions, 859–861

Dalfopristin, antibiotic resistance, 681
Damped oscillating systems, in blood pressure monitoring, 963–965
Damping, time response, compromise between, in blood pressure monitoring, 969–970
Data measurement/interpretation, 961–994
　blood pressure monitoring, 963–972
　cardiac output, 973–980
　respiratory monitoring, 981–994
D-dimer assay, in venous thromboembolism, 449
DDVAP. *See* Desmopressin
Deamino-arginine vasopressin, preoperative administration, 148
Debridement of burns, 91
Decannulation, accidental
　as complication of tracheostomy, 481
　procedure for avoiding, 481–482
Decision-making capacity of patient, 161–163
　defined, 162
　patients without, 163
Decontamination of digestive tract, 553–554
Deep tendon reflexes, with spinal cord injury, 248
Deep vein thrombosis, 443, 822
　prophylaxis, 824t
　with spinal injury, 260–261
Defibrillator devices, 358
Degenerative disorder, as cause of seizure, 209
Delayed traumatic intracerebral hematoma, 237
Delayed wound healing, with malnutrition, 43
Delirium, nursing management, 180–181
Delivery-dependent lactate production, in oxygen transport, 26–27
Delivery-dependent oxygen consumption, in oxygen transport, 24–25
Denial of patient, with spinal cord injury, 264
Depressed skull fracture, 233
　risk factors for, 220
　seizure with, 233
Dermatomal diagram, 249

Designer drugs, as cause of fulminant hepatic
   failure, 608
Desipramine, 787
Desmopressin, transfusion therapy and, 848
Developmental disorders, as cause
   of seizure, 209
Dexmedetomidine, 778–779
   dosing, 779
   precautions, 779
Diabetes. *See also* Diabetes insipidus;
      Diabetes mellitus
   with cardiovascular disease, 103
   nephrogenic, 666–667
   stroke and, 270
   uncontrolled, syndromes of, 639
Diabetes insipidus, 666–667
   diagnosis of, 666
Diabetes mellitus
   airway management with, 477
   with anion gap acidosis, 518
   in encephalopathy, 303
   in immunocompromised patient, 731
   radiocontrast medium-induced acute renal
      failure, risk factor, 145
   renal failure, 139–140
   surgical risks with, 98
Diabetic ketoacidosis, 639–641, 640t
   abdominal pain with, 600
   lactic acidosis, 36
   management of, 640t
Dialysis, 536, 539–543, 621, 654, 656
   bleeding, uncontrollable, 539
   blood urea nitrogen
      factors affecting value, 542t
      indicators of dialysis adequacy, 540
   with chronic renal failure, 147
   continuous venovenous
      hemofiltration with, 543
   creatinine, factors affecting, 542t
   creatinine concentrations, indicators of
      dialysis adequacy, 540
   dialyzer, 540
      anaphylactic reaction, 541
   fluid overload, 539
   fluid removal, 542–543
   hyperalimentation, 541–542
   hyperkalemia, 539
   with hyperkalemia, 535
   hypotension, 541
      causes of, 542t
   hypotension during,
      causes of, 542t

   hypoxemia, 541
   indications for, 536t
   medications, 541–542
   solute removal, 539–540
   urine output, increase by diuretic use, 543
   water removal, 539
   withdrawal of, 171
Dialysis orders, 541t
Dialyzer
   anaphylactic reaction to, 541
   in hemodialysis, 540
Diamox, 518
   with metabolic acidosis, 518
Diaphoresis
   with anaphylaxis, 804
   mechanical ventilator support and, 489
Diaphragmatic dysfunction, 152
Diarrhea
   Clostridium difficile, 553
   nursing management, 180
Diastolic dysfunction, 317–318
   treatment of, 317t
Diazepam, 223
   with increased intracranial
      pressure, 242
Didanosine, for HIV, 709
Difficult airway, 473–474
Diffuse pulmonary infection, with acute
      respiratory distress syndrome, 423
Digestive tract decontamination, 553–554
Digitalis
   as antiarrhythmic, 338
   sustained ventricular tachycardia, 356
   toxicity, 345–347
   ventricular tachycardia with, 358
Digoxin
   as antiarrhythmic, 337
   with atrial fibrillation, 334
   with bradyarrhythmias, 324
   serum concentration monitoring, 755
   systolic dysfunction, 315
Dilantin, as cause of fulminant
      hepatic failure, 608
Dilated cardiomyopathy, 314–317
Diltiazem, with atrial fibrillation, 335
Dilution concentration curve, normal
      cardiac output, 976
Dipylidium, as cause of fulminant hepatic
      failure, 608
Dipyridamole thallium scan, 102
Disability, in injured patient, initial
      approach, 67–68

Discontinuation of mechanical
     ventilation, 501–510
  arterial blood gas determination, 503
  current recommendations, 505
  decreased inspiratory muscle strength, 508
  duration of, 504
  hemodynamic stability, 503
  hypoxemia, causes of, 506t
  increased dead space ventilation, 506
  oxygenation, 503
  oxygenation failure, 506
  pressure-support ventilation, 502–503
  protocol weaning, 503–504
     criteria for, 504t
  rapid shallow breathing index, 502
  spontaneous breathing trials, 501, 504–505
  synchronized intermittent mandatory
     ventilation, 502–503
  tapered support, 502–503
  T-piece, 502, 504
  T-piece trials, 502
  uncompensated respiratory acidemia, 508
  ventilatory failure, 506–508
     algorithm, 507
  weaning
     American College of Chest Physicians
        definition, 501
        criteria, 502–503t
     weaning criteria, 502
     weaning failure, 505–508
Disopyramide, serum concentration
     monitoring, 755
Disseminated intravascular coagulation,
     826–828
  conditions associated with, 826t
  laboratory findings, 827t
  mediators of, 827t
  transfusion therapy and, 847
Distal hemodialysis access, as contraindication
     to subclavian vein catheterization, 916
Diuresis, 427
Diuretics, systolic dysfunction, 315
Divalent ions, 647–659
Diverticular disease, lower gastrointestinal
     hemorrhage with, 563
Dizziness, with sustained ventricular
     tachycardia, 355
DNR order. See Do not resuscitate order
Dobutamine, 764–765
  dosing, 764–765
  precautions, 765
Dobutamine stress echo, 102–104

Doctrine of implied consent, 163
Dofetilide, 787
  as antiarrhythmic, 338
  with atrial fibrillation, 340
Do not resuscitate order, 124–125, 164–165
  case study, 164–165
  defined, 165
Dopamine, 120
  in cardiac arrest, 120
  dosing, 754–764
  with renal failure, 534
Doppler-guided catheterization, 925
Dorsalis pedis artery, catheterization,
     923–924
Down's syndrome, difficult endotracheal
     intubation and, 475
Dressings, 179–179t
  for burns, 91
Droperidol, 787
Drug doses, 745–782. See also under
     specific drug
  absorption, 745–746
  antihypertensive therapy, 767–776
  bioavailability, defined, 745
  combination therapy, 767
  creatinine clearance, 747–748
  cyanide toxicity, 768
  dexmedetomidine, 779
  distribution, 746
  dobutamine, 764–765
  dopamine, 754–764
  enalaprilat, 775
  epinephrine, 765–766
  esmolol, 775–776
  excretion, 747–748
  fenoldopam, 774–775
  with hepatic failure, 748
  high-extraction drugs, 747
  hypotension, drug dosing with, 768
  inotropic therapy, 754–766
     cardiac, vascular effects, 761–763t
  intravenous analgesic, 777t
  intravenous sedative, 778t
  isoproterenol, 766
  labetalol, 773–774
  low-extraction drugs, 747
  metabolism, 746–747
  milrinone, 765
  narcotic analgesic therapy, 759–760t
  neuromuscular blocking therapy, 757–758t
  nitroglycerin, 773
  nitroprusside, 768–773

norepinephrine, 766
oral antihypertensive therapy,
    pharmacodynamics, 771–772t
parenteral antihypertensive
    therapy, pharmacodynamics,
    769–770t
pharmacokinetic relations, 753
phenylephrine, 767
propofol, 776–779
with renal failure, 536
with renal impairment, 749–752t
renal insufficiency,
    effects of, 747
sedative therapy, 776–779
serum concentration, 748–749
    monitoring, 755–756t
vasoactive drugs, 754–767
vasopressin, 766–767
vasopressors, 766–767
Drug-induced renal failure, 145–146
Drug interactions, 783–798
    See also under specific drug
Drugs
    adverse reactions, 783–798
        See also under specific drug
    illicit, as cause of seizure, 208
Dryness of skin, in burns, 93
Dual chamber pacing, with
    bradyarrhythmias, 329
Dubin-Johnson syndrome, 588
Duplex ultrasonography in
    trauma patient, 77–78
Dural vascular structures,
    laceration of, 233
Dynamical systems,
    use of, 1005–1008
Dysarthria, with stroke, 275
Dysfibrinogenemia, 823
    transfusion therapy and, 856–857
Dysmenorrhea, abdominal
    pain with, 600
Dysmetria, with stroke, 276
Dysreflexia with spinal injury, 261
Dysrhythmia
    as complication of percutaneous central
        venous catheterization, 917
    encephalopathy and, 303
    with pulmonary artery
        catheterization, 922
    surgical risks with, 98
Dystonia, in differential diagnosis
    of seizure, 212

Early ambulation, nursing care for, 176
Echocardiography, in trauma patient, 73
Eclampsia, as cause of hypertensive
    crisis, 386
Eclamptic seizures, 215
Ectasy (drug), as cause of fulminant
    hepatic failure, 608
Efavirenz, for HIV, 709
Elective cardioversion, with atrial
    fibrillation, 340
Electrical burns, 87
Electrical cardioversion, with atrial
    fibrillation, 334–336
Electrical injury, 93–94
    cardiac dysrhythmias from, 93
    muscle damage in, 93
    serum creatinine kinase in, 93
Electrical stimulation, for wounds, 179
Electroencephalography
    coma and, 195
    with seizure, 219
Electrolyte abnormalities
    with nutritional deficiency, 51
    precipitating factors, 323
Electrolytes
    assessment, with renal failure, 144
    causes of encephalopathy, 300–303
    in coma evaluation, 195
    disturbance, as cause of
        seizure, 208
    hepatic function and, 135
    serum concentrations of, with
        nutritional support, 54
Elevated factor VIII level, 823
Elevated filling pressures, 314
Embolectomy, pulmonary, 461
Embolic risk, with atrial flutter, 342
Embolism, abdominal pain with, 600
Emergency department
    thoracotomy, 74
    pericardial tamponade, 74
Emergency Medical Treatment and Active
    Labor Act, 167
Empowerment issues in nursing, 175
Enalaprilat, 775
    dosing, 775
    with hypertensive emergencies, 391
    pharmacodynamics of, 770
    precautions, 775
Encephalitis
    as cause of seizure, 208
    herpes simplex, 201

Encephalopathy, 297–308
  airway, 298
  anoxic, prognosis, 199–200
  breathing, 298
  cardiovascular causes, 303–304
    dysrhythmias, 303
    myocardial infarction, 303
    on-pump CAB, 303–304
  as cause of seizure, 208
  causes of, 298t–299t
  cerebrovascular accident, 298–299
  circulation, 298
    cardiac dysfunction, 298
  defined, 297
  disability, 298–299
  emergency causes of, 298–306, 298t, 299–306
  endocrine causes, 303
    Addison's disease, 303
    Cushing's syndrome, 303
    diabetes mellitus, 303
    hypothyroidism, 303
  hemorrhagic stroke, 300
  hepatic causes, 304–305, 606–607
    cirrhosis, 304
    grades of, 607t
    liver failure, 304
    neurologic, 606–607
    portal hypertension, 304
    portal-systemic bypass, 304
    psychiatric, 606
  hepatic function and, 131
  hypercarbic breathing, 298
  hypoglycemia, 299
  hypoxia, 298
  iatrogenic causes, 304
    anesthetics, 304
    lights, 304
    narcotics, 304
    sedatives, 304
    sleep deprivation, 304
    steroids, 304
  ischemic stroke, 299–300
  meningitis, 300
  mental status changes, 299–300
  metabolic/electrolyte causes, 300–303
    hypercalcemia, 302
    hypernatremia, 302
    hypocalcemia, 302
    hyponatremia, 300–301
    osmolar abnormalities, 302–303
    thiamine deficiency, 303
  sepsis, 299
  septic encephalopathy, 305–306
    mental status, 305
    respiratory alkalosis, 305
    tachypnea, 305
  uremic encephalopathy, 306
    aluminum neurotoxicity, 306
    asterixis, 306
    diagnosis of exclusion, 306
    dialysis disequilibrium syndrome, 306
Endobronchial obstruction, 434
Endocrine causes of encephalopathy, 303
  Addison's disease, 303
  Cushing's syndrome, 303
  diabetes mellitus, in encephalopathy, 303
  hypothyroidism, 303
Endocrine disturbance, as cause of seizure, 208
Endocrine emergencies, 629–646
  adrenal insufficiency, 629–634
    adrenal crisis, treatment of, 631–632
    adrenal function, biochemical tests of, 631
    clinical features, 630
    diagnosis, 630–631
    etiology of, 629–630
    glucocorticoid potencies, 630t
    prior steroid therapy, 630–631
  glucocorticoid supplementation, perioperative, 634t
  glucose homeostasis disorders, 639–641
    adrenal insufficiency, 641
    diabetic ketoacidosis, 639–641, 640t
    hyperglycemic hyperosmolar nonketotic syndrome, 639–641, 640t
    normoglycemia, 639
    thyroid disorders, 642
  thyroid dysfunction, 634–638
    management, 635t
    myxedema coma, 637–638
    sick-euthyroid syndrome, 638
    thyroid storm, 634–636
Endocrine system, 629–674
  chemical homeostasis, 661–674
  divalent ions, 647–659
  emergencies, 629–646
End of life issues, 169–171
  pain control, 169–170
  rule of double effect, 170
  withdrawal of life-sustaining treatment, 170–171
    food/fluids, forgoing, 171

Index

ventilator withdrawal, 170–171
withdrawal of dialysis, 171
withdrawal of other treatments, 171
World Health Organization Analgesic
 Ladder, 169
Endometriosis, abdominal pain with, 600
Endometritis, abdominal pain with, 600
Endoscopic ablation, with liver failure, 614
Endoscopic biliary drainage, hepatic function
 and, 132
Endoscopic coagulation, as cause of
 gastrointestinal hemorrhage, 559
Endoscopic retrograde
 cholangiopancreatography
 hepatic function and, 135
 pancreatitis and, 569
Endoscopic sclerotherapy, gastrointestinal
 hemorrhage, 560–561
Endoscopic transpapillary sphincterotomy,
 587
Endoscopic variceal ligation, 560–561
Endothelial cell regulation, 814t
 coagulation, 814t
Endothelins, endothelial cell regulation, 814
Endotoxin
 gut, 550
 signaling receptor complex for, 10–11
Endotracheal intubation, 114, 469
 in burn, 90
 complications of, 472
 difficult, congenital syndromes with, 475t
 head position for, 474
 indications for, 469
 route of, 469–471
 with spinal cord injury, 260
 standard approaches, 471–473
 successful, confirmation of, 474–477
Endotracheal tube, 469
 aspiration, 1009–1010
 blind, 473
 confirmation of placement, 478t
 cuffed, *vs.* noncuffed, 480–481
 inner cannula, 481
 misplaced, 479t
 selection, 469–471
 size, 479t
Enteral nutrition, 48–51, 92, 180
 aspiration during, 50
 in pancreatitis, 578
Enteric bacteria, gut, 549
Enteritis, abdominal pain with, 600
Enterobacter, antibiotic resistance, 676

Enterobacter aerogenes, peritonitis, 700
Enterobacter cloacae, peritonitis, 700
Enterobacter species, 684–685
 as cause of peritonitis/abscess, 696
 control/prevention, 685
 epidemiology, 684
 therapy, 685
Enterococcus
 antibiotic resistance, 676
 as cause of peritonitis/abscess, 696
 tertiary peritonitis, 700
Enterocyte, lipid membrane, 547–548
Enterostomal nurses, certified, 178–179
Entropy in thermal physics, similarity of
 ratios, 1014
Environmental reservoirs, antibiotic
 resistance, 683
Enzymatic barriers, gut, 548
Epididymitis, abdominal pain with, 600
Epidural hematoma, 233–235
 seizure with, 234–235
Epiglottis, 476
 airway management with, 476
 as cause of respiratory acidosis, 523
Epilepsy, 208, 210t, 286. *See also* Status
 epilepticus
 abdominal pain with, 600
 syndromes, 209–210t
Epinephrine, 117–119, 765–766, 805
 in bronchospasm, 436–437
 in cardiac arrest, 117–119
 dosing, 765–766
 use of, 115
Epivir, for HIV, 709
Epstein-Barre virus, as cause of fulminant
 hepatic failure, 608
Eptifibatide, in myocardial infarction, 372
ERCP. *See* Endoscopic retrograde
 cholangiopancreatography
Ertapenem, antibiotic resistance, 684–685
Erythromycin, 787, 794
 as cause of fulminant hepatic failure, 608
 gut motility enhancement, 552
 with hepatic failure, 748
Escharotomy, 91
 placement, 92
Escherichia coli
 antibiotic resistance, 676
 as cause of peritonitis/abscess, 696
 causing intra-abdominal infection, 696
 in immunocompromised patient, 728
 peritonitis, 700

Escherichia coli (*Contd.*)
   tertiary peritonitis, 700
   third-generation cephalosporin-resistant, 676
Esmolol, 343, 775–776
   with atrial fibrillation, 335
   with atrial flutter, 343
   dosing, 775–776
   with hypertensive emergencies, 391
   in nonparoxysmal junctional tachycardia, 347
   pharmacodynamics of, 770
Esophageal obturator airways, 473
Esophageal-tracheal Combitube, in trauma patient, 64
Esophageal varices, 559–561
Estrogen, 823
Ethanol intoxication, lactic acidosis, 36
Ethical issues, surgical intensive care, 161–174
   best interest standard, 163
   clinical judgment, made by physician, 161
   competency, legal term, made by judge, 161
   decision-making capacity, 161–163
      defined, 162
      patients without, 163
   doctrine of implied consent, 163
   do not resuscitate order, 164–165
      case study, 164–165
      defined, 165
   Emergency Medical Treatment and Active Labor Act, 167
   end of life issues, 169–171
      food/fluids, forgoing, 171
      pain control, 169–170
      rule of double effect, 170
      suffering, relief of, 169–170
      ventilator withdrawal, 170–171
      withdrawal of dialysis, 171
      withdrawal of life-sustaining treatment, 170–171
      withdrawal of other treatments, 171
      World Health Organization Analgesic Ladder, 169
   futility, medical, 166–168
      case study, 167–168
      defined, 167
      resolving conflicts over, 168–169
   hierarchy of decision-makers, 163
   indefinite continuation of treatment, limitations to, 165
   informed consent, 161
   limits to other types of care, issues, 166
   perseverence of life, 166
   physician-assisted suicide, 171–172
   professional integrity, 168–169
   substituted judgment, principle of, 163
Ethosuximide, serum concentration monitoring, 755
Ethylene glycol
   anion gap acidosis from, 518
   lactic acidosis from, 35–36
Excision of burns, 92–93
Excretion of drugs, 747–748
Exercise, allergic reaction, 801
Expired gas sampling, cardiac output measurement, 974
Expired minute ventilation, in mechanical ventilator support, 490
Explanation of procedures by nursing staff, 178
Expressive aphasia, with stroke, 275
Extended-spectrum β-lactamase-producing *Klebsiella pneumoniae,* 685–686
   control/prevention, 685–686
   epidemiology, 685
Extracellular fluid, 661
   volume status, with renal failure, 144–144t
Extremity
   examination of, in trauma patient, 70
   fracture of, 66
   injured patient, examination of, 70
Extubation, 477–479
Eye movements in coma, 193

Facial edema, 91
Facial palsy, with stroke, 275
Facial seborrheic dermatitis, with HIV/AIDS, 711
Factor IX deficiency. *See* Hemophilia B
Factor VII deficiency, transfusion therapy and, 865
Factor VIII deficiency. *See* Hemophilia A
Factor V Leiden mutation, 823
Familial Mediterranean fever, abdominal pain with, 600
Family communication with patient in spinal cord injury, 264
FAST. *See* Focused Assessment for Sonographic examination of Trauma Patient
Fat embolism, as cause of respiratory acidosis, 523

Index

Fatty liver of pregnancy
  as cause of fulminant hepatic failure, 608
  coagulation disorder with, 826
Febrile illness, with neutropenia, 729t
Febrile nonhemolytic transfusion reactions,
    transfusions, 857–859
Febrile seizures, 208
Feeding tubes, 48–51. *See also* Nutritional
    support
Femoral artery, catheterization, 924
Fenoldopam, 774–775
  dosing, 774–775
  pharmacodynamics of, 770
Fentanyl, 759–760
  adverse reactions, 790–791
  analgesic therapy, 790–791
  pharmacodynamics of, 777
Fever
  as cause of respiratory disorder, 524
  CT scanning, 218
  in immunocompromised patient, 735–736
  with pulmonary embolism, 446
Fialuridine, as cause of fulminant hepatic
    failure, 608
Fiberoptic bronchoscopy, 471–473, 905
  indications for, 906t
Fiberoptic laryngoscopy, 473, 483
  with spinal cord injury, 255
Fibrillatory waves, with atrial fibrillation, 332
Fibrinogen, 818
Fibrinolytic therapy
  antiplatelet therapy, combination,
      ST-segment elevation myocardial
      infarction, 371–372
  with stroke, 281
Fick principle, 25, 974–977, 1000
Fine needle aspiration
  with acute abdomen, 597
  in pancreatitis, 574
First-degree burns, 87
Flail chest, 67
  as cause of respiratory acidosis, 523
Flaviviridae, transfusion therapy and, 875
Flecainide, 787
Flexible fiberoptic bronchoscopy, 905
  indications for, 906t
Flexion-extension radiographs, in trauma
    patient, 72
Flow-dependent lactate production, oxygen
    transport and, 26
Flow-dependent oxygen consumption, 1001
  oxygen transport and, 25

Fluconazole, 794
Flucytosine, serum concentration
    monitoring, 755
Fluid and electrolyte therapy. *See* Fluid
    homeostasis
Fluid homeostasis, 661–674
  body compartments, 661–662
  colloid solutions, 664t
  crystalloid solutions, 664t
  electrolytes, distribution of, 661–662
  fluid balance, normal state, 662t
  gastrointestinal secretions,
      composition of, 662t
  goal of fluid and electrolyte therapy, 664
  hormonal response, 663–664
  hypernatremia, 664–672
    causes, treatment of, 668t
  hyperosmolality, 664–672
  hypertonicity, 664–672
  hyponatremia, 668–669
    cause, treatment of, 669t
  hypo-osmolality, 668–669
  normal state, 662t
  in normal state, 662t
  potassium, 670–672
  with renal failure, 534
  stress of surgery, effect of,
      662–664
  trauma, effect of, 662–664
  water, distribution of, 661–662
Fluid overload, with hemodialysis, 539
Fluid resuscitation, 66, 426
  in burns, 89–90
Fluoroquinolones
  in pancreatitis, 576
  resistance, 676, 685
Flutamide, as cause of fulminant hepatic
    failure, 608
FNTHR. *See* Febrile nonhemolytic
    transfusion reactions
Focal cortical dysplasia, as cause
    of seizure, 209
Focal neurologic examination,
    CT scanning, 218
Focused Assessment for Sonographic
    Examination of Trauma
    Patient, 67, 74–76
Foley catheter placement
  in burn patient, 89
  in trauma patient, 68
Fondaparinux, in pulmonary
    embolism, 460

Food additives
  allergic reaction, 801
  effect on platelet function, 815
Foods
  allergic reaction to, 801
  patient forgoing, 171
Foreign body
  anaphylaxis and, 804
  bronchoscopy with, 908
  as cause of hemoptysis, 484
  as cause of respiratory acidosis, 523
Foreign tissue, in multiple organ failure, 10–11
Foscarnet, 794
Fosphenytoin, 223
  with epilepsy, 216
Foville syndrome, 276
Fractures. *See also under* specific fracture
  in blunt multiple trauma, 81–86, 82t
  cerebral perfusion pressure, 93
  coagulopathy, 84
  diagnostic tests, 81
  early fracture stabilization, advantages of, 82
  femur fractures, plates, 83t
  hemothorax, 93
  hypothermia, 84
  initial survey, 81
  intracranial pressure, 93
  management of, 84–85
  mean arterial pressure, intracranial pressure, relationship between, 83
  multi-disciplinarian nature of, 84–85
  plates for femur fractures, 83t
  pulmonary contusion, treatment of, 82–83
  resuscitation, 81
  severe pelvic injury, 84
  skull, 231–234
    basilar skull fractures, 233–234
    depressed skull fractures, 233
    linear nondisplaced skull fractures, 231–232
  treatment, 84–85
Frequency ratio, in blood pressure monitoring, 963–964
Fresh frozen plasma
  transfusion therapy and, 846–847
  warfarin-related bleeding, 896
Frostbite, 94–95
  amputation, risk for, 95
  morbidity, 94
  treatment protocol, 95

Fructose, lactic acidosis, 36
Fugue states, in differential diagnosis of seizure, 212
Fulminant hepatic failure, 605–628
  acute-on-chronic liver failure, 605–606
  bioartificial livers for, trials, 622t
  causes of, 608t–609t
  definitions, 605–607
  hepatic encephalopathy, 606–607
  hybrid bioartificial liver
    hybrid bioartificial livers, 622–623
    mechanical obstruction, 609–610
    pathologic supply dependency, 610–611
    role of nitric oxide, 610
    trials, 622t
  lactic acidosis, 36
Fungal overgrowth, gut, prevention of, 553
Fungus ball, as cause of hemoptysis, 484
Furosemide, with increased intracranial pressure, 241
Fusion inhibitors, with HIV/AIDS, 717
Fusobacterium species, causing intra-abdominal infection, 696
Futility, medical, 166–168
  case study, 167–168
  defined, 167
  resolving conflicts over, 168–169

Gallstones, pancreatitis and, 569–570
γ irradiation guidelines, 871–872
Ganciclovir, 794
Gangrene, venous, 414–415
Gardner-Wells tongs, use of, with spinal cord injury, 254–255
Gas exchange
  in mechanical ventilation, 489–490
  respiratory monitoring, 987–989
Gastric aspiration, as cause of respiratory acidosis, 523
Gastric atony, with spinal cord injury, 261
Gastric emptying, delayed, 50
Gastritis, 561–562
  abdominal pain with, 600
Gastroesophageal reflux, 50
Gastrointestinal bleeding, 557–568
  antacids, 561
  balloon tamponade, as cause of gastrointestinal hemorrhage, 559
  causes of, 559–563, 565t
  Child–Pugh class A cirrhosis, 559
  Child–Pugh class C cirrhosis, 559

Index

colon cancer, lower gastrointestinal hemorrhage with, 563
colonic polyps, lower gastrointestinal hemorrhage with, 563
diverticular disease, lower gastrointestinal hemorrhage with, 563
duodenal ulcers, 557
endoscopic coagulation, as cause of gastrointestinal hemorrhage, 559
endoscopic sclerotherapy, 560–561
endoscopic variceal ligation, 560–561
endoscopy, 557–559
esophageal varices, 557, 559–561
gastric ulcer, 557
gastritis, 561–562
gastrotomy, as cause of gastrointestinal hemorrhage, 559
hemorrhage, 557–559, 563–565
hemorrhoids, lower gastrointestinal hemorrhage with, 563
with HIV/AIDS, 711
H2-receptor antagonists, 561–562
inflammatory bowel disease, lower gastrointestinal hemorrhage with, 563
ischemic colitis, lower gastrointestinal hemorrhage with, 563
Mallory-Weiss lesion, 559
  as cause of gastrointestinal hemorrhage, 559
Meckel's diverticulum, with lower gastrointestinal hemorrhage, 563
patient evaluation, 563–565
peptic ulcer disease, 562–563
  proton pump inhibitors, 562
  surgical treatment, 562–563
rectal cancer, lower gastrointestinal hemorrhage with, 563
Sengstaken-Blakemore tube, protocol for use, 560t
stigmata of recent hemorrhage, 558–559
stress ulcer prophylaxis, 561–562
sucralfate, 561
treatment, 558, 564
vascular ectasias, lower gastrointestinal hemorrhage with, 563
vasoconstrictor therapy, 560
Gastrointestinal secretions, 662
composition of, 662t
Gastrointestinal tract, as source for bacteria, 700
Gastrotomy, as cause of gastrointestinal hemorrhage, 559

Gatifloxacin, 787
Generalized convulsive status epilepticus, 222–223, 223t
evaluation/management of, 222–223
nonconvulsive status epilepticus, compared, 224
Generalized tonic-clonic seizures, 209–210
Genito-urinary injury
initial approach to, 76
in trauma patient, 76
  CT scan, 76
  intravenous pyelogram, 76
  retrograde urethrogram, 76
Gentamicin
antibiotic resistance, 684
serum concentration monitoring, 755
Gerstman's syndrome, with stroke, 275
GFR. *See* Glomerular filtration rate
Gilbert's syndrome, 588
Glanzmann's thrombasthenia, 816, 818
Glasgow Coma Scale, 192–193t
in head injury, 229–230
Glasgow Outcome Scale, 199–199t
Global cerebral dysfunction, nursing care, 181
Global cerebral hypoperfusion, 211–212
Globus hystericus, with anaphylaxis, 804
Glomerular filtration rate, 140–141
estimation of, 141–143
Gloves, for contact precautions, 681
Glucocorticoids, 631, 633–634
perioperative supplementation, 634t
potencies, 630t
Glucose
in coma evaluation, 195
with hyperkalemia, 535
Glucose homeostasis disorders, 639–642
adrenal insufficiency, 641
diabetic ketoacidosis, 639–641, 640t
hyperglycemic hyperosmolar nonketotic syndrome, 639–641, 640t
normoglycemia, 639
thyroid disorders, 642
Glucose intolerance, modification of nutritional regimen with, 52
Glucose-6-phosphatase deficiency, lactic acidosis, 36
Glutamate, 612
Glycolysis, lactic acidosis, 34
Glyconeogenic amino acids, deamination of, lactic acidosis, 34

Glycoprotein IIb/IIIa antagonists, 373–374
  effect on platelet function, 815
  in myocardial infarction, 371–374
Glycyrrhizinic acid, 520
Gold
  as cause of fulminant hepatic failure, 608
  thrombocytopenia with, 853
Goldenhar's syndrome, difficult endotracheal intubation and, 475
Goodpasture's syndrome, as cause of hemoptysis, 484
Gowns, for contact precautions, 681, 683
Graduated compression stockings, in venous thromboembolism, 454
Grafting of burn, 92–93
Graft-vs-host disease, transfusion-associated, 869–872
  γ irradiation guidelines, 871–872
  implicated blood components, 871
  prevention, 871
Gram-negative sepsis, as cause of respiratory disorder, 524
Grand mal seizures, 209–210
Granulocyte transfusions, in immunocompromised patient, 729–730
Granulomatous angiitis, brain, as cause of seizure, 209
Gray platelet syndrome, 818
Grey Turner's sign, 601
Guidewire embolus, as complication of percutaneous central venous catheterization, 917
Guidewire exchange, 934
Guillain-Barre syndrome, 201
  as cause of respiratory acidosis, 523
Gut failure, defined, 554
Gut function, 547–556
  antibiotic prophylaxis, 553–554
  bacteriologic barrier, 549–550
  chemical barrier, 548
  Clostridium difficile colitis, 549–550
  digestive tract decontamination, 553–554
  enzymatic barrier, 548
  gut failure, defined, 554
  immunologic barrier, 548–549
  local barrier, 548
  mechanical barrier, 547–548
  motility, enhancing, 552
  mucosal barrier, 547–550
  multiple system organ failure, 550–551
  nutritional support, 552
  oxygen transport, 551
  physical barrier function, 547–548
  prophylaxis, antibiotics, 553–554
  stress ulcer prophylaxis, 552–553
  supporting barrier function, 551–554
  systemic barrier, 548–549
Gut translocation hypothesis of shock, 15

HAART. See Highly active antiretroviral therapy
Haemophilus influenzae, in immunocompromised patient, 730, 733
Haloperidol, 787
Halo vests, use with spinal cord injury, 254–255
Hand carriage, 683
Hand hygiene, 680–681, 683–684
  antiseptic handrub, 680
  handwashing, 680
Handrub, antiseptic, 680
Handwashing, 680
Harris-Benedict equations, energy expenditure estimation by, 46–47
Head injury, 71–72, 219–220, 229–245.
    See also Coma
  CT scanning, 71, 218
    indications for, 71t
  epidural hematoma, 234–235
  examination, 69
    Glasgow Coma Scale, 69–70t
  hematoma, 234–237
    subdural, 235–236
  hypertensive crisis with, 386
  initial approach to, 71–72
  intracerebral hematoma, delayed, 237
  intracranial pressure management, 238–241
  pathophysiology, 237–238
  posttraumatic seizures, 241–242
  seizure with, 209
  skull fractures, 231–234
    basilar skull fractures, 233–234
    depressed skull fractures, 233
    linear nondisplaced skull fractures, 231–232
  transtentorial herniation, 71
  traumatic intracerebral hematoma, 236–237
Head position for endotracheal intubation, 474
Heart block, with pulmonary artery catheterization, 922
Heart failure
  clinical features, 316t
  pathophysiology of, 314–318

Index

Heart rate, 309–310
 dysrhythmias, 309
 sinus tachycardia, 309–310
Heat exposure, as cause of respiratory disorder, 524
Heat stroke, as cause of fulminant hepatic failure, 608
Helical computed tomography
 in pancreatitis, 571
 in venous thromboembolism, 448
Helicobacter pylori. See also Peptic ulcer
 in peptic ulcer disease, 562
Heliox, bronchospasm, 438
Hemangiomas, coagulation disorder, 826
Hematologic malignancies, lactic acidosis, 36–37
Hematoma, 234–237
 as cause of seizure, 208
 with coma, 189
 delayed traumatic intracerebral, 237
 epidural, 234–235
 intracerebral
  delayed, 237
  risk factors for, 220
  seizure with, 236–237
  traumatic, 236–237
 seizure with, 234–237
 subdural, 235–236
  risk factors for, 220
Hemiballismus, 276
Hemiparesis, with stroke, 275
Hemochromatosis, abdominal pain with, 600
Hemodiabsorption, as liver assist device, 621
Hemodialysis, 539–543
 bleeding, uncontrollable, 539
 blood urea nitrogen
  factors affecting, 542t
  indicators of dialysis adequacy, 540
 continuous venovenous hemofiltration, comparison, 543–544
 continuous venovenous hemofiltration and, 543
 creatinine, factors affecting, 542t
 creatinine concentrations, indicators of dialysis adequacy, 540
 dialyzer, 540
  anaphylactic reaction, 541
 fluid overload, 539
 fluid removal, 542–543
 hyperalimentation, 541–542
 hyperkalemia, 539
 hypotension, 541
  causes of, 542t
 hypoxemia, 541
 lactic acidosis, 39
 as liver assist device, 621
 medications, 541–542
 orders, 541t
 solute removal, 539–540
 urine output, increase by diuretic use, 543
 water removal, 539
Hemodynamic stability, in discontinuation of mechanical ventilation, 503
Hemodynamic variables
 in diagnosis of sepsis, 5
 normal ranges, 313t
Hemofiltration, as liver assist device, 621
Hemoglobin concentration, transfusion therapy and, 834–835, 837–838
Hemoglobin saturation
 in oxygen transport, 25
 in transfusion therapy, 834–835
Hemolytic uremic syndrome, 529
Hemophilia A, 816
 transfusion therapy and, 848, 863–864
Hemophilia B, 816
 transfusion therapy and, 863–864
Hemopneumothorax with spinal cord injury, 259
Hemoptysis, 484–486
 bronchoscopy with, 907–908
 massive, causes of, 484
 with pulmonary embolism, 446
 treatment, 486
Hemorrhage
 as cause of seizure, 208
 cerebellar, coma with, 189–190
 cerebral, 271
 as complication of transbronchoscopic procedure, 912
 gastrointestinal, 557–568
  antacids, 561
  balloon tamponade, as cause of gastrointestinal hemorrhage, 559
  causes of, 559–563
  Child–Pugh class A cirrhosis, 559
  Child–Pugh class C cirrhosis, 559
  colon cancer, lower gastrointestinal hemorrhage with, 563
  colonic polyps, lower gastrointestinal hemorrhage with, 563
  diverticular disease, lower gastrointestinal hemorrhage with, 563

Hemorrhage (Contd.)
  duodenal ulcers, 557
  endoscopic coagulation, as cause of gastrointestinal hemorrhage, 559
  endoscopic sclerotherapy, 560–561
  endoscopic variceal ligation, 560–561
  endoscopy, 557–559
  esophageal varices, 557, 559–561
  gastric ulcer, 557
  gastritis, 561–562
  gastrotomy, as cause of gastrointestinal hemorrhage, 559
  hemorrhoids, lower gastrointestinal hemorrhage with, 563
  H2-receptor antagonists, 561–562
  inflammatory bowel disease, lower gastrointestinal hemorrhage with, 563
  ischemic colitis, lower gastrointestinal hemorrhage with, 563
  lower gastrointestinal hemorrhage, 557, 563–565, 565t
  Mallory-Weiss lesion, 559
  Meckel's diverticulum, with lower gastrointestinal hemorrhage, 563
  patient evaluation, 563–565
  peptic ulcer disease, 562–563
  rectal cancer, lower gastrointestinal hemorrhage with, 563
  Sengstaken-Blakemore tube, protocol for use, 560t
  stigmata of recent hemorrhage, 558–559
  stress ulcer prophylaxis, 561–562
  sucralfate, 561
  treatment, 558, 564
  upper gastrointestinal hemorrhage, 557–559
  vascular ectasias, lower gastrointestinal hemorrhage with, 563
  vasoconstrictor therapy, 560
 in hypertensive emergency, 393
 intracerebral, 280
  as cause of seizure, 208
 intracranial, as cause of hypertensive crisis, 386
 parenchymatous, 271
 petechial, in hypertensive emergency, 393
 pulmonary, 484–486
  angiography/embolization, 485
  balloon tamponade, 485
  bronchoscopy, 485
  radionuclear scanning, 485
  surgery, 485–486

  treatment, 486
 subarachnoid, 271
  as cause of hypertensive crisis, 386
  as cause of seizure, 208
  coma with, 189
  prognosis, 200
 supratentorial, coma with, 189
 thalamic, coma with, 189
Hemorrhagic diatheses, pathophysiology of, 814
Hemorrhagic stroke, encephalopathy and, 300
Hemorrhagic telangiectasia, hereditary, 816
Hemorrhoids, lower gastrointestinal hemorrhage with, 563
Hemosiderosis, pulmonary, as cause of hemoptysis, 484
Hemostatic defect, patient management, 817–820
Hemostatic problems prior to surgery, treatment options, 819t
Hemothorax
 with catheter use, 51
 as cause of respiratory acidosis, 523
 in multiple blunt trauma, 93
 with percutaneous central venous catheterization, 917
Hemotympanum, 233
Henderson-Hasselbalch equation, 515, 520
 bicarbonate buffer system, 513–514
 respiratory acidosis, 521–522
Heparin
 low-dose, in venous thromboembolism, 452–453
 low-molecular-weight, in venous thromboembolism, 453
 with myocardial infarction, 376
 with pulmonary embolism, 457, 459
 with spinal cord injury, 260
 with stroke, 282–283
 thrombocytopenia with, 823, 828–829, 829t, 853
Heparinoid, for venous thromboembolism prevention, 825
Hepatic dysfunction, with malnutrition, 44
Hepatic encephalopathy, 606–607, 611–613, 618–619
 grades of, 607t
 hepatic function and, 133, 135
 neurologic, 606–607
 psychiatric, 606
Hepatic failure, 605–628
 acute-on-chronic liver failure, 605–607

causes of, 607–609, 608t–609t
coagulopathy with, 619–620
definitions, 605–607
dose reduction with, 748
drug dosing, 748
fulminant hepatic failure, 606–609
hepatic encephalopathy, 606–607, 611–613, 618–619
   grades, 607t
hybrid bioartificial liver
   hybrid bioartificial livers, 622–623
   mechanical obstruction, 609–610
   pathologic supply dependency, 610–611
   role of nitric oxide, 610
   trials, 622t
infection with, 619
kidney failure with, 617–618
liver assist devices, 621–622
management, 613–624
metabolic complications with, 620
pathophysiologic features, 609–613
patient transfer, 614–615
respiratory failure with, 618
systemic circulation with, 616–617
tissue hypoxia, 609–611
before transfer to liver center, 613–614
in transplantation, 616, 620–621
   complications, 616–620
   patient selection, 616t
   survival rates after, 615t
treatment of, 614
Hepatic function, 129–138, 547–628
alanine aminotransferase, increases in, 130
albumin, 131–132
alcoholism, 131
anesthesia, effects of, 129–130
ascites, 131–132, 135
aspartate aminotransferase, increases in, 130
bariatric surgery, 133
bilirubin, 131
   for primary biliary cirrhosis, 131
biochemical measurements-, 131
blood flow reduction, 129
branched-chain amino acids, 133–134
central venous pressure monitoring, 135
Child–Pugh class, 131
Child's classification, 131–132
Child–Turcotte–Pugh system, 131–132
chronic hepatitis, 130
cirrhosis, 130–133
   surgical mortality, 132t

encephalopathy, 131
endoscopic biliary drainage, 132
endoscopic retrograde cholangiopancreatography, 135
hepatic encephalopathy, 133
   presence of, 135
hepatic reserve, importance of, 133
hepatitis, 130
hepatitis B infection, common causes of, 131
history, 134
infection, 132
laboratory evaluation, 134
liver biopsy, 135
liver disease, irreversible stage of, 130
metabolic support, indications for, 133–134
monitoring of serum electrolytes, 135
nutrition, 131
operative procedures, major risk factors for, 132–133
physical examination, 134
preoperative assessment, 134–135
preoperative metabolic support, 133–134
prothrombin time, 131–132
Pugh's modification, 131
risk factors for surgery, 130–133
scoring, 131
surgical risk, with cirrhosis, 131t
ultrasonography, 135
Hepatic reserve, hepatic function and, 133
Hepatic transaminases, in pancreatitis, 573–574
Hepatitic ischemia, 588
Hepatitis, 130, 588
abdominal pain with, 600
as cause of fulminant hepatic failure, 608
effect on hepatic function, 130
hepatic failure, 607
hepatic function and, 130
viral, hepatic failure, 607
Hepatitis B, 874–875
hepatic function and, 131
transfusion therapy and, 874–875
Hepatitis C, 875
transfusion therapy and, 875
Hepatobiliary, with HIV/AIDS, 711
Hepatobiliary complications, with catheter use, 51
Herbal remedies, as cause of fulminant hepatic failure, 608
Herpes simplex, as cause of fulminant hepatic failure, 608

Herpes simplex encephalitis, 201
Herpes zoster, abdominal pain with, 600
HHNS. *See* Hyperglycemic hyperosmolar nonketotic syndrome
Hibernating myocardium, 367
Hierarchy of decision-makers, 163
High-extraction drugs, 747
High-frequency ventilation, 497–498
Highly active antiretroviral therapy, with HIV/AIDS, 712
　variables associated with, 703
Hip fracture, 843
　surgery, venous thromboembolism with, 455
　transfusion therapy and, 842–843
Hip replacement, venous thromboembolism with, 455
Hirudin, in pulmonary embolism, 459–460
Histamine H_2 blockers, thrombocytopenia with, 853
HIV. *See* Human immunodeficiency virus
HLA-matched platelets, matching for, 854t
Hormones, as cause of respiratory disorder, 524
Horner's syndrome, as complication of percutaneous central venous catheterization, 917
Hospital antibiotic restriction, 678
Host defenses
　changes throughout human development, 726
　in immunocompromised patients, 726–728
HPA axis. *See* Hypothalamic-pituitary-adrenal axis
Human immunodeficiency virus (HIV), 703–724
　antiretroviral therapy, 712–717
　　highly active, 712
　　lactic acidosis with, 36
　as cause of seizure, 209
　clinical presentation to surgeon, 711t
　complications, 717–718
　epidemiology, 704–705
　ethical issues, 718–719
　highly active antiretroviral therapy, 703, 712
　legal issues, 718–719
　needle stick, 706–707
　occupational, prevention of, 708–710
　outcome of surgery, 717–718
　postexposure prophylaxis, 708–710, 709t
　recognizing, 710–712
　regimens against, 709t
　risk to surgeon, 703–724, 707t
　transfusion therapy and, 860, 875
　transmission
　　from surgeon, 707–708
　　to surgeon, 705–707, 707t
Hybrid bioartificial liver, 622–623
　biologic component, 622–623
　mechanical obstruction, 609–610
　pathologic supply dependency, 610–611
　role of nitric oxide, 610
　synthetic substrate, 622
Hydralazine
　with hypertensive emergencies, 391
　pharmacodynamics of, 769
Hydration, with spinal cord injury, 260
Hydrochloric acid, with metabolic acidosis, 518
Hydrochlorothiazide, thrombocytopenia with, 853
Hydrocortisone, 632
Hydromorphone, 759–760
　adverse reactions, 790–791
　analgesic therapy, 790–791
　pharmacodynamics of, 777
Hydronephrosis, with metabolic acidosis, 518
Hydrostatic pulmonary edema, as cause of hypoxemia, 506
Hydrothorax, with catheter use, 51
Hydroxychloroquine, as cause of fulminant hepatic failure, 608
Hymenoptera stings, allergic reaction, 801
Hyperalimentation, with hemodialysis, 541–542
Hyperbicarbonatemia, 519
Hyperbilirubinemia, 586. *See also* jaundice
Hypercalcemia, 520, 650–651, 657
　bisphosphonates, 650–651
　cardiovascular symptoms, 650
　encephalopathy and, 302
　forced diuresis, 650
　hypovolemia, 650
　neuromuscular symptoms, 650
　symptomatic, 650
　treatment, 651
Hypercapnia
　bronchospasm, 440
　coma, 189
Hypercarbic breathing, in encephalopathy, 298
Hypercoagulable states, 823t
Hyperfibrinolysis, 821
Hyperglycemia, 51, 639
　as cause of seizure, 208, 215

Index

Hyperglycemic hyperosmolar nonketotic syndrome, 639–641, 640t
Hyperhomocysteinemia, 823
Hyperinflation, intrinsic, 398. *See also* Auto-positive end-expiratory pressure
Hyperkalemia, 641
  with anion gap acidosis, 518
  as complication, with renal failure, 535
  with hemodialysis, 539
  as indication for dialysis, 536
  symptoms of, 671
  treatment, 535t, 672
Hyperlactatemia, lactic acidosis, 33–35
Hypermagnesemia, 653–654, 657
  as cause of respiratory acidosis, 523
  renal failure, 653
Hypermetabolism, 3
Hypernatremia
  causes, 668t
  encephalopathy and, 302
  treatment, 668t
Hyperosmolal ionic contrast therapy, radiocontrast medium-induced acute renal failure, 145
Hyperosmolar coma. *See* Hyperglycemic hyperosmolar nonketotic syndrome
Hyperosmolar hyperglycemic hyperosmolar nonketotic syndrome, 639
Hyperparathyroidism, 520, 600
  pancreatitis and, 569
Hyperperfusion syndrome, with carotid endarterectomy, 417
Hyperphosphatemia, 535, 648, 655–656, 658
  absorption of phosphates, controlling, 656
  hemodialysis, 656
  renal failure, 655
  treatment, 656
Hyperpigmentation of skin, in burns, 93
Hyperpyrexia, in thyroid dysfunction, 634
Hyper reninism, 520
Hypertension
  with atrial fibrillation, 330
  mechanical ventilator support and, 489
  in renal failure, 140
  stroke and, 270
  surgical risks with, 98
Hypertensive crisis, 385–394
  antihypertensive therapy, 388–391
  causes of, 386t
  initial evaluation, 387t
  management of, 388
  parenteral medications, 390t

  types of, 385–386
Hypertensive emergencies, 385–394
  antihypertensive therapy, 388–391
    fenoldopam, 389
    fentanyl, 388
    midazolam, 388
    nitroprusside, 389
    sodium nitroprusside, 389
  aortic dissection, 392–393
  blood pressure, reduction of, 388
  cardiac/vascular complications, 392–393
  causes of, 385–386t
  central nervous system complications, 393
  cerebral edema, 393
  coronary artery bypass surgery, 393
  heart rate, importance of, 392
  hypertensive urgency, 385–386
    differentiating between, 386
  initial evaluation, 386–387, 387t
  labetalol, 393
  laboratory data, 387
  management of, 388
  microinfarcts, 393
  nitroprusside, 393
  parenteral medications, 390t
  patient history, 386
  petechial hemorrhages, 393
  physical examination, 387
  severe left ventricular dysfunction, 392
  tachycardia, problem of, 392
  types of, 385–386
Hypertensive encephalopathy, as cause of seizure, 208
Hypertensive heart disease, 314–317
Hypertensive urgency, 385–386
  hypertensive emergency, differentiating between, 386
Hyperthermia, 635–636
Hyperthyroidism, with atrial fibrillation, 330
Hypertonic saline, with cerebral edema, 285
Hypertransfusion, for emergency resuscitation, 423
Hypertriglyceridemia, 51
  modification of nutritional regimen with, 52
  pancreatitis and, 569
Hyperventilation
  with cerebral edema, 284
  in coma, 232
  in differential diagnosis of seizure, 212
  in head injury, 239–240
  with liver failure, 619

Hyperventilation syndrome,
    anaphylaxis and, 804
Hypoadrenalism, 629–630
Hypoalbuminemia, 518
Hypoaldosteronism, with metabolic
    acidosis, 518
Hypocalcemia, 648–650, 657
    as complication, with renal failure, 535
    encephalopathy and, 302
    pancreatitis, association, 648
    transfusion therapy and, 873
    treatment, 649
Hypochlorhydria, in immunocompromised
    patient, 732
Hypofibrinogenemia, transfusion
    therapy and, 856–857
Hypogammaglobulinemia, transfusion
    therapy and, 848
Hypoglycemia
    with anaphylaxis, 804
    as cause of seizure, 208
    in encephalopathy, 299
Hypokalemia, 518
    symptoms of, 670
Hypokalemic paralysis, as cause of respiratory
    acidosis, 523
Hypomagnesemia, 648, 652–653, 657
    ECG changes, 652
    forced diuresis, 654
    hemodialysis, 654
    magnesium equilibrates, 653
    neurologic disturbances, 652
    serum magnesium concentration, 652–653
    treatment of, 653
Hyponatremia
    as cause of respiratory disorder, 524
    as complication, with renal failure, 535
    encephalopathy and, 300–301
    as indication for dialysis, 536
    treatment of, 669t
Hypophosphatemia, 654–655, 657–658
    as cause of respiratory acidosis, 523
    glucose tolerance, 655
    insulin resistance, 655
    intravenous phosphate preparations, 655
Hyposplenism, in immunocompromised
    patient, 730
Hypotension
    with anaphylaxis, 803
    with carotid endarterectomy, 417
    as cause of respiratory disorder, 524
    during dialysis, causes of, 542t

with dialysis, 542t
    drug dosing, 768
    with hemodialysis, 541
    in multiple organ failure, 9
    pancreatitis, differential diagnosis, 573
    with spinal cord injury, 257–258
    transfusion therapy and, 873
Hypothalamic lesions, in head injury, 230
Hypothalamic-pituitary-adrenal axis, 629
Hypothermia, 94–95, 638
    emergency treatment of, 94
    morbidity, 94
    in multiple blunt trauma, 84
    transfusion therapy and, 873
Hypothyroidism, 638
    airway management with, 477
Hypotonic water loss, 665–666
Hypoventilation, as cause of respiratory
    acidosis, 523
Hypovolemia, 1005
Hypovolemic shock, with anaphylaxis, 804
Hypoxemia
    in bronchospasm, 433
    as cause of respiratory disorder, 524
    causes of, 506t
    with dialysis, 541
    lactic acidosis, 36
Hypoxia, 427
    in encephalopathy, 298
Hysteria, as cause of respiratory disorder, 524

Ibutilide, 787
    with atrial fibrillation, 340
ICD. *See* Implantable defibrillator
ICF. *See* Intracellular fluid
ICHD. *See* Inter-Society Commission on Heart
    Disease Resources
ICP. *See* Intracranial pressure
Idiogenic osmols, 665
Idiopathic seizures, 207, 209
    treatment, 215
Ileostomy, 662
Ileus
    abdominal pain with, 600
    with spinal cord injury, 261
Illicit drug use
    as cause of hypertensive crisis, 386
    as cause of seizure, 208
Imipenem, 794
    resistance to, 676, 684–685
Immobilization of head/neck with spinal cord
    injury, 245–246

Index

Immune-enhancing nutritional formulas, 48
Immune host defenses,
    in immunocompromised patients, 725–728
Immune paralysis hypothesis of shock, 15
Immune system depression,
    with malnutrition, 43
Immunocompromised patient,
    infection in, 725–742
  altered microbial flora, 732–733
  antibody deficiency, 733
  asplenia, 730
  CMI defects, 733
  complement deficiency, 730
  defects in immunity, 733–735
  diabetes mellitus, 731
  febrile illness, with neutropenia, 729t
  fever, 735–736
  hypochlorhydria, 732
  infection-induced immune dysfunction, 733–734
  innate defects, 728–733
  malignancy, 731
  malnutrition, 731
  management, 737–738
  neurological dysfunction, 731–732
  neutropenia, 728–730
  prevention, 738–739
  splenic dysfunction, 730
  stress, 732
  tobacco use, 732
  transplantation, 734–735
Immunomodulation, with transfusion, 861–863, 874
Immunosuppression, in acute abdomen, 601
Impaired immune competence,
    with malnutrition, 44
Impaired wound healing, with malnutrition, 44
Implantable defibrillator
  with premature ventricular contractions, 353
  with sustained ventricular tachycardia, 357
Inborn errors of metabolism
  as cause of seizure, 209
  lactic acidosis, 36
Indefinite continuation of treatment,
    limitations to, 165
Indinavir, for HIV, 709
Indocyanine green dye, time-concentration curve, in cardiac output measurement, 974–976
Infarct extension, in myocardial infarction, 379

Infection-induced immune dysfunction in immunocompromised patient, 733–734
Infectious disease, 675–744
  AIDS, 703–724
  antibiotic resistance, 675–692
  defined, 4
  diagnostic criteria, 5t
  HIV, 703–724
  immunocompromised patient, 725–742
  intra-abdominal infection, 693–702
Infectious disease specialists, 680
Infectious risks of transfusions, 833–894
  bacteria, 876–877
  West Nile virus, 875
Inferior myocardial infarction, 327
Inflammatory bowel disease
  abdominal pain with, 600
  lower gastrointestinal hemorrhage with, 563
Inflammatory cytokines, transfusion therapy and, 857–858
Inflammatory process, controls, 10
Inflammatory response syndrome, pancreatitis and, 577
Inflammatory variables in diagnosis of sepsis, 5
Informed consent, 161
Infratentorial infarcts, surgery, 287
Infratentorial lesion, 194–195
  in coma, 194–195
Initial approach to injured patient, 63–80
  abdomen, 69–70, 74–76
  airway, 63–64
  breathing, 64–65
  chest, 69, 72–73
  circulation, 65–67
  disability, 67–68
  emergency department thoracotomy, 74
  evaluation, 68–69
  extremities examination, 70
  genito-urinary injuries, 76
  head, 69, 71–72
  management, 63–68
  multiple blunt trauma, 81
  musculoskeletal injuries, 76–78
  neck, 69, 72
  physical examination, 69–70
  stabilization, 63–68
  treatment, 68–69
  ventilation, 64–65
Initiation of nutritional support,
    timing of, 51–52

Injured patient, 63-96. *See also* Trauma
  abdominal injuries, 74-76
  airway, 63-64
  blunt multiple trauma, fractures in, 81-86
  breathing, 64-65
  burns, 87-93
  chest injuries, 72-73
  circulation, 65-67
  disability, 67-68
  electrical injury, 93-94
  emergency department thoracotomy, 74
  evaluation, 68-69
  frostbite, 94-95
  genito-urinary injuries, 76
  head injury, 71-72
  hypothermia, 94-95
  initial approach to, 63-80
  management, initial, 63-68
  musculoskeletal injuries, 76-78
  neck injury, 72
  physical examination, 69-70
    abdomen, 69-70
    chest, 69
    extremities, 70
    head, 69
    neck, 69
  stabilization, 63-68
  treatment, initial, 68-69
  ventilation, 64-65
Innate defects, in immunocompromised patient, 728-733
Innate host defenses, in immunocompromised patients, 725-728
Inotropic therapy
  cardiac, vascular effects, 761-763t
  drug dosing, 754-766
  systolic dysfunction, 315
Inspiratory muscle strength, in discontinuation of mechanical ventilation, 508
Inspired gas, oxygen concentration in, 495
Insulin, with hyperkalemia, 535
Insulin-mediated glucose transport, hypokalemia, 670
Integrilin, 372
Integrity of physician, 161-174
  best interest standard, 163
  clinical judgment, made by physician, 161
  competency, legal term, made by judge, 161
  decision-making capacity, 161-163
    defined, 162
    patients without, 163
  doctrine of implied consent, 163
  do not resuscitate order, 164-165
    case study, 164-165
    defined, 165
  Emergency Medical Treatment and Active Labor Act, 167
  end of life issues, 169-171
    food/fluids, forgoing, 171
    pain control, 169-170
    rule of double effect, 170
    suffering, relief of, 169-170
    ventilator withdrawal, 170-171
    withdrawal of dialysis, 171
    withdrawal of life-sustaining treatment, 170-171
    withdrawal of other treatments, 171
    World Health Organization Analgesic Ladder, 169
  futility, medical, 166-168
    case study, 167-168
    defined, 167
    resolving conflicts over, 168-169
  hierarchy of decision-makers, 163
  indefinite continuation of treatment, limitations to, 165
  informed consent, 161
  limits to other types of care, issues, 166
  perseverence of life, 166
  physician-assisted suicide, 171-172
  substituted judgment, principle of, 163
Interactions, drug, 783-798. *See also under specific drug*
Interdisciplinary approach to quality care, 175
Interleukin-1
  with acute respiratory distress syndrome, 423
  in peritoneal response to infection, 694
Interleukin-6, with acute respiratory distress syndrome, 423
Interleukin-8
  with acute respiratory distress syndrome, 423
  in peritoneal response to infection, 694
Intermittent mandatory ventilation, 494
  synchronized, in discontinuation of mechanical ventilation, 502-503
Internal jugular vein catheterization, contraindications to, 918
Interpretation of data, 961-994
Inter-Society Commission on Heart Disease Resources, three-position letter code, 329

Interstitial lung disease
    as cause of respiratory acidosis, 523
    as cause of respiratory disorders, 524
Intra-abdominal abscess, 698–699
    antibiotic therapy, 697t
    bacteria causing, 696
    diagnosis, 698–699
    management, 699
Intra-abdominal infection, 693–702
    anatomy, abdominal cavity, 693
    antibiotic therapy, 697t
    diagnosis, 695–700
    intra-abdominal abscess, 698–699
        bacteria causing, 696
        diagnosis, 698–699
        management, 699
    management, 695–700
    peritoneal infection
        cytokines and, 694t
        defense against, 694–695
        local response, 694–695
        systemic response, 695
    peritonitis
        bacteria causing, 696
        diagnosis, 695–696
        management, 696–698
        microbiology, 700t
        secondary, 695–698
        tertiary, 699–700
    physiology of abdominal cavity, 693
Intra-arterial thrombolysis, 282
Intracellular fluid, 661
Intracellular hemoglobin
        buffer system, 512–513
Intracerebral hematoma, 237
    risk factors for, 220
Intracerebral hemorrhage, 280
    as cause of seizure, 208
Intracranial hemorrhage, as cause of
        hypertensive crisis, 386
Intracranial pressure
    elevated, as source of cerebral ischemia, 272
    in head injury, 238–241
    pharmacologic control of, 241t
    reduction, in trauma patient, 64–65
    with seizure, 238–241
Intractable shock, cause of, 66
Intraoperative evaluation, 97–186
Intrathoracic pressure, 397
    cardiorespiratory function, interaction
        between, 986–987
    changes in, 397–399

Intrathoracic trauma, with acute respiratory
        distress syndrome, 423
Intravascular hemolysis in renal failure, 140
Intravascular volume
    repletion, transfusion therapy and, 848
    significance of, 108
Intravenous access in critically ill patient,
        65–66
Intravenous drug delivery
    amiodarone, 378
    analgesics, 777t
    esmolol, 343
    recombinant tissue plasminogen
        activator, 281
    sedatives, 778t
    vitamin K, 801
Intravenous pyelogram, 76
Intrinsic acute renal failure, 531–532
    acute tubular necrosis, 531
    causes, 531–532
    nephrotoxicity, 531–533
    prolonged renal hypoperfusion, 531
Intrinsic hyperinflation, 398, 401–402. See
        also Auto-positive end-expiratory
        pressure
    weaning, 399–400
Intubation
    bronchoscopy, 909–912
    bronchospasm, 438–440
    difficult, 908
    laryngeal mask airway, in trauma patient, 64
Intubation tube, 469–471
Invasive monitoring, complications with,
        415–416
    access complications, 416
    axillary artery catheterization, 415
    brachial artery complications, 415
    radial artery catheterization, 415
Iodinated radiocontrast dyes, allergic reaction,
        800–801
Ionized calcium concentration, 647–648
    total serum calcium concentration,
        relationship between, 647
Ions, divalent, 647–659
Ipsilateral eye deviation, with stroke, 275
Iron overload, transfusion therapy and, 874
Ischemia, cerebral
    physiology of, 272–273
    sources of, 272t
    vasospasm-related, 280
Ischemic colitis, lower gastrointestinal
        hemorrhage with, 563

Ischemic heart disease, 103, 314–317
  multivariate predictors, 103t
Ischemic hepatitis, as cause of fulminant
    hepatic failure, 608
Ischemic stroke
  encephalopathy and, 299–300
  venous thromboembolism, 456
Isolated factor XIII deficiency, transfusion
    therapy and, 857
Isoniazid, lactic acidosis, 36
Isoproterenol, 120, 766
  in cardiac arrest, 120
  dosing, 766
  precautions, 766
Itching of burns, 93
IVP. *See* Intravenous pyelogram

Japanese encephalitis, in transfusion
    therapy, 875
Jaundice, 7–8
  with acute renal failure, 537
  initial evaluation, 586
  nonobstructive, 587–589
    cholangitis, 586–589
    hemolysis, 588–589
    hepatocellular dysfunction, 587–588
  obstructive, cholangitis, 586–589
    Charcot's triad, 587
    endoscopic retrograde
      cholangiography, 587
    endoscopic transpapillary
      sphincterotomy, 587
    percutaneous transhepatic
      cholangiography, 587
Joint probabilities, 1008–1011

Kartagener's syndrome, as cause of
    hemoptysis, 484
Kasabach-Merritt syndrome, 826.
    See also Hemangioma
Kernohan's notch phenomenon,
    in head injury, 231
Ketoacidosis, 518, 639–641, 640t
  abdominal pain with, 600
  management of, 640t
Ketoconazole
  with acute respiratory distress
    syndrome, 429
  as cause of fulminant hepatic failure, 608
Kidney disease, stages of, 141t
Kidney function. *See also* Renal failure
  preoperative evaluation of, 140–144

King's College Hospital, criteria, 615
Klebsiella
  as cause of peritonitis/abscess, 696
  in immunocompromised patient, 728
Klebsiella oxytocia, peritonitis, 700
Klebsiella pneumoniae, 700
  antibiotic resistance, 676
  peritonitis, 700
Klippel-Feil syndrome, difficult endotracheal
    intubation and, 475
Knee replacement, venous
    thromboembolism with, 455
Kupffer cell
  gut, macrophage bed, 548
  in hepatic failure, 609
  neutrophils, 588
Kussmaul's sign, 402
Kyphoscoliosis, as cause of respiratory
    acidosis, 523

Labetalol
  dosing, 773–774
    precautions, 774
  with hepatic failure, 748
  with hypertensive emergency, 391, 393
  pharmacodynamics of, 769
Lactate acidosis, 36
Lactate production, delivery-dependent,
    oxygen transport and, 26–27
Lactate-pyruvate ratio, in oxygen transport, 26
Lactic acidosis, 33–42
  acetaminophen overdose, 36
  alkali therapy, 39
  anemia, 36
  with anion gap acidosis, 518
  antiretroviral therapy with HIV, 36
  associated acidemia, 35
  asthma exacerbation, 36
  biguanides, 36
  biotin, 36
  blood oxygen content, 37
  carbon monoxide poisoning, 36
  cardiac performance, 37
  cellular hypoxia, 33
  clinical correlates, 37
  Cori cycle, glyconeogenesis via, 34
  cyanide poisoning, 36
  diabetic ketoacidosis, 36
  ethanol intoxication, 36
  ethylene glycol, 35
    poisoning, 36
  etiologies of, 36t

Index

etiology of, 35–37
fructose, 36
fructose-1,6-diphosphatase deficiency, 36
fulminant liver failure, 36
glucose-6-phosphatase deficiency, 36
glycolysis, 34
glyconeogenic amino acids,
 deamination of, 34
hematologic malignancies, 36–37
hemodialysis, 39
hepatic extraction, 34
hyperlactatemia, 33–35
hypoxemia, 36
hypoxia, 35
 evidence of, 35
inborn errors of metabolism, 36
ischemia, 35–36
isoniazid, 36
lactate clearance, 34–35
lactate dehydrogenase, 33
lactate metabolism, 34
lactic acidosis, 37
mitochondrial dysfunction, 35
mitochondrial oxidative
 phosphorylation, 33
oxidative phosphorylation, congenital
 disorders of, 36
pathogenesis, 33–35
peritoneal dialysis, 39
propylene glycol, 35–36
pyruvate, effect of, 34
pyruvate carboxylase deficiency, 36
pyruvate dehydrogenase complex, 34
pyruvate dehydrogenase deficiency, 36
regional perfusion, 37
renal excretion, 34–35
salicylate overdose, 36
seizures, 36
serum lactate, elevated, etiology of, 38–39
shock, 35–36
short bowel syndrome, 36
small cell carcinoma, 37
sugar alcohols, 36
thiamine deficiency, 36
tissue oxygen delivery, inadequate, 36
treatment of, 37–39
Type A, 36
Type B, 35–36
Lactobacillus species, as cause of
 peritonitis/abscess, 696
Lactoferrin, gut, 548
Lacunar infarction, 275

Lacunar syndromes, 275t
Lamivudine plus stavudine, for HIV, 709
Lamotrigine, with epilepsy, 217
Lanoteplase, with myocardial infarction, 371
Laparoscopy, with acute abdomen, 597
Large-volume paracentesis, with
 liver failure, 614
Laryngeal edema
 airway management with, 476
 postintubation, as cause of respiratory
  acidosis, 523
Laryngeal fracture, airway
 management with, 476
Laryngeal mask airway, in trauma patient, 64
Laryngoscopy
 classification of views, 478
 direct, 471–472
Laryngospasm, as cause of respiratory
 acidosis, 523
Laryngotracheitis, as cause of respiratory
 acidosis, 523
Late organ failure, 8
Latex allergy, allergic reaction, 801
Lead poisoning, abdominal pain with, 600
Left ventricular dilation, with sepsis, 320
Left ventricular dysfunction, 108
 in hypertensive emergency, 392
Left ventricular hypertrophy, 317
Lepiota helvella poisoning, as cause of
 fulminant hepatic failure, 608
Leukemia
 abdominal pain with, 600
 fulminant hepatic failure with, 608
Leukocyte-associated DNA virus, transfusion
 therapy and, 859
Leukocyte reduction of blood components,
 transfusion therapy and, 855–856
Leukoreduced blood components,
 transfusions, 857–863
 cytomegalovirus, 859–861
 febrile nonhemolytic transfusion
  reactions, 857–859
 immunomodulation, 861–863
LeVeen shunt, 826
Levetiracetam, with epilepsy, 217
Lev–Lenegre's disease, 327
Levofloxacin, antibiotic resistance, 684
Liddle's syndrome, 520
Lidocaine, 121–122
 with atrial fibrillation, 335–336
 with cardiac arrest, 121–122
 with hepatic failure, 748

Lidocaine (Contd.)
  with myocardial infarction, 378
  serum concentration monitoring, 755
  with sustained ventricular tachycardia, 357
Life support, in cardiac arrest, 113–128
Ligands, in multiple organ failure, 11t
Lights, effect of, in encephalopathy, 304
Linear nondisplaced skull fractures, 231–232
  seizure with, 231–232
Linezolid, 794
  antibiotic resistance, 681–682
Lipopolysaccharide, 10–11
Lisofylline, with acute respiratory distress syndrome, 429
Lithium carbonate, with bradyarrhythmias, 325
Liver assist devices, 621–622
Liver biopsy, hepatic function and, 135
Liver disease. See also Liver failure
  coagulation disorders, 820–822
  with renal failure, 139
  transfusion therapy and, 847, 865–866
Liver enzyme profiles, 586
Liver failure, 605–628
  acute-on-chronic liver failure, 605–607
  algorithm for initial approach, 617
  causes of, 607–609, 608t–609t
  coagulopathy with, 619–620
  definitions, 605–607
  encephalopathy and, 304
  fulminant hepatic failure, 606–609
    See also Fulminant hepatic failure
  hepatic encephalopathy with, 606–607, 611–613, 618–619
    grades of, 607t
  hybrid bioartificial liver, 622–623
    mechanical obstruction, 609–610
    pathologic supply dependency, 610–611
    role of nitric oxide, 610
    trials, 622t
  infection with, 619
  kidney failure with, 617–618
  liver assist devices, 621–622
  management, 613–624
  metabolic complications with, 620
  modification of nutritional regimen with, 52–53
  pathophysiologic features, 609–613
  patient transfer, 614–615
  respiratory failure with, 618
  systemic circulation with, 616–617
  tissue hypoxia, 609–611
  before transfer to liver center, 613–614
  in transplantation, 616, 620–621
    complications, 616–620
    patient selection, 616t
    survival rates after, 615t
Liver function tests, in coma evaluation, 195
Liver transplantation, 616, 620–621
  complications, 616–620
  contraindications to, 621
  with HIV infection, 717
  infectious diseases after, 727
  orthotopic, 621
  patient selection, 616t
  survival rates after, 615t
LMWH. See Low molecular weight heparin
Localization-related seizure, 209
Locked-in syndrome, 201, 276
Long QT associated ventricular tachycardia, therapy for, 358
Loop diuretics, with renal failure, 533–534
Lorazepam, 223, 778
  with epilepsy, 216
  with increased intracranial pressure, 241–242
Lovastatin, as cause of fulminant hepatic failure, 608
Low birth weight, transfusion therapy and, 861
Lower extremity ischemia, 411–413
  arterial thromboembolism, 412
  arterial thrombosis, 412
  clinical presentation, 411–412
  differential diagnosis, 412
  Doppler probe, 411
  following aortic procedures, 416
  history, 411
  medical, surgical treatment, 412–413
  non-occlusive ischemia, 412
  physical examination, 411
Lower gastrointestinal hemorrhage, 557, 563–565
  causes of, 565t
  patient evaluation, 563–565
  treatment, 564
Low-extraction drugs, 747
Low molecular weight heparin, 457–458, 897–899
  with spinal cord injury, 260
Lumbar puncture, 947–950
  anatomy, 947
  bleeding with, 949
  coma and, 195
  complications of, 949–950

Index

CSF analysis, 948–949
  headache with, 950
  lumbar puncture positions, 949
  paramedian approach, 948
  paresthesias with, 949
  positioning, 947
  procedure, 947–948
  vertebral ligaments, 948
Lund and Browder chart, burn size, 88–89
Lung abscess, as cause of hemoptysis, 484
Lung contusion, with acute respiratory distress syndrome, 423
Lung injury, acute. *See* Acute lung injury
Lung volume, gas flow, relation between, 981
Lupus anticoagulant, 823
Lymphadenopathy, with HIV/AIDS, 711
Lymphocytes, transfusion therapy and, 870
Lymphoid tissue reduction, gut-associated, with malnutrition, 44
Lymphoma
  as cause of fulminant hepatic failure, 608
  as cause of hemoptysis, 484
Lymphopenia, with HIV/AIDS, 711
Lysine chloride, with metabolic acidosis, 518
Lysozyme, gut, 548

Magnesium, 651–654
  atomic absorption spectroscopy, 651
  with chronic renal failure, 148–149
  deficiency, 520
  hypermagnesemia, 653–654, 657
  hypomagnesemia, 652–653, 657
  intravenous, bronchospasm, 437
  ultrafiltration, 651
Major vessel thrombosis, 275
Malaria
  abdominal pain with, 600
  transfusion therapy and, 875
Malignancy, 823
  in immunocompromised patient, 731
Malignant hypertension, 529
Mallory-Weiss lesion, 559
  as cause of gastrointestinal hemorrhage, 559
Malnutrition, 731
  in immunocompromised patient, 731
  mouth feeding, 731
  parenteral nutrition, 731
  physiologic consequences of, 43–44, 44t
  pulmonary complications of surgery with, 154
  risk factors for, 44t
  tube feeding, 731

Mandatory exploration, in trauma patient, 72
Mandibular injury, airway management with, 476
Man-in-the-barrel syndrome, 276
Mannitol, 240
  with increased intracranial pressure, 241
  with liver failure, 619
  with renal failure, 533–534
MAP. *See* Mean arterial pressure
Massive transfusion, transfusion therapy and, 847
MAST. *See* Pneumatic anti-shock garment
Mastectomy, as contraindication to subclavian vein catheterization, 916
Mastocytosis, with anaphylaxis, 804
Maxillary injury, airway management with, 476
Maximum inspiratory pressure, 984
Mean arterial pressure, intracranial pressure, relationship between, 83
Measles
  abdominal pain with, 600
  in immunocompromised patient, 734
Measurement of data, 961–994
Mechanical ventilation, 427–428, 489–500
  airway pressure release ventilation, 497
  arterial blood, 490t
  arterial blood gas determination, 503
  assist-control ventilation, 493–494
  in bronchospasm, 438–440
  as cause of respiratory disorder, 524
  control mode ventilation, 493
  criteria for instituting, 491
  current recommendations, 505
  decreased inspiratory muscle strength, 508
  detrimental effects of, minimizing, 400t
  duration of, 504
  gas exchange, 489–490
  hemodynamic stability, 503
  high-frequency ventilation, 497–498
  hypoxemia, causes of, 506t
  increased dead space ventilation, 506
  initial settings, 497t
  inspired gas, oxygen concentration in, 495
  intermittent mandatory ventilation, 494
  mechanical ventilation, 497–498
  modes of ventilation, 491–498
  oxygenation, 503
    failure of, 506
  positive end-expiratory pressure, 495
  pressure-support ventilation, 497, 502–503
  protocol weaning, 503–504

Mechanical ventilation (Contd.)
  rapid shallow breathing index, 502
  resolution of original indication of, 503
  respiratory mechanics, 490–491
  respiratory rate, 495
  safety features, 496–497
  spontaneous breathing trials, 501, 504–505
  suctioning of patients on, 177–178
  synchronized intermittent mandatory ventilation, 502–503
  tapered support, 502–503
  tidal volume, 495–496
  T-piece, 502, 504
  trigger sensitivity, 496
  uncompensated respiratory acidemia, 508
  ventilation failure, 506–508
  ventilator flow patterns, 496
  ventilatory failure, algorithm for investigating, 507
  weaning, 501–510
    American College of Chest Physicians definition, 501
    approaches, 502–505
    criteria, 502–503t
    protocol, 504t
  weaning failure, 505–508
Meckel's diverticulum, with lower gastrointestinal hemorrhage, 563
Mefexamide, with metabolic acidosis, 518
Meningitis
  as cause of seizure, 208
  encephalopathy and, 300
Mental status, poor progression, CT scanning, 218
Mental status changes, 299–300
  cardiovascular causes, 303–304
    dysrhythmias, 303
    myocardial infarction, 303
    on-pump CAB, 303–304
  in encephalopathy, 299–300
  endocrine causes, 303
    Addison's disease, 303
    Cushing's syndrome, 303
    diabetes mellitus, 303
    hypothyroidism, 303
  hemorrhagic stroke, 300
  hepatic causes, 304–305
    cirrhosis, 304
    liver failure, 304
    portal hypertension, 304
    portal-systemic bypass, 304
  iatrogenic causes, 304

    anesthetics, 304
    lights, 304
    narcotics, 304
    sedatives, 304
    sleep deprivation, 304
    steroids, 304
  ischemic stroke, 299–300
  meningitis, 300
  metabolic/electrolyte causes, 300–303
    hypercalcemia, 302
    hypernatremia, 302
    hypocalcemia, 302
    hyponatremia, 300–301
    osmolar abnormalities, 302–303
    thiamine deficiency, 303
  septic encephalopathy, 305–306
    mental status, 305
    respiratory alkalosis, 305
    tachypnea, 305
  in thyroid dysfunction, 634
  uremic encephalopathy, 306
    aluminum neurotoxicity, 306
    asterixis, 306
    diagnosis of exclusion, 306
    dialysis disequilibrium syndrome, 306
Mental status examination, 192–193
  in coma, 192–193
Meperidine, 759–760
  adverse reactions, 790–791
  analgesic therapy, 790–791
Mercury, abdominal pain with, 600
Meropenem, antibiotic resistance, 684–685
Mesenteric adenitis, abdominal pain with, 600
Mesenteric ischemia, 400–401, 414, 599–601
  angiography, 414
  clinical presentation, 414
  contrast-enhanced computed tomography, 414
  differential diagnosis, 414
  medical, surgical management, 414
  mesenteric artery thrombosis, 414
  mesenteric venous thrombosis, 414
  non-occlusive mesenteric ischemia, 414
  superior mesenteric artery emboli, 414
  thrombectomy, 414
Metabolic acid–base disorders, 516–519
Metabolic acidemia
  lactic acidosis, 33
Metabolic acidosis, 514, 518

Index

Metabolic alkalosis, 514, 518–519
   as cause of respiratory acidosis, 523
   classification of, 520
   factors contributing to, 520
Metabolic causes of encephalopathy, 300–303
Metabolic support
   in burns, 92
   in pancreatitis, 578–579
Metabolism of drugs, 746–747.
   See also specific drug
Metastatic disease, as cause of hemoptysis, 484
Methanol intoxication
   anion gap acidosis from, 518
   in lactic acidosis, 36
Methicillin-resistant *Staphylococcus aureus,* 676, 681–682
   control/prevention, 681–682
   epidemiology, 681
   therapy, 681
Methylxanthines, bronchospasm, 437
Metoclopramide, gut motility enhancement, 552
Metoprolol, with hepatic failure, 748
Metronidazole, 794
MI. *See* Myocardial infarction
Microbes, in multiple organ failure, 10–11
Microbial flora, in immunocompromised patient, 732–733
Microbiology tertiary peritonitis, peritonitis, 700t
Microinfarcts, in hypertensive emergency, 393
Micronutrient deficiency syndromes, 43
   with malnutrition, 44
Micronutrient requirements, 47–48
   deficiency syndromes from failure to provide, 51
Midazolam, 778
   with epilepsy, 216
Migraine, in differential diagnosis of seizure, 212
Millard-Gubler syndrome, 276
Milrinone, 765
   dosing, 765
MIP. *See* Maximum inspiratory pressure
Misplaced endotracheal tube, 479t
Mitochondrial dysfunction, lactate acidosis, 35
Mitochondrial oxidative phosphorylation, 33
Mitral regurgitation, 379
Mitral stenosis, as cause of hemoptysis, 484
Mitral valve replacement, with atrial fibrillation, 339

Mittelschmerz, abdominal pain with, 600
Modification of nutrition regimen, 52–54
   conditions requiring, 52–54
Modified Allen's test, in arterial catheterization, 923
Molecular weight heparin, 896
Monro-Kellie doctrine, 237–241
Morganella morganii
   intra-abdominal infection with, 696
   peritonitis/abscess with, 696
Morphine, 759–760
   pharmacodynamics of, 777
Motility of gut, enhancing, 552
Motor examination, 194
   in coma, 194
   grading system for, 246
Movement disorders, in differential diagnosis of seizure, 212
Moxifloxacin, 787
Mucor fungi, in immunocompromised patient, 728
Mucosal atrophy, with malnutrition, 44
Mucosal barrier, gut, 547–550
   bacteriologic barrier, 549–550
      Clostridium difficile colitis, 549–550
   immunologic barrier, 548–549
      local barrier, 548
      systemic barrier, 548–549
   physical barrier function, 547–548
      chemical barrier, 548
      enzymatic barrier, 548
      mechanical barrier, 547–548
Mucosal immune hypothesis, gut, 548–549
Mucous membrane impairment, in immunocompromised patients, 725–726
Multifocal atrial tachycardia, 344–345
   acute therapy, 345
   amiodarone therapy, 345
   calcium channel blockers, 345
   clinical presentation, 344
   etiology of, 344
   ventricular rhythm, 344
Multiple invasive devices, antibiotic resistance, 675
Multiple myeloma, radiocontrast medium-induced acute renal failure, risk factors, 145
Multiple organ failure. *See also* Multiple organ failure syndrome
   defined, 3

Multiple organ failure syndrome, 5–13
  acute lung injury, 7
  autonomic nervous system, 8–13
    activation of, 9
  blood sugar control, 15
  cardiovascular system, 6
  clinical features, 5–8
  clinical progress, 15
  coagulation cascade, 12–13
  corticosteroid administration, 15
  counter inflammatory response, 11–12
  defined, 5–6t
  down-regulation, activated neutrophils, 11
  endotoxin, signaling receptor
    complex for, 10–11
  energy expenditure, increase of, 8
  final common pathway, existence of, 8
  foreign tissue, 10–11
  gut, 548, 550–551
    translocation hypothesis, shock, 15
  hematologic system, 6
  hepatic system, 6
  hypotension, 9
  immune paralysis hypothesis, shock, 15
  inflammatory process, controls on, 10
  jaundice, 7–8
  late organ failure, transition to, 8
  lipopolysaccharide, 10–11
  microbes, 10–11
  neurologic system, 6
  neuropeptides, release of, 9
  number of organ systems in failure,
    survival rates, 6t
  pathophysiology, 8–13
  peripheral tissue inflammation, 9
  PIRO model, 16
  procoagulant, anticoagulant, homeostatic
    balance, 13
  progression of, 5–6
  pro-inflammatory products, transformation
    to anti-inflammatory lipoxins, 9–10
  renal system, 6
  respiratory system, 6
  sepsis, pathogenesis of organ failure in,
    10–13
  shock, pathogenetic networks in, 14
  Shwartzman reaction, 10
  signal amplification, 11
    pro-inflammatory cytokines, 11
  survival, discriminators of, 7t
  systemic inflammatory response
    syndrome, 7
  tissue factor, 12–13
  tissue hypoxia, 15
  toll-like receptors, ligands, 11t
  two-hit hypothesis, shock, 14
Multiple sclerosis
  abdominal pain with, 600
  as cause of respiratory acidosis, 523
  as cause of seizure, 209
Mumps, abdominal pain with, 600
Muscle group testing, in spinal
    cord injury, 247t
Muscular dystrophy, as cause of respiratory
    acidosis, 523
Musculoskeletal injury
  angiography, 76–78
  duplex ultrasonography, 77–78
  initial approach to, 76–78
  plain X-rays, 76–77
  pneumatic anti-shock garment, 76
  in trauma patient, 76–78
Mushroom poisoning
  abdominal pain with, 600
  as cause of fulminant hepatic failure, 608
Myasthenia gravis, 201
  as cause of respiratory acidosis, 523
Myasthenic crisis, as cause of respiratory
    acidosis, 523
Myeloproliferative syndromes, 823
Myocardial contusion in trauma patient, 73
Myocardial infarction, 97, 99t
  abdominal pain with, 600
  alveolar pulmonary edema, 100
  with anaphylaxis, 804
  anatomy of, 367–368
  angioplasty in, 374–375
    indications for, 374–375
  antiplatelet therapy, 371–372
  cardiac risk index, 100
  chronic stable angina, 100
  combination fibrinolytic, 371–372
  complications of, 379–380
    cardiogenic shock, 380
    infarct extension, 379
    mitral regurgitation, 379
    right ventricular infarction, 379–380
    ventricular free wall rupture, 379
    ventricular septal rupture, 379
  coronary stenting, 373–374
    glycoprotein IIb/IIIa antagonists,
      373–374
  defined, 367
  diagnosis of, 368–369

encephalopathy and, 303
glycoprotein IIb/IIIa receptor antagonists, 372
    abciximab, 372
    tirofiban, 372
ischemia, 100
major coronary arteries, distributions of, 368
medical therapy for, 375–378
    angiotensin-converting enzyme inhibitors, 377
    antiarrhythmics, 378
    aspirin, 375
    β-blockers, 377
    calcium antagonists, 378
    heparin, 376
    nitrates, 376–377
    thienopyridines, 375–376
multivariate analysis, 100
pathogenesis, 367–368
percutaneous intervention, 372–375
    vs. thrombolytic therapy, 374t
stepwise logistic regression, 100
surgical risks with, 98–100
thrombolytic therapy, 369–372
    contraindications, 370t
    indications, 370t
    reteplase, 370
    streptokinase, 370
    tenecteplase, 371
    tissue plasminogen activator, 370
venous thromboembolism in, 456
Myocardial ischemia
    with anaphylaxis, 803
    precipitating factors, 323
Myocardial lactate production, transfusion therapy and, 839
Myocarditis, abdominal pain with, 600
Myoclonic seizures, 210–211
Myoclonus
    continuous, 199
    in differential diagnosis of seizure, 212
Myxedema
    as cause of respiratory acidosis, 523
    coma and, 637–638

Nafcillin, with hepatic failure, 748
Nalbuphine, 759–760
Narcotic analgesic therapy, 759–760t
    dosing, 759–760t
Narcotics
    effect on platelet function, 815

    in encephalopathy, 304
    withdrawal, abdominal pain with, 600
Narrow QRS complex, with atrioventricular nodal re-entry, 348
Nasal intubation
    blind, 471–472
    tubes, 49
Nasogastric suction, hypokalemia, 670
Nasogastric tube
    in burn victim, 90
    placement, 256
    in trauma patient, 68
Nasopharyngeal airway, 470
Nasotracheal intubation, 469
    orotracheal intubation, compared, 471t
National Institutes of Health Stroke Scale, 293–296
National Kidney Foundation, clinical practice guidelines, 140–141
Near drowning, 259
    with acute respiratory distress syndrome, 423
Nebulized albuterol, bronchospasm, 435–436
Neck injury, 72
    airway management with, 476
    CT scan, 72
    examination, 69
    flexion-extension radiographs, 72
    initial approach to, 72
    magnetic resonance scanning, 72
    mandatory exploration, 72
    selective exploration, 72
Needle stick, with HIV/AIDS, 706–707. *See also* Acquired immune deficiency syndrome; Human immunodeficiency virus
Negative-pressure ventilation, in mechanical ventilator support, 491–492
Neisseria gonorrhea, in immunocompromised patient, 730
Neisseria meningitidis,
    in immunocompromised patient, 730, 733
Nelfinavir, for HIV, 709
Neoplasms, with HIV/AIDS, 711
Nephrogenic diabetes, 666–667
Nephropathy, in renal failure, 145
Nephrotic syndrome, 823
Nephrotoxic therapy, in renal failure, 140
Neurological dysfunction, in immunocompromised patient, 731–732

Neurological syndromes following spinal cord injury, 251–254
Neurologic disability, prevention of, in trauma patient, 67–68
Neurologic examination
　in coma, interpretation of, 194–195
　in head injury, 229–230
　interpretation of, 194–195
Neuromuscular blocking therapy, 757–758t
　allergic reaction, 801
　bronchospasm, 440
　dosing, 757–758t
Neuropeptide release, in multiple organ failure, 9
Neurotoxins, as cause of respiratory acidosis, 523
Neutropenia
　febrile illness with, 729t
　in immunocompromised patient, 728–730
Neutrophils
　with acute respiratory distress syndrome, 423
　down-regulation, in multiple organ failure, 11
　dysfunction, in immunocompromised patient, 728
Nicardipine, with hypertensive emergencies, 391
Nicotine, as cause of respiratory disorder, 524
Nicotinic acid, as cause of fulminant hepatic failure, 608
Nifedipine, with hypertensive emergencies, 391
Nimodipine, with hypertensive emergencies, 391
Nitrates
　in myocardial infarction, 376–377
　systolic dysfunction, 315
Nitric acid, endothelial cell regulation, 814
Nitric oxide, with acute respiratory distress syndrome, 429
Nitrofurantoin, as cause of fulminant hepatic failure, 608
Nitroglycerin, 773
　dosing, 773
　with hypertensive emergencies, 391
　pharmacodynamics of, 769
　precautions, 773
Nitroprusside, 768–773
　dosing, 768–773
　in hypertensive emergency, 393
　pharmacodynamics of, 769
　systolic dysfunction, 315
NNRTIs. *See* Nonnucleoside reverse transcriptase inhibitors
Non-β lactam antibiotics, allergic reaction, 801
Nonconvulsive status epilepticus, 223–224, 223t
　generalized convulsive status epilepticus, compared, 224
Nonimmune hemolysis, transfusion therapy and, 873
Nonnucleoside reverse transcriptase inhibitors, with HIV/AIDS, 712
Nonobstructive jaundice, 587–589
　cholangitis, 586–589
　hemolysis, 588–589
　hepatocellular dysfunction, 587–588
Nonocclusive mesenteric insufficiency, abdominal pain with, 600
Nonoliguric renal failure, defined, 529
Non-opioid therapy, adverse reactions, 791–795
Nonparoxysmal junctional tachycardia, 346–347
　accelerated junctional rhythm, 346
　acute myocardial infarction, 347
　acute therapy, 347
　atrial pacing, 347
　cannon A waves, 347
　cardiac surgery, 347
　clinical presentation, 347
　digitalis toxicity, 346–347
　esmolol, 347
　etiology of, 346–347
　pulmonary embolization, 347
　sepsis, 347
Nonsteroidal antiinflammatory drugs
　as cause of fulminant hepatic failure, 608
　effect on platelet function, 815
　thrombocytopenia with, 853
Nonstructural pathologies, 191
Non-ST-segment elevation myocardial infarction, 367
Nonsustained ventricular tachycardia, 352–353
Norepinephrine, 119–120, 766
　in cardiac arrest, 119–120
　dosing, 766
　with spinal cord injury, 258
Normoglycemia, 639
NRTIs. *See* Nucleoside reverse transcriptase inhibitors

NSAIDs, 897
   allergic reaction, 801
   radiocontrast medium-induced acute renal failure, risk factors, 145
NSTEMI. *See* Non-ST-segment elevation myocardial infarction
NSVT. *See* Nonsustained ventricular tachycardia
Nucleoside reverse transcriptase inhibitors, with HIV/AIDS, 712–717
Nursing surgical critical care, 175–184
   acute respiratory distress syndrome, patient care, 178
   airway management, 176–178
   certified enterostomal nurses, 178–179
   chronic health evaluation, 175
   cognition impairment, 181
   collaboration in, 175
   comfort of patient, 178
   defined, 176
   delirium management, 180–181
   diarrhea, 180
   dressings, 179
      selection of, 179t
   early ambulation, 176
   electrical stimulation, wounds, 179
   empowerment, 175
   enteral feeding, 180
   explaining procedures, 178
   global cerebral dysfunction, 181
   in intensive care unit care, 176–177
   interdisciplinary approach to quality care, 175
   mechanical ventilation, suctioning of patients on, 177–178
   positioning techniques, 178
   pressure ulcers, 178–180
   repositioning, 176–177
   role of, 176
   therapeutic touch, 178
   topical oxygen for wounds, 179
   ultrasound for wounds, 179
   vacuum-assisted closure of wounds, 179
   ventilator management, 176–178
   warmth therapy, for wounds, 179
   wound management, 178–180
Nutrition. *See also* Nutritional support
   hepatic function and, 131
   in immunocompromised patients, 726
   modification of regimen, conditions requiring, 52–54
   with renal failure, 536

Nutritional assessment, 44–46, 46t
Nutritional support, 43–60, 51t, 55
   caloric requirements, 46–47
   enteral nutrition, 48–51
   following spinal injury, 261–262
   formulations, 48
   gut function and, 552
   immune-enhancing formulas, 48
   initiation of, timing, 51–52
   malnutrition, physiologic effects of, 43–44
   micronutrient requirements, 47–48
   modification of nutrition regimen, 52–54
   monitoring adequacy of, 54–55
   nutritional assessment, 44–46
   parenteral delivery route, 48–51
   parenteral nutrition, 50–51
   preoperative, 55
   protein requirements, 47

Obesity
   airway management with, 477
   as cause of respiratory acidosis, 523
   pulmonary complications of surgery with, 154
Obstructive jaundice, cholangitis, 586–589
   Charcot's triad, 587
   endoscopic retrograde cholangiography, 587
   endoscopic transpapillary sphincterotomy, 587
   percutaneous transhepatic cholangiography, 587
Obstructive lung disease, 981, 984
Obstructive sleep apnea, as cause of respiratory acidosis, 523
Obstructive uropathy, with renal failure, 140
Octreotide
   as cause of fulminant hepatic failure, 608
   in pancreatitis, 578
Oliguric renal failure, 529, 537
On-pump CAB, 303–304
Open, closed peritoneal tap and lavage, 957–958
Open cardiac massage, 115
Open peritoneal tap and lavage, 957–958
Opiates. *See also* specific opiate
   allergic reaction to, 801
Optimum red cell mass, transfusion therapy and, 837
Oral antihypertensive therapy, pharmacodynamics, 771–772t
Oral contraceptives, stroke and, 271

Oral intubation, blind, 471–472
Orchitis, abdominal pain with, 600
Organ dysfunction variables in diagnosis of sepsis, 5
Organ failure. *See* Multiple organ failure syndrome
Orogastric tube, in trauma patient, 68
Oropharyngeal airway, 114, 470
Orotracheal intubation, 114, 469
   nasotracheal intubation, compared, 471t
   in trauma patient, 64
Orotracheal tube, changing of, 477
Orthotopic liver transplant, 621
Osler-Rendu-Weber syndrome, 816
Osmolal gap, 667
Osmolality
   defined, 664
   tonicity, distinction between, 665
Osmolar abnormalities in encephalopathy, 302–303
Osmotic therapy, with cerebral edema, 284
Osteomyelitis, abdominal pain with, 600
Ovarian cyst, abdominal pain with, 600
Over-inflated alveoli, in acute respiratory distress syndrome, 428
Oxacillin, antibiotic resistance, 681
Oxidative phosphorylation, congenital disorders of, 36
Oxygenation
   arterial blood, 490t
      variables affected by, 490t
   in mechanical ventilator support, 489–490
Oxygen consumption, transfusion therapy and, 841–842
Oxygen content of blood, 834–836
Oxygen delivery
   consumption, relationship between, 998–1000
   tissue oxygen demand, gap between, 26
   transfusion therapy and, 838
Oxygen dissociation curves under different conditions, transfusion therapy and, 835
Oxygen supply, demand, components of, 22t
Oxygen transport, 21–32, 551, 577–578, 839, 973
   adequacy of, 24–27
   aerobic glycolysis, 27
   afterload, cardiac output and, 23
   blood flow, 22–24
   cardiac index, 25
   cardiac output, determinants of, 23t

delivery-dependent lactate production, 26–27
delivery-dependent oxygen consumption, 24–25
DVO_2-arterio-venous oxygen content differences, 25
Fick principle, 25
flow-dependent lactate production, 26
flow-dependent oxygen consumption, 25
global extraction, limitation to, 26
hemoglobin
   arterial saturation of, 25
   concentration, 25
inotropic support, 24
   cardiac output, 23–24
lactate-pyruvate ratio, 26
oxygen delivery, tissue oxygen demand, gap between, 26
oxygen supply, demand, 21–22
   components of, 22t
   hemoglobin, target for saturation of, 22
in pancreatitis, 577–578
preload, cardiac output and, 23–24
pulmonary artery catheter, monitoring with, 27–29
pulmonary capillary wedge pressure, cardiac output, 23
restoration of, 27–29, 577–578
shock, defined, 24
systemic vascular resistance, 23
treatment, 27–29
volume loading, unloading in vascular system, relationship, 23
VO_2-oxygen consumption, 25

Pacemaker code, 329–330
Pacemaker syndrome, 329
Pain control. *See also under* specific medication
   at end of life, 169–170
Palpitation, with sustained ventricular tachycardia, 355
Pancreatic secretions, 662
Pancreatitis, 569–582, 601, 1006
   abdominal pain with, 600
   antibiotics, 576–577
   debridement, 575–576
   diagnosis, 571–574
   drainage, 575–576
   etiology of, 569–570
   fine needle aspiration, 574
   with HIV/AIDS, 711

Index

hypocalcemia, association, 648
laboratory data, 573–574
metabolic support, 578–579
   antisecretory, 578–579
   nutritional, 578
nutritional regimen modification with, 53
oxygen transport restoration, 577–578
   cardiovascular support, 577
   pulmonary support, 577–578
   renal support, 578
pathology, 570–571
pathophysiology, 569–571
patient history, 571–573
physical information, 571–573
prognostic indicators, 571t
radiologic data, 574
source control, 575
treatment, 575–579
Pancuronium, 757–758
Panic attacks, in differential diagnosis of seizure, 212
Papillomatosis, airway management with, 476
Paracentesis, 955–956
   complications, 956
   diagnostic tests, 956
   procedure, 955–956
   sites for, 956
Paradoxical breathing, bronchospasm, 434–435
Paraldehyde, anion gap acidosis from, 518
Paralytic ileus, 593
Paraneoplastic syndrome, as cause of seizure, 209
Parasitic infestations, as cause of hemoptysis, 484
Parasomnias, in differential diagnosis of seizure, 212
Paraventricular thalamic nuclei, in head injury, 230
Parenchymatous hemorrhage, 271
Parenteral antihypertensive therapy, pharmacodynamics, 769–770t
Parenteral delivery route, 48–51
Parenteral medications. *See also* specific medication
   in hypertensive emergency, 390t
Parenteral nutrition, 48–51, 578. *See also* Nutritional support
Parenteral steroid preparations, allergic reaction, 801
Parkland formula, burns, 90
Paroxysmal nocturnal hemoglobinuria, 823

Parvovirus B19
   as cause of fulminant hepatic failure, 608
   transfusion therapy and, 875
Pathophysiologic conditions, 185–742
   cardiovascular function, 309–420
   central nervous system function, 187–308
   endocrine system, 629–674
   gastrointestinal function, 547–628
   hepatic function, 547–628
   infectious diseases, 675–742
   pulmonary function, 421–510
   renal function, 185–742
Patient transfer with liver failure, 614–615
PCWP. *See* Pulmonary capillary wedge pressure
PEEP. *See* Positive end-expiratory pressure
Pelvic fractures, 66
Penicillin, 794
   effect on platelet function, 815
Pentamidine, 787
Pentasaccharide, for venous thromboembolism prevention, 825
Pentobarbital, with increased intracranial pressure, 241
Peptic ulcer, 557, 562–563
   Helicobacter pylori in, 562
   prophylaxis, 561–562
   proton pump inhibitors, 562
   surgical treatment, 562–563
Peptide hormones, allergic reaction, 801
Peptococcus, as cause of peritonitis/abscess, 696
Peptostreptococcus, as cause of peritonitis/abscess, 696
Percutaneous central venous catheterization, complications of, 917
Percutaneous tracheostomy, 937–946
   bronchoscope, age of, 940
   bronchospasm, 943
   catheter, placement of, 940
   contraindications, 938
   equipment, 939
   guiding catheter, 940
   indications, 938
   location, 938–939
   method, 939–943
   personnel, 939
   pitfalls of, 943
   positioning, 940
   premature extubation, 943
   safety of, 938

Percutaneous tracheostomy (*Contd.*)
    technique, 938–943
    tracheal stenosis, 943
Perfusion pressure with renal failure, 146
Pericardial tamponade, 67, 74, 318–320
    form of diastolic dysfunction, 319
    pericardial effusions, 319
Pericarditis
    abdominal pain with, 600
    as indication for dialysis, 536
Periorbital ecchymoses, in head injury, 233–234
Peripheral tissue inflammation, in multiple organ failure, 9
Peripheral vascular disease
    radiocontrast medium-induced acute renal failure, risk factors, 145
    surgical risks with, 98
Peritoneal dialysis, lactate acidosis, 39
Peritoneal lavage
    criteria for, 75t
    in trauma patient, 74–75
Peritonitis, 695–700, 700t
    antibiotic therapy, 697t
    bacteria causing, 696
    diagnosis, 695–696
    management, 696–698
    microbiology, 700t
Permanent pacing, 329
Pernicious anemia, abdominal pain with, 600
Peroxidase, gut, 548
Persistent headache, CT scanning, 218
Persistent vegetative state, 202–203
Petechial hemorrhages, in hypertensive emergency, 393
Peyer's patches, gut, 548
Pharmacology, 745–810. *See also under specific drug*
    anaphylaxis, 799–810
    drug dosing, 745–782
    drug interactions, 783–798
Phenobarbital, 223
    serum concentration monitoring, 755
Phentolamine mesylate, with hypertensive emergencies, 391
Phenylephrine, 767
    dosing, 767
Phenytoin, 216–217, 221, 223
    as cause of fulminant hepatic failure, 608
    with epilepsy, 216–217
    with increased intracranial pressure, 242
    serum concentration monitoring, 756

Pheochromocytoma
    with anaphylaxis, 804
    as cause of hypertensive crisis, 386
Philadelphia collar, use of, with spinal cord injury, 254
Phlegmasia alba dolens, 414
Phlegmasia cerulea dolens, 414–415
Phosphorus, 654–656
    with chronic renal failure, 148–149
    hyperphosphatemia, 655–656, 658
    hypophosphatemia, 654–655, 657–658
Physical examination of trauma patient, 69–70
Physician-assisted suicide, 171–172
Pierre Robin syndrome, difficult endotracheal intubation and, 475
Pilomotor erection, with anaphylaxis, 804
Pimozide, 787
Pindolol, with hepatic failure, 748
Piperacillin, antibiotic resistance, 683
PIRO model, in multiple organ failure, 16
Plain X-rays in trauma patient, 76–77
Plasma clotting factors, 818t
Plasma exchange, as liver assist device, 621
Plasma expanders, effect on platelet function, 815
Plasma perfusion, as liver assist device, 621
Plasma transfusion, 846–848
    contraindications, 848
    indications, 847–848
Plasminogen activators, effect on platelet function, 815
Platelet alloimmunization, 855–856
Platelet count increment, calculation of, 851
Platelet function
    defects, transfusion therapy and, 867
    drugs affecting, 815t, 852t
Platelets
    crossmatching, transfusion therapy and, 855
    pheresis, transfusion therapy and, 848, 876
    replacement of, in trauma patient, 66
    role of, 811–812
Platelet transfusion, 848–856
    bone marrow hypoplasia, 850
    invasive procedures, 850–851
    platelet destruction, 851
    platelet selection, 848–849
    refractoriness, 851–855
Plates for femur fractures, 83t
Pleurisy, abdominal pain with, 600
Pleuritic chest pain, with pulmonary embolism, 446

Index

Pneumatic anti-shock garment, for trauma patient, 76
Pneumatic compression devices, use of, with spinal cord injury, 260
Pneumococcal meningitis, 201
Pneumonia
  abdominal pain with, 600
  airway management with, 476
  bronchoscopy with, 906–907
  as cause of hypoxemia, 506
  as cause of respiratory acidosis, 523
  as cause of respiratory disorder, 524
  diagnosis of, 1009
  in immunocompromised patient, 734
Pneumothorax
  abdominal pain with, 600
  with catheter use, 51
  as cause of respiratory acidosis, 523
  as complication of percutaneous central venous catheterization, 917
  as complication of transbronchoscopic procedure, 912
Poikilothermia with spinal injury, 262
Poliomyelitis, as cause of respiratory acidosis, 523
Polymyxin B, antibiotic resistance, 686
Porphyria, abdominal pain with, 600
Portal hypertension, in encephalopathy, 304
Portal-systemic bypass, in encephalopathy, 304
Positive airway pressure mask, use of, with spinal cord injury, 259
Positive end-expiratory pressure, 396–397, 495, 981–983
  in acute respiratory distress syndrome, 426–427
  in mechanical ventilator support, 491
Positive-pressure inspiration, 398–399
Posterior fossa infarctions, 276
Postexposure prophylaxis, HIV/AIDS, 708–710
Posthypocapnic acidosis, 518
Posttransfusion purpura, transfusion therapy and, 874
Posttraumatic seizures, 219–221, 241–242
  diagnosis, 220–221
  epidemiology, defined, 219–220
  risk, 220
  treatment of, 221
Potassium
  depletion, 520
  in hypokalemia, deficit of, 671

Prazosin, with hepatic failure, 748
Prearrest factors in cardiac arrest, 123
  age, effect of, 123
  associated disease, 123
  gender, 123
Preeclampsia/eclampsia, as cause of hypertensive crisis, 386
Pregnancy, 669
  fatty liver of, 608, 826
  transfusion therapy and, 860
  venous thromboembolism with, 456–457
Preload, cardiac, 310–312
  carbon monoxide, relationship, 310
  central venous pressure, 310–312
  compliance, 310
  defined, 310
  Frank-Starling principle, 310–312
  left ventricular pressure-volume loops, 311
  pulmonary artery occlusion pressure, 311
  right atrial pressure, 310
Premature atrial impulse, with atrioventricular nodal re-entry, 347
Premature ventricular contractions, 352–353
  acute, chronic therapy, 352–353
  cannon A waves, 352
  clinical presentation, 352
  etiology of, 352
Prerenal acute renal failure, 527–531
  acute tubular necrosis, 527
    contrasted, 531t
    distinguished, 531
  causes, 527–530
  central pressure, monitoring, 530
  diagnosis, 530–531
  differential diagnosis of, 529t
  glomerular filtration rate, 527
  patient evaluation, 530t
  treatment, 531
Pressure limited ventilation, in mechanical ventilator support, 493
Pressure-support ventilation, 497, 502–503
Pressure ulcers
  nursing care and, 179–180
  prevention of, 178–180
Priapism, with spinal cord injury, 251
Primary generalized seizure, 209
Probucol, 787
Procainamide, 122, 787
  as antiarrhythmic, 337
  in cardiac arrest, 122
  serum concentration monitoring, 755
  with sustained ventricular tachycardia, 357

Procoagulant, anticoagulant, homeostatic balance, 13
Progesterone, as cause of respiratory disorder, 524
Pro-inflammatory products, transformation to anti-inflammatory lipoxins, 9–10
Prone positioning, in acute respiratory distress syndrome, 428
Propafenone, as antiarrhythmic, 337
Prophylactic component therapy, transfusion therapy and, 868
Propofol, 776–779
 bronchospasm, 440
 dosing, 776
 with epilepsy, 216
 precautions, 776
Propranolol, with hepatic failure, 748
Proprioception, with spinal cord injury, 248
Propylene glycol, 35–36
Prostaglandins, with acute respiratory distress syndrome, 429
Prostatitis, abdominal pain with, 600
Protamine sulfate, dosing schedules, 897
Protease inhibitors, with HIV/AIDS, 712–717
Protein analysis, with nutritional support, 55
Protein calorie deficiency, 43
Protein C deficiency, 823
Protein malnutrition, transfusion therapy and, 848
Protein requirements, 47. *See also* Nutrition
Protein S deficiency, 823
Protein serum concentrations, measurement of, 44–46
Proteinuria, 141t
 defined, 141t
Proteus species, as cause of peritonitis/abscess, 696
Prothrombin complex concentrate, warfarin-related bleeding, 896
Prothrombin 20210 G-A polymorphism, 823
Prothrombin time, hepatic function and, 131–132
Proton pump inhibitors, for stress ulcer prophylaxis, 552–553
Pruritus, with anaphylaxis, 803–804
Pseudomonas aeruginosa, 683–684
 antibiotic resistance, 676
 as cause of peritonitis/abscess, 696
 control/prevention, 684
 epidemiology, 683
 in immunocompromised patient, 728
 intra-abdominal infection with, 696

 peritonitis, 700
 tertiary peritonitis, 700
 therapy, 683
Pseudo-obstruction, abdominal pain with, 600
Pseudoseizures, in differential diagnosis of seizure, 212
Psychiatric disorders, 214
Psychological impact of burns, 93
Psychological impact of spinal injury, 263–264
Psychosis, abdominal pain with, 600
Psychotropic drugs, effect on platelet function, 815
Puget Sound Blood Center, algorithm approach, transfusion therapy and, 868–869
Pugh's modification, hepatic function, 131
Pulmonary arterial access, 920–923
 complications of, 921–922
 technique, 920–921
 wedge pressure interpretation, 922–923
Pulmonary artery catheterization
 catheter placement, 104–109, 975
  thermistor-equipped, 975
 catheter removal, 932
 complications of, 922
 monitoring oxygen delivery, 27–29
Pulmonary artery perforation, with pulmonary artery catheterization, 922
Pulmonary artery tracing, blood pressure monitoring, 968
Pulmonary capillary wedge pressure, 108
 oxygen transport, 23
Pulmonary complications with surgery, 151–160
 active respiratory infections, 155
 analgesia, postoperative, 156
 anesthesia, 154–155
 assessment, preoperative, 153–154
 atelectasis, 152
 bronchodilators, with pulmonary complications, 156
 cardiopulmonary exercise testing, preoperative, 153
 cardiopulmonary risk assessment, preoperative, 154
 closing volume, 152
 diaphragmatic dysfunction, 152
 functional residual capacity, 152
 incision, 155
 intraoperative complications, 156
 malnutrition, 154

Index

obesity, 154
perioperative, 151–160
postoperative, incidence of, 151–152
preoperative risks, 155–156
pulmonary disease
   chronic obstructive disease, preoperative, 154
   respiratory infections, preoperative, 154
pulmonary pathophysiology, postoperative, 152–153
radiospirometry, preoperative, 153
respiratory infections, 155
respiratory therapy, 156–157
   postoperative, 154, 156–157
risk factors, 154–155
smoking, 154
   cessation of, 156
spirometry, preoperative, 153
split lung function studies, 153
thoracotomy, 152–153
Pulmonary contusion
   with spinal cord injury, 259
   in trauma patient, 73
   treatment of, 82–83
Pulmonary diffusion abnormality, as cause of respiratory disorder, 524
Pulmonary disease
   chronic obstructive disease, preoperative, 154
   respiratory infections, preoperative, 154
Pulmonary edema
   as cause of respiratory acidosis, 523
   with spinal cord injury, 259
Pulmonary embolectomy, 461
Pulmonary embolism, 434
   abdominal pain with, 600
   with anaphylaxis, 804
   as cause of hypoxemia, 506
   as cause of respiratory acidosis, 523
   as cause of respiratory disorder, 524
   clinical manifestations of, 446t
   in nonparoxysmal junctional tachycardia, 347
   precipitating factors, 323
   scope of problem of, 444
   with spinal injury, 260–261
   test results, 449
   ventilation perfusion lung scan, 451
Pulmonary hemorrhage, 484–486
   angiography/embolization, 485
   balloon tamponade, 485
   bronchoscopy, 485

radionuclear scanning, 485
surgery, 485–486
treatment, 486
Pulmonary hypertension, as cause of hemoptysis, 484
Pulmonary infarction, with pulmonary artery catheterization, 922
Pulmonary infection with spinal cord injury, 260
Pulmonary shunts, as cause of respiratory disorder, 524
Pulmonary vascular resistance, 396–397
Pulseless electrical activity, guidelines for, 117
Pulse oximetry for respiratory monitoring, 989–990
Pulsus paradoxus, bronchospasm, 434
Pupillary light reflexes, in coma, 199
Pupils, in coma, 193
Pure diastolic dysfunction, pure systolic dysfunction, contrasted, 318
PVCs. *See* Premature ventricular contractions
Pyelonephritis, abdominal pain with, 600
Pyogenic abscess, as cause of seizure, 208
Pyruvate, lactate acidosis, 34
Pyruvate carboxylase deficiency, lactate acidosis, 36
Pyruvate dehydrogenase deficiency, lactate acidosis, 36
Pyruvate metabolism
   in lactic acidosis, 34

QRS synchronized DC cardioversion, with atrial flutter, 342–343
QT interval, drugs prolonging, 787t
Quadriplegia, fear of, with spinal cord injury, 263
Quetiapine, 787
Quinidine, 787
   as antiarrhythmic, 337
   with hepatic failure, 748
   serum concentration monitoring, 756
Quinine, thrombocytopenia with, 853
Quinolones, 793
Quinupristin, 794
   antibiotic resistance, 681–683

Raccoon eyes. *See* Periorbital ecchymoses
Radial artery catheterization, 415, 923
   Allen's test, 415
   complications associated with, 415
   Doppler test, 415

Radiation therapy
  airway management with, 476
  for burns, 87
Radioactive filtration markers, urinary clearance, 142
Radiocontrast medium-induced acute renal failure, 144–145, 145t, 532
  prevention of, 146t
  risk factors, 145t
Radiographic contrast therapy
  administration in high-risk patients, 807
  effect on platelet function, 815
Radionuclide cholescintigraphy, 584
Radiospirometry, preoperative, 153
Rales, with pulmonary embolism, 446
Ranitidine, for stress ulcer prophylaxis, 552
Ranson's criteria, pancreatitis, 570–571
Rapid shallow breathing index, 502
RBCs. See Red blood cell transfusion
Recombinant concentrates, transfusion therapy and, 848
Recombinant factor VIIa, transfusion, 848, 863–869
  massive transfusion, 867–868
  red cell transfusions, 868–869
Recombinant tissue plasminogen activator, 281, 460. See also Tissue plasminogen activator
  patient eligibility criteria, 281t
Rectal cancer, lower gastrointestinal hemorrhage with, 563
Rectal diazepam, with epilepsy, 216
Rectal examination, with spinal cord injury, 248
Rectus sheath hematoma, abdominal pain with, 600
Red blood cell transfusion, 833–846
  benefit from, 845
  oxygen delivery, consumption, 834–846
Refeeding alkalosis, 520
Refeeding syndrome, 54, 655
  modification of nutritional regimen with, 54
Refractory tachyarrhythmias, in thyroid dysfunction, 634
Rehabilitation
  after spinal injury, 263–264
  after stroke, 279
Remote symptomatic seizures, 207–209
  causes of, 209t
  treatment, 215
Renal cortical atrophy, with malnutrition, 44

Renal disease. See also Renal failure
  coagulation disorders with, 822
Renal excretion, lactate acidosis, 34–35
Renal failure, 139–150, 527–538. See also Acute renal failure
  abdominal aortic aneurysm surgery, 140
  acute, 139–150, 527–538
  albuminuria, 141t
  anemia, 148
  anesthesia, 147–148
  with anion gap acidosis, 518
  aortic surgery, 147
  assessment of volume status, 143–144
  bleeding disorders, 148
  blood flow, adequacy of, 146
  calcium, 148–149
  cardiopulmonary bypass, 140
  cardiovascular surgery, 146–147
  chronic renal failure, 139, 147–149
  complications of, 534t
  contrast nephropathy, 145
  Counahan-Barratt equation, use with children, 143
  deamino-arginine vasopressin, preoperative administration of, 148
  defined, 529
  development of, 140t
  diabetes mellitus with, 139
  dialysis, 147
  differential diagnosis of, 529t
  drug dosing, 749–752t
  drug-induced, 145–146
  duration of bypass, severity of renal failure, correlation, 146
  electrolytes, assessment of, 144
  evaluation of patient with, 530t
  extracellular fluid, volume status, 144–144t
  factors associated with development of, 140t
  glomerular filtration rate, 140–141
    estimation of, 141–143
  kidney function evaluation, 140–144
  liver disease with, 139
  magnesium, 148–149
  magnesium levels, 148–149
  National Kidney Foundation, clinical practice guidelines, 140–141
  obstructive uropathy with, 140
  patient history, 140
  perfusion pressure, 146
  phosphorus, 148–149
  phosphorus levels, 148–149

Index

physical examination, 140
precipitating conditions, 139–140
proteinuria, 141t
radiocontrast medium-induced, 144–145, 145t
   prevention of, 146t
   risk factors, 145t
r-HuEPO therapy, 148
risk factors, 139–140
Schwartz equation, use with children, 143
sepsis with, 139
serum creatinine
   increased, causes of, 142t
   measurement of, 141–142
severity of disease, 139–140
stages of, 140–141, 141t
surgery, 139–140
underlying medical conditions, 139–140
Renal function support, 539–547
   continuous venovenous hemofiltration, 543
   dialysis, continuous venovenous hemofiltration with, 543
   hemodialysis, 539–543
   renal replacement method, 543–544
Renal infarct, abdominal pain with, 600
Renal insufficiency, effects of, 747
Renal tubular acidosis, 518
Renal tubular cell, 513
Renovascular hypertension, as cause of hypertensive crisis, 386
Repetitive seizures, CT scanning with, 218
Repositioning of patient, by nursing staff, 176–177
Resin perfusion, as liver assist device, 621
Resonance, in blood pressure monitoring, 963–966
Respiration, disruption of muscles of, with spinal cord injury, 259
Respiratory acid–base disorders, 519–524
   respiratory acidosis, 521–522
   respiratory alkalosis, 522–524
Respiratory acidemia, in discontinuation of mechanical ventilation, 508
Respiratory acidosis, 521–522
   causes of, 523
Respiratory alkalosis, 514, 522–524
   causes of, 524
   in septic encephalopathy, 305
Respiratory distress, in bronchospasm, 438
Respiratory distress syndrome, acute. *See* Acute respiratory distress syndrome

Respiratory failure, clinical signs of, in trauma patient, 63
Respiratory infections, 155
   pulmonary complications of surgery with, 155
Respiratory insufficiency
   with malnutrition, 43–44
   modification of nutritional regimen with, 52
Respiratory mechanics, 490–491
Respiratory monitoring, 981–994
   airway resistance, 983
   alveolar gas equation, 987–988
   alveolar oxygen tension, arterial oxygen tension, differences between, 987–988
   auto-PEEP, defined, 983
   auto-PEEP effect, measurement, 983
   Bohr equation, 991
   capnogram, normal, phases of, 992
   capnograph waveforms, examples of, 984
   capnography, 992t
   capnometry, limitations of, 990–991
   dynamic compliance, 985–986
   gas exchange monitoring, 987–989
   gas flow, lung volumes, relation between, 981
   during general anesthesia, 991t
   intrathoracic pressure, cardiorespiratory function, interaction, 986–987
   lung volume monitoring, 984–987
   maximum inspiratory pressure, 984
   obstructive lung disease, 981, 984
   positive end-expiratory pressure, 981–983
   pressure, 981
   respiratory terms, 982t
   restrictive lung disease, 984
   shunt fraction, 987
   square-wave flow pattern, 983
   static lung compliance, 985–986
   tissue oxygen delivery, 26, 36, 227, 610–611, 987
   ventilator spirometers, 964–965
   zero flow requirement, 981
Respiratory therapy, postoperative, 156–157
Response variables, control variables, distinguished, 998–1005
Restrictive lung disease, 984
Resuscitation
   in cardiac arrest, 122–124
   duration of, 123
   hypertransfusion for, 423
Reteplase, with myocardial infarction, 370

Reticular activating system, in head injury, 229–230
Retrograde cholangiopancreatography, pancreatitis and, 569
Retrograde urethrogram, in trauma patient, 76
Retrovir plus lamivudine, for HIV, 709
Reye's syndrome, as cause of fulminant hepatic failure, 608
Rhabdomyolysis, hyperkalemia, 670
Rheumatic fever, abdominal pain with, 600
Rheumatoid arthritis, airway management with, 476
r-HuEPO therapy, with chronic renal failure, 148
Rifampin, with hepatic failure, 748
Right ventricular ejection pressure load, 396
Right ventricular infarction, 379–380
Risperidone, 787
RLD. See Restrictive lung disease
Rocky mountain spotted fever, abdominal pain with, 600
Rocuronium, 757–758
Rotor syndrome, 588
rtPA. See Recombinant tissue plasminogen activator
Rubber nasopharyngeal airway, 114
Rule of double effect, in end of life issues, 170
Rule of nines, 88
  inaccuracy of, with children, 89
Rule of palm, 88
Rules of combination, 1013

Safety features in mechanical ventilation, 496–497
Salicylates
  allergic reaction, 801
  anion gap acidosis from, 518
  as cause of respiratory disorder, 524
  overdose, lactate acidosis, 36
Saliva, composition of, 662
Salmonella, in immunocompromised patient, 730
Salpingitis, abdominal pain with, 600
Sarafloxacin, 787
Sarcoidosis
  airway management with, 476
  as cause of seizure, 209
Scheduled antibiotic changes, antibiotic resistance, 683
Schwartz equation, use with children, 143
Scleroderma, airway management with, 476

Screening laboratory tests, effect on platelet function, 815–816
Sea anemone stings, as cause of fulminant hepatic failure, 608
Seborrheic dermatitis, with HIV/AIDS, 711
Second-degree burns, 87
  deep, 87
  superficial, 87
Sedatives. See also under specific medication
  adverse reactions, 788–790
  comparison, 778t
  dosing, 776–779
  in encephalopathy, 304
  intravenous delivery, 778t
  overdose, as cause of respiratory acidosis, 523
Seizure, 207–228
  absence seizures, 210
  acute symptomatic, 207
  alcohol withdrawal seizures, 215
  with anaphylaxis, 804
  anticoagulation, 218
  antiepileptic drugs, 215–217
    in acute setting, 216
    long-term management, 217
    pharmacologic considerations, 216–217
  causation of, 207–209
  coma with, 189
  complex partial, 211
  convulsive, 209–210
  cryptogenic, 207
  defined, 207–208
  depressed skull fracture, risk factors for, 220
  diazepam, 223
  differential diagnosis, 211–214, 212t, 213–214
  eclamptic, 215
  emergency CT scanning, 218t
  epilepsy, 208
  epilepsy syndromes, 209–210t
  first seizure evaluation, 218–219
    electroencephalogram, 219
    imaging, 218–219
    laboratory evaluation, 218
    patient history, 218
    work-up, 222
  fosphenytoin, 223
  generalized convulsive status epilepticus, 222–223, 223t
    evaluation/management of, 222–223
    nonconvulsive status epilepticus, compared, 224

generalized tonic-clonic, 209–210
global cerebral hypoperfusion, 211–212
grand mal, 209–210
head injury, 219–220
hematomas, 234–237
   delayed traumatic intracerebral
      hematoma, 237
   epidural hematoma, 234–235
   subdural hematoma, 235–236
   traumatic intracerebral hematoma,
      236–237
hyperglycemic, 215
idiopathic, 207, 209
   treatment, 215
intracerebral hematoma, risk factors for, 220
intracranial pressure management, 238–241
with lactate acidosis, 36
localization-related, 209
lorazepam, 223
myoclonic, 210–211
nonconvulsive status epilepticus, 223–224
pathophysiology, 237–238
phenobarbital, 223
phenytoin, 216–217, 221, 223
postictal phase, 210
poststroke, mechanisms of, 285
posttraumatic, 219–221, 241–242
   diagnosis, 220–221
   epidemiology, defined, 219–220
   risk, 220
   treatment, 221
primary generalized, 209
psychiatric disorders, 214
remote symptomatic, 207
   treatment of, 215
simple partial, 211
skull fractures, 231–234
   basilar skull fractures, 233–234
   depressed skull fractures, 233
   linear nondisplaced skull fractures,
      231–232
status epilepticus, 221–224
   epidemiology, defined, 221–222
   generalized convulsive status epilepticus,
      clinical features of, 222
with stroke, 285–286
subdural hematoma, risk
   factors for, 220
symptomatic, 208
   causes of, 208t–209t
   remote, 208–209
   treatment, 215

syncope, 211–212 (*See also* Global
   cerebral hypoperfusion)
tonic phase, 209–210
transient ischemic attacks, 212–214
treatment of, 215
types of, 209–211
valproate, 217, 221, 223
Semi-open peritoneal tap and lavage, 958
Sengstaken-Blakemore tube, protocol
   for use, 560t
Sepsis
   in acute respiratory distress
      syndrome, 422
   catheter-related, 51, 929–930
   defined, 4
   diagnostic criteria, 5t
   in encephalopathy, 299
   increased oxygen delivery,
      consumption in, 999
   in nonparoxysmal junctional
      tachycardia, 347
   pathogenesis of organ failure in, 10–13
   with renal failure, 139–140
Sepsis-induced hypotension, 4
Septal injury in trauma patient, 73
Septicemia, in immunocompromised
   patient, 730
Septic encephalopathy, 305–306
   mental status, 305
   respiratory alkalosis, 305
   tachypnea, 305
Septic shock, 320
   with anaphylaxis, 804
Sequential compression devices, in venous
   thromboembolism, 454
Serum lactate, elevated,
   etiology of, 38–39
Serum sodium concentration, water balance,
   relationship of, 664–665
Settings for mechanical ventilation, 497t
Seventeen-hydroxycorticosteroid
   response, 663
Severe sepsis, defined, 4
Shallow breathing index, 502
Shock
   clinical variables to assess, 1000–1004
   coma with, 189
   defined, 24
   in lactate acidosis, 35–36
   pancreatitis and, 569
   pathogenetic networks in, 14
   as source of cerebral ischemia, 272

Short bowel syndrome
  lactate acidosis, 36
  modification of nutritional
    regimen with, 53–54
Shunt fraction
  in acute respiratory distress syndrome, 425
  in respiratory monitoring, 987
Shunts, with liver failure, 614
Shwartzman reaction, in multiple organ
    failure, 10
SIADH. See Syndrome of inappropriate
    antidiuretic hormone
Sick-euthyroid syndrome, 638
Sickle cell anemia, abdominal pain with, 600
Sick sinus syndrome, 329
Sidestream capnometer, mainstream,
    compared, 993
Silver sulfadiazine, for burns, 90
Simple partial seizures, 211
SIMV. See Synchronized intermittent
    mandatory ventilation
Sinus node dysfunction, 324
Sirolimus, serum concentration
    monitoring, 756
SIRS. See Systemic inflammatory response
    syndrome
Size of burn, Lund and Browder chart, 88–89
Skeletal muscle wasting,
    with malnutrition, 43–44
Skin
  breakdown of, with spinal injury, 262
  burn depth, 88
  dryness, in burns, 93
  hyperpigmentation, in burns, 93
Skull fractures, seizure with, 231–234
  basilar skull fractures, 233–234
  depressed skull fractures, 233
  linear nondisplaced skull
    fractures, 231–232
Sleep
  deprivation, in encephalopathy, 304
  disorders of, in differential diagnosis of
    seizure, 212
Small cell carcinoma
  lactate acidosis, 36–37
  lactic acidosis and, 36
Smoke inhalation, bronchoscopy with, 908
Smoking
  cessation of, pulmonary
    complications and, 156
  pulmonary complications of
    surgery with, 154

stroke and, 270
Snake bite, as cause of respiratory
    acidosis, 523
Snap test, in blood pressure monitoring, 966
Sodium, water balance, relationship, 664–665
Sodium bicarbonate, 120–121
  with cardiac arrest, 120–121
  with hyperkalemia, 535
Solute removal, with hemodialysis, 539–540
Somatosensory evoked potentials,
    in coma, 199
Somatostatin, in pancreatitis, 578
Sorbitol, lactate acidosis, 36
Sotalol, 787
  as antiarrhythmic, 337
  with sustained ventricular tachycardia, 358
Speech, with stroke, 279
Spider bite, abdominal pain with, 600
Spinal cord injury, 245–268
  acute respiratory distress
    syndrome with, 259
  anterior cord syndrome, 254
  anteroposterior cervical spine
    radiograph, 250
  antiplatelet therapy with, 260
  aspiration with, 259
  atelectasis, 259
  autonomic dysreflexia, 261
  bilaterally-locked facets, 251
  bladder distention, cause of, 261
  bowel distention, cause of, 261
  bradycardia with, 257–258
  bronchoscopy, 255
  Brown-Sequard syndrome, 251–254
  C1-C2 complex, 250
  central cord syndrome, 254
  cervical spinal cord anatomy, 248
  clinical assessment, 245–249
  compression fractures, cervical
    vertebrae, 251
  continuously oscillating beds, 260
  cricothyroidotomy, 255
  deep tendon reflexes, 248
  deep venous thrombosis, 260–261
  denial of patient with, 264
  dermatomal diagram, 249
  dynamic flexion/extension views, 249–250
  endotracheal intubation, 260
  family communication in, 264
  fiber-optic laryngoscopy, 255
  Gardner-Wells tongs, use of, 254–255
  gastric atony, 261

gastrointestinal management, 261–262
halo vests, use of, 254–255
hemodynamics, 257–258
hemopneumothorax with, 259
heparin, 260
hydration, 260
hypotension, 257–258
ileus, 261
immobilization of head/neck with, 245–246
incomplete lesions, 253
low molecular weight heparin, 260
medical management, 256–261
monitoring, 256
motor examination, 246
  grading system for, 246
muscle group testing, 247t
muscles of respiration, disruption of, 259
nasogastric tube placement, 256
near drowning, 259
neurological syndromes following, 251–254
neurologic examination with, 245
nitrogen needs, 262
norepinephrine, 258
nutritional support following, 261–262
open mouth odontoid view, 251
pain sensation with, 246
patient history, 245
Philadelphia collar, use of, 254
plain cervical spine films, 250
pneumatic compression devices, use of, 260
poikilothermia, 262
positive airway pressure mask, use of, 259
priapism, 251
prophylactic therapy, duration of, 260
prophylaxis, 261
proprioception, 248
psychological factors, 263–264
pulmonary contusion, 259
pulmonary edema with, 259
pulmonary emboli, 260–261
pulmonary infection, 260
quadriplegia, fear of, 263
radiographic assessment, 249–251
rectal examination, 248
rehabilitation, preparation for, 263–264
respiratory system, 258–260
sensory examination, 246–249
skin breakdown, 262
stabilization of injured spine, 254–256
steroids, 256–257
thoracolumbosacral braces, use of, 254
three-view cervical spine series, 249
urinary tract management, 262–263
Spirometry, preoperative, 153
Splenectomy, in immunocompromised patient, 730
Splenic dysfunction, in immunocompromised patient, 730
Split lung function studies, 153
Spondylitis, as cause of respiratory acidosis, 523
Spontaneous inspiration, 397–398
  trials, in discontinuation of mechanical ventilation, 501
Square-wave
  in blood pressure monitoring, 968–969
  flow pattern in respiratory monitoring, 983
Stabilization of patient, initial approach to, 63–68
Stab wound victim, transfusion therapy and, 865
Staphylococcus aureus
  antibiotic resistance, 676
  in immunocompromised patient, 728
  methicillin-resistant, 681–682
Staphylococcus epidermidis
  in immunocompromised patient, 728
  peritonitis, 700
  transfusion therapy and, 876
Staphylokinase, with myocardial infarction, 371
Starvation, with anion gap acidosis, 518
Static lung compliance, 985–986
  in acute respiratory distress syndrome, 425
Statistical ensembles, 1011–1016
Status epilepticus, 221–224, 286
  CT scanning, 218
  epidemiology, defined, 221–222
  generalized convulsive status epilepticus, clinical features of, 222
  nonconvulsive, 223t
Steal syndromes, 272
STEMI. *See* ST-segment elevation myocardial infarction
Stenting with stroke, 282
Steroids
  with acute respiratory distress syndrome, 429
  with adrenal insufficiency, 630–631
  with cerebral edema, 284
  encephalopathy, 304

Steroids (*Contd.*)
  head injury and, 241
  with spinal cord injury, 256–257
Stomach secretions. *See* Gastrointestinal secretions
Storage pool deficiency, 818
Streptococci
  as cause of peritonitis/abscess, 696
  in immunocompromised patient, 728
Streptococcus pneumoniae, in immunocompromised patient, 730, 733
Streptokinase
  allergic reaction, 801
  with myocardial infarction, 370
  in pulmonary embolism, 460
Stress, in immunocompromised patient, 732
Stress response, 3–20
Stress ulcer prophylaxis, 552–553, 561–562
Stroke, 269–296
  anticoagulation, 282–283
  blood pressure, 279–281
  brainstem syndromes, 276t
  cardiac risk factors, 271
  as cause of seizure, 208–209
  cerebral edema
    barbiturate coma, 285
    hypertonic saline, 285
    hyperventilation, 284
    management of, 284–285
    osmotic therapy, 284
    steroids, 284
  diabetes, 270
  diagnosis, 274–278
    posterior fossa infarctions, 276
    watershed infarcts, 276
  epidemiology, 269–271
  etiology of, 271t
  hypertension, 270
  infratentorial infarcts, surgery, 287
  intensive care therapy, 278–279
    cardiac, 278
    electrolytes/laboratory examination, 279
    fever, 278–279
    hemodynamic optimization, 279
    nutrition/speech, 279
    pulmonary, 278
    rehabilitation, 279
  lacunar infarction, 275
  lacunar syndromes, 275t
  major vessel thrombosis, 275
  medical therapy, 278–286
  modifiable risk factors, 270

National Institutes of Health scale, 293–296
neurointerventional therapy, 282
  angioplasty, 282
  intra-arterial thrombolysis, 282
  stenting, 282
neuroprotection, 281
oral contraceptives, 271
pathophysiology, 271–274
  cerebral autoregulation, 273–274
  cerebral blood flow, 273
  cerebral ischemia, 272–273, 272t
  etiologies of, 271t
radiological/laboratory diagnosis, 277–278
rtPA, patient eligibility criteria, 281t
seizure prophylaxis, 285–286
smoking, 270
supratentorial infarcts, surgery, 287
surgical management, 287
systemic thrombolytic therapy, 281–282
tissue plasminogen activator, patient eligibility criteria, 281t
unmodifiable risk factors, 270
venous thromboembolism, 456
Structural pathologies, 191
ST-segment elevation myocardial infarction, 367
  associated with fibrin-rich clot, 368
  fibrinolytic, antiplatelet therapy, combination, 371–372
Stunned myocardium, 367
Subarachnoid hemorrhage, 271
  as cause of hypertensive crisis, 386
  as cause of seizure, 208
  coma with, 189
  prognosis, 200
Subclavian artery pseudoaneurysm, as complication of percutaneous central venous catheterization, 917
Subclavian vein catheterization, contraindications to, 916
Subcutaneous β-agonists, in bronchospasm, 436–437
Subdural hematoma, 235–236
  as cause of seizure, 208
  risk factors for, 220
  seizure with, 235–236
Substituted judgment, principle of, 163
Substrate intolerance, with nutritional support, 54
Sucking chest wound in trauma patient, 72–73

Index

Sucralfate
    gastrointestinal hemorrhage, 561
    for stress ulcer prophylaxis, 552
Suction catheter, changing tracheostomy tube over, 483
Suctioning of patients on mechanical ventilation, 177–178
Sudden cardiac death, 367
Sugar alcohols, lactate acidosis, 36
Suicide, physician-assisted, 171–172
Sulbactam, antibiotic resistance, 686
Sulfamethoxazole
    as cause of fulminant hepatic failure, 608
    in immunocompromised patient, 735
Sulfamylon, with metabolic acidosis, 518
Sulfasalazine, as cause of fulminant hepatic failure, 608
Sulfur toxicity, with metabolic acidosis, 518
Superior vena cava, perforation of, with catheter use, 51
Supratentorial hemorrhages, coma with, 189
Supratentorial infarcts, surgery, 287
Supratentorial mass lesion, with transtentorial herniation, 194
Supraventricular tachycardia, with pulmonary embolism, 446
Surfactant therapy, with acute respiratory distress syndrome, 429
Survival, discriminators of, defined, 4
Sustained ventricular tachycardia.
    See Ventricular tachycardia
Sustiva, for HIV, 709
Sympatholytic antihypertensive therapy, with bradyarrhythmias, 324
Symptomatic seizures, 208
    treatment, 215
Synchronized intermittent mandatory ventilation, 494
    in discontinuation of mechanical ventilation, 502–503
Syncope, 211–212. *See also* Global cerebral hypoperfusion
    with atrioventricular nodal re-entry, 348
    in differential diagnosis of seizure, 212
Syndrome of inappropriate antidiuretic hormone, 668
Synthetic oxygen carrying solution, Fluosol DA, transfusion therapy and, 840
Systemic arterial catheterization, 923–925
    complications, 924–925
    technique, 924
Systemic inflammatory response syndrome, 7
    defined, 4
    pancreatitis and, 577
Systemic lupus erythematosis, as cause of seizure, 209
Systemic vascular resistance, 23
Systolic dysfunction, 314–317
    diastolic dysfunction, distinguished, 317–318
    treatment of, 317t
Systolic pressure variation, 402–403

Tabes dorsalis, abdominal pain with, 600
Tachyarrhythmias, 330–347
    antiarrhythmic therapy classification, 335t
    atrial fibrillation, 330–340
        antiarrhythmic drugs, 337t
        anticoagulation, 339
        β-blocker therapy, 332
        chronic therapy, 336–339
        classification of antiarrhythmic therapy, 335t
        clinical presentation, 332–334
        elective cardioversion, 340
        etiology of, 330–331
        treatment, 334–336
    atrial flutter, 340–344
        acute therapy, 342–343
        chronic therapy, 343–344
        clinical presentation, 340–342
        etiology of, 340
    multifocal atrial tachycardia, 344–345
        acute therapy, 345
        clinical presentation, 344
        etiology of, 344
    nonparoxysmal junctional tachycardia, 346–347
        acute therapy, 347
        clinical presentation, 347
        etiology of, 346–347
    primary atrial tachycardias, 345–346
        acute therapy, 345–346
        chronic therapy, 345–346
        clinical presentation, 345
        etiology of, 345
Tachycardia
    with anaphylaxis, 803
    with atrial fibrillation, 331
    in hypertensive emergency, 392
    mechanical ventilator support and, 489
    multifocal atrial, 344–345
        acute therapy, 345

Tachycardia (*Contd.*)
    clinical presentation, 344
    etiology of, 344
    nonparoxysmal junctional, 346–347
        acute therapy, 347
        clinical presentation, 347
        etiology of, 346–347
    pancreatitis, differential diagnosis, 573
    primary atrial, 345–346
        acute therapy, 345–346
        chronic therapy, 345–346
        clinical presentation, 345
        etiology of, 345
    with pulmonary embolism, 446
Tachycardia-bradycardia syndrome, 324
Tachypnea
    mechanical ventilator support and, 489
    pancreatitis, differential diagnosis, 573
    with pulmonary embolism, 446
    in septic encephalopathy, 305
Tacrolimus, serum concentration monitoring, 756
Talk and deteriorate syndrome, 189. *See also* Coma
Tamponade, pericardial, 74
Tapered support, in discontinuation of mechanical ventilation, 502–503
Telangiectasia, hemorrhagic, hereditary, 816
Temporary pacing, 328–329
Temporomandibular joint syndrome, airway management with, 476
Tenecteplase, with myocardial infarction, 371
Tension hemothorax, 67
Tension pneumothorax, 67, 440
Terbutaline, in bronchospasm, 436–437
Tetanus, airway management with, 476
Tetracycline, as cause of fulminant hepatic failure, 608
Thalamic hemorrhage, coma with, 189
Thallium imaging, 103
Theophylline, serum concentration monitoring, 756
Therapeutic plasma exchange, transfusion therapy and, 848
Therapeutic touch, use of by nursing staff, 178
Thermal burns, 87
Thermal physics, entropy in, similarity of ratios, 1014
Thermistor-equipped pulmonary artery catheter placement, 975
Thermodilution, 973–974

Thiamine deficiency
    in encephalopathy, 303
    lactate acidosis and, 36
Thienopyridines, in myocardial infarction, 375–376
Thioridazine, 787
Third-degree burns, 87
Third-generation cephalosporin resistance, 676
Thoracentesis, 950–951
    complications, 951
    fluid analysis, 951
    procedure, 950–951
    seated position for, 950
Thoracic aortic aneurysm, as cause of hemoptysis, 484
Thoracic duct injury, as complication of percutaneous central venous catheterization, 917
Thoracic electrical impedance, 977
Thoracic pump therapy, 115
Thoracolumbosacral braces, use of, with spinal cord injury, 254
Thoracostomy, 951–955
    abdominal visceral injury, 953
    bleeding, 953
    collection system, mechanical problems, 953
    complications, 953
    drainage systems, 954–955
        three-bottle system, 954–955
    infection, 953
    lung injury, 953
    malpositioning of tube, 953
    procedure, 951–953
    reexpansion pulmonary edema, 953
Threatened abortion, abdominal pain with, 600
Three-position ICHD code, 329t
Thrombin inhibitor, for venous thromboembolism prevention, 825
Thrombocytopenia
    drugs implicated, 853t
    heparin-associated, 828–829, 829t
    transfusion therapy and, 866–867
Thromboembolism
    arterial, 142–143 (*See also* Arterial thromboembolism)
    venous, 443–468, 823, 917 (*See also* Venous thromboembolism)
Thrombolytic therapy
    with myocardial infarction, 370–371
    lanoteplase, 371

Index

reteplase, 370
staphylokinase, 371
streptokinase, 370
tenecteplase, 371
tissue plasminogen activator, 370
risk of bleeding complications, 283
with stroke, 281–282
Thrombomodulin, endothelial cell regulation, 814
Thrombophlebitis, with pulmonary embolism, 446
Thrombosis
catheter-related, 934
causes of, 600
major vessel, 275
Thrombotic diatheses, pathophysiology of, 814
Thrombotic dysfunction, 822–826
Thrombotic thrombocytopenic purpura, transfusion therapy and, 847–848
Thromboxane synthesis, drugs inhibiting, 852
Thyroid dysfunction, 634–638, 642
abdominal pain with, 600
management of, 635t
myxedema coma, 637–638
sick-euthyroid syndrome, 638
thyroid storm, 634–636
Thyroid function tests, in coma evaluation, 195
Thyroid hormone
as cause of respiratory disorder, 524
replacement therapy, 638
Thyroid storm, 634–636
Thyromegaly, airway management with, 477
TIA. *See* Transient ischemic attack
Ticarcillin, antibiotic resistance, 683
Ticlopidine, in myocardial infarction, 375
Tics, in differential diagnosis of seizure, 212
Tidal volume, in mechanical ventilation, 495–496
Tirofiban, in myocardial infarction, 372
Tissue factors
endothelial cell regulation, 814
in multiple organ failure, 12–13
Tissue hypoxia, 35, 609–611
in lactic acidosis, 35
with liver failure, 609–611
in multiple organ failure, 15
Tissue oxygen delivery
in respiratory monitoring, 26, 36, 227, 610–611, 987

Tissue oxygen demand, oxygen delivery, gap between, 26
Tissue perfusion variables in diagnosis of sepsis, 5
Tissue plasminogen activator, 814
endothelial cell regulation, 814
with liver failure, 814
with myocardial infarction, 370
with stroke, patient eligibility criteria, 281t
TNF. *See* Tumor necrosis factor
Tobacco use, in immunocompromised patient, 732
Tobin and Yang, rapid shallow breathing index, 502
Tobramycin, 756
antibiotic resistance, 684
serum concentration monitoring, 756
Toll-like receptors, in multiple organ failure, 11t
Tongue, in airway obstruction, 113
Tonicity, osmolality, distinction between, 665
Topical antibiotics in burns, 90
Topical oxygen for wounds, 179
Topiramate, with epilepsy, 217
Torsades de pointes, with sustained ventricular tachycardia, 356
Total body surface area burn, 87
Toxic inhalation, with acute respiratory distress syndrome, 423
Toxoplasmosis, in immunocompromised patient, 734
t-PA. *See* Tissue plasminogen activator
T-piece, in discontinuation of mechanical ventilation, 502, 504
Tracheal gas insufflation, 428
Tracheal perforation, as complication of percutaneous central venous catheterization, 917
Tracheal stimulation, limiting duration of, 324
Tracheobronchial disruption, suspected, bronchoscopy with, 908
Tracheostomy, 479–484
accidental decannulation with, 481
bronchoscope, age of, 940
bronchospasm, 943
catheter, placement of, 940
complications of, 480
contraindications, 938
equipment, 939
guiding catheter, 940
indications, 938
location, 938–939

Tracheostomy (Contd.)
  method, 939–943
  percutaneous, 937–946
  personnel, 939
  pitfalls of, 943
  positioning, 940
  premature extubation, 943
  safety of, 938
  technique, 938–943
  tracheal stenosis, 943
  in trauma patient, 64
Tracheostomy tube, 469
  changing, 482–484
    over suction catheter, 483
    indications for tube change, 482
    procedure, 482–484
Tranquilizer overdose, as cause of respiratory acidosis, 523
Transbronchoscopic procedures, complications of, 912t
Transcranial Doppler, in coma, 202
Transcutaneous feeding tubes, 49
Transesophageal echocardiography
  with atrial fibrillation, 340
  with atrial flutter, 344
  in trauma patient, 73
Transfusion in Critical Care trial, red cell transfusion, 843–845
Transfusion therapy, 833–894
  contraindications to, 856
  cryoprecipitate transfusion, 856–857
    indications, 856–857
  graft-vs-host disease, transfusion-associated, 869–872
    γ irradiation guidelines, 871–872
    implicated blood components, 871
    prevention, 871
  HLA-matched platelets, matching for, 854t
  infectious risks, 833–894
    bacteria, 876–877
    west Nile virus, 875
  leukoreduced blood components, 857–863
    cytomegalovirus, 859–861
    febrile nonhemolytic transfusion reactions, 857–859
    immunomodulation, 861–863
  noninfectious risks, 872–874
    acute, 872–873
    delayed, 874
  plasma transfusion, 846–848
    contraindications, 848
    indications, 847–848
  platelets, 848–856
    alloimmunization, 855–856
    function, drugs affecting, 852t
    refractoriness, 851–855
    response to, 853t
    selection, 848–849
  prophylactic platelet transfusion, 849–851
    bone marrow hypoplasia, 850
    invasive procedures, 850–851
    platelet destruction, 851
  recombinant factor VIIa, 863–869
    massive transfusion, 867–868
    red cell transfusions, 868–869
  red blood cell transfusion, 833–846
    oxygen delivery, consumption, 834–846
  thrombocytopenia, drugs implicated, 853t
Transient global amnesia, in differential diagnosis of seizure, 212
Transient ischemic attack, 212–214
  in differential diagnosis of seizure, 212
Transjugular intrahepatic shunts, with liver failure, 614
Translaryngeal intubation, 480
Transmural left ventricular ejection pressure, defined, 398
Transtentorial herniation, 71
  with supratentorial mass lesion, 194
Transvenous pacemaker, as contraindication to subclavian vein catheterization, 916
TRAP. See Trial to Reduce Alloimmunization to Platelets
Trauma, 63–96
  abdominal injuries, 74–76
  airway, 63–64
  blunt multiple trauma, fractures in, 81–86
  breathing, 64–65
  burns, 87–93
  as cause of hemoptysis, 484
  as cause of respiratory acidosis, 523
  as cause of respiratory disorder, 524
  as cause of seizure, 208
  chest injuries, 72–73
  circulation, 65–67
  coma with, 189–190
    differential diagnosis, 189–190
    prognosis, 200
  disability, 67–68
  electrical injury, 93–94
  emergency department thoracotomy, 74
  evaluation of, 68–69
  frostbite, 94–95
  genito-urinary injuries, 76

head injury, 71–72
hypothermia, 94–95
initial approach, 63–80
intracerebral hematoma, 236–237
  seizure with, 236–237
management, initial, 63–68
musculoskeletal injuries, 76–78
neck injury, 72
physical examination, 69–70
  abdomen, 69–70
  chest, 69
  extremities, 70
  head, 69
  neck, 69
stabilization, 63–68
treatment, initial, 68–69
venous thromboembolism with, 456
ventilation, 64–65
Treacher Collins syndrome
  difficult intubation with, 475
Tremor, with stroke, 276
Trendelenburg position, vascular
  access and, 916, 918
Trial to Reduce Alloimmunization
  to Platelets, transfusion
  therapy and, 855–856
TRICC. *See* Transfusion in Critical Care
Tricyclics
  as cause of fulminant hepatic
    failure, 608
  effect on platelet function, 815
Trigger sensitivity, in mechanical
  ventilation, 496
Trimethoprim
  as cause of fulminant hepatic failure, 608
  in immunocompromised patient, 735
Troponin I elevation, elevation of, 369
Trousseau's sign, 649
Trypanosoma cruzi, transfusion
  therapy and, 875
Tuberculosis, as cause of hemoptysis, 484
Tuberous sclerosis, as cause
  of seizure, 209
Tumor necrosis factor
  with acute respiratory distress
    syndrome, 423
  in hepatic failure, 609
  in peritoneal response to
    infection, 694
Turner's syndrome, difficult
  intubation with, 475
Two-hit hypothesis of shock, 14

Ulcer
  peptic, 557, 562–563
    prophylaxis, 561–562
  stress, prophylaxis, 552–553
Ultrasound examination
  of abdomen, 74–76, 586
  of cardiac output, 977
  duplex, 77–78
  of hepatic function, 135
  of musculoskeletal injury, 77–78
  of trauma patient, 74–76
  of venous thromboembolism, 448–449
  of wounds, 179
Ultra-violet B irradiation, transfusion
  therapy and, 855–856
Uncal herniation, 230–231
  lateralizing signs in, 232
Undrained foci of infection,
  consequence of, 700
Unfractionated heparin, 897–899
  in pulmonary embolism, 457
  for venous thromboembolism
    prevention, 825
Unstable angina pectoris, 367
Upper airway obstruction, 434
  with anaphylaxis, 805
Upper airway tumors, airway management
  with, 476
Upper extremity ischemia, 413
  arterial thromboembolism, 413
  arterial thrombosis, 413
  clinical presentation, 413
  differential diagnosis, 413
  medical, surgical treatment, 413
  vasospasm or non-occlusive ischemia, 413
Upper gastrointestinal
  hemorrhage, 557–559
  duodenal ulcers, 557
  endoscopy, 557–559
  esophageal varices, 557
  gastric ulcer, 557
  stigmata of recent hemorrhage, 558–559
  treatment of, 558
Uremia
  as indication for dialysis, 536
  platelet dysfunction with, 857
Uremic bleeding, as indication for dialysis,
  536
Uremic encephalopathy, 306
  aluminum neurotoxicity, 306
  asterixis, 306
  dialysis disequilibrium syndrome, 306

Ureteral diversions, with metabolic
    acidosis, 518
Ureterosigmoidostomy, with metabolic
    acidosis, 518
Urinalysis, in trauma patient, 68
Urinary catheters
  in immunocompromised patients, 739
  indwelling, 739
Urinary tract management with
    spinal injury, 262–263
Urine output, increase by diuretic use, 543
Urine toxicology screen, in coma
    evaluation, 195
Urokinase, in pulmonary embolism, 460
Urolithiasis, abdominal pain with, 600
Uropathy
  obstructive, renal failure and, 140
  renal failure with, 140
Urticaria, with anaphylaxis, 803–804
UVB. *See* Ultra-violet B

Vacuum-assisted closure of wounds, 179
Valproate, 216–217, 221, 223
Valproic acid
  as cause of fulminant hepatic failure, 608
  serum concentration monitoring, 756
Valsalva maneuver, with atrioventricular
    nodal re-entry, 349
Valvular heart disease, 314–317, 328
  with atrial fibrillation, 330
  surgical risks with, 98
Valvular injury
  with pulmonary artery catheterization, 922
  in trauma patient, 73
VanA phenotype, antibiotic resistance, 682
VanB phenotype, antibiotic resistance, 682
Vancomycin resistance, 676, 681–683
    control/prevention, 683
    epidemiology, 682
    therapy, 682–683
Van der Pol's oscillator, 1007–1008
Varicella, as cause of fulminant hepatic
    failure, 608
Vascular access, 915–928
    axillary artery, 924
    brachial artery, 924
    central venous access, 915–920
      complications of catheterization, 917
      femoral vein cannulation, 919–920
      indications for catheterization, 915–916
      internal jugular approach, 918–919
      subclavian vein catheterization, 916–917

Doppler-guided catheterization, 925
    dorsalis pedis artery, 923–924
    femoral artery, 924
    internal jugular vein catheterization,
      contraindications to, 918
    pulmonary arterial access, 920–923
      complications, 921–922
      complications of, 922
      technique, 920–921
      wedge pressure interpretation, 922–923
    subclavian vein catheterization,
      contraindications to, 916
    systemic arterial catheterization, 923–925
      complications, 924–925
      technique, 924
Vascular catheters, in immunocompromised
    patients, 739
Vascular complication management, 392–393
Vascular disease
  coma, differential diagnosis, 188–189
  prognosis, 200
  in renal failure, 140
Vascular ectasias, lower gastrointestinal
    hemorrhage with, 563
Vascular emergencies, 411–420
  arterial insufficiency, 411–413
    arterial thromboembolism, 412–413
    arterial thrombosis, 412–413
    clinical presentation, 411–413
    differential diagnosis, 412–413
    lower extremity, 411–413
    medical, surgical treatment, 412–413
    non-occlusive ischemia, 412
    upper extremity, 413
    vasospasm or non-occlusive
      ischemia, 413
  carotid endarterectomy, 416–417
    cervical hematoma, 417
    hyperperfusion syndrome, 417
    hypotension/hypertension, 417
  invasive monitoring, complications
      with, 415–416
    access complications, 416
    axillary artery catheterization, 415
    brachial artery complications, 415
    radial artery catheterization, 415
  mesenteric ischemia, 414
    clinical presentation, 414
    differential diagnosis, 414
    medical, surgical management, 414
  phlegmasia cerulea dolens, 414–415
  vascular procedure complications, 416

Index

aortic procedures, 416
   perioperative bleeding, 416
   colon ischemia following abdominal aneurysm repair, 416
   lower extremity ischemia following aortic procedures, 416
   venous gangrene, 414–415
Vascular endothelium, role of, 813–814
Vasculitis
   as cause of hemoptysis, 484
   as cause of seizure, 209
   complications of, 272
Vasoactive therapy
   adverse reactions, 787–788
   cardiac, vascular effects, 761–763t
   dosing, 754–767
Vasoconstrictor therapy, 560
Vasopressin, 119, 766–767
   in cardiac arrest, 119
   dosing, 766–767
   precautions, 767
Vasopressors, 66, 766–767
   dosing, 766–767
Vasospasm
   cerebral ischemia with, 280
   as source of cerebral ischemia, 272
Vasovagal syncope, with anaphylaxis, 804
Vecuronium, 757–758
   with increased intracranial pressure, 241
Vegetative state, 202–203
Vena cava interruption, in venous thromboembolism, 454
Venlafaxine, 787
Veno-arterial extracorporeal membrane oxygenation, 429
Venous gangrene, 414–415
Venous thromboembolism, 443–468, 823. *See also* pulmonary embolism
   anticoagulation, 457–460
      new therapy, 459–460
   clinical manifestations, 446t
   D-dimer assay, 449
   diagnosis, 445–450
   diagnostic test combinations, 449–450
   general surgery, 455
      higher-risk patients, 455
      low-risk patients, 455
      moderate-risk patients, 455
      very high-risk patients, 455
   graduated compression stockings, 454
   gynecologic surgery, 455
   helical computed tomography, 448
   incidence, 443
   ischemic stroke, 456
   low-dose heparin, 452–453
   low-molecular-weight heparin, 453
   medical conditions, 456
   myocardial infarction, 456
   neurosurgery, 456
   oral anticoagulants, 453
   orthopedic surgery, 455
      elective hip replacement, 455
      elective knee replacement, 455
      hip fracture surgery, 455
   pregnancy, 456–457
   prevention regimens, 825t
   prophylaxis, 450–457
   pulmonary angiography, 447
   pulmonary embolectomy, 461
   regimens to prevent, 825t
   risk factors, 443–445
   sequential compression devices, 454
   spinal cord injury, 456
   with spinal injury, 260–261
   thrombolytic therapy, 460–461
   trauma, 456
   treatment of, 457–461
   ultrasonographic examination, 448–449
   urologic surgery, 455
   vena cava interruption, 454
   V/Q scanning, 447–448
Veno-venous low frequency positive pressure ventilation, 429
Ventilation, 64–65, 114, 1012, 1015–1016. *See also* Breathing; Ventilator
   airway management in, 65t
   airway pressure release ventilation, 497
   American College of Chest Physicians, definition of weaning, 501
   approaches to, weaning criteria, 502
   arterial blood, 490t
      gas determination, 503
      variables affected by, 490t
   assist-control ventilation, 493–494
   in bronchospasm, 438–440
   in cardiac arrest, 114
   as cause of respiratory disorder, 524
   control mode ventilation, 493
   current recommendations, 505
   decreased inspiratory muscle strength, 508
   detrimental effects of, minimizing, 400t
   duration of, 504
   effect on cardiac function, 396t
   gas exchange, 489–490

Ventilation (*Contd.*)
   hemodynamic effects of, 397t
   hemodynamic stability, 503
   high-frequency ventilation, 497–498
   hypoxemia, causes of, 506t
   increased dead space ventilation, 506
   initial approach, 64–65
   initial settings, 497t
   inspired gas, oxygen concentration in, 495
   intermittent mandatory ventilation, 494
   intracranial pressure reduction, 64–65
   mechanical, 427–428, 489–500
   modes of ventilation, 491–498
   mouth-to-mask, 114
   mouth-to-mouth, 114
   oxygenation, 503
   oxygenation failure, 506
   positive end-expiratory pressure, 495
   pressure-support ventilation, 497, 502–503
   protocol weaning, 503–504
      criteria for, 504t
   rapid shallow breathing index, 502
   resolution of original indication of, 503
   respiratory mechanics, 490–491
   respiratory rate, 495
   safety features, 496–497
   spontaneous breathing trials, 501, 504–505
   suctioning of patients on, 177–178
   synchronized intermittent mandatory ventilation, 502–503
   tapered support, 502–503
   tidal volume, 495–496
   T-piece
      in discontinuation, 502, 504
   trigger sensitivity, 496
   uncompensated respiratory acidemia, 508
   ventilator flow patterns, 496
   ventilatory failure, 506–508
      algorithm for investigating, 507
   weaning failure, 505–508
   weaning from, 170–171, 501–510
      approaches to, 502–505
      criteria for, 502–503t
Ventilation-perfusion abnormalities, as cause of respiratory disorder, 524
Ventilation-perfusion lung scan, in pulmonary embolism, 451
Ventilator
   in acute lung injury, 428–429
   in acute respiratory distress syndrome, complications, 427
   flow patterns, in mechanical ventilation, 496
   management of, 910
   by nursing staff, 176–178
   optimization of support, 1011–1017
   withdrawal, 170–171, 501–510
Ventilator spirometer, 964–965
Ventricular arrhythmias, 352–358
   nonsustained ventricular tachycardia, 352–353
   premature ventricular contractions, 352–353
   sustained ventricular tachycardia, 353–358
   ventricular fibrillation, 353–358
Ventricular dilation, with sepsis, 320
Ventricular dysfunction, 108
   in hypertensive emergency, 392
   in thyroid dysfunction, 634
Ventricular ectopy, postoperative ischemic event risk, 103
Ventricular ejection pressure load, 396
Ventricular fibrillation, 353–358
Ventricular free wall rupture, 379
Ventricular hypertrophy, 317
Ventricular infarction, 379–380
Ventricular interdependence, 399
Ventricular septal rupture, 379
Ventricular tachycardia, 119, 353–358
   abnormal QRS morphology, 355
   with abnormal QRS morphology, 355
   acute therapy, 356–357
   American Heart Association Advanced Cardiac Life Support, guidelines, 357
   amiodarone, 357
   angina, 355
   angiography, 357
   chronic therapy, 357–358
   clinical presentation, 355–356
   digitalis-associated, 356, 358
   dizziness, 355
   implantable cardioverter-defibrillator, 357
   lidocaine, 357
   long QT associated, therapy for, 358
   palpitation, 355
   procainamide, 357
   severity of underlying coronary disease, 357
   sotalol, 358
   symptoms of heart failure, 355
   synchronized DC cardioversion, 356
   torsades de pointes, 356
   twelve-lead ECG, 354
   weakness, 355
   wide QRS complex tachycardia, 355–356

Index

Ventriculostomy catheter,
  placement of, 240
Vertebral artery pseudoaneurysm,
  as complication of percutaneous
  central venous catheterization, 917
Vertebral ligaments, lumbar
  puncture and, 948
Vertigo, with stroke, 276
Vicodin, as cause of fulminant
  hepatic failure, 608
Videx, for HIV, 709
Viracept, for HIV, 709
Viral cirrhosis, 605
Viral hepatitis, 588. *See also* Hepatitis
  hepatic failure, 607
Visceral protein analysis
  measurements, 44–46
  with nutritional support, 55
Vital signs, in coma, 192
Vitamin K
  antagonist, for venous thromboembolism
    prevention, 825
  deficiency of, 821–822
  intravenous delivery, 801
  nonbleeding patient, 895–896
  transfusion therapy and, 847
  warfarin, differences in
    half-lives, 895–897
Vocal cord paralysis, as cause of respiratory
  acidosis, 523
Volume depletion, in renal failure, 140
  radiocontrast medium-induced, 145
Volume limited ventilation, in mechanical
  ventilator support, 492
Volume loading in vascular system,
  unloading, relationship
  between, 23
Von Willebrand disease, 814, 816–818
  transfusion therapy and, 847–848
Von Willebrand factor, endothelial cell
  regulation, 814
Voriconazole, 794

Wallenberg syndrome, 276
Warfarin, 895–897
  as antiarrhythmic, 337
  with atrial fibrillation, 339–340
  drug interactions, 795
  overdose, 895–897
  in pulmonary embolism, 453, 458–459
  vitamin K, differences in half-lives,
    895–897

Warmth therapy, for wounds, 179
Water balance, serum sodium
  concentration, relationship of,
  664–665
Watershed infarcts, 276
Weaning from mechanical ventilation
  American College of Chest Physicians
    definition, 501
  criteria, 502–503t
  failure of, 505–508
  protocol, 503–504
    criteria for, 504t
  T-piece, 502, 504
Weber syndrome, 276
West Nile virus, with transfusions, 875
Wheezing
  with anaphylaxis, 803
  in bronchospasm, 434
  differential diagnosis, 434
Wide complex tachycardia
  with atrial fibrillation, 332
  with sustained ventricular tachycardia,
    355–356
Wilson's disease, 614
  as cause of fulminant hepatic
    failure, 608
Winter's formula, metabolic acidosis, 517
Wiskott-Aldrich syndrome, 816, 818
Withdrawal of life-sustaining
    treatment, 170–171
  food/fluids, forgoing, 171
  ventilator withdrawal, 170–171
  withdrawal of dialysis, 171
  withdrawal of other treatments, 171
Wolff-Parkinson-White Syndrome, 335,
  349–352
World Health Organization Analgesic
  Ladder, 169
Wound dressings, 179–179t
Wound healing, with HIV
  infection, 717–718
Wound management by nursing
  staff, 178–180

Xanthines, as cause of respiratory
  disorder, 524
Ximelagatran, in pulmonary
  embolism, 460
X-ray evaluation of trauma
  patient, 67–68
Xylitol
  in lactic acidosis, 36

Library Service
VA Medical Center
830 Chalkstone Avenue
Providence, RI 02908